BASIC SCIENCE FOR SURGEONS

A REVIEW

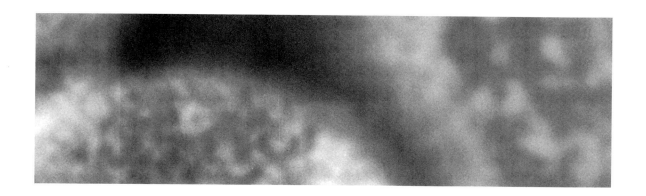

BASIC SCIENCE FOR SURGEONS

A REVIEW

Louis C. Argenta, M.D.

Professor and Chairman
Department of Plastic and Reconstructive Surgery
Wake Forest Medical Center
Winston-Salem, North Carolina

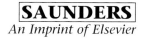
SAUNDERS
An Imprint of Elsevier

Saunders

An Imprint of Elsevier Inc.

The Curtis Center
Independence Square West
Philadelphia, Pennsylvania 19106

BASIC SCIENCE FOR SURGEONS: A REVIEW　　　　　ISBN 0–7216–9074–2

Notice

Medicine is an ever-changing field. Standard safety precautions must be followed, but as new research and clinical experience broaden our knowledge, changes in treatment and drug therapy may become necessary or appropriate. Readers are advised to check the product information currently provided by the manufacturer of each drug to be administered to verify the recommended dose, the method and duration of administration, and contraindications. It is the responsibility of the treating physician, relying on experience and knowledge of the patient, to determine dosages and the best treatment for each individual patient. Neither the Publisher nor the editor assume any liability for any injury and/or damage to persons or property arising from this publication.

THE PUBLISHER

Printed in the United States of America

Last digit is the print number:　9　8　7　6　5　4　3　2　1

Dedication

To my wife, Ginger, beloved inspirational companion and mother of our eight children.

To my teachers, Jeremiah Turcotte, William C. Grabb, Reed O. Dingman, and Paul Tessier, men whose lifetimes were devoted to advancing patient care and the science of medicine.

Contributors

Maria D. Allo, M.D.
Chair, Department of Surgery, Santa Clara Valley
Medical Center, San Jose, California
Endocrine Physiology and Dysfunction

Harry L. Anderson, III, M.D., F.A.C.S., F.C.C.M.
Associate Professor of Surgery, Division of Trauma and
Critical Care, Department of Surgery, University of
Massachusetts Medical School; Attending Surgeon,
UMass Memorial Medical Center, Worcester,
Massachusetts
Respiratory Insufficiency, Failure, and Support

Juan D. Arenas, M.D.
Assistant Professor of Surgery, University of Michigan, and
University of Michigan Health System, Ann Arbor,
Michigan
*The Immunologically Compromised and Transplant
Surgery Patient*

Louis C. Argenta, M.D.
Professor and Chairman, Department of Plastic and
Reconstructive Surgery, Wake Forest Medical Center,
Winston-Salem, North Carolina
Abnormal Wound Healing

Peter A. Argenta, M.D.
Assistant Professor of Obstetrics and Gynecology,
University of Minnesota, Minneapolis, Minnesota
Reproductive Physiology and Dysfunction

Donald Armstrong, M.D.
Professor Emeritus, Weill Medical College of Cornell
University, and Memorial Sloan-Kettering Cancer Center,
New York, New York
Fungal Infection

Rebekah C. Austin, M.D.
Chief Resident, Wake Forest University Baptist Medical
Center, Winston-Salem, North Carolina
Fundamentals of Neurophysiology and Neurodysfunction

Philip S. Barie, M.D., M.B.A., F.C.C.M., F.A.C.S.
Professor of Surgery and Public Health, and Chief,
Division of Critical Care and Trauma, Weill Medical
College of Cornell University; Director, Anne and
Max A. Cohen Surgical Intensive Care Unit,
New York-Presbyterian Hospital, New York, New York
Bacterial Infection

Anthony J. Bleyer, M.D.
Associate Professor, Section on Nephrology, Wake Forest
University School of Medicine, Winston-Salem,
North Carolina
*Perioperative Renal Dysfunction and Failure: Diagnosis
and Management*

R. Randal Bollinger, M.D., Ph.D., M.B.A.
Professor of Surgery and Immunology,
Duke University, and Chief of General Surgery,
Duke University Medical Center, Durham,
North Carolina
Principles and Practice of Transplantation

Loren J. Borud, M.D.
Instructor in Surgery, Harvard Medical School; Attending
Surgeon, Division of Plastic Surgery, Beth Israel
Deaconess Medical Center, Boston, Massachusetts
Applied Embryology of the Extremities

David L. Bowton, M.D.
Professor, Anesthesiology (Critical Care) and Internal
Medicine (Pulmonary and Critical Care), Wake Forest
University School of Medicine; Professor and Head,
Section on Critical Care, Department of Anesthesiology,
Wake Forest University Baptist Medical Center,
Winston-Salem, North Carolina
Physiology of Normal and Abnormal Respiration

Peter C. Brath, M.D.
Anesthesiologist, Piedmont Anesthesia and Pain
Consultants, Winston-Salem, North Carolina
Acute Cardiopulmonary Resuscitation

Margaret F. Brock, M.D.
Assistant Professor of Anesthesiology and Anesthesiology Residency Program Director, Wake Forest University School of Medicine, Winston-Salem, North Carolina
Perioperative Fever and Hypothermia

Jason M. Budde, M.D.
Fellow in Cardiothoracic Surgery, Department of Cardiothoracic Surgery, Emory University School of Medicine, Atlanta, Georgia
Cardiac Physiology and Dysfunction

Alphonse R. Burdi, Ph.D.
Professor of Cell and Developmental Biology, University of Michigan Medical School; Research Scientist, Center for Human Growth and Development, University of Michigan, Ann Arbor, Michigan
Applied Neuroembryology

Randy W. Calicott, M.D.
Assistant Professor, and Medical Director, Inpatient Operting Room, Wake Forest University School of Medicine, Baptist Medical Center, Winston-Salem, North Carolina
General Anesthesia

Darrell A. Campbell, Jr., M.D.
Henry King Ransom Professor of Surgery and Chief of Clinical Affairs, University of Michigan Hospitals and Health Centers, Ann Arbor, Michigan
The Immunologically Compromised and Transplant Surgery Patient

Leopoldo C. Cancio, M.D.
Director, United States Army Burn Center, United States Army Institute of Surgical Research, Fort Sam Houston, Texas
Thermal Injury

Mark A. Carlson, M.D.
Assistant Professor, Department of Surgery, University of Nebraska Medical Center, Omaha, Nebraska
The Cell: Structure and Function

Michael J. Casey, M.D.
Fellow, Section on Nephrology, Wake Forest University School of Medicine, Winston-Salem, North Carolina
Perioperative Renal Dysfunction and Failure: Diagnosis and Management

Michael C. Chang, M.D., F.A.C.S.
Director, Trauma Services, and Associate Professor of Surgery, Wake Forest University Health Sciences, Winston-Salem, North Carolina
Alternatives in Physiologic Monitoring; Shock: Differential Diagnosis and Management

Herbert Chen, M.D.
Assistant Professor of Surgery, University of Wisconsin; Chief of Endocrine Surgery, University of Wisconsin Hospitals and Clinics, Madison, Wisconsin
Principles of Tumor Biology

Gloria A. Chin, M.D., M.S.
Assistant Professor, Division of Plastic Surgery, Department of Surgery, University of Florida College of Medicine; Chief, Plastic Surgery Section, Malcom Randall VA Medical Center, Gainesville, Florida
Growth Factors and Cytokines

Walter J. Chwals, M.D., F.A.C.S., F.A.A.P.
Professor of Surgery and Pediatrics, Case Western Reserve School of Medicine; Rainbow Babies and Children's Hospital, Cleveland, Ohio
The Pediatric Surgical Patient

Bridget L. Colvin, B.S.
Graduate Student/ Ph.D. Candidate in Immunology, University of Pittsburgh, Pittsburgh, Pennsylvania
Immune System and Transplant Immunology

Sheila M. Coogan, M.D.
Assistant Professor of Surgery, Stanford University School of Medicine, Stanford; Vascular Surgeon, Stanford University Hospital, Stanford; Chief, Endovascular Surgery, Palo Alto VA Hospital, Palo Alto, California
Physiology of Arterial Venous and Lymphatic Systems

Robert A. Cowles, M.D.
Fellow in Pediatric Surgery, Children's Hospital of New York-Presbyterian and Columbia University College of Physicians and Surgeons, New York, New York
Gastrointestinal Failure and Liver Failure

Tiffany K. Danton, M.D.
Resident in Plastic Surgery, Division of Plastic and Reconstructive Surgery, Stanford University School of Medicine, Stanford, California
Fetal Wound Healing

Bonnie J. Dattel, M.D.
Professor and Assistant Dean, Division of Maternal-Fetal Medicine, Department of Obstetrics and Gynecology, Eastern Virginia Medical School, Norfolk, Virginia
The Pregnant Surgical Patient

Lisa R. David, M.D.
Assistant Professor, Department of Plastic and Reconstructive Surgery, Wake Forest University Baptist Medical Center, Winston-Salem, North Carolina
Applied Embryology of the Head and Neck

Anthony J. DeFranzo, Jr., M.D.
Associate Professor, Wake Forest University School of Medicine; North Carolina Baptist Hospital, Winston-Salem, North Carolina
Skin and Adnexal Structures

Allan F. deGuzman, Ph.D.
Assistant Professor of Radiation Oncology, Wake Forest University Medical School, Winston-Salem, North Carolina
Radiation Therapy and Radiation Injury

Osvaldo Delbono, M.D., Ph.D.
Associate Professor, Department of Physiology and Pharmacology, Wake Forest University School of Medicine, Winston-Salem, North Carolina
Skeletal Muscle Physiology: Injury and Repair

Lisa S. Dresner, M.D., F.A.C.S.
Associate Professor of Surgery, Director of Surgical Clerkship, and Co-Director, Medical-Surgical Intensive Care, SUNY Downstate, Brooklyn, New York
The Elderly Surgical Patient

Linda Dvali, M.D., M.Sc., F.R.C.S.(C)
Assistant Professor, University of Toronto; University Health Network, Toronto Western Hospital, Toronto, Ontario, Canada
Peripheral Nerve: Anatomy, Injury, and Repair

Mariano S. Dy-Liacco, M.D.
Clinical Instructor, University of Louisville, and University of Louisville School of Medicine, Louisville, Kentucky
Principles and Practice of Transplantation

Soumitra R. Eachempati, M.D., F.A.C.S.
Associate Professor of Surgery, Weill Medical College of Cornell University; Director, Trauma Quality Assurance, New York-Presbyterian Hospital, New York, New York
Bacterial Infection

Frederic E. Eckhauser, M.D.
Professor of Surgery, Johns Hopkins School of Medicine; Director of Surgical Sciences, Johns Hopkins Bayview Medical Center, Baltimore, Maryland
Gastrointestinal Failure and Liver Failure

Samir M. Fakhry, M.D., F.A.C.S.
Chief of Trauma Services, Inova Regional Trauma Center; Associate Chair for Research and Education, Department of Surgery, Inova Fairfax Hospital, Falls Church, Virginia
Hematology and Hemostasis

Josef E. Fischer, M.D.
Mallinckrodt Professor of Surgery, Harvard School of Medicine; Chairman, Department of Surgery, Beth Israel Deaconess Medical Center, Boston, Massachusetts
Nutrition

David M. Fitzgerald, M.D.
Associate Professor of Medicine, Cardiology Section, Wake Forest University School of Medicine, Winston-Salem, North Carolina
Recognition and Treatment of Perioperative Arrhythmias

Donald E. Fry, M.D.
Professor and Chairman, Department of Surgery, University of New Mexico School of Medicine; Chief of Surgery, University of New Mexico Hospital, Albuquerque, New Mexico
Viral Infections

Cleon W. Goodwin, M.D.
Professor of Surgery, Department of Surgery, Johns Hopkins University School of Medicine; Professor of Surgery, and Director, Baltimore Regional Burn Center, Baltimore, Maryland
Thermal Injury

A. Gerson Greenburg, M.D., Ph.D.
Professor of Surgery, Brown Medical School; Surgeon-in-Chief, and Chief, Medical Quality Management, The Miriam Hospital, Providence, Rhode Island
Transfusion and Replacement Therapy

Mark A. Grevious, M.D.
Assistant Professor of Surgery, Division of Plastic, Reconstructive and Cosmetic Surgery, University of Illinois College of Medicine at Chicago, Chicago, Illinois
Physicochemical Injuries

David N. Herndon, M.D.
Professor, Departments of Surgery and Pediatrics, and Jesse H. Jones Distinguished Chair in Burn Surgery, University of Texas Medical Branch; Chief of Staff and Director of Research, Shriners Hospitals for Children, Galveston, Texas
Metabolic Response to Trauma

Michael H. Hines, M.D.
Associate Professor, Cardiothoracic Surgery and Pediatrics, Wake Forest University School of Medicine; Director, Congenital Heart Surgery, Brenner Children's Hospital of Wake Forest University/Baptist Medical Center, Winston-Salem, North Carolina
Applied Cardiac Embryology

Warren Holshouser, M.D.
Fellow, Cardiovascular Electrophysiology, Wake Forest
University School of Medicine, Winston-Salem,
North Carolina
  Recognition and Treatment of Perioperative Arrhythmias

Pamela A. Howard, M.D.
Director, Western States Burn Center, Greeley, Colorado
  Thermal Injury

Timothy D. Howard, Ph.D.
Assistant Professor, Wake Forest University School of
Medicine, Winston-Salem, North Carolina
  The Fundamentals of Molecular Genetics

John Hoyle, M.D.
Assistant Professor of Medicine, Wake Forest University
School of Medicine, Winston-Salem, North Carolina
  Recognition and Treatment of Perioperative Arrhythmias

T. William Huang, M.D., Ph.D.
Assistant Professor, Department of Radiation Oncology,
Wake Forest University School of Medicine,
Winston-Salem, North Carolina
  Radiation Therapy and Radiation Injury

Kirsten Huber, M.D., Ph.D.
General Surgeon, Department of Surgery, Inova Fairfax
Hospital, Falls Church, Virginia
  Hematology and Hemostasis

Christopher P. Johnson, M.D.
Professor of Surgery, Division of Transplantation, Medical
College of Wisconsin; Froedtert Memorial Lutheran
Hospital, Milwaukee, Wisconsin
  The Diabetic Surgical Patient

Gordon L. Kauffman, Jr., M.D.
Professor of Surgery and Cellular and Molecular
Physiology, and Chief, Division of General Surgery,
Penn State University College of Medicine, Hershey,
Pennsylvania
  Gastrointestinal and Hepatic Physiology and Dysfunction

Jeffrey S. Kelly, M.D., F.A.C.E.P.
Associate Professor of Anesthesiology (Critical Care) and
Clinical Instructor in Emergency Medicine, Wake Forest
University School of Medicine, Winston-Salem,
North Carolina
  Acute Cardiopulmonary Resuscitation

Mark Knower, M.D.
Ochsner Clinic, Mandeville, Louisiana
  Physiology of Normal and Abnormal Respiration

Costas Koumenis, Ph.D.
Assistant Professor, Section of Radiation Biology,
Department of Radiation Oncology, Wake Forest
University School of Medicine, Winston-Salem,
North Carolina
  Radiation Therapy and Radiation Injury

W. Thomas Lawrence, M.P.H., M.D., F.A.C.S.
Professor of Surgery (Plastic), University of Kansas
Medical School; Chief, Section of Plastic Surgery, Kansas
University Medical Center, Kansas City, Kansas
  The Normal Wound Healing Process

Raphael C. Lee, M.D., Sc.D., Ph.D.
Professor, Departments of Plastic Surgery, Dermatology,
Molecular Medicine and Anatomy (Biomechanics),
University of Chicago, Chicago, Illinois
  Physicochemical Injuries

Robert W. Letton, Jr., M.D., F.A.C.S., F.A.A.P.
Assistant Professor of Surgery and Pediatrics, Wake Forest
University School of Medicine; Pediatric Surgeon, Wake
Forest University Baptist Medical Center, Winston-Salem,
North Carolina
  The Pediatric Surgical Patient

Jayme E. Locke, M.D.
Resident, Department of Surgery, Johns Hopkins Medical
Institutions, Baltimore, Maryland
  The Morbidly Obese Surgical Patient

Michael T. Longaker, M.D., F.A.C.S.
Deane P. and Louise Mitchell Professor, and Director,
Children's Surgical Research, Stanford University,
Stanford, California
  Fetal Wound Healing

Todd J. Lucas, M.D.
Attending Physician, Moncrief Army Community
Hospital, Columbia, South Carolina
  Transfusion and Replacement Therapy

Susan E. Mackinnon, M.D.
Shoenberg Professor of Surgery, and Chief, Division of
Plastic and Reconstructive Surgery, Washington University
School of Medicine; Barnes-Jewish Hospital, St. Louis,
Missouri
  Peripheral Nerve: Anatomy, Injury, and Repair

Mark A. Malangoni, M.D., F.A.C.S.
Professor of Surgery, Case Western Reserve University;
Chair, Department of Surgery, MetroHealth Medical
Center, Cleveland, Ohio
  Electrolytes and Electrolyte Dysfunction

Joshua M.V. Mammen, M.D.
Assistant Resident, General Surgery, University of Cincinnati, Cincinnati, Ohio
   Nutrition

Albert T. McManus, Ph.D.
Professor of Surgery, Department of Surgery, University of Texas Health Science Center, San Antonio; Retired, Chief Scientist, Institute of Surgical Research, Fort Sam Houston, Texas
   Thermal Injury

James O. Menzoian, M.D., F.A.C.S.
Boston University School of Medicine; Chief, Section of Vascular Surgery, Boston Medical Center, Boston, Massachusetts
   Thromboembolic Disease

William H. Messerschmidt, M.D.
Professor of Surgery, Quillen College of Medicine, East Tennessee State University, Johnson City; Attending, Johnson City Medical Center, Johnson City; Attending, Bristol Regional Medical Center, Bristol, Tennessee
   Myocardial Insufficiency, Failure, and Support

Christopher P. Michetti, M.D., F.A.C.S.
Trauma/Critical Care Surgeon, Department of Surgery, Inova Fairfax Hospital; Assistant Professor of Surgery, Virginia Commonwealth University School of Medicine, Inova Campus, Falls Church, Virginia
   Hematology and Hemostasis

Lyle L. Moldawer, Ph.D.
Professor of Surgery, Department of Surgery, University of Florida College of Medicine, Gainesville, Florida
   Growth Factors and Cytokines

Cullen D. Morris, M.D.
Fellow in Cardiothoracic Surgery, Department of Cardiothoracic Surgery, Emory University School of Medicine, Atlanta, Georgia
   Cardiac Physiology and Dysfunction

Michael J. Morykwas, M.S., Ph.D.
Associate Professor, Department of Plastic and Reconstructive Surgery, Wake Forest University School of Medicine, Winston-Salem, North Carolina
   Abnormal Wound Healing

Lawrence J. Mulligan, M.S., Ph.D.
Principal Clinical Trial Leader, Heart Failure Management, Medtronic, Inc., Minneapolis, Minnesota
   Cardiac Physiology and Dysfunction

Noriko Murase, M.D.
Associate Professor of Surgery, University of Pittsburgh, and T.E. Starzl Transplantation Institute, University of Pittsburgh Medical Center, Pittsburgh, Pennsylvania
   Immune System and Transplant Immunology

Thomas E. Nelson, Ph.D.
Professor Emeritus, Wake Forest University School of Medicine, Winston-Salem, North Carolina
   Perioperative Fever and Hypothermia

John E. Niederhuber, M.D.
Professor, Departments of Oncology and Surgery, University of Wisconsin, Madison, Wisconsin
   Principles of Tumor Biology

Irene O'Shaughnessy, M.D.
Acting Chief, Division of Endocrinology, Medical College of Wisconsin, Milwaukee, Wisconsin
   The Diabetic Surgical Patient

John M. Park, M.D.
Assistant Professor of Urology, and Chief, Division of Pediatric Urology, University of Michigan Medical School, Ann Arbor, Michigan
   Applied Urinary and Reproductive Embryology

Suzanne E. Patton, M.D., Ph.D.
Private Practice, Hematologist-Oncologist, Northwest Georgia Oncology Centers, Austell, Georgia
   Cancer Therapy Alternatives

Erle E. Peacock, Jr., M.D., J.D.
Clinical Professor of Surgery, University of North Carolina School of Medicine, Chapel Hill, North Carolina; Visiting Professor, University of Virginia School of Medicine, Charlottesville, Virginia
   Legal Medicine, Medical Ethics, and Professional Behavior

Ziv M. Peled, M.D.
Post-Doctoral Research Fellow, Children's Surgical Research Program, Stanford University School of Medicine, Stanford, California; Resident in Plastic Surgery, Harvard University School of Medicine, Boston, Massachusetts
   Fetal Wound Healing

D. Glenn Pennington, M.D.
Professor of Surgery, Department of Surgery, Quillen College of Medicine, East Tennessee State University, Johnson City; Attending, Johnson City Medical Center, Johnson City; Attending, Bristol Regional Medical Center, Bristol, Tennessee
   Myocardial Insufficiency, Failure, and Support

Walter J. Pories, M.D., F.A.C.S.
Professor of Surgery and Biochemistry, Brody School of
Medicine, East Carolina University; Attending Surgeon,
Pitt County Memorial Hospital, Greenville, North Carolina
The Morbidly Obese Surgical Patient

Basil A. Pruitt, Jr., M.D.
Professor of Surgery, Uniformed Services University of the
Health Sciences, Bethesda, Maryland; Clinical Professor
of Surgery, University of Texas Health Science Center at
San Antonio, San Antonio, Texas
Thermal Injury

Joseph D. Raffetto, M.D., F.A.C.S.
Assistant Professor of Surgery, Boston Medical Center,
Boston University School of Medicine, Boston,
Massachusetts
Thromboembolic Disease

Suzanne M. Russo, M.D.
Assistant Professor, University of Alabama at Birmingham,
Birmingham, Alabama
Radiation Therapy and Radiation Injury

Matthew Sackett, M.D.
Fellow, Cardiovascular Electrophysiology, Wake Forest
University School of Medicine, Winston-Salem,
North Carolina
*Recognition and Treatment of Perioperative
Arrhythmias*

Amar Safdar, M.D., M.B.B.S.
Associate Professor of Medicine, University of Texas, and
M.D. Anderson Cancer Center, Houston, Texas
Fungal Infection

Gregory Schultz, Ph.D.
Professor, Department of Obstetrics and Gynecology,
University of Florida, Gainesville, Florida
Growth Factors and Cytokines

Vandana Shashi, M.B.B.S., M.D.
Assistant Professor, Wake Forest University School of
Medicine, and North Carolina Baptist Hospital,
Winston-Salem, North Carolina
The Fundamentals of Molecular Genetics

Edward G. Shaw, M.D.
Professor and Chairman, Department of Radiation
Oncology, Wake Forest University School of Medicine,
Winston-Salem, North Carolina
Radiation Therapy and Radiation Injury

Jeffrey S. Shilt, M.D.
Assistant Professor, Department of Orthopaedic Surgery,
Wake Forest University Baptist Medical Center,
Winston-Salem, North Carolina
Bone and Cartilage

Marcus Spies, M.D.
Instructor in Plastic Surgery, and Staff Surgeon,
Department of Plastic, Hand and Reconstructive Surgery,
Medizinische Hochschule Hannover, Hannover,
Germany
Metabolic Response to Trauma

Volker W. Stieber, M.D.
Assistant Professor, Department of Radiation Oncology,
Wake Forest University School of Medicine, and Wake
Forest University Baptist Medical Center, Winston-Salem,
North Carolina
Radiation Therapy and Radiation Injury

Jack W. Strandhoy, Ph.D.
Professor of Physiology and Pharmacology, Associate in
Medicine (Nephrology), and Associate in Surgical
Sciences (Hypertension Center), Wake Forest University
School of Medicine, Winston-Salem, North Carolina
Renal Physiology and Dysfunction

Angus W. Thomson, Ph.D., D.Sc.
Professor of Surgery and Immunology, and Director of
Transplant Immunology, Thomas E. Starzl
Transplantation Institute, University of Pittsburgh Medical
Center, Pittsburgh, Pennsylvania
Immune System and Transplant Immunology

Frank M. Torti, M.D., M.P.H.
Charles L. Spurr Professor of Medicine, Wake Forest
University School of Medicine; Chairman, Department of
Cancer Biology, and Director, Comprehensive Cancer
Center of Wake Forest University, Winston-Salem,
North Carolina
Cancer Therapy Alternatives

George Tsoulfas, M.D.
General Surgery Resident, University of Iowa Hospitals
and Clinics, Iowa City, Iowa
Immune System and Transplant Immunology

Joseph Upton, M.D.
Associate Clinical Professor of Surgery, Harvard Medical
School; Attending Surgeon, Children's Hospital, Beth
Israel Deaconess Medical Center, Boston, Massachusetts
Applied Embryology of the Extremities

Alex B. Valadka, M.D., F.A.C.S.
Associate Professor of Neurosurgery, Baylor College of Medicine; Chief of Neurosurgery, Ben Taub General Hospital, Houston, Texas
Central Nervous System Impairment, Seizure, Coma, and Death

Ravi Veeramasuneni, M.D.
Fellow, Plastic and Reconstructive Surgery, Section of Plastic and Reconstructive Surgery, Department of Surgery, Temple University School of Medicine, Fox Chase-Temple Cancer Center, Philadelphia, Pennsylvania
Respiratory Insufficiency, Failure, and Support

Jakob Vinten-Johansen, M.S., Ph.D.
Professor, Division of Cardiothoracic Surgery, Department of Surgery, and Associate Professor, Department of Physiology, Emory University School of Medicine, Atlanta, Georgia
Cardiac Physiology and Dysfunction

Lawrence X. Webb, M.D.
Professor, and Director, Orthopaedic Traumatology, Department of Orthopaedic Surgery, Wake Forest University Baptist Medical Center, Winston-Salem, North Carolina
Bone and Cartilage

Robert S. Weller, M.D.
Associate Professor of Anesthesiology, Wake Forest University School of Medicine; Attending Physician, North Carolina Baptist Medical Center, Winston-Salem, North Carolina
Sedation and Regional Anesthesia

Deborah M. Whelan, M.D.
Assistant Professor, Department of Anesthesiology, Wake Forest University School of Medicine, and Wake Forest University Baptist Medical Center, Winston-Salem, North Carolina
General Anesthesia

Marcus G. Williams, M.D.
Professor of Surgery, Department of Surgery, Quillen College of Medicine, East Tennessee State University, Johnson City; Attending, Johnson City Medical Center, Johnson City; Attending, Bristol Regional Medical Center, Bristol; Attending, Veterans Administration Medical Center, Mountain Home, Tennessee
Myocardial Insufficiency, Failure, and Support

John A. Wilson, M.D.
Associate Professor of Neurosurgery, Wake Forest University School of Medicine; Attending Physician, Wake Forest University Baptist Medical Center, Winston-Salem, North Carolina
Fundamentals of Neurophysiology and Neurodysfunction

Charles J. Yowler, M.D., F.A.C.S.
Associate Professor of Surgery, Case Western Reserve University; Director, Comprehensive Burn Care Center, and Surgical Critical Care Fellowship, MetroHealth Medical Center, Cleveland, Ohio
Electrolytes and Electrolyte Dysfunction

Christopher K. Zarins, M.D.
Chidester Professor of Surgery, Stanford University School of Medicine; Chief, Division of Vascular Surgery, Stanford University Medical Center, Stanford, California
Physiology of Arterial Venous and Lymphatic Systems

Michael E. Zenilman, M.D., F.A.C.S.
Professor of Surgery, SUNY Downstate Medical Center; Clarence and Mary Dennis Professor and Chairman of Surgery, and Program Director, Surgical Residency Program, SUNY Downstate, Brooklyn, New York
The Elderly Surgical Patient

Marya Zlatnik, M.D.
Assistant Clinical Professor, Department of Obstetrics, Gynecology, and Reproductive Sciences, University of California San Francisco, San Francisco, California
The Pregnant Surgical Patient

Preface

Meaningful education of medical students and residents has become increasingly complex over the past 15 years. The massive amount of information at the basic science level continues to grow exponentially with the advent of genomics, molecular medicine, and biomedical discovery. The mass of knowledge that is presented to the medical student in the first 2 years has reached an almost indigestible volume. The ability to retain and apply this information in clinical practice has become progressively more difficult. Of greatest concern is the attitude that the amount of basic information is so great that the student should "simply wait to get some of it after you have chosen your specialty field."

Concomitant with this growth has been the progressive fragmentation of the surgical subspecialties and the progressive contraction of general surgery to an intra-abdominal specialty. Previously residents spent 3 to 5 years in general surgery handling an extremely wide variety of patients and problems before becoming subspecialists. Residents now spend 1 to 3 years in general surgery and are then passed into subspecialty training, where the greatest emphasis is on technical and operative skills. The amount of time available to the resident to reexamine the basic science of a surgical disease has become markedly truncated and compromised.

The purpose of this book is to provide a bridge from medical school into surgical training before the resident subspecializes. It is meant to reemphasize the basic physiologic, embryologic, and pathophysiologic processes that are relevant to surgery in general rather than just general surgery. It is meant to expand and refocus the learner's basic understanding of principles that transcend all of surgery. Ideally, this book should be read by a senior medical student once he or she has made the decision to enter surgery, and then reread during the first 2 years of resident training so as to broaden and deepen the scope of knowledge.

The scope of surgical subspecialties is so diverse that some redundancy in such a book is inevitable. Some of the chapters may not apply to a specific subspecialty, but the basic physiology and pathophysiology provide a common philosophy that should encompass all specialties. Chapters have been written by individuals who are specialists in these fields.

The editors have learned an extraordinary amount just in the process of preparing this text. This process has reemphasized in our minds the need for periodic review of our fundamental knowledge base. As sophistication in patient care increases, the need for all surgeons to be familiar with fundamental scientific components justifiably continues. We all owe our patients the most up-to-date and comprehensive care possible.

Louis C. Argenta

Plate 1

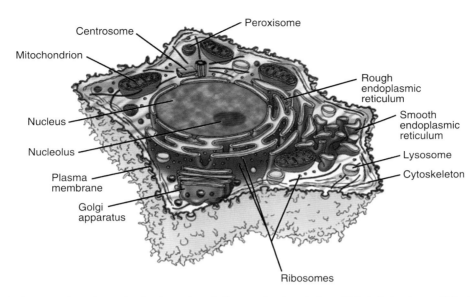

FIGURE 1–1 Cross section of an animal eukaryotic cell. See text for description of labeled structures. (Adapted from Cooper GM: The Cell: A Molecular Approach [2nd ed]. Washington, DC: ASM Press, 2000, with permission.)

FIGURE 1–2 Space-filling model of phosphatidylcholine, a typical phospholipid of the plasma membrane. This molecule consists of a three-carbon backbone (glycerol) to which two fatty acids (nonpolar region) and one phosphate group (polar region) are esterified; a choline group is esterified to the phosphate. **Inset.** Polar and nonpolar regions of the molecule. (Adapted from Alberts B, Bray D, Lewis J, et al: Molecular Biology of the Cell [2nd ed]. London: Garland Science Publishing, 1989. Reproduced by permission of Routledge, Inc., part of The Taylor & Francis Group.)

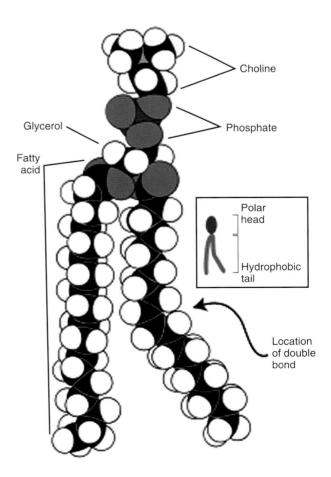

Plate 2

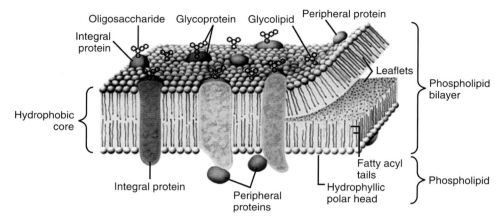

FIGURE 1–3 Phospholipid bilayer membrane and membrane-associated proteins. See text for details. (Adapted from Lodish H, Berk A, Zipursky SL, et al: Molecular Cell Biology [4th ed]. New York: WH Freeman, 2000, with permission.)

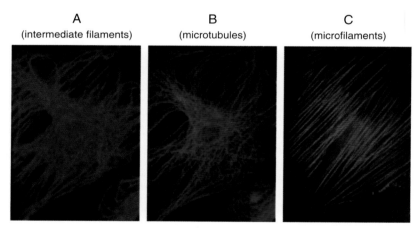

FIGURE 1–4 Immunofluorescence micrographs of the fibroblast cytoskeleton. **A,** Intermediate filaments. **B,** Microtubules. **C,** Microfilaments. (Adapted from Lodish H, Berk A, Zipursky SL, et al: Molecular Cell Biology [4th ed]. New York: WH Freeman, 2000, with permission.)

Plate 3

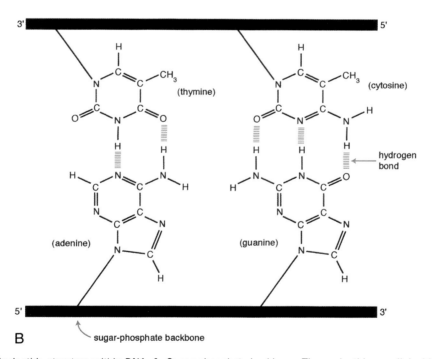

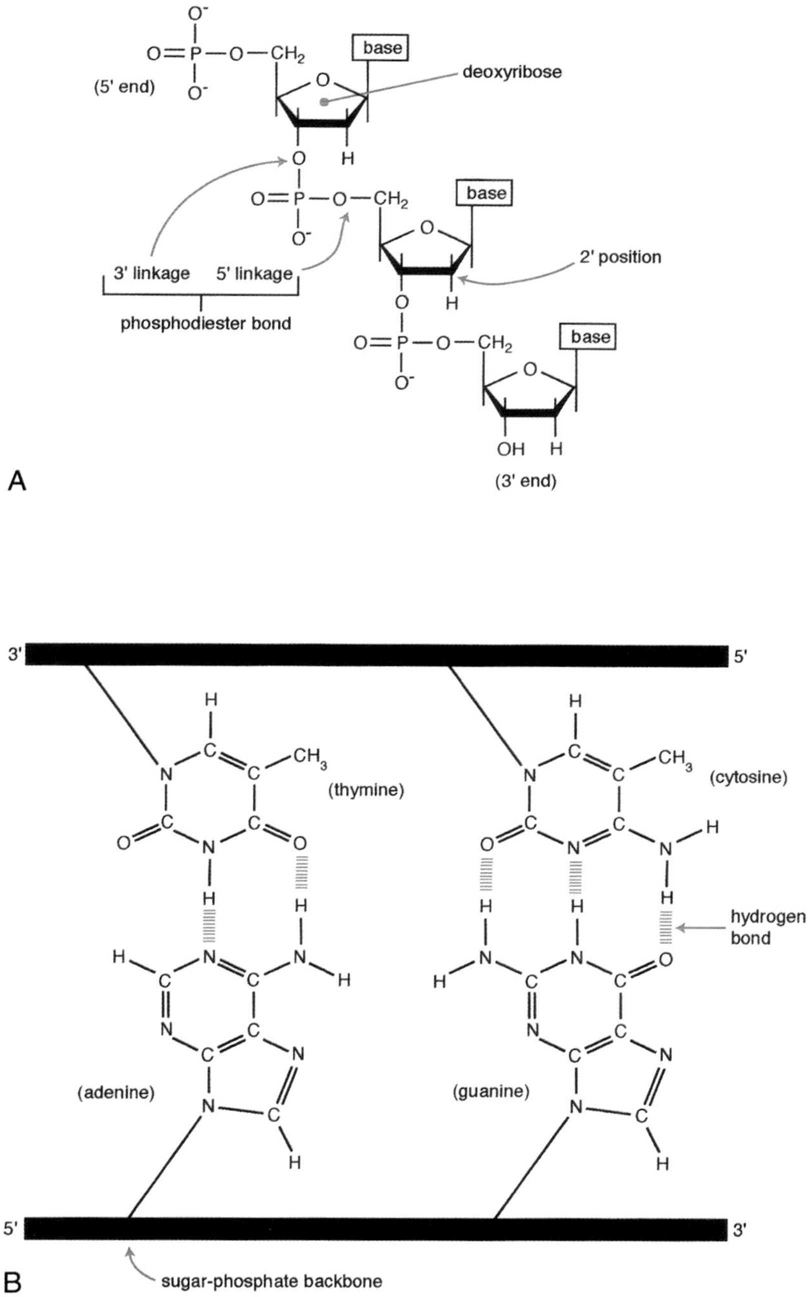

FIGURE 1–5 Nucleotide structure within DNA. **A,** Sugar-phosphate backbone. The nucleotides are linked in a polymer by 3′-5′-phosphodiester bonds. **B,** Nitrogenous bases of DNA and the base-pairing relationships. Thymine pairs with adenine and cytosine pairs with guanine via hydrogen bonds (*dashed red lines*). The sugar-phosphate backbone illustrated in **A** is represented here by the *solid black line.* (Adapted from Alberts B, Bray D, Lewis J, et al: Molecular Biology of the Cell [2nd ed]. London: Garland Science Publishing, 1989. Reproduced by permission of Routledge, Inc., part of The Taylor & Francis Group.)

Plate 4

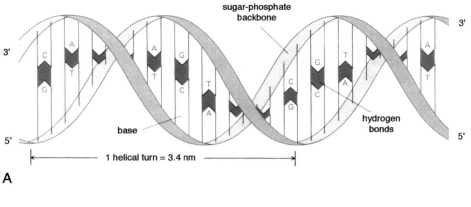

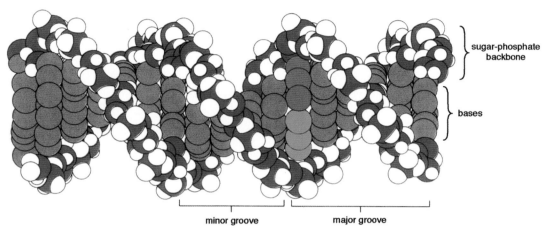

A

B

FIGURE 1–6 Double helix structure of DNA. **A,** The sugar-phosphate illustrated in Figure 1–5 occupies the external surface of the DNA polymer; the bases are turned inward, which facilitates base-pairing. **B,** Space-filling model. Two base-paired nucleotides are colored purple and green. (Adapted from Alberts B, Bray D, Lewis J, et al: Molecular Biology of the Cell [2nd ed]. London: Garland Science Publishing, 1989. Reproduced by permission of Routledge, Inc., part of The Taylor & Francis Group.)

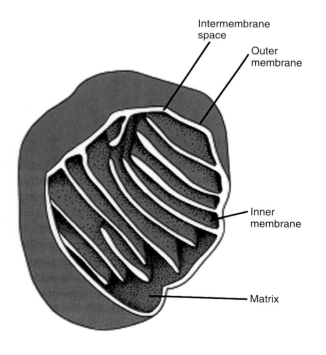

FIGURE 1–7 Mitochondrion. The inner membrane forms invaginations (cristae) in the organelle's interior, which greatly increases the surface area (and thus the metabolic capacity) of the inner membrane. (Adapted from Alberts B, Bray D, Lewis J, et al: Molecular Biology of the Cell [2nd ed]. London: Garland Science Publishing, 1989. Reproduced by permission of Routledge, Inc., part of The Taylor & Francis Group.)

Plate 5

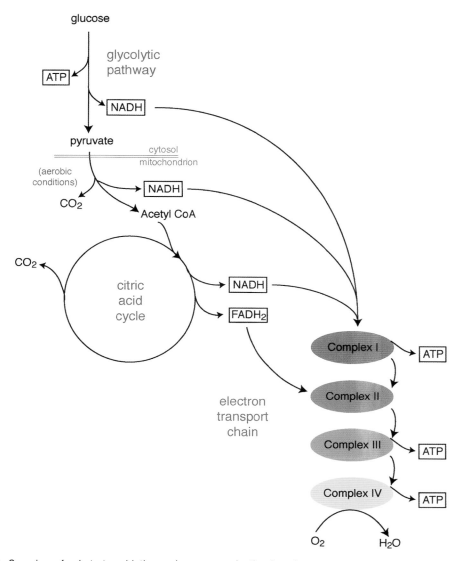

FIGURE 1–8 Overview of substrate oxidation and energy production in eukaryotes: a nonstoichiometric representation. This is the general pathway of glucose utilization under aerobic conditions. Note that the glycolytic pathway is located in the cytosol, and the rest of the reactions take place in the mitochondrion. See text for details.

FIGURE 1–9 The four phases of the eukaryotic cell cycle: G_1, S, G_2, and M. The G_0 state is a resting condition associated with the G_1 phase. See text for details. (Adapted from Lodish H, Berk A, Zipursky SL, et al: Molecular Cell Biology [4th ed]. New York: WH Freeman, 2000, with permission.)

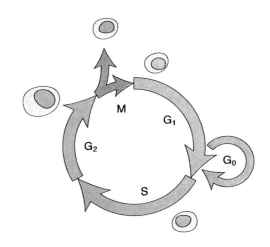

Plate 6

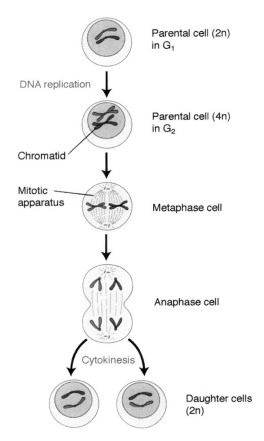

FIGURE 1–10 Mitosis. This sequence begins with the cell in G_1 phase **(top)**, proceeds through the S phase into G_2, and then begins the formal steps of mitosis. See text for details. (Adapted from Lodish H, Berk A, Zipursky SL, et al: Molecular Cell Biology [4th ed]. New York: WH Freeman, 2000, with permission.)

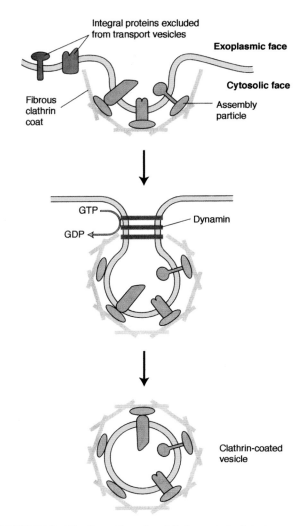

FIGURE 1–11 Formation of a clathrin-coated pit during receptor-mediated endocytosis. See text for details. (Adapted from Lodish H, Berk A, Zipursky SL, et al: Molecular Cell Biology [4th ed]. New York: WH Freeman, 2000, with permission.)

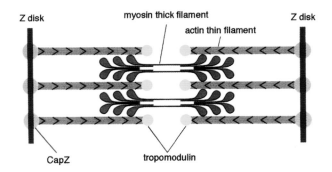

FIGURE 1–12 Actin-myosin contractile complex of skeletal muscle. Each muscle cell is packed with myofibrils, which are bundles of filaments that traverse the length of the cell and are oriented in the direction of contraction. Each filament is composed of sarcomere units strung end-to-end; an individual sarcomere is diagrammed. The Z disks (also called Z lines) mark the ends of an individual sarcomere. The Z disk functions to anchor the actin thin filaments; this anchorage is facilitated by CapZ, an actin-capping protein, and α-actinin. Tropomodulin caps the opposite end of each thin filament. The thick filaments are composed of myosin II and interdigitate with the thin filaments. Muscle contraction occurs when the heads of the myosin II protein walk along the thin filaments in an ATP-dependent process; this action draws the Z disks together, which shortens the sarcomere. (Adapted from Lodish H, Berk A, Zipursky SL, et al: Molecular Cell Biology [4th ed]. New York: WH Freeman, 2000, with permission.)

Plate 7

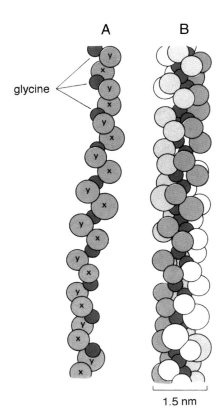

FIGURE 1–13 Structure of type I collagen. Each sphere represents an amino acid residue. **A,** Single-strand polymer. **B,** Each molecule of collagen is composed of three such strands arranged in a triple helix, which also is known as a collagen fibril. The amino acid residue represented by "y" typically is proline or hydroxyproline; "x" can be any residue. (Adapted from Alberts B, Bray D, Lewis J, et al: Molecular Biology of the Cell [2nd ed]. London: Garland Science Publishing, 1989. Reproduced by permission of Routledge, Inc., part of The Taylor & Francis Group.)

glycine

1.5 nm

A Endocrine signaling

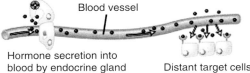

Blood vessel

Hormone secretion into blood by endocrine gland

Distant target cells

B Paracrine signaling

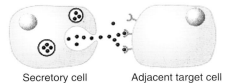

Secretory cell   Adjacent target cell

C Autocrine signaling

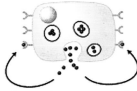

Key:
- • Extracellular signal
- Y Receptor
- ꭥ Membrane-attached signal

Target sites on same cell

D Juxtacrine signaling

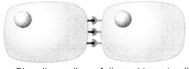

Signaling cell   Adjacent target cell

FIGURE 1–14 Basic signaling mechanisms: endocrine (**A**); paracrine (**B**); autocrine (**C**); and juxtacrine (**D**). See text for details. (Adapted from Lodish H, Berk A, Zipursky SL, et al: Molecular Cell Biology [4th ed]. New York: WH Freeman, 2000, with permission.)

Plate 8

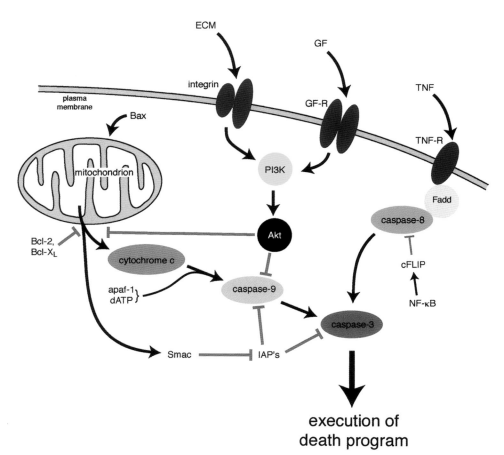

FIGURE 1–15 Overview of signaling during apoptosis. A typical cell receives multiple inputs, such as ligation of integrin receptors to the ECM or activation of growth factor receptors (GF-R), which tend to promote survival via activation of intracellular survival pathways. The phosphatidylinositol-3-kinase (PI3K)/Akt sequence is a prominent survival pathway activated by both growth factors and ECM anchorage. Activated Akt promotes survival through multiple mechanisms, such as by inhibition of cytochrome *c* release and inhibition of caspase-9. The pro-survival members of the Bcl-2 family typically inhibit release of cytochrome *c* from the mitochondria. Cell death usually is initiated through one of two major pathways: mitochondria-dependent or death receptor-dependent. A number of pro-apoptotic stimuli induce cytochrome *c* release from the mitochondria via the action of pro-apoptotic Bcl-2 proteins, such as Bax. Once in the cytosol, cytochrome *c* complexes with apaf-1, dATP, and caspase-9 (the apoptosome). This complex results during caspase-9 activation, which cleaves (and thus activates) caspase-3. Activation of caspase-3 generally is considered to be the final common pathway for execution of the apoptotic program. The activity of caspase-9 and caspase-3 is inhibited by the IAP family of proteins. If the cell receives an apoptotic stimulus, however, the protein Smac is released from the mitochondrion; Smac inhibits the IAPs, which relieves inhibition of the caspases. Smac release therefore is pro-apoptotic. Caspase-3 also can be activated by caspase-8, which is activated by the death receptor complex. Here, TNF initiates the death receptor complex by ligating the TNF receptor, which subsequently binds the adapter protein Fadd. Caspase-8 is held in check by cFLIP, which is turned on by the action of NF-κB. The transcription factor NF-κB has context-dependent effects of cell survival; in this scenario NF-κB is pro-survival. Not shown is another protein, AIF (apoptosis-inducing factor), which can be released from mitochondria. It can initiate apoptosis in an apparently caspase-independent pathway, which is incompletely characterized.

Plate 9

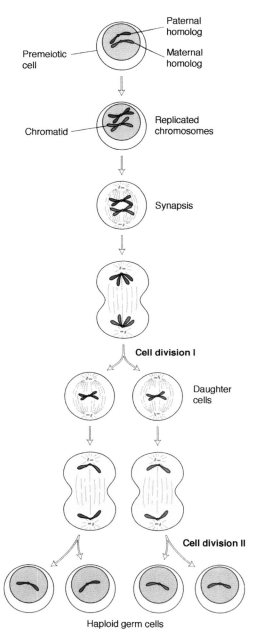

FIGURE 1–16 Meiosis. See text for details. (Adapted from Lodish H, Berk A, Zipursky SL, et al: Molecular Cell Biology [4th ed]. New York: WH Freeman, 2000, with permission.)

Plate 10

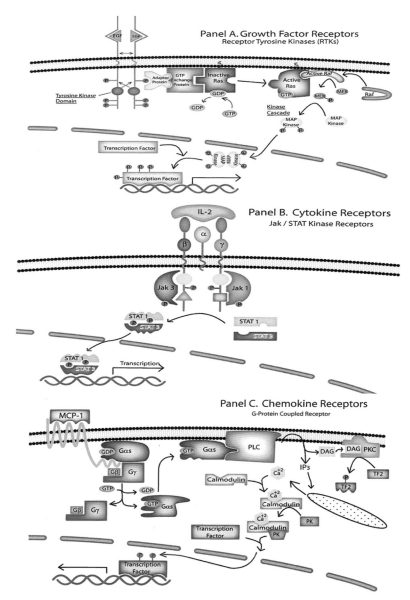

FIGURE 2–1 Typical receptor structures and signal transduction pathways for growth factors, cytokines, and chemokines. **A,** Receptors for growth factors typically are receptor tyrosine kinases (RTKs) that dimerize after binding the growth factor and autophosphorylate key tyrosines in the cytoplasmic domain of the receptors. Adaptor proteins bind at the phosphotyrosine sites, and GTP-exchange factors (GEF) dock with the adaptor proteins, which then promote exchange of GTP on Ras-GDP. Active Ras-GTP initiates a kinase cascade (Raf, Mek) that phosphorylates and activates MAP kinase, which dimerizes, translocates to the nucleus where it phosphorylates, and activates transcription factors leading to expression of selected genes. **B,** Receptors for cytokines typically consist of homo- or heteromultimeric subunits that aggregate after binding the cytokine, which permits Jak kinases bound to the cytoplasmic segments of the receptors close to phosphorylate each other when they are brought into close apposition. The activated Jak kinases phosphorylate and activate Stat transcription factors, which dimerize, translocate to the nucleus, and promote transcription of selected genes. **C,** Chemokine receptors are all 7-transmembrane spanning receptors that are coupled to G-protein trimer subunit complexes. After binding the chemokine, the receptor promotes exchange of GTP on the $G_{s\alpha}$-GDP subunit, which then dissociates from the G_β-G_δ subunits; the $G_{s\alpha}$-GTP subunit then binds with and activates the phospholipase C (PLC) enzyme located in the plasma membrane. Active PLC generates two important second messengers: diacylglycerol (DAG), which activates protein kinase C (PKC), and inositol trisphosphate (IP$_3$), which stimulates release of Ca^{2+} from cytoplasmic stores and activates calmodulin. Both PKC and calmodulin activate transcription factors that selectively stimulate transcription of genes.

Contents

PART XII
Legal and Ethical Conduct

PART I

Biologic Basis of Disease

CHAPTER 1

The Cell: Structure and Function

Mark A. Carlson, M.D.

In lay terms, the *cell* commonly is defined as the smallest form of life; this definition leads to the nebulous topic of the definition of life. Alternatively, the biologic definition of *cell* may be reduced to an entity that (1) is microscopic in size; (2) is membrane-bound; (3) contains the necessary instructions (i.e., DNA) for and is capable of reproduction; (4) consumes substrates; and (5) synthesizes molecules. There are two general cell types: *eukaryotes*, which possess a nucleus; and *prokaryotes*, which do not have a nucleus. In addition, there are four types of eukaryotes: animals, plants, fungi, and protozoa. The primary goal of this chapter is to describe the essential components of animal eukaryotic cell structure and function. The description of each component is short, with a minimal number of figures. The reader is directed to specialized textbooks for more comprehensive reading and illustrations of a given topic.

Cell Structure

Membrane

The cell membrane is the outer layer that divides the cell interior (*cytoplasm* or *cytosol*) from the exterior (*extracellular space*) (Fig. 1–1). The cell membrane consists of two layers of phospholipid (i.e., a *phospholipid bilayer*, which is the basic structure of biologic membranes). A phospholipid molecule consists of a three-carbon backbone (glycerol) to which two fatty acyl chains and a phosphate group are attached; the phosphate group can be further esterified to another entity (e.g., choline) to create, for example, the phospholipid known as phosphatidylcholine (Fig. 1–2). Phospholipids are *amphipathic*; that is, they have hydrophilic (phosphate group) and hydrophobic (fatty acyl chains) components in one molecule. The phospholipid bilayer is organized such that the hydrophobic acyl chains face and intermingle with one another, whereas the phosphate groups are turned outward to face the aqueous environment (Fig. 1–3). This produces a barrier, which is relatively impermeable to polar molecules.

Embedded in the phospholipid bilayer membrane are proteins and cholesterol molecules (Fig. 1–3). Membrane-associated proteins fall under a general classification as either *integral* (contained within the membrane) or *peripheral*. Most integral proteins also are transmembrane in that they completely span the membrane, having cytoplasmic, transmembrane, and extracellular domains. Peripheral proteins attach to the membrane surface with ionic (noncovalent) forces. Typically, membrane proteins on the outer leaflet are extensively glycosylated, which is important for receptor–ligand interactions (especially with regard to immune recognition of self and non-self). Most protein and lipid components of a phospholipid bilayer are relatively free to move within the plane of the membrane, which is the basis for the concept of *membrane fluidity*. Components of a biologic membrane are not fixed in location; on the

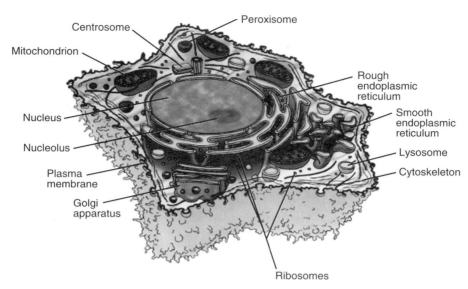

FIGURE 1–1 Cross section of an animal eukaryotic cell. See text for description of labeled structures. (Adapted from Cooper GM: The Cell: A Molecular Approach [2nd ed]. Washington, DC: ASM Press, 2000, with permission.) *See Color Plate 1.*

contrary, the membrane is analogous to the surface of an ocean, on which "ships" (e.g., integral membrane proteins) are floating about. This dynamic situation is vital for the assembly of various membrane and extra-membrane components to generate enzymatic reactions, membrane pores, focal adhesions, and other membrane-localized events, as discussed below. The degree of membrane fluidity is determined in part by: (1) the number of desaturations (double bonds) in the fatty acyl chains of the membrane phospholipids (increasing the number of desaturations increases fluidity); (2) the length of the fatty acyl chains (increasing the length decreases the fluidity); (3) temperature (an elevation increases fluidity); and (4) cholesterol (decreases fluidity). *Cholesterol* is a weakly polar molecule that incorporates its hydrophobic portion into the membrane, thereby reducing the "packing" of fatty acyl chains and filling the spaces created by acyl chain desaturation.

Cytoskeleton

The cytoskeleton is an intracellular physical framework that enables a cell to change its shape, migrate, perform vesicular transport, and organize intracellular organelles. Additionally, the cytoskeleton appears to function as a biochemical *scaffold* for some enzymatic pathways. A biochemical scaffold facilitates an enzymatic reaction by drawing the participants in proximity to one another. The three primary constituents of the cytoskeleton are microtubules, microfilaments, and intermediate filaments. A microtubule is a rigid, cylindrical polymer consisting of stacked rings of the protein *tubulin*; each ring contains

13 copies of tubulin arranged in a 25 nm circle. Microtubules are polarized by the designation of *plus* and *minus* ends; typically, tubulin proteins are added to the former and removed from the latter.

Microtubule organization in the cell is coordinated by the *centrosome* (also known as the *microtubule organizing center*, or MTOC), an organelle near the nucleus from which microtubules emanate outward (leading with their plus ends) until they connect to the plasma membrane (Fig. 1–4). Microtubules may be conceptualized as *struts*, which support the shape of the plasma membrane. This is not a static arrangement, however; there is continual extension and retraction of microtubules in an ongoing, GTP-dependent process known as *dynamic instability*. This arrangement allows the cell to respond morphologically to specific stimuli, such as during migration or cell division. Microtubule stability can be enhanced in differentiated cells (e.g., neurons, which need to maintain a stable axonic structure of up to 1 meter in length) by various *microtubule-associated proteins* (MAPs), which inhibit microtubule depolymerization and enhance microtubule binding to organelles.

Actin microfilaments are another primary component of the cytoskeleton. Actin is a globule-shaped protein that exists either in a free cytosolic pool or as a linear, helical actin polymer (the microfilament); actin is one of the most common proteins in the cell (ranging from 1% to 10% of total cell protein, depending on the cell type). Similar to microtubules, the actin polymer has plus and minus ends, also known as the *barbed* and *pointed* ends, respectively. In general, the plus end adds actin subunits from the cytosolic

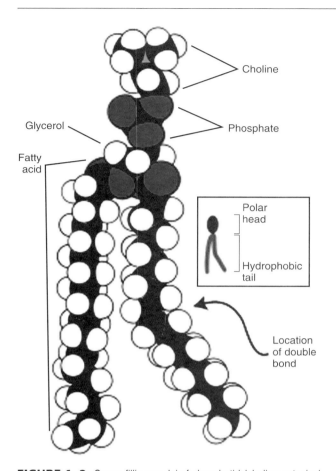

FIGURE 1–2 Space-filling model of phosphatidylcholine, a typical phospholipid of the plasma membrane. This molecule consists of a three-carbon backbone (glycerol) to which two fatty acids (nonpolar region) and one phosphate group (polar region) are esterified; a choline group is esterified to the phosphate. **Inset.** Polar and nonpolar regions of the molecule. (Adapted from Alberts B, Bray D, Lewis J, et al: Molecular Biology of the Cell [2nd ed]. London: Garland Science Publishing, 1989. Reproduced by permission of Routledge, Inc., part of The Taylor & Francis Group.) *See Color Plate 1.*

pool (*actin polymerization*), which sets up a situation similar to that in microtubules in that the microfilament is in a state of regulated dynamic instability (i.e., the polymers can lengthen or shorten depending on the signaling environment). Actin polymerization is energy-requiring (ATP-dependent) and is maintained in check by a number of *actin-binding proteins* (ABPs), of which profilin, gelsolin, and thymosin-β4 are typical examples. Actin microfilaments also can be cross-linked (and thus stabilized) by proteins such as α-actinin or filamin. The actin cytoskeletal network is organized in three general patterns: (1) as parallel bundles (plus ends all pointing in the same direction); (2) as contractile bundles (plus ends pointing in both directions); and (3) as a crisscrossing network. In general, microfilaments extend from one membrane structure to another, such as from one side of the plasma membrane to the other (Fig. 1–4), or from the plasma membrane to the nucleus; microfilaments are most densely populated, however, in the region just underneath the cell membrane (the *cortex*). The role of microfilaments in the cytoskeleton can be conceptualized as "cables" or "guy wires" strung between membranous structures. The combination of microtubules (rigid struts) and actin microfilaments (guy wires) describes a cytoskeletal network in which the struts are held in place by the tension of the wires, similar to the way a tall relay tower is secured in the upright position by tension cables. This theory of struts and wires, which describes the cytoskeletal support of the cell shape, is called *tensegrity*.

Actin microfilaments also play a prominent role in cell motility and anchorage. Some cells can move across or through the extracellular matrix (ECM) (i.e., migrate) if appropriately signaled. A cell migrates by extending itself in the direction of migration; the protruding portion of the membrane in this process is termed a *lamellipodia*. A cell also can send out thin membranous extensions known as

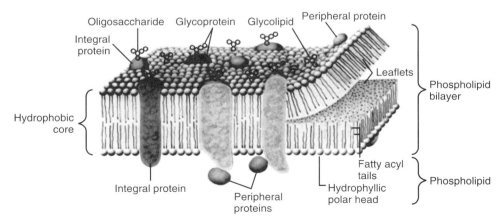

FIGURE 1–3 Phospholipid bilayer membrane and membrane-associated proteins. See text for details. (Adapted from Lodish H, Berk A, Zipursky SL, et al: Molecular Cell Biology [4th ed]. New York: WH Freeman, 2000, with permission.) *See Color Plate 2.*

A
(intermediate filaments) B
(microtubules) C
(microfilaments)

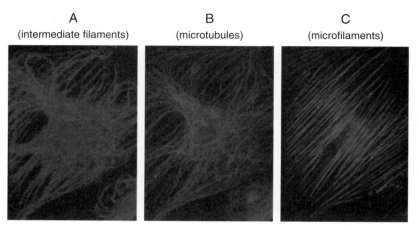

FIGURE 1–4 Immunofluorescence micrographs of the fibroblast cytoskeleton. **A,** Intermediate filaments. **B,** Microtubules. **C,** Microfilaments. (Adapted from Lodish H, Berk A, Zipursky SL, et al: Molecular Cell Biology [4th ed]. New York: WH Freeman, 2000, with permission.) *See Color Plate 2.*

microspikes or *filopodia.* The generation of both lamellipodia and filopodia is driven by polymerization of parallel bundles of actin in the developing structure and is under the control of two small Rho GTPases, Rac and Cdc42. A cell migrates by extending these processes out from its leading edge in the direction of motion while retracting processes at the rear of the cell. Actin *stress fibers* form to a varying degree in cells that are anchored to a substratum. Stress fibers, which have a contractile bundle configuration, attach to the plasma membrane at *focal adhesion contacts* (see further discussion below); these contacts are complexes of multiple proteins that form at sites of attachment to the ECM in nonmigratory cells (e.g., a confluent monolayer of fibroblasts cultured on fibronectin).

Intermediate filaments, the third component of the cytoskeleton, are so named because their diameter falls between that of the thicker microtubules and the thinner microfilaments. Intermediate filaments are found only in multicellular organisms. The cellular organization of intermediate filaments is somewhat similar to that of microtubules (Fig. 1–4); the former also is a major component of the nuclear skeleton. In general, intermediate filaments are more stable than the dynamic microfilaments and microtubules. An intermediate filament consists of multiple protein chains wrapped together in a complex helical structure; each chain is a polymer that can contain up to three subunit types. In general, there are *four classes* of intermediate filaments: (1) *keratins* (which are in part responsible for the physical characteristics of hair and epidermis); (2) *vimentins* (including desmin and vimentin, which are the most widely expressed intermediate filaments); (3) *neurofilaments* (which traverse the entire length of a neuron and axon, giving the latter tensile strength); and (4) *lamins* (which form a meshwork just underneath the nuclear membrane).

Nucleus

The nucleus houses the genetic material, or *DNA,* of the cell. DNA is a polymer of *deoxyribonucleic acids*; a unit (nucleotide) of the polymer consists of a five-carbon sugar core molecule (2-deoxyribose) onto which a phosphate group and an organic base (adenine, guanine, cytosine, or thymine) are attached at the 5' and 1' positions, respectively (Fig. 1–5). The 5'-phosphate forms an ester linkage with the 3'-hydroxyl group of another nucleotide, which is the basis for constructing a polymer of DNA. Two single strands combine to generate a double helix of DNA, in which the phosphate groups are positioned toward the outside, forming a "sugar–phosphate backbone" (Fig. 1–6); the organic base residues are turned inward and form hydrogen bonds with the bases on the opposite strand, a phenomenon called *base pairing.* Typically, adenine pairs with thymine, and guanine pairs with cytosine. The structure of mRNA is similar, except the core sugar molecule is ribose instead of 2-deoxyribose, and the base uracil is substituted for thymine. The entire human DNA complement, or genome, contains about 3×10^9 base pairs; and the genome is organized into 23 individual DNA polymers, or *chromosomes.* Each nucleus has two copies of each chromosome, for a total of 46 chromosomes per nucleus. If strung end-to-end, the chromosomes from a single nucleus would be several meters in length. To package them into a nucleus, which is in the range of 5 μm in diameter (i.e., about a million-fold reduction in length), the DNA is coiled tightly around DNA-binding proteins called *histones.*

The nucleus is bounded by a bilaminar membrane (i.e., a double phospholipid bilayer); the cell itself is bounded by a single phospholipid bilayer (Fig. 1–1). The inner membrane is supported by a meshwork of nuclear lamins and contains the *nucleoplasm* (an aqueous environment

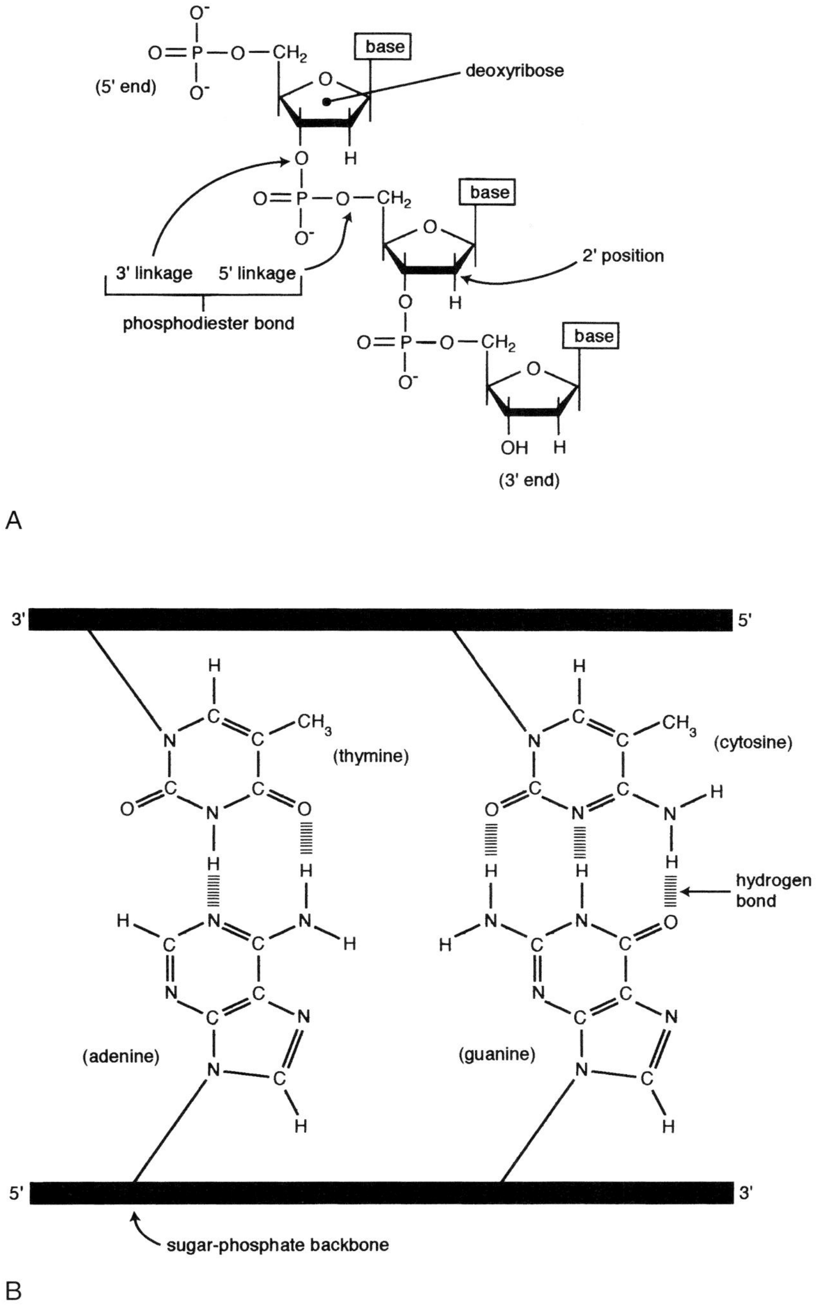

FIGURE 1–5 Nucleotide structure within DNA. **A,** Sugar-phosphate backbone. The nucleotides are linked in a polymer by 3′-5′-phospho-diester bonds. **B,** Nitrogenous bases of DNA and the base-pairing relationships. Thymine pairs with adenine and cytosine pairs with guanine via hydrogen bonds (*dashed red lines*). The sugar-phosphate backbone illustrated in **A** is represented here by the *solid black line*. (Adapted from Alberts B, Bray D, Lewis J, et al: Molecular Biology of the Cell [2nd ed]. London: Garland Science Publishing, 1989. Reproduced by permission of Routledge, Inc., part of The Taylor & Francis Group.) *See Color Plate 3.*

analogous to the cytoplasm that is the location of the DNA); the outer membrane is continuous with the endoplasmic reticulum (ER) in the cytoplasm (a connection that facilitates transport of molecules and complexes between the nucleus and the ER). Transport across the nuclear membrane occurs in part through the *nuclear pore complex*

(NPC), which consists of about 200 proteins (for a combined weight of approximately 124,000 kDa) and forms an opening approximately 10 nm in diameter across the nuclear membrane, allowing passive diffusion of molecules less than 9 kDa in size. Molecules larger than 9 kDa that need to be transported into the nucleus require a nuclear

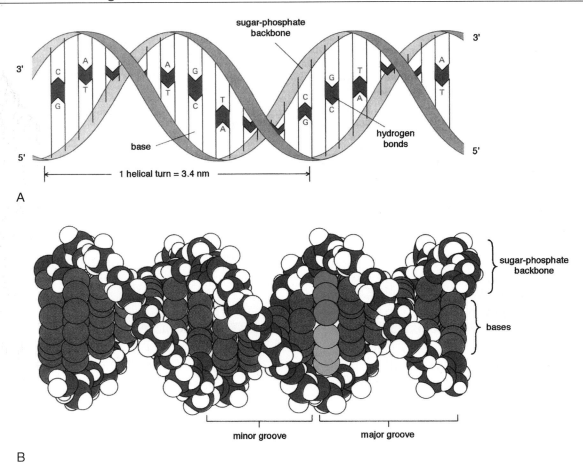

FIGURE 1–6   Double helix structure of DNA. **A,** The sugar-phosphate illustrated in Figure 1–5 occupies the external surface of the DNA polymer; the bases are turned inward, which facilitates base-pairing. **B,** Space-filling model. Two base-paired nucleotides are colored purple and green. (Adapted from Alberts B, Bray D, Lewis J, et al: Molecular Biology of the Cell [2nd ed]. London: Garland Science Publishing, 1989. Reproduced by permission of Routledge, Inc., part of The Taylor & Francis Group.) *See Color Plate 4.*

localization signal (a short peptide attached to an end to the protein that identifies it as a nuclear import target), a transport facilitator protein called *importin*, and GTP (a source of energy). The nucleus also is the site of *transcription*, in which DNA is transcribed into messenger RNA (mRNA) by RNA polymerase I; the mRNA subsequently directs protein synthesis in ribosomes associated with the endoplasmic reticulum (see below). Transcription occurs in the *nucleolus* (Fig. 1–1), a nuclear organelle that is not bounded by a membrane. Ribonucleoproteins, the building blocks of ribosomes, also are synthesized in the nucleolus.

Organelles

Mitochondria

The mitochondrion, typically about 1 μm in length, produces high-energy molecules that the cells utilize during energy-requiring processes. Similar to the nucleus, the mitochondrion is membrane-bound by a double phospholipid bilayer (Figs. 1–1 and 1–7). The outer membrane contains *porin*, a protein that forms pores, allowing molecules less than 5 kDa in size to diffuse freely in an out of the intermembrane space. The intermembrane space (located, as the name suggests, between the outer and inner membranes) contains enzymes that phosphorylate substrates (sugars and nucleotides) as they diffuse into the space. The mitochondrial inner membrane has numerous invaginations, or *cristae*, which greatly increase the surface area of the inner membrane; this membrane also is enriched in *cardiolipin*, which increases membrane impermeability to water. The inner membrane contains enzymes critical for the production of ATP, the primary high-energy molecule of the cell. Within the inner membrane is the *mitochondrial matrix*, which houses enzymes important for lipid and carbohydrate oxidation, including the proteins involved in the tricarboxylic acid (TCA) cycle. Mitochondria also have their own DNA in the matrix; it is believed that mitochondria were once independent organisms that invaded eukaryotes and established a symbiotic relationship.

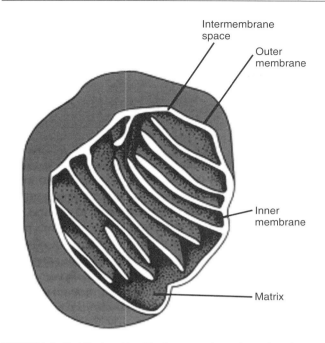

Intermembrane
space

Outer
membrane

Inner
membrane

Matrix

FIGURE 1–7 Mitochondrion. The inner membrane forms invaginations (cristae) in the organelle's interior, which greatly increases the surface area (and thus the metabolic capacity) of the inner membrane. (Adapted from Alberts B, Bray D, Lewis J, et al: Molecular Biology of the Cell [2nd ed]. London: Garland Science Publishing, 1989. Reproduced by permission of Routledge, Inc., part of The Taylor & Francis Group.) *See Color Plate 4.*

The mitochondrial DNA complement is small (in humans it is approximately 10^{-5} the size of the nuclear genome); yet the mitochondrion synthesizes some of its own proteins from mitochondrial DNA, utilizing transcriptional and translational machinery contained within the mitochondrial matrix. Most mitochondrial proteins, however, are imported from the cytosol.

Endoplasmic reticulum

The endoplasmic reticulum (ER) is the major site of protein and lipid synthesis. It is bounded by a single phospholipid bilayer, which is continuous with the outer nuclear membrane (Fig. 1–1). The ER forms a perinuclear labyrinthic network that has *rough* and *smooth* regions. The rough ER is so named because its membranes are studded with ribosomes. A ribosome is a complex of protein and ribosomal RNA; the ribosome complex is assembled in two subunits, 40S and 60S (the labels refer to relative migration in a centrifugation density gradient). mRNA from the nucleus is transported to the ribosome, where the mRNA is translated into protein, which is secreted directly into the ER lumen. Proteins synthesized in the ER have a final destination other than the cytosol; that is, they will be membrane-bound or secreted into the extracellular matrix.

A number of posttranslational protein modifications occur in the lumen of the ER, including glycosylation, disulfide bond formation, protein folding, and subunit assembly. Newly synthesized proteins must undergo appropriate folding to attain the correct three-dimensional conformation; otherwise they cannot function or, even worse, are harmful to the cell.

Protein folding is aided by *chaperones*, which are proteins in the ER lumen that bind to polypeptide chains as they emerge from the ribosome and direct subsequent folding. Improperly ER-processed proteins (i.e., those with inappropriate glycosylation, disulfide bonding, folding, or subunit assembly) are targeted for degradation and usually do not make it out of the ER. The smooth ER lacks ribosomes; it is the primary location for lipid and sterol synthesis, and it is a major storage site for intracellular calcium. In addition, the smooth ER is the location of the P-450 enzyme system, which is active in detoxification.

Golgi apparatus

The Golgi apparatus is the location of further processing, packaging, and routing for membrane-bound proteins. The Golgi, which is bounded by a single phospholipid bilayer, is juxtaposed to the ER and consists of multiple discoid *cisternae*, which are packed one on top of another, having the cross-sectional appearance of a stack of coins or pancakes (Fig. 1–1). The periphery of each cisterna is thickened, and transport vesicles bud and fuse in this region. The *cis* side of each cisterna faces the ER and is the side where vesicles fuse; the *trans* side faces away from the ER and is the side where vesicles bud. Proteins destined for membrane residence are synthesized and begin posttranslational modification in the ER; they subsequently are transported to the Golgi, where the posttranslational modification is completed. The finished proteins then are sorted into destination-specific membrane-bound vesicles, which bud from the *trans* Golgi and transport the proteins to their final residence.

Lysosomes

The lysosome is a major site for degradation and digestion of substrate. The lysosome is bounded by a single phospholipid bilayer (Fig. 1–1); the organelle interior is maintained acidic (pH 5) by proton pumps in the organelle's membrane. The lysosome contains a number of digestive enzymes (*hydrolases*), which function optimally in an acidic environment; if leaked into the cytosol (pH ~ 7.2), these enzymes are ineffective. All lysosomal proteins are synthesized in the ER, processed in the Golgi, and transported by vesicle to the lysosome using a specific lysosomal targeting address. The inner leaflet of the lysosomal membrane appears to be protected from autodigestion by extensive glycosylation of integral membrane proteins. Substrate for lysosomal digestion includes internalized receptor–ligand complexes, lipoproteins (i.e., cholesterol turnover), dysfunctional cellular organelles, and phagocytized material such as bacteria. The breakdown products of lysosomal digestion (e.g., amino acids) are recycled back into the cytosol for cellular utilization.

Peroxisomes

The peroxisome (Fig. 1–1), a single membrane-bound organelle, contains enzymes that oxidize fatty acids and amino acids. Hydrogen peroxide is produced during these degradation reactions; this product is further metabolized to H_2O in an O_2-consuming reaction by catalase, an enzyme within the peroxisome. Peroxisomal fatty acid oxidation is not coupled to ATP generation, as is the case in mitochondria—there is no electron transport chain in the peroxisome (see later in the chapter). The energy generated from peroxisomal oxidation reactions is released as heat, and the acetyl coenzyme A (CoA) likewise generated is transported back to the cytosol for utilization during synthesis.

Cellular Functions

Energy Metabolism

The primary location of energy metabolism in the cell is the mitochondrion (the cell's "power house"), and the primary high-energy molecule generated by mitochondria, which fuels energy-requiring cellular processes, is *ATP*. The overall scheme of ATP production (also known as *oxidative phosphorylation*) involves oxidation of substrate (carbohydrate, lipid, and to a lesser extent protein) in the mitochondrial matrix (Fig. 1–8), which provides energy via an *electron transport chain* for *proton pumps* to establish a proton gradient between the intermembrane space and the matrix. The backflow of protons down this electrochemical gradient and across the inner membrane provides the energy for an enzyme, *ATP synthase* (an integral protein of the inner membrane), to combine ADP and inorganic phosphate (P_i) to form ATP.

Glucose, a six-carbon sugar, is the typical substrate utilized to fuel ATP production. After transport from the cell exterior into the cytoplasm, glucose is partially metabolized by cytosolic enzymes in the *glycolytic pathway* (alternatively known as *glycolysis* or the *Embden-Meyerhof pathway*) to pyruvate, a three-carbon molecule (Fig. 1–8). Each molecule of glucose consumed by glycolysis results in the net production of two ATP molecules and two molecules of *NADH* (the reduced form of nicotinamide adenine dinucleotide, or NAD). NADH can donate electrons to the electron transport chain, which can drive ATP production. Pyruvate is transported into the mitochondrial matrix, where the molecule is oxidized to *acetyl CoA*, a carrier for the two-carbon molecule. Acetyl CoA also is

generated from the β-oxidation of fatty acids in the mitochondrial matrix. Acetyl CoA is completely oxidized in the matrix to CO_2 in the *Krebs cycle* (alternatively known as the *citric acid, tricarboxylic acid,* or *TCA* cycle), which generates NADH and *FADH$_2$* (the reduced form of flavin adenine dinucleotide, FAD) (Fig. 1–8). These molecules donate electrons to the electron transport chain in a process that ultimately consumes O_2. If oxygen is not available for the electron transport chain, glycolysis becomes *anaerobic*; pyruvate is converted to lactate, which is excreted from the cell. Anaerobic glycolysis produces ATP in the absence of oxygen (a relatively inefficient process); a side effect is the production of lactate, which can result in systemic acidosis.

The electron transport chain (also known as the *respiratory chain*) is a series of enzymes in the inner mitochondrial membrane that accepts electrons from the above donors and transports them down an energy gradient to the final electron acceptor, molecular oxygen (O_2), which is converted to H_2O (Fig. 1–8). The transport of electrons down the chain releases energy, which is utilized by proton pumps in the inner membrane to pump protons out of the matrix and into the intermembrane space. The proton extrusion powered by the electron transport chain creates an electrochemical gradient. ATP synthase, a large (500 kDa) nine-subunit complex embedded in the inner membrane (which is impermeable to H^+), translocates protons from the intermembrane space back into the matrix. This translocation releases energy the synthase enzyme utilizes to drive ATP production. The whole process in which energy derived from the oxidative phosphorylation of substrate is coupled to ATP production via the generation of an electrochemical gradient is called *chemiosmotic coupling*. Once a molecule of glucose enters the glycolytic pathway it is metabolized to pyruvate and then is completely oxidized to CO_2 and H_2O in the Krebs cycle/electron transport chain; it can liberate enough energy to generate 36 molecules of ATP.

Transcription

Transcription is the process by which the genetic code, DNA, is converted (transcribed) to a message (RNA), which in the case of mRNA can be read (translated) by the cell's synthetic machinery to generate specific proteins. Gene expression (i.e., the sum of the process from transcription through translation, with new protein as the end result) requires tight, careful regulation so the right protein is synthesized at the right time during the cell's life span. Dysregulated gene expression can be disastrous, leading to premature cell death or transformation. Transcription is performed by *RNA polymerases*, of which there are three types, designated I, II, and III. Polymerase I synthesizes precursor rRNA for the manufacture of ribosomes;

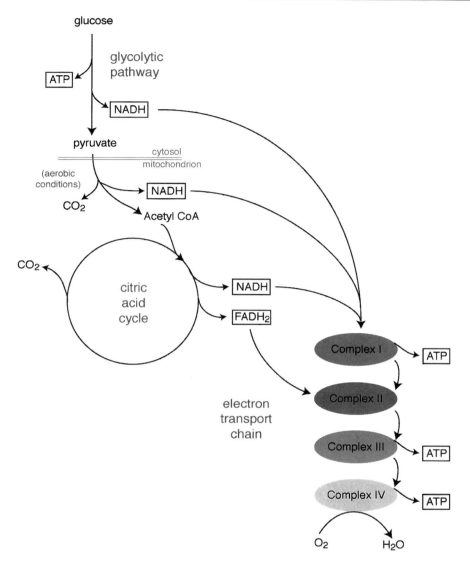

FIGURE 1–8 Overview of substrate oxidation and energy production in eukaryotes: a nonstoichiometric representation. This is the general pathway of glucose utilization under aerobic conditions. Note that the glycolytic pathway is located in the cytosol, and the rest of the reactions take place in the mitochondrion. See text for details. *See Color Plate 5.*

polymerase II synthesizes mRNA for protein translation (and hence is the critical polymerase for gene expression); and polymerase III generates both tRNA and rRNA.

Eukaryotic gene expression is regulated primarily at the level of transcription initiation—commonly through the effect of *transcription control regions*, which are segments of DNA that regulate the binding of RNA polymerase II (Pol II) to transcription initiation sequences. The transcription control regions act in a *cis* fashion; that is, they regulate transcription of a DNA segment located on the same gene as the control regions (contrast this with *trans* action, in which the regulator and the target can be on separate genes). Transcription control regions, which are relatively close to the target DNA (within 200 bp

upstream of the transcription start site), are known as *promoters* (of which the TATA box is the most common sequence); regions that are relatively distant from the target (potentially many kilobases up- or downstream) are known as *enhancers*. Proteins known as *transcription factors* bind to promoter and enhancer regions and either activate or repress transcription. For Pol II to initiate transcription, a sequence of binding involving the polymerase enzyme, DNA, and a series of polypeptides known as the *TFII transcription factors* must generate the Pol II transcription-initiation complex, which ultimately may contain up to 70 polypeptides.

After eukaryotic mRNA transcription has begun, 7-methylguanosine is added to the beginning of the nascent chain (i.e., the 5′ end) in a processing step called *capping*. As the nascent mRNA chain grows, it is bound by heterogeneous ribonucleoprotein particles (hnRNPs), which assist in further mRNA processing and transport. Transcription is halted (in the case of mRNA synthesis) after a cleavage and polyadenylation signaling sequence appears at the end of the nascent mRNA chain. The mRNA subsequently is cleaved from the Pol II complex, and a polymer of 200 to 250 adenylate residues is added to the 3′ end of the mRNA (*polyadenylation*). mRNA also is processed by *splicing*, in which segments of RNA called *introns* are removed by a large ribonucleoprotein complex called the *spliceosome*, and the remaining RNA segments (*exons*) are rejoined (spliced) to generate the processed mRNA, which is translated.

Translation

Translation is the process of mRNA-directed protein synthesis. Each mRNA transcript contains a *genetic code* that specifies the order in which amino acids are added to a nascent polypeptide chain in the ribosome. The code consists of three-nucleotide sequences called *codons* (or triplets); it follows that there are $4^3 = 64$ possible codons, 61 of which specify a particular amino acid (Table 1–1). Because there are only 20 amino acids, however, the genetic code is *degenerate* (i.e., redundant) in that some amino acids are specified by more than one codon. Leucine, serine, and arginine, for example, may each be specified by one of six redundant codons; on the other hand, tryptophan and methionine each has only one codon. All protein synthesis begins at the amino-terminus with a methionine residue, the codon for which is AUG (the *start*, or initiator, codon; equivalent to ATG in DNA). Translation is halted at the carboxy-terminus by one of three *termination* (or halt) codons (UAA, UGA, or UAG — the three codons of the 64 that do not specify an amino acid). The series of triplet sequences that begins at the start codon and ends at the termination codon is called the *reading frame*; it follows that each mRNA has three potential reading frames.

Table 1–1
Amino acids (n = 20) with their symbols and codons

Full Name	Three-Letter Symbol	One-Letter Symbol	Codon
Alanine	Ala	A	GCA, GCC, GCG, GCU
Arginine	Arg	R	AAC, AAU
Asparagine	Asn	N	AAC, AAU
Aspartic acid	Asp	D	GAC, GAU
Cysteine	Cys	C	UGC, UGU
Glutamic acid	Glu	E	GAA, GAG
Glutamine	Gln	Q	CAA, CAG
Glycine	Gly	G	GGA, GGC, GGG, GGU
Histidine*	His	H	CAC, CAU
Isoleucine*	Iso	I	AUA, AUC, AUU
Leucine*	Leu	L	UUA, UUG, CUA, CUC, CUG, CUU
Lysine*	Lys	K	AAA, AAG
Methionine*	Met	M	AUG
Phenylalanine*	Phe	F	UUC, UUU
Proline	Pro	P	CCA, CCC, CCG, CCU
Serine	Ser	S	AGC, AGU, UCA, UCC, UCG, UCU
Threonine*	Thr	T	ACA, ACC, ACG, ACU
Tryptophan*	Trp	W	UGG
Tyrosine	Tyr	Y	UAC, UAU
Valine*	Val	V	GUA, GUC, GUG, GUU

*Essential amino acid (n = 9).
Adapted from Alberts B, Bray D, Lewis J, et al: Molecular Biology of the Cell (2nd ed). London: Garland Science Publishing, 1989. Reproduced by permission of Routledge, Inc., part of The Taylor & Francis Group.

Translation of the mRNA outside the correct reading frame usually results in premature termination secondary to the early appearance of a halt codon in the incorrect reading frame.

Translation occurs in the ribosome, which can be located in the rough ER or the cytosol (Fig. 1–1). The 5′ end of the mRNA complexes with a 40S ribosomal subunit and other translation-initiation proteins; the 60S subunit then binds to the complex to complete the ribosome assembly, and translation proceeds from the 5′ end to the 3′ end of the mRNA, adding amino acids to the nascent polypeptide chain at about three residues per second. As one ribosome begins translation and travels down the mRNA, another ribosome can initiate translation at the 5′ end; in this fashion, a typical mRNA can be occupied by 10 or more ribosomes, each translating at various points along the mRNA chain. This complex of ribosomes and mRNA is known as a *polysome*.

The synthesis of a peptide as directed by the mRNA template is mediated by transfer RNA (tRNA) subunits. Each tRNA particle has a specific *anticodon* that can base-pair with the codons of the ribosome-bound mRNA, and each tRNA carries a specific amino acid residue. For example, the start codon AUG is recognized by the tRNA that contains the anticodon CAU; this tRNA carries a methionine residue. The next codon is read by the appropriate tRNA, which adds its amino acid residue to the methionine already in place; this process repeats until the stop codon is read. A protein synthesized by an ER ribosome takes up final residence in a membrane; a protein synthesized by a cytosolic ribosome remains in the cytosol. Membrane proteins are synthesized with a hydrophobic *signal peptide* on the end of the emerging nascent chain; this peptide is bound by a *signal recognition particle* (SRP) in the lumen of the ER. The SRP directs the ribosome to an ER membrane complex called the *translocon*, which directs the nascent polypeptide chain into the ER lumen, in which further processing and packaging may be accomplished to ensure transport to the appropriate destination.

Cell Replication

The overriding goal of cell replication is to produce two copies of the cell's DNA and then segregate each copy into the two daughter cells. Cell replication (also known as cell division) occurs in the context of the *cell cycle*, which may be described as a sequence of four phases (Fig. 1–9). The G_1 (gap) phase begins at completion of the previous cell division (i.e., at the end of the previous M phase) and ends at the onset of DNA synthesis, which, by definition is the beginning of the S (synthetic) phase. After a new complement of DNA has been synthesized during the S phase, the cell cycle enters the G_2 phase, in which final cellular preparations are made before beginning the

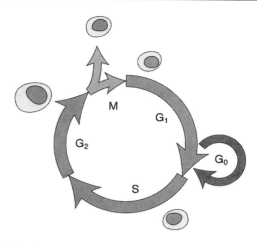

FIGURE 1–9 The four phases of the eukaryotic cell cycle: G_1, S, G_2, and M. The G_0 state is a resting condition associated with the G_1 phase. See text for details. (Adapted from Lodish H, Berk A, Zipursky SL, et al: Molecular Cell Biology [4th ed]. New York: WH Freeman, 2000, with permission.) *See Color Plate 5.*

division process. The beginning of cell division marks the end of the G_2 phase and the beginning of the M (mitotic) phase. Two daughter cells are produced during the M phase; these cells subsequently enter the G_1 phase, and a new cell cycle begins.

In rapidly dividing human cells an entire cell cycle requires about 24 hours, of which the G_1 phase is (approximately) 9 hours, the S phase is 10 hours, the G_2 phase is 4.5 hours, and the M phase is 0.5 hour. Under certain conditions a cell can remain in the G_1 phase for an indefinite time, during which the cell can assume specialized functions and synthesize proteins specific for these functions. This process is called *differentiation*, and the extended G_1 phase in which it occurs is known as the G_0 *phase*. Most cells (e.g., cardiac, neuronal, connective tissue) in the adult human are in the G_0 phase, but there are notable exceptions (e.g., stem cells in the epidermis, gut epithelium, and bone marrow) in which the cells cycle continuously throughout the life span of the organism. There are some cells (e.g., cardiac and neuronal) that, under in vivo conditions, do not reenter the cell cycle after passing into the G_0 phase (in the recent literature this paradigm does not appear to be immutable); that is, these cells have undergone *terminal differentiation*. Other cells (e.g., the fibroblast) can move in and out of the G_0 phase repeatedly.

Mitosis is the phase of the cell cycle in which chromosomes condense, segregate, and migrate into the new daughter cells (Fig. 1–10). The first stage of mitosis is *prophase*, in which each chromosome (around 45 mm long if straightened) along with its copy (generated during the S phase) is condensed onto a chromosome scaffold

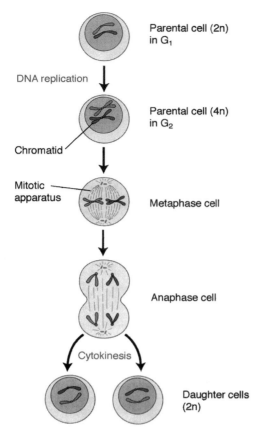

Parental cell (2n)
in G_1

DNA replication

Parental cell (4n)
in G_2

Chromatid

Mitotic
apparatus

Metaphase cell

Anaphase cell

Cytokinesis

Daughter cells
(2n)

FIGURE 1–10 Mitosis. This sequence begins with the cell in G_1 phase **(top)**, proceeds through the S phase into G_2, and then begins the formal steps of mitosis. See text for details. (Adapted from Lodish H, Berk A, Zipursky SL, et al: Molecular Cell Biology [4th ed]. New York: WH Freeman, 2000, with permission.) *See Color Plate 6.*

(several micrometers in length). The next stage of mitosis is *metaphase*, in which the condensed DNA on the chromosomal scaffolds are aligned at the center of the cell; by this time the nuclear membrane has been broken down. Each *metaphase chromosome* consists of two copies of a given chromosome (also known as *sister chromatids*) held together near their midpoint by the *centromere*. During *anaphase* the sister chromatids separate and migrate toward opposite poles of the cell to the *mitotic apparatus*, or spindle, which forms in each future daughter cell. The chromatid migration of anaphase results in an identical chromosomal complement for each daughter cell. The final phase of mitosis is *telophase*, in which a new nuclear envelope forms around the segregated chromatids, which decondense into conventional chromosomes. Occurring in conjunction with telophase is *cytokinesis*, which is the pinching off of cytoplasm between the two daughter nuclei to complete the physical separation of the daughter cells.

The primary regulators of the cell cycle are the family of *cyclin-dependent kinases* (Cdks). A Cdk forms a heterodimer

with its regulatory subunit (a member of the cyclin family), with the Cdk having no activity in the absence of the cyclin. Cyclin levels rise and fall in synchrony with the cell cycle. There are three general types of cyclin-Cdk heterodimers: G_1-, S-, and M-phase Cdk complexes. The substrate specificity of a given Cdk is regulated in part by the particular cyclin that binds to it. Broadly speaking, substrate phosphorylation by Cdk results in cell cycle progression.

Commitment to cell cycle progression usually occurs between the G_1 and S phases (known as the G_1/S phase transition or, alternatively, as the *restriction point*). For example, a fibroblast in G_0 (the extended G_1 phase) stimulated with a *mitogen* (an agent such as a soluble growth factor that stimulates cell division) increases the expression of G_1-phase Cdk complexes, which among other actions phosphorylate the *Rb* (retinoblastoma) *protein*. Nonphosphorylated Rb protein is an inhibitor of the E2F family of transcription factors; Rb phosphorylation disinhibits the E2F transcription factors, which subsequently promote expression of proteins necessary for commencement of the S phase. Rb phosphorylation is coincident with passage through the restriction point. Prior to the restriction point, continuous mitogen stimulation is required to maintain cell cycle progression; after the restriction point is passed, however, the cells progress through the replication cycle regardless of mitogen presence or absence.

E2F influence results in the formation of S-phase Cdk complexes, which initiate DNA synthesis by phosphorylating (and thereby activating) DNA *prereplication complexes*, which proceed with DNA synthesis. The M-phase Cdk complex is activated upon completion of DNA synthesis; it first directs assembly of the chromosomes at the metaphase plate and then activates the *anaphase-promoting complex* (APC). This complex promotes loss of the protein connections between sister chromosomes at the metaphase plate, which permits chromosome segregation and anaphase to progress. The APC also promotes degradation of the M-phase Cdk complex; loss of the complex allows the separated chromosomes to be enveloped by new nuclear membranes and promotes cytokinesis.

Progression of the cell cycle can be regulated by the p53, p21, or p15/p16 proteins. The p53 protein (also known as "the guardian of the genome") is a transcription factor that is activated in the presence of DNA damage (e.g., secondary to ultraviolet irradiation) and arrests the cell cycle in the G_1 phase. If the DNA can be repaired, p53 inhibition is lifted after repairs are complete, and the cell cycle is allowed to continue. If the DNA damage is irreparable, the cell may be driven into apoptosis. Perpetuation of cells with genetic mutations secondary to DNA damage is prevented in part by the p53 protein; not surprisingly, p53 is inactivated in many forms of cancer, allowing damaged DNA to replicate. The p21 family of proteins binds and inhibits the cyclin-Cdks and DNA polymerase; p21 expression is increased by p53. The p15 and p16 protein families bind to the cyclins and Cdks, thereby preventing their association and subsequent Cdk activation.

Molecule Transport

Membrane vesicle trafficking (the *secretory pathway*) is the primary mechanism by which proteins and lipids are transported in the cell; the secretory pathway is conserved through the phyla. The pathway follows this basic scheme: Transport vesicles move from the ER → *cis* Golgi → *trans* Golgi → the target membrane. Vesicular transport can be regulated or constitutive; the latter type is present in all cells, delivers a continuous supply of vesicles via the Golgi apparatus, and does not depend on external signaling or calcium. During regulated vesicular transport, regulated proteins are stored in submembrane *dense secretory granules* (named after their electron microscopic appearance), which fuse with a membrane to release their contents when cytosolic Ca^{2+} is momentarily raised to ~1 μM (i.e., an order of magnitude increase above baseline). An example of regulated vesicular transport is neurotransmitter release into the synaptic cleft during transmission of an impulse.

The process of vesicular budding is facilitated by *coatomers* (or COP complexes), which coat a vesicle formed by the Golgi apparatus, thereby regulating the direction of vesicle movement. Coatomers contains ADP ribosylation factor (*ARF*), which is a small GTP-binding protein essential for vesicular budding. A vesicle coated with COP-1 is budded in a retrograde direction (i.e., Golgi → ER), which is useful for recycling chaperones and other ER proteins. COP-2 directs budding in an antegrade direction (i.e., Golgi → target membrane). Prior to fusing with the target (acceptor) membrane, the coatomer coat is shed; the vesicle fusion is mediated in part by SNARE proteins; SNARE-v (located on the vesicular membrane) and SNARE-t (located on the target membrane) facilitate accurate targeting of specific vesicles with specific target membranes. Rab is a small GTP-binding protein that associates with SNARE-v on the vesicular membrane. If SNARE-v and SNARE-t interact (as happens immediately prior to membrane fusion), Rab hydrolyzes its GTP and fusion ensues. Specific Rabs exist for each subcellular location, which assists the process of specific targeting.

Vesicles also transport material from the cell membrane into the cell interior; the general term for this process is *endocytosis*. There are three general mechanisms of endocytosis: pinocytosis, receptor-mediated endocytosis, and phagocytosis. Pinocytosis is a continuous, non-receptor-mediated generation of relatively small vesicles from the plasma membrane into the cytosol. Invaginations form in the plasma membrane and pinch off into the cell as a

vesicle, carrying in water, proteins, ions, and other extracellular molecules in a nonspecific fashion. This process can transport a relatively large volume of material because the high frequency of pinocytotic vesicle formation can turn over the entire plasma membrane mass in as little as 1 hour. Once inside the cell, pinocytotic vesicles coalesce to form *early endosomes*, which then fuse with lysosomes to form *late endosomes*, and the vesicle contents subsequently are digested.

During receptor-mediated endocytosis (Fig. 1–11), extracellular ligands are bound by specific membrane receptors; this event recruits a protein called *clathrin* to the cytosolic portion of the receptor, which in association with the *adaptin complex* mediates an invagination of the plasma membrane containing the receptor–ligand complexes into a newly formed *clathrin-coated pit*.

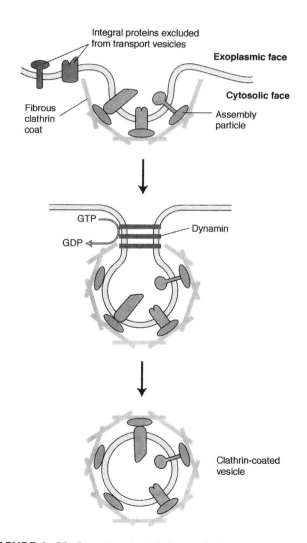

FIGURE 1–11 Formation of a clathrin-coated pit during receptor-mediated endocytosis. See text for details. (Adapted from Lodish H, Berk A, Zipursky SL, et al: Molecular Cell Biology [4th ed]. New York: WH Freeman, 2000, with permission.) *See Color Plate 6.*

Clathrin is a hexamer that complexes with other clathrins to form a cage-like structure (the pit) around invaginating receptor–ligand vesicles. The protein *dynamin* polymerizes at the neck of the vesicle, and the vesicle pinches off in a GTP-dependent process. The pinched-off vesicle is engulfed by the clathrin "cage" as the vesicle enters the cytosol. The fate of the vesicle derived from receptor-mediated endocytosis is fusion with a lysosome and recycling or degradation of the ligand–receptor complexes. Growth factor and lipoproteins are common examples of ligands, which the cell internalizes via receptor-mediated endocytosis. *Transcytosis* is a specialized form of receptor-mediated endocytosis in which an endocytized material is brought into the cell, transported to another area of the cell membrane, and then released into the extracellular space. This mechanism is used, for example, in neonatal intestinal epithelial cells to absorb maternal immunoglobulin.

The third type of endocytosis, phagocytosis, involves binding a large particle (e.g., a bacterium or an apoptotic body) to membrane receptors, with the subsequent engulfment of the particle by the cell; there is no involvement of clathrin. Typically, a particle that has been opsonized (covered) with host antibodies is bound to a phagocytic cell (commonly a neutrophil or macrophage, although many other cell types can phagocytize) via *Fc receptors*, which recognize the Fc portion of the antibody. A signal transduction event involving Src kinase then occurs that results in the extension of pseudopodia around the particle (i.e., membrane engulfment). The pseudopodia extension is driven by actin polymerization; phagocytosis therefore is dependent on the actin cytoskeleton. After the particle has been ingested by the cell it becomes a *phagosome*, which subsequently fuses with lysosomes to become a *phagolysosome*; degradation of the phagocytized material ensues.

Vesicular transport within the cell is mediated by a variety of *molecular motors*, of which *dyneins* and *kinesins* are two common families. The head of one of these large (300 kDa) motor proteins binds to microtubules, and the tail binds to the membrane-bound structure to be transported. The head migrates along the microtubule in an ATP-dependent process; in general, dynein motors move toward the minus end of the microtubule (i.e., toward the centrosome), and the kinesin motors move toward the plus end (i.e., toward the plasma membrane). Actin-based molecular motors, also known as *myosins*, can transport vesicles along actin filaments (myosin-I) and generate skeletal muscle contraction (yosin-II) (Fig. 1–12).

Cell–Cell and Cell–Matrix Connections

Most cells in the body are integrated into various tissues, where the cells perform specialized functions. The structure and function of a particular tissue is due in large part to the organization of the cells in the tissue; this organization is defined by cell–cell and cell–matrix interactions. Cells attach to other cells via *cell-adhesion molecules* (CAMs), which are surface membrane receptors that can bind cells of the same (*homophilic* interaction) or different (*heterophilic* interaction) type. The cadherin family of proteins and the immunoglobulin CAMs (also known as N-CAMs) are the major components of homophilic cell–cell binding; binding of the former and latter is calcium-dependent and calcium–independent, respectively. E-cadherin maintains the cell–cell connections of epithelial sheets, such as in the intestinal mucosa. This type of adherence is reinforced by the formation of *adherens junctions* and *desmosomes*, which are specific cell–cell contact points where cadherins are concentrated. N-CAMs participate in neural cell–cell connections. The selectin protein family and mucin-like CAMs allow cells of differing types to adhere during heterophilic binding; for example, *P-selectin* on the surface of leukocytes allows these cells to bind to the endothelium of blood vessels and extravasate. *Gap junctions* are a specialized form of cell–cell contact in which the 12 copies of the protein *connexin* form a channel between the cytoplasm of the two cells in contact. This allows small molecules to travel back and forth between cells, which facilitates metabolic coupling of neighboring cells.

The extracellular matrix provides a scaffold for organ structure and anchorage points for individual cells, which is vital for specialization of cellular functions. The ECM

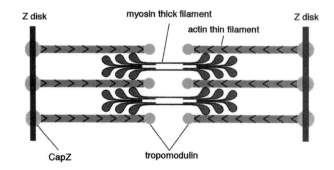

FIGURE 1–12 Actin-myosin contractile complex of skeletal muscle. Each muscle cell is packed with myofibrils, which are bundles of filaments that traverse the length of the cell and are oriented in the direction of contraction. Each filament is composed of sarcomere units strung end-to-end; an individual sarcomere is diagramed. The Z disks (also called Z lines) mark the ends of an individual sarcomere. The Z disk functions to anchor the actin thin filaments; this anchorage is facilitated by CapZ, an actin-capping protein, and α-actinin. Tropomodulin caps the opposite end of each thin filament. The thick filaments are composed of myosin II and interdigitate with the thin filaments. Muscle contraction occurs when the heads of the myosin II protein walk along the thin filaments in an ATP-dependent process; this action draws the Z disks together, which shortens the sarcomere. (Adapted from Lodish H, Berk A, Zipursky SL, et al: Molecular Cell Biology [4th ed]. New York: WH Freeman, 2000, with permission.) *See Color Plate 6.*

also provides the basis for the rigidity and incompressibility of bone and for the tensile strength of tendons and ligaments. The composition of the ECM varies from tissue to tissue but usually contains a mixture of *collagen, fibronectin, proteoglycans,* and *polysaccharides.* These molecules are all synthesized and modified intracellularly and then are secreted into the ECM, where they can undergo further modification (e.g., collagen fibril cross-linking, which increases strength and stability) and subunit assembly. Collagen, a fibrous protein, is the major constituent of the ECM. To date, there are about 19 types of collagen, but 80% to 90% of the collagen in the body consists of types I, II, III, and IV. Types I, II, and III form collagen fibrils; the structure of type I collagen triple helix fibril is shown in Figure 1–13. Type IV collagen and laminin, a large heterotrimeric protein, form the planar-shaped basement membrane. The fibronectins are a group of more than 20 proteins, all dimers, and are generated from a single fibronectin gene with alternative splicing of the fibronectin transcript. The primary function of the fibronectins is to bridge the connection between cells and the collagen ECM; fibronectins therefore play a critical role in processes involving cell–ECM interactions, such as cellular migration or anchorage-dependent survival. The proteoglycans, such as heparin or chondroitin sulfate, consist of long repeating disaccharide polymers (*glycosaminoglycans*) surrounding a protein core. These molecules are heavily hydrated, and they cushion cells from mechanical forces; proteoglycans also bind and serve as a reservoir for various growth factors and cytokines. *Hyaluronan* (or *hyaluronic acid* or *hyaluronate*) is an ECM polysaccharide that is not linked to a protein; it also is heavily hydrated and forms a viscous substance that resists compressive forces and inhibits cell–cell adhesion.

The primary mediator of cell–matrix connections is the *integrin* family of membrane receptors. Integrins are integral transmembrane heterodimers consisting of an α subunit and a β subunit. Various combinations of α and β subunits generate the more than 20 identified integrins; each integrin has its own ECM binding specificity, which usually is defined as a peptide recognition sequence. An important recognition sequence for integrin-mediated anchorage to the ECM is RGD (arginine-glycine-aspartate). The RGD sequence occurs multiple times in fibronectin, and the primary integrin that binds fibronectin (via RGD recognition) is $\alpha_5\beta_1$. In general, integrins bind ECM proteins with relatively low affinity; however, because the integrin receptor concentration is relatively high (10^3 to 10^4 per cell), integrin-mediated ECM binding is able to maintain cell anchorage. During the course of binding to ECM proteins, integrins cluster at membrane surface sites called *focal adhesions* or *focal contacts.* This clustering recruits numerous proteins with various enzymatic and adapter functions to the cytoplasmic side of the focal adhesion. Focal adhesions are linked to the actin cytoskeleton, thereby forming a continuous mechanical link between the ECM, integrin receptor, and cytoskeleton. This relationship promotes cell survival and can facilitate entrance into the cell cycle. Anchorage-dependent cells therefore are dependent on integrin function for their homeostasis. Loss of anchorage dependence on survival is one criterion of malignant transformation.

Signal Transduction

Signal transduction is the process in which a cell receives, integrates, and responds to signals from its environment. The evolving picture of signal transduction is an increasingly complex, intersecting collection of pathways that involve receptors, enzymes, cofactors, protein adaptors and scaffolds, and small messenger molecules. Functioning as a unit, these entities receive a signal (commonly but not exclusively a secreted molecule in the extracellular space) and translate it into an appropriate response, which could be the opening of ion gates, shortening of contractile units,

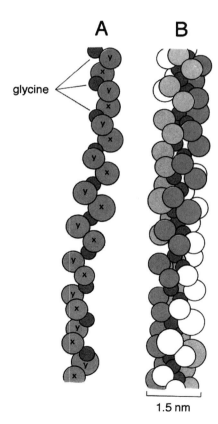

FIGURE 1–13 Structure of type I collagen. Each sphere represents an amino acid residue. **A,** Single-strand polymer. **B,** Each molecule of collagen is composed of three such strands arranged in a triple helix, which also is known as a collagen fibril. The amino acid residue represented by "y" typically is proline or hydroxyproline; "x" can be any residue. (Adapted from Alberts B, Bray D, Lewis J, et al: Molecular Biology of the Cell [2nd ed]. London: Garland Science Publishing, 1989. Reproduced by permission of Routledge, Inc., part of The Taylor & Francis Group.) *See Color Plate 7.*

extension of filopodia, augmentation or inhibition of specific gene expression, or initiation of the cell cycle, among others. Signal transduction may be organized into three components: (1) the signal; (2) the signal receptor; and (3) the postreceptor pathway that produces the effect.

Signal component

The nature of a secreted signal can be *endocrine* (a secreted signaling molecule travels through the extracellular space and affects a distant cell—also known as *hormonal*); *paracrine* (the signaling molecule affects a cell nearby or a neighbor of the secreting cell); *juxtacrine* (the signal is transmitted between two cells by direct physical contact of their cell surface ligands and receptors); or *autocrine* (the cell responds to its own secreted signaling molecules) (Fig. 1–14). Alternatively, the signal can consist of mechanical force, heat, light, oxygen tension, or other unconventional sources. A partial listing of signaling agents and their associated transduction mechanism is shown in Table 1–2.

Receptor component

Signal receptors may be grouped into five basic categories: (1) intracellular receptors, which require transport of the signal across the plasma membrane before receptor ligation can occur; (2) transmembrane receptors with intrinsic enzymatic activity, which act on intracellular substrates after ligating an extracellular signal; (3) transmembrane receptors, which are linked to intracellular kinases; (4) transmembrane receptors linked to an intracellular second messenger; and (5) transmembrane receptors, which regulate ion gates.

INTRACELLULAR RECEPTORS. *Cortisol* and *thyroxine* are typical molecules that signal via intracellular receptors. After crossing the plasma membrane, the signaling molecule ligates its receptor, which can be located in either the cytosol or the nucleus. The receptor–ligand complex ends up in the nucleus, where it regulates transcription. The effect from this type of signal transduction can take hours to days to set in because the mechanism involves modulation of protein synthesis.

RECEPTORS WITH INTRINSIC ACTIVITY. Ligation of molecules such as platelet-derived growth factor (PDGF) or insulin to their receptor activates *receptor tyrosine kinase* (RTK) activity on the cytoplasmic portion of the receptor. The activated RTK phosphorylates additional tyrosine residues on the cytoplasmic portion of RTKs (*autophosphorylation*) and on RTK-associated proteins (*transphosphorylation*). These phosphorylation events generally activate protein–protein binding sites, upregulate enzymatic activity of RTK substrates, or both; this process

is the basis of RTK signal transduction. Alternatively, molecules such as atrial natriuretic factor (ANF) activate receptor guanosine cyclase activity, which generates cGMP from GTP at the cytoplasmic portion of the receptor; the cGMP then functions as a second messenger.

RECEPTORS LINKED TO KINASES. A receptor linked to kinases lacks intrinsic enzymatic activity; but upon ligation of the signaling molecule (e.g., an *interferon* or *growth hormone*) the receptor activates cytosolic tyrosine kinases. Phosphorylation of tyrosine residues transmits signals in a fashion similar to that of the RTK mechanism (see above). *Integrin receptors*, which bind ECM proteins, are another example of kinase-linked receptors. For example, upon binding the ECM protein fibronectin the $\alpha_5\beta_1$ integrin activates *focal adhesion kinase*, a cytosolic tyrosine kinase that has downstream effects on cell adhesion, cell survival, the cell cycle, and other intracellular events.

RECEPTORS LINKED TO SECOND MESSENGERS. The prime example of the receptor subtype that is linked to second messengers is the family of GTP-binding proteins. There are two general types of GTP-binding proteins: monomeric GTPases and trimeric G *proteins* (consisting of α, β, and γ subunits). There are five common subfamilies of monomeric GTPases, listed here with their regulatory function: Ras (growth and differentiation; see below); Rho (cytoskeletal regulation and integrin activation); Rab (vesicular transport); ARF (vesicle formation); and Ran (nuclear transport). Trimeric G proteins transmit signals from signaling molecules such as the *catecholamines* and *glucagon*. The binding of a signaling molecule to a G *protein-linked receptor* (an integral membrane protein with seven transmembrane domains) induces receptor association with an inactive G protein, which subsequently is activated by the binding of GTP to G_α subunit. This subunit dissociates from the β and γ subunits and activates a membrane-associated effector enzyme such as adenylyl cyclase or phospholipase C. The effector generates a second messenger, such as cAMP, ITP, or DAG, which has context-dependent effects (see below). Trimeric G proteins also are known by the term *molecular switch*, because their activity varies depending on whether they bind GTP (switched on) or GDP (switched off).

ION GATE RECEPTORS. Ligand binding by an ion gate receptor typically induces a conformational change in the receptor, which results in the opening of a receptor-associated channel through the membrane that permits select ions (e.g., Na^+, K^+, or Ca^{2+}) to travel in the direction of their electrochemical gradient. A notable member of this receptor category is the *nicotinic acetylcholine receptor*, which is a complex of five subunits located on

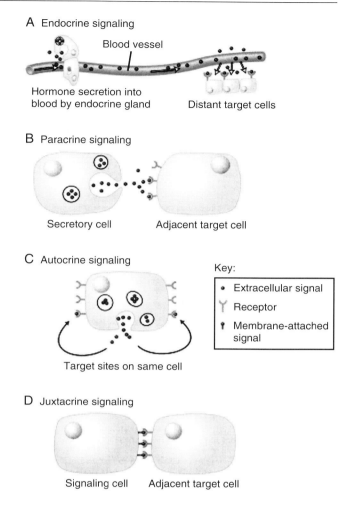

A Endocrine signaling

Blood vessel

Hormone secretion into
blood by endocrine gland

Distant target cells

B Paracrine signaling

Secretory cell   Adjacent target cell

C Autocrine signaling

Key:

• Extracellular signal

Y Receptor

ⵎ Membrane-attached
signal

Target sites on same cell

D Juxtacrine signaling

Signaling cell   Adjacent target cell

FIGURE 1–14 Basic signaling mechanisms: endocrine (**A**); paracrine (**B**); autocrine (**C**); and juxtacrine (**D**). See text for details. (Adapted from Lodish H, Berk A, Zipursky SL, et al: Molecular Cell Biology [4th ed]. New York: WH Freeman, 2000, with permission.) *See Color Plate 7.*

the postsynaptic membrane. Upon binding of the neuro-transmitter acetylcholine, an ion gate for Na^+ opens in the center of the receptor, and the influx of Na^+ perpetuates the action potential in the postsynaptic membrane.

Postreceptor component

The postreceptor component of signal transduction is an increasingly complex maze of messenger molecules, protein kinases and phosphatases, and adapter molecules. Two prominent topics are briefly discussed here: the second messenger concept, and a specific kinase pathway (Ras/MAPK).

SECOND MESSENGERS. The second messenger concept typically involves receptor-mediated generation of an intracellular molecule (the "second" messenger) after receptor activation by the extracellular signaling molecule (the "first" messenger). The second messenger then modulates various intracellular processes. The net effect depends on the specific messenger and the cellular

context. Some common second messengers along with their associated receptors and downstream effects are described in Table 1–3.

RAS/MAP KINASE PATHWAY. One of the primary targets of tyrosine kinase signaling is the monomeric GTPase Ras. For example, autophosphorylation of an RTK can result in the binding of Grb2, an adapter protein, via SH2 (Src homology) domains to the cytoplasmic portion of the RTK. Grb2 functions to bring upstream and downstream members of a signaling pathway into proximity, thereby promoting transduction of the signal. The RTK–Grb2 complex subsequently binds to the Sos protein via SH3 homology domains, which also are located on Grb2. The bound Sos then binds Ras, which promotes Ras-GTP binding, thus turning on the Ras molecular switch. Activated Ras turns on the *mitogen-activated protein kinase* (MAPK) cascade. The MAPKs comprise a disparate family of protein kinases, the common members of which are extracellular

Table 1–2
Partial list of agents involved in signal transduction

Agent	Abbreviation	Predominant Signaling Mechanism	Receptor/Second Messenger
Epinephrine	–	Paracrine, endocrine	β-Adrenergic receptor→G protein→adenylyl cyclase→cAMP
Atrial natriuretic factor	ANF	Endocrine	Receptor guanosine cyclase activity→cGMP
Platelet-derived growth factor	PDGF	Autocrine, paracrine	Receptor tyrosine kinase
Insulin	–	Endocrine	
Nerve growth factor	NGF	Autocrine, paracrine	
Epidermal growth factor	EGF	Autocrine, paracrine	
Transforming growth factor-β	TGFβ	Autocrine, paracrine	TGFβ receptor→receptor multimerization→Ser/Thr kinase activity→SMAD transcription factor activation
Hedgehog	Hh	Paracrine	Complex with the Ptc and Smo receptors→activation of the Ci transcription factor
Prostacyclin	PGI_2	Autocrine, paracrine	IP receptor→G protein→adenylyl cyclase→cAMP
Thyroxine	T_4	Endocrine	Intracellular receptor→hormone-receptor complex→transcription regulation
Cortisol	–	Endocrine	
Tumor necrosis factor-α	TNFα	Paracrine, endocrine	TNFα receptor→FADD→caspase cascade
Interleukin-1	IL-1	Paracrine, endocrine	IL-1 receptor→IRAK-1→NF-κB
Acetylcholine	Ach	Paracrine (synaptic)	Nicotinic ACh receptor→Na^+/K^+ ion channel
Growth hormone	GH	Autocrine, paracrine, endocrine	Membrane receptor→receptor dimerization→receptor-linked tyrosine kinase activity
Interferons	IFN		
Shear stress	–	Transfer of mechanical force	Integrin receptor→focal adhesion formation→FA-associated tyrosine kinase activity
Oxygen partial pressure	Po_2	"Endocrine"	Carotid body chemoreceptor→O_2^- sensitive K^+ channel
Major histocompatibility complex antigens	MHC	Juxtacrine	T-cell receptor→CD3 complex→tyrosine kinase activity→IL-2 production

Note that some agents have similar classifications. Many adapter proteins that participate in transduction have not been included in this table.

regulated kinase (ERK), p38, and c-Jun N-terminal kinase (JUNK). Activated MAPKs generally translocate to the nucleus, where they regulate gene expression. The effect of MAPK activation is context-dependent; possible effects are survival promotion, cell cycle entry, stimulation of motility, or even activation of the cell death program. Activation of Ras and the MAP kinases can occur through inputs other than RTKs, including second messengers generated by G protein signaling.

Survival and Apoptosis

Certain biologic processes involve a massive turnover of cell number. In the adult human, for example, tissues

Table 1-3
Partial list of second messenger molecules with their typical path of generation and downstream effects

Second Messenger	Typical Generation Path	Typical Downstream Effect
Cyclic AMP (camp)	G protein-linked receptor→G protein→adenylyl cyclase	Activation of protein kinase A→cell-dependent effects
Phosphoinositides	Activation of phosphoinositide kinases/ phosphatases via RTKs or G protein-linked receptors → phosphorylation/dephosphorylation of membrane phosphatidylinositol	Membrane phosphoinositides function as adapter/scaffold molecules to facilitate/ stimulate various enzymatic reactions (e.g., activation of Akt)
Diacylglycerol (DAG)	Activation of phospholipase C via RTKs or G protein-linked receptors→cleavage of phosphatidylinositols	Activation of protein kinase C → cell-dependent effects
Inositol triphosphate (IP$_3$)	Activation of phospholipase C via RTKs or G protein-linked receptors→cleavage of phosphatidylinositols	Release from intracellular Ca^{2+} stores and opening of membrane Ca^{2+} gates → increased cytosolic $[Ca^{2+}]$
Calcium (Ca^{2+})	Increased cytosolic concentration by IP$_3$ action	Activation of protein kinase C → cell-dependent effects
Nitric oxide (NO)	Calcium-dependent NO synthase	Activation of cytosolic guanylate cyclase
Cyclic GMP (cGMP)	ANF receptor with intrinsic guanylate cyclase activity or NO-dependent cytosolic guanylate cyclase	Smooth muscle relaxation

Akt, protein kinase B; RTK, receptor tyrosine kinase.

such as the epidermis and gut epithelium are constantly regenerating. If injured, most tissues in the body respond with either a healing or regenerative response. In the fetus, numerous structures evolve early only to regress by the time of birth. If the enormous amount of cell replication in the above processes is not balanced by an appropriate amount of cell deletion, organism development and homeostasis would be disrupted. Furthermore, most cells, whether progressing through the cell cycle or in G_0, die if removed from their native environment (i.e., their substratum, or ECM). The point of all these examples is that the survival of any cell from one moment to the next is not happenstance; on the contrary, cell survival is a tightly, continuously regulated process.

The physiologic opposite to cell survival in vivo is a form of cell death called *apoptosis*, also known as programmed cell death. Apoptosis can be thought of as "cell suicide" in which a cell, under the proper stimuli, can activate proteolytic pathways that produce ordered destruction of that individual cell. This process must be distinguished from *necrosis*, a form of cell death that may be thought of as "cell murder." Necrosis usually occurs after some catastrophic cell injury (e.g., anoxia) and appears to be the end result of gross disruption of the cell's metabolic machinery. The distinction between apoptosis and necrosis is easy to make in textbooks, but in vivo these two seemingly separate processes are difficult to distinguish and may

coexist. With myocardial infarction, for example, features of necrosis (cellular swelling with an acute inflammatory component) and apoptosis (cell shrinkage and nuclear pyknosis without inflammation) can appear in the same histologic section.

Finally, there is at least one additional type of cell death that is nonphysiologic and distinguishable from apoptosis or necrosis: the rapid cessation of metabolism that occurs with histologic fixatives. Promotion of survival in normal, nonhematologic cells typically requires two conditions: cell anchorage and soluble trophic factors. *Cell anchorage* is the condition of attachment of the cell to the ECM, which generally is mediated by members of the integrin family of receptors (membrane proteins that bind ECM molecules). Soluble trophic factors usually are protein or lipid molecules (including growth factors, cytokines, and hormones), which after secretion into the extracellular space, influence cell survival via autocrine, paracrine, or hormonal mechanisms (Fig. 1-14). The requirements for growth factors and anchorage vary according to the cell type. For example, epithelial cells are particularly prone to apoptosis after loss of anchorage to the basement membrane, whereas fibroblasts are more tolerant to such loss and trophic factor withdrawal. The regulation of survival and death is an active area of research; some of the prominent pathways involved in this regulation are illustrated in Figure 1-15.

Reproduction and Regeneration

Animals reproduce by first generating and then combining *gametes* (sperm and egg cells). The *germ cells* that generate gametes undergo a reduction in chromosomes from 2*n* (*diploid*) to 1*n* (*haploid*), so the embryo that results from the union of the egg and sperm contains the proper complement (2*n*) of chromosomes. The process through which a germ cell undergoes two divisions to generate haploid

gametes is called *meiosis* (Fig. 1–16). During the first step, DNA synthesis occurs in the germ cell, which produces a 4*n* chromosome complement. The replicated chromosomes condense into chomatids and align themselves with their homologous partner at the cell equator in a condition called *synapsis*. This physical arrangement sets up the opportunity for *genetic recombination*, in which two homologous chromosomes can exchange various segments of DNA. Recombination is one method organisms employ

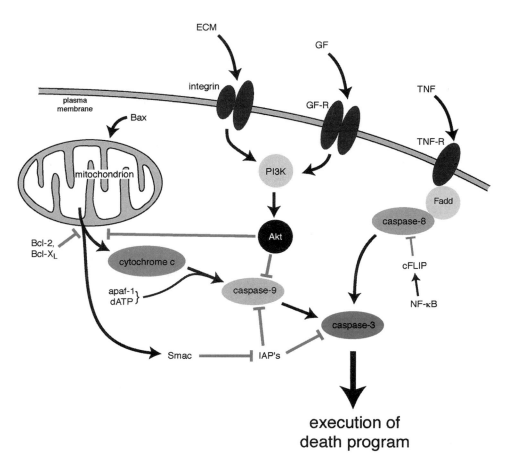

FIGURE 1–15 Overview of signaling during apoptosis. A typical cell receives multiple inputs, such as ligation of integrin receptors to the ECM or activation of growth factor receptors (GF-R), which tend to promote survival via activation of intracellular survival pathways. The phosphatidylinositol-3-kinase (PI3K)/Akt sequence is a prominent survival pathway activated by both growth factors and ECM anchorage. Activated Akt promotes survival through multiple mechanisms, such as by inhibition of cytochrome *c* release and inhibition of caspase-9. The pro-survival members of the Bcl-2 family typically inhibit release of cytochrome *c* from the mitochondria. Cell death usually is initiated through one of two major pathways: mitochondria-dependent or death receptor-dependent. A number of pro-apoptotic stimuli induce cytochrome *c* release from the mitochondria via the action of pro-apoptotic Bcl-2 proteins, such as Bax. Once in the cytosol, cytochrome *c* complexes with apaf-1, dATP, and caspase-9 (the apoptosome). This complex results during caspase-9 activation, which cleaves (and thus activates) caspase-3. Activation of caspase-3 generally is considered to be the final common pathway for execution of the apoptotic program. The activity of caspase-9 and caspase-3 is inhibited by the IAP family of proteins. If the cell receives an apoptotic stimulus, however, the protein Smac is released from the mitochondrion; Smac inhibits the IAPs, which relieves inhibition of the caspases. Smac release therefore is pro-apoptotic. Caspase-3 also can be activated by caspase-8, which is activated by the death receptor complex. Here, TNF initiates the death receptor complex by ligating the TNF receptor, which subsequently binds the adapter protein Fadd. Caspase-8 is held in check by cFLIP, which is turned on by the action of NF-κB. The transcription factor NF-κB has context-dependent effects of cell survival; in this scenario NF-κB is pro-survival. Not shown is another protein, AIF (apoptosis-inducing factor), which can be released from mitochondria. It can initiate apoptosis in an apparently caspase-independent pathway, which is incompletely characterized. *See Color Plate 8.*

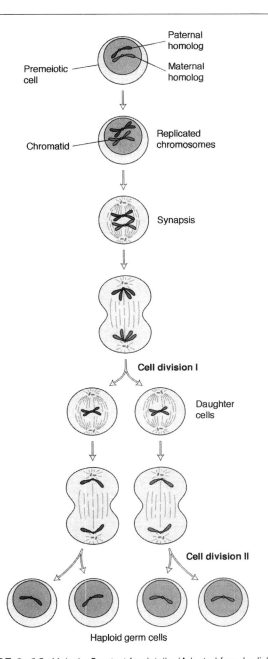

FIGURE 1–16 Meiosis. See text for details. (Adapted from Lodish H, Berk A, Zipursky SL, et al: Molecular Cell Biology [4th ed]. New York: WH Freeman, 2000, with permission.) *See Color Plate 9.*

to increase genetic diversity. After the 4n complement of chromosomes aligns during synapsis, the first meiotic cell division occurs, producing two diploid (2n) daughter cells. These diploid daughter cells undergo a second meiotic division (without further DNA synthesis), producing four haploid (1n) gametes. During the second meiotic division, the chromosomes sort randomly (*independent assortment*) to the gametes; this is another method organisms employ to increase genetic diversity. Thus, meiosis begins with one 2n germ cell and finishes with four

haploid gametes. The gametes from male and female (i.e., the sperm and egg) combine to generate a diploid embryo during *fertilization*, yet another method to increase genetic diversity.

Reproduction *generates* new organisms from two parental organisms. An individual organism, however, can regenerate new tissue in response to tissue loss from injury, disease, or normal physiologic turnover. Tissue regeneration secondary to stem cell biology currently is a topic of intense interest. A stem cell is an undifferentiated, renewable source of new cells; cells produced from stem cells can differentiate and specialize in function (i.e., they can become part of the tissue in which they were produced). For example, stem cells located in the basal layer of the epidermis and in the small intestinal crypts generate new epidermal and epithelial cells that replace cells that have undergone physiologic sloughing from the outer epidermis and villous tips, respectively. Mitosis of a stem cell produces two daughter cells; one daughter remains an undifferentiated stem cell, and the other differentiates according to the local environment. In this manner stem cells are self-perpetuating and typically are not susceptible to *replicative senescence*. In contrast, other wild-type cell strains (e.g., dermal fibroblasts) stop replicating in vitro after 60 to 90 cell divisions (i.e., the cells become senescent). Stem cells function throughout the life of the organism; to use the previous example, human epidermis and intestinal mucosa generate new cells continuously, regardless of the person's age.

Stem cells have been demonstrated in a wide range of adult tissues, including muscle and neural tissue, which traditionally were considered incapable of regeneration; the distribution of stem cells may well extend to all tissues. Stem cells vary in their *potency*, or the range of daughter cell types the stem cell is able to produce. An embryo is *totipotent* in that all cells in an organism ultimately derive from this one stem cell. A bone marrow stem cell is *pluripotent* because it can give rise to a number of hematologic cells. Stem cells may differ in the extent of their pluripotency (from oligopotency to multipotency); in fact, it has been suggested that adult stem cells from one tissue might give rise to cells of a different tissue (e.g., neural cells from hematologic stem cells). The epidermal stem cells referred to above are *unipotent* in that they give rise to one type of differentiated daughter cell.

The intense interest in stem cell research derives from the potential advances in health care that could result from stem cell biology. Artificial organs could be engineered using the patient's own stem cells, producing tissue that theoretically would not undergo immunologic rejection. Potential applications of such bioengineering are the treatment of juvenile diabetes, spinal cord injury, and ischemic heart disease, and there are many other examples. There are associated ethical concerns about stem cell research, however, particularly with respect to the use of stem cells derived from human embryos, which essentially are totipotent. Researchers have a keen interest in experimenting with totipotent cell lines, but because each of these cells has the theoretical potency to develop into a human there has been opposition to the use of human embryologic stem cells.

An alternative to the use of embryologic stem cells is to employ adult stem cells; presently it is not clear, however, if adult stem cells are "as potent" as their embryologic equivalents. It has been shown, nevertheless, that the transfer of an adult mammalian nucleus into an egg cytoplast reprograms the nucleus so a totipotent stem cell is produced. This is precisely what was done when cloning the sheep "Dolly" in 1997. This type of nuclear reprogramming traditionally was thought to be not feasible because it had been believed that the DNA in differentiated cells had undergone irreversible modification that prevented dedifferentiation back to a totipotent embryo. Apparently this is not the case, and totipotent adult stem cells may be feasible. Whether embryos (or tissue) derived from adult animal cells

can produce animals (or tissue) with normal life spans without increased susceptibility to disease, however, remains to be seen.

Bibliography

Alberts B, Bray D, Johnson A, et al: Essential Cell Biology: An Introduction to the Molecular Biology of the Cell. London: Garland Science Publishing, 1998.

Alberts B, Bray D, Lewis J, et al: Molecular Biology of the Cell (3rd ed). London: Garland Science Publishing, 1994.

Cooper GM: The Cell: A Molecular Approach (2nd ed). Washington, DC: ASM Press, 2000.

Fuller GM, Shields D: Molecular Basis of Medical Cell Biology. Stamford, CT: Appleton & Lange, 1998.

Goodman SR: Medical Cell Biology. Philadelphia: JB Lippincott, 1994.

Lewin B: Genes VII. Oxford: Oxford University Press, 1999.

Lodish H, Berk A, Zipursky SL, et al: Molecular Cell Biology (4th ed). New York: WH Freeman, 2000.

CHAPTER 2

Growth Factors and Cytokines

Gloria A. Chin, M.D., M.S., Gregory Schultz, Ph.D., and Lyle L. Moldawer, Ph.D.

Historical Overview of Growth Factors, Cytokines, and Chemokines

In 1962 a small polypeptide was isolated from the mouse submaxillary gland that promoted early eruption of incisors and eyelid opening in neonatal mice. Further studies demonstrated that this polypeptide stimulated epidermal cells to proliferate continuously in chemically defined culture medium containing essential nutritional factors (i.e., adequate levels of vitamins, essential amino acids, and cofactors). Prior to these discoveries, no single, biochemically defined agent was known that could promote continuous cycles of cell division in vitro under conditions of complete nutritional sufficiency. Based on these properties, the polypeptide was named epidermal growth factor (EGF). These results firmly established the concept of the regulation of cell proliferation and differentiation by a specific protein. The field of cell growth and differentiation factors has grown to include other classes of regulatory molecules including cytokines and chemokines. Collectively, their actions include essentially all types of cells and span from the earliest phases of embryonic development to regulation of the most highly specialized, terminally differentiated tissues. Today, several hundred growth factors, cytokines, and chemokines have been identified, and their impact on biology and medicine was recognized by the 1986 Nobel Prize in Physiology or Medicine awarded to Dr. Rita Levi-Montalcini and Dr. Stanley Cohen for their pioneering work in the discovery and characterization of growth factors and their receptors.

The nomenclature of growth factors and cytokines evolved in an inconsistent manner, often resulting in confusing and misleading terminology. Historically, growth factors were named based on the type of cell that was stimulated [e.g., fibroblast growth factor (FGF) or EGF], the source of the growth factor (e.g., platelet-derived growth factor, PDGF), the structure of the protein (e.g., insulin-like growth factor-I, IGF-I), or the action of protein on cultured cells (e.g., transforming growth factor-β, TGF-β). Six major families of growth factors are presented in Table 2–1. Proteins that were identified by their ability to regulate leukocyte and lymphocyte proliferation and differentiation were initially named interleukins (e.g., interleukin-2, IL-2), and other proteins were named based on their regulation of the differentiation of precursor inflammatory cells (e.g., granulocyte/macrophage

Table 2–1
Major growth factor families

Growth Factor Family	Cell Source	Actions

Transforming growth factor-β: TGF-β1, TGF-β2, TGF-β3	Platelets, fibroblasts, macrophages	Fibroblast chemotaxis and activation
		ECM deposition
		    ↑Collagen synthesis
		    ↑TIMP synthesis
		    ↓MMP synthesis
		Reduces scarring
		    ↓Collagen
		    ↓Fibronectin

Platelet-derived growth factor: PDGF-AA, PDGF-BB, VEGF	Platelets, macrophages, keratinocytes, fibroblasts	Activation of immune cells and fibroblasts
		ECM deposition
		    ↑Collagen synthesis
		    ↑TIMP synthesis
		    ↓MMP synthesis
		Angiogenesis

Fibroblast growth factor: acidic FGF, basic FGF, KGF	Macrophages, endothelial cells, fibroblasts	Angiogenesis Endothelial cell activation Keratinocyte proliferation and migration ECM deposition
Insulin-like growth factor: IGF-I, IGF-II, insulin	Liver, skeletal muscle, fibroblasts, macrophages, neutrophils	Keratinocyte proliferation Fibroblast proliferation Endothelial cell activation Angiogenesis ↑Collagen synthesis ECM deposition Cell metabolism
Epidermal growth factor: EGF, HB-EGF, TGF-α, amphiregulin, betacellulin	Keratinocytes, macrophages	Keratinocyte proliferation and migration ECM deposition
Connective tissue growth factor (CTGF)	Fibroblasts, endothelial cells, epithelial cells	Mediates action of TGF-β on collagen synthesis

colony-stimulating factor, GM-CSF) or their ability to suppress viral infections (e.g., interferon-alfa, IFN-α). Further research on these regulatory proteins, however, invalidated the initial concept that growth factors and cytokines were produced by, or acted on, a narrow range of target cells. This led to the adoption of the more general term, cytokine (Latin: *cyto* meaning cell and *kine* meaning action or motion) to describe these regulatory proteins, as they shared the ability to regulate the proliferation and differentiation of cells.

In several cases, there has been a trend to revise the nomenclature for many of these growth factors and cytokines. One such example is the effort to standardize the nomenclature for members of the tumor necrosis factor (TNF) and TNF receptor superfamilies (ligands being call TNFS and a number, and the receptors called TNFSR and a number). In this chapter, however, we use the more historical basis for grouping these regulatory

proteins, and the term *growth factor* is used to describe the mitogenic proteins listed in Table 2–1 and the term *cytokine* to indicate protein mediators listed in Table 2–2 that have major regulatory effects on inflammatory cells. A third important group of small regulatory proteins, listed in Table 2–3, has been identified; they are collectively named *chemokines* based on a contraction of "chemo-attractive cytokine(s)." The structural and functional similarities among chemokines were not initially appreciated, and this has led to an idiosyncratic nomenclature consisting of many acronyms that were based on their biologic functions [e.g., monocyte chemoattractant protein 1 (MCP-1), macrophage inflammatory protein 1, MIP-1], their source for isolation (platelet factor 4, PF-4), or their biochemical properties [interferon-inducible protein of 10 kDa (IP-10) or regulated upon activation normal T-cell expressed and secreted, RANTES].

Table 2–2
Cytokine activity in wound healing

Cytokine	Cell Source	Biologic Activity
Proinflammatory cytokines		
TNF-α	Macrophages	PMN margination and cytotoxicity; $\pm$ collagen synthesis; provides metabolic substrate
IL-1	Macrophages, keratinocytes	Fibroblast and keratinocyte chemotaxis; collagen synthesis
IL-2	T lymphocytes	Increases fibroblast infiltration and metabolism
IL-6	Macrophages, PMNs, fibroblasts	Fibroblast proliferation, hepatic acute-phase protein synthesis
IL-8	Macrophages, fibroblasts	Macrophage and PMN chemotaxis, keratinocyte maturation
IFN-γ	T lymphocytes, macrophages	Macrophage and PMN activation; retards collagen synthesis and cross-linking; stimulates collagenase activity
Anti-inflammatory cytokines		
IL-4	T lymphocytes, basophils, mast cells	Inhibition of TNF, IL-1, IL-6 production; fibroblast proliferation; collagen synthesis
IL-10	T lymphocytes, macrophages, keratinocytes	Inhibition of TNF, IL-1, IL-6 production; inhibits macrophage and PMN activation

Table 2–3
Chemokine families

Chemokines	Cells Affected
α-Chemokines (CXC) *with* glutamic acid-leucine-arginine near the N-terminal Interleukin-8 (IL-8)	Neutrophils
α-Chemokines (CXC) *without* glutamic acid-leucine-arginine near the N-terminal Interferon-inducible protein of 10 kDa (IP-10) Monokine induced by interferon-γ (MIG) Stromal-cell-derived factor 1 (SDF-1)	Activated T lymphocytes
β-Chemokines (CC) Monocyte chemoattractant proteins (MCPs): MCP-1, -2, -3, -4, -5 Regulated upon activation, normal T-cell expressed and secreted (RANTES) Macrophage inflammatory protein (MIP-1α) Eotaxin	Eosinophils, basophils, monocytes, activated T lymphocytes
β-Chemokines (C) Lymphotactin	Resting T lymphocytes
δ-Chemokines (CXXXC) Fractalkine	Natural killer cells

As their biochemical properties were established, it was recognized that the approximately 40 chemokines could be grouped into four major classes based on the pattern of cysteine residues located near the N-terminus. In fact, there has been a recent trend to reestablish a more organized nomenclature system based on these four major classes. In general, chemokines have two primary functions: (1) they regulate the trafficking of leukocyte populations during normal health and development, and (2) they direct the recruitment and activation of neutrophils, lymphocytes, macrophages, eosinophils, and basophils during inflammation.

Receptors and Signal Transduction Pathways for Growth Factors, Cytokines, and Chemokines

All growth factors, cytokines, and chemokines affect cells by activating receptors that are integral membrane proteins. In general, both the specificity and affinity of the receptors for their ligands is high, with K_d values in the range of 10^{-9} to 10^{-12} M. A physiologically significant effect is often generated by occupancy of a low percentage of receptors ($<10\%$), which can cause cells to respond to very low levels of growth factors, cytokines, and chemokines. Also, the expression of many receptors for growth factors, cytokines, and chemokines may be regulated by another cytokine or even the same cytokine, which permits positive amplification or negative feedback inhibition.

The principal function of all receptor proteins is to convert an extracellular signal (i.e., the specific binding of the growth factor, cytokine, and chemokine by the receptor) into intracellular signals, which then trigger physiologic responses in the target cell. However, receptors for growth factors, cytokines, and chemokines utilize different transduction pathways to generate their intracellular signals. Receptors for growth factors typically have intrinsic tyrosine kinase activity that is activated when a specific ligand is bound. This initiates a cascade of signal-transduction steps that eventually causes changes in the target cell's physiology (e.g., mitosis, migration, apoptosis, or synthesis of specialized proteins such as collagen). These changes result from alterations in basic processes in the responding cell, such as ion fluxes, microfibril polymerization, or transcription of genes.

The EGF receptor (EGF-R) and its signal-transduction system have been studied extensively and provide an excellent example of how receptor tyrosine kinases (RTKs) generate changes in cells. As shown in Figure 2–1A, target cells typically have about 10,000 specific, high-affinity,

monomeric EGF-R molecules in their plasma membrane. After binding EGF, the EGF-R monomers rapidly dimerize, and the kinase domain autophosphorylates selected tyrosine side chains in the cytoplasmic segment of the companion EGF-R protein. Adaptor proteins in the cytoplasm (e.g., GRB2) bind the specific phosphotyrosine residues that are generated on the activated EGF-R. Guanine nucleotide-exchange (GEF) proteins (e.g., Sos) then bind to specific domains on the adaptor protein, generating a trimeric complex of the EGF-R, the adaptor protein, and the guanine nucleotide-exchange protein. The primary function of the GEF protein is to induce an exchange of GTP with GDP bound on GDP-Ras protein. The activated GTP-Ras protein then initiates a kinase cascade by activating two kinases (Raf and Mek), which culminates in the phosphorylation and activation of the serine/threonine kinase activity of a key regulatory protein, mitogen-activated protein (MAP) kinase. After dimerizing, activated MAP kinase translocates to the nucleus, where it phosphorylates specific sites on various transcription factors (e.g., serum response factor, SRF; ternary complex factor, TCF), which then associate and bind to specific DNA sequences (e.g., serum response element, SRE) that regulate expression of specific genes. Phosphorylation of various transcription factors by MAP kinase can produce multiple effects on gene expression, thereby producing distinct effects by different growth factors on different cells.

Several mechanisms act to limit activation of an RTK signal transduction system. Protein phosphatase enzymes in the cytosol rapidly inactivate signal transduction proteins by removing phosphate groups that were added to tyrosine, serine, and threonine side chains by the kinase enzymes. Many growth factor–receptor complexes are rapidly internalized and degraded in lysozomes, which limits the duration of the initiating step of the signal transduction pathway. Also, the key transduction protein Ras has intrinsic GTPase activity, which limits the duration of the GTP–Ras complex. It remains active by limiting the time the GTP–Ras persists before the GTP is hydrolyzed to GDP.

Cytokine receptor proteins differ substantially from RTK proteins (Fig. 2–1B). They typically consist of homodimers, heterodimers, or heterotrimers of α-, β-, and γ-type transmembrane proteins, and all lack intrinsic kinase activity. A general model for cytokine receptor signaling proposes that signaling is initiated when ligand binding causes aggregation of receptor subunits. These receptor aggregates become the structural framework for the interaction with either docking proteins or kinases. The receptors for many families of cytokines, such as the IL-2, IL-6, and IL-10 families, interact noncovalently with a family of tyrosine kinases called Jak kinases (*Janus* kinases) through specialized regions of the cytoplasmic segments of receptor subunits. The Jaks phosphorylate each other

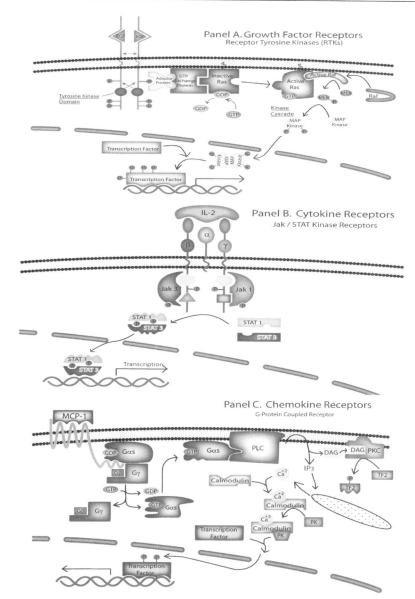

FIGURE 2–1 Typical receptor structures and signal transduction pathways for growth factors, cytokines, and chemokines. **A,** Receptors for growth factors typically are receptor tyrosine kinases (RTKs) that dimerize after binding the growth factor and autophosphorylate key tyrosines in the cytoplasmic domain of the receptors. Adaptor proteins bind at the phosphotyrosine sites, and GTP-exchange factors (GEF) dock with the adaptor proteins, which then promote exchange of GTP on Ras-GDP. Active Ras-GTP initiates a kinase cascade (Raf, Mek) that phosphorylates and activates MAP kinase, which dimerizes, translocates to the nucleus where it phosphorylates, and activates transcription factors leading to expression of selected genes. **B,** Receptors for cytokines typically consist of homo- or heteromultimeric subunits that aggregate after binding the cytokine, which permits Jak kinases bound to the cytoplasmic segments of the receptors close to phosphorylate each other when they are brought into close apposition. The activated Jak kinases phosphorylate and activate Stat transcription factors, which dimerize, translocate to the nucleus, and promote transcription of selected genes. **C,** Chemokine receptors are all 7-transmembrane spanning receptors that are coupled to G-protein trimer subunit complexes. After binding the chemokine, the receptor promotes exchange of GTP on the $G_{s\alpha}$-GDP subunit, which then dissociates from the G_{β}-G_{δ} subunits; the $G_{s\alpha}$-GTP subunit then binds with and activates the phospholipase C (PLC) enzyme located in the plasma membrane. Active PLC generates two important second messengers: diacylglycerol (DAG), which activates protein kinase C (PKC), and inositol trisphosphate (IP_3), which stimulates release of Ca^{2+} from cytoplasmic stores and activates calmodulin. Both PKC and calmodulin activate transcription factors that selectively stimulate transcription of genes. *See Color Plate 10.*

when they are brought into close apposition upon aggregation of the receptor subunits. Phosphorylation of Jaks greatly increases their catalytic activity, and they further phosphorylate themselves and tyrosines in the cytoplasmic tails of the aggregated cytokine receptor subunits. These receptor phosphotyrosines form sites where latent cytoplasmic transcription factors, called Stats (signal *t*ransducers and *a*ctivators of *t*ranscription), dock and are activated by phosphorylation of a single tyrosine by the Jaks. The phosphorylation step releases the Stats from the receptor–Jak complex, and the Stats dimerize and translocate to the nucleus, where they bind to specific sequences of DNA and initiate gene transcription. Thus the Jaks provide the cytokine receptors with tyrosine kinase activity that generates all the downstream signaling of cytokines.

In the IL-2 and IL-6 superfamilies, specificity for cytokine signaling is determined by the composition of the subunits comprising the receptor complex, the four known Jaks that bind the receptor, and the seven known Stats that are phosphorylated. The activity of the cytokine receptor Jak/Stat signaling system is limited by protein phosphatase enzymes, as noted for the growth factor RTK signaling system. In addition, the concentration of biologically active protein for some cytokines in blood is modulated by the presence of soluble receptors (e.g., TNF-α, IL-1, IL-6) that are generated by proteolytic cleavage of membrane receptors and act as sinks, or by natural competitive inhibitors (e.g., IL-1ra).

Chemokine receptors (Fig. 2–1C) and their signal transduction mechanism comprise a third type of system. All chemokine signaling receptors are 7-transmembrane spanning proteins, and they generate intracellular signals by interacting with trimeric G protein-coupled systems that are functionally linked to phospholipases. Although most chemokine receptors bind more than one chemokine, the four known CXC receptors (CXCR 1–4) bind only CXC chemokines (α family of chemokines), the eight known CC receptors (CCR 1–8) bind only CC chemokines (β family of chemokines), and the one known CXXXC receptor (CX$_3$CR1) binds the only member of the CX$_3$C family member, fractalkine (δ family of chemokines).

Many cell-surface receptors are coupled to trimeric, signal-transducing, G protein complexes including the chemokines, epinephrine, glucagon, ACTH, and prostaglandin E$_1$ (PGE$_1$), and all utilize a similar post-receptor signaling pathway. Binding of a chemokine to its receptor produces conformational changes in the cytoplasmic segments of the receptor, which generate a binding site for the GDP-G$_s$ subunit of the trimeric G protein complex. Interaction of the GDP-G$_s$ subunit with the chemokine–receptor complex promotes displacement of GDP by GTP in the G$_s$ subunit and dissociation of the GTP-G$_s$ subunit from the G$_\beta$ and G$_\gamma$ subunits.

The GTP-G$_s$ subunit then docks with and activates phospholipase-C (PLC), a key enzyme in the cytoplasmic leaflet of the plasma membrane. Active PLC cleaves a phosphate ester bond of the membrane lipid phosphoinositol 4,5-bisphosphate (PIP$_2$), which generates two important signal transduction molecules: the water-soluble molecule inositol trisphosphate (IP$_3$) and the lipid-soluble molecule diacylglycerol (DAG). DAG molecules activate the membrane-bound enzyme protein kinase-C (PKC), which phosphorylates and activates various transcription factors that influence gene expression. IP$_3$ molecules diffuse through the cytosol and interact with IP$_3$-sensitive Ca^{2+} channels in the membrane of the endoplasmic reticulum, causing release of stored Ca^{2+} ions. The localized increase in the Ca^{2+} ion concentration triggers various responses, including activation of the small cytosolic protein called calmodulin. The Ca^{2+}-calmodulin molecule can bind and activate several kinases that phosphorylate and activate various transcription factors, leading to changes in the profile of mRNAs and proteins synthesized by target cells.

Although the three receptor models present distinct signal transduction pathways for prototypical growth factor, cytokine, and chemokine receptor systems, the situation is more complex because interaction (cross-talk) occurs between the pathways. For example, the cytoplasmic regions of RTK receptors can interact directly with Jak proteins leading to phosphorylation and activation of Stat transcription factors. The G–protein-coupled receptors of the chemokine receptors also can activate adenylate cyclase, the enzyme that generates cyclic AMP (cAMP), which is a major second messenger that influences multiple cellular processes. Although most of the major effects of growth factors, cytokines, and chemokines result from the signal transduction pathways that are presented, other signal transduction pathways, such as the Smads, are involved in mediating the effects of growth factors, especially transforming growth factor-β (TGF-β).

Local Versus Systemic Actions of Growth Factors, Cytokines, and Chemokines

The hallmark property of growth factors, cytokines, and chemokines is their ability to regulate the migration, differentiation, and proliferation of cell populations during inflammation and tissue repair. Their effect on cells depends to a certain extent on their mode of production. Some growth factors, cytokines, and chemokines are released into the bloodstream and produce a systemic effect, resembling classic endocrine hormones that are synthesized in specialized tissues and released into the bloodstream to act on distant target organs. Interleukins IL-6 and IL-10 are examples of cytokines that appear systemically in the circulation and regulate the hepatic acute-phase and acquired immune responses, respectively. In contrast, cytokines such as tumor necrosis factor-α (TNF-α) and IL-1α are primarily membrane-associated and are released locally to induce tissue inflammation. Their appearance in the bloodstream is infrequent, but when it does occur they can mediate the systemic inflammatory response syndrome (SIRS) response. However, most growth factors, cytokines, and chemokines exert their physiologic effects locally on neighboring cells (a *paracrine* action) or on the same cell that synthesized and released it (an *autocrine* action).

It has been recognized that some growth factors and cytokines are present in the plasma membrane of cells as integral membrane pro-proteins [e.g., TNF-α and transforming growth factor-α (TGF-α)] and are able to bind receptors on adjacent cells through a *juxtacrine* interaction. Futhermore, some growth factors and cytokines produce their effects on cells while still within the cytoplasm after synthesis by a process called *intracrine* action. Additionally, many growth factors, cytokines, and chemokines have the ability to enhance or suppress their own production by a direct autoregulatory feedback mechanism. In summary, growth factors, cytokines, and chemokines typically act locally through *paracrine, autocrine, juxtacrine, and intracrine* mechanisms and are key regulators in inflammation and surgical wound healing.

Key Growth Factors

Growth factors share the important characteristic of acting as a direct mitogen for target cells. Although they play essential roles in embryonic development, their importance for surgeons focuses more on their key roles in normal cell turnover and in the response of tissues to injury. They are synthesized and secreted by many differentiated cells involved in wound healing, including platelets, inflammatory cells, fibroblasts, epithelial cells, and vascular endothelial cells. Growth factors typically are grouped into major families based on their biochemical structure: epidermal growth factor (EGF), TGF-β, insulin-like growth factor (IGF), platelet-derived growth factor (PDGF), fibroblast growth factor (FGF), and recently connective tissue growth factor (CTGF).

Epidermal Growth Factor Family

The epidermal growth factor family comprises four mammalian proteins: EGF, TGF-α, amphiregulin, heparin-binding epidermal growth factor (HB-EGF), and betacellulin. These peptides are similar in structure, bind to the same cell membrane receptor, and have similar but not identical biologic effects. EGF, the most thoroughly studied member of the family, is synthesized as a large transmembrane glycoprotein precursor molecule that is proteolytically cleaved to release a small biologically active 53-amino-acid fragment. It is folded into a triple loop structure that is stabilized by disulfide bonds, is required for biologic activity, and distinguishes all members of the EGF family from other families of growth factors.

Platelets contain a substantial amount of EGF (approximately 500 pmol/10^{12} platelets). After clotting, the local concentration of EGF in the interstitial fluid rises to levels sufficient to induce mitosis and migration of cells, suggesting a role for EGF during the early phase of wound healing. EGF is secreted by keratinocytes and, in an autocrine fashion, directs epithelialization. EGF is synthesized by several tissues, including kidney, lacrimal gland, submandibular gland, Brunner's gland, and megakaryocytes; it is found in many secretions such as saliva, tears, and urine.

Reports on clinical trials with EGF have noted that repeated topical application of EGF accelerated the rate of epidermal regeneration of partial-thickness dermatome wounds, enhanced healing of chronic wounds, and promoted epithelial regeneration of corneal injuries. EGF promotes healing in these wounds presumably by stimulating migration and division of epithelial cells and by increasing synthesis of proteins such as fibronectin, which aid in cell attachment and migration. Although EGF does not efficiently induce synthesis of mRNA for extracellular matrix proteins such as collagen, EGF presumably increases the numbers of fibroblasts in wounds through chemotaxis and mitosis, resulting in more total collagen production.

Transforming growth factor-α is synthesized by a large variety of normal cells including activated macrophages, eosinophils, hepatocytes, keratinocytes, gastrointestinal cells, brain cells, and placental cells. TGF-α and EGF have many similar effects on cells. Both factors stimulate mitosis of keratinocytes and fibroblasts, suppress gastric acid secretion, and accelerate healing of epidermal injuries. Although the role of heparin-binding EGF in wound healing is not known, its production by macrophages and its ability to bind a component of the extracellular matrix (heparin sulfate) suggest that it may be involved in wound healing. Both heparin-binding EGF and EGF are mitogens for keratinocytes and fibroblasts, but heparin-binding EGF, unlike EGF, is not a mitogen for vascular endothelial cells. The mitogens amphiregulin and betacellulin were isolated from tumor cells (human colon carcinoma cells and mouse pancreatic beta cell tumors) and share the three-disulfide, triple-loop structure characteristic of EGF family members. They also bind, albeit more weakly, to the EGF receptor (EGF-R).

Transforming Growth Factor-β Family

Three distinct TGF-β varieties have been identified in humans: TGF-β1, TGF-β2, and TGF-β3. All are synthesized as latent 28-kDa dimers that appear to be activated by proteolytic cleavage in a complex process involving the binding of latent TGF-β by the mannose-6-phosphate receptor and cleavage by plasmin. TGF-β1 was initially isolated and sequenced from platelets; and like TGF-α, it was named for its ability to stimulate reversibly the growth of normal fibroblasts in soft agar. The TGF-βs are synthesized by a wide variety of cell types, including platelets, macrophages, lymphocytes, fibroblasts, bone cells, and keratinocytes. Nearly all cells have TGF-β receptors. Thus, TGF-βs are probably the most broadly acting of all the families of growth factors. A distinguishing characteristic of the TGF-β family of proteins is their ability to inhibit the growth of a number of cell types, particularly cells derived from the ectoderm such as keratinocytes and leukocytes. There are three distinct TGF-β receptor proteins, designated types I, II, and III, that interact in a complex fashion to generate the cellular signal transduction pathway. The type II receptor appears to bind TGF-β and then aggregate with the type I receptor protein, which activates the serine/threonine kinase domain in the cytoplasmic region of the type I receptor, leading to phosphorylation of Smad transcription factors present in the cytoplasm. A balance of Smad-3, Smad-4, and Smad-7 actions leads to transcription of TGF-β-responsive genes. The type III TGF-β receptor probably does not participate in signal transduction directly but may act as a reservoir for TGF-β.

The TGF-βs have similar but not identical biologic actions on cells. All three of the TGF-β isomers can stimulate chemotaxis of inflammatory cells and stimulate production of extracellular matrix through increased synthesis of collagens and proteoglycans. In addition, TGF-βs downregulate synthesis of the matrix metalloproteinases (MMPs) in fibroblasts and upregulate synthesis of the natural inhibitors of MMPs, the tissue inhibitors of metalloproteinases (TIMPs). These properties make TGF-βs important regulators of the deposition and removal of extracellular matrix. It is not surprising that incisional wound healing can be accelerated by addition of exogenous TGF-β protein or by transfection of the wound incision by plasmids expressing the TGF-β gene. However, excess or prolonged action of TGF-βs have been implicated in several fibroproliferative diseases, such as scleroderma, hepatic sclerosis, and interstitial pulmonary fibrosis. Studies on keloid and hypertrophic scars showed increased expression of TGF-β1 mRNA in the tissues. Experiments in animal models suggest that blocking TGF-β1 and TGF-β2 with injections of neutralizing antibodies reduces scarring in skin incisions; and TGF-β3, in some animal models, suppresses scarring. Other important members of the TGF-β superfamily include the bone morphogenic proteins (BMPs) and the activin and inhibin hormones. Although this chapter focuses primarily on the role of growth factors, cytokines, and chemokines in soft tissue, BMPs clearly play key roles in the normal maintenance and repair of cartilage and bone injuries.

Insulin-like Growth Factor Family

Insulin-like growth factor I (IGF-I) and insulin-like growth factor II (IGF-II) have substantial amino acid sequence homology to proinsulin. Both IGF-I and IGF-II are synthesized as large precursor molecules (195 and 156 amino acids) that are proteolytically cleaved to release the biologically active monomeric proteins (70 and 67 amino acids). Although IGF-I and IGF-II are synthesized by a wide range of adult tissues, IGF-II is synthesized predominantly during fetal development, whereas IGF-I synthesis remains high in a wide range of adult tissues including liver, heart, lung, kidney, pancreas, cartilage, brain, and muscle. Many of the biologic actions originally attributed to growth hormone are mediated in part by IGF-I, which is also known as somatomedin C. IGF-I stimulates skeletal, cartilage, and bone growth. However, combinations of growth hormone and IGF-I are more effective than either hormone alone.

This led to the dual effector theory of growth hormone and IGF-I action: Growth hormone initiates cell differentiation and increases the production of IGF-I, which then promotes cell division. The IGF-I receptor is a tyrosine kinase, as is the insulin receptor. However, the IGF-II receptor is not a kinase; it is also called the mannose-6-phosphate (M6P) receptor because of its ability to bind mannose-6-phosphate groups that are part of the carbohydrate structures of glycoproteins. The signal transduction pathway for the IGF-II receptor is not understood.

Unlike other peptide growth factors, plasma contains substantial levels of IGF-I, which primarily reflects hepatic synthesis. IGF-I is reversibly bound by high-affinity IGF-binding proteins in plasma. At least six IGF binding proteins have been identified, and most tissues that synthesize IGFs also synthesize IGF-binding proteins. Because the IGFs are inactive while bound to their binding proteins, the dynamic balance between free and bound IGFs has a substantial influence on the effects of IGFs during wound healing. IGF-I is found in substantial levels in platelets and is released during clotting along with the other growth factors present in platelets. IGF-I is a chemotactic agent for vascular endothelial cells and may stimulate angiogenesis under certain conditions. IGF-I also stimulates mitosis of many cells in vitro, such as fibroblasts, osteocytes, and chondrocytes. It may also act synergistically with PDGF to enhance epidermal and dermal regeneration.

Platelet-Derived Growth Factor Family

The PDGF family comprises two major proteins of interest for surgeons: PDGF and vascular endothelial growth factor (VEGF). PDGF and VEGF have similar structures, but they act through different receptors and stimulate different actions. PDGF is primarily mitogenic for mesenchymal cells, whereas VEGF is almost exclusively a mitogen for vascular endothelial cells. PDGF is composed of two polypeptide chains (A and B) combined in three disulfide-linked dimeric isoforms (AA, AB, BB). It is secreted by a variety of cells important for wound healing, including placental cells, fibroblasts, vascular smooth muscle cells, and vascular endothelial cells. Macrophages also synthesize a PDGF-like protein that binds to PDGF receptors. The macrophage-derived PDGF-like protein together with PDGF-AA isoform are present in human wound fluids for several days after surgery. The PDGF receptor is a tyrosine kinase formed by two subunits, designated α and β. The α receptor subunit recognizes both the A and B subunits of PDGF, whereas the β receptor subunit recognizes only the B subunit of PDGF. Because all three PDGF receptor types (αα, αβ, ββ) are expressed by different cell types, treatment with the PDGF-BB isoform generally has the broadest effect.

Significantly decreased levels of all three PDGF isomers and its receptors were demonstrated in chronic, nonhealing wounds. The treatment of acute and chronic wounds with PDGF-BB resulted in elevation of PDGF-AA in both types of wounds. The topical application of recombinant PDGF-BB to acute wounds in animal models resulted in improved wound-breaking strength and healing times. Clinical studies using topical recombinant PDGF-BB on chronic, nonhealing diabetic ulcers have also demonstrated decreased healing times and an increased percentage of wounds that go on to heal compared to untreated controls. The recombinant human PDGF-BB isoform (Regranex) is the only recombinant growth factor medication approved by the U.S. Food and Drug Administration (FDA) for the treatment of chronic wounds, specifically diabetic foot ulcers.

A heparin-binding, disulfide-linked, homodimeric protein, VEGF was originally isolated from pituitary cell cultures. It is secreted mainly by keratinocytes but is also produced by macrophages and fibroblasts. It is a potent mitogen for endothelial cells and has minimal mitogenic effect on cells that are responsive to PDGF, including fibroblasts and vascular smooth muscle cells. In addition to its ability to stimulate mitosis of cultured endothelial cells, VEGF was found to be angiogenic in vivo. Although little is known about the role VEGF may play in wound healing, its selective mitogenic action on vascular endothelial cells, its ability of bind to heparin, and its angiogenic action in vivo suggests that it may be an important factor in wound healing.

Fibroblast Growth Factor Family

The FGF family consists of 14 homogeneous, heparin-binding, 28 kDa proteins that appear to play important roles in regulating key aspects of embryonic development and wound healing. Two members, named acidic FGF (aFGF) and basic FGF (bFGF) are closely related proteins with isoelectric points of pH 5.6 and 9.6, which are reflected in their names. Neither the aFGF nor the bFGF precursor proteins contain a typical leader sequence, which is found in essentially all secreted proteins, so it is unclear how they are released from cells. Nevertheless, substantial amounts of FGF are found bound to proteoglycans such as heparan sulfate in the extracellular matrix, especially in the basement membrane of capillaries. Their association with the extracellular matrix may serve to protect FGF from proteolytic degradation by functioning as a storage depot, with the liberation of FGF through matrix-degrading enzymes such as heparinase or cathepsin D following injury. FGF receptors are tyrosine kinases, and binding of FGFs require the combined action of heparan sulfate proteoglycans and the FGF receptors, of which there are multiple forms that have varying specificity for the FGFs.

The FGFs appear to play a major role in wound healing. They stimulate proliferation of all the major cell types involved in wound healing including vascular endothelial cells, fibroblasts, keratinocytes, and other specialized cell types such as chondrocytes and myoblasts. Many of the cells that respond to FGF also synthesize the peptide, including fibroblasts, astrocytes, endothelium, smooth muscle cells, chondrocytes and osteoblasts. The FGFs may have their most important effect in wound healing by stimulating angiogenesis through inducing endothelial cell migration and proliferation. Studies using a topical application of recombinant bFGF on diabetic ulcers demonstrated improved healing. In a phase III trial in China using a topical application of recombinant bFGF on burns, surgical incisions and chronic dermal ulcers showed an accelerated rate of wound closure; moreover, healing time decreased by an average of 3 to 4 days, and the wound closure rate was higher than 90% for all of the groups. Recombinant bFGF was also shown to improve healing of chronic pressure sores when given alone or in sequential treatment with granulocyte/macrophage colony-stimulating factor (GM-CSF).

Keratinocyte growth factor (KGF or FGF-7) is another important member of the FGF family. KGF is a 22.5 kDa glycoprotein that shares about 40% amino acid sequence identity with aFGF and bFGF; it contains a hydrophobic N-terminal secretory signal sequence and has two major isoforms, KGF-1 and KGF-2. In contrast to FGFs, synthesis of KGF is restricted to fibroblasts; and, most importantly, KGF stimulates mitosis almost exclusively of keratinocytes. This has led to the concept that KGF is a paracrine effector of epithelial cell growth. The role of KGF in wound healing is not fully understood, but it is highly upregulated in the dermis during wound healing. Because it selectively stimulates mitosis of keratinocytes, it is logical to assume that KGF would be useful for treating partial-thickness burns or meshed skin grafts. Topical KGF treatment of explanted meshed human skin grafts in athymic animals has been shown to accelerate closure of interstices; and studies using topical recombinant KGF-2 on chronic venous stasis ulcers have demonstrated improved wound closure. Phase III studies are currently in progress. The KGF receptor is a tyrosine kinase that is an isoform of the *FGFR-2* gene.

Connective Tissue Growth Factor

Connective tissue growth factor (CTGF), a cysteine-rich, 38 kDa protein, is a member of the recently described CCN family, which includes CTGF, *cysteine-rich 61 (cyr61), neuroblastoma overexpressed (nov)*, elm 1, Cop-1, and WISP-3. CTGF was first identified in medium conditioned by cultured human vascular endothelial cells due to a fortuitous cross-reactivity of a polyclonal antiserum to PDGF with CTGF. CTGF is produced by a variety of cells including fibroblasts, vascular endothelial cells, vascular smooth muscle cells, chondrocytes, and glioblastoma cells. Interestingly, physiologic levels of the coagulation cascade protease thrombin upregulates expression of CTGF mRNA in fibroblasts, suggesting that the coagulation process promotes CTGF formation during normal tissue repair. The CTGF receptor has not been biochemically identified.

From a surgical viewpoint, the most important biologic effect of CTGF is its ability to promote formation of scar tissue. CTGF is mitogenic and chemotactic for fibroblasts, and it strongly stimulates synthesis of type I collagen and fibronectin. It has been implicated in a variety of fibrotic disorders, such as systemic and localized sclerosis, keloids, and Dupuytren's contractures. Furthermore, studies have shown important links between TGF-β and CTGF. TGF-β directly upregulates expression of CTGF mRNA and protein in cultured fibroblasts; levels of TGF-β and CTGF mRNAs are coordinately expressed during wound repair; and CTGF transcripts are induced in skin fibroblasts at the site of epidermal injections of TGF-β in neonatal mice. Most importantly, neutralizing antibodies to CTGF or antisense oligonucleotides targeting CTGF block the induction of collagen synthesis by TGF-β, which indicates that CTGF functions as a downstream mediator of TGF-β action on fibroblasts. Therapies that selectively inhibit CTGF action may be useful for reducing fibrosis in numerous pathologic conditions.

Key Cytokines

Historically, the term cytokine was used to describe proteins that regulated mitosis and differentiated the functions of immune system cells (e.g., T and B lymphocytes, macrophages, polymorphonuclear leukocytes, and tumor cell lines). However, as it became clear that cytokines could also influence nonimmune system cells (e.g., fibroblasts, endothelial cells, epidermal cells) and that some of the classic growth factors could influence important functions of immune system cells (e.g., migration, proliferation), separation of the proteins into cytokines and growth factors became blurred. Hence the more generic term cytokine was frequently used to describe both groups of regulatory proteins. In this chapter, we use the term cytokine in its more original context to describe proteins that are involved in the immune response to inflammation and/or tissue injury, and we emphasize their importance in processes that are important for surgeons.

Pro-inflammatory Cytokines

Tumor necrosis factor-α

The activity of most cytokines can often be categorized as being proinflammatory or anti-inflammatory depending on their role in the host immune response and their involvement in local and systemic inflammation. One of the earliest proinflammatory cytokines identified was TNF-α. TNF-α was induced unintentionally during the 1880s when a New York surgeon, William Coley, injected a preparation of gram-positive and gram-negative bacteria, "Coley's toxins", into patients with inoperable neoplastic disease. In some of the patients treated with the bacterial cocktail, hemorrhagic necrosis developed in the tumors, which in certain cases progressed to complete tumor resolution.

Historically called cachectin, TNF-α is produced by macrophages and other cells from the monocyte lineage in response to microbial pathogens, tumors, hemorrhagic shock, and tissue injury. It acts in a paracrine fashion to initiate the innate immune response by stimulating production of other proinflammatory cytokines and by stimulating the influx of inflammatory cells. TNF-α also plays a significant role in the development of a Th1 response and serves as a communication link between the innate and acquired immune responses. Another significant role of TNF-α is in early wound healing, where it modulates angiogenesis, suppresses proliferation of vascular endothelial cells, and induces the production of IL-1, IL-3, G-CSF, and GM-CSF. TNF-α also stimulates fibroblast proliferation and inhibits their synthesis of collagen; and it induces fibroblasts to produce matrix metalloproteinases (MMPs), IL-1, IL-6, and leukocyte inhibitory factor (LIF).

Normal wound healing requires the release of TNF-α at the appropriate times and in adequate levels. Excessive activation of immune cells can lead to tissue damage through the production of reactive oxygen species, proteolytic enzymes, and arachidonic acid metabolites. Studies have shown that rats with chronically elevated TNF-α levels had impaired wound healing compared to controls. More recently, studies have reported elevated levels of TNF-α in nonhealing versus healing chronic venous ulcers, although no cause-and-effect relation has been established. Systemically, excessive levels of circulating TNF-α has been associated with multisystem organ failure and increased morbidity and mortality during inflammatory disease states.

Interleukin-1

The general term interleukin was originally used to refer to the molecules that signaled between cells in the immune system. It was later determined that interleukins have many more functions. They are currently designated by the order in which they are identified. They are used to define the class of mediators that regulate specific components of immune signaling between leukocytes and somatic cell subpopulations.

Interleukin-1, originally known as lymphocyte-activating factor and as an endogenous pyrogen, is actually a family of at least three proteins that are primarily secreted by activated macrophages. Two forms of IL-1 (IL-1α and IL-1β) are agonists; the third (IL-1 receptor antagonist, or IL-1ra), is a pure receptor antagonist. IL-1β is processed from an inactive precursor and is readily secreted, whereas IL-1α exists primarily as a membrane-associated form. Members of the IL-1 superfamily are produced by a variety of other cells, including B and T lymphocytes, neutrophils, natural killer (NK) cells, fibroblasts, endothelial cells, epithelial cells, smooth muscle cells, and vascular tissues in response to trauma, infection, or exposure to antigens.

Interleukin-1 is involved in the escalation of local and systemic inflammatory responses. As an inducer of the innate immune response, IL-1α and IL-1β directly stimulate fibroblasts and vascular endothelial cells. IL-1 enhances local inflammation through secondary cytokine production and acts in an endocrine fashion to induce liver hepatocytes to produce acute-phase proteins, fibrinogen, C-reactive protein, and haptoglobin, which are mediators of systemic inflammation. IL-1 is also involved in acquired immunity, primarily as an adjuvant and a co-mitogen for proliferating T cells.

Interleukin-1α is found in large quantities in the skin, where it is presumed to serve as a regulator of growth and proliferation. IL-1 is important in wound healing because it increases the expression of proinflammatory genes.

It has the ability to initiate and sustain the production of MMPs and suppress the production of tissue inhibitor metalloproteinases (TIMPs), thereby modifying the extracellular matrix to aid in cell migration. Another important proinflammatory property of IL-1 is its ability to increase the expression of adhesion molecules such as intercellular adhesion molecule-1 (ICAM-1) on endothelial and other cell surfaces. This property promotes the infiltration of inflammatory and immunocompetent cells into the extravascular space.

Interleukin-2

Interleukin-2 is primarily a T cell growth factor. It induces growth and differentiation of T-cells, NK cells, some B lymphocytes, and lymphokine-activated killer cells. Activation of NK cells by IL-2 results in increased interferon-γ (IFN-γ) production and increased cytotoxic effects against tumor targets. Clinical trials have studied the use of IL-2 to treat some human cancers. Although IL-2 has high toxicity (in part through the induction of TNF-α), it has been approved for the treatment of patients with metastatic melanoma. Patients infected with human immunodeficiency virus type 1 (HIV-1) with low CD4 T cell counts following IL-2 therapy developed increased numbers of circulating T cells.

Interleukin-2 appears to be essential for sustaining the postinjury repair response during wound healing. IL-2 activates monocytes to produce cytokines, particularly TNF-α. In a study involving rats treated with doxorubicin, IL-2 administration increased the infiltration of inflammatory cells and fibroblasts into the wounds, resulting in increased wound-breaking strength. This action is most important in wounds in immunocompromised hosts, as IL-2 did not increase wound strength in normal control rats.

Interleukin-6

Interleukin-6 (IL-6), a pleiotropic cytokine, is unique in that it has both proinflammatory and anti-inflammatory characteristics. IL-6 has numerous biologic activities that can be divided into effects on regulation of the hematopoietic system and those involved in activation of the innate or acute-phase immune response. Similar to other proinflammatory cytokines, IL-6 is predominantly produced by macrophages and cells from the monocyte lineage. Locally, within the wound, it is secreted by polymorphonuclear neutrophils (PMNs) and fibroblasts. Its concentration in the wound directly parallels the number of PMNs. IL-6 has been shown to be a potent inducer of fibroblast proliferation. It is also able to suppress proinflammatory responses by down-regulating TNF-α and IL-1, which are potent inducers of IL-6 expression. It reduces chemokine expression as well.

Unlike most cytokines, IL-6 has a significant endocrine component and is rapidly released into the circulation in response to inflammation. The systemic effects of IL-6 on nonimmune cells are closely tied to activation of the innate immune system, activation of the hypothalamic-pituitary-adrenal axis, and induction of the hepatic acute-phase protein response. IL-6 has also been shown to be pyrogenic. Burn patients and patients with acute bacterial infections have elevated plasma IL-6 concentrations, which have been shown to be occasionally predictive of the outcome of patients with sepsis or SIRS. Studies have documented that IL-6 is produced by synovial fibroblasts in the presence of rheumatoid arthritis, and several studies have shown elevated serum IL-6 concentrations in patients with this disease, frequently correlating with disease severity.

Interleukin-8

Interleukin-8 (IL-8), a proinflammatory cytokine, is a member of the CXC chemokine family. It appears to exert its effects early in acute wounds. IL-8 is primarily secreted by macrophages and fibroblasts and is chemotactic for neutrophils and monocytes. It has been shown to increase neutrophil degranulation and the expression of endothelial cell adhesion molecules. IL-8 is found in highest concentrations during the first day of an injury and appears to be important in promoting keratinocyte maturation and margination. Elevated levels of IL-8 have been identified in fibroblasts from patients with psoriasis compared to normal controls, implicating it in the pathogenesis of the psoriatic wound-healing phenotype. The expression of IL-8 mRNA in fetal fibroblasts is significantly less than in adult control fibroblasts, indicating that the diminished proinflammatory response in fetal tissue may contribute to the scarless healing seen in utero.

Interferon-γ

Interferon-γ (IFN-γ), primarily produced by T lymphocytes and macrophages, activates macrophages and PMNs and increases their cytotoxicity. IFN-γ is involved in tissue remodeling during healing. It has been shown to reduce wound contraction by retarding collagen production and lattice cross-linking while increasing collagenase production. In experimental wound models, treatment with IFN-γ has been shown to impair reepithelialization and wound disruption strength in a dose-dependent fashion when applied locally or given systemically.

Anti-inflammatory Cytokines

Interleukin-4

Interleukin-4, predominantly produced by T lymphocytes and to a lesser extent by mast cells and basophils, activates B-lymphocyte proliferation and immunoglobulin E (IgE) antibody-mediated immunity. Its most significant role in

wound healing is its anti-inflammatory effects: its ability to inhibit macrophage production of the proinflammatory cytokines TNF-α, IL-1, and IL-6. It promotes healing through stimulating fibroblast proliferation and collagen synthesis, and it is able to stimulate fibroblasts directly to synthesize proteoglycans.

Interleukin-10

Interleukin-10 is an important anti-inflammatory cytokine produced by T lymphocytes, monocytes, and epithelial cells. IL-10 has been shown to suppress a spectrum of cytokines: the proinflammatory cytokines, IL-1, TNF-α, IL-6, IL-8, and IL-12; the hematopoietic growth factors GM-CSF, G-CSF, and M-CSF; and IL-10 itself. Additionally, it inhibits the synthesis of MMPs, gelatinase, and collagenase. Using neutralizing antibodies, Sato et al. were able to demonstrate the inhibitory effects of IL-10 on PMN and macrophage infiltration and on proinflammatory cytokine expression. Elevated IL-10 levels were identified in chronic venous stasis ulcers, indicating a contribution to the nonhealing state.

Key Chemokines

Chemokines are a complex family of at least 40 low-molecular-weight (6 to 14 kDa) secreted proteins with varying cellular targets and biologic responses. Four major chemokine families have been identified at the present time. The families are distinguished by the pattern of conserved cysteine residues located near the N-terminus. The CXC family members (also known as α-chemokines) have a single noncysteine amino acid situated between the two N-terminal cysteine disulfide residues. The CXC chemokines can be further divided into those that contain the sequence glutamic acid-leucine-arginine (E-L-R) near the N-terminal preceding the CXC sequence and those that do not. The CXC chemokines (e.g., IL-8) that contain the E-R-L sequence are generally chemotactic for neutrophils, whereas those that do not contain the sequence (e.g., interferon-inducible protein 10, or IP10, and monokine induced by IFN-γ, or MIG) act on lymphocytes. The CC family members (also known as β-chemokines) have two adjacent cysteine disulfide residues near the N-terminus (no amino acids intervene). The C family members (also known as γ-chemokines) have a single N-terminal cysteine disulfide bond. The single member of the CXXXC family (also known as a δ-chemokine), fractalkine, has three amino acids residues intervening between the two N-terminal cysteine disulfide bonds.

Chemokines can also be defined as being either homeostatic or inflammatory. Homeostatic chemokines are those that are constitutively expressed during development or other normal physiologic processes, whereas inflammatory chemokines are those that are strongly upregulated in response to inflammatory or immune stimuli. An example of a homeostatic chemokine is secondary lymphoid organ cytokine (SLC, CCL21). Mice with spontaneous mutations preventing expression of functional SLC were observed to have a severe depletion of lymph node T cells.

There is growing appreciation that a large number of chemokines and chemokine receptors are essential for fine-tuning the trafficking and recruitment of leukocyte populations to lymphoid tissues and to the sites of tissue injury and inflammation. Chemokines are the dominant factors that control the attraction of leukocytes to tissues during inflammation. They play a significant role in sepsis and particularly in the development of adult respiratory distress syndrome. In addition, chemokines also play key roles in regulating normal T-cell, B-cell, and NK-cell development. The coordinated synthesis of chemokines together with changes in the expression of cell surface adhesion molecules is primarily responsible for the selective trafficking of leukocyte populations from intravascular to extravascular compartments. In addition, chemokines play a predominant role in the activation of these leukocyte populations upon their extravasation into extravascular compartments and provide paracrine signaling for angiogenesis.

The primary inducers of chemokine synthesis are the proinflammatory cytokines IL-1 and TNF-α. There is also growing evidence that cellular adhesion per se can activate the expression of several chemokines. In particular, recruited leukocytes interacting with adhesion molecules on endothelial cells, basement membranes, extracellular matrix, and fibroblasts often induce the expression of various chemokines, including IL-8 (CXCL8). This augmentation of chemokine synthesis by recruited leukocyte populations as they traverse cell-to-cell or cell-to-matrix contact may promote autocrine feedback loops that stimulate a chemokine cascade in the local microenvironment.

Several members of this superfamily are mitogenic for keratinocytes, which is of obvious importance in wound healing. Similarly, chemokines can be both angiogenic and antiangiogenic. As becomes readily evident, the biologic properties of chemokines far exceed their chemotactic or chemokinetic properties. Only during the past few years has the role of chemokines in lymphoid development and in T-helper (Th1, Th2) cell responses been identified. Much of the interest in chemokines and lymphocyte function resulted from the discovery that CD4+ cells express chemokine receptors and that the entry of HIV-1 is dependent on the chemokine receptors CXCR4 and CCR5, which serve as co-receptors (with CD4) for HIV-1 entry. This observation has resulted in an explosion of interest in chemokines and their receptors in T-cell biology distinct from their role in the recruitment and

activation of inflammatory cells. More importantly, these findings have led to greater exploration for the role of chemokines in directing the acquired immune response to bacterial and viral pathogens.

Role of Growth Factors, Cytokines, and Chemokines in Normal Wound Healing

Wound healing is a precisely orchestrated sequence of events that includes migration, maturation, and activation of various cell populations during the three phases of wound healing: inflammation, fibroplasia, and scar maturation. Although it is not within the scope of this chapter to discuss wound healing in depth, it is important for the surgeon to have a general understanding of the role of growth factors, cytokines, and chemokines in the regulation of each phase of healing.

Inflammation

Tissue repair begins after an injury has occurred whether the result of physical trauma, chemical exposure, or an antigen–antibody response. The sequence and magnitude of cellular events that occur after an injury depend to a large extent on the wound conditions and the presence of tissue and cellular debris, infection, and foreign bodies. Tissue debris and bacterial agents, in particular, induce a more severe inflammatory response.

A skin laceration illustrates the early events leading to inflammation. The body's initial response to stop the bleeding involves the synergistic effects of platelet aggregation and activation of the clotting cascade. Once platelet aggregation has developed, the preformed α-granules in the cytoplasm degranulate, releasing PDGF, TGF-β, TGF-α, platelet-derived epidermal growth factor (PDEGF), and platelet-derived endothelial cell growth factor (PDECGF). In addition to these proteins, α-granules release factor V, fibrinogen, fibronectin, plasminogen, and platelet factor-4 (PF-4, or CXCL4). These cytokines and proteins are involved early in coagulation and in inflammation. The intrinsic clotting cascade, initiated by exposure to damaged tissue, together with platelet aggregation accelerates the conversion of prothrombin to thrombin in the presence of factor V. Thrombin participates in the conversion of fibrinogen to fibrin to provide a network for clot formation and a significant component for the provisional matrix important for healing to continue. As coagulation progresses, the inflammatory response continues to escalate. Local factors, histamine, prostaglandin E2, PDGF, and PF-4 are chemotactic for neutrophils. Monocytes are also stimulated to migrate from the capillaries into the extravascular space by chemotactic factors, including collagen fragments, fibronectin fragments, elastin from damaged matrix, PF-4, and TGF-β. Once in the wound, neutrophils and macrophages serve as scavengers to remove foreign material, infectious agents, and cellular debris. In addition to its phagocytic activity, neutrophils have been found to produce proinflammatory cytokines, which provide the early chemotactic signals for local fibroblasts and keratinocytes.

Repair and Collagen Synthesis

Macrophages are a major source of cytokines that regulate fibroblast proliferation, collagen production, and scar remodeling. As inflammation progresses, macrophages further increase their numbers through their secretion of colony-stimulating factor 1 (CSF-1). Macrophages also secrete collagenases and elastase to remove the damaged matrix while cell migration, proliferation, and extracellular matrix (ECM) production continue. Fibroblasts then migrate into the provisional matrix under the influence of chemotactic cytokines such as PDGF, TGF-β, EGF, and lymphokines. The movement of cells through the wounded area is made possible by their ability to bind and release fibronectin, fibrin, and vitronectin molecules via their cell surface integrin receptors. Both PDGF and TGF-β have been demonstrated to upregulate integrin receptors on fibroblasts. As they migrate, one pole of the fibroblast remains fixed, whereas at the opposite pole lamellipodia extend in search of the correct ECM molecule to which they can attach. Once the initial fixed pole releases, the cell moves while attached to the new site. The direction of movement is guided by the presence of integrin receptors and by the alignment of the fibrils in the preliminary wound matrix, where fibroblasts have been demonstrated to migrate along, not across, matrix fibers. Migration is facilitated by large quantities of hyaluronic acid in the provisional matrix, permitting easier penetration by migratory cells.

Matrix metalloproteinases are a group of enzymes that can cleave a path through the lattice to further facilitate fibroblast migration through the matrix. Enzymes involved in this process include MMP-1, gelatinase (MMP-2), stromelysin (MMP-3), and plasminogen activator, which generates plasmin through the breakdown of plasminogen. These enzymes share a common catalytic domain containing a zinc ion, and they target matrix proteins (collagen, fibronectin, laminin, gelatin) as their substrates. The induction and expression of MMPs is mainly under the regulatory control of proinflammatory cytokines such as IL-1, TNF-α, and EGF, but they can be induced by cellular debris and antigen-antibody complexes as well. MMPs also contribute to scar remodeling during the final stage of healing.

Transforming growth factor-β may be the most potent stimulator of collagen synthesis. By decreasing protease activity, it contributes to collagen accumulation. Specific antibodies to TGF-β have been demonstrated to limit collagen accumulation in wounds. As previously mentioned in the growth factor section, CTGF is the downstream mediator for TGF-β production of collagen and proteoglycans in the extracellular matrix. The PDGF isoforms have different effects on collagen synthesis. PDGF-AB has been shown to increase expression of procollagen mRNA, whereas PDGF-BB downregulates it. FGF and EGF stimulate collagen synthesis, and glucocorticoids inhibit collagen production.

Angiogenesis

Endothelial cell migration and capillary tube formation are facilitated by changes in the matrix in the capillary wall induced by collagenases. The advancing endothelial cells synthesize fibronectin to modify the matrix to facilitate their own migration. The cells also must express various integrins to allow their migration. Many of the macrophage-derived cytokines directly and indirectly stimulate the endothelial cell migration and proliferation required for angiogenesis. Basic fibroblast growth factor (bFGF, FGF2) is a potent angiogenic stimulant. Endothelial cells can synthesize and respond to bFGF (FGF2). Multiple growth factors and cytokines have been identified as angiogenic stimulants, including TGF-α, EGF, TGF-β, TNF-α, PDECGF, VEGF, and angiogenin.

Epithelialization

Epithelialization begins as early as 24 to 48 hours after injury. For injuries that include a damaged basement membrane, the cells migrate over a provisional matrix that includes fibrin, fibronectin, and vitronectin. The epithelial cells themselves add components to the provisional matrix if the substances are not already present. Cells continue to migrate until contact inhibition occurs; then the cell monolayer differentiates into more basal-like cells. Migration and proliferation of epithelial cells are stimulated by EGF. It is found in a wide variety of tissues, and most cells have receptors for EGF. TGF-α is also a potent stimulant of epithelial cell migration and proliferation. Other factors that stimulate epithelial cell proliferation include heparin-binding epidermal growth factor (HB-EGF), IGF, KGF, and bFGF. The two processes, cell migration and proliferation, are regulated at least to some degree independently; cytokines such as TGF-β can stimulate migration but not proliferation. Epithelial cells are an important source of PDGF-6, TGF-β, and TGF-α. Keratinocytes at the advancing wound edge have the ability to secrete MMPs, which facilitate their migration and penetration through eschar in a wound.

In open wounds, wound contraction proceeds until complete epithelization has occurred or the defect has been surgically closed. Contraction is a cell-directed process that requires cell division but not collagen synthesis. TGF-β stimulates collagen lattice contraction and is a mediator of wound contraction. It also facilitates the transition of fibroblasts to myofibroblasts. Myofibroblasts attached to the collagen lattice are stimulated to shorten their actin and myosin-like filaments to contract. PDGF can also stimulate contraction of matrices by a TGF-β independent mechanism.

Scar Maturation

Scar remodeling is the hallmark of the final period of healing. At approximately 21 days following injury the net accumulation of wound collagen becomes stable. Collagen synthesis is most likely downregulated through a mechanism involving IFN-γ and collagen matrix. TNF-α also downregulates collagen synthesis, possibly by downregulating TGF-β expression. This occurs despite the fact that TGF-β may still be present. As more collagen is synthesized, fibronectin is broken down. IFN-γ downregulates synthesis of fibronectin as well as collagen.

During this remodeling phase, there is a continual turnover of collagen molecules as old collagen is broken down and new collagen is synthesized in a denser, more organized fashion along lines of stress. Several of the MMPs that degrade collagen and proteoglycans have been identified: MMP-1 (interstitial collagenase); MMP-2 (gelatinase); MMP-3 (stromelysin). They are found in both scar tissue and normal connective tissues. In their role as regulators of healing, macrophages are able to control both the synthesis of collagen and proteoglycans and their degradation through release of metalloproteinase tissue inhibitors (TIMPs). Other enzymes, such as hyaluronidase, are also involved in scar remodeling. The activities of these enzymes and their inhibitors are under the influence of cytokines such as TGF-β, PDGF, IL-1, and EGF.

Abnormal Wound Healing

The healing process in chronic wounds is generally prolonged or incomplete and uncoordinated, resulting in a poor anatomic and functional outcome. In clinical practice, the most common chronic wounds are chronic venous stasis ulcers, diabetic ulcers, and chronic wounds resulting from pressure. Chronic nonhealing wounds are a prime clinical example of the importance of the wound cytokine profile and the critical balance necessary for normal healing to proceed.

Several studies have demonstrated a difference in the microenvironment of acute versus chronic wounds. Falanga and colleagues (Bucalo et al.) demonstrated stimulation of the proliferation of human dermal fibroblasts and endothelial cells in exudates from healing wounds (partial-thickness skin donor sites). In contrast, an inhibitory effect on cell proliferation was noted in fluids obtained from chronic wounds (venous ulcers). This difference in acute and chronic wounds was also noted by Bennett and Schultz, who reported that mastectomy drainage fluids exhibited cell proliferation enhancement, whereas exudates from chronic wounds showed cell proliferation inhibition.

To determine why these differences occurred, studies were done to determine the levels of certain growth factors and their receptors. Using dextranomer beads to recover endogenous growth factors in wounds, levels of PDGF and TGF-β were determined to be significantly lower in chronic wounds than in acute wounds. Using a rat model, both PDGF and PDGF receptors were found to be downregulated in impaired wounds.

In general, most chronic wounds exhibit a decrease in growth factor expression and, in some cases, growth factor receptors as well. The precise pattern of growth factor expression in the various types of chronic wound is not yet known. The absolute levels of growth factors may not be as important as the relative concentrations necessary to replace the specific deficiencies in the tissue repair processes. For the treatment of chronic wounds, Robson proposed that growth factor therapy be tailored to the deficiency in the repair process. Effectiveness of therapy is predicated on adequate growth factor levels and the expression of their receptors. Excessive degradation of receptors and binding of growth factors by macromolecules such as macroglobulin and albumin would reduce the effectiveness of therapy.

The mechanisms involved in the creation and perpetuation of chronic wounds are varied and depend on the individual wounds. In general, the inability of chronic venous stasis ulcers to heal appears to be related to impaired wound epithelialization. Microscopically, the wound edges show hyperproliferative epidermis, even though further immunohistochemical studies revealed optimal conditions for keratinocyte recruitment, proliferation, and differentiation. The ECM and the expression of integrin receptors by keratinocytes that allow it to translocate play an important regulatory role in epithelialization. After receiving the signal to migrate, epidermal cells begin by disassembling its attachments from the basement membrane and neighboring cells. They then travel over a provisional matrix containing fibrinogen, fibronectin, vitronectin, and tenascin; they stop when they encounter laminin. During this process, keratinocytes are producing fibronectin and continue to do so until the epithelial cells establish contact, at which time they again begin manufacturing laminin to regenerate the basement membrane.

There is evidence that the interaction between the integrin receptors on keratinocytes and the ECM transforms resting cells to a migratory phenotype. Integral to this transformation is an alteration in the pattern of the integrin receptors expressed. After epithelialization is complete, integrin expression reverts back to the resting pattern. To complicate this process further, growth factors are involved in mediating keratinocyte activation and integrin expression and in alterations in the matrix. Growth factors are able to affect these processes differentially; for example, TGF-β is able to promote epithelial migration while inhibiting proliferation. Although TGF-β induces the integrin expression necessary for migration, the cells behind those at the leading edge have little proliferative ability, so epithelial coverage of the wound is inhibited. Some chronic wounds may be deficient in TGF-β and its receptors.

Chronic wounds have also been demonstrated to have elevated matrix-degrading enzymes and decreased levels of inhibitors for these enzymes. Unlike chronic venous stasis ulcers, pressure ulcers appear to have difficulty healing, which is likely related to impaired ECM production. Studies have indicated that the neutrophil elastase present in chronic wounds can degrade peptide growth factors and is responsible for degrading fibronectin. Pressure ulcers have also shown an increase in MMPs and plasminogen activators in tissue. Chronic wound fluids demonstrate increased levels of the gelatinases MMP-2 and MMP-9. Levels of MMP-1 and MMP-8 were also found to be higher in pressure ulcers and venous stasis ulcers than in acute healing wounds. In addition, several of the endogenous proteinase inhibitors were shown to be decreased in chronic wounds. Proteinase inhibitors serve a regulatory role in matrix degradation by containing matrix-degrading enzymes. Factors that promote MMP production or activation could counteract the effectiveness of proteinase inhibitors (e.g., the destruction of TIMP by neutrophil elastase). The MMP-9/TIMP-1 levels ratio may indicate an imbalance, which contributes to the chronic nature of the wound.

Conditions that promote the chronicity of wounds are repeated trauma, foreign bodies, pressure necrosis, infection, ischemia, and tissue hypoxia. These wounds share a chronic inflammatory state characterized by an increased number of neutrophils, macrophages, and lymphocytes, which produce inflammatory cytokines (e.g., TNF-α) and the chemokines IL-1 and IL-6. In vitro studies have shown these cytokines to induce the expression of MMPs in a variety of cells including macrophages, fibroblasts, keratinocytes, and endothelial cells. They are also involved in the downregulation of TIMP expression. Although there may be a relative excess of MMPs in the wound, they are secreted as proenzymes, which require activation for matrix degradation to occur. Serine proteinases degrade matrix components and activate MMPs. Neutrophil elastase, also present in increased concentrations in chronic wounds, is important for orchestrating matrix-degrading events. Although the inflammatory profile differs for the various types of chronic ulcer, the general relation is an increase in inflammatory cytokines, which leads to the activation of proteinases and MMPs and a decrease in tissue inhibitors, resulting in a degradative state and wound chronicity. Nwomeh and colleagues described this common pathway as a self-perpetuating environment of oxygen metabolites and degradative enzymes that overwhelm the equilibrium to destroy the endogenous protease inhibitors, thereby establishing a chronic wound.

Bibliography

Alfano M, Poli G: Cytokine and chemokine based control of HIV infection and replication. Curr Pharm Des 2001;7: 993-1013.

Arai K, Lee F, Miyajima A, et al: Cytokines: coordinators of immune and inflammatory responses. Annu Rev Biochem 1990;59:783-836.

Attisano L, Tuen Lee-Hoeflich S: The Smads. Genome Biol 2001;2:3010.

Baggiolini M, Loetscher P, Moser B: Interleukin-8 and the chemokine family. Int J Immunopharmacol 1995;17:103-108.

Beer HD, Longaker MT, Werner S: Reduced expression of PDGF and PDGF receptors during impaired wound healing. J Invest Dermatol 1997;109:132-138.

Bennett NT, Schultz GS: Growth factors and wound healing: biochemical properties of growth factors and their receptors. Am J Surg 1993;165:728-737.

Bennett NT, Schultz GS: Growth factors and wound healing. Part II. Role in normal and chronic wound healing. Am J Surg 1993;166:74-81.

Blum WF, Ranke MB: Insulin-like growth factor binding proteins (IGFBPs) with special reference to IGFBP-3. Acta Paediatr Scand Suppl 1990;367:55-62.

Border WA, Noble NA: Transforming growth factor β in tissue fibrosis. N Engl J Med 1994;10:1286-1292.

Bradham DM, Igarashi A, Potter RL, Grotendorst GR: Connective tissue growth factor: a cysteine-rich mitogen secreted by human vascular endothelial cells is related to the SRC-induced immediate early gene product CEF-10. J Cell Biol 1991;114:1285-1294.

Brigstock DR: The connective tissue growth factor/cysteine-rich 61/nephroblastoma overexpressed (CCN) family. Endocr Rev 1999;20:189-206.

Brown GL, Curtsinger L, Jurkiewicz MJ, et al: Stimulation of healing of chronic wounds by epidermal growth factor. Plast Reconstr Surg 1991;88:189-194.

Brown GL, Nanney LB, Griffen J, et al: Enhancement of wound healing by topical treatment with epidermal growth factor. N Engl J Med 1989;321:76-79.

Bucalo B, Eaglstein WH, Falanga V: Inhibition of cell proliferation by chronic wound fluid. Wound Repair Regen 1993;1: 181-186.

Carpenter G, Cohen S: Epidermal growth factor. J Biol Chem 1990;265:7709-7712.

Centrella M, Horowitz MC, Wozney JM, McCarthy TL: Transforming growth factor-β gene family members and bone. Endocr Rev 1994;15:27-39.

Chambers RC, Leoni P, Blanc-Brude OP, et al: Thrombin is a potent inducer of connective tissue growth factor production via proteolytic activation of protease-activated receptor-1. J Biol Chem 2000;275:35584-35591.

Clauss M: Molecular biology of the VEGF and the VEGF receptor family. Semin Thromb Hemost 2000;26:561-569.

Cohen S: Isolation of a mouse submaxillary gland protein accelerating incisor eruption and eyelid opening in the newborn animal. J Biol Chem 1962;237:1555-1562.

Cohen S: The stimulation of epidermal proliferation by a specific protein (EGF). Dev Biol 1965;12:394-407.

Cooper DM, Yu EZ, Hennessey P, et al: Determination of endogenous cytokines in chronic wounds. Ann Surg 1994;219:688-692.

Cordon-Cardo C, Vlodavsky I, Haimovitz-Friedman A, et al: Expression of basic fibroblast growth factor in normal human tissues. Lab Invest 1990;63:832-840.

Daniele S, Frati L, Fiore C, Santoni G: The effect of the epidermal growth factor (EGF) on the corneal epithelium in humans. Graefes Arch Clin Exp Ophthalmol 1979;210:159-165.

Davidson JM, Krieg T, Eming SA: Particle-mediated gene therapy of wounds. Wound Repair Regen 2000;8:452-459.

Dinarello CA: Interleukin-1, interleukin-1 receptors and interleukin-1 receptor antagonist. Int Rev Immunol 1998;16: 457-499.

Dinarello CA, Moldawer LL: Chemokines and their receptors. In Dinarello CA, Moldawer LL (eds): Proinflammatory and Anti-inflammatory Cytokines in Rheumatoid Arthritis (2nd ed). Thousand Oaks, CA: Amgen Inc, 2000: 99-110.

Dinarello CA, Moldawer LL: Proinflammatory and anti-inflammatory cytokines in rheumatoid arthritis. 2000;1: 1-282.

DiPietro LA: Wound healing: the role of the macrophage and other immune cells. Shock 1995;4:233-240.

Duncan MR, Frazier KS, Abramson S, et al: Connective tissue growth factor mediates transforming growth factor beta-induced collagen synthesis: down-regulation by cAMP. FASEB J 1999;13:1774-1786.

Ehrlich HP: The physiology of wound healing: a summary of normal and abnormal wound healing processes. Adv Wound Care 1998;11:326-328.

Fantl WJ, Johnson DE, Williams LT: Signalling by receptor tyrosine kinases. Annu Rev Biochem 1993;62:453-481.

Finch PW, Rubin JS, Miki T, et al: Human KGF is FGF-related with properties of a paracrine effector of epithelial cell growth. Science 1989;245:752-755.

Frazier K, Williams S, Kothapalli D, et al: Stimulation of fibroblast cell growth, matrix production, and granulation tissue formation by connective tissue growth factor. J Invest Dermatol 1996;107:404-411.

Fu X, Shen Z, Chen Y, et al: Randomised placebo-controlled trial of use of topical recombinant bovine basic fibroblast growth factor for second-degree burns. Lancet 1998;352:1661-1664.

Gillitzer R, Goebeler M: Chemokines in cutaneous wound healing. J Leukoc Biol 2001;69:513-521.

Grotendorst GR: Connective tissue growth factor: a mediator of TGF-beta action on fibroblasts. Cytokine Growth Factor Rev 1997;8:171-179.

Heldin CH, Westermark B: Mechanism of action and in vivo role of platelet-derived growth factor. Physiol Rev 1999;79:1283-1316.

Igarashi A, Nashiro K, Kikuchi K, et al: Connective tissue growth factor gene expression in tissue sections from localized scleroderma, keloid, and other fibrotic skin disorders. J Invest Dermatol 1996;106:729-733.

Johnson GR, Saeki T, Gordon AW, et al: Autocrine action of amphiregulin in a colon carcinoma cell line and immunocytochemical localization of amphiregulin in human colon. J Cell Biol 1992;118:741-751.

Katz MH, Alvarez AF, Kirsner RS, et al: Human wound fluid from acute wounds stimulates fibroblast and endothelial cell growth. J Am Acad Dermatol 1991;25:1054-1058.

Ksontini R, MacKay SL, Moldawer LL: Revisiting the role of tumor necrosis factor alpha and the response to surgical injury and inflammation. Arch Surg 1998;133:558-567.

Lawrence WT: Physiology of the acute wound. Clin Plast Surg 1998;25:321-340.

Lee RC, Doong H: Control of matrix production during tissue repair. In Lee RC, Mostoe TA, Siebert JW (eds): Advances in Wound Healing and Tissue Repair. New York: World Medical Press, 2000:1-25.

Li L, Dixon JE: Form, function, and regulation of protein tyrosine phosphatases and their involvement in human diseases. Semin Immunol 2000;12:75-84.

Luster AD: Chemokines—chemotactic cytokines that mediate inflammation. N Engl J Med 1998;338:436-445.

Luther SA, Cyster JG: Chemokines as regulators of T cell differentiation. Nat Immunol 2001;2:102-107.

Massague J: TGF-β signal transduction. Annu Rev Biochem 1998;67:753-791.

Massague J: Transfroming growth factor-α. J Biol Chem 1990;265:21393-21396.

Mast BA, Schultz GS: Interactions of cytokines, growth factors, and proteases in acute and chronic wounds. Wound Repair Regen 1996;4:411-420.

Matsuoka J, Grotendorst GR: Two peptides related to platelet-derived growth factor are present in human wound fluid. Proc Natl Acad Sci USA 1989;86:4416-4420.

McGee GS, Broadley KN, Buckley A, et al: Recombinant transforming growth factor beta accelerates incisional wound healing. Curr Surg 1989;46:103-106.

Moussad EE, Brigstock DR: Connective tissue growth factor: what's in a name? Mol Genet Metab 2000;71:276-292.

Mustoe TA, Galiano RD: Mediators of wound healing, including the role of growth factors. *In* Lee RC, Mustoe TA, Siebert JW (eds): Advances in Wound Healing and Tissue Repair. New York: World Medical Press, 2000;29:55.

Nwomeh BC, Yager DR, Cohen IK: Physiology of the chronic wound. Clin Plast Surg 1998;25:341-356.

Olson MF, Marais R: Ras protein signalling. Semin Immunol 2000;12:63-73.

Phillips LG, Abdullah KM, Geldner PD, et al: Application of basic fibroblast growth factor may reverse diabetic wound healing impairment. Ann Plast Surg 1993;31:331-334.

Robson MC: The role of growth factors in the healing of chronic wounds. Wound Repair Regen 1997;5:12-17.

Robson MC, Hill DP, Smith PD, et al: Sequential cytokine therapy for pressure ulcers: clinical and mechanistic response. Ann Surg 2000;231:600-611.

Robson MC, Phillips LG, Lawrence WT, et al: The safety and effect of topically applied recombinant basic fibroblast growth factor on the healing of chronic pressure sores. Ann Surg 1992;216:401-408

Rubin JS, Osada H, Finch PW, et al: Purification and characterization of a newly identified growth factor specific for epithelial cells. Proc Natl Acad Sci USA 1989;86:802-806.

Rumalla VK, Borah GL: Cytokines, growth factors, and plastic surgery. Plast Reconstr Surg 2001;108:719-733.

Samelson LE, Klausner RD: Tyrosine kinases and tyrosine-based activation motifs: current research on activation via the T cell antigen receptor. J Biol Chem 1992;267:24913-24916.

Sato S, Nagaoka T, Hasegawa M, et al: Serum levels of connective tissue growth factor are elevated in patients with systemic sclerosis: association with extent of skin sclerosis and severity of pulmonary fibrosis. J Rheumatol 2000;27:149-154.

Schultz GS, White M, Mitchel R, et al: Epithelial wound healing enhanced by transforming growth factor-α and vaccinia growth factor. Science 1987;235:350-352.

Shah M, Foreman DM, Ferguson MWJ: Neutralisation of TGF-β1 and TGF-β2 or exogenous addition of TGF-β3 to cutaneous rat wounds reduces scarring. J Cell Sci 1995; 108: 985-1002.

Shah M, Foreman DM, Ferguson MW: Neutralising antibody to TGF-beta 1,2 reduces cutaneous scarring in adult rodents. J Cell Sci 1994;107:1137-1157.

Shing Y, Christofori G, Hanahan D, et al: Betacellulin: a mitogen from pancreatic beta cell tumors. Science 1993;259: 1604-1607.

Shoyab M, Plowman GD, McDonald VL, et al: Structure and function of human amphiregulin: a member of the epidermal growth factor family. Science 1989;243:1074-1076.

Siebert JW, Cabera RC, Longaker MT: Scarless healing: lessons from fetal wounds. 2000;57-74.

Smith PD, Polo M, Soler PM, et al: Efficacy of growth factors in the accelerated closure of interstices in explanted meshed human skin grafts. J Burn Care Rehabil 2000;21:5-9.

Steed DL, Diabetic Ulcer Study Group: Clinical evaluation of recombinant human platelet-derived growth factor for the treatment of lower extremity diabetic ulcers. J Vasc Surg 1995;21:71-81.

Subramaniam PS, Torres BA, Johnson HM: So many ligands, so few transcription factors: a new paradigm for signaling through the stat transcription factors. Cytokine 2001;15: 175-187.

Tarnuzzer RW, Schultz GS: Biochemical analysis of acute and chronic wound environments. Wound Repair Regen 1996;4:321-325.

Ward SG, Westwick J: Chemokines: understanding their role in T-lymphocyte biology. Biochem J 1998;333:457-470.

Werner S, Peters KG, Longaker MT, et al: Large induction of keratinocyte growth factor expression in the dermis during wound healing. Proc Natl Acad Sci USA 1992;89: 6896-6900.

Zlotnik A, Yoshie O: Chemokines: a new classification system and their role in immunity. Immunity 2000;12:121-127.

CHAPTER 3

The Normal Wound Healing Process

W. Thomas Lawrence, M.P.H., M.D., F.A.C.S.

When tissue is injured, the body is obligated to repair the damage. The ideal response to tissue injury would be to regenerate damaged structures and precisely recreate the pre-injury condition. Unfortunately, humans are incapable of a regenerative response and instead respond to injury by producing a patch of scar. Scar formation requires that a series of biologic processes occur in a carefully orchestrated sequence. In this chapter, these processes are reviewed as they occur in skin. Though the healing response varies slightly in different tissues, healing in skin is fairly typical of how healing occurs in tissues throughout the body.

Wound healing is a biologic process and, therefore, occurs as a continuum of biologic activity lasting at least 6 to 12 months. In order to simplify consideration of the process, it has been broken down into stages, though one stage does not abruptly stop as the next one starts. The stages are also not independent in that the products of one stage frequently are involved in subsequent ones (Fig. 3–1).

Early Wound Healing Events

Creation of Hemostasis

When vascular endothelium is intact, platelet aggregation and thrombosis are limited by several mechanisms.

Endothelial cells synthesize prostacyclin, which is a potent inhibitor of platelet aggregation, and protein C, which degrades coagulation factors V and VII. In addition, circulating thrombin is bound by antithrombin III, limiting its activity. Any injury that penetrates the dermis creates vascular damage. This results in disruption of the normally smooth layer of endothelial cells lining blood vessels.

When a blood vessel is disrupted, several things occur. Vasoconstriction is stimulated by circulating catecholamines (epinephrine), the sympathetic nervous system (norepinephrine), and prostaglandins released by injured cells. In addition, platelets adhere to exposed subendothelial elements as a result of interactions between glycoprotein receptors on the platelets and subendothelial proteins. Platelet adherence requires fibrinogen and von Willebrand factor. Additional proteins such as laminin, thrombospondin, and vitronectin also may be involved. When platelets adhere to the subendothelium, they release the contents of alpha granules, dense bodies, and lysosomes within their cytoplasm. The alpha granules contain albumin, platelet thrombospondin, plasminogen, fibrinogen, fibronectin, platelet factor 4, von Willebrand factor, β-thromboglobulin, immunoglobulin G, coagulation factors V and VIII, and a variety of cytokines. The cytokines include platelet-derived growth factor (PDGF), transforming growth factor-β (TGF-β), transforming growth factor-α (TGF-α), fibroblast growth factor (FGF)-2, platelet-derived epidermal growth factor (EGF), and platelet-derived endothelial cell growth factor. The dense granules contain ADP, ATP, calcium, and serotonin. The lysosomes include digestive proteases required for inter- and intracellular functions. Many of these factors stimulate additional platelet aggregation as well as the coagulation cascades. Some cytokines contribute to early wound healing events, while others are not involved until later in the wound healing process.

Fibrin is the end product of the coagulation cascades, and it stabilizes the initial platelet plug. The coagulation cascade, like platelet aggregation, is triggered by exposure to subendothelial elements. Subendothelial cells release a "tissue factor" that binds an activated form of factor VII in plasma, initiating the extrinsic coagulation cascade.

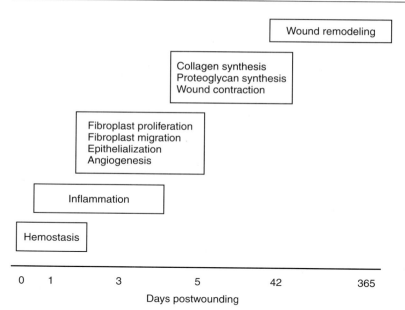

FIGURE 3–1 Primary wound healing activities.

The cascade results in the production of thrombin, which catalyzes the formation of fibrin from fibrinogen. The alternative intrinsic coagulation pathway is initiated by activation of factor XII and also results in fibrin formation. This pathway is not essential and is not specifically triggered by injury.

The clot that forms after injury therefore consists of aggregated platelets and red blood cells enmeshed within a fibrin lattice. This lattice contributes to hemostasis and also forms the early "provisional" matrix within the wound (Table 3–1). Cytokines released at the time of injury are bound to the lattice, which serves as a reservoir for these factors as healing progresses. Additional proteins derived from both plasma and local cells also are bound. The fibronectins are particularly important such proteins.

Fibronectins are a class of glycoproteins that facilitate cellular attachment. They are synthesized by fibroblasts and epithelial cells, and play roles in both early healing and mature tissues. Within the provisional matrix, fibronectins facilitate the attachment of various cell types to fibrin and thereby contribute to cellular migration within the wound. The attachment of cells to fibronectin involves the binding of one of nearly a dozen binding sites on the fibronectin molecule with integrins on the cell membrane. Integrins are a group of over 20 cell membrane molecules. They primarily bind extracellular matrix and have α and β subunits. Different cells express different integrins, and individual cells can express different integrins at different times. The expression of specific

Table 3–1

Predominant wound matrix characteristics at different phases of healing

	Early "Provisional" Matrix	Mature Matrix
Time period where predominant	First postwounding week	Subsequent weeks
Primary lattice components	Fibrin	Collagen
	Fibronectin	Fibronectin
		Proteoglycans
Primary cellular elements	Red blood cells	Fibroblasts
	Platelets	
	Inflammatory cells	
Vascular supply	Forming capillaries	More mature vessels
Epithelial cover	Advancing monolayer	Multilaminated epidermis

integrin receptors by various cells is influenced by cytokines. In addition to contributing to cell adhesion, the interaction of matrix proteins with integrin receptors can stimulate specific cellular functions such as cellular migration.

When stimulated to migrate, cells anchored to fibronectin develop lamellipodia that reach out until they find another appropriate binding site. They then attach to the new site, release the old site, and pull themselves in the desired direction. Fibronectin fragments have been demonstrated to be chemotactic for fibroblasts and therefore can facilitate migration by this mechanism as well. Inflammatory cell migration throughout the wound is vital in that cytokines derived from these cells are essential for angiogenesis, epithelialization, and other wound healing activities.

Inflammation

The body responds to injury by producing an inflammatory response. The first signs of inflammation are seen within minutes of wounding. Hunter described the physical signs of inflammation in 1794. They include erythema, edema, heat, and pain.

The physiologic changes that generate these signs occur primarily in 10- to 15-μ-diameter microvenules within the capillary bed. Within 10 to 15 minutes after injury, the initial vasoconstriction that contributed to hemostasis is replaced by a vasodilatory response. This vasodilation generates erythema and heat. As the microvenules dilate, gaps form between the endothelial cells lining the vessels. Plasma passively leaks through the gaps into the extravascular space, generating edema. The edema contributes to the pain that characterizes inflammation, as does ischemia related to vascular damage and noxious tissue breakdown products.

Kinins are one of the mediators of the vasodilatory response. Kinins are a family of peptides nine amino acids in length. They are released from protein-binding molecules in the plasma by activation of kallikrein, another by-product of the clotting cascade. Additional factors such as leukotrienes, which are mast cell derived, and endothelial products contribute to vasodilation. Histamine and prostaglandins produced by mast cells in the injured area contribute to both vasodilation and increased vascular permeability. Thrombin and possibly neutrophil factors also increase vascular permeability.

Leukocytes play a number of critical roles during the inflammatory phase of healing. They all require activation to perform these functions. After activation, both neutrophils and macrophages engulf and digest foreign material and bacteria utilizing hydrolytic enzymes and oxygen radicals. Phagocytic cells have receptors on their surface that allow them to recognize, bind, and engulf foreign material.

Macrophage-binding receptors include the CD14 receptor, which is an immunoglobulin-type adhesion molecule that binds bacterial lipopolysaccharide, and the α_1-β_2 integrin, also known as CD11b/CD18. The release of oxygen radicals and proteases involved in phagocytosis is an additional inflammatory stimulus.

Macrophages are critical mediators of the entire healing process and have many functions in addition to phagocytosis. Unlike neutrophils, they have been demonstrated to be essential for normal healing. They are a key source of matrix metalloproteinases (MMPs) such as collagenase and elastase that break down damaged matrix. Most importantly, macrophages are a primary source of cytokines required for fibroblast proliferation, collagen production, and other aspects of healing. Among these are PDGF, TGF-β, TGF-α, interleukin (IL)-1, insulin-like growth factor-1, and FGF-2. Macrophages also produce prostaglandins and arginine, which are additional important regulators of the healing process. Though phagocytosis was thought for some time to be the only function of neutrophils, they may also produce proinflammatory cytokines that activate fibroblasts and keratinocytes.

Like macrophages, lymphocytes have been demonstrated to be essential for healing. The vital lymphocytes are T cells in that there is no evidence that B cells are involved in the healing process. T cells appear in experimental wounds in large numbers on day 5 after wounding and peak in numbers on day 7. Different T-cell subsets have different effects on the healing process. CD4+ T-helper cells promote healing. Depletion of the CD8+ subset of lymphocytes improves healing, suggesting that this subset of T lymphocytes downregulates the healing process. Lymphocytes are also vital for cellular immunity, though this has limited importance in minor trauma.

Lymphocytes, like macrophages, are a source of cytokines. Lymphocyte-derived cytokines include heparin-binding EGF, a form of FGF-2; TGF-β; interferon-γ; interleukins IL-1, IL-2, and IL-6a; TNF-α; and fibroblast activating factor. Cytokines derived from macrophages contribute to lymphocyte activation, which is essential for cytokine release.

Eosinophils are only present in the peripheral circulation in limited numbers under normal circumstances and also are represented to a limited degree in the wound milieu. They can produce TGF-α, though their role in healing is most likely limited.

The migration of leukocytes into the wound milieu is stimulated by a variety of chemotactic factors. Bacterial products, complement factors, histamine, prostaglandin E$_2$, leukotrienes, PDGF, TNF-α, and fibrin breakdown products all have been demonstrated to be chemotactic for leukocytes. Additional factors such as platelet factor 4 have been demonstrated to be specifically chemotactic for neutrophils, while collagen fragments, fibronectin fragments, elastin, complement components, thrombin, and TGF-β have been demonstrated to be chemotactic for macrophages.

Neutrophil migration into the extravascular space requires upregulation of the α_1-β_2 integrin (CD11/CD18) on the neutrophil surface. Initially, neutrophils loosely adhere to capillary walls and roll along the walls in a process mediated by selectins on the endothelial cells' surface. They subsequently firmly adhere to the endothelial cells in a process involving the intercellular adhesion molecules (ICAMs), which are expressed during inflammation by endothelial cells. The primary ICAM involved is ICAM-1, which binds to the β_2 component of the leukocyte integrin. After firmly adhering to the vessel walls, the cells actively transmigrate between endothelial cells into the extravascular space. Neutrophils produce elastase and collagenase in response to chemoattractant stimulation, and these enzymes are involved in migration through the vascular wall as well.

Monocytes within the peripheral circulation migrate through capillaries in a fashion similar to neutrophils. The monocytes transform into macrophages during the transmigration in a process mediated by serum factors and fibronectin, and are subsequently activated. Activating factors include PDGF, IL-2, and interferon-σ from T lymphocytes, fibronectin, collagen, and bacterial or viral stimuli. The exact manner in which macrophages differentiate is determined by the activating stimulus. Some macrophages may be activated to primarily produce metalloproteinases or be phagocytic, whereas others may differentiate into primarily cytokine producers.

Though neutrophils predominate in wounds for the first 24 to 48 hours, their numbers subsequently diminish rapidly. Cells trapped within clot are sloughed, and the remaining cells gradually become senescent and are phagocytosed by macrophages. Macrophages and lymphocytes to a lesser degree remain in the wounded area for 5 to 7 days and then gradually diminish in numbers unless foreign bodies or infectious agents elicit a more prolonged inflammatory response.

Intermediate Wound Healing Events

Forty-eight hours after wounding, hemostasis has been accomplished, the acute signs of inflammation are dying down, and the wounded area is filled with a fibrin-fibronectin matrix. Cellular elements within the provisional matrix include primarily inflammatory cells and some residual erythrocytes. Significant changes occur in the wound matrix over the ensuing 2 to 3 days. Mesenchymal cells migrate into the wound matrix and proliferate. Angiogenesis initiates revascularization of the injured area. The disrupted epithelial surface begins to regenerate itself.

Fibroblasts are the primary mesenchymal cell in intact dermis. Cells are lost or damaged in any injury, and the wound area must be repopulated with cells for normal biologic functions to occur. Undifferentiated mesenchymal cells in the vicinity of the wound may differentiate into fibroblasts when stimulated by cytokines released in the wound milieu. In addition, a variety of chemotactic factors stimulate fibroblasts from the wound periphery to migrate into the wound. These include PDGF, TGF-β, and EGF as well as fibronectin.

Fibroblast migration requires the upregulation of cell membrane integrin receptors that bind fibronectin and fibrin in the provisional wound matrix. PDGF and TGF-β stimulate upregulation of these integrins. Fibroblasts then migrate in the manner previously described. As one pole of the fibroblast remains fixed to the matrix through its integrin-binding site, lamellipodia extend out until another binding site in the matrix is identified. When one is found, the initially bound site is released, the new site is bound, and the cell moves. The direction of movement is guided not only by the orientation of the binding proteins but also by the alignment of the fibrils in the preliminary wound matrix. Cells preferentially migrate along fibers and not across them. Concentrations of hyaluronic acid also may modulate the direction of cellular migration.

The fibroblasts may need to cleave a path through the provisional matrix. They have the ability to produce proteolytic enzymes to facilitate this migration, including matrix metalloproteinase-1 (MMP-1), gelatinase (MMP-2), and stromelysin (MMP-3). Synthesis and release of these enzymes may be modulated in part by TGF-β.

The fibroblast population is further expanded by proliferation of both resident and newly arrived cells. A large number of cytokines have been demonstrated to stimulate fibroblast proliferation, including PDGF and TGF-β.

Angiogenesis

Dermal matrix includes a web of blood vessels that provides essential elements for tissue metabolism. This web is disrupted by wounding and must be regenerated. Vascular disruption contributes to the high lactate levels, acidic pH, and decreased oxygen tension within wounded tissue. All of these factors stimulate angiogenesis. As a first step in angiogenesis, small sprouts of vascular endothelial cells bud from microvenules at the wound periphery. Proliferation of endothelial cells at the bud base combined with cellular migration results in elongation of the bud. The cells take on a more curved orientation and eventually form a lumen as they migrate. The buds grow until they contact other buds. The buds then interconnect, forming a vascular loop, and the budding process begins anew.

The migration of endothelial cells involves many of the same features discussed previously. Endothelial cells bind to fibrin and fibronectin within the provisional matrix using integrin-binding domains and then pull themselves over the matrix. Upregulation of the α-β_3 integrins is specifically associated with initiation of revascularization and is a vital component of the angiogenic response. Endothelial cells also have the ability to produce MMPs to break down collagen and plasminogen activator to facilitate breakdown of fibrin when needed. They also generate a neo–basement membrane consisting of fibronectin and proteoglycans as they migrate. The migration and proliferation of endothelial cells as required for angiogenesis are stimulated by a variety of cytokines. Basic fibroblast growth factor, or FGF-2, is a powerful angiogenic stimulant, and heparin is an important cofactor facilitating its activity. Vascular endothelial growth factor is another key angiogenic stimulant. Stimulatory cytokines diminish in number when an area is completely revascularized. The flux in concentrations of angiogenic factors may stimulate maturation of the vascular system.

Epithelialization

The epithelium provides an impervious barrier between the outside environment and the body, and re-establishment of this barrier after injury is vital. Within the first day after epithelium has been violated, re-epithelialization begins. Basal cells at the wound edge elongate and begin to migrate. They migrate essentially as a monolayer in a leapfrog fashion. Additional suprabasilar cells also may migrate and contribute to the monolayer. Epithelial appendages such as hair follicles and sweat glands also can generate an advancing epithelial monolayer if they are preserved within the wound bed. Migrating epithelial cells have the capacity to secrete MMPs to aid in penetrating eschar or scab as well a plasminogen activator to break down fibrin. Migrating basal cells generally migrate in the direction of the underlying matrix fibers. After migration is initiated, basal cells at the wound edge thicken and begin to proliferate. Proliferation is initiated 48 to 72 hours after wounding.

Changes occur within epithelial cells as they elongate and become migratory. Actin filaments 40 to 80 Å in width appear within the cytoplasm. Desmosomes that link the epithelial cells together and hemidesmosomes that link the cells to the underlying basement membrane both disappear. The integrins that facilitate attachment are downregulated in the cell membrane, and several other integrins that facilitate migration are expressed. The lag between wounding and the initiation of migration results from the interval required for these intracellular changes to occur. The precise signal that induces these changes is unknown, though decreased calcium concentrations or increased magnesium concentrations may be involved.

If the epidermal basement membrane is intact, the epithelial cells simply migrate over it. If it has been damaged, as occurs in most substantial wounds, epithelial cells migrate over the provisional matrix of fibrin and fibronectin. The migrating cells contribute additional elements to the neo–basement membrane, including tenascin, vitronectin, and collagens type I and V. Cells migrate until they reach cells migrating from a different direction. They then cease migrating as a result of "contact inhibition," which also results in cessation of enzyme secretion. At this point, the basal epithelial cells become more basaloid and hemidesmosomes that fix the cells to the underlying basement membrane reform.

Additional cellular proliferation regenerates a more normal multilaminated epithelium covered by keratin. The new epithelium is similar to normal epithelium, though it is slightly thinner, and the basement membrane is flatter in that the rete pegs of epidermis that normally penetrate the dermis are not seen.

Cytokines primarily involved in epithelial migration and proliferation include EGF, TGF-α, and keratinocyte growth factor, which is also known as FGF-7. Some of the cytokines derive from inflammatory cells and some derive from the epithelial cells themselves.

Late Wound Healing Events

Four to 5 days after wounding, the fibrin-fibronectin provisional matrix has been repopulated with fibroblasts. At this point many of the fibroblasts undergo a phenotypic change in order to initiate synthetic activity. They develop a more prominent rough endoplasmic reticulum and Golgi apparatus.

The primary protein synthesized by fibroblasts is collagen. Collagen makes up 25% of the protein in the body and more than 50% of the protein in scar tissue. Collagen synthesis continues at an accelerated rate for 2 to 4 weeks in most wounds and subsequently begins to slow. Cytokines involved in the stimulation of collagen synthesis include TGF-β, PDGF, and EGF. The rate of collagen synthesis is affected by a number of factors, including age, tension, pressure, and stress. As more collagen is synthesized, it begins to replace fibrin as the primary component of the wound matrix. Fibronectin, however, remains a key matrix component facilitating cellular attachment and migration (see Table 3–1).

There are at least 19 types of collagen, each with slight differences in the polypeptide chains. Type I collagen makes up 80% to 90% of the collagen normally found in dermis. Type III is the second most common type and makes up 10% to 20% of dermal collagen. Increased concentrations of type III are seen embryologically and in the early phases of healing, though the reason for this is unclear. Type II collagen is seen almost exclusively in cartilage, while type IV collagen is a key component of basement membranes. Type V is seen in the media of blood vessels, and type VII forms the anchoring fibrils of epidermal basement membrane. The remaining collagen types are found in small concentrations in specific parts of the body.

Type I collagen consists of three polypeptide chains wrapped around each other to form a triple helix. The polypeptide chains are individually synthesized and align themselves into their characteristic orientation within the endoplasmic reticulum in a process facilitated by terminal peptides on the polypeptide chains. Another key activity that occurs after release of the polypeptide chains into the endoplasmic reticulum is hydroxylation of lysine and proline moieties within the polypeptide chains. Hydroxylysine formation, in particular, is critical because it is essential for subsequent cross-link formation. Hydroxyproline is found almost exclusively in collagen and serves as a marker of the quantity of collagen in tissue. The hydroxylation process requires the specific enzymes prolyl and lysyl hydroxylase, as well as essential cofactors oxygen, vitamin C, α-ketoglutarate, and ferrous iron. Deficiencies of vitamin C or oxygen, or suppression of enzymatic activity by corticosteroids, can lead to underhydroxylated collagen that is incapable of generating strong cross-links.

After the collagen molecule is synthesized, it is secreted into the extracellular space. The terminal peptides that facilitated triple helix formation interfere with the aggregation of collagen molecules into fibrils. These peptides are cleaved by specific enzymes in the extracellular space. After this occurs, the more compact molecules align themselves in a staggered fashion in bundles of four or five molecules. The orientation of the molecules is determined by electrostatic bonds, with approximately 25% of the length of the molecules overlapping. This produces a characteristic banding pattern when the molecules are viewed by electron microscopy. In addition to combining in a side-to-side fashion, the bundles of molecules orient themselves in an end-to-end fashion to form fibrils and fibers.

The electrostatic cross-links that initially bind the molecules together are subsequently replaced by more stable covalent bonds. The bonds occur between residues of lysine and lysine, lysine and hydroxylysine, and hydroxylysine and hydroxylysine. The strongest cross-links form between two hydroxylysine residues.

Dermal extracellular connective tissue matrix contains various proteins in addition to collagen and fibronectin, including proteoglycans and elastin. Proteoglycans, like collagen, are synthesized by fibroblasts and consist of a protein core covalently linked to one or more glycosaminoglycans. Proteoglycan synthesis increases in response to injury, and proteoglycans are an important component of the mature wound matrix. Dermatan sulfate,

chondroitin sulfate (in cartilage), heparin and heparin sulfate, keratan sulfate, and hyaluronic acid are more common proteoglycans. Though the precise biologic function of many of the proteoglycans is not completely understood, their primary function is to bind proteins and alter their orientation in a manner that influences their activity. Chondroitin sulfate and dermatan sulfate, for example, help orient collagen molecules in a manner that facilitates fibril formation. The increase in dermatan sulfate concentration in a wound parallels the increase in collagen. Hyaluronic acid may be a particularly important proteoglycan. It is a prominent component of both early and more mature matrix. It contributes to skin's viscoelastic properties in that it is extremely hygroscopic and it is a potent modulator of cellular migration. Heparin is a critical cofactor of FGF-2 in angiogenic stimulation. Other proteoglycans also may have a significant impact on healing through interactions with cytokines.

Elastin is a third component of normal dermal matrix, and it gives skin its characteristic elasticity. It is not synthesized in response to injury and is not found in scar. Scar is therefore much stiffer and less elastic than normal dermis.

Wound Contraction

Wound contraction, like collagen synthesis, begins 4 to 5 days after wounding. It continues most actively for approximate 2 weeks, though it will continue for longer periods if wound closure is not accomplished. Though the average rate of wound contraction is 0.6 to 0.7 mm/day, the rate of wound contraction varies significantly in different anatomic locations. In areas where the skin is tight, such as the pretibial area or scalp, it will proceed more slowly than in areas of skin laxity, such as the buttock. Wound shape also affects the rate of contraction, with square wounds contracting more quickly than circular wounds. This explains why circular intestinal stomas better maintain patency.

Wound contraction across a joint surface can produce a contracture that limits joint excursion, leading to deleterious functional results. Such contractures commonly are seen after burn wounds to the neck, axillae, and other joint surfaces.

Contracting wounds are characterized by the presence of myofibroblasts at their periphery. Myofibroblasts are slightly modified fibroblasts with defining characteristics that can be identified only on electron microscopy. First described in 1971, their defining characteristics include actin-rich microfilaments in the cytoplasm, a multilobulated nucleus, and abundant rough endoplasmic reticulum. It is thought that myofibroblasts pull wounds together in a "picture frame" fashion from the wound periphery. They bind to each other as well as the wound edge through desmosomes and maculae adherens to facilitate this process.

This concept has been supported by experiments in which excisional wounds were created and allowed to begin contraction prior to excision of either the central or peripheral portions of the wound. The wounds from which central portions were excised were unaffected, whereas those from which peripheral elements were removed stopped contracting completely. Myofibroblasts appear in a wound 4 to 6 days after wound formation and disappear after 4 weeks through apoptosis.

Based on experiments utilizing collagen lattices, others alternatively believe that fibroblasts in the wound center play a critical role in wound contraction. They suggest that the fibroblasts pull the matrix centripetally through retraction of their fibropodia. Proponents of this theory point out that the time course of expression of actin microfilaments shows a peak that corresponds more closely to cellular apoptosis than maximum contraction. They point out that the time periods during which myofibroblasts are seen in the wound do not necessarily correlate with peaks in wound contraction activity. Both groups agree that the process is cell mediated, but does not require collagen synthesis. TGF-β is a potent stimulant of wound contraction in experimental models, and other cytokines may be involved as well.

As mentioned, wound contraction is not always desirable, and, at times, inhibition of the process is preferred. Clinically, this can be achieved by closing the wound with a skin graft, though skin graft placement does not completely prevent additional contraction. Full-thickness grafts with a greater complement of dermis inhibit the process more effectively than split-thickness grafts. Grafts placed soon after wounding inhibit contraction more effectively than those placed at later time points. Splints can be effective deterrents of contraction, but they must be utilized for months to be effective. If utilization is terminated early, wounds respond with accelerated contraction.

Terminal Wound Healing Events

The primary terminal wound healing event is scar remodeling, and it becomes the predominant wound healing activity beginning approximately 21 days after wounding. Stimulation of collagen synthesis is downregulated in a process that most likely involves interferon-γ, TNF-α, and the collagen matrix itself. As the rate of collagen synthesis decreases, it reaches a level similar to the rate of collagen breakdown. Collagen breakdown is catalyzed by the MMPs previously mentioned.

The MMPs represent a family of enzymes that break down extracellular matrix. There are at least 25 MMPs that affect different substrates. MMPs are produced by a variety of cell types, and different enzymes often are produced by different cells. MMP activity is modulated by tissue inhibitors of metalloproteinase (TIMPs). Four isoforms of TIMPs have been described. The balance of MMPs and TIMPs is particularly important during the remodeling phase of healing, and it is regulated by cytokines, including TGF-β, PDGF, and IL-1.

The result of ongoing collagen turnover during remodeling is a denser, more organized collagen matrix with fibers oriented along lines of stress. The number of intra- and intermolecular cross-links involving collagen molecules increases dramatically during this phase of healing as well. As collagen remodeling occurs, the wound matrix becomes less cellular through apoptosis of multiple cell types involved in the healing process. The quantity of water and proteoglycans in the wound matrix diminishes as well. The collagen matrix never obtains quite the level of organization of intact dermis, however.

The result of these activities is a marked gain in wound strength. Three weeks after wounding, when this phase of healing begins, wound bursting strength is only 15% of normal skin. As scar remodeling proceeds most actively between 3 and 6 weeks after wounding, the wound rapidly gains strength. By 6 weeks after wounding, the wound has reached 80% to 90% of its eventual strength (Fig. 3–2). The bursting strength of a wound never reaches the strength of unwounded skin, and peaks at approximately 80% of normal skin breaking strength at 6 months. In addition to increasing wound strength, scar remodeling is visible to the surgeon as a change in the texture, thickness, and color of the healing wound. These changes can occur for up to 12 months after a wound is created.

Epilogue

What has been described in this chapter is the sequence of events that occurs in a representative wound in a normal patient. The process can be thrown awry by local events, such as infection or foreign bodies, as well as systemic problems, such as diabetes, malnutrition, cancer, and even old age. Congenital problems such as Ehlers-Danlos syndrome also can alter the process. Some patients, for poorly understood reasons, produce excessive scar in response to injury, resulting in hypertrophic scars or keloids.

In addition, not all wounds are the same. Different aspects of the healing process are more important in some types of wounds than others. For an abrasion or partial-thickness burn, epithelialization is the wound healing activity of primary importance, and collagen synthesis has limited impact. For large open wounds extending into the subcutaneous layer or deeper, wound contraction and epithelialization are the paramount wound healing activities. Alternatively, for an incisional wound that has been surgically closed, epithelialization and wound contraction are of limited importance and collagen synthesis is the primary concern.

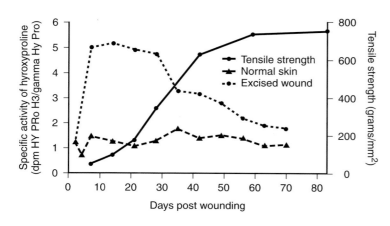

FIGURE 3–2 Graphs depicting tensile strength as well as collagen synthetic activity (specific activity of hydroxyproline) in healing wounds and unwounded skin at different time points after wounding. (Adapted from Peacock EE Jr: Wound Repair [3rd ed]. Philadelphia: WB Saunders, 1984:111.)

Though one or more of these additional features may need to be considered for a specific wound in an individual patient, the basic elements of the healing process will not change and must be understood in order to manage the problem optimally.

Bibliography

Adams DO, Hamilton DA: The cell biology of macrophage activation. Annu Rev Immunol 1984;2:283.

Ahlen K, Rubin K: Platelet-derived growth factor-BB stimulates synthesis of the integrin alpha$_2$-subunit in human diploid fibroblasts. Exp Cell Res 1994;215:347.

Albelda SM, Buck CA: Integrins and other cell adhesion molecules. FASEB J 1990;4:2868.

Ammeland E, Prasad CM, Raymond RM, et al: Interactions among inflammatory mediators on edema formation in the canine forelimb. Circ Res 1981;49:298.

Ansprunk DH, Falterman K, Folkman J: The sequence of events in the regression of corneal capillaries. Lab Invest 1978;38:284.

Assoian RK, Fleurdelys BE, Stevenson HC, et al: Expression and secretion of type β transforming growth factor by activated human macrophages. Proc Natl Acad Sci U S A 1987;84:6020.

Assoian RK, Grotendorst GR, Miller DM, et al: Cellular transformation by coordinated action of three peptide growth factors from human platelets. Nature 1984;309:804.

Atkinson YH, Marasco WA, Lopez AF, et al: Recombinant human tumor necrosis factor alpha. J Clin Invest 1988;81:759.

Baird A, Mormede P, Bohlen P: Immunoreactive fibroblast growth factor in cells of peritoneal exudate suggests its identity with macrophage growth factor. Biochem Biophys Res Commun 1985;126:358.

Barbul A, Breslin RJ, Woodard JP, et al: The effect of in vivo T helper and T suppressor lymphocyte depletion on wound healing. Ann Surg 1989;209:479.

Bar-Shavit R, Kahn A, Fenton JW, et al: Chemotactic response of monocytes to thrombin. J Cell Biol 1983;96:282.

Beezhold DH, Personius C: Fibronectin fragments stimulate tumor necrosis secretion by human monocytes. J Leukoc Biol 1992;51:59.

Bently JP: The role of chondroitin sulfate formation in wound healing. Ann Surg 1967;165:186.

Berry DP, Harding KG, Stanton MR, et al: Human wound contraction: collagen organization, fibroblasts and myofibroblasts. Plast Reconstr Surg 1998;102:124.

Bisgaard H, Kristensen J, Sondergaared J: The effect of leukotriene C4 and D4 on cutaneous blood flow in humans. Prostaglandins 1982;23:797.

Blotnick S, Peoples GE, Freeman MR, et al: T-lymphocytes synthesize and export heparin-binding epidermal growth factor-like growth factor and basic fibroblast growth factor, mitogens for vascular cells and fibroblasts: differential production and release by CD4[+] and CD8[+] T cells. Proc Natl Acad Sci U S A 1994;91:2890.

Brew K, Kinakarpandian D, Nagase H: Tissue inhibitors of metalloproteinases: evolution, structure and function. Biochim Biophys Acta 2000;1477:267.

Buck M, Houglum K, Chojkier M: Tumor necrosis factor-alpha inhibits collagen alpha a (I) gene expression and wound healing in a murine model of cachexia. Am J Pathol 1996;149:195.

Carter SB: Cell movement and cell spreading: a passive or an active process? Nature 1970;255:858.

Caterson B, Lowther DA: Changes in the metabolism of the proteoglycans from sheep articular cartilage in response to mechanical stress. Biochim Biophys Acta 1978;540:412.

Cavani A, Zambruno G, Marconi A, et al: Distinctive integrin expression in the newly formed epidermis during wound healing in humans. J Invest Dermatol 1993;101:600.

Chapman JA, Kellgren JH, Steven FS: Assembly of collagen fibrils. Fed Proc 1966;25:1811.

Chen WYJ, Abatangelo G: Functions of hyaluronan in wound repair. Wound Repair Regen 1999;7:79.

Cherry PD, Furchgott RF, Zawadzki JV, et al: Role of endothelial cells in relaxation of isolated arteries by bradykinin. Proc Natl Acad Sci U S A 1982;72:2106.

Cines DB, Pollack ES, Buck CA, et al: Endothelial cells in physiology and in the pathophysiology of vascular disorders. Blood 1998;91:3627.

Circolo A, Welgus HG, Pierce G, et al: Differential regulation of the expression of proteinases/antiproteinases in fibroblasts: effects of interleukin-1 and platelet-derived growth factor. J Biol Chem 1991;266:12283.

Clark RAF, DellaPelle P, Manseau E, et al: Blood vessel fibronectin increases in conjunction with endothelial cell proliferation and capillary ingrowth during wound healing. J Invest Dermatol 1982;79:269.

Clark RAF, Folkvord JM, Hart CE, et al: Fibronectin as well as other extracellular matrix proteins mediate human keratinocyte adherence. J Invest Dermatol 1985;84:378.

Clark RAF, Lanigan JM, DellaPelle P, et al: Fibronectin and fibrin provide a provisional matrix for epidermal cell migration during wound re-epithelialization. J Invest Dermatol 1982;70:264.

Clark RAF, Nielsen LD, Welch MP, et al: Collagen matrices attenuate the collagen synthetic response of cultured fibroblasts to TGF-β. J Cell Sci 1995;108:1251.

Dahlback B: Blood coagulation. Lancet 2000;355:1627.

Desmouliere A, Redard M, Darby I, et al: Apoptosis mediates the decrease in cellularity during the transition between granulation tissue and scar. Am J Pathol 1995;146:56.

Deuel TF, Senior RM, Huang JS, et al: Chemotaxis of monocytes and neutrophils to platelet-derived growth factor. J Clin Invest 1982;69:1046.

Dunlap MK, Donaldson DJ: Inability of colchicine to inhibit newt epidermal cell migration or prevent concanavalin-A mediated inhibition of migration studies. Exp Cell Res 1978;116:15.

Ehrlich HP: Wound closure: evidence of cooperation between fibroblasts and collagen matrix. Eye 1988;2:149.

Ezekowitz RAB, Williams DJ, Koziel H, et al: Uptake of *Pneumocystis carinii* mediated by the macrophage mannose receptor. Nature 1991;351:155.

Fishel RS, Barbul A, Beschorner WE, et al: Lymphocyte participation in healing: morphologic assessment using monoclonal antibodies. Ann Surg 1987;206:25.

Folkman J, Klagsbrun M: Angiogenic factors. Science 1987;235:442.

Ford-Hutchinson AW, Bray MA, Doig MV, et al: Leukotriene B, a potent chemokinetic and aggregating substance released from polymorphonuclear leukocytes. Nature 1980;286:264.

Forrester JC, Zederfeldt BH, Hayes TL, et al: Wolff's law in relation to the healing skin wound. J Trauma 1970;10:770

Fukai N, Apte SS, Olsen BR: Nonfibrillar collagens. *In* Ruoshalahti E, Enfvall E (eds):Extracellular Matrix Components. San Diego: Academic Press, 1994:3.

Gabbiani G, Chapponnier C, Huttner I: Cytoplasmic filaments and gap junctions in epithelial cells and myofibroblasts during wound healing. J Cell Biol 1978;76:561.

Gabbiani G, Ryan GB, Majno G: Presence of modified fibroblasts in granulation tissue and their possible role in wound contraction. Experientia 1971;27:549.

Gailit J, Xu J, Bueller H, et al: Platelet-derived growth factor and inflammatory cytokines have differential effects on the expression of integrins alpha₁β1 and alpha₅β1 by human dermal fibroblasts in vitro. J Cell Physiol 1996;169:281.

Garlick JA, Taichman LB: Fate of human keratinocytes during reepithelialization in an organotypic culture model. Lab Invest 1994;70:916.

Gillman T: Healing of cutaneous abrasions and of incisions closed with sutures or plastic adhesive tape. Med Proc 1958;4:751.

Gipson IK, Spurr-Michaud SJ, Tisdale AS: Hemidesmosomes and anchoring fibril collagen appear synchronously during development and wound healing. Dev Biol 1988;126:253.

Gospodarowicz D, Abraham J, Schilling J: Isolation and characterization of a vascular endothelial cell mitogen produced by pituitary-derived follicular stellate cells. Proc Natl Acad Sci U S A 1989;86:7311.

Gospodarowicz D, Neufeld G, Schweigerer L: Fibroblast growth factor: structural and biologic properties. J Cell Physiol 1987;5(Suppl):15.

Granstein RD, Murphy GF, Margolis RJ, et al: Gamma interferon inhibits collagen synthesis in vivo in the mouse. J Clin Invest 1987;79:1254.

Griffith TM, Edwards DH, Lewis MJ, et al: The nature of the endothelium derived vascular relaxant factor. Nature 1984;308:645.

Grinnell F: Fibronectin and wound healing. J Cell Biochem 1984;25:107.

Grinnell F: Wound repair, keratinocyte activation and integrin modulation. J Cell Sci 1992;101:1.

Grzesiak HH, Piershbacher MD: Shifts in concentrations of magnesium and calcium in early porcine and rat wound fluids activate the cell migratory response. J Clin Invest 1995;95:227.

Hassel JR, Kimura JH, Hascall VC: Proteoglycan core protein families. Annu Rev Biochem 1986;55:539.

Hennings H, Michail D, Cheng D, et al: Calcium regulation of growth and differentiation of mouse epidermal cells in culture. Cell 1980;19:245.

Hering TM, Marchant RE, Anderson JM: Type V collagen during granulation tissue development. Exp Mol Pathol 1983;39:219.

Holund B, Clemmenonn I, Junker P, et al: Fibronectin in experimental granulation tissue. APMIS Suppl 1982; 90:159.

Hsieh P, Chen LB: Behavior of cells seeded on isolated fibronectin matrices. J Cell Biol 1983;96:1208.

Hubner G, Griseldi S: Differential regulation of pro-inflammatory cytokines during wound healing in normal and glucocorticoid-treated mice. Cytokine 1996;8:548.

Hynes RO: Fibronectins. Sci Am 1986;254:42.

Hynes RO: Integrins: a family of cell surface receptors. Cell 1987;48:549.

Hynes RO: Integrins: versatility, modulation and signaling in cell adhesion. Cell 1992;69:11.

Ignotz RA, Massaugue J: Transforming growth factor-beta stimulates the expression of fibronectin and collagen and their incorporation into the extracellular matrix. J Biol Chem 1986;261:4337.

Jackson A, Friedman S, Zhan X, et al: Heat shock induces release of FGF1 from NIH 3T3 cells. Proc Natl Acad Sci U S A 1992;89:10691.

Keshar S, Stein M: The versatility of macrophages [review]. Clin Exp Allergy 1992;22:19.

Leibovich SJ, Ross R: The role of the macrophage in wound repair: a study with hydrocortisone and antimacrophage serum. Am J Pathol 1975;78:71.

Levenson SM, Geever EF, Crowley LV, et al: The healing of rat skin wounds. Ann Surg 1965;161:293.

Lewis T, Grant R: Vascular reactions of the skin to injury. Part II. The liberation of a histamine-like substance in injured skin; the underlying cause of factitious urticaria and of wheals produced by burning, and observations upon the nervous control of certain skin reactions. Heart 1924;11:209.

Ley K: Leukocyte adhesion to vascular endothelium. J Reconstr Microsurg 1992;8:495.

Loedam JA, Meijers JCM, Sixma JJ, et al: Inactivation of human factor VIII by activated protein C: cofactor activity of protein S and protective effect of von Willebrand factor. J Clin Invest 1988;82:1236.

Mackie EJ, Halfter W, Liverani D: Induction of tenascin in healing wounds. J Cell Biol 1988;107:2757.

Madden JW, Peacock EE Jr: Studies on the biology of collagen during wound healing. I. Rate of collagen synthesis and deposition in cutaneous wounds of the rat. Surgery 1968;64:288.

Marasco WA, Phan SH, Krutzsch H, et al: Purification and identification of formyl-methionyl-leucyl-phenylalanine as the major peptide neutrophil chemotactic factor produced by Escherichia coli. J Biol Chem 1984;259:5430.

Martin CW, Muir IFK: The role of lymphocytes in wound healing. Br J Plast Surg 1990;43:655.

Menger MD, Vollmar B: Adhesion molecules as determinants of disease: from molecular biology to surgical research. Br J Surg 1996;83:588.

Musson RA: Human serum induces maturation of human monocytes in vitro. Am J Pathol 1983;111:331.

Nanney LB, Magid M, Stoscheck C, et al: Comparison of epidermal growth factor binding and receptor distribution in normal human epidermis and epidermal appendages. J Invest Dermatol 1984;83:385.

Newman SL, Henson JE, Henson PM: Phagocytosis of senescent neutrophils by human monocyte derived macrophages and rabbit inflammatory macrophages. J Exp Med 1982;156:430.

Niall M, Ryan GB, O'Brien BM: The effect of epidermal growth factor on wound healing in mice. J Surg Res 1982;33:164.

Nielson EG, Phillips SM, Jimenez S: Lymphokine modulation of fibroblast proliferation. J Immunol 1982;128:1484.

Nimmi ME: Collagen: its structure and function in normal and pathological connective tissues. Semin Arthritis Rheum 1974;4:95.

Norris DA, Clark RAF, Swigart LM, et al: Fibronectin fragment(s) are chemotactic for human peripheral blood monocytes. J Immunol 1982;129:1612.

Odland G, Ross R: Human growth repair. I. Epidermal regeneration. J Cell Biol 1968;39:135.

Oh E, Pierschbacher M, Ruoslahti E: Deposition of fibronectin in tissue. Proc Natl Acad Sci U S A 1981;78:3218.

Overall CM, Wrana JJ, Sodek J: Independent regulation of collagenase, 72kD progelatinase, and metalloendoproteinase inhibitor expression in human fibroblasts by transforming growth factor-β. J Biol Chem 1989;264:1860.

Parks WC: Matrix metalloproteinases in repair. Wound Repair Regen 1999;7:423.

Parsons SL, Watson SA, Brown PD, et al: Matrix metalloproteinases. Br J Surg 1997;84:160.

Peacock EE Jr: Wound Repair (3rd ed). Philadelphia: WB Saunders, 1984:3.

Peterson JM, Barbul A, Breslin RJ, et al: Significance of T-lymphocytes in wound healing. Surgery 1987;102:300.

Postlethwaite AE, Kang AH: Collagen- and collagen peptide-induced chemotaxis of human blood monocytes. J Exp Med 1976;143:1299.

Postlethwaite AE, Keski-Oja J, Balian G, et al: Induction of fibroblast chemotaxis by fibronectin: localization of the chemotactic region of a 140,000 molecular weight non-gelatin-binding fragment. J Exp Med 1981;153:494.

Postlethwaite AE, Keski-Oja L, Moses HL, et al: Stimulation of the chemotactic migration of human fibroblasts by transforming growth factor-β. J Exp Med 1987;165:251.

Proveddini DM, Deftos LJ, Manolagas SC: 1,25-Dihydroxyvitamin D3 promotes in vitro morphologic and enzymatic changes in normal human monocytes consistent with their differentiation into macrophages. Bone 1986;7:23.

Rao AK: Congenital disorders of platelet function: disorders of signal transduction and secretion. Am J Med Sci 1998;316:69.

Rappolee DA, Mark D, Banda MJ, et al: Wound macrophages express TGF-alpha and other growth factors in vivo: analysis by mRNA phenotyping. Science 1988;241:708.

Regan M, Efron J, Kirk S, et al: The role of macrophages/monocytes in normal wound healing. Wound Repair Regen 1993;1:120.

Roberts AB, Anzano MA, Wakefield LM, et al: Type β transforming growth factor: a bifunctional regulator of cellular growth. Proc Natl Acad Sci U S A 1985;82:119.

Ross R: The role of T lymphocytes in inflammation. Proc Natl Acad Sci U S A 1994;91:2879.

Ross R, Benditt EP: Wound healing and collagen formation: fine structure in experimental scurvy. J Cell Biol 1962;12:533.

Ross R, Everett NB, Tyler R: Wound healing and collagen formation. VI. The origin of the wound fibroblast studied in parabiosis. J Cell Biol 1970;44:645.

Rudolph R: The effect of skin graft preparation on wound contraction. Surg Gynecol Obstet 1976;142:49.

Rudolph R: Location of the force of wound contraction. Surg Gynecol Obstet 1979;148:547.

Rutherford RB, Ross R: Platelet factors stimulate fibroblasts and smooth muscle cells quiescent in plasma serum to proliferate. J Cell Biol 1976;69:196.

Sakai L, Keene DR, Morris NP, et al: Type VII collagen is a major structural component of anchoring fibrils. J Cell Biol 1986;103:1577.

Schaffer M, Barbul A: Lymphocyte function in wound healing and following injury. Br J Surg 1998;85:444.

Senior RM, Griffin GL, Mecham RP, et al: Val-Gly-Val-Ala-Pro-Gly, a repeating peptide in elastin is chemotactic for fibroblasts and monocytes. J Cell Biol 1984;99:870.

Seppä H, Grotendorst GR, Seppä S, et al: Platelet-derived growth factor is chemoattractant for fibroblasts. J Cell Biol 1982;92:584.

Shing Y, Folkmann J, Sullivan R, et al: Heparin affinity: purification of a tumor-derived capillary endothelial cell growth factor. Science 1984;223:1296.

Simpson DM, Ross R: The neutrophilic leukocyte in wound repair: a study with antineutrophil serum. J Clin Invest 1972;51:2009.

Singer I, Scott S, Kawka DW, et al: Cell surface distribution of fibronectin and vibronectin receptors depends on substrate composition and extracellular matrix accumulation. J Cell Biol 1988;106:2171.

Snyderman R, Phillips J, Mergenhagen SE: Polymorphonuclear leukocyte chemotactic activity in rabbit serum and guinea pig serum treated with immune complexes: evidence for C5a as the major chemotactic factor. Infect Immun 1970;1:521.

Sporn MB, Roberts AB: Transforming growth factor β: recent progress and new challenges. J Cell Biol 1992;119:1017.

Stern DM, Naworth PP, Marcum J, et al: Interactions of antithrombin III with bovine aortic segments. J Clin Invest 1985;75:272.

Stiernberg J, Redin WR, Warner WS, et al: The role of thrombin and thrombin receptor activating peptide (TRAP-508) in initiation of tissue repair. Thromb Haemost 1993;70:158.

Stricklin GP, Nanney LB: Immunolocalization of collagenase and TIMP in healing human burn wounds. J Invest Dermatol 1994;103:488.

Sullivan DJ, Epstein WS: Mitotic activity of wounded human epidermis. J Invest Dermatol 1963;41:39.

Todd R, Donoff BR, Chiang T, et al: The eosinophil as a cellular source of transforming growth factor alpha in healing cutaneous wounds. Am J Pathol 1991;138:1307.

Tonnesen MG, Smedly LA, Henson PM: Neutrophil-endothelial cell interactions: modulation of neutrophil adhesiveness induced by complement fragments C5a and C5a des arg and formyl-methionyl-leucyl-phenylalanine in vitro. J Clin Invest 1984;745:1581.

Tzeng DY, Deuel TF, Huang JS, et al: Platelet-derived growth factor promotes human peripheral monocyte activation. Blood 1985;66:179.

Veis A, Averey J: Modes of intermolecular crosslinking in mature insoluble collagen. J Biol Chem 1965;240:3899.

Vu TH, Werb Z: Matrix metalloproteinases: effectors of development and normal physiology. Genes Dev 2000; 14:2123.

Wahl SM, Hunt DA, Wakefield LM, et al: Transforming growth factor-β induces monocyte chemotaxis and growth factor production. Proc Natl Acad Sci U S A 1987;84:5788.

Werb Z, Banda MJ, Jones PA: Degradation of connective tissue matrices by macrophages I. Proteolysis of elastin, glycoproteins and collagen by proteinases isolated from macrophages. J Exp Med 1980;152:1340.

Werb Z, Tremble P, Damsky CH: Regulation of extracellular matrix degradation by cell-extracellular matrix interactions. Cell Differ Dev 1990;32:299.

Werner S, Peters KG, Longaker MT, et al: Large induction of keratinocyte growth factor expression in the dermis during wound healing. Proc Natl Acad Sci U S A 1992;89:6896.

Westermark B, Blomquist W: Stimulation of fibroblast migration by epidermal growth factor. Cell Biol Int Rep 1980;4:649.

White JG, Gerrard JM: Ultrastructural features of abnormal platelets: a review. Am J Pathol 1976;83:589.

Williams TJ, Peck MJ: Role of prostaglandin-mediated vasodilation in inflammation. Nature 1977;270:530.

Williamson LM, Sheppard K, Davies JM, et al: Neutrophils are involved in the increased vascular permeability produced by activated complement in man. Br J Haematol 1986;64:375.

Wright SD, Meyer BC: Fibronectin receptor of human macrophages recognizes sequence Arg-Gly-Asp-Ser. J Exp Med 1985;162:762.

Wright SD, Ramos RA, Tobias PS, et al: CD14, a receptor for complexes of lipopolysaccharide (LPS) and LPS-binding protein. Science 1995;249:1431.

CHAPTER 4

Abnormal Wound Healing

Louis C. Argenta, M.D. and Michael J. Morykwas, M.S., Ph.D.

Factors in Abnormal Wound Healing

The vast majority of patients, even those with debilitating disease, usually heal without difficulty following surgery. However, because of the great complexity of immunologic, hormonal, and cellular interactions that occur in the process of wound healing, the potential for impaired healing exists for all surgical specialties (Boxes 4–1 and 4–2). Problems in wound healing result from abnormalities intrinsic to the patient (the patient's age, pre-existing physical condition, and disease and its stage); abnormalities extrinsic to the patient (normal effects of medications and treatments, as well as their complications and side effects); and combinations of both. The arbitrary division of intrinsic versus extrinsic factors is often unclear.

Infection

Infection is the most common cause of impaired wound healing. Delayed healing may be the first sign of infection. Bacterial counts in wounds progress from colonization to critical colonization to clinical infection. Concentrations of 10^5 organisms per gram of tissue adversely affect almost every stage of wound healing. The inflammatory phase is usually prolonged when significant numbers of bacteria are present. Collagen deposition, wound contraction, and epithelization rates are adversely affected. Bacterial metalloproteinases and antitoxins result in abnormal and prolonged inflammatory response with progressive tissue destruction.

It is generally accepted that concentrations of bacteria greater than 10^5 bacteria per gram of tissue result in clinical infection for most bacteria. However, only 10^2 organisms of a β-hemolytic streptococcus are sufficient to cause clinical infection. Tissue biopsy cultures are 95% to 100% accurate for clinical infection as opposed to swabs, which are 60% to 80% accurate.

Control of infection begins with débridement of necrotic tissue to reduce the bioburden. All devitalized tissue should be removed, as well as any foreign body within the wound. When the viability of tissue is questionable, repeated serial débridement is required. Active surgical débridement is preferable to enzymatic and other passive débridements.

Appropriate antimicrobials should be administered systemically. Topical antimicrobials, including silver dressings, cedexomar iodine, and topical antibiotics, also help control bacterial infections.

Wounds heal more rapidly in a moist environment rather than a dry one. Moisture prevents desiccation and helps create a barrier to outside bacteria, thus promoting repair of dermis. A moist environment is facilitated with dressings that block the passage of air and provide an appropriate amount of occlusion. Gauze moistened with saline, Dakin's solution, or antibiotic solution should be changed two to three times a day to avoid "wet-to-dry" injury.

Box 4–1

Systemic Factors Producing Abnormal Wound Healing

Genetic connective tissue disease
- Marfan syndrome
- Ehlers-Danlos syndrome

Systemic inflammatory disease
- Polyarteritis nodosa
- Behçet's syndrome

Nutritional deficiency
- Protein
- Essential amino acids
- Vitamins
- Trace elements

Advanced age

Diabetes mellitus

Uremia

Chronic liver disease
- Alcoholism
- Jaundice

Medications

Neoplasms and chemotherapy

Atherosclerosis

Immune suppression

Medical prostheses and indwelling devices present special problems because of the development of microbial biofilms on these devices. Extracellular polymeric materials, primarily polysaccharides, encapsulate bacteria adjacent to the prosthesis and make systemic antibiotic

Box 4–2

Local Wound Factors Producing Abnormal Wound Healing

- Infection
- Devitalized tissue
- Foreign body
- Irradiation
- Smoking
- Tissue ischemia
  - Arterial insufficiency
  - Chronic venous insufficiency

treatment much less effective. Removal of prostheses and medical devices, particularly if they are loose, must be considered. Prosthesis coverage and closure of adjacent dead space with blood-bearing tissue, such as muscle flaps, also should be considered.

Tissue Ischemia

Appropriate tissue oxygenation is required for the aerobic metabolism necessary for wound healing. Neurophil function, especially in bacterial killing, cannot proceed without adequate levels of oxygen. Formation of stable collagen requires the hydroxylation of proline and lycine, processes that are critically dependent on appropriate oxygen levels.

Tissue oxygen levels below 35 mm Hg are associated with poor healing. Wound fibroblasts are unable to replicate normally at low oxygen tensions, and collagen production is impaired. Factors that contribute to ischemia include poor arterial inflow, poor venous outflow, smoking, radiation, diabetes, vasculitis, and fibrosis. Uncomplicated anemia rarely results in tissue ischemia. Poor arterial inflow secondary to arthrosclerosis or trauma can be corrected by vascular bypass. Correction of functional cardiac abnormalities that impair cardiac output also should be addressed.

Impaired wound healing frequently occurs with chronic venous insufficiency. Diffusion of oxygen from capillaries to the surrounding tissue is impaired by proteinaceous exudates that accumulate around capillaries. Over time, scar develops around capillaries, making diffusion of oxygen difficult, and small wounds progressively occur. Control of edema secondary to venous insufficiency with compression garments is helpful if the patient remains compliant.

Age

Delays in wound healing can be related to age, but age rarely results in nonhealing. The elderly heal at a slower rate and with less scarring for similar wounds than the young. A study during World War I demonstrated a relationship between scarring and increasing age in soldiers. The addition of age-related comorbidities such as diabetes, malnutrition, poor neurologic function, and peripheral vascular disease contribute to this intrinsic delay.

Wound healing is delayed in the elderly as a result of abnormalities in all three stages of wound healing: inflammation, proliferation, and remodeling. The inflammatory response is progressively attenuated with age, as is the proliferative potential of fibroblast endothelial cells. The elderly demonstrate decreased stimulation and production of macrophages, B lymphocytes, and monocytes in the proliferative stages. Cells migrate more slowly, and the proliferation and maturation of fibroblasts are decreased.

This results in a decrease in extracellular matrix formation. Animal studies have demonstrated reduced oxygen consumption and a decrease in glucose metabolism with progressive age. Collagen production and wound contracture are decreased with age. The elderly patient rarely forms excessive scarring, even in races prone to do so.

Diabetes Mellitus

Approximately 5% of the U.S. population at present will be diagnosed with diabetes at some time in their life. With the ongoing epidemic of obesity, the incidence of type 2 diabetes is expected to increase significantly. Diabetes mellitus interferes with almost every phase of wound healing. Local tissue ischemia secondary to vascular end-organ damage at the microcirculation level is significant in both ulcerated and nonulcerated tissues. The basement membrane thickens in diabetes, resulting in microaneurysms and irregular flow patterns, thus diminishing local blood flow. Hypoperfusion results in tissue ischemia and a decreased local oxygen level, predisposing tissue to impaired healing.

Diabetics have abnormal collagen metabolism with decreased levels of hydroxyproline. Granulation tissue formation is abnormal because of decreased fibroblast growth, decreased matrix formation, and abnormalities in local angiogenesis. Keratinocytes are poorly stimulated, resulting in impaired epithelialization. Abnormal and decreased wound strength encourages late breakdown of wounds considered to be healed. Diabetics also demonstrate increased wound collagenase levels that result in unstable collagen over time. Abnormal collagen cross-linking results in decreased wound strength and decreased wound contraction.

The ability to resist infection is significantly compromised in diabetics. Granulocytes have impaired chemotaxis and reduced ability to phagocytize bacteria. Control of diabetes with serum glucose levels below 250 mg/dL improves granulocyte function. Hemoglobin A_{1c} measurements are effective in monitoring long-term control of diabetes. A value of 0.07% represents good control of glucose levels over the previous 90-day period, whereas values over 0.12% indicate poor control. Control of diabetes and stabilization of hemoglobin A_{1c} levels should be accomplished prior to elective surgery.

Diabetic wounds frequently harbor gram-positive organisms, and studies demonstrate that diabetics have a reduced number of gram-negative organisms. Diabetics are particularly prone to fungal infections, which further compromise wound healing.

Smoking

Smoking and the use of nicotine patches have an adverse effect on healing secondary to vasoconstriction. One cigarette will decrease local oxygen by 30% for 1 hour. Nicotine increases the risk of thrombus formation in small vessels because of increased platelet adhesion. Over time, nicotine also inhibits proliferation of fibroblasts, macrophages, and red blood cells.

Systemically, smoking elevates carboxyhemoglobin levels, resulting in competition with oxygen for transport of the hemoglobin molecule. Hydrogen cyanide, a by-product of burning tobacco, selectively inhibits oxidative metabolism and oxygen transport at the cellular level. Cellular respiration is therefore decreased. Smoking increases wound complications in the skin and subcutaneous tissue, as well as in bone and bowel. Smokers demonstrate a fourfold incidence of fractures compared to nonsmokers from equal trauma. These fractures have an increased risk of nonunion and delayed union.

Patients who electively stop smoking 2 weeks before surgical intervention have healing rates no different than nonsmokers. Hyperbaric oxygen also may be of benefit in people who have recently smoked.

Tissue Irradiation

Tissues that have been irradiated for treatment of malignancy demonstrate fibrosis and progressive obliteration of vessels over time. Radiation has both acute and chronic effects on tissue that may impair healing or result in later breakdown of healed tissue. Radiation permanently impairs fibroblast and keratinocyte proliferation in the treated field. Acutely, radiation produces severe inflammation in the dermis. Collagen is degraded and breaking strength decreased. If fibroblasts cannot proliferate adequately, progressive injury and ulceration occur. Irradiated tissues are chronically hypoxic secondary to endarteritis obliterans in the microcirculation. Endothelial proliferation and angiogenesis are severely impaired in irradiated tissue, resulting in the inability to form meaningful granulation tissue.

Acutely irradiated tissue demonstrates inflammation, erythema, edema, and desquamation of skin. Late effects include fibrosis and thickening of skin and subcutaneous tissue, changes in pigmentation, and telangiectasias. Minor injuries can result in late tissue breakdown and ulceration. Healing complications may occur long after irradiation therapy. Perioperative radiation leads to delayed healing in the surgery area and increased potential for later breakdown. Areas that have been irradiated previously, and particularly those that demonstrate hypopigmentation, should be avoided for elective surgical incisions. Nonhealing wounds in irradiated sites are best treated by introduction of flaps carrying new blood supply into the area.

Pharmacologic Agents

Many drugs commonly used in clinical practice can result in impaired wound healing.

Glucocorticosteroids

Glucocorticosteroids inhibit normal wound healing by their immunosuppressive and anti-inflammatory mechanisms. Glucocorticoids stabilize lysosomal membranes, inhibiting the release of cytokines and enzymes. This results in a decrease in the inflammatory response needed for normal healing. New capillary formation is decreased, as is fibroblast proliferation. Formation of granulation tissue and laying down of extracellular matrix is decreased in these individuals. Epithelialization and contraction are affected in a dose-related manner.

After delayed wound healing occurs in these patients, there is a persistent decrease in tensile strength. The dermis remains attenuated and is prone to injury with even minor shearing forces.

Some of the anti-inflammatory effects of steroids can be reversed with the administration of vitamin A. Vitamin A reverses the inhibitory effects of glucocorticoids on the inflammatory phase of wound healing. The effect of steroids on wound closure is time and dose related. Patients who receive chronic steroids may have delayed healing time for up to 1 year after cessation of the drug. Low doses of steroids for short periods of time do not significantly affect wound healing.

Nonsteroidal anti-inflammatory agents probably do not have significant effects on wound healing. Extremely high doses in animals have been implicated in problems with healing, but these are usually beyond therapeutic doses.

Chemotherapeutic agents

Chemotherapy given for the treatment of neoplasms results in injury to rapidly dividing cells groups, and in particular bone marrow suppression. Impaired formation of lymphocytes and monocytes compromises the inflammatory phase of wound healing. Chemotherapeutic drugs also affect the inflammatory phase by interfering with the vascular response during this phase. Delays in cellular infiltration of the wound result in decrease in fibrin deposition and ultimately in poor healing. Cytotoxic agents most significantly impair the proliferative phase of healing because of interference with DNA and RNA synthesis. In addition, systemic neutropenia renders the patient more prone to further impairing healing.

Alkylating agents, antimetabolites, anti-tumor antibodies, and corticosteroids given preoperative probably interfere with healing more than do the same drugs given postoperatively. Drugs such as methotrexate, 5-fluorouracil, and 6-mercaptopurine are considered less detrimental, particularly if they are given 3 weeks after surgery.

Immunosuppressive agents given to prevent rejection after organ transplantation adversely affect wound healing. Agents such as azathioprine, cyclosporine, FK-506, and prednisone are commonly used, and all interfere in the inflammatory phase of healing. The use of these drugs in immunosuppressed patients must be weighed against potential healing problems. Because there are few viable alternatives at this time, wound complications in these patients are common.

Nutritionally Compromised Wound Healing

Because wound healing is an anabolic process, energy is required for normal healing. Patients who have been chronically and significantly malnourished may demonstrate impaired wound healing. In the United States, such levels of protein depletion are unusual, except for the chronically debilitated and patients with long-term systemic disease. Serum albumin levels greater than 3.5 g/dL usually reflect adequate protein stores and positive nitrogen balance. Albumin levels of less than 3 g/dL should arouse suspicion for potential wound complications. Recent studies, however, show that potentially normal wound healing can occur with albumin levels as low as 2.0 g/dL. Because serum albumin does not respond immediately to catabolic processes, levels of serum transferrin or serum prealbumin, which has a shorter half-life, have been suggested as better indicators of adequate nutrition.

Trauma, sepsis, nephrotic syndrome, liver disease, and burns can result in poor oral intake of protein. Protein deficiency results in a decreased fibroblast proliferation, decreased angiogenesis, and a decreased synthesis and remodeling of collagen. Protein supplementation given by feeding tube or intravenously can improve wound healing in chronically malnourished patients even if positive nitrogen balance cannot be maintained.

Patients who have been clinically ill, have been unable to eat orally for a week, or have suffered severe injuries should receive multivitamin supplementation by a feeding tube or intravenously. U.S. Department of Agriculture (USDA) levels are recommended rather than megadoses.

Vitamin Deficiencies

Vitamin A

Deficiency of vitamin A influences almost all stages of wound healing. Macrophage and monocyte stimulation, fibronectin deposition, and cellular adhesion are all adversely affected in vitamin A deficiencies. Vitamin A supplementation can improve wound healing in steroid-impaired animals. Supplementation levels and duration of vitamin A therapy should be monitored carefully because vitamin A is fat soluble and has a well-described toxic state. Oral doses of 25,000 IU/day or topical application of 200,000 IU ointment three times a day should be sufficient in most adults.

Vitamin C

Vitamin C deficiency resulting in scurvy has been classically described as causing problems in wound healing. Impaired healing of wounds may occur without any of the other systemic signs of scurvy. Vitamin C is a necessary cofactor in the hydroxylation of lysine and proline in collagen synthesis and cross-linking. In addition, ascorbic acid increases the patient's ability to resist infection by facilitating leukocyte migration into the wound. Deficiencies are treated with 100 to 1000 g of vitamin C orally per day.

Vitamin E

Vitamin E is an antioxidant with anti-inflammatory properties. Excessive intake of vitamin E decreases collagen production and decreases inflammation. Large doses can interfere with normal wound healing. Patients taking large doses of vitamin E as antiaging therapy can have significant problems after surgery.

Trace Element Deficiencies

Trace elements are important for proper wound healing and are often-overlooked factors in patients with wound healing problems. Mineral supplements commonly are administered to the chronically ill. Therapy should be administered at USDA-recommended levels because supraphysiologic levels of trace elements will not accelerate wound healing.

Zinc

Zinc is involved in more than 100 enzymatic reactions in the body and is an essential cofactor for normal cellular growth and replication. Zinc directly influences epithelialization and fibroblast proliferation and is involved in many immunologic responses, including phagocytosis and bacteriocidal activities. Zinc deficiencies can occur in chronic alcoholism, severe surgical trauma, large burns, psoriasis, and gastrointestinal fistulas. Oral supplementation with 500 mg of zinc is usually therapeutic.

Iron

Iron is required for deoxyribonucleotide production. It is also a cofactor required for conversion of hydroxyproline to proline. Clinically, however, patients with acute or chronic iron deficiency anemia rarely have significant wound healing problems. If perfusion is sufficient, tissue oxygenation usually can be maintained, even at very low hemoglobin levels.

Keloids and Hypertrophic Scars

Most vertebrates heal by scar formation. A scar is never a restoration of structural integrity, but is rather a patch. Periodically in healing, the production of an abnormal and excessive amount of connective tissue results in the formation of hypertrophic scars or keloids. Overabundant scar tissue was first described several thousand years ago in the Edwin Smith Surgical Papyrus. Despite the long history of such tissue having been recognized as an abnormal entity, the causative factors and optimal therapies have not been identified yet.

Hypertrophic scarring and keloids generally are accepted as being two separate conditions, although they are histologically difficult to distinguish. *Hypertrophic scars* are erythematous, pruritic lesions elevated above the surrounding skin level but staying within the confines of the original wound. Almost any surgical scar may have such an appearance immediately after surgery. Between 2 and 6 months after wound closure, normal scars regress in size and redness. Hypertrophic scars remain firm, red, pruritic, and elevated for an indefinite period of time, and may then regress. Hypertrophic scars normally develop in areas of movement and tension, such as the neck, shoulder, chest wall, and flexor surfaces. *Keloids* are benign dermal fibroproliferative tumors unique to humans. In addition to being raised above the level of surrounding skin, they invade the dermis surrounding subcutaneous tissue. They may develop months to years after the initial injury, and have been reported to develop without an identified injury. Keloids have true genetic patterns. They generally are less correctable by treatment because they tend to recur often.

Keloids more frequently occur on the shoulders, chest, upper arms, cheeks, and earlobes, although they also may occur in other anatomic locations. Keloid tissue is histologically characterized by a haphazard deposition of thick collagen bundles that have a hyalinized appearance, and that form nodules containing mast cells, eosinophils, plasma cells, and lymphocytes. The nodules are surrounded by numerous vessels, although the nodules proper contain few vessels. Transforming growth factor-β1 has been postulated to be implicated in the pathogenesis of both keloids and hypertrophic scars. There may be familial tendencies for keloid formation, with both autosomal dominant and autosomal recessive patterns of inheritance reported. There also may be an endocrine association, with keloid formation being associated with abnormal thyroid, parathyroid, and hypothalamus function.

Hypertrophic scars histologically also exhibit increased collagen bundles, although the collagen does not exhibit the hyalinized appearance that is present in keloidal tissue.

The collagen is deposited parallel to the surface as with uninjured skin. Nodules are not present in hypertrophic scars as they are in keloidal tissue.

The incidence of keloids and hypertrophic scars varies with ethnic background, age, anatomic location, and causative injury. More data are available for keloid formation, with the highest incidence occurring between 10 and 30 years of age and with a greater predilection among individuals with greater levels of melanin. The male-to-female ratio is approximately 1:1. Reports of varying degrees of formation between sexes may be skewed by the fact that more females have their ears pierced than males.

Many treatment modalities have been tried, particularly with keloids. Surgical excision is one of the oldest reported treatments for keloids, but, without adjunct therapy, recurrence is the rule. Currently, surgery is used with an adjunctive therapy such as pressure/compression, postoperative injection of steroids, pressure with silicone sheeting, or oral medications. Radiation with a 4-MeV electron-beam linear accelerator totaling 15 Gy administered over 3 days after surgery is currently a widely accepted treatment with acceptable results. Local pressure is useful both for prophylactic treatment in high-risk situations and for treatment of established lesions. Compression garments are standard prophylactic treatments following burn injury. Proposed mechanisms of pressure therapy include decreased local blood flow, localized hypoxia resulting in fibroblast and collagen degradation, increased collagen degradation associated with decreased levels of chondroitin 4-sulfate, and decreased scar hydration.

Intralesional injections of corticosteroids (e.g., Kenalog-10) can be administered as initial therapy in small lesions or as an adjunct after surgical excision. Injections are given monthly until a quiescent state is reached. These injections may be accompanied by pain, with additional side effects including skin atrophy, hypopigmentation or depigmentation, telangiectasia, ulceration, and necrosis.

CO_2 laser ablation has been proposed as effective, but recurrence rates are similar to those with surgical excision. Argon lasers produce more nonspecific thermal damage than CO_2 lasers, but also are associated with high levels of recurrence. Lasers with wavelengths specific for vessel ablation (yttrium-aluminum-garnet and pulsed dye lasers) have shown early promise.

A wide variety of other pharmacologic and adjuvant modalities have been tried, with mostly anecdotal reports of success. Those reported include topical retinoic acid and systemic colchicines, lathyrogenic agents, methotrexate, antihistamines, interferon (α, β, and γ), and bleomycin. Side effects of all of these pharmacologic agents are significant and severely compromise long-term therapy. Physical modalities such as ultrasound, massage, and static electric field induction have anecdotal reports of success.

Chronic Wounds

A chronic wound is a wound that does not respond to standard care and remains unhealed at 3 months. There are an estimated 6 million people with chronic wounds in the United States, with an estimated treatment cost of $5 to $7 billion per year. The pathophysiology of a chronic wound is usually multifactorial (Box 4–3). Immunosuppression, malnutrition, ischemia, edema, bacterial contamination, and necrotic tissue are frequent predisposing triggers. Correction or control of as many predisposing factors as are amenable to treatment is required before wound healing can occur. Sharp débridement of necrotic material decreases bacterial load and improves cytokine interactions. Serial débridements are usually necessary until viable tissue is achieved. Systemic antibiotic therapy is based on quantitative tissue biopsy rather than swabs. Most chronic wounds are able to withstand a bacterial load that would cause clinical infection in acute wounds. Topical antiseptics and antibiotics should be chosen carefully because many of these agents will impair wound healing. Arterial revascularization is frequently helpful to increase local tissue oxygenation. Compression dressings are important in decreasing edema to improve circulation in patients with edema. Control of diabetes and other systemic factors should be initiated as quickly as possible.

Wounds that do not demonstrate progressive healing once treatable comorbidities have been remedied may benefit from surgical procedures, including grafts and flaps.

Pressure Sores

The fundamental pathology of all pressure sores is prolonged pressure over a bony prominence. Local microcirculation is occluded by tissue pressure that exceeds capillary filling pressure of 25 mm Hg. Neurologic impairment, the duration of pressure, the amount of pressure, shear forces, and local moisture influence the ability of tissue to recover. Most pressure sores occur over the trochanter, sacrum, ischium, or heel. If unrelieved by frequent turning, pressures in the sacral area can rapidly approach 80 mm Hg in recumbent patients.

Pressure sores usually begin in the underlying subcutaneous or fat tissue, which is less resistant to ischemia than is skin. Small cutaneous ulcers develop over much larger areas of underlying necrotic tissue. Treatment of pressure sores is multifactorial. Relief of pressure with air flotation beds, débridement of necrotic tissue, adequate nutrition supplementation, and frequently surgical

---

Box 4-3
Pathophysiology of Chronic Wounds

Pressure Sores
Decubiti

Vascular Disorders
Chronic venous insufficiency
Arthrosclerosis
Chronic lymphedema

Infection
Bacterial
Fungal
Parasitic

Hematologic Disorders
Sickle cell disease
Hypercoagulopathies
Polycythemia

Neoplastic Conditions
Marjolin's ulcer
Kaposi's sarcoma
Metastatic and primary neoplasm

Inflammatory Disorders
Vasculitis
Necrobiosis lipoidica diabeticus
Pyoderma gangrenosum

Metabolic Disorders
Diabetes
Gout

Trauma
Radiation
Burn
Factitious ulcer

---

intervention are required to correct these problems. The long-term prognosis of pressure sores relates directly to the patients' ability to modify their physical activities.

Diabetic Foot Ulcers

Chronic ulcers are the leading cause of amputation in diabetic patients. Diabetic ulcers are usually secondary to pressure over bony prominences, complicated by neuropathy. The long-held small vessel disease theory has not been substantiated by blinded studies. Lack of sensation of the toes and feet in diabetics allows progressive painless ischemia. Abnormalities in diabetic red blood cells result in increased blood viscosities, decreased microvascular flow, capillary sludging, and thrombosis. Diabetic ulcers constantly demonstrate increased thickness of the basement membrane in adjacent muscle.

Correction of diabetic ulcers requires diabetic control, surgical débridement, control of local infection, and, if possible, the correction of infrapopliteal occlusive disease. Control of hyperglycemia has been shown to reverse nerve dysfunction. Long-term success involves chronic pressure relief and appropriate orthotic shoes, once healing is achieved. Daily examination of the feet by diabetics is helpful. Nonetheless, the incidence of ulcers resulting in amputations remains alarmingly high in diabetic patients.

Leg Ulcers

Ulcers of the lower extremities are probably the most common form of chronic ulcer. Multiple etiologic factors may exist. Chronic venous insufficiency, secondary to valvular incompetence, accounts for approximately 85% of leg ulcers. Venous hypertension also may arise from deep vein thrombosis or calf muscle dysfunction. Increased venous pressure results in microvascular thrombosis and increased permeability to microlymphatics. An insoluble perivascular fibrin cuff forms that impairs diffusion of oxygen and nutrients to tissue, leading to cell death and ulceration.

Treatment of leg ulcers secondary to venous insufficiency requires daily active treatment by the patient or caregiver. Elevation and compression dressings such as an Unna boot, three-layer dressings, or elastic support stockings are critical. Débridement of necrotic material, control of local infection, and occasionally wide surgical excision may be necessary. The long-term prognosis of ulcers secondary to venous insufficiency is totally related to chronic control of the edema with long-term use of pressure garments.

Arterial insufficiency and vasculitis are other sources of chronic leg ulcers. Ulcers secondary to chronic esoteric bacterial and parasitic infections are extremely rare in the Western world. Identification of treatment of the underlying diseases is critical. Once systemic disease is controlled, local wound therapy is usually successful.

Bibliography

Blackburn WR, Cosman B: Histologic basis of keloid and hypertrophic scar differentiation: clinicopathologic correlation. Arch Pathol 1966;82:65.

Breasted JH: The Edwin Smith Surgical Papyrus. Chicago: University of Chicago Press, 1930.

Carell A, Ebeling AH: Age and multiplication of fibroblast. J Exp Med 1921;34:599.

Chernoff RS, Milton KY, Lipschitz D: The effect of a very high-protein liquid formula on decubitus ulcer healing in long-term tube-fed institutional patients [abstract]. J Am Diet Assoc 1990;90:1.

Crandon JH, Lind CC, Dill DB: Experimental human scurvy. N Engl J Med 1940;223:353.

Daly JM, Reynolds J, Sigal RK, et al: Effect of dietary protein and amino acids on immune function. Crit Care Med 1990;18:S86.

Dow G, Brown A, Sibbald RG (Ed.): Infection in chronic wounds: controversial diagnosis and treatment. Ost Wounds Manage 1999;45:23.

Ehrlich HP, Hunt TK: Effects of cortisone and vitamin A on wound healing. Ann Surg 1968;167:324.

Ehrlich HP, Hunt TK: The effects of cortisone and anabolic steroids on the tensile strength of healing wounds. Ann Surg 1969;170:203.

Ferguson MK: The effect of antineoplastic agents on wound healing. Surg Gynecol Obstet 1982;154:421.

Fowler SA: Wound healing in the corneal epithelium in diabetic and normal rats. Exp Eye Res 1980;31:167.

Goodson WH III, Hunt TK: Wound healing in experimental diabetes mellitus: importance of early insulin therapy. Surg Forum 1978;29:95.

Goodson WH III, Hunt TK: Deficient collagen formation by obese mice in a standard wound model. Am J Surg 1979;138:692.

Heikkinen E, Aalto M, Vihersaari T, Kulonen E, et al: Age factor in the formulation and metabolism of experimental granulation tissue. J Gerontol 1971;26:294.

Hinman CD, Maibach H: Effect of air exposure and occlusion on experimental human skin wounds. Nature 1963;200:377.

Hunt TK: Distribution of oxygen and its significance in healing tissue. In Longacre JJ (ed): The Ultrastructure of Collagen. Springfield, IL: Charles C Thomas, 1976:177.

Hunt TK, Zederfeldt B, Goldstick TK: Oxygen and healing. Am J Surg 1969;118:521.

Jensen JA, Goodson WH, Hopf HW: Cigarette smoking decreases tissue oxygen. Arch Surg 1991;26:1131.

Kischer CW, Shetlar MR: Collagen and mucopolysaccharides in the hypertrophic scar. Connect Tissue Res 1974;2:205.

Kyro A, Usenius JP, Aarnio M, et al: Are smokers a risk group for delayed healing of tibial shaft fractures? Ann Chir Gynaecol 1993;82:254.

Marino H: Biologic excision: its value in treatment of radionecrotic lesions. Plast Reconstr Surg 1967;40:180.

Oqawa R, Mitsuhashi K, Hyakusoku H, Miyashita T: Postoperative electron-beam irradiation therapy for keloids and hypertrophic scars: retrospective study of 147 cases followed for more than 18 months. Plast Reconstr Surg 2003;111:547.

Peacock EE, Madden JW, Trier WC: Biological basis for the treatment of keloids and hypertrophic scars. South Med J 1970;63:755.

Reus WF 3d, Colen LB, Straker DJ: Tobacco smoking and complications in elective microsurgery. Plast Reconstr Surg 1992;89:490.

Robson MC: Wound infection. Surg Clin North Am 1997;77:637.

Robson MC, Lea CE, Dalton JB, Heggers JP: Quantitative bacteriology and delayed wound closure. Surg Forum 1968;19:501.

Robson MC, Stenberg BD, Heggers JP: Wound healing alterations caused by bacteria. Clin Plast Surg 1990;3:485.

Witte MB, Barbul A: General principles of wound healing. Surg Clin North Am 1997;77:509.

CHAPTER 5

Fetal Wound Healing

Ziv M. Peled, M.D., Tiffany K. Danton, M.D., and Michael T. Longaker, M.D., F.A.C.S.

- ▶ The Biology of Fetal Wound Healing
    - Inflammation
    - The Cytokine Milieu
    - The Extracellular Matrix
    - The External Fetal Environment
    - Additional Characteristics
- ▶ Novel Technologies and Potential Applications
- ▶ Bibliography

It has been over a decade since scientists first noted the capability for early gestational age human fetal skin to heal in a scarless fashion. This observation stood in stark contrast to postnatal cutaneous healing that resulted in scar formation. Since the first clinical observations of scarless repair, investigators have been working to uncover the biomolecular mechanisms responsible for this phenomenon. A testament to the significant interest in this field is the number of animal models that have been developed to study this phenomenon. In fact, scarless repair has now been documented in numerous animal models, including the rabbit, sheep, rat, mouse, monkey, and human. The field has expanded tremendously as a result of scientific interest and will continue to improve for this reason and because of improvements in investigative technology.

This chapter reviews what is currently known about the biology of fetal wound healing. The various animal models that have been used to study fetal repair and the characteristics of in utero wound healing are discussed. Novel advances in technology that might improve our ability to study this process are presented. A more global view of scarless healing and analysis of how our understanding of this process may have important applications in other fields of medicine completes this chapter.

The Biology of Fetal Wound Healing

The healing of cutaneous fetal wounds differs in many ways from that of their adult counterparts (Table 5–1).

As we analyze what is currently known about fetal repair, the differences from the adult process can be viewed along several important parameters. First, the fetus displays a distinctive inflammatory response to wounding. Second, the fetal wound is exposed to a unique cytokine milieu upon injury. Third, the composition of the extracellular matrix (ECM) and the rate at which the ECM is produced and degraded in a fetal wound differ from that of the adult. Finally, the external environment surrounding a cutaneous fetal wound differs markedly from that of the adult cutaneous wound. We discuss each of these differences individually and examine how each might contribute to the scarless phenotype.

Inflammation

Cutaneous repair in the postnatal mammal takes place in a series of distinct, yet overlapping stages. The first such stage often is referred to as the inflammatory phase. In the cutaneous fetal wound, the degree as well as the quality of the inflammatory response differs from that seen in the adult. A fetal lamb animal model has demonstrated a minimal acute inflammatory response to wounding. The inflammatory response to phlogistic agents becomes more robust with advancing gestational age. These findings may relate to a fetal immune system that is immature. Early gestational age fetal neutrophils do not respond as effectively as later gestational age fetal neutrophils to chemotactic stimuli. Furthermore, it has been shown that polymorphonuclear leukocytes from early third-trimester fetal lambs fail to phagocytose *Staphylococcus aureus* secondary to both a primary defect in phagocytic capability and the inability of fetal plasma to effectively opsonize the bacteria. Fetal rabbit wounds exhibit a paucity of neutrophils and a relative abundance of macrophages in the first 4 days after wounding. Given that inflammatory cells elaborate a number of different cytokines and that the cellular acute inflammatory response to wounding differs in the fetus as compared to the adult, it is not unreasonable to postulate that the cytokine milieu elaborated after wounding in the fetus would also differ from the adult.

Table 5–1
Healing characteristics of adult and fetal wounds

	Adult	Fetal
Acute inflammation	Greater	Less
Angiogenesis	Greater	Less
TGF-β, bFGF	Greater	Less
Matrix formation	Slow	Rapid
Epithelization	Slow	Rapid
Keratin formation	Mature	Immature
Cell proliferation	Slow	Rapid
Rate of wound closure	Slow	Rapid
Scab	Present	Absent
Scar	Present	Absent

bFGF, basic fibroblast growth factor, TGF-β, transforming growth factor-β.

The Cytokine Milieu

During cutaneous adult wound healing, numerous cytokines and growth factors are released. These molecules play critical roles in determining the phenotypic outcome, which is invariably a scar. In studying the biomolecular processes underlying scarless fetal repair, scientists have focused their attention on those cytokines thought to be important in the adult wound repair process to examine how their biology differs in the fetus. The cytokine that has received perhaps the most attention is transforming growth factor-β (TGF-β).

TGF-β is one member of a superfamily of polypeptide growth factors that modulate a wide array of cellular processes ranging from wound repair to embryonal development to cell motility and cell death. With respect to human disease, TGF-β has been associated with a variety of fibroproliferative disorders. These clinical entities include scleroderma, glomerulonephritis, cirrhosis, pulmonary fibrosis, hypertrophic scar formation, and keloid pathogenesis. In addition, TGF-β plays a prominent role in normal adult wound healing, where it is known primarily for its profibrotic properties. For example, TGF-β is known to be chemotactic for fibroblasts and to promote fibroblast synthesis of collagen. In vivo, a dramatic increase occurs in fibrosis when TGF-β is exogenously added to fetal rabbit wounds. In contrast, in situ hybridization studies have demonstrated a paucity of TGF-β1 mRNA expression in fetal wounds as compared to their adult counterparts. Neutralizing antibodies to TGF-β1 and TGF-β2 administered to adult rodent wounds can reduce scarring. However, not all isoforms of TGF-β

may be profibrotic. Exogenous TGF-β3 added to adult murine cutaneous wounds resulted in a diminished mononuclear cell infiltrate as well as reduced scarring. It seems likely that TGF-β3 may have some antifibrotic properties, whereas TGF-β1 and TGF-β2 may play predominantly profibrotic roles.

In studying the potential role of TGF-β in fetal wound healing, we have made use of a Sprague-Dawley animal model. Work with this animal model in our laboratory has demonstrated that a transition from a scarless to a scar-forming phenotype occurs in cutaneous repair between days 16 and 18 of gestation. Using this model, we subsequently investigated the ontogeny of TGF-β1 and TGF-β3 as well as TGF-β receptor I (TβRI) and TGF-β receptor II (TβRII) expression as a function of gestational age at time points representing both the scarless and scar-forming periods of rat gestation. Our results have demonstrated that unwounded fetal skin has a much higher ratio of TGF-β3 to TGF-β1 at 14 and 16 days of gestation, when wound healing is scarless in the fetal rat model. The ratio of TGF-β3 to TGF-β1 was markedly lower by days 18 and 21 (periods during rat gestation when wounds heal with scarring), mostly as a result of a decrease in TGF-β3 expression. Similar results were noted in fetal dermal fibroblasts harvested at the same gestational ages, suggesting that the findings in unwounded fetal skin may be largely secondary to changes in fibroblast gene expression. Unwounded fetal skin exhibited relatively greater gene expression levels of both TβRI and TβRII at 14 and 16 days of gestation, suggesting increased signaling of what may be a predominantly antifibrotic signal (i.e., TGF-β3). Reverse transcriptase–polymerase chain reaction has shown that TGF-β1 levels did not change between days 16 and 18 of gestation, whereas TGF-β3 and TβRII expression was twofold higher at day 16. The levels of fibromodulin, a proteoglycan known to have a strong affinity for TGF-β1, were greater than threefold higher at day 16 as compared to day 18 of gestation. These data suggest the possibility of even lower TGF-β1 activity during the scarless period of rat gestation secondary to reduced TGF-β1 bioavailability.

The TGF-β family of cytokines are not the only molecules known to play a role in adult wound healing and hence are unlikely to be the sole determinants of the scarless phenotype in fetal wound repair. Epidermal growth factor (EGF) and platelet-derived growth factor (PDGF), among other cytokines, also are thought to play roles in adult wound repair, yet their potential roles in scarless fetal repair remain to be characterized. We have demonstrated that gene expression for both EGF and PDGF-B is markedly elevated in fetal rat skin early in gestation when healing is scarless (days 14 and 16), as compared to later in gestation (days 18 and 21) when healing results in scar formation. Collectively, however, all of these results only begin to scratch the tip of the proverbial iceberg when it comes to understanding the cytokine milieu of scarless repair because relatively few studies characterizing these cytokines have been done in fetal wounds themselves. One such study did demonstrate a paucity of TGF-β protein as detected by immunohistochemistry in fetal mouse lip wounds as compared to similar neonatal or adult wounds, yet clearly more investigation into this area is needed before any definitive conclusions can be reached. Therefore, at this time, the definitive roles of "wound growth factors" in scarless fetal healing remain to be elucidated.

The Extracellular Matrix

There are a number of differences between the ECM of fetal and adult wounds. In both the fetal sheep and rabbit models, elevated and persistent deposition of hyaluronic acid (HA) has been observed. These findings may be important in that HA is a component of the ECM that is thought to perhaps promote an orderly deposition of collagen secondary to its high coefficient of hydration that may, in turn, facilitate a homogeneous migration of fibroblasts into the provisional matrix. HA has been shown to down-regulate both platelet aggregation and platelet-induced cytokine release. The presence of HA modulates not only cell movement but the inflammatory cascade as well, and may have an important role in the phenotypic response to wounding.

Fibronectin is another important ECM component with a myriad of roles in wound repair, including acting as a chemoattractant for mesenchymal cells, promoting opsonization of microorganisms, and acting as a scaffold for cellular migration. Human fetal skin contains higher levels of this ECM component as compared to neonatal or adult human skin. In a fetal sheep model, it was demonstrated that fibronectin is present earlier in fetal as compared to adult wounds. By immunohistochemistry, tenascin, another ECM component whose actions oppose those of fibronectin with respect to cell adhesion, also was found to be deposited earlier in fetal wounds as compared to neonatal or adult wounds. Perhaps the rapid deposition of tenascin and fibronectin along with the presence of high amounts of EGF early in gestation help mediate the efficient and rapid epithelialization seen in fetal wounds.

Certainly one of the most abundant ECM molecules, and one of the most relevant to wound repair, is collagen. It is not surprising that the endogenous collagen profile as well as the rate of collagen deposition after wounding differ between the fetus and adult. For example, fetal skin has a greater percentage of type III collagen (~20%) than adult skin (~10%). Collagen is also laid down more rapidly in the fetal wound as compared to the adult wound. Fetal fibroblasts likely are involved in these phenomena, and investigators have demonstrated that prolyl hydroxylase, an enzyme that catalyzes an important step in collagen synthesis, is present in higher amounts in fetal fibroblasts as compared to adult fibroblasts until 20 weeks of gestation, when activity falls to adult-like levels. Recent data demonstrate that fetal fibroblasts produce higher levels of the novel collagen receptor discoidin domain receptor (DDR)-1 at time points during gestation when cutaneous healing is scarless. Although the precise role of the DDR family of receptors in wound healing remains a mystery, it is known that the binding of collagen type I to a specific isoform, DDR2, can induce the expression of interstitial collagenase, an enzyme known to be important for keratinocyte migration after wounding. Taken together, all of these factors may play a critical role in modulating the rate and type of collagen deposition and, therefore, in mediating the scarless phenotype of early gestation fetal skin wounds.

The External Fetal Environment

Initially, it was believed that the unique phenotypic response of the early gestation fetus to cutaneous wounding was a result of the fetal environment. There can be no doubt that the external environment surrounding the fetus is very different from the external environment that surrounds the postnatal animal. First, the fetal environment is sterile. Second, the fetus is bathed in amniotic fluid (AF) that is rich in a number of growth factors known to play a role in wound repair. AF also contains molecules that serve important functions in the ECM, such as fibronectin and tenascin. Enzymes believed to play important roles in wound remodeling, such as matrix metalloproteinases and their tissue inhibitors, also have been isolated from AF.

Fetal tissues are also hypoxic in comparison to adult tissues. Although this finding seems paradoxical to efficient, let alone successful, wound healing, it must be kept in mind that hypoxia has been shown to induce the production of potent cytokines such as vascular endothelial growth factor. One must also bear in mind that this hypoxic environment occurs in the context of a distinctive inflammatory response to wounding, a unique cytokine milieu, and perhaps less differentiated fibroblasts.

Although the unique external environment of the fetus may play a role in scarless wound repair, it is not absolutely essential. One research group has established that adult sheep skin grafted onto an early gestation fetal lamb and subsequently wounded still heals with a scar, despite being in the uterine environment and being perfused with fetal blood. Conversely, another group demonstrated that fetal tissues have the capacity to heal in a scarless fashion outside of the fetal environment. The exact role of the fetal environment in determining the phenotypic response of the fetus to wounding remains to be elucidated.

Additional Characteristics

Several other important points regarding fetal wound healing must be stated for completeness. These characteristics relate to the specificity of the scarless phenotype in terms of gestational age of the animal, species of the animal, size of the wound, and tissue that is wounded.

As alluded to above, several animal models used in the study of fetal repair exhibit a transition from a scarless phenotype early in gestation to a scar-forming phenotype later in gestation. In the Sprague-Dawley rat, this transition occurs between days 16 and 18 of gestation. In fetal sheep, the transition occurs between days 100 and 120 of gestation, and in the rhesus monkey, the transition occurs between days 85 and 100 of gestation. Interestingly, in the rhesus monkey, a "transition wound" in which the collagen architecture was similar to that of unwounded dermis, but which lacked hair follicles and sebaceous glands, was noted during the transition period to adult-type healing. In short, an animal is more likely to demonstrate an "adult-like" process of wound repair with a scar the later in gestation that animal is wounded.

Scarless fetal repair also depends on the tissue that is wounded. The initial descriptions of scarless cutaneous repair also noted significant intraperitoneal adhesions when further surgery was performed. The fetal diaphragm, intestine, and stomach all scar upon wounding. Scarring in these tissues occurs at time points during gestation when a cutaneous wound would heal in a scarless manner. Hence, not all fetal tissues possess the capability for scarless healing.

The fetal wound repair process is also species specific. For example, two groups of investigators independently demonstrated that wounds made in fetal rabbits do not contract, whereas others have noted wound contraction after wounding using a fetal sheep model. Finally, the ability to heal without a scar also depends on the size of the wound defect. In an elegant study, excisional wounds greater than 4 mm in diameter were shown to heal with a histologic scar 50% of the time, even at early time points of gestation.

In summary, the scarless fetal wound healing phenotype is very likely a result of the interplay of a number of different factors. These include not only characteristics intrinsic to the fetal cells, but also characteristics of the wound itself and perhaps even components of the external fetal environment.

Novel Technologies and Potential Applications

Although we have learned much about the molecular biology of scarless wound healing, there is much more that we do not understand. Until recently, one of the primary rate-limiting steps has been the use of individual candidate gene approaches. These approaches were necessary secondary to the lack of an automated technology to study gene expression on a larger scale. At this point in time, however, this limitation no longer applies secondary to the advent of microarray technology.

Using relatively standardized protocols, complementary DNA arrays now can be used to analyze the expression of thousands of genes in a short period of time. The sensitivity of this technology also has progressed to the point where we can reliably detect gene transcripts present at only a few copies per cell. In addition, because this technology is computerized and automated, it allows incredible flexibility in, access to (e.g., over the Internet), and organization of the large amounts of data collected.

In an effort to obtain functional information at the nucleic acid level, several approaches can be utilized. The most common and straightforward is large-scale comparative expression analyses aimed at determining patterns of gene expression. This approach already has been used in attempting to understand how resistance and sensitivity to certain chemotherapeutic agents used in the treatment of human cancers relate to variations in gene transcript levels in different tumor cell lines. Moreover, this approach can lead to the discovery of novel proteins in other species as well as in humans. Incredibly, this technology has yet to be applied to the study of fetal wound healing. With its vast potential, the day may not be far off when microarrays will enable us to characterize the gene expression motifs of cell types and tissues that heal in a scarless manner. This information will be a quantum leap forward in helping us to decipher the biomolecular blueprint for scarless repair.

In addition to advances in gene expression technology, advances in cellular biology may impact our understanding of the scarless healing paradigm. A significant portion of the wound healing literature has focused on the fibroblast as the cell primarily responsible for modulating repair. Recent studies have demonstrated that keratinocytes derived from keloid specimens can affect the proliferation as well the collagen secretory characteristics of normal human dermal fibroblasts. These studies highlight the importance of epithelial-mesenchymal interactions in keloid pathogenesis, but also beg the question of whether similar interactions are occurring in fetal skin.

The ultimate goal of research into fetal wound healing is to be able to manipulate the postnatal wound healing process to recapitulate a scarless phenotype. However, scarring is not only skin deep. The knowledge gained through the study of early gestation, scarless, cutaneous fetal healing may have widespread applications in a number of different medical fields. A good analogy that illustrates the far-reaching impact that fetal wound healing research could have on other aspects of medicine is that of space research technology. Although very few people have ever been in space, the National Aeronautics and Space Administration has touched the lives of many people both in the United States and around the world. For example, the same technology used in placing people into outer space now launches the satellites that help us predict the weather and make the convenience of cellular phones possible. In an analogous manner, our understanding of the biomolecular processes underlying scarless repair may enable us to ameliorate other disorders.

A prime example, then, of the translational potential for research in fetal wound healing is the problem of keloids and hypertrophic scarring. These clinical entities represent a worldwide biomedical burden with several billion people at risk. These "overhealing" syndromes can be viewed as one end of a spectrum of healing phenotypes, with skin "regeneration" (i.e., scarless fetal healing) at the other end. If this is indeed the case, the knowledge gained in studying the fetal wound healing paradigm potentially could be used in studying these lesions. As a result, a biologically based therapy could be designed to treat these entities, which lack an effective treatment modality today. Another relevant example of how the knowledge of fetal repair has potential medical applications relates to the fact that not all fetal tissues heal in a scarless fashion. For example, many organs in the fetal gastrointestinal tract heal with scar formation during early gestation, even when cutaneous wounds would heal in a scarless manner. Perhaps our understanding of the mechanisms of scarless cutaneous repair could be applied to attenuating scarring in other organs. Such knowledge potentially could help minimize intraperitoneal adhesions postoperatively, reduce scarring after infarction, and even perhaps treat systemic fibrotic disorders such as scleroderma. With continued efforts in both research and technology, one day it may even be possible to eliminate scarring completely.

Bibliography

Adzick NS, Harrison MR, Glick PL, et al: Comparison of fetal, newborn, and adult wound healing by histologic, enzyme-histochemical, and hydroxyproline determinations. J Pediatr Surg 1985;20:315.

Adzick NS, Longaker MT: Animal models for the study of fetal tissue repair. J Surg Res 1991;51:216.

Athayde N, Romero R, Gomez R, et al: Matrix metalloproteinases-9 in preterm and term human parturition. J Matern Fetal Med 1999;8:213.

Bennett NT, Schultz GS: Growth factors and wound healing: biochemical properties of growth factors and their receptors. Am J Surg 1993;165:728.

Bennett NT, Schultz GS: Growth factors and wound healing: Part II. Role in normal and chronic wound healing. Am J Surg 1993;166:74.

Border WA, Noble NA: Transforming growth factor beta in tissue fibrosis. N Engl J Med 1994;331:1286.

Border WA, Noble NA: TGF-beta in kidney fibrosis: a target for gene therapy. Kidney Int 1997;51:1388.

Border WA, Ruoslahti E: Transforming growth factor-beta in disease: the dark side of tissue repair. J Clin Invest 1992;90:1.

Bracaglia R, Montemari G, Rotoli M, Petrosino R: Variation in acute phlogistic reactions in the skin of rabbit fetuses. Ann Plast Surg 1982;9:175.

Broekelmann TJ, Limper AH, Colby TV, McDonald JA: Transforming growth factor beta 1 is present at sites of extracellular matrix gene expression in human pulmonary fibrosis. Proc Natl Acad Sci U S A 1991;88:6642.

Burrington JD: Wound healing in the fetal lamb. J Pediatr Surg 1971;6:523.

Cass DL, Bullard KM, Sylvester KG, et al: Wound size and gestational age modulate scar formation in fetal wound repair. J Pediatr Surg 1997;32:411.

Castilla A, Prieto J, Fausto N: Transforming growth factors beta 1 and alpha in chronic liver disease: effects of interferon alfa therapy [see comments]. N Engl J Med 1991;324:933.

Chin G, Lee S, Hsu M, et al: Discoidin domain receptors and their ligand collagen are temporally regulated in fetal rat fibroblasts in vitro. Plast Reconstr Surg 2001;107:769.

Clark RA: Potential roles of fibronectin in cutaneous wound repair. Arch Dermatol 1988;124:201.

DePalma RL, Krummel TM, Durham LAD, et al: Characterization and quantitation of wound matrix in the fetal rabbit. Matrix 1989;9:224.

Diehn M, Eisen MB, Botstein D, Brown PO: Large-scale identification of secreted and membrane-associated gene products using DNA microarrays. Nat Genet 2000;25:58.

Duggan DJ, Bittner M, Chen Y, et al: Expression profiling using cDNA microarrays. Nat Genet 1999;21:10.

Fisher DA, Lakshmanan J: Metabolism and effects of epidermal growth factor and related growth factors in mammals. Endocr Rev 1990;11:418.

Garner WL, Karmiol S, Rodriguez JL, et al: Phenotypic differences in cytokine responsiveness of hypertrophic scar versus normal dermal fibroblasts. J Invest Dermatol 1993;101:875.

Glat P, Longaker M: Wound healing. In Aston SJBR, Thorne CHM (eds): Grabb and Smith's Plastic Surgery. Philadelphia: Lippincott–Raven, 1997:3.

Gruschwitz M, Muller PU, Sepp N, et al: Transcription and expression of transforming growth factor type beta in the skin of progressive systemic sclerosis: a mediator of fibrosis? J Invest Dermatol 1990;94:197.

Harrison MR, Langer JC, Adzick NS, et al: Correction of congenital diaphragmatic hernia in utero, V. Initial clinical experience. J Pediatr Surg 1990;25:47; discussion 56.

Harwood FL, Goomer RS, Gelberman RH, et al: Regulation of alphaV-B3 and alpha5-B1 integrin receptors by basic fibroblast growth factor and platelet-derived growth factor-BB in intrasynovial flexor tendon cells. Wound Repair Regen 1999;7:381.

Hildebrand A, Romaris M, Rasmussen LM, et al: Interaction of the small interstitial proteoglycans biglycan, decorin and fibromodulin with transforming growth factor beta. Biochem J 1994;302:527.

Hsu M, Peled ZM, Chin GS, et al: Ontogeny of expression of transforming growth factor-beta 1 (TGF-beta 1), TGF-beta 3, and TGF-beta receptors I and II in fetal rat fibroblasts and skin. Plast Reconstr Surg 2001;107:1787; discussion 1795.

Ihara S, Motobayashi Y, Nagao E, Kistler A: Ontogenetic transition of wound healing pattern in rat skin occurring at the fetal stage. Development 1990;110:671.

Iocono JA, Ehrlich HP, Keefer KA, Krummel TM: Hyaluronan induces scarless repair in mouse limb organ culture. J Pediatr Surg 1998;33:564.

Iocono JA, Krummel TM, Keefer KA, et al: Repeated additions of hyaluronan alter granulation tissue deposition in sponge implants in mice. Wound Repair Regen 1998;6:442.

Jennings RW, Adzick NS, Longaker MT, et al: Ontogeny of fetal sheep polymorphonuclear leukocyte phagocytosis. J Pediatr Surg 1991;26:853.

Krummel TM, Michna BA, Thomas BL, et al: Transforming growth factor beta (TGF-beta) induces fibrosis in a fetal wound model. J Pediatr Surg 1988;23:647.

Krummel TM, Nelson JM, Diegelmann RF, et al: Fetal response to injury in the rabbit. J Pediatr Surg 1987;22:640.

Lander ES: Array of hope. Nat Genet 1999;21:3.

Lawrence WT: Wound healing biology and its application to wound management. In O'Leary JP (ed): The Physiologic Basis of Surgery. Baltimore: Williams & Wilkins, 1996:118.

Lee TY, Chin GS, Kim WJ, et al: Expression of transforming growth factor beta 1, 2, and 3 proteins in keloids. Ann Plast Surg 1999;43:179.

Lim IJ, Phan TT, Bay BH, et al: Induction of keloid-like collagen secretory characteristics in normal fibroblasts co-cultured with keloid-derived keratinocytes. Am J Physiol 2002 in press.

Lim IJ, Phan TT, Song C, et al: Investigation of the influence of keloid-derived keratinocytes on fibroblast growth and proliferation in vitro. Plast Reconstr Surg 2001;107:797.

Lin RY, Sullivan KM, Argenta PA, et al: Exogenous transforming growth factor-beta amplifies its own expression and induces scar formation in a model of human fetal skin repair. Ann Surg 1995;222:146.

Longaker MT, Adzick NS: The biology of fetal wound healing: a review. Plast Reconstr Surg 1991;87:788.

Longaker MT, Chiu ES, Adzick NS, et al: Studies in fetal wound healing. V. A prolonged presence of hyaluronic acid characterizes fetal wound fluid. Ann Surg 1991;213:292.

Longaker MT, Harrison MR, Crombleholme TM, et al: Studies in fetal wound healing: I. A factor in fetal serum that stimulates deposition of hyaluronic acid. J Pediatr Surg 1989;24:789.

Longaker MT, Whitby DJ, Adzick NS, et al: Studies in fetal wound healing, VI. Second and early third trimester fetal wounds demonstrate rapid collagen deposition without scar formation. J Pediatr Surg 1990;25:63, discussion 68.

Longaker MT, Whitby DJ, Ferguson MW, et al: Adult skin wounds in the fetal environment heal with scar formation. Ann Surg 1994;219:65.

Longaker MT, Whitby DJ, Ferguson MW, et al: Studies in fetal wound healing: III. Early deposition of fibronectin distinguishes fetal from adult wound healing. J Pediatr Surg 1989;24:799.

Longaker MT, Whitby DJ, Jennings RW, et al: Fetal diaphragmatic wounds heal with scar formation. J Surg Res 1991;50:375.

Lorenz HP, Adzick NS: Scarless skin wound repair in the fetus. West J Med 1993;159:350.

Lorenz HP, Longaker MT, Perkocha LA, et al: Scarless wound repair: a human fetal skin model. Development 1992;114:253.

Lorenz HP, Whitby DJ, Longaker MT, Adzick NS: Fetal wound healing: the ontogeny of scar formation in the non-human primate. Ann Surg 1993;217:391.

Mackool RJ, Gittes GK, Longaker MT: Scarless healing: the fetal wound. Clin Plast Surg 1998;25:357.

Martin P: Wound healing—aiming for perfect skin regeneration. Science 1997;276:75.

Massague J: TGF-beta signal transduction. Annu Rev Biochem 1998;67:753.

Mast B, Cohen I: Normal wound healing. In Achauer BM, Eriksson E, Guyuron B, et al (eds): Plastic Surgery: Indications, Operations, and Outcomes, Vol I. St. Louis: Mosby, 2000:37.

Mast BA, Albanese CT, Kapadia S: Tissue repair in the fetal intestinal tract occurs with adhesions, fibrosis, and neovascularization. Ann Plast Surg 1998;41:140; discussion 144.

Meuli M, Lorenz HP, Hedrick MH, et al: Scar formation in the fetal alimentary tract. J Pediatr Surg 1995;30:392.

Mulvihill SJ, Stone MM, Fonkalsrud EW, Debas HT: Trophic effect of amniotic fluid on fetal gastrointestinal development. J Surg Res 1986;40:291.

Olutoye OO, Barone EJ, Yager DR, et al: Hyaluronic acid inhibits fetal platelet function: implications in scarless healing. J Pediatr Surg 1997;32:1037.

Peled ZM, Rhee SJ, Hsu M, et al: The ontogeny of scarless healing II: EGF and PDGF-B gene expression in fetal rat skin and fibroblasts as a function of gestational age. Ann Plast Surg 2001;47:417.

Pierce GF, Brown D, Mustoe TA: Quantitative analysis of inflammatory cell influx, procollagen type I synthesis, and collagen cross-linking in incisional wounds: influence of PDGF-BB and TGF-beta 1 therapy. J Lab Clin Med 1991;117:373.

Pierce GF, Mustoe TA, Senior RM, et al: In vivo incisional wound healing augmented by platelet-derived growth factor and recombinant c-sis gene homodimeric proteins. J Exp Med 1988;167:974.

Raghow B, Irish P, Kang AH: Coordinate regulation of transforming growth factor beta gene expression and cell proliferation in hamster lungs undergoing bleomycin-induced pulmonary fibrosis. J Clin Invest 1989;84:1836.

Raghunathan R, Faust J, Misra S, Miller ME: Ontogeny of neutrophil chemotaxis in fetal lambs. Pediatr Res 1986;20:265.

Roberts AB, Sporn MB, Assoian RK, et al: Transforming growth factor type beta: rapid induction of fibrosis and angiogenesis in vivo and stimulation of collagen formation in vitro. Proc Natl Acad Sci U S A 1986;83:4167.

Sakura M, Nakabayashi M, Takeda Y, Sato K: Elevated fetal fibronectin in midtrimester amniotic fluid is involved with the onset of preeclampsia. J Obstet Gynaecol Res 1998;24:73.

Schena M, Heller RA, Theriault TP, et al: Microarrays: biotechnology's discovery platform for functional genomics [see comments]. Trends Biotechnol 1998;16:301.

Schena M, Shalon D, Davis RW, Brown PO: Quantitative monitoring of gene expression patterns with a complementary DNA microarray [see comments]. Science 1995;270:467.

Scherf U, Ross DT, Waltham M, et al: A gene expression database for the molecular pharmacology of cancer [see comments]. Nat Genet 2000;24:236.

Shah M, Foreman DM, Ferguson MW: Neutralising antibody to TGF-beta 1,2 reduces cutaneous scarring in adult rodents. J Cell Sci 1994;107:1137.

Shah M, Foreman DM, Ferguson MW: Neutralisation of TGF-beta 1 and TGF-beta 2 or exogenous addition of TGF-beta 3 to cutaneous rat wounds reduces scarring. J Cell Sci 1995;108:985.

Sherlock G, Hernandez-Boussard T, Kasarskis A, et al: The Stanford Microarray Database. Nucleic Acids Res 2001;29:152.

Singer AJ, Clark RA: Cutaneous wound healing. N Engl J Med 1999;341:738.

Smith LT, Holbrook KA, Madri JA: Collagen types I, III, and V in human embryonic and fetal skin. Am J Anat 1986;175:507.

Somasundaram K, Prathap K: Intra-uterine healing of skin wounds in rabbit foetuses. J Pathol 1970;100:81.

Soo C, Hu FY, Zhang X, et al: Differential expression of fibromodulin, a transforming growth factor-beta modulator, in fetal skin development and scarless repair. Am J Pathol 2000;157:423.

Southern E, Mir K, Shchepinov M: Molecular interactions on microarrays. Nat Genet 1999;21:5.

Steinbrech DS, Longaker MT, Mehrara BJ, et al: Fibroblast response to hypoxia: the relationship between angiogenesis and matrix regulation. J Surg Res 1999;84:127.

Sudbeck BD, Parks WC, Welgus HG, Pentland AP: Collagen-stimulated induction of keratinocyte collagenase is mediated via tyrosine kinase and protein kinase C activities. J Biol Chem 1994;269:30022.

Tonnesen MG, Jenkins D Jr, Siegal SL, et al: Expression of fibronectin, laminin, and factor VIII-related antigen during development of the human cutaneous microvasculature. J Invest Dermatol 1985;85:564.

Vogel W, Gish GD, Alves F, Pawson T: The discoidin domain receptor tyrosine kinases are activated by collagen. Mol Cell 1997;1:13.

Whitby DJ, Ferguson MW: The extracellular matrix of lip wounds in fetal, neonatal and adult mice. Development 1991;112:651.

Whitby DJ, Ferguson MW: Immunohistochemical localization of growth factors in fetal wound healing. Dev Biol 1991;147:207.

Whitby DJ, Longaker MT, Harrison MR, et al: Rapid epithelialisation of fetal wounds is associated with the early deposition of tenascin. J Cell Sci 1991;99:583.

Xu J, Clark RA: Extracellular matrix alters PDGF regulation of fibroblast integrins. J Cell Biol 1996;132:239.

Yamamoto T, Noble NA, Miller DE, Border WA: Sustained expression of TGF-beta 1 underlies development of progressive kidney fibrosis. Kidney Int 1994;45:916.

Zhang K, Garner W, Cohen L, et al: Increased types I and III collagen and transforming growth factor-beta 1 mRNA and protein in hypertrophic burn scar. J Invest Dermatol 1995;104:750.

CHAPTER 6

The Fundamentals of Molecular Genetics

Timothy D. Howard, Ph.D. and Vandana Shashi, M.B.B.S., M.D.

Basics of Molecular Genetics

In order to understand the mutations and variations associated with genetic diseases, it is essential to understand the normal structure, function, and regulation of mammalian genes. Toward this end, the first section of this chapter provides an overview of the basic structure of DNA and the process of protein synthesis from human genes.

The entire basis of molecular genetics, and inheritance in general, is determined by the order of four nitrogen-containing bases that comprise a DNA strand. These four bases, adenine, cytosine, guanine, and thymine (commonly denoted as simply A, C, G, and T, respectively), make up the genes in all living organisms, and determine the structure and function of protein molecules that carry out the role of any given cell type. With the exception of mature erythrocytes, all cells in the human body contain DNA in the form of chromosomes. Each chromosome consists of a single, linear double strand of DNA tightly coiled upon a protein scaffolding. The complex folding pattern allows for approximately five linear feet of DNA to be efficiently and compactly packaged into each cell.

DNA exists in human cells as two linear strands of DNA, coupled together through hydrogen bonding. These two strands intertwine to form a characteristic helical structure, referred to as a double helix. Each strand consists of a string of nucleotides made up of the four nitrogenous bases and a deoxyribose sugar molecule linked through a covalent phosphodiester bond (Fig. 6–1).

Several properties of DNA enable it to replicate accurately and encode for the thousands of proteins in the human body. First, the two individual strands of DNA are coupled together by a base-pairing pattern that is conserved between almost all living organisms. The unique chemical structure of each of the four bases encourages two hydrogen bonds to form between adenine and thymine (A : T) and three between cytosine and guanine (C : G) (see Fig. 6–1). The hydrogen bonding is weak for a given pair of bases, but, along the entire strand of DNA, the cumulative effect of the binding is quite strong. This binding pattern is important for the exact duplication of DNA during mitosis and meiosis and the encoding of proteins from the gene sequence. Second, each strand of DNA is directional, meaning that it is "read" from the 5′ phosphate end to the 3′ hydroxyl end (referred to as

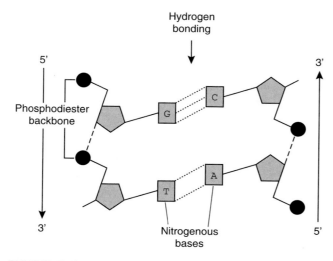

FIGURE 6–1 The basic structure of DNA, composed of two linear strands of nucleotides held together by specific patterns of hydrogen bonding. The A : T base pairings are held together by two hydrogen bonds, whereas the C : G base pairings are held together by three. The two strands form an antiparallel double helix.

simply 5′-to-3′). Proteins that are encoded from a specific gene are generated from this 5′-to-3′ sequence of the four bases. Because of the specific base pairing of the two linear DNA strands, a double-helical structure is formed in which the two strands are antiparallel, meaning that the 5′-to-3′ orientation is in the opposite direction on each strand. Genes may be encoded on either of the two strands.

Because of tissue development, growth, and cell turnover, replication of DNA occurs routinely as a part of mitosis. Therefore, DNA must have a mechanism for exact duplication of each chromosome. This replication occurs with a unique collection of enzymes that use each of the two DNA strands as a template to construct two new strands, following the base-pairing rule (A : T and C : G). The resulting new double helices therefore consist of one old and one new strand, each containing the exact DNA sequence as the original parent strand.

For each cell to carry out the functions of its specific tissue or organ, a unique combination of genes must be activated or inactivated. For genes to be "expressed," the DNA sequence corresponding to that gene must first be "transcribed" to a separate molecule similar to DNA, called RNA (ribonucleic acid). A polymerase enzyme recognizes a sequence of specific DNA bases that indicate where transcription should begin. The DNA sequence is then used as a template to construct messenger RNA (mRNA), with additional DNA sequences determining where transcription should end. Further processing of the mRNA removes sequences that are not needed to construct the desired protein (referred to as introns), and the

processed mRNA leaves the nucleus and moves into the cytoplasm.

Just as the DNA contains sequences that indicate where transcription of the mRNA is to begin, the mRNA contains specific sequences of bases that indicate where the protein should begin to be produced, or "translated." In this case, every three mRNA bases (referred to as a codon) encode for a single amino acid, the basic building block of proteins. Amino acids are linked together by covalent bonds, dependent on the three-base pattern, to eventually form a single protein chain. The chains then may act individually or in protein complexes to carry out the functions of the cell.

Inheritance Patterns

The inheritance of genetic disorders can be classified into three major categories: chromosomal, single gene, and complex (multifactorial). This section is devoted to elucidating the principles of single-gene inheritance. A discussion of the other traditional inheritance patterns listed above and unusual mechanisms such as genomic imprinting, mosaicism, and mitochondrial mutations can be found in the excellent textbooks on genetics listed in the Bibliography.

Single-gene disorders are caused by mutations within an individual (single) gene. Each entity is rare, but, as a group, they affect about 2% of the general population, chiefly in the pediatric age group, with approximately 6% to 8% of hospitalized children having a single-gene disorder. Often referred to as Mendelian disorders, over 9000 single-gene disorders have been described according to the Online Mendelian Inheritance in Man (OMIM) database. The patterns of inheritance in single-gene disorders depend on the chromosomal location of the gene (autosome or sex chromosome) and whether the disorder is dominant or recessive.

Because genetic disorders are inherited in several complex ways, pedigree analysis remains the cornerstone of determining the pattern of inheritance both in the diagnostic process and for purposes of genetic counseling, despite the technological advances that enable molecular testing for a host of genetic disorders. However, several factors can be misleading when interpreting a pedigree. Contiguous gene syndromes (caused by a microdeletion on a chromosome, resulting in a loss of several genes in close proximity to one another) can be inherited in a manner suggestive of a dominant single-gene disease. If the age of onset of a disease is late or variable, a family history may be deceptively normal. Similarly, the occurrence of a new mutation in a family must be considered when other family members appear to be unaffected. Two other factors affecting pedigree analysis are locus heterogeneity (mutations at different genes or loci causing the same disease) and allelic heterogeneity (different mutations at the same locus).

Autosomal Dominant Inheritance

Autosomal dominant (AD) disorders are disorders in which the gene is located on an autosome and the condition is expressed in heterozygotes (individuals with one abnormal allele). AD diseases tend to be more severe in homozygotes than in heterozygotes. An example is the common skeletal dysplasia achondroplasia, which in the homozygous form is fatal in the first year of life, whereas the heterozygous form is compatible with a fairly normal life. AD disorders comprise about half of all single-gene disorders and thus are the most common Mendelian disorders.

AD conditions have some typical features:

1. The disease is seen in every generation, with an affected person having an affected parent. An exception to this is *nonpenetrance* (no expression of the condition in a person who has the gene mutation).

2. An affected person has a 50% risk of passing on the gene mutation with each pregnancy.

3. Males and females are equally likely to be affected and to transmit the condition to their offspring of either sex. On pedigree analysis, recognition of male-male transmission of a disorder confirms that the disorder is autosomal dominant in inheritance.

4. A large number of individuals with AD diseases represent new mutations, and in those instances the pedigree would show no other affected members. The AD craniosynostosis syndromes, such as Apert's syndrome and Crouzon's disease, are typical examples of conditions with a high new mutation rate. Reduced fitness in these conditions leads to a preponderance of new mutations.

5. *Reduced penetrance*, defined as the failure to express the phenotype in 100% of individuals with the mutant allele, is common in AD disorders. These disorders also can show *variable expressivity*, with affected members (even within a family) showing variation in the severity of manifestations. The mechanisms responsible for variable expressivity are poorly understood and, with the focus of research on gene expression and function, there may better understanding in the future.

6. *Pleiotropy*, which is the occurrence of diverse manifestations caused by a single-gene mutation, is another feature of AD disorders. Every gene has a primary function of directing the production of a protein that may have multiple effects. Again, as with variability, pleiotropy is poorly understood.

Several of the features seen in AD disorders are illustrated by the study of Saethre-Chotzen syndrome, an AD syndrome with craniosynostosis, facial asymmetry, and digital abnormalities. Affected members within a given family can have significant variability of manifestations, although it is a highly penetrant condition (Figs. 6–2 through 6–5). Craniosynostosis affects the coronal suture frequently but can be absent in some individuals. Surgical intervention is needed for the craniosynostosis and in some instances for the cutaneous syndactyly of the second and third fingers. Intelligence is usually normal. Mutations in the *TWIST* gene are responsible for most cases of Saethre-Chotzen syndrome, and molecular testing is available on a clinical basis. Some patients with features of Saethre-Chotzen syndrome may have mutations in the fibroblast growth factor receptor-3 (*FGFR3*) gene,

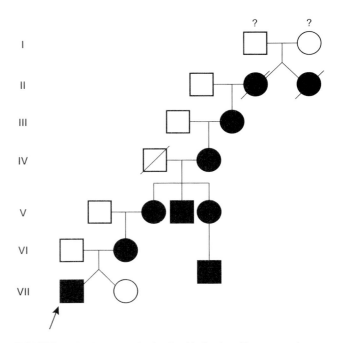

FIGURE 6–2 Pedigree of a family with Saethre-Chotzen syndrome, an autosomal dominant (AD) craniosynostosis syndrome, with variable manifestations. Note that, in this family, pedigree analysis alone would not be sufficient to distinguish between AD inheritance and X-linked recessive inheritance because there has been no male-to-male transmission. The *arrow* indicates the proband (first affected family member coming to medical attention).

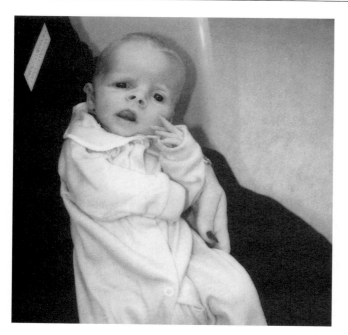

FIGURE 6–3 Frontal view of proband with Saethre-Chotzen syndrome (see pedigree in Fig. 6–2) exhibiting cranial asymmetry as a result of unilateral craniosynostosis, facial asymmetry, and low-set ears in the newborn period.

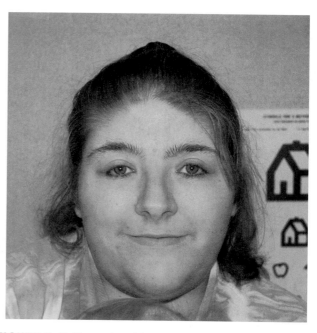

FIGURE 6–5 The mother of the proband in Figure 6–2 is also affected with Saethre-Chotzen syndrome, with a low frontal hairline, ptosis of the eyelids, and facial asymmetry. Note the variability in manifestations between the mother and son.

illustrating locus heterogeneity (mutations in different genes causing similar phenotypes, a feature seen not uncommonly in AD disorders).

Autosomal Recessive Inheritance

Autosomal recessive (AR) disorders are rarer than AD conditions, and occur in individuals who are homozygous for a particular mutation, with no normal allele at that locus.

The abnormal alleles are inherited from the parents, one from each (new mutations are rare). The heterozygote (carrier) parents are asymptomatic because their other normal allele is able to compensate for the presence of the abnormal allele. AR disorders share a few common characteristics:

1. Other affected individuals in a family usually are seen in the same generation as the proband, not in the parents or offspring.

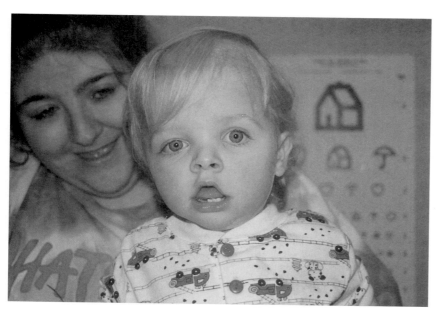

FIGURE 6–4 Frontal view of the same patient after surgical correction of the craniosynostosis.

2. Carriers (heterozygotes) are usually healthy, showing no symptoms or signs of the disorder.

3. The recurrence risk for parents of an affected child is 25% because both parents would be carriers. Consanguineous matings increase the risk of AR disorders. Belonging to certain ethnic groups also may increase the carrier frequency for some genetic disorders, such as Tay-Sachs disease in Ashkenazi Jewish individuals, cystic fibrosis in Caucasian populations, and sickle cell disease in populations of African descent.

4. Males and females are equally likely to be affected.

5. Incomplete penetrance, variable expressivity, and new mutations are uncommon in AR disorders, in contrast to AD disorders.

The gene carrier frequency in certain populations enables geneticists to provide risk calculations for couples at risk for AR diseases, based on their ethnicity, even without a family history. Such risk estimations enable accurate genetic counseling, prenatal diagnosis, and prevention. The American College of Obstetrics and Gynecology recommends screening for AR diseases such as hemoglobinopathies, Tay-Sachs disease, and recently cystic fibrosis based upon the ethnic origin of the parents. Although rare, AR diseases form the majority of conditions that are routinely screened for in newborns, because of their significant morbidity and mortality.

X-linked Inheritance

Genes on the X chromosome are unequally distributed among males and females, with males being hemizygous and females being either heterozygous or homozygous for a particular locus. However, the quantity of the protein product formed by the single allele in the male is equal to the product produced by the female. This dosage compensation is due to inactivation of an X chromosome in females, as outlined in the Lyon hypothesis. The principle of this hypothesis is that, in somatic cells in the female, only one X chromosome is transcriptionally active, with the other X chromosome being inactivated early in the embryonic stage, in a random fashion. This permanent inactivation of the X chromosome results in functional mosaicism at every locus and influences expression of X-linked phenotypes in females who carry X-linked recessive disease gene mutations.

According to the OMIM database, over 400 genetic diseases have been determined to be due to X-linked inheritance; these are divided into X-linked dominant and X-linked recessive disorders. In X-linked recessive inheritance, all males who inherit the mutation have manifestations of the condition. In females the disease is manifested in the homozygous state (when the father is affected and the mother is a carrier), although this is an unusual occurrence because most X-linked conditions are rare. Another mechanism that causes females who carry X-linked recessive mutations to have manifestations of the condition is skewed X inactivation, with preferential inactivation of the normal X chromosome in a majority of cells. This has been reported in disorders such as Duchenne's muscular dystrophy and hemophilia type A.

The typical features of X-linked recessive disorders are as follows:

1. More males are affected than females. Heterozygous females can be variably affected, depending on the pattern of X inactivation.

2. All female offspring of an affected male will be carriers of the condition. Female carriers have a 50% chance of having an affected son or a carrier daughter. All the affected males in a family are related through the females.

3. There is no male-to-male transmission of the condition.

4. Isolated cases frequently can be due to new mutations.

In X-linked dominant inheritance, both heterozygous females and hemizygous males show phenotypic manifestations. The distinguishing feature between X-linked dominant inheritance and AD inheritance is that, in the former, all the daughters of an affected male are affected, but there is no male-to-male transmission. With an affected female, the pattern of transmission may seem similar to an AD disorder because 50% of her offspring, male or female, will be affected. X-linked dominant disorders are rare. Some can be lethal in affected males, thus resulting in a preponderance of affected females who survive as a result of less severe manifestations. Examples of X-linked dominant disorders are X-linked hypophosphatemic rickets, wherein there is failure to reabsorb phosphorus from the renal tubules, resulting in rickets, and incontinentia pigmenti, which is characterized by lethality in affected males and a blistering rash, cognitive abnormalities, seizures, and teeth anomalies in females.

The Human Genome Project

The Human Genome Project is a major initiative to gain a better understanding of the genetics of human diseases and basic biology. As a result of the rapid improvements in technology, the groups working on the project were able to surpass the initial goals set for the period of 1993 to 1998. Most of these initial goals were to generate a better map of the human genome, which includes identifying a substantial portion of the DNA base sequence that comprises all human genes. The government-funded Human Genome Project, along with Celera Genomics, a privately funded company attempting to achieve similar goals, announced in the summer of 2000 that a "rough draft" of the human DNA sequence was completed. Although this genetic information is not the complete sequence of the human genome (there are still sequence gaps to be filled), it is a valuable resource for scientists searching for disease genes.

Currently, one of the primary goals of the Human Genome Project is to identify the natural genetic variation that exists among individuals. Clearly, there are differences among individuals that do not present as a disease or disabling trait. These changes are due to slight variations in gene expression that fall within some "normal" range, and lead to differences in height, hair color, eye color, and even personality traits. Changes that occur outside of this range may lead to either disease or a strong predisposition to disease. The normal variations that occur are referred to as *polymorphisms*, while DNA sequence changes that cause a pronounced phenotype are referred to as *mutations*. However, there is some degree of ambiguity in many cases as to when a genetic change that causes a predisposition to a disease is considered a mutation, because it may occur in the general population with a high frequency. Typically polymorphisms occur in regions between genes that do not have an effect on a gene's function, or cause subtle changes that may have slight or cumulative effects. Although polymorphisms may contribute to the susceptibility to a disease, an environmental exposure may be required for the disease to be fully expressed. One extreme example of this situation would be variations that predispose to lung cancer, but only in individuals who smoke.

Mutation Concepts

Specific types of variations may occur within a given DNA sequence, independent of whether they are polymorphisms or mutations (Fig. 6–6). Some of these changes occur on a scale that can be detected at the chromosome level, whereas

Silent	Met His Tyr Pro Arg ATG CAT TAT CCT CGT	→	Met His Tyr Pro Arg ATG CAT TAC CCT CGT
Missense	Met His Tyr Pro Arg ATG CAT TAT CCT CGT	→	Met His His Pro Arg ATG CAT CAT CCT CGT
Nonsense	Met His Tyr Pro Arg ATG CAT TAT CCT CGT	→	Met His STOP ATG CAT TAG CCT CGT
Insertion/deletion	Met His Tyr Pro Arg ATG CAT TAT CCT CGT	→	Met His Tyr Leu Val ATG CAT TAC CTC GTA

FIGURE 6–6 Types and consequences of genetic mutations. For each type of mutation, the DNA sequence is shown below and the amino acid sequence is shown above. The site of the mutation is underlined in both sequences.

others can be detected only by examining the DNA at the molecular level. In addition, although a single gene may be responsible for a specific genetic condition, many different types of gene mutations (allelic heterogeneity) may be responsible for altering or eliminating the function of that gene. For example, in the first two published papers describing mutations in the *TWIST* gene leading to Saethre-Chotzen syndrome, 10 different mutations were identified in 11 different individuals. Although these mutations themselves were each unique, each would presumably lead to a loss of function of the TWIST protein, which would in turn lead to the Saethre-Chotzen characteristic phenotype.

Missense Mutations

Single-base changes, commonly a C to a T or an A to a G, are referred to as missense mutations or single nucleotide polymorphisms, depending on their role in disease. These variations are extremely common and occur frequently throughout the genome. The vast majority of these changes probably have little or no effect because they occur between genes or within the noncoding portions of genes. However, these polymorphisms also are studied extensively in single-gene disorders as well as genetically complex diseases such as diabetes, asthma, prostate cancer, and cardiovascular disease. Missense mutations may occur within the protein-coding region of a gene with little or no effect, or they may lead to completely altered gene function, depending on their location.

Nonsense Mutations

Any type of variation that leads to a premature stop codon in the protein is referred to as a nonsense mutation.

This premature stop typically leads to a truncated protein product that cannot perform its function in the cell appropriately. These truncated products also may interfere with the normal products to prevent them from functioning properly as well.

Insertions and Deletions

These changes may be of any size, and range from single bases to large chromosomal abnormalities. Small insertions and deletions within the coding region of a gene may result in "frameshift" mutations. Because proteins are encoded from the mRNA in three-nucleotide codons, any change in this pattern, or reading frame, will result in the production of a different sequence of amino acids, and therefore a different protein. Therefore, small mutations that insert or delete nucleotides that are not multiples of three will shift the reading frame. The new protein product typically will have no function, an abnormal function, or an interference with the normal gene product.

Molecular Genetic Testing

For research purposes and clinical diagnosis, detection of mutations or polymorphisms is a primary focus of molecular genetics laboratories. Several methods have been used routinely to detect mutations and polymorphisms at the molecular level, the most common of which are restriction fragment length polymorphism (RFLP) analysis, allele-specific oligonucleotide (ASO) hybridization, and

direct DNA sequencing. All of these techniques require the use of the polymerase chain reaction (PCR), which has become a staple in molecular genetics. PCR utilizes the directionality and base-pairing code of DNA replication, and results in the exponential amplification of a specific DNA fragment from within the entire genomic background. These amplified products then can be used in later processes to determine the genetic variations that are present in this smaller fragment. Because of the exponential amplification, very little genomic DNA (several nanograms) is required for the test. Therefore, DNA can be obtained from newborn blood spots, swabs from the inside of the cheek, or a drop of blood from a finger stick.

Restriction Fragment Length Polymorphisms

As part of their host defense mechanism, bacteria have enzymes that digest specific DNA sequences, mostly to protect the bacterial genome from viral infection. These enzymes have been isolated and purified from the bacteria, and are used routinely as a valuable tool in molecular genetics. Each enzyme recognizes a specific sequence along the DNA strand and digests the DNA within or near that sequence (Fig. 6–7). Restriction enzymes only cut the DNA sequences that are identical to their target sequence. Therefore, a missense mutation may either create or abolish a restriction enzyme site. To test for this type of mutation in the lab, the genomic DNA from the patient sample is amplified by PCR, using DNA primers that flank the mutated site. The resulting PCR products then are digested

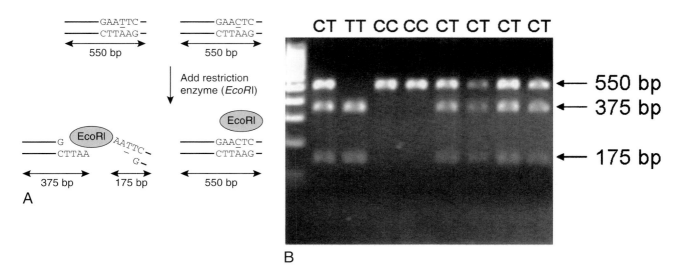

FIGURE 6–7 Detection of a missense mutation using RFLP analysis. **A,** The T-to-C mutation is underlined in the double-stranded 550-bp DNA sequence shown at the top. After exposure to the *EcoR*I restriction enzyme, the T allele is digested while the C allele is not. The resulting fragments from the digestion are 375 and 175 bp in length. **B,** Agarose gel electrophoresis of the restriction enzyme digested fragments. Heterozygous (CT) individuals have three bands (one for the C and two for the T allele), whereas homozygous CC individuals have only the 550-bp fragment and homozygous TT individuals have only the 375- and 175-bp fragments.

with the specific restriction enzyme that recognizes the mutated site. If the site is present, the enzyme will cut the DNA at its recognition sequence. If the recognition site is not present (because of the mutation), the enzyme will not cut the DNA fragment. The fragments from the restriction enzyme digestion reaction then are separated using gel electrophoresis, which separates DNA fragments based on their size (i.e., number of nucleotides). Individuals without the mutation will have only one fragment, and therefore one "band," on the gel. Individuals with two copies of the mutation will have two bands, consisting of the two pieces of the digested fragment. Individuals with a mutation on only one chromosome will have three bands, consisting of a combination of the fragments described above. RFLPs are useful in the detection of known mutations, such as those that occur frequently in a population. However, if the mutation is not known, RFLP analysis cannot be used.

Allele-Specific Oligonucleotide Hybridization

In instances in which RFLP analysis cannot be utilized (e.g., restriction enzyme sites are not changed), ASO hybridization commonly is used (Fig. 6–8). This method is based on the base-pairing specificity of DNA, and is dependent on the fact that "mismatched" base pairing will not occur under optimal conditions. For this assay, the region encompassing the mutation is amplified from genomic DNA using PCR. For each patient to be tested, the PCR product is covalently bound to a membrane and denatured so that it is single stranded. Two specific DNA oligonucleotides of 15 to 20 base pairs (corresponding to the normal and mutant sequence) are synthesized commercially and labeled with a radioactive tag. Both oligonucleotides are combined with the membrane containing the patient DNA, allowing the labeled probes to hybridize with the target sequence. Only the probes that are an exact match to the target will hybridize, while the remaining probes will be washed away. By exposing the membrane to radiographic film, it can be determined if the patient sequences contain the normal sequence, the mutant sequence, or both. As with RFLP analysis, ASO hybridization is only useful for the detection of known mutations.

DNA Sequencing

For many genetic disorders, a spectrum of mutations may be present within the defective gene. Furthermore, a given mutation may occur rarely or only in a single family, making it difficult to accomplish large-scale screening for these genes. DNA sequencing is required to first identify the novel mutation, which then can be screened using either RFLP or ASO hybridization analysis in additional

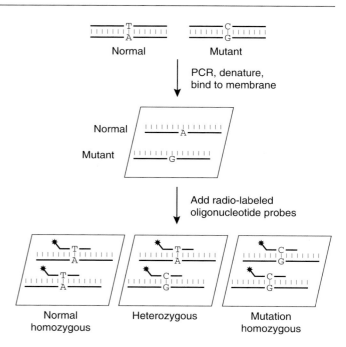

FIGURE 6–8 Detection of a missense mutation using ASO hybridization. The normal and mutant sequences are amplified by PCR, denatured, and covalently bound to a membrane. Radioactively labeled probes are combined individually with the membrane, and identical sequences will hybridize. A radioactive signal with an allele-specific probe indicates the presence of that allele.

family members. DNA sequencing has gone through many changes since it was originally described in the late 1970s. The current standard for DNA sequencing involves the use of specifically modified, fluorescent-labeled nucleotides (referred to as dideoxynucleotide triphosphates [ddNTPs]), which, in addition to the typical nucleotides, are added to a growing DNA strand using a target DNA sequence as a template (Fig. 6–9). When a ddNTP is added to the growing strand, the reaction no longer extends the growing chain. Using a combination of all four nucleotides, each labeled with a different color of fluorescent dye, the entire sequence of a region can be determined. Although the surrounding sequence must be known for the original sequencing primers to be designed, a mutation can be identified by comparing a patient's sequence with a known normal control sequence. Ideally, sequencing would be used to screen and detect mutations in all instances. However, because of the expense of the sequencing components and the necessary equipment, sequencing is utilized only when necessary or for research purposes.

Gene Therapy

Traditional strategies utilized to treat genetic disorders involved dietary restriction of a precursor substance,

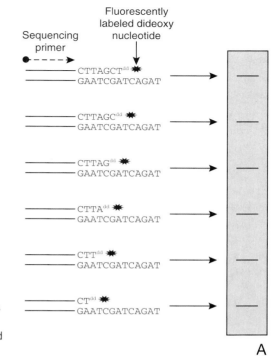

FIGURE 6–9 Detection of a missense mutation using DNA sequencing. **A,** The sequence is determined using fluorescently labeled ddNTPs, which stop the growing DNA strand. Each new fragment will have a unique size (and fluorescent color) that can be easily identified with gel or capillary electrophoresis. **B,** Sequence data from an automated DNA sequencer, showing the three possible genotypes for a specific missense mutation.

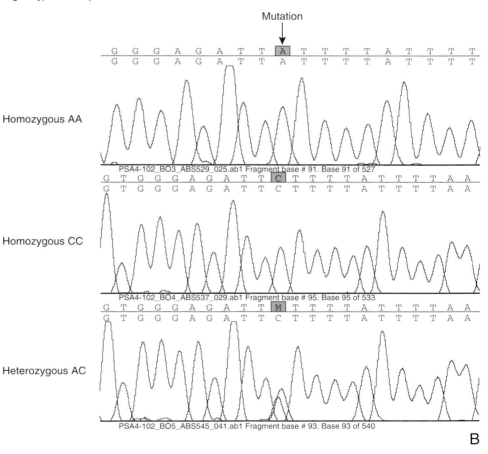

replacement of a metabolite or cofactor, pharmacologic diversion of metabolites, and depletion of a harmful compound from the body. In recent years, efforts to increase the residual activity of the mutant protein have resulted in enzyme replacement treatments in disorders such as Gaucher's disease and adenosine deaminase deficiency. Organ transplantation, regarded as a form of gene transfer therapy, leads to a modification of the somatic genotype by providing tissue with a normal genotype in a particular tissue or organ, resulting in production of a normal protein in an individual who carries a mutation in a gene encoding a particular protein. The outcomes vary according to the disorder and carry, in addition, the disadvantages of significant mortality and morbidity related to the transplantation and immunosuppressive treatments. Examples include bone marrow transplantation for leukodystrophies and liver transplantation for α_1-antitrypsin deficiency. This chapter does not address gene replacement therapy by organ transplantation, but rather focuses on replacement of a single gene.

With the advent of advanced genetic technologies and the hope that gene therapy will provide the definitive therapeutic approach for a myriad of genetic disorders, there has been unprecedented interest in gene therapy studies in both human and animal models in the last 15 years. Introduction of a single gene into target cells to correct the mutant phenotype should, in principle, be a permanent cure for genetic diseases. Although several clinical trials to determine safety and efficacy are underway, there has been no disorder that has been "cured" by gene therapy. Nevertheless, gene therapy holds great promise for the treatment of human genetic diseases, and there have been more than 400 clinical trials involving gene therapy, with approximately 4000 patients having participated.

General Principles

The transfer of DNA/RNA to target cells is carried out in *somatic* cells, with the intention of correcting the DNA mutation in those cells. *Germline* gene therapy, which involves the modification of the genotype of the fertilized egg, is fraught with ethical and technical difficulties, carries the risk of introduction of new mutations, and is not permitted in any country currently.

The two main approaches to gene therapy are in vivo and ex vivo approaches. In the in vivo approach, the new gene is delivered directly into the target cells, often injected into the patient's blood stream. The advantage of this approach is that it is easy, but the challenge is in being able to reach the target cells in the body, and thus the in vivo approach is not used widely in clinical trials. A specialized type of in vivo gene therapy is in situ gene therapy, in which the gene is placed directly into the

affected tissue. An example of this is the injection of a vector carrying the dystrophin gene directly into the muscle of an individual with Duchenne's muscular dystrophy.

In ex vivo gene therapy, the target cells are removed from the body, genetically modified and amplified, and reintroduced into the body. This approach is advantageous because the modified cells can be selected for in culture, but it can be used only in conditions in which the target cells can be removed from the body. A classical example of this type of gene therapy is the treatment of X-linked severe combined immunodeficiency disease (SCID) by inserting a complementary DNA (cDNA) of the gene γc cytokine receptor subunit (carried in a retroviral vector) into autologous bone marrow stem cells, which then are transfused back into the patient. Ten months after the gene transfer, the two patients who received the therapy were still expressing the transgene, and the T, B, and natural killer cell counts and function were normal and matched those of age-matched healthy controls. Dramatic clinical improvement occurred, with restoration of normal growth and development. This represents the first possibility of a cure of a genetic condition by gene therapy, although considerable caution has to be exercised to make sure that the effects of therapy are permanent.

Purposes

The goal of gene therapy is to achieve one of three purposes, depending on the disease being treated:

1. Compensation for a mutant gene that results in a loss-of-function phenotype, such as increased phenylalanine levels in phenylketonuria. Introduction of a normal copy of the gene would correct the phenotype. The transferred gene would need cofactors and other molecules necessary for its function. The mutant gene would coexist along with the transferred normal gene.

2. Replacing or inactivating a dominant mutant gene whose product causes the disease. This is much more difficult to perform because the abnormal gene would have to be functionally silenced (removed) and replaced by the normal gene. An example is osteogenesis imperfecta, wherein the abnormal proα (1) collagen causes the phenotype and laboratory studies are designed to degrade the mRNA from the mutant allele.

3. Causing a pharmacologic effect to counteract the effects of an abnormal gene. Gene therapy in cancer is an example of this purpose.

There are certain requirements for gene therapy with any disorder. These are that the responsible gene be identified or the biochemical basis be known, that a cDNA clone or the gene itself be available, that the risk-benefit ratio be favorable compared to alternative treatments, that an appropriate target cell be available, and that there be data from animal studies that indicate efficacy of gene therapy for that disorder. It is also necessary that an alternative efficacious method of therapy be unavailable. Gene therapy protocols are still in the research phase, and thus approval from institutional review boards is necessary prior to initiating a trial.

Methods of Gene Transfer

A carrier molecule, called the vector, is used to transfer the gene into the target cell. An ideal vector would be one that is safe, manufactured without difficulty, and introduced easily into the target cell and that would induce lifelong production of the gene product within the target tissue. In reality, there is no such ideal vector for any of the disorders that have been treated with gene therapy. The most widely used vectors are derived from viruses, such as retroviruses and adenoviruses. Retroviruses have only three genes, and thus it is technically easy to remove and replace these with the gene to be transferred. They allow large inserts (~8 kb) and enter virtually any target cell. However, they do not integrate their DNA into a nonreplicating cell, which is a disadvantage. To overcome this shortcoming, newer trials are using lentiviruses, the class of retroviruses that includes the human immunodeficiency virus, because they are capable of DNA integration in nondividing cells. Adenoviral vectors allow smaller inserts (~5 kb) and thus may not be suitable for a number of disorders in which the gene is larger. They are expressed only for a few weeks and elicit a very strong inflammatory response, but offer the advantages of being able to infect a wide variety of cells and having the ability to integrate their DNA into host cells that are not replicating.

Nonviral vectors do not carry the biologic risk that viral vectors do, but the shortcoming is that the DNA introduced is taken up by the lysosomes and degraded and not taken up by the nucleus. Nonviral vectors include naked DNA and DNA packaged in liposomes, with protein and artificial chromosomes (DNA packaged with the functional elements of a chromosome). Human gene therapy trials that have used nonviral vectors have had limited success.

Adverse Effects

There has been much publicity of the recent death of a patient in a gene therapy trial as a result of an adverse reaction to an adenoviral vector. Although the scientific community had been cognizant of the potential adverse effects, the demise of a patient has highlighted the need for carefully scrutinizing the scientific and ethical judgment of investigators, the state of the science of viral vectors, and the need for closer oversight by regulatory bodies such as the National Institutes of Health and the Food and Drug Administration.

A reaction to the vector is prime among the concerns in gene therapy. This risk can be minimized by animal safety studies and carefully conducted preliminary human studies. Another concern is that the transferred gene may disrupt normal cellular function by insertion into and disruption of an essential gene or by causing activation of an oncogene, leading to malignancies. This concern is less of a realistic threat, but all these issues need to be addressed before embarking on gene therapy for a specific disorder.

Future Directions

Gene therapy trials have been performed for diseases including single-gene disorders such as SCID and cystic fibrosis; cancers such as gliomas and ovarian carcinomas, in which "suicide" gene therapy is carried out by introducing genes that increase chemosensitivity of the target cells; cardiovascular diseases such as hypercholesterolemia caused by low-density lipoprotein receptor deficiency; and infectious diseases such as acquired immunodeficiency syndrome. Thus far, the results have not shown that gene therapy has been curative for any disorder, although preliminary results have been encouraging in the instance of SCID. The field of gene therapy has been criticized for promising too much and not achieving much. However, it should be noted that major technologies take long periods of time to develop, and more basic and clinical research will be needed to fully determine if gene therapy will live up to its expectations. No other area of medicine holds such promise of curing a myriad of disorders.

Bibliography

Aase JM, Smith DW: Facial asymmetry and abnormalities of palms and ears: a dominantly inherited developmental syndrome. J Pediatr 1970;76:928.

Anderson WF: Gene therapy: the best of times, the worst of times. Science 2000;288:627.

Bianchi E, Arico M, Podesta AF, et al: A family with the Saethre-Chotzen syndrome. Am J Med Genet 1985; 22:649.

Blau HM, Springer ML: Gene therapy—a novel form of drug delivery. N Engl J Med 1995;333:1204.

Bunnell BA, Morgan RA: Gene therapy for infectious diseases. Clin Microbiol Rev 1998;11:42.

Candotti F, Blaese RM: Gene therapy of primary immunodeficiencies. Springer Semin Immunopathol 1998;19:493.

Cavazzana-Calvo M, Hacein-Bey S, de Saint Basile G, et al: Gene therapy of human severe combined immunodeficiency (SCID)-X1 disease. Science 2000;288:669.

Chotzen F: Eine eigenartige familiaere Entwicklungsstoerung (Akrocephalosyndaktylie. Dysotosis craniofacialis und hypertelorismus). Monatsschr Kinderheikd 1932;55:97.

Collins FS, Patrinos A, Jordan E, et al: New goals for the U.S. Human Genome Project: 1988–2003. Science 1998;282:682.

El Ghouzzi V, Le Merrer M, Perrin-Schmitt F, et al: Mutations of the TWIST gene in the Saethre-Chotzen syndrome. Nat Genet 1997;15:42.

Howard TD, Paznekas WA, Green ED, et al: Mutations in TWIST, a basic helix-loop-helix transcription factor, in Saethre-Chotzen syndrome. Nat Genet 1997;15:36.

Kaye EM: Lysosomal storage diseases. Curr Treat Options Neurol 2001;May 3:249.

Mankin HJ, Rosenthal DI, Xavier R: Gaucher disease: new approaches to an ancient disease. J Bone Joint Surg Am 2001;83:748.

National Center for Biotechnology Information: OMIM: Online Mendelian Inheritance in Man. Available at *www.ncbi.nlm.nih.gov/omim*

Paznekas WA, Cunningham ML, Howard TD, et al: Genetic heterogeneity of Saethre-Chotzen syndrome, due to TWIST and FGFR mutations. Am J Hum Genet 1998;62:1370.

Rimoin DL, Connor JM, Pyeritz RE: Emory and Rimoin's Principles and Practice of Medical Genetics (3rd ed). Edinburgh: Churchill Livingstone, 1997.

Rosenberg LE, Schecter AN: Gene therapist heal thyself. Science 2000;287:1751.

Saethre M: Ein Beitrag zum Turmschaedelproblem (Pathogenese Erblichkeit und Symptomatologic). Dtsch Z Nervenheilkd 1931;119:533.

Schmidt-Wolf GD, Schmidt-Wolf LGH: Cancer and gene therapy. Ann Hematol 1996;73:207.

Scriver CR, Beaudet AL, Sly WS, Valle D (eds): The Metabolic and Molecular Basis of Inherited Disease (8th ed). New York: McGraw-Hill, 2000.

Staff AC: An introduction to gene therapy and its potential prenatal use. Acta Obstet Gynecol Scand 2001;80:485.

Thompson JS, Thompson MW: Genetics in Medicine (6th ed). Philadelphia: WB Saunders, 2001.

Vogel F, Motulsky AG: Human Genetics: Problems and Approaches (3rd ed). New York: Springer-Verlag, 1997.

Yla-Herttuala S, Martin JF: Cardiovascular gene therapy. Lancet 2000;355:213.

CHAPTER 7

Immune System and Transplant Immunology

George Tsoulfas, M.D., Bridget L. Colvin, B.S., Noriko Murase, M.D., and Angus W. Thomson, Ph.D., D.Sc.

Embryologic Origin and Function of the Organs of the Immune System

The basis for the functional diversity of the immune system is set early in life during embryonic development by differentiation of the various cell populations. Stem cells are first formed in the embryonic yolk sac of the developing embryo. Some of these cells migrate at the sixth week of gestation to the liver, where they begin hematopoietic activity. By the 12th week there is a small contribution by stem cells in the spleen. By 20 weeks of gestation, the bone marrow (BM), thymus, and lymph nodes (LNs) all contribute to hematopoiesis, with the BM becoming the main hematopoietic center at 38 weeks (the liver maintains some hematopoietic activity in the neonate and teenager).

The lymphoid organs can be divided into primary (central) ones, where lymphocytes are produced, and secondary (peripheral) ones, to which lymphocytes migrate and in which they interact with nonlymphoid cells to mature and initiate immune responses. The primary lymphoid organs are the thymus and bone marrow; secondary lymphoid organs are the spleen, LNs, and lymphoid tissue distributed in the mucosa of the upper respiratory tract (bronchial-associated lymphoid tissue, or BALT) and the intestines (gut-associated lymphoid tissue, or GALT).

Thymus

The thymus plays a central role in the differentiation of T lymphocytes and the induction of tolerance to self. It develops in the embryo as an epithelial outgrowth of the third and fourth pharyngeal pouches, together with the parathyroid glands. During the sixth week of gestation, this epithelial structure is seeded by primitive mesenchymal and neural crest cells. The thymus is active during childhood and involutes during adolescence. It is divided by trabeculae, extending from its capsule into lobules. Each lobule has a cortex and a medulla. The cortex consists primarily of immature T-lymphocyte aggregates as well as a smaller number of epithelial and dendritic cells (DCs), whereas the less populated medulla has a higher epithelial cell/lymphocyte ratio.

The thymus is an organ of intense cell proliferation and death, with only 1% of cells generated eventually migrating to the peripheral tissues. The interaction between the T lymphocytes and the epithelial cells leads to the elimination or inactivation of self-reactive T-cell clones (negative selection) and to differentiation of the surviving ones. Thymic hormones such as thymosin, thymopoietin, and thymic humoral factor are believed to play a role in this process.

Bone Marrow

Toward the end of gestation hematopoietic stem cells migrate from the liver to the BM, the long bones, and the axial skeleton (pelvis, rib cage, vertebrae). In the adult, however, few remain in the long bones; most are in the axial skeleton. The BM is the site where all the cellular elements of the immune system are produced by progenitor cells. These, in turn, give rise to hematopoietic precursors with more limited potential. The most primitive are the hematopoietic stem cells, which divide to produce the common lymphoid and myeloid progenitors. The lymphoid progenitor gives rise to the B lymphocyte [which differentiates upon activation in the lymphoid tissue to antibody (Ab)-producing plasma cells] and the T lymphocyte (which migrates to the thymus for further differentiation). In turn, the myeloid progenitors give rise to erythroblasts, megakaryocytes, and leukocytes.

Spleen

The spleen develops from mesenchymal tissue between the stomach and the pancreas during the fifth week of gestation. In about 20% of normal individuals incomplete fusion of this mesenchymal tissue can lead to the presence of accessory spleens. The structure of the spleen is central to its multiple functions. It is divided into red and white pulp, with the former being the area where blood is filtered

and senescent or diseased erythrocytes, bacteria, parasites, and particulate matter are removed. This process is augmented by the presence of opsonins, some of which (e.g., tuftsin, properdin, fibronectin) are produced in the spleen to activate complement and to stimulate granulocyte and macrophage motility and phagocytosis. The white pulp contains lymphoid aggregates called *lymphoid follicles* and the *periarteriolar lymphoid sheaths* (PALS). The latter contain mostly T cells, whereas the former are B cell-dominated. With this unique anatomy, the spleen functions as a prime center for antigen (Ag) processing and presentation. In the PALS, presentation of Ag by DCs and macrophages to CD4$^+$ T-helper (Th) cells leads to activation of the cell-mediated immune response. Ags in the germinal centers are presented to B lymphocytes by germinal center Ag-presenting cells (APCs) and stimulate the synthesis of Abs. The spleen is the largest producer of immunoglobulin M (IgM).

The spleen deserves special mention as its involvement in a great variety of immunologic processes often makes it a target for surgical resection. Splenectomy is used as a therapeutic measure in certain diseases, such as hereditary spherocytosis, hereditary elliptocytosis, warm (IgG) acquired immune hemolytic anemia, and Felty's syndrome or when medical treatment fails (e.g., for hairy cell leukemia or immune thrombocytopenic purpura). In other cases, such as chronic lymphocytic leukemia, chronic myeloblastic leukemia, non-Hodgkin's lymphoma, multiple myeloma, thrombotic thrombocytopenic purpura, Gaucher's disease (where partial splenectomy may be the procedure of choice). Moreover, splenectomy has a palliative role for the hematologic consequences of hypersplenism or symptomatic splenomegaly.

An important consideration for the surgeon performing splenectomy for congenital or acquired anemias is to ensure that all the splenic tissue is removed. Accessory spleens are seen in 15% to 30% of patients, most frequently in the hilum, which can lead to the persistence of symptoms postoperatively. If any concerns exist, successful splenectomy can be confirmed postoperatively by the presence of abnormally formed erythrocytes and cytoplasmic inclusions (e.g., Heinz, Pappenheimer, or Howell-Jolly bodies in the circulation.

Complications following splenectomy range from those that are perioperative, such as bleeding, injury to the tail of the pancreas (the main indication for leaving a drain following splenectomy), and subdiaphragmatic abscess, to those related to the immunologic role of the spleen. Following splenectomy, thrombocytosis with platelet levels up to 1 million/mm^3 and leukocytosis are frequently seen, although the clinical significance of these two conditions remains undetermined. Postsplenectomy sepsis (PSS), although rare, represents the most significant complication. It manifests as increased susceptibility to usually gram-positive encapsulated bacteria, eventually leading to sepsis. The incidence ranges from 0.6% to 4.0% in children and 0.3% to 1.0% in adults. In children it occurs more frequently following splenectomy for congenital or acquired anemias, whereas in adults splenectomy for malignancies appears to be a more prominent cause. Mortality can be as high as 50%, and the symptoms (e.g., malaise, fever, headaches) are initially nonspecific and followed within 24 to 72 hours by the signs and symptoms of overwhelming sepsis. The organisms most frequently involved are *Streptococcus pneumoniae*, *Haemophilus influenzae*, and *Neisseria meningitidis*.

To prevent this significant complication, an effort is made to postpone splenectomy until a child is 4 years old. Also, if possible, vaccinations, especially against *S. pneumoniae* are given prior to the surgery. There is some debate regarding the role of prophylactic antibiotics, although they are frequently used in children less than 10 years old and in immunosuppressed patients. However, all these measures may be insufficient, underlying the importance of advising patients and their families about this complication and the need to seek urgent medical care when any of the initial symptoms occur.

The importance of PSS has led to a change in our thinking about splenic injury due to trauma, in which case every effort is made to apply nonoperative treatment or splenic repair instead of resection. Nevertheless, given the rare occurrence of PSS, these considerations should not compromise the overall welfare of the trauma patient. Other attempts to avoid PSS consist of autotransplantation following splenectomy. This has not been shown to have much success, however, partly because at least 30% to 50% of splenic tissue is needed and, more importantly, because it appears that the presence of intact splenic circulation is necessary to achieve the benefits of adequate splenic function, including prevention of PSS.

Lymph Nodes

Because of their anatomic locations throughout the body, LNs play an important "role in the induction of the immune response. Their function as transit stations for lymphatic flow also allows various Ags to pass continuously through them. B lymphocytes are localized in the follicles found in the cortex, and, subsequent to Ag and helper cell stimulation, part of these areas become germinal centers. T cells are found in the paracortical areas of LNs, where their interactions with APCs, such as DCs and macrophages, lead to their activation and proliferation. The activated cells can then reenter the circulation through the efferent lymphatics, reach the periphery, and mediate the immune response.

GALT and BALT

For the surgical specialist, the immunologic role of the intestine cannot be understated. The gut has a passive role in protecting the individual from infection by acting as a mechanical and physiologic barrier (with peristalsis and the resident microbial flora). It also undertakes an active role in the form of the GALT (which includes the tonsils, adenoids, Peyer's patches, and appendix); here Ag is collected and presented to B cells in the follicles and germinal centers as well as to T cells. In addition to its role in Ag presentation, the GALT is one of the main producers of secretory IgA. A similar, but less organized aggregate of lymphoid tissue, known as BALT, exists in the respiratory epithelium.

Cellular Components of the Immune System

Innate versus Adaptive Immunity

The immune system can be divided into the innate, or nonspecific, immune system and the adaptive, or specific, immune system. The former consists of cells and their products that operate against a variety of pathogens and inflammatory stimuli, whereas the latter consists of cells and mechanisms directed against specific insults. It should be noted that the separation is not strict, as cells or mediators may have roles in both systems.

Innate immune system

The innate immune system can be thought of as having three components. The first comprises the defense of an organism with mechanical barriers (intact skin, mucus coating of epithelial cells, cilia of the respiratory tract, fluids such as saliva, tears, or sweat, which inhibit pathogen adhesion), chemical barriers (e.g., the low pH in the stomach), and physiologic conditions (e.g., body temperature and oxygen tension). The second component consists of humoral factors, such as complement, which when activated are able to participate in the destruction of pathogens through the *classic* and *alternative* pathways. They can also promote the immune response by recruiting other effector cells. The final component of the innate immune system consists of its effector cells, a brief overview of which can be seen in Table 7–1. These cells perform their function mainly but not exclusively by phagocytosis. This process consists of several phases, including *chemotaxis, attachment, degranulation, intracellular killing* (through oxygen-dependent or oxygen-independent mechanisms), and *intracellular digestion*.

Table 7–1

Cells of the innate immune system

Cells	Origin	Characteristics	Location	Function
Neutrophils or PMNs	Myeloid progenitor in bone marrow (BM)	60–70% of WBCs; diameter 10–12 µm; basophilic cytoplasm, azurophilic granules, and peroxisomes; immature cells (bands) have kidney-shaped nucleus, whereas mature ones (segmented) have two- or three-lobed nuclei	Blood; migrates to tissues when inflammation present	Phagocytosis, activation of bactericidal mechanisms
Eosinophils	Myeloid progenitor in BM	3% of WBCs; diameter 9–12 µm with large bilobed or indented nucleus; granules stain pink/red with eosin and contain eosinophilic cationic protein and major basic protein	Blood	Defense against parasites
Basophils	Myeloid progenitor in BM	<1% of WBCs; diameter 8–10 µm with large, round nucleus; ovoid granules stain intensely with basic dyes and contain histamine, heparin	Blood; enter tissues when activated and become mast cells	High-affinity receptors for IgE; role in allergic reactions
Monocytes/ macrophages	Myeloid progenitor in BM	Diameter 9–15 µm for monocytes and 20–25 µm for macrophages; nucleus oval with prominent nucleoli; large number of lysosomes and mitochondria; enzyme markers include peroxidase and lysozyme	Leave BM and go to tissues where may undergo morphologic changes (e.g., Kupffer cells in liver, Langerhans cells in skin)	Phagocytosis; antigen presentation
Dendritic cells (DCs)	Myeloid and lymphoid progenitor in SM	Distinctive branch morphology; irregularly shaped, often multilobed; nuclei abundant; cytoplasm has few granules	DCs in nonlymphoid tissue (e.g., heart, liver, skin, kidney) are immature APCs, whereas DCs in secondary lymphoid tissue (spleen and LNs) are mature, as they present Ag and have co-stimulatory ability	Phagocytosis; antigen presentation; delivery of activating signals
Natural killer (NK) cells	Lymphoid progenitor in SM	Non-T, non-B lymphocytes with granular morphology	Activation is not MHC-restricted	Involved in defense against viruses, intracellular pathogens, tumor cells antibody-dependent cell-mediated cytotoxicity; possible role in autoimmunity

Natural killer (NK) cells represent another cell type that acts against virus-infected cells and tumor cells by releasing lytic granules. These cells play a role in innate immunity. Finally, as in any discussion of the immune system, special mention should be made of the DCs.

These are rare, branched leukocytes that function as highly specialized professional APCs. Immature DCs trap Ags in the periphery, direct them to regional lymphoid tissue, and subsequently present them to T cells while at the same time delivering the second signal (co-stimulation)

Table 7–2
Lymphocyte subtypes

Cell type	Function
B cells: humoral response	Activated B cells that produce immunoglobulins and direct the humoral response;
Plasma cells	participate in allergic/hypersensitivity reactions and hyperacute and chronic rejection
Memory cells	Responsible for a more rapid response in a future encounter with the same pathogen, which is the basis for immunizations
T cells: cell-mediated response	Control viral and intracellular bacterial infections; participate in acute and chronic
Cytotoxic Tc cells (CD8+)	rejection, delayed-type hypersensitivity reactions, and cytokine release
Helper Th cells (CD4+)	Provide co-stimulatory signal for B cell activation
Suppressor (Ts) or regulatory T cells	Controversy exists about their exact function but they probably downregulate the immune response by controlling T cell activation; possible role in tolerance induction

required for T cell activation. The importance of this presentation and co-stimulation for the specific immune response makes the DC an appealing candidate cell for cancer and infectious disease therapy. On the other hand, blocking their normal immunostimulatory function could promote allograft survival.

Adaptive immune system

The main effector cells of specific immunity are the lymphocytes. They are small, round cells with a large nucleus and thin cytoplasm. Their primary subdivision is into B and T cells. B (bursal) lymphocytes are so named because of functionally similar cells that originate from the bursa of Fabricius in birds. As this organ does not exist in mammals, B cells in mammals are those that originate in the liver during fetal life and in the BM after birth. T cells originate in the BM as well but migrate to the thymus to complete their maturation.

Both types of cells remain "dormant" while circulating in the blood and lymph until they encounter an Ag in the peripheral lymphoid tissues and bind to it through their Ag-specific receptor. For B cells this receptor is, in essence, membrane-bound immunoglobulin, whereas for T cells it is the T cell Ag–receptor complex (TCR). Although each cell has a specific receptor for a given Ag, somatic gene rearrangements ensure an immune system able to deal with many potential pathogens. After binding of the Ag, a process of natural selection occurs. Lymphocytes that recognize an Ag and have been activated undergo clonal expansion and proliferation, whereas those that recognize an Ag without being activated undergo apoptosis. This process, which explains the specific nature of adaptive immunity, is also responsible for the several-day delay in its activation.

Both types of lymphocyte have their own subdivision of labor, as shown in Table 7–2. The subtypes of B cells are differentiated by the distinct Ig class on their surface (discussed later in the chapter). T cells, on the other hand,

are differentiated by the cluster of differentiation (CD4 or CD8) Ag on their surface.

Antibodies

Antibodies or immunoglobulins are glycoproteins produced by plasma cells (B cells activated by an Ag). Abs can be thought of as a bridge that serves to bring together the various Ags with the effector cells of the immune response. As such, their structure is closely related to their function. As seen in Figure 7–1, each Ab consists of two light chains (κ or λ) and two heavy chains (α, β, γ, δ, or ε). In any one Ab, the two heavy chains and the two light chains are identical, and they are linked to each other with disulfide bonds. The *constant region* is preserved among Abs of the same isotype, whereas the *variable region* differs and accounts for the Ag specificity. Even within the variable regions there are areas of increased variability called

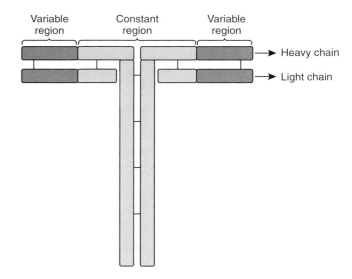

FIGURE 7–1 Basic structural elements of an antibody.

hypervariable regions, which, when the Ab folds, form the Ag-binding site, a surface complementary to a specific Ag. The immune system is able to generate Abs of different specificities by combining different variable heavy and light chains through the process of *combinatorial diversity*. This process is further enhanced by somatic recombination, a process of rearrangements at the genomic DNA level. There are five heavy-chain classes that determine specific functional characteristics of each Ab, as can be seen in Table 7–3.

Complement

Complement is a group of proteins present in low concentration in normal serum but that form a potent enzymatic cascade with significant amplification when activated. There are two pathways of complement activation by different signals that lead to the same common mechanism of action, as can be seen in Figure 7–2.

One way complement participates in immune defense is by inserting the membrane attack complex (MAC) into a target cell, resulting in subsequent membrane damage and lysis of the cell by osmotic swelling. This mode of attack is useful against intracellular organisms and thin-walled pathogens. A more important action of complement is its role as an opsonin through C3b, which leads to phagocytosis of offending organisms. Also, C3a and C5a,

known as anaphylatoxins, are responsible for mast cell and basophil degranulation and neutrophil production of reactive oxygen intermediates. In addition, C5a acts as a chemoattractant on the vascular endothelium. Finally, complement plays a role in the elimination of Ag–Ab complexes, a process central to type III hypersensitivity, which is discussed later.

Cytokines

Cytokines (some of which are referred to as "interleukins") are proteins or glycoproteins produced by monocytes (monokines), lymphocytes (lymphokines), and a wide variety of other cell types. They exert their effect on cells of the immune system and as such are key mediators of the immune response, the stress response, inflammation, infection, sepsis, allergic reactions, and graft rejection. The key producers and functions of cytokines are summarized in Table 7–4.

Interleukin-1 (IL-1) and IL-2 play a key role in the activation and proliferation of T lymphocytes and for this reason are targets for certain immunosuppressive medications such as glucocorticoids (IL-1) and the calcineurin inhibitors cyclosporin and tacrolimus (IL-2). The particular group of cytokines produced by a cell in a given situation can lead to different types of immunologic responses. More specifically, CD4+ T cells have

Table 7–3
Immunoglobulin classes

Class of Antibody	Percent of Serum Pool	Characteristics	Function
IgG	75	Four subclasses (IgG 1–4) based on H chain differences; half-life 21 days; monomer	Major Ig in secondary immune response; complement activation; protection of newborn as only Ig to cross the placenta; opsonization
IgA	15	Exists as serum IgA (IgA1) and secretory IgA (IgA2) in saliva, tears, colostrum, intestinal secretions; secretory component protects from protease; half-life in serum 6 days; monomer or dimer	Secretory; interferes with pathogen adhesion; opsonization
IgM	10	Half-life 10 days; pentamer	Predominant antibody (Ab) in primary immune response; predominant Ab produced by fetus; complement activation
IgD	1	Half-life 2–3 days; monomer	Possible role in B cell activation
IgE	Trace	Half-life 2–3 days	Great affinity for basophils and mast cells; involved in atopic reactions (anaphylaxis, asthma); defense against parasites

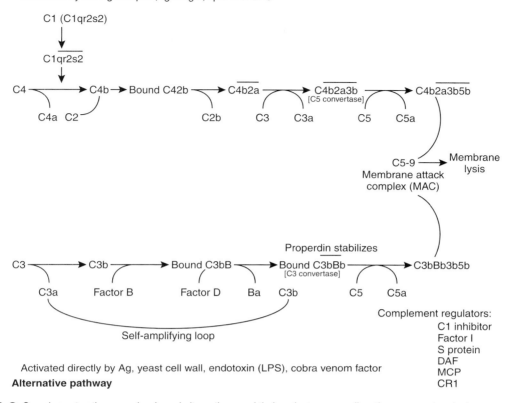

Classical pathway
Activated by Ab-Ag complex, IgM>IgG, lipid A of LPS

Activated directly by Ag, yeast cell wall, endotoxin (LPS), cobra venom factor
Alternative pathway

FIGURE 7–2 Complement pathways—classic and alternative—and their activators, as well as the common terminal sequence to which they lead. There is also a self-amplifying loop to augment the effect of this enzymatic cascade as well as several regulators to mediate it. DAF, decay accelerating factor; MCP, membrane cofactor protein, protein S (also called vitronectin).

been subdivided into two groups: Th1 and Th2 cells. It is believed that Th1 cells produce interferon-γ (IFN-γ) and IL-2, leading to cytotoxic T-cell activation and proliferation and eventually to target cell destruction (such as occurs during acute allograft rejection). On the other hand, Th2 cells produce IL-4 and IL-10 and can promote tolerance, or at least Ag-specific anergy, to the transplanted allograft. The potential to manipulate the immune response by using or targeting cytokines or their receptors or the cells that produce them is an area of great interest in the field of transplantation. Furthermore, cytokines such as IL-1 and tumor necrosis factor-α (TNF-α) have been shown to play a key role in mediating the systemic effects seen with sepsis (e.g., fever and hypotension). This has led to the possibility of using Abs or other antagonist molecules against these cytokines to control the harmful sequelae of sepsis. Unfortunately, the clinical studies conducted have not yet met with much success. Another area where cytokines have shown some promise is as biologic response modifiers in malignancy. IFN-γ and IL-2 have been used to stimulate the production of lymphokine-activated killer (LAK) cells with a 10% to 15% improvement

in survival in cases of metastatic melanoma and renal carcinoma.

Chemokines

Another important group of cellular mediators are the chemokines. They are small (8 to 14 kDa) molecules that regulate trafficking of various cell types of leukocytes through interactions with a subset of seven transmembrane, G protein-coupled receptors. Their discovery is the result of improved investigational tools, as the development of expressed sequence tag (EST) databases and bioinformatics (computer-assisted sequence analysis) have led to rapid identification of many novel genes. More than 50 chemokines have been found, with many more probably yet to come.

Chemokines, along with adhesion molecules, have been reported to be responsible for the timely recruitment of specific leukocyte populations to areas of tissue damage during the inflammatory response. Chemokine receptors have been found to act as co-receptors for human immunodeficiency virus (HIV) infection. These chemoattractive

Table 7–4
Cytokines

Cytokine	Produced by	Function
IL-1	Monocytes, DCs, Langerhans, endothelial, microglial cells	Induce expression of IL-12 rec by I cells; release of hepatic acute-phase proteins; involvement in sepsis; cytokine synthesis; influences B cells and macrophage activation
IL-2	Activated T cells (CD4+)	Proliferation of activated T cells; B-cell, macrophage, and NK cell activation
IL-3	Activated T cells, mast cells	Granulopoiesis and lymphopoiesis
IL-4	Activated T cells, mast cells, and basophils	Inhibits macrophage activation; MHC-II induction
IL-5	T cells (CD4+)	Eosinophil colony-stimulating factor; B-cell differentiation factor
IL-6	T and B cells, macrophages, fibroblasts, astrocytes, keratinocytes	B-cell differentiation; acute-phase reaction (liver); lymphocyte activation
IL-7	BM, spleen	T-cell differentiation; promotes immune effector functions in T cells, NK cells, and macrophages; modulates quantity and quality of immune responses; possible therapeutic role in transplantation, immunotherapy, and infectious diseases
IL-8	T cells, macrophages	Leukocyte chemotaxis and PMN activation; first member of chemokine family to be identified
IL-9	TH2 lymphocytes	Mast cell proliferation; T and B cell and hematopoietic progenitor cell proliferation
IL-10	T cells	Inhibits cytokine production by T and NK cells by inhibiting macrophage/ DC activation; limits inflammatory response
IL-11	BM stromal cells and several types of tissue	Mobilization of progenitor stem cells; pleiotropic effects on bone remodeling, neurons, adipocytes and GI and bronchial epithelium; anti-inflammatory effects by downregulation of TNF and other mediators
IL-12	Monocytes/macrophages, DCs, Langerhans, neutrophils, keratinocytes, microglia, astrocytes	Promotes the release of IFN-γ from T and NK cells and facilitates a Th1-type immune response; candidate for multicomponent vaccine for cancer and infectious diseases
IL-13	T cells, mast cells, keratinocytes, basophils	Modulates phenotype of B cells; role in IgE production in allergic responses; deactivating effect on monocytes with implications for autoimmune diseases
IL-15	Wide variety of cells and tissues, but not in normal T, B, or NK cells	Plays a role in protective immune responses, allograft rejection, and the pathogenesis of autoimmune disorders
IL-16	T cells, fibroblasts	Chemotactic factor for CD4 cells and eosinophils; prime resting CD4 cells for IL-2; involved in asthma and bullous pemphigoid, HIV
IL-17	T cells	Blockade of IL-17 shown to increase cardiac allograft survival; promotes synovial inflammation and cartilage degradation
IL-18	Adrenal cortex, Kupffer cells, keratinocytes, osteoblasts, epithelial cells	IFN-γ induction; apoptosis induction through the Fas ligand; possible antitumor effects
IFN	IFN-α by leukocytes; IFN-β by fibroblasts; IFN-γ by T cells	Antitumorigenic; NK cell activation; lymphocyte proliferation; antiviral effect; macrophage stimulation; DTH regulation
TNF-$\alpha\beta$	Various cells including monocytes and NK, B, and T cells	Activates macrophages and PMNs; nitric oxide (NO) production and increased vascular permeability; fever and shock mediators; role in apoptosis
GM-CSF	Various cells including T and B cells, macrophages, fibroblasts, keratinocytes, endothelial cells, mast cells	Proliferation and differentiation; control of infection; wound-healing promotion; potentiates IL-2-driven T cell cytotoxicity; apoptosis inhibition; reconstitution of immune system after irradiation, as during bone marrow transplant (BMT); neutropenia reversal
TGF-β	Platelets; various cell types	Mitogenic and proliferative effects depending on the cell; immunomodulatory potential with immunosuppressive action; both a tumor promoter and tumor suppressor
Flt3 ligand	Widely expressed in many tissues and cell types	Development of hematopoietic progenitor cells; key regulator of DCs; possible role in stem cell mobilization and immunotherapy by its effect on DCs

cytokines have also been shown to play a role in DC maturation and B and T cell development. Furthermore, they appear to be involved in infections, angiogenesis, tumor growth, and metastasis. An exciting area of chemokine research with applications to the field of transplantation is the finding that certain chemokine receptors are associated with the Th1 or Th2 phenotype. The implication is that the gradient and type of chemokines produced by these cells can affect their migration to different areas and the differentiation of specific leukocytes, thereby influencing the type of immune responses against an allograft. Finally, chemokines may prove significant therapeutic targets, leading to selective modulation or prevention of cellular interactions in the immune system through disruption of ligand binding to the G protein-coupled receptors.

Major Histocompatibility Complex

To mount a successful immune response, the APCs must present Ag to the T and B lymphocytes in conjunction with a glycoprotein known as the major histocompatibility Ag. This group of Ags is part of the major histocompatibility complex (MHC), which in essence is what makes individuals different in the context of graft acceptance and rejection. The requirement for this interaction is called MHC restriction. The MHC is encoded by a group of genes in the short arm of chromosome 6. Several loci exist for the three classes of gene products, as can be seen in Table 7–5. The ability of the immune system to respond to a variety of stimuli is based on the fact that MHC molecules are both polygenic (several genes exist for each MHC class) and polymorphic (different alleles exist for each gene).

Each individual inherits a set of MHC genes (haplotype) from each parent. The haplotypes that appear to be the most important in terms of matching in the field of transplantation are the A, B, and DR loci. An effort is made to match the donor and the recipient. MHC matching is not an absolute requirement, however, because for transplantation of some organs (liver) MHC matching does not appear to be a major determinant of rejection; with others (heart), time considerations do not allow this flexibility. The advent of improved immunosuppression

has decreased the importance of MHC matching. Furthermore, rejection may still be seen even with a perfect match (identical siblings) owing to the effect of numerous not yet well defined minor histocompatibility Ags. Despite these considerations, for organs such as the kidney and pancreas if a "perfect" match between the donor and recipient is found (six-antigen match) anywhere in the country the organ goes to its matched recipient.

Immune Response

In its quest to gain entry to the organism, an offending pathogen first must overcome a multitude of mechanical, chemical, and biologic barriers, some of which have been described previously in this chapter. If the efforts of the pathogen are successful, the pathogen is then faced with the innate, or nonspecific, immune system. Attempts to control the offending organism by the innate immune system lead eventually to inflammation, with its four principal characteristics: *rubor, calor, dolor,* and *tumor.* However, the most important task of the innate immune system is to set the stage for activation of adaptive immunity. This is done through the release of cytokines and, more importantly, through involvement of the APCs, particularly DCs and macrophages.

After the pathogen gains entry, it travels via the afferent lymphatics or the blood to various points in the body, where it comes in contact with APCs. APCs, in turn, process and present Ags of the pathogen to the effector cells of the immune system, mainly T and B lymphocytes. T and B lymphocytes have receptors specific for a certain Ag, the result of genetic combinatorial diversity; therefore through a process called the *clonal selection theory* each Ag activates a specific subset of lymphocytes.

More specifically, B cells are able to deal with Ags in the blood and extracellular spaces. There, the Ag binds to Igs on the surface of the B cell and Abs are released, representing humoral immunity. The functions of these Abs are multiple: (1) they neutralize the pathogen by binding to it, thereby blocking access to the cells; (2) they act by coating the pathogen, a process called opsonization, making the

Table 7–5 MHC classes			
Class	**Type**	**Expressed by**	**Recognized by**
I	HLA-A, -B, -C	All nucleated cells and platelets	CD8+ cells
II	HLA-DR, -DQ, -OP	B lymphocytes, activated T cells, macrophages, dendritic cells	CD4+ cells, B cells
III	Complement cascade	Complement	Cells with complement receptors

pathogen vulnerable to phagocytic cells; (3) they activate complement, which derives its name from its primary function of enabling phagocytes to destroy pathogens; and (4) they present T cells with one of the two signals they need for activation. In addition, a subset of B cells is transformed into memory cells. Memory B cells constitute the basis of immunization and enable an organism to respond in a prompt way to a later infection by the same pathogen.

Cell-mediated immunity begins when a pathogen infects the cell or is engulfed by a phagocyte and the Ag is displayed on the cell surface in association with MHC molecules (described above). This is the first signal required for T cell activation. The second is provided by professional APCs such as DCs, macrophages, and B cells. T cells exist as different subsets with different roles. Cytotoxic T cells are able to kill infected cells and hence play a central role in combating intracellular infections by bacteria, viruses, and parasites. Another subset is the helper T (Th) cells, which provide the co-stimulatory signal to naive B cells. A third, less well defined type of T cell is the regulatory/suppressor T cell, which probably controls the immune response and may therefore play a role in the quest for tolerance induction in the fields of transplantation and autoimmune diseases.

The immune response is complex. Each effector cell is equipped to control the pathogen itself. It also interacts with the other cells of the immune system, leading to a well orchestrated and significantly augmented response.

Hypersensitivity Reactions

There are situations where the immune response to an Ag can become excessive, and the effector functions activated become a threat to the host rather than a means of defense. These reactions are grouped together under the heading "hypersensitivity reactions." What further distinguishes these reactions is the fact that the "challenger" may be an otherwise innocuous Ag found in the environment or even in the host.

The reactions are the result of previous activation; and as the secondary immune responses they represent, they occur a short time after exposure. There are four major types of hypersensitivity reaction (I to IV), based on the characteristics of the immune response. Some of the basic features of these reactions are summarized in Table 7–6.

Table 7–6
Hypersensitivity reactions

Type	Basic Mechanism	Examples	Detection	Therapy
I: immediate-type hypersensitivity	Allergen binds to IgE Basophil and mast cell degranulation	Asthma, insect bites, allergic rhinitis, anaphylactic shock	Skin test; radioallergoabsorbent test, measuring level of IgE Abs specific for a particular allergen	Avoidance Hyposensitization Medications such as antihistamines, mast cell- and basophil-stabilizing (cromolyn, theophyline, epinephrine), anti-inflammatory
II: antibody-dependent cytotoxic hypersensitivity	Cell-bound antigen binds to IgG or IgM Ab-mediated cellular toxicity IgG opsonization IgM agglutination Complement activation	Goodpasture's syndrome, autoimmune hemolytic anemia, rheumatic fever, erythroblastosis fetalis	Immunofluorescence for antibodies; indirect hemagglutination assay (Coombs)	Diuretics and alkalinization of urine for transfusion reactions UV light Steroids Splenectomy for IgG (warm) hemolytic anemia
III: immune complex hypersensitivity	Complex formed by soluble antigen and IgG or IgM Complement activation	Poststreptococcal glomerulonephritis, SLE, serum sickness	Immunofluorescence for antibodies	Avoidance Corticosteroids Anti-inflammatory agents
IV: delayed-type hypersensitivity	Antigen binding to T-cell receptor Cytotoxicity as a Th1 response	Contact dermatitis, tuberculosis, viral infections	Skin test, tuberculin PPD	Avoidance Antibiotics for the infectious causes

Type I Hypersensitivity

Type I, or immediate, hypersensitivity is also known as anaphylaxis, allergy, or atopy. It occurs when the allergen responsible comes into contact with Ag-specific IgE on the surface of mast cells and basophils in a presensitized host. This eventually leads to mast cell and basophil degranulation and an amplified immune response. Because of the speed with which this occurs (seconds to minutes), this type of reaction is also known as immediate hypersensitivity. Although usually local, there are cases where the Ag obtains access to the circulation, leading to a systemic response of generalized inflammation, capillary dilation with increased vascular permeability, and smooth muscle contraction. The resulting symptoms—swelling of the upper respiratory tract, bronchoconstriction with respiratory distress, hypotension—can be rapidly fatal unless reversed, usually with epinephrine, antihistamines, and/or corticosteroid use. This condition is known as *anaphylactic shock*.

Type II Hypersensitivity

The type II hypersensitivity reaction involves binding of preformed IgG or IgM Abs with cell-bound Ags. This binding gives rise to effector mechanisms such as activation of the classic complement pathway, Ab-mediated cytotoxicity through the activation of NK cells, opsonization by IgG, and agglutination by IgM.

Type III Hypersensitivity

Also known as immune complex hypersensitivity, type II hypersensitivity reactions are initiated by formation of complexes between soluble Ag and preformed IgG or IgM Abs that are not easily cleared by the immune system. This Ag–Ab complex formation leads to activation of the complement system, especially the anaphylatoxins C3a and C5a, which act as vasodilators and chemoattractants for neutrophils, which further damage the local tissue.

Type IV Hypersensitivity

Often referred to as delayed-type hypersensitivity (DTH), the type IV reaction takes about 24 to 72 hours to develop. It results from the interaction of Ag with presensitized T cells. It is a major part of the body's response to intracellular microorganisms. DTH can also occur secondary to substances coming into contact with the skin, resulting in contact dermatitis. Some of these substances (e.g., metal ions) act as haptens, which must bind to host protein first to elicit the T-cell response.

Inheritable Syndromes of Defective Immunity

Knowledge of the mechanisms of the immune system is central to understanding the clinical syndromes caused by the many inheritable syndromes. Table 7–7 provides a list of the more important ones. The significance of these syndromes for the surgeon cannot be overemphasized, as their presence can alter the expected clinical presentation and the patient's response to many surgical diseases. They should be considered in patients with a relevant family history of nonresolving infections, poor responses to antibiotic treatment appropriate for the organism, or, most importantly, poor responses to infections caused by opportunistic organisms.

Pregnancy and the Immune System

A special note should be made about the periods of gestation and early life. During these periods the immune system is immature, as it has not had the opportunity to be exposed to immunogenic stimuli. The placenta acts as a barrier for the fetus against exposure to the many Ags to which the mother may be exposed while playing a central role as a lifeline for the fetus in terms of nutrition and oxygenation. The placenta is also responsible for the active transport of maternal IgG Abs to the fetus while the fetal immune system is unable to synthesize its own. After birth, the amount of maternal IgG decreases as the newborn starts to produce its own, with complete replacement of maternal Abs by 4 to 6 months of life. This increased Ab production continues until normal levels are achieved sometime during adolescence.

The low Ab levels during early life mean that the immune response may not be strong. This is especially true in the case of prematurity, where IgG levels are even lower than they would normally be, making these infants particularly susceptible to a variety of infections. The passage of IgG through the placenta is also responsible for hemolytic disease of the newborn (erythroblastosis fetalis), which occurs when a presensitized mother is carrying an Rh$^+$ fetus. An advantage of the immaturity of the immune system is that transplants undertaken early in life (despite the technical challenges and the scarcity of size-appropriate organs) may have an improved chance of achieving donor-specific tolerance through a process of chimerism.

Despite the fact that the fetus is a semiallogeneic graft, no rejection is seen during normal gestation. Various theories have been proposed to explain this phenomenon, including the existence of the placenta as

Table 7–7

Inheritable immune deficiency diseases

Disease	Mode of Transmission	Defect	Symptoms	Treatment
Chronic granulomatous disease	Heterogeneous group of disorders, with some X-linked recessive (I, Ia, IV) and some autosomal recessive (II, III)	Most frequent defect in cytochrome b leading to impaired generation of antimicrobial oxidizing substances (H_2O_2) during phagocytosis	Disseminated abscesses and lymphadenopathy, splenomegaly early in life followed later by suppurative granulomas in lungs, spleen, bones	Antibiotics, abscess drainage, IFN-γ, neutrophil infusion from family members as temporary measure
Chediak-Higashi disease	Autosomal recessive	Altered chemotactic function and degranulation of neutrophils, decreased NK activity	Increased susceptibility to pyogenic infections and lymphoma	Antibiotics, most patients die during childhood
Bruton's X-linked hypogammaglobu-linemia	X-linked	B cells and serum Ig low or absent, plasma cells not seen, intact T cell function	Manifests 6–12 months after birth, recurrent pyogenic infections (S. aureus, H. influenzae, S. pyogenes)	Injection of pooled human gamma globulin monthly, FFP administration, antibiotics
Common variable hypogammaglobu-linemia or immunodeficiency	Unknown, MHC-linked			Same as for Bruton's X linked hypo-gammaglobulinemia
Congenital thymic aplasia, DiGeorge syndrome	Autosomal inheritance, associated with maternal alcohol use	Failure in embryogenesis of third and fourth pharyngeal pouch from which the thymus and parathyroids arise	First symptoms secondary to hypocalcemia, increased susceptibility to infections by intracellular pathogens	Treatment of hypocalcemia, transplantation of fetal thymic tissue (controversial procedure), condition may improve by 5–6 years of age
Wiskott-Aldrich syndrome	X-linked	Lack of antibody response to polysaccharide antigens, anomalous isotype production with increased IgA and IgE and low IgM	Associated with thrombocytopenia and eczema; bleeding disorder at 6 months; susceptibility to infections by CMV, varicella, herpes simplex	Platelet transfusion for bleeding, administration of IV Ig and antibiotics, bone marrow transplantation
Severe combined immunodeficiency disorder	X-linked recessive or autosomal recessive	Both humoral and cell-mediated immunity; subtypes include ADA and PNP deficiency	Overwhelming microbial infection	Gene therapy for ADA; antibiotics and Ig; bone marrow transplantation: transplantation of fetal liver and thymus (controversial); patients usually die within 1–2 years

Table continued on opposite page

Table 7–7
Inheritable immune deficiency diseases—*Continued*

Disease	Mode of Transmission	Defect	Symptoms	Treatment
Ataxia-telangiectasia	Autosomal recessive	Selective IgA deficiency	Involves nervous system with uncoordinated muscle movements (ataxia), vascular system with dilatation of small blood vessels (telangiectasia), and sinopulmonary infections	Antibiotics for infections, treatment of complications
Complement deficiencies	Many	Classic pathway and C3 → wide range of pyogenic infections as defective opsonization and phagocytosis; C5–9 → *Neisseria* susceptibility as cannot effect extracellular lysis; C1, C2, C4 → inability to eliminate immune complexes leading to autoimmune diseases (i.e., SLE); C1 inhibitor deficiency → uncontrolled activation of classic pathway with increased activation of vasoactive C2a, leading to hereditary angioneurotic edema	Supportive care and antibiotics

ADA, adenosine deaminase; PNP, purine nucleotide phosphorylase.

an immune-privileged site, where the trophoblastic layer represents an immunologic barrier by not exhibiting full MHC expression. Another hypothesis is that a state of tolerance is achieved by production of anti-inflammatory cytokines from the trophoblasts, such as IL-4, IL-10, and TGF-β, which lead to a predominantly Th2 response.

Transplantation

Terminology

At this point in the chapter we turn our attention to transplantation. It represents an exciting field with continuous progress that challenges the surgeon in terms of technical skill and his or her knowledge of immunology. Before proceeding further, it is useful to review some of the terms widely used in the transplantation field. The organ to be transplanted is known as the *graft*. Grafts that are placed in a different anatomic position in the same individual, such as parathyroid tissue following a parathyroidectomy, are known as *autografts*. When the transplant is between genetically identical individuals (identical twins), it is referred to as an *isograft* or *syngeneic graft*. Grafts between individuals of the same species are known as *allografts* or *homografts*, whereas those between members of different species are known as *xenografts* or *heterografts*. The type of graft determines to a large extent its acceptance by the

recipient: Xenografts are prone to hyperacute (within minutes) rejection, whereas isografts can be readily accepted with minimal if any immunosuppression. Another subdivision is between solid organ transplantation (heart, kidney, liver, pancreas, lung, small bowel) and that involving cells alone, such as bone marrow transplantation (BMT) and pancreatic islet cell transplantation.

The low availability of donors for most types of transplantation has led to some innovations. More specifically, the scarcity of livers and the need for smaller grafts for the pediatric population has led to *reduced-size* and *split liver* transplantation. For reduced-size grafts, the graft is downsized usually to a lobe, thereby allowing less time to find a suitable donor and in effect decreasing pretransplant mortality. Patient survival at 1 year has ranged between 70% and 80%, which is similar to that associated with conventional liver transplantation. In the case of the split liver, precluding any vascular or biliary anomalies of the graft, the liver is divided into one part that includes segments 2, 3, and 4 and another that involves the rest. Thus two recipients, usually an adult and a pediatric patient, can benefit from a single donor. Another method has been the use of *living-related donors* for kidney and livers (using the left lateral segment) with results that equal or surpass those with cadaveric donations, again increasing the pool of potential donors. Finally, the use of *living-unrelated* or *"emotionally related"* donors for renal grafts with outcomes similar to those with three Ag matches has served to underscore the importance of a short ischemia period and decreased preservation injury. Advantages of living-related and living-unrelated donation, apart from the apparently decreased risk of rejection, include less immunosuppression and a shorter time on the waiting list, which translates into fewer complications arising from the recipient's own organ failure. The main disadvantage is the fact that a healthy donor must undergo major surgery, something that makes maximum care when handling tissues a priority.

Grafts can also be divided according to their anatomic placement in the recipient. Those placed in the same position as the recipient's diseased organ are known as *orthotopic transplants* (e.g., liver, heart). Often grafts are placed in a different position because (1) there is no benefit in removing the recipient's own organ and further complicating an already challenging procedure and (2) it allows easier access for future biopsies of the grafts. These replacements are known as *heterotopic transplantation*; they include renal and pancreatic grafts and pancreatic islet transplants, where the islets are infused through the portal vein via a minimally invasive but not always successful procedure. However, in the case of islet transplantation there is renewed hope, as a group from the University of Alberta in Canada has shown that in patients with type 1 diabetes islet transplantation can result in insulin independence with excellent metabolic control when glucocorticoid-free immunosuppression is combined with infusion of an adequate islet mass.

Immunologic Testing

A battery of immunology tests are required prior to transplantation to determine the suitability of the graft for the recipient. This includes *ABO testing*, which follows the rules of blood transfusions in that type O recipients can receive only type O grafts, whereas AB recipients can receive grafts of all types. *Histocompatibility testing* and its implications have been discussed previously in the chapter. It should be noted that LILA typing is not in and of itself an indication that the graft will be accepted, as it should be determined whether the recipient has Abs against the donor. This is done by the *cytotoxic crossmatch*, where serum of the recipient is incubated with lymphocytes of the potential donor. A positive crossmatch is liable to lead to hyperacute rejection. The extensive reticuloendothelial system of the liver makes crossmatching less of a necessity, as Abs may be phagocytized by Kupffer cells. For the heart, crossmatching is not always practiced because of the time constraints, although it has been shown to have some effect. Finally, the sera of potential recipients are tested periodically against a panel of the most frequent Ags to determine the *percent panel-reactive antibody* (% PRA). This provides a measure of the reactivity of the recipient, and the higher number in the case of renal allografts makes finding a suitable donor more difficult. This can change over time as the patient is exposed to different Ags (e.g., with transfusions or pregnancies) and is thus done periodically while the potential recipient is on the waiting list.

Rejection Phenomena

As a result of transplantation, donor hematolymphoid cells migrate from the allograft to the recipient's lymphoid and nonlymphoid tissues simultaneously with an influx of recipient cells into the allograft. This interaction between donor and recipient cells causes bidirectional allostimulation of T cells. If there is failure to reach a "balance" between these two immunologic "rivals," rejection occurs. As can be seen in Table 7–8, there are various types of rejection, each with its own characteristics.

Table 7–8
Types of allograft rejection

Type	Timing	Mediators	General Histology
Hyperacute	Minutes to hours, usually in the operating room	Preformed antibodies, usually seen with xenografts; complement and cloning cascade activation with blood vessel thrombosis	Ischemic thrombosis of the graft
Acute	Weeks to months	Th1 activation, involvement of IL-2, IFN-γ, TNF-α, IL-3, and chemokines	Arterial inflammation or necrosis, interstitial hemorrhage
Chronic	Months to years	CD4-Th2 cells combined with antibody- and cell-mediated components	Obliterative arteriopathy, patchy interstitial inflammation, fibrosis and associated parenchymal atrophy, depletion of organ-specific lymphoid tissue

Factors that influence rejection include preformed Abs as a result of pregnancy, prior transplantation or transfusion, or the presence of ABO or MHC incompatibility. As with MHC, any degree of mismatching results in progressive attrition of graft function over time, especially with heart, kidney, lung, and pancreas grafts. Prolonged cold ischemia time, use of marginal donors, and preservation injury to the graft have been shown to stress the allograft and increase its immunogenicity. Other factors that influence rejection include the adequacy of immunosuppression and donor age. Specifically for acute rejection, age, sex, and race have been shown to have a small influence, as younger, healthier, female, black recipients show increased responsiveness to the donor organ. Chronic rejection in turn has been shown to have an association with prior viral infections, such as from a cytomegalovirus (CMV)-positive donor to a CMV-negative recipient. Also, chronic rejection appears more frequently in the setting of severe or persistent episodes of acute rejection, raising the hypothesis of repetitive injury to the organ. A donor with atherosclerosis and a recipient with conventional risks of atherosclerosis have also been associated with an increased risk of chronic rejection.

Overall, identification of rejection and its severity consists of a combination of histopathologic evaluation, radiologic testing (ultrasonography, computed tomography, magnetic resonance imaging), and the presence of symptoms indicating declining organ function. Diagnostic tools to guide immunosuppressive therapy, in addition to the patient's signs and symptoms, vary according to the organ(s), although biopsy is a constant aid. More specifically, apart from the use of biopsy, coronary angiography is used for the heart, and pulmonary function tests are useful for the lung. Possible indicators of rejection are assays to measure serum creatinine for the kidney; bilirubin, γ-glutamyl transferase (GGT), transaminases, and alkaline phosphatase for the liver; urinary amylase or serum amylase, lipase, and glucose for the pancreas; and endoscopy for the small bowel.

Treatment of acute rejection consists mainly of adjusting the immunosuppressive regimen, with the patient usually responsive. Much less success has been seen with chronic rejection, where the main strategy has been to increase or change the baseline immunosuppression. Unfortunately, it is too late in most cases to stop either the accumulated immunologic injury or the functional decline of the organ.

Graft-Versus-Host Disease

Graft-versus-host disease (GVHD) represents a special situation in the fight between the donor's and the recipient's immune systems, where engrafted immunocompetent donor T lymphocytes, stimulated mainly by DCs, respond to alloantigens on the host cells and threaten the immuno-compromised host. This is seen mainly in BM and small bowel transplantation, as in both cases the graft carries a significant number of donor-derived passenger leukocytes. The incidence of GVHD is 50% to 70% when an HLA-matched sibling is the donor for BM transplantation; the figure increases in cases of partial MHC mismatches.

In its acute form, GVHD includes a maculopapular skin rash, hepatitis, enteritis, and delayed hematologic reconstitution. A mononuclear cell infiltrate with CD8+ T and NK cells is seen in the epithelium of the oropharynx, the crypts of the intestine, and the periportal areas of the liver. In its chronic form, GVHD presents with sclerodermic changes of the skin, xerostomia, xerophthalmia, malabsorption, and skin and joint contractures. Pathologically, there is no mononuclear cell infiltrate but, rather, marked collagen deposition and fibrosis in the dermis, lamina propria of the intestine, and portal triad. These changes are thought to be the result of uncontrolled action of host-responsive T cells with a helper phenotype that stimulate fibroblast proliferation and collagen synthesis through the elaboration of a proinflammatory cytokine environment.

Prevention of GVHD has mainly consisted of (1) modifying the graft by depleting it of alloreactive T cells or some subpopulations of passenger leukocytes through the use of irradiation or (2) using immunosuppressive agents such as methotrexate, prednisone, or cyclosporine. Treatment of GVHD consists mainly of immunosuppression and is more successful with acute than with chronic GVHD.

Therapeutic Immunomodulation

Some of the main strategies to combat rejection include the use of immunosuppressive medication as well as efforts to induce acceptance of the graft. The main immunosuppressive medications and their mechanisms, effects, and toxicities are shown in Table 7–9. These medications are used as part of a combination to increase their therapeutic effectiveness by intervening at more than one stage of the immune pathway and to decrease toxicity from any one agent.

Another way to prevent rejection is to achieve immunologic tolerance of the graft by the recipient's immune system. This represents the "holy grail" of transplantation, as achieving immunologic tolerance would translate to long-term donor Ag-specific graft acceptance without the maintenance and adverse effects of immunosuppression. Although several strategies are being actively investigated, none has yet to meet with uniform success and acceptance.

Hematopoietic chimerism associated with, and as a basis for, transplantation tolerance represents the

Table 7–9
Immunosuppressive medications

Medication	Mechanism of Action	Effect during Transplantation	Side Effects/Toxicity
Corticosteroids	Bind intracellular receptors and inhibit DNA and RNA synthesis	Inhibit IL-1, primary immunosuppression	Hypertension, peptic ulcer disease, striae, buffalo hump, obesity, hyperglycemia, hypernatremia, avascular necrosis of femoral head, osteoporosis, psychosis
Cyclosporine (CsA)	Cyclic peptide of fungal origin that binds to intracellular T cell receptors; cyclophillin, which inhibits calcineurin	Suppresses T-cell activation by blocking IL-2; primary immunosuppression	Hirsutism, neurotoxicity, nephrotoxicity, hyperglycemia, hepatotoxicity, hyperkalemia, gingival hyperplasia
Azathioprine	Antimetabolite that inhibits conversion of inosine monophosphate (IMP) to essential purines	Inhibits cell proliferation in nonspecific manner; in the past, primary immunosuppression	Severe bone marrow suppression, hepatotoxicity
OKT3	Anti-CD3 monoclonal Ab that binds to the T cell receptor complex	Induction therapy and rejection not responsive to standard regimen; rapid sensitization	Pulmonary edema shortly after administration of dose, fever, chills
Antilymphocyte globulin (ALG)	Polyclonal serum obtained by injecting human lymphocytes into various species	Acts against mature T cells; used as induction and for acute rejection	Fever, thrombocytopenia, leukopenia, anemia
Tacrolimus (FK506)	Macrolide antibiotic of fungal origin; different structure from CsA but same mechanism of blocking FKB-binding protein and inhibiting calcineurin	Inhibits T cell activation and maturation by blocking IL-2; 500 times more potent than CsA; primary immunosuppression	Nephrotoxicity, hyperglycemia, tremors, headache
Mycophenolate mofetil(MMF)	Modified eater of mycophenolic acid; blocks de novo purine synthesis	Inhibits B and T cell proliferation selectively; primary immunosuppression	Nausea, emesis, diarrhea
Sirolimus (rapamycin)	Macrolide antibiotic of fungal origin with mechanism similar to FK506, including same receptors	Inhibits activated cell proliferation induced by IL-2 and IL-4; synergistic with CsA; antiproliferative effect	Thrombocytopenia, leukopenia, hyperlipidemia
Daclizumab (Xenapax)	IgG monoclonal Ab to the Tac subunit of IL-2, which functions as an IL-2 receptor antagonist	Inhibits IL-2-mediated lymphocyte activation; used in prevention of acute rejection during renal transplantation in combination with other medications, such as CsA and steroids	Hypersensitivity reactions, gastrointestinal symptoms
Deoxyaspergualin (DSG)	Unknown; possibly through binding of HSP-70	Inhibits differentiation of B and T cells into fully mature cells; inhibits macrophage IL-1 production; reduces preformed Abs in xenografts; useful in combination regimen	Paresthesias, sporadic myelosuppression, gastrointestinal toxicity

coexistence of the donor's and recipient's immune systems. The premise was first shown in the seminal work by Owen and then Medawar in nonidentical cattle and mice twins. Its significance became obvious with the groundbreaking work of Starzl, who analyzed a small group of fortunate liver allograft recipients who had achieved long-term graft acceptance without the need for immunosuppression. He found that the recipients and the grafts were both chimeras through a postulated process of reciprocal clonal expansion and depletion of immune cells in graft and recipient, something referred to as the "two-way paradigm." To achieve this chimerism in the immunocompetent host, recipient preconditioning such as irradiation and/or cytoreductive chemotherapy combined with T cell-depleting Abs and/or conventional immunosuppression may be needed. After creating this suitable environment, donor BM infusion is used to induce the state of chimerism. The mechanisms involved are thought to include central deletion as well as peripheral mechanisms. Several centers are currently evaluating clinical protocols whereby vascularized organ allograft recipients are given donor BM infusions at the time of transplantation.

Efforts to induce tolerance through the process of microchimerism have centered on the effect of passenger leukocytes on the recipient's immune system. Prominent among these donor-derived cells are DCs, which play a key role in both the direct and indirect pathways of allorecognition. When stimulated to mature, they upregulate surface levels of MHC Ags, T cell co-stimulatory molecules (CD4O, CD8O, CD86), and intercellular adhesion molecules involved in DC–T cell interaction. They migrate to T-cell areas in the LNs or the spleen. There has been a need to reexamine the ontogeny of DCs, as research has shown that, apart from those developing from the myeloid progenitor (myeloid DC), there is another group developing from committed lymphoid precursors. The significance of this lies in the fact that although the two DC subsets when mature are equally efficient at priming naive T cells, the responses they induce may indeed be different. One type of DC may promote a Th1 response, whereas the other may result in a Th2 or mixed Th1/Th2 response.

The fact that molecular signaling between DC and naive (THO) cells in a specific cytokine environment directs their differentiation into Th1 or Th2 cells has significant implications for transplantation. It has recently been shown that certain cytokines (e.g., IL-10) can inhibit IL-12 production by DCs and lead to the predominance of Th2 or likely regulatory T cells, with potential for establishing donor cell microchimerism and tolerance. Experimental DC-targeted approaches for treating organ allograft rejection include administration of co-stimulatory blocking agents together with donor DCs or genetic engineering of DCs to express "tolerogenic" molecules

such as cytotoxic T leukocyte antigen-4–Ig (CTLA4-Ig), IL-10, or transforming growth factor-β1 (TGF-β1).

Complications

The technical and immunologic challenges the transplant team and the patient encounter mean that there is a significant number of complications of which both need to be aware. These complications can be broadly subdivided into those associated with the surgical procedure itself and those that are unique to the immunosuppressed patient. It should be stressed that this subdivision is not as clear in practice as in theory, and the clinician faced with worsening function of a graft should consider both technical and immunologic problems such as rejection.

Surgical complications

As with most types of surgery, wound infections, seçomas, and hematomas can occur. The immunosuppressed and often malnourished patient is at a disadvantage dealing with these complications, and special care is needed during the operation when handling tissues and achieving hemostasis. Lymphoceles deserve special mention as they can occur with relative frequency, especially following renal transplantation. They can cause problems in terms of infection compression of the vascular supply to the graft.

Any time multiple anastomoses are required, there is the potential for leaks or thrombosis. Some examples include urinary leaks secondary to increased tension or due to the tenuous vascular supply of the transplanted ureter. Such leaks can often be treated by stenting; if this does not resolve the leak, reoperation with creation of a neoureterocystostomy or pyeloureterostomy to the host ureter may be required. In the case of the kidney, renal vein thrombosis can present with proteinuria, whereas in a pancreatic graft arterial or venous thrombosis may present early with increased blood glucose levels. The latter is responsible for 20% of graft losses. With liver transplantation, hepatic artery thrombosis predisposes the graft to hepatic abscess formation and often leads to the need for retransplantation.

As with any type of surgical patient, special attention by the anesthesiologist is required. Good communication with the surgeon is needed to prevent or manage complications, such as the coagulopathy of the anhepatic phase during liver transplantation and possible fluid overload. The latter can easily compromise the newly placed liver and its function. In the case of renal transplantation, medications cleared by the kidney, such as certain muscle relaxants, should be avoided.

Complications unique to the transplant patient

Rejection represents a great threat to the graft and necessitates continuous monitoring by the clinician. It can occur at any point following transplantation, as was previously described with the various types of rejection. Any change in graft function or overall health of the patient should lead, in addition to consideration of a biopsy, to tests that would potentially uncover rejection: serum creatinine for the kidney; transaminases, alkaline phosphatase, bilirubin, and GGT for the liver; and urinary amylase (if bladder drainage is employed) or serum glucose (an increase is a late finding) for the pancreas. For some organs, such as the heart and the small bowel, the best way to identify rejection promptly is periodic biopsies, as other indicators have not proven as successful. Efforts to treat rejection consist of either adjusting the dose of the primary immunosuppressive regimen or changing to different types of medication. The use of immunosuppression has its own potential toxicities, as can be seen in Table 7–9.

Another severe, often life-threatening complication is infection, which can occur during the early postoperative period as well as throughout the life of the recipient. Transplant patients are extremely susceptible to infections because of the immunosuppression. These infections can present insidiously, with mild, often nonspecific symptoms (e.g., fever, headache, general malaise) at the onset. They include the common bacterial infections as well as infection with other opportunistic organisms, such as fungal (*Candida albicans* and *Aspergillus*), protozoan (*Pneumocystis carinii*), and viral (cytomegalovirus, herpes simplex, herpes zoster) pathogens. In many cases they become rapidly systemic, necessitating a decrease in the immunosuppressive regimen with potential graft loss. Often the symptoms mimic those of rejection, presenting the clinician with a diagnostic challenge with very different or, more accurately, exactly the opposite modes of treatment for each case. Management of these infections consists of antibiotic prophylaxis as well as treatment appropriate for each infection.

Progress has been made with the use of agents such as hyperimmune serum and ganciclovir for CMV and acyclovir for viral infections. Another important group, especially considering that hepatitis C represents the most common indication for liver transplantation, is the one where reactivation of hepatitis is seen following transplantation. Reactivation can occur 7 to 10 years after transplantation for both hepatitis B and hepatitis C. With the progression to cirrhosis, the patient returns to the waiting list. Given the chronic organ shortage, this situation has raised the issue in some centers of using grafts from HCV carriers for HCV-positive recipients.

Other complications include primary nonfunction of the graft, which occurs for livers at a rate of 5% to 10%. This is the result mainly of severe preservation injury or the use of a marginal donor, and it contributes to significant morbidity and mortality. Liver graft preservation injury is related to the cold ischemia time. Pathologic features include sinusoidal endothelial cell damage and hepatocellular edema. Complement and other mediators, such as platelets, adhesion molecules, cytokines, reactive oxygen intermediates, and eicosanoid products have been implicated. Prominent among them appears to be nitric oxide (NO), the discovery of which led to a Nobel Prize in Medicine in 1998. NO has been recognized to play critical roles during infection, inflammation, and rejection; and it has recently been shown to have at least moderate beneficial effects in several models of liver injury.

Finally, transplant patients show an increased risk for certain malignancies, including lymphoma, skin cancer (basal and squamous cell mainly), and cervical cancer, and for the development of the post-transplant lymphoproliferative disorders (PTLD). The latter represent polyclonal B-cell lymphoproliferative disorders, which appear to be a consequence of heavy immunosuppression and in some cases are associated with Epstein-Barr virus infection. Lymphomas constitute 20% of cancers in transplant patients compared with only 5% in the general population. PTLD has a higher incidence of central nervous system involvement, which is again rare in the general population. Some possible explanations for this increased incidence of malignancy following transplantation include decreased immunosurveillance and susceptibility to viral infections. Management includes treatment appropriate for the malignancy and a decrease in, or even termination of, the immunosuppression.

Conclusions

For the surgical specialist, immunology provides important insights into the pathogenesis of allograft rejection. Moreover, improved understanding of the role of specific molecules and cell populations in immunologically mediated events provides a rational basis for the design of novel therapies that are likely to lead to improved outcomes in organ transplantation. However, what probably makes the field of transplantation most appealing is the rapid and continuing evolution of the field, leaving us with the belief that the best is yet to come.

Bibliography

Alard P, Matriano JA, Socarras S, et al: Detection of donor-derived cells by polymerase chain reaction in neonatally tolerant mice: microchimerism fails to predict tolerance. Transplantation 1995;60:1125-1130.

Barber WH, Mankin JA, Laskow DA, et al: Long-term results of a controlled prospective study with transfusion of donor-specific bone marrow in 57 cadaveric renal allograft recipients. Transplantation 1991;51:70-75.

Beatty PG, Hansen JA: Bone marrow transplantation for the treatment of hematologic diseases: status in 1992. Leukemia 1993;7:1123-1129.

Bell D, Young JW, Banchereau J: Dendritic cells. Adv Immunol 1999;72:255-324.

Billingham RE, Lampkin GH, Medawar PB, et al: Tolerance to homografts, twin diagnosis, and the freemartin condition in cattle. Heredity 1952;6:201.

Blaese RM, Culver KW, Miller AD: T lymphocyte-directed gene therapy for ADA-SCID: initial trial results after 4 years. Science 1995;270:475-480.

Blakolmer K, Seaberg EC, Batts K, et al: Analysis of the reversibility of chronic liver allograft rejection implications for a staging schema. Am J Surg Pathol 1999;23:1328-1339.

Bodey B, Bodey B, Siegel SE, et al: Molecular biological ontogenesis of the thymic reticulo-epithelial cell network during the organization of the cellular microenvironment. In Vivo 1999;13:267-294.

Broelsch CE, Emond JC, Whitington PF, et al: Application of reduced-size liver transplants as split grafts, auxiliary orthotopic grafts, and living related segmental transplants. Ann Surg 1990;212:368-377.

Chao NJ, Schmidt GM, Niland JC, et al: Cyclosporine, methotrexate and prednisone compared with cyclosporine and prednisone for prophylaxis of acute graft-versus-host disease. N Engl J Med 1993;329:1225-1230.

Delmas S, Picot MC, Vergnes C, et al: Risk factors of chronic rejection in kidney transplantation, results of a single center study. Nephrologie 1999;20:153-158.

Doranz BJ, Grovit-Ferbas K, Sharron MP, et al: A small-molecule inhibitor directed against the chemokine receptor CXCR4 prevents its use as an WV-i coreceptor. J Exp Med 1997;186:1395-1400.

European FK506 Multicentre Liver Study Group: Randomised trial comparing tacrolimus (FK506) and cyclosporin in prevention of liver allograft rejection. Lancet 1994;344:423-428.

Feng Y, Broder CC, Kennedy PE, et al: HIV-1 entry cofactor: functional cDNA cloning of a seven-transmembrane, G protein-coupled receptor. Science 1996;272:872-877.

Forster R, Enrich T, Kremmer E, et al: Expression of the G-protein-coupled receptor BLR1 defines mature, recirculating B cells and a subset of T-helper memory cells. Blood 1994;84:830-840.

Garcia-Morales R, Carreno M, Mathew J, et al: Continuing observations on the regulatory effects of donor-specific bone marrow cell infusions and chimerism in kidney transplant recipients. Transplantation 1998;65:956-965.

Gingrich RD, Ginder GD, Goeken D, et al: Allogeneic marrow grafting with partially mismatched, unrelated donors. Blood 1988;71:1375-1381.

Grattan MT, Moreno-Cabral CE, Starnes VA, et al: Cytomegalovirus infection is associated with cardiac allograft rejection and atherosclerosis. JAMA 1989;261:3561-3566.

Guirao X, Lowry SF: Biologic control of injury and inflammation: much more than too little or too late. World J Surg 1996;20:437-446.

Hartley SB, Cooke MP, Fulcher DA, et al: Elimination of self-reactive B lymphocytes proceeds in two stages-arrested development and cell death. Cell 1993;72:325-335.

Hayry P, Mennander A, Yilmaz S, et al: Towards understanding the pathophysiology of chronic rejection. Clin Invest 1992;70:780-790.

Hyde RM: Immunology (3rd ed). Malvern: Williams and Wilkins, 1995:226-238.

Ildstad ST, Sachs DH: Reconstitution with syngeneic plus allogeneic or xenogeneic bone marrow leads to specific acceptance of allografts or xenografts. Nature 1984;307:168-170.

Ildstad ST, Wren SM, Bluestone JA, et al: Characterization of mixed allogeneic chimeras: immunocompetence, in vitro reactivity, and genetic specificity of tolerance. J Exp Med 1985;162:231-244.

International Working Party: Terminology for hepatic allograft rejection. Hepatology 1995;22:648-654.

Janeway CA, Travers P: Immunobiology: The Immune System in Health and Disease, 3M edition. London and New York, Current Biology and Garland Publishing, 1997:5.15-5.28.

Kalinski P, Hilkens CM, Wierenga EA, et al: T-cell priming by type-1 and type-2 polarized dendritic cells: the concept of a third signal. Immunol Today 1999;20:561-567.

Kasiske BL: Clinical correlates to chronic renal allograft rejection. Kidney 1997;63(Suppl):S71-S74.

Kinoshita T: Biology of complement: the overture. Immunol Today 1991;12:291-295.

Kobayashi H, Nonami T, Kurokawa T, et al: Role of endogenous nitric oxide in ischemia reperfusion injury in rat liver. J Surg Res 1995;59:772-779.

Kobel DE, Friedl A, Cerny T, et al: Pneumococcal vaccine in patients with absent or dysfunctional spleen. Mayo Clin Proc 2000;75:749-753.

Lafferty LU, Gazda LS: Tolerance: a case of self/not-self discrimination maintained by clonal deletion? Hum Immunol 1997;52:119-126.

Lynch AM, Kapila R: Overwhelming postsplenectomy infection. Infect Dis Clin North Am 1996;10:693-707.

Margolin KA: Interleukin-2 in the treatment of renal cancer. Semin Oncol 2000;27:194-203.

Monaco Ap, Burke IF, Ferguson RM, et al: Current thinking on chronic renal allograft rejection: issues, concerns, and recommendations from a 1997 roundtable discussion. Am J Kidney Dis 1999;33:150-160.

Morelli AE, Thomson AW: Role of dendritic cells in the immune response against allografts. Curr Opin Nephrol Hypertens 2000;9:607-613.

Murakami T, Nakajima T, Koyanagi Y, et al: A small molecule CXCR4 inhibitor that blocks T cell line-tropic HIV-1 infection. J Exp Med 1997;186:1389-1393.

Ober C: The maternal-fetal relationship in human pregnancy: an immunogenetic perspective. Exp Clin Immunogenet 1992;9:1-14.

O'Connell PJ, Morelli AE, Logar AJ, et al: Phenotypic and functional characterization of mouse hepatic CD8a+ lymphoid-related dendritic cells. J Immunol 2000;165: 795-803.

Ohmori H, Dhar DK, Nakashima Y, et al: Beneficial effects of FK409, a novel nitric oxide donor, on reperfusion injury of rat liver. Transplantation 1998;66:579-585.

Opal SM, Fisher CJ, Dhainaut IF, et al: Confirmatory interleukin-1 receptor antagonist trial in severe sepsis: a phase III, randomized, double-blind, placebo-controlled, multicenter trial: the Interleukin-1 Receptor Antagonist Sepsis Investigator Group. Crit Care Med 1997;25: 1115-1124.

O'Reilly RJ, Papadopoulos E, Boulad F: Allogeneic bone marrow transplantation. *In* Bach FH, Auchincloss H Jr (eds): Transplantation Immunology. New York: Wiley-Liss, 1995:161.

Owen RD: Immunogenetic consequences of vascular anastomoses between bovine twins. Science 1945;102:400-401.

Pachter HL, Grau J: The current status of splenic preservation. Arch Surg 2000;34:137-174.

Philip PA, Flaherty L: Treatment of malignant melanoma with interleukin-2. Semin Oncol 1997;24(Suppl 4):S32-S38.

Pulendran B, Smith IL, Caspary G, et al: Distinct dendritic cell subsets differentially regulate the class of immune response in vivo. Proc Natl Acad Sci USA 1999;96:1036-1041.

Reyes J, Gerber D, Mazariegos GV, et al: Split-liver transplantation: a comparison of ex-vivo and in situ techniques. J Pediatr Surg 2000;35:283-289.

Rissoan MC, Soumelis V, Kadowaki N, et al: Reciprocal control of T helper cell and dendritic cell differentiation. Science 1999;283:1183-1186.

Rogiers X, Malago M, Habib N, et al: In situ splitting of the liver in the heart-beating cadaveric organ donor for transplantation in two recipients. Transplantation 1995;59: 1081-1083.

Roncarolo MG, Levings MK: The role of different subsets of T regulatory cells in controlling autoimmunity. Curr Opin Immunol 2000;12:676-683.

Sallusto F, Mackay CR, Lanzavecchia A: Selective expression of the eotaxin receptor CCR3 by human T helper 2 cells. Science 1997;277:2005-2007.

Schols D, Struyf S, Van Damme J, et al: Inhibition of T-tropic FIIV strains by selective antagonization of the chemokine receptor CXCR4. J Exp Med 1997;186:1383-1388.

Seaman WE: Natural killer cells and natural killer T cells. Arthritis Rheum 2000;43:1204-1217.

Shapiro AMJ, Lakey JRT, Ryan EA, et al: Islet transplantation in seven patients with type 1 diabetes mellitus using a glucocorticoid-free immunosuppressive regimen. N Engl J Med 2000;343:230-238.

Shapiro R, Rao AS, Fontes P, et al: Combined simultaneous kidney-bone marrow transplantation. Transplantation 1995;60:1421-1425.

Sozzani S, Allavena P, D'Amico G, et al: Differential regulation of chemokine receptors during dendritic cell maturation: a model for their trafficking properties. J Immunol 1998;161:1083-1086.

Starzl TE, Demetris AJ: Transplantation milestones: viewed with one- and two-way paradigms of tolerance. JAMA 1995;273:876-879.

Starzl TE, Demetris AJ, Murase N, et al: Cell migration, chimerism, and graft acceptance. Lancet 1992;339:1579-1582.

Strieter RM, Polverini PJ, Arenberg DA, et al: Role of C-X-C chemokines as regulators of angiogenesis in lung cancer. J Leukoc Biol 1995;57:752-762.

Swinnen U: Diagnosis and treatment of transplant-related lymphoma. Ann Oncol 2000;11(Suppl 1):45-48.

Terasaki P1, Cecka JM, Gjerston DW, et al: High survival rates of kidney transplants from spousal and living unrelated donors. N Engl J Med 1995;333:333-336.

Thomson AW, Lu L: Are dendritic cells the key to liver transplant tolerance? Immunol Today 1999;20:27-32.

Thomson AW, Lu L: Dendritic cells as regulators of immune reactivity: implications for transplantation. Transplantation 1999;68:1-8.

Tkayama T, Nishioka Y, Lu L, et al: Retroviral delivery of viral interleukin-10 into myeloid dendritic cells markedly inhibits their allostimulatory activity and promotes the induction of T-cell hyporesponsiveness. Transplantation 1998;66:1567-1574.

Tuczu EM, Hobbs RE, Rincon G, et al: Occult and frequent transmission of atherosclerotic coronary disease with cardiac transplantation: insights from intravascular ultrasound. Circulation 1995;91:1706-1713.

Van Saase IL, Van der Woude FJ, Thorogood J, et al: The relation between acute vascular and interstitial renal allograft rejection and subsequent chronic rejection. Transplantation 1995;59:1280-1285.

Vetro SW, Bellanti JA: Fetal and neonatal immunoincompetence. Fetal Ther 1989;4(Suppl 1):82-91.

Vicari AP, Figueroa DJ, Hedrick JA, et al: TECK: a novel CC chemokine specifically expressed by thymic dendritic cells and potentially involved in T cell development. Immunity 1997;7:291-301.

Weir DM, Stewart J: Immunology (8th ed). Edinburgh: Churchill Livingstone, 1997:285-293.

Whitehead B, Rees P, Sorensen K, et al: Incidence of obliterative bronchiolitis after heart-lung transplantation in children. J Heart Lung Transplant 1993;12:903-908.

Winters GL, Kendall TJ, Radio SJ, et al: Posttransplant obesity and hyperlipidemia: major predictors of severity of coronary arteriopathy in failed human heart allografts. J Heart Transplant 1990;9:364-371.

Zlotnik A, Yoshie O: Chemokines: a new classification system and their role in immunity. Immunity 2000;12:121-127.

CHAPTER 8

Principles and Practice of Transplantation

R. Randal Bollinger, M.D., Ph.D., M.B.A.
and Mariano S. Dy-Liacco, M.D.

From its modest beginnings, solid organ transplantation has developed into a standard medical and surgical therapy for end-stage organ failure. It is a field that combines surgical innovation with clinical immunology. The replacement of human tissue with that from other living creatures has long been a goal of health care providers but only recently has been realized clinically. The reality of establishing vascular anastomosis as accomplished by Alexis Carrel in 1902, and his early work on kidney transplantation, began the modern era of transplantation. Carrel suspected that attempts at allotransplantation failed without exception because of immunologic mechanisms, but he did not pursue these mechanisms as a part of his later research efforts. In 1942, Peter Medawar and Thomas Gibson published their landmark paper on skin homografts. Their observations of sequential skin grafts in burned aviators firmly established rejection as an immunologic phenomenon. From these humble beginnings followed delineations of human histocompatibility antigens, tissue typing, and their effects on kidney graft survival. Joseph Murray showed the surgical viability of organ transplantation in 1954 when he performed the first successful renal transplant between identical twins, an accomplishment that garnered him a Nobel Prize. The development of surgical techniques for liver transplantation by Thomas Starzl in the late 1960s, and the introduction of antithymocyte globulin as well as the new immunosuppressive agent cyclosporine in 1983, revolutionized the modern era of transplantation.

Currently, transplantation of the kidney, liver, pancreas, heart, and lung are clinical realities for patients with end-stage organ failure. Survival rates for these organs all exceed 75% at 1 year. Postoperatively, the majority of patients stay in the hospital less than a week in some centers and enjoy an uneventful postoperative recovery. The care of transplant patients is truly a multidisciplinary specialty. Physicians with backgrounds in internal medicine, surgery, infectious diseases, and critical care all participate in the care of these very complex but rewarding patient populations. In this chapter, fundamental immunology of transplanted organs is discussed, as well as basic immunotherapy regimens to prevent rejection postoperatively. Specific drugs and their mechanisms of action are described. The essential elements of a pretransplant work-up as well as the common postoperative complications are covered. This chapter will be useful for the education of surgical subspecialists, house officers, and students involved in the care of these fascinating transplant patients.

Immunology of Organ Transplantation

The compatibility of a donor organ with the recipient is the basis of organ survival. In humans, compatibility is determined to a large extent by the red blood cell ABO antigens and the major histocompatibility complex (MHC) antigens. These two groups of antigens are thought to be the main determinants of immune response to a transplanted organ. MHC antigens, encoded on chromosome 6, are present on all nucleated cells. In humans, these antigens are referred to as human leukocyte antigens (HLAs). The HLA locus consists of at least seven regions: DP, DQ, DR, class III, B, C, and A. The HLA-A, -B, and -C loci encode class I molecules, expressed on all nucleated cells. The HLA-DR, -DQ, and -DP loci encode class II molecules, expressed on B lymphocytes, monocytes, macrophages, and some T cells. Class III molecules include complement and cytokines.

The histocompatibility of a transplant refers to antigens shared between donor and recipient. Donor organs are matched to recipients first on the basis of ABO blood type. Kidneys and pancreata, which tend to be less tolerant of rejection, also undergo HLA typing. Transplantation based on blood type follows the rules for blood transfusion; for example, a type O recipient can receive only a type O organ, whereas a type AB recipient can receive any ABO-type organ. In practice, recipients usually receive a graft with the same blood type as their own.

HLA matching involves the A, B, and DR loci, which appear to play a major role in graft histocompatibility. These loci are highly polymorphic; that is, they have a number of variants at each gene locus. A child will inherit one set of A, B, and DR gene loci, referred to as a haplotype, from each parent. Consequently, a potential transplant recipient has two A/B/DR haplotypes, one inherited from each parent, which encode for a total of six antigens. Donor and recipient A/B/DR antigens are compared to determine the HLA match, which can range anywhere between zero and six antigens. Thus a six-antigen match refers to shared histocompatibility antigens, rather than a perfect genetic match. Because cadaver kidney six-antigen matches have significantly better long-term survival, any such matches (from a nationwide database of potential recipients) are first offered to the identified recipient anywhere in the United States. Otherwise, kidneys typically are distributed on a regional basis.

The presence of preformed antibodies to a donor organ will result in immediate (hyperacute) rejection of a transplanted kidney, pancreas, heart, or lung. For kidney and pancreas transplants, a complement-dependent lymphocytotoxicity crossmatch to test for these antibodies is performed by mixing donor lymphocytes with recipient serum and then adding complement. Lysis of the donor lymphocytes constitutes a positive crossmatch. A potential recipient must have a negative crossmatch, indicating no preformed antibodies to the donor organ, to proceed with the transplant. Heart and lung transplant recipients do not undergo a crossmatch because of time constraints. Liver transplants do not seem to be significantly affected by these antibodies, and a crossmatch is not done.

The immune response to a transplant begins with detection of donor antigens by T and B lymphocytes, a stimulus termed *signal one*. Lymphocyte proliferation requires activation of co-stimulatory receptors on the cell surface, termed *signal two*. Cytokines induce a major part of the resulting response, in addition to direct activation of T and B cells by antigen. Macrophages called antigen-presenting cells (APCs) process antigen, then interact with T-helper cells, resulting in release of interleukin-1 (IL-1). IL-1 stimulates proliferation of T-helper cells, which secrete interleukin-2 (IL-2). Circulating IL-2 activates cytotoxic T cells that target the donor organ. Secreted IL-2 also causes B-cell growth and differentiation into plasma cells, which in turn produce antibodies directed against the graft.

Immunosuppression

Current immunosuppressive therapy is a far cry from the whole-body irradiation that was once the only available modality. In the early 1950s, the first drug therapy available consisted of huge steroid doses that often caused death from infection. Today corticosteroids are still used, but in much lower doses and in conjunction with highly effective immunosuppressive agents (Table 8–1). Patients typically are placed on a regimen of two or three immunosuppressive drugs. These *maintenance therapy* regimens are supplemented perioperatively with additional immunosuppression in the form of either high-dose steroids or additional, more powerful immunosuppressive agents. This practice is referred to as *induction therapy*, which helps dampen the initial immune response to the transplanted organ. Similarly high doses of potent drugs are used for *rejection therapy*.

Corticosteroids

Corticosteroids reduce IL-1 secretion. This in turn inhibits proliferation of T-helper cells, minimizing the production of IL-2 and blunting the cytotoxic T-cell response. Normally, a steroid taper using methylprednisolone (Solu-Medrol) is begun at the time of transplant. This is then converted to a maintenance dose of prednisone, generally in the range of 20 to 30 mg/24 hr. The initial maintenance dose is itself often tapered over the long term. Common side effects include weight gain, cushingoid facies, delayed wound healing, and hyperglycemia.

Table 8–1
Transplant medications

	Mechanism of Action	Indications	Side Effects
Prednisone	Inhibits IL-1 secretion and T-cell proliferation	Maintenance immunotherapy	Weight gain, HTN, myopathy, bone loss, hirsutism
Cyclosporine	Suppresses IL-2 production and T-cell activation	Maintenance immunotherapy	Renal dysfunction, HTN, hirsutism, CNS effects, hyperlipidemia
Tacrolimus	Suppresses IL-2 production and T-cell activation	Maintenance immunotherapy	Renal dysfunction, diabetes, CNS effects, HTN
Sirolimus	Blocks T- and B-cell response to IL-2	Maintenance immunotherapy	Myelosuppression, $\uparrow$ triglycerides
Azathioprine	Interferes with DNA and RNA synthesis	Maintenance immunotherapy	Myelosuppression
Mycophenolate mofetil	Blocks T- and B-cell differentiation and proliferation	Synergistic with cyclosporine or tacrolimus	GI upset, myelosuppresion
OKT3	Monoclonal mouse antibody to T cell CD3 receptor	Induction therapy, steroid-resistant rejection	Fever/chills, pulmonary edema, serum sickness, chest pain, tachycardia, HTN
Antithymocyte globulin	Polyclonal rabbit or horse serum antibodies to human lymphocytes	Induction therapy, steroid-resistant rejection	Fever/chills, thrombocytopenia, serum sickness
Daclizumab and Basiliximab	IL-2 receptor antagonists	Induction therapy	Minor GI problems, CNS effects

CNS, central nervous system; GI, gastrointestinal; HTN, hypertension; IL-1, interleukin-1; IL-2, interleukin-2.

Azathioprine

Azathioprine (Imuran) is a purine analog that inhibits cell division. This effectively suppresses B- and T-cell proliferation. Patients must be monitored carefully for aplastic anemia, neutropenia, and thrombocytopenia when using azathioprine. This drug is rapidly being replaced by newer immunosuppressants with less toxic side effects.

Mycophenolate mofetil

Mycophenolate mofetil (CellCept), or "MMF," inhibits the de novo pathway for purine synthesis. Because B and T cells depend more on the de novo purine synthesis pathway, versus the salvage pathway, MMF acts in a more selective manner than azathioprine in suppressing proliferation of lymphocytes. Gastrointestinal side effects are common, especially diarrhea and/or nausea. Gastrointestinal disturbances often resolve with a reduction in dosage. MMF can cause leukopenia and anemia, and should not be used with azathioprine.

Cyclosporine

Cyclosporine (Sandimmune, Neoral) blocks IL-2 production by T cells. Cyclosporine forms a complex with an intracellular binding protein, and this complex inhibits calcineurin, an enzyme in the intracellular pathway for T-cell secretion of IL-2. Cyclosporine typically is used in conjunction with prednisone and CellCept for "triple-drug therapy," or sometimes with prednisone alone. Drug dosing is adjusted using serum trough levels. Nephrotoxicity can result from too high a level. Other side effects include tremors, headaches, hirsutism, and hypertension. Many transplant centers are replacing cyclosporine with tacrolimus as the cornerstone of their immunosuppressive regimens.

Tacrolimus

Tacrolimus (Prograf), although structurally different from cyclosporine, also inhibits calcineurin, preventing T-cell secretion of IL-2. Tacrolimus, also referred to as FK506, normally is used in combination with prednisone and CellCept. Side effects include neurotoxicity, nephrotoxicity, hyperglycemia, hyperkalemia, and hypertension.

Sirolimus

Sirolimus (Rapamune) is structurally similar to tacrolimus, and binds to the same intracellular protein. However, it does not inhibit cytokine release; instead it blocks the response of T and B cells to IL-2. Sirolimus was approved by the Food and Drug Administration in 1999 for use in renal transplantation, in combination with cyclosporine and prednisone. Several centers have been using it for liver transplantation as well. The optimal use of sirolimus in clinical transplantation is still under investigation, both for prophylaxis of rejection and for treatment of refractory rejection. Reported side effects include myelosuppression and hypertriglyceridemia; the drug does not appear to be nephrotoxic.

Muromonab-CD3

Muromonab-CD3 (OKT3) is a murine monoclonal antibody directed against the T-cell CD3 complex. OKT3 blocks the T-cell response to an allograft; therapy often is monitored by following a patient's white cell count and CD3 cell count. A powerful immunosuppressant, OKT3 typically is reserved for induction therapy in pancreas or kidney-pancreas transplants and repeat kidney transplants. In addition, this drug is used for treating steroid-refractory rejection. Patients can develop anti-OKT3 antibodies, which make repeat usage (for further episodes of rejection) ineffectual. Administration of OKT3 causes a cytokine release syndrome that can result in severe pulmonary edema with the first or second dose. A pretreatment chest radiograph should be checked and dialysis used if necessary to remove excess fluid. Other side effects include fevers and chills as well as neurologic sequelae ranging from a mild headache to severe encephalopathy.

Polyclonal antibodies

Polyclonal antibodies, made by injecting other species with human lymphocytes, are used for both induction therapy and treatment of rejection. Two versions currently are used: antithymocyte globulin (Thymoglobulin) and antithymocyte gamma globulin (ATGAM). Immunizing rabbits with human thymocytes produces Thymoglobulin; ATGAM is the equine version. Administration of polyclonal antibodies results in lysis and immune clearance of T and B cells, and is reflected by a lowered lymphocyte count. Premedication with Solu-Medrol, diphenhydramine (Benadryl), and acetaminophen helps alleviate the flu-like symptoms experienced by many patients. Thymoglobulin is preferred by many centers because of its milder side effects compared to ATGAM.

Daclizumab and basiliximab

Daclizumab (Zenapax) and basiliximab (Simulect) are two newer agents often used for induction therapy. They have similar mechanisms of action because each of them is an IL-2 receptor antagonist. Side effects are minimal, with no nephrotoxicity. Patients with a high immunologic risk for graft rejection and patients with expected delayed graft function are typical candidates for these drugs. These agents appear to be equally effective, and the choice of which to use is a matter of transplant center preference.

Rejection

Maintaining graft function without undue side effects to the patient is the ongoing goal of transplant physicians. Careful monitoring for rejection is a standard part of patient care. Rejection typically is divided into three types: hyperacute, acute, and chronic.

Hyperacute Rejection

Hyperacute rejection occurs when the recipient has circulating antibodies to donor antigen. These antibodies attack the donor vascular endothelium, causing vascular occlusion of the graft, with immediate failure. Hyperacute rejection usually occurs upon perfusion of the graft, although it can take several hours for complete graft failure. Treatment consists of graft removal. A pretransplant positive crossmatch using donor lymphocytes and recipient sera predicts, and therefore prevents, hyperacute rejection in most situations. The crossmatch is used for kidney and pancreas transplantation. Heart, lung, and small bowel transplants all are susceptible to hyperacute rejection, but there is insufficient time between procurement and implantation of these organs to run a crossmatch. Liver transplants commonly are not subject to hyperacute rejection.

Acute Rejection

Acute rejection is primarily cell mediated, though antibody sometimes may play a role. T-cell–mediated (*cellular*) rejection is characterized by a lymphocytic infiltrate typical of an inflammatory reaction. Damage to vascular endothelium is seen with antibody-mediated (*humoral*) rejection. Acute rejection typically occurs within a few days to a few months after transplant, though it may occur at any time in the life of the graft. Rejection episodes at later times often are due to a failure to take immunosuppressive medications.

Chronic Rejection

Chronic rejection refers to a gradual process of endothelial, epithelial, and interstitial fibrosis thought to be caused by antibodies. Graft loss usually occurs over a period of several years. It manifests itself as bronchiolitis obliterans in the lung, vanishing bile duct syndrome in the liver, accelerated atherosclerosis in the heart, and glomerulosclerosis in the kidney.

Organ Procurement

Once a potential donor is identified, donor management is handled by the local organ procurement organization (OPO). An OPO is a nonprofit organization responsible for identification and care of organ donors. They work closely with the procurement team to manage organ retrieval, preservation, transportation, and data follow-up regarding cadaveric organ donors.

Cadaver donors are brain dead, with artificial support of ventilation and circulation. This permits a controlled procurement in the operating room with optimal preservation of donor organs. Separate thoracic and abdominal teams procure the respective organs. After initial dissection, organs are infused with cold (4°C) preservation solution via aortic cannulas, with aortic cross-clamps placed just above the celiac axis and on the ascending aorta. The thoracic and abdominal cavities are cooled with an icy slush of sterile saline solution. After removal from the donor, the organs are packaged with ice in coolers and transported to the recipient hospitals.

The physiologic changes associated with brain death may influence donor organ quality and transplantation outcomes. Cerebral ischemia and brainstem herniation produce a massive sympathetic outflow with associated poor peripheral organ perfusion and hypertension. The tissue ischemia in this early phase causes oxygen free radical production, further damaging the donor organs. After this initial hypertensive phase, a drop in sympathetic outflow is accompanied by a drop in blood pressure. The loss of autonomic tone leads to persistent hypotension with resultant poor end-organ perfusion. Coagulopathies, pulmonary edema, hypothermia, and electrolyte abnormalities develop during this second phase. Clinical management includes maintaining intravascular volume and perfusion pressure to minimize ischemic damage to donor organs.

Hypothalamic-pituitary axis dysfunction during brain death often leads to a neurogenic diabetes insipidus from decreased vasopressin production. Although animal models show a decrease in thyroid hormones and cortisol, this has not been conclusively shown in brain-dead human donors. Whether hormonal changes during brain death affect transplant organ outcomes is still uncertain.

The time between aortic cross-clamping and reperfusion of an organ in the recipient is called the cold ischemia time. Each organ has an accepted cold ischemia time beyond which acceptable graft function is unlikely (Table 8–2).

Ischemia-Reperfusion Injury

Transplanted organs all have some degree of ischemia-reperfusion injury caused by the interruption of blood flow during the time of ischemia. This ischemic period consists of (1) the initial normothermic ischemia during organ harvesting (i.e., "warm ischemia time"); (2) hypothermic preservation (i.e., "cold ischemia time"); and (3) the time needed for revascularization (i.e., "rewarming time"). Ischemia will precipitate changes in cell metabolism and structure (Box 8–1).

During tissue ischemia, metabolism becomes anaerobic, resulting in decreased ATP as well as cellular acidosis. The cell membrane ATP-dependent ionic pumps are affected, leading to intracellular buildup of sodium cations; this causes cellular swelling. The anaerobic pathway also leads to increased hypoxanthine levels.

Reperfusion of ischemic tissue will further increase intracellular sodium as well as calcium, causing further cellular swelling. The excess hypoxanthine is converted by

Table 8–2
Maximum recommended cold ischemia times for transplanted organs

Organ	Max. Cold Ischemia (hr)
Kidney	36
Pancreas	20
Liver	18
Small bowel	12
Lung	6
Heart	4

Box 8–1
Cellular Effects of Ischemia

- Altered membrane potential
- Altered ion distribution (↑ intracellular calcium/sodium)
- Cellular swelling
- Cytoskeletal disorganization
- Increased hypoxanthine
- Decreased ATP
- Decreased phosphocreatine
- Decreased glutathione
- Cellular acidosis

From Collard CD, Gelman S: Pathophysiology, clinical manifestations, and prevention of ischemia-reperfusion injury. Anesthesiology 2001; 94:1133, with permission.

xanthine oxidase to uric acid, releasing reactive oxygen free radicals.

Ischemia-reperfusion also causes complement and leukocyte activation, resulting in an inflammatory response that can cause further damage to cells. In particular, leukocyte–endothelial cell adhesion along with platelet aggregation may result in thrombosis with organ dysfunction or failure.

Currently, attempts at minimizing ischemia-reperfusion injury in transplants focus mainly on (1) minimizing the ischemic period, (2) inducing hypothermia to reduce metabolic activity during the ischemic time, and (3) using preservation solutions that minimize the metabolic effects of ischemia.

Pretransplant Work-up

Potential recipients are first screened on the basis of whether the intended transplant would improve their quality of life and life expectancy. Certain comorbidities (e.g., malignancy, severe vascular disease, drug addiction, active infection) can preclude transplantation. A thorough psychosocial evaluation is necessary, because psychiatric stability and social support are factors that influence a patient's ability to comply with lifelong monitoring and immunosuppressive therapy.

The preoperative work-up includes blood chemistries, a complete blood count, coagulation profile, liver function tests, a chest radiograph, and an electrocardiogram. In addition to these standard preoperative studies, serology studies are needed. A hepatitis panel and human immuno-deficiency virus and cytomegalovirus (CMV) titers will screen for diseases that can affect transplant outcomes.

Additional testing will depend on the organ involved and the patient's medical history. Thoracic organ transplant recipients require extensive cardiac and pulmonary preoperative evaluations. Most centers routinely include a dobutamine echocardiogram in their work-up of abdominal organ transplant recipients; pulmonary function tests are indicated for a history of smoking or lung disease. A voiding cystourethrogram is indicated in diabetics slated for renal transplantation, to check for bladder dysfunction that may require an intermittent bladder catheterization regimen after the transplant.

Intraoperative Considerations

Careful coordination with an experienced anesthesia team is necessary for optimal patient management during the operation. Patients requiring transplantation typically have altered physiology requiring a tailored anesthetic approach.

The reperfusion of an organ during transplantation sometimes is associated with physiologic changes resulting from the systemic flushing of preservation solution and metabolites, as well as intrinsic preservation damage. Reperfusion of the liver can result in a transient hyperkalemia, hypocalcemia, metabolic acidosis, depressed cardiac output with hypotension, right heart dysfunction with pulmonary hypertension, and fibrinolysis. Kidneys, probably because of their relatively smaller size, usually do not incur any clinically significant reperfusion effects during surgery. Pancreas transplant reperfusion sometimes can cause hypotension and arrhythmias as a result of a massive release of pancreatic hormones and enzymes. Lung reperfusion will cause pulmonary edema, which may require increased positive end-expiratory pressure and diuresis. Cardiac transplants depend on successful weaning from cardiopulmonary bypass, that is, optimizing heart rate and rhythm, volume status, contractility, and afterload.

Postoperative Complications

Complications tend to fall into one of three categories: (1) surgical complications, (2) medication side effects, and (3) overimmunosuppression. However, underimmunosuppression leads to the complication of acute allograft rejection.

Surgical complications may be due not only to poor technique, but also to the underlying disease of the organ failure patient. They include bleeding, wound infection, vascular strictures and thromboses, breakdown of bowel anastomoses, biliary anastomotic strictures, and leaking bronchial anastomoses. Delayed graft function from long rewarming times (as well as prolonged cold ischemia) can significantly impair a patient's recovery.

Transplant medications can have significant, deleterious side effects. Nephrotoxicity from the calcineurin inhibitors cyclosporine and FK506 is a common complication and can lead to chronic renal insufficiency if not treated. The calcineurin inhibitors, prednisone, and OKT3 all can affect the central nervous system, with symptoms ranging from a mild headache to profound mental status changes. One must keep in mind that drugs that affect the cytochrome P-450 enzyme system (e.g., azole antifungals, diltiazem, verapamil, dilantin, phenobarbital, rifampin) will affect levels of cyclosporine, FK506, and sirolimus, which are metabolized by the P-450 enzyme system.

Although necessary for allograft acceptance, immunosuppression can predispose an individual to a myriad of infections. Common bacterial, viral, and fungal flora that inhabit the human body can become pathogens with a depressed immune system. Patients normally receive prophylactic medication for oral thrush and *Pneumocystis carinii* pneumonia postoperatively. Cytomegalovirus infection is a common occurrence (usually 1 or more months after the transplant), and patients deemed to be at high risk for CMV infection receive prophylactic antivirals. Cytomegalovirus infections in the immunosuppressed transplant population can lead to death if not treated in time. Patients often walk a fine line between too much immunosuppression, leading to infection, and too little, with ensuing acute rejection. In the face of a serious infection, many transplant physicians will decrease immunosuppression and tolerate some degree of rejection. Long-term immunosuppression increases a patient's risk of malignancy; excess immunotherapy often can lead to post-transplant lymphoproliferative disorder.

Treatment of Rejection

The diagnosis of acute rejection in a transplanted organ is based on clinical parameters of organ dysfunction, elevated lab indices, and tissue biopsies (Table 8–3).

Treatment of cellular acute rejection consists of a temporary increase in immunotherapy. Initial treatment is usually a 3- to 5-day course of high-dose steroids (e.g., Solu-Medrol 500 mg IV each day). Rejection that does not respond to steroid therapy is next treated with a course of either polyclonal (Thymoglobulin, ATGAM) or mono-clonal (OKT3) antibodies. Antibody treatment can have serious side effects, and should not be started without a tissue diagnosis of rejection.

Hyperacute and accelerated acute rejection are pri-marily humoral (i.e., antibody mediated). Although rare compared to cellular rejection, humoral acute rejection is found most commonly in renal transplant patients, especially those recipients sensitized by previous transplants. Treatment is by plasmapheresis, which filters off plasma proteins, including antibodies. A 3- to 5-day course of plasmapheresis often is followed by a dose of intravenous immune globulin (Gamimune N), which serves to neutralize the allograft-directed antibodies.

Chronic rejection is currently untreatable. Efforts at preventing or delaying chronic rejection include (1) avoid-ing acute rejection, (2) minimizing ischemia-reperfusion injury, (3) improving preprocurement management of cadaveric donors, and (4) inducing allograft tolerance.

The Future of Transplantation

Although organ transplantation has become an accepted therapy, allograft rejection and complications of immunotherapy continue to be significant problems. Transplantation tolerance is a venue that is being explored aggressively. Tolerance refers to acceptance of the allograft by the recipient without the need for long-term immunosuppression. Proposed methods for inducing tolerance include (1) T-cell co-stimulatory blockade and (2) induction of chimerism.

T-cell activation by foreign antigen begins when the T-cell receptor (TCR) binds to antigen on the APC. However, T-cell proliferation and differentiation will not occur unless co-stimulatory molecules on the T-cell surface are activated. Among the co-stimulatory pathways

Table 8–3
Indicators of acute rejection

Organ	Diagnostic Tests	Clinical Signs	Biopsy Histology
Kidney	↑ Creatinine	↓ In urine Fever	T-cell infiltrate around and within tubules
Pancreas	↑ Amylase, lipase ↑ Glucose	Pain around graft	Lymphocyte infiltrate involving septa and acinar tissue
Liver	↑ LFTs, ↑ PT	Fever, ascites ↓ In bile	Portal lymphocyte infiltrate
Small bowel	Endoscopy reveals inflammation and ulceration	Fever, diarrhea ↑ Stomal output Abdominal pain Nausea, vomiting	↑ Apoptotic figures ↑ Lymphocytes in lamina propria ↓ Villus height ↓ Goblet cells ulceration
Heart	ECG changes	Fatigue, arrhythmias	Perivascular lymphocyte infiltrate
Lung	↓ Pao_2, ↓ FEV_1 CXR infiltrate	Fever, malaise	Perivascular mononuclear infiltrate

CXR, chest radiograph; ECG, electrocardiogram; FEV_1, forced expiratory volume measured over first second of exhalation; LFTs, liver function tests; Pao_2, partial pressure of arterial oxygen; PT, prothrombin time.

that have been identified, the B7/CD28 pathway appears to be critical for full T-cell activation. CD28 is a T-cell surface molecule that binds the B7-1 and B7-2 ligands found on APCs. This pathway can be blocked with CTLA4-immunoglobulin (Ig), a fusion protein of human CTLA4 and IgG that competes for the B7 binding sites. (CTLA4 is a T-cell surface molecule that appears to have an inhibitory role.) Transplantation tolerance has been induced in some animal models with CTLA4-Ig blockade of the B7/CD28 pathway.

The CD40-CD40 ligand (CD154) pathway also has been identified as critical to T-cell activation. Stimulation of this pathway induces B7 molecules on APCs. Blockade with an anti-CD154 monoclonal antibody in murine models has been shown to result in long-term graft survival. One group has used CTLA4-Ig in combination with anti-CD154 monoclonal antibody to prevent renal allograft rejection in primates.

The co-stimulatory pathways can be thought of as a "two-signal" model of T-cell activation (Fig. 8–1). The antigen-dependent signal one occurs when the TCR binds alloantigen presented by an APC. Signal two, which is independent of antigen, consists of the co-stimulatory signaling mediated by the T-cell surface molecules and is therefore termed the "cosignal" in Figure 8–1. Signal one without signal two results in T-cell anergy and hence tolerance.

Another approach to transplant tolerance is to induce chimerism of donor lymphocytes in the recipient, whose immune system then will recognize the donor antigens as "self" antigens. A chimera is a composite of genetically distinct individuals. Transplantation chimerism refers to the presence in the transplant recipient of a population of circulating donor lymphocytes that coexist with the recipient's native lymphocytes. The host and donor lymphocyte populations confer immunologic characteristics of both to the host. Current attempts involve simultaneously transplanting donor bone marrow along with the donor organ. Some researchers believe intrathymic clonal deletion is pivotal to establishing chimerism-associated tolerance. Transplanting donor thymus to help induce tolerance is under investigation.

An ongoing problem in transplantation is the shortage of donor organs. Xenotransplantation could provide the solution to this shortage, as well as possibly address the issue of transplant tolerance. One significant problem with xenotransplantation to humans is the presence in humans of preformed antibodies to the α-galactose moiety found on the surface of nearly all cells in subhuman species. These naturally occurring antibodies are in the circulation of all humans after a few months of life and react immediately with antigens of all mammalian species except Old World primates. Complement-mediated hyperacute rejection occurs unless the immune systems of the donor and

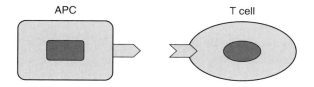

First Signal		
MHC Class I	Recognition	CD8
Class II		CD4
Ag-Peptide		CD3/TCR
Cosignal		
CD11a/CD18(LFA-1)	Adhesion	CD54(ICAM-1)
CD54(ICAM-1)		CD11a/CD18(LFA-1)
CD58/59(LFA-3)		CD2
CD106/(VCAM-1)		CD49d/CD29(VLA-4)
CD80(B7-1)	Costimulation	CD28
CD86(B7-2)		CD28
OX40L	Th2 differentiation	CD134(OX40)
4-1BBL	Th1 differentiation	CD137(4-1BB)
CD80(B7-1)	Inhibition	CD152(CTLA4)
CD86(B7-2)		CD152(CTLA4)
CD40	Upregulation of B7 molecules; Th1 differentiation	CD154(CD40L)
CD95(Fas)	Apoptosis	CD95L(FasL)
		CD95(Fas)

FIGURE 8–1 T cell co-signalling molecules and their immunological role. (From Tanaka J, Asaka M, Imamura M: T-cell co-signalling molecules in graft-versus-host disease. Ann Hematol 2000;79:283. © Springer-Verlag.)

recipient are altered. Genetic engineering of porcine donors has partially ameliorated the rejection response. Use of organs from transgenic pigs, which have human complement regulatory molecules, and, most recently, cloned pigs, which lack the enzyme to form the α-galactose target moiety on their cells, has eliminated hyperacute rejection and may reduce acute vascular rejection as a barrier to xenogeneic transplantation.

Perhaps the newest frontier in transplantation science is the rethinking of the conceptual framework of the immune system. It is becoming increasingly clear that the many immune processes in the body form a complex, integrated network of interacting systems. This constantly adapting network depends more on patterns of interaction than on any one element. Attempts at immunosuppression to date have been based on the science of controlling one element in an immune pathway. Theoretical immunologists are developing a new model of the immune system, based on a nonlinear and complex systems perspective.

An interdisciplinary approach involving immunology, mathematical theory, and computer modeling is playing a pivotal role in the development of this model. This radically new understanding of the immune system may well be the sword that cuts the Gordian knot of transplant rejection.

Selected References

Belzer FO, Southard JH: Principles of solid-organ preservation by cold storage. Transplantation 1988;45:673.

This is Folkert Belzer's classical paper that introduced his now widely used University of Wisconsin (UW) preservation solution. The paper provides a succinct and still very relevant description of the principles of organ preservation for transplantation.

Ginns LC, Cosimi AB, Morris PJ: Transplantation. Malden, MA: Blackwell Science, 1999.

This comprehensive text covers both the clinical practice and basic science of organ transplantation.

Norman DJ, Turka LA: Primer on Transplantation (2nd ed). Malden, MA: Blackwell Science, 2001.

This text provides a good clinical overview of abdominal and thoracic organ transplantation.

Roitt I, Brostoff J, Male D: Immunology (6th ed). St. Louis: Mosby, 2001.

A classical textbook of immunology, well written and thorough.

Stuart FP, Abecassis MM, Kaufman DB (eds): Organ Transplantation. Georgetown, TX: Landes Bioscience, 2000.

A clear description of surgical techniques for all types of organ transplantation.

Bibliography

Bumgardner GL, and the Phase III Daclizumab Study Group: Results of 3-year Phase III clinical trials with daclizumab prophylaxis for prevention of acute rejection after renal transplantation. Transplantation 2001;72:839.

Converse JM: Alexis Carrel: the man, the unknown. Plast Reconstr Surg 1981;68:629.

DeWolf A, Kang Y, Sherman L: Anesthesia for organ transplantation. *In* Stuart FP, Abecassis MM, Kaufman DB (eds): Organ Transplantation. Georgetown, TX: Landes Bioscience, 2000:329.

Gibson T, Medawar P: The fate of skin homografts in man. J Anat 1942;77:299.

Hancock WW, Sayegh MH, Zheng XG, et al: Costimulatory function and expression of CD40 ligand, CD80, and CD86 in vascularized murine cardiac allograft rejection. Proc Natl Acad Sci U S A 1996;93:13967.

Hanto DW, Whiting JF, Valente JF: Transplantation of the liver and intestine. *In* Norton JA, Bollinger RR, Chang AE, et al (eds): Surgery: Basic Science and Clinical Evidence. New York: Springer-Verlag, 2001:1484.

Health Services and Resources Administration, Office of Special Programs, Department of Transplantation, and United Network of Organ Sharing (UNOS). 2000 Annual Report of the U.S. Scientific Registry for Transplant Recipients and the Organ Procurement and Transplantation Network: Transplant Data: 1990–1999. Rockville, MD, and Richmond, VA: U.S. Department of Health and Human Services and UNOS, 2000.

Kirk AD, Harlan DM, Armstrong NN, et al: CTLA4-Ig and anti-CD40 ligand prevent renal allograft rejection in primates. Proc Natl Acad Sci U S A 1997; 94:8789.

Mathew JM, Garcia-Morales R, Fuller L, et al: Donor bone marrow-derived chimeric cells present in renal transplant recipients infused with donor marrow. I. Potent regulators of recipient antidonor immune responses. Transplantation 2000;70:1675.

McDevitt HO: Discovering the role of the major histocompatibility complex in the immune response. Annu Rev Immunol 2000;18:1.

Moore R: Simulect: redefining immunosuppressive strategies. Transplant Proc 2000;32:1460.

Murray JE, Merrill JP, Harrison JH: Kidney transplantation between seven pairs of identical twins. Ann Surg 1958; 148:343.

Orosz CG: Complexity and transplantation. Graft 1999; 1(5):175.

Parker DC, Greiner DL, Phillips NE, et al: Survival of mouse pancreatic islet allografts in recipients treated with allogeneic small lymphocytes and antibody to CD40 ligand. Proc Natl Acad Sci U S A 1995;92:9560.

Pratshcke J, Wilhelm MJ, Kusaka M, et al: Brain death and its influence on donor organ quality and outcome after transplantation. Transplantation 1999; 67:343.

Remuzzi G: Cellular basis of long-term organ transplant acceptance: pivotal role of intrathymic clonal deletion and thymic dependence of bone marrow microchimerism-associated tolerance. Am J Kidney Dis 1998; 31:197.

Stahelin H: Cyclosporin: historical background. Prog Allergy 1986;38:19.

Starzl TE, Marchioro TL, Von Kaulla KN, et al: Homotransplantation of the liver in humans. Surg Gynecol Obstet 1963;117:659.

Stratta RJ, Alloway RR, Lo A, Hodge E: A multicenter trial of two daclizumab dosing strategies versus no antibody induction in simultaneous kidney-pancreas transplantation: interim analysis. Transplant Proc 2001;33:1692.

Tanaka J, Asaka M, Imamura M: T-cell co-signalling molecules in graft-versus-host disease. Ann Hematol 2000;79:283.

Terasaki PI, Vredevoe DL, Porter KA, et al: Serotyping for homotransplantation. V. Evaluation of a matching scheme. Transplantation 1966;4:688.

Van Rood JJ, Eernisse JG, Van Leeuwen A: Leucocyte antibodies in sera from pregnant women. Nature 1958;181:1735.

Wang CY, Pinsky DJ: Contribution of inflammation to reperfusion injury. J Card Surg 2000;15:149.

Yamada K, Shimizu A, Ierino FL, et al: Allogeneic thymo-kidney transplants induce stable tolerance in miniature swine. Transplant Proc 1999;31:1199.

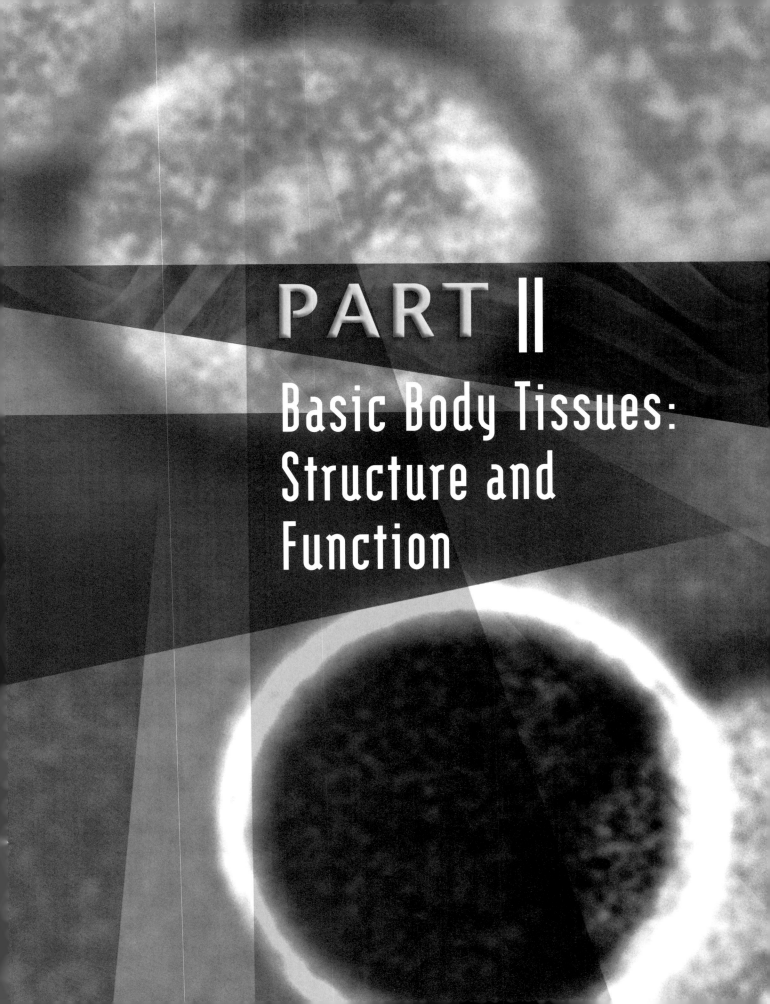

PART II
Basic Body Tissues: Structure and Function

CHAPTER 9

Skin and Adnexal Structures

Anthony J. DeFranzo, Jr., M.D.

The skin is the largest organ of the body by weight. It is divided anatomically into epidermis, dermis, and hypodermis. The epidermis is a specialized epithelial layer that varies widely over various parts of the body; the dermis is a collagen matrix accounting for greater than 90% of skin thickness; and the hypodermis is a subcutaneous layer of adipose tissue. All these layers have multiple functions that are well integrated. The skin is frequently injured, and its important barrier function is largely unappreciated. It is simply assumed that the skin is a perfect container and will protect the body from the environment and will repair and regenerate itself for a lifetime. Protection from heat, cold, ultraviolet radiation, microorganisms, and chemicals and prevention of loss of essential bodily fluids go largely unnoticed. Loss of barrier function in a major burn reminds us of how important the function of the skin is to life. Yet the skin is much more than a container. It has multiple sensory receptors, provides temperature regulation, and functions as an immunologic screen. Each of these functions is provided by a specialized cell, cellular organelle, or adnexal structure. The structural and functional analysis of the skin has improved remarkably over the last two decades with advances in immunology, microbiology, and electron microscopy. This chapter provides a comprehensive analysis of skin structure and illustrates how the details of this structure provide an understanding of skin function.

Epidermis

The epidermis consists of stratified squamous epithelium divided into four keratinocyte layers: from deep to superficial, the stratum germinativum, the stratum spinosum, the stratum granulosum, and the stratum corneum. The keratinocytes of the epidermis continually renew themselves and differentiate into the keratinized cells of the outermost stratum corneum. Eighty percent or more of the cells that constitute the epidermis are keratinocytes. All keratinocytes display keratin filaments in their cytoplasm and form desmosomes or modified desmosomal junctions with neighboring cells. Approximately 30 different keratins have been described. Interspersed within the epidermis are three other cell types: melanocytes, Langerhans' cells, and Merkel cells. Also, the epidermis produces skin appendages such as hair follicles, sebaceous glands, nails, and sweat glands (Fig. 9–1).

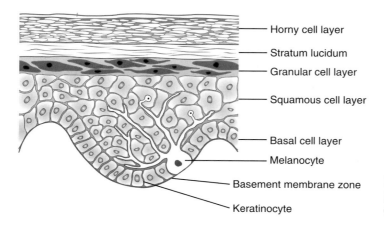

Horny cell layer

Stratum lucidum

Granular cell layer

Squamous cell layer

Basal cell layer

Melanocyte

Basement membrane zone

Keratinocyte

FIGURE 9–1 The epidermis. (From Sams WM Jr, Lynch PJ [eds]: Principles and Practice of Dermatology [2nd ed]. London: Churchill Livingstone, 1996:2, with permission.)

Layers of the Epidermis

Progressive differentiation of keratinocytes leads to the formation of terminally differentiated or keratinized keratinocytes of the stratum corneum. The process is genetically controlled and involves the following changes in cell morphology:

1. Cells flatten and increase in size.

2. New cellular organelles appear and organelles reorganize.

3. General cellular metabolism shifts to a keratinization metabolism.

4. Changes occur in the plasma membrane, cell surface antigens, and receptors.

5. Loss of all cellular organelles occurs.

6. Dehydration occurs.

At the completion of keratinization, a terminally differentiated keratinocyte contains keratin and a protein-reinforced plasma membrane with surface-associated lipids.

Stratum germinativum (Basal cell layer)

In this layer, the keratinocytes are attached to the basement membrane. They are columnar in shape and are very mitotically active. These basal cells have a large nucleus and nucleolus. Their cytoplasm contains typical cellular

organelles, Golgi apparatus, rough endoplasmic reticulum, mitochondria, lysosomes, ribosomes, and melanosome vacuoles, phagocytized from melanocytes. Basal keratinocytes in this layer have fine bundles of keratin filaments around the nucleus that insert into desmosomes and hemidesmosomes. Microfilaments of actin, myosin, and α-actinin are also found in basilar keratinocytes and participate in the outward migration of epidermal cells. All cells in the basal layer are not actively dividing. Stem cells, transient amplifying cells, and postmitotic cells are found in the basal layer. The stem cell presides within a group of mitotically active basal cells, transient amplifying cells, and postmitotic cells. This organization of cells is termed an *epidermal proliferative unit*. Columns of organized cells are thought to migrate from the basal stratum germinativum to the outer stratum corneum.

Stratum spinosum (Squamous cell or Prickle cell layer)

The cells of the stratum spinosum have a spinelike cell border under the microscope. These "spines" of the cells in the stratum spinosum are numerous desmosomes. Desmosomes are special calcium-dependent cell membrane structures that bind cells together and counteract mechanical stress. The cells of the inner stratum spinosum have a rounded nucleus and a polyhedral shape. Cells of the outer stratum spinosum are flatter and larger and display new organelles called lamellar granules. Lamellar granules consist of glycoprotein, glycolipids, phospholipids, free sterols, and acid hydrolases (lipases, proteases, acid phosphatase, and glycosidases). Although lamellar granules develop in the stratum spinosum, they act primarily at the junction between the stratum granulosum and stratum corneum. All cells of the stratum spinosum contain large bundles of keratin filaments. These keratin filaments surround the nucleus concentrically and insert into desmosomes peripherally just as in the stratum germinativum.

Stratum granulosum (Granular cell layer)

The most prominent new feature of the cells of the stratum granulosum is the appearance of prominent basophilic keratohyalin granules. These granules are chiefly composed of an electron-dense protein, pro-filaggrin, and keratin intermediate filaments. Loricrin, another important protein found in keratohyalin granules, is also present in the stratum corneum. As a granular cell differentiates into a cornified cell, pro-filaggrin is converted to filaggrin (the name is derived from *fi*lament *agg*regation prote*in*). This process occurs by proteolysis with three or more proteases and by dephosphorylation. Filaggrin is the matrix protein that enables the aggregation and disulfide bonding of keratin filaments. This process produces the dense keratinization of the cells of the inner stratum corneum.

Lamellar granules are seen first in the outer stratum spinosum. Later they become active at the junction between the stratum granulosum and stratum corneum. In the cells of the outer stratum granulosum, lamellar granules aggregate in clusters, bond to cell membranes, and, by exocytosis, empty into the intercellular space. The contents of the lamellar granules are folded or stacked into disks within the granule and secreted in the same configuration. The hydrolytic enzymes are discharged from the lamellar granules along with the lipids and protein. The action of these enzymes results in the formation of sheets of intercellular lamellae of barrier lipids. These lipids create a barrier that is hydrophobic at the junction between the stratum granulosum and stratum corneum. Water loss through the skin is decreased and the passage of external polar compounds is blocked by this barrier.

Cells of the stratum granulosum complete the terminal differentiation to keratinized cells with an abrupt change that is not completely understood. The granular cell loses its nucleus and almost all cellular contents. The keratin filaments and filaggrin matrix are the only remaining cellular contents. Multiple enzymes have been categorized in the granular cell and are responsible for its terminal differentiation. These enzymes include proteases, phosphatases, esterases, acid hydrolases, DNAse, RNAse, and plasminogen activator.

Stratum corneum (Horny cell layer)

The cornified cells of the stratum corneum are flat, polyhedron-shaped cells that are the largest cells of the epidermis. However, the terminal differentiation from granular to cornified cell results in a 45% to 86% loss of dry weight. The cornified cell consists of 80% high-molecular-mass keratin held together by disulfide bonds. The rest of the cellular content consists of an electron-dense matrix surrounding the keratin filaments (thought to be filaggrin). Enzymes are still active within the cytoplasm of the cornified cell. These enzymes continue to act on lipids as they did at the granular cell–cornified cell junction, where they formed an intercellular lamella or sheet of barrier lipids. Lipids are covalently bonded to the cell surface in the stratum corneum. Enzymes also play a role in promoting desquamation. A lectin associated with the cell membrane is also in part responsible for adhesion versus desquamation as the cornified cell moves to the surface within the stratum corneum.

Both the morphology and function of cornified cells change as they migrate through the stratum corneum. The cells of the inner layer of the stratum corneum are thick and have a dense parallel arrangement of keratin filaments. These cells are tightly adherent, with modified desmosomes and superior-inferior interlocking ridges and villi. This layer within the stratum corneum has been called the *stratum compactum*. Cells in this layer have less ability to bind water than cells in the middle and outer layers. Cells in the middle layer of the stratum corneum have the highest water-binding capacity and the highest concentration of free amino acids. Cells of the outermost stratum corneum undergo proteolytic degradation of desmosomes, making this layer prone to desquamation. This outer layer of the stratum corneum has been called the *stratum disjunctum*. It must be understood that the stratum corneum is not a metabolically inactive layer of "dead" cells. Cellular metabolic activity continues to augment barrier function and regulate desquamation.

Epidermal Nonkeratinocytes: Melanocytes, Merkel Cells, and Langerhans' Cells

Melanocytes

The purpose of melanocytes is to synthesize and distribute melanin to protect the skin from ultraviolet radiation. Melanocytes are found chiefly in the stratum germinativum. Their cell body may be noted below the stratum germinativum but always external to the lamina densa. Microscopically, melanocytes have an ovoid nucleus, pale-staining cytoplasm, and pigmented melanosomes. The melanocyte migrates from the neural crest and is first seen in the epidermis of the developing fetus around day 50. Melanocytes may migrate to the epidermis by using integrin receptors. They are not found at random in the epidermis but are integrated among keratinocytes in a very organized manner. Melanocytes have an interesting dendritic configuration; their dendrites extend to multiple keratinocytes in the stratum germinativum and fewer keratinocytes in the other more external epidermal layers. Desmosomal junctions between melanocytes and keratinocytes are not found. Melanocytes are melanin pigment–synthesizing cells that form epidermal melanin units with keratinocytes. An estimated 36 keratinocytes within and external to the stratum germinativum establish a functional unit. Each melanocyte delivers pigment to the cells in its unit. Pigment is delivered to keratinocytes by melanocyte-keratinocyte cell membrane fusion and breakdown, or keratinocyte phagocytosis of melanocytic dendrites containing melanosomes (Fig. 9–2).

The melanosome is the functionally distinguishing organelle of the melanocyte. Melanosome metabolism is complex and race dependent. The melanosome is an ovoid organelle that produces melanin by a series of reactions catalyzed by enzymes mediated by receptors and regulated by hormones (melanocyte-stimulating hormone and sex hormones), inflammatory mediators, and vitamin D synthesized in the epidermis. The keratinocyte is thought to synthesize soluble factors that influence melanocyte division, dendrite proliferation, and melanin production. Melanocytes ordinarily divide at a rate that matches keratinocyte division. Melanosomes are distributed in the keratinocyte separately or in membrane-bound aggregates termed *melanosome complexes*, and this distribution varies by race. Melanosomes that synthesize brown or black pigments are elliptical and display longitudinal concentric lamellae. Melanosomes that synthesize red or yellow pigment are varied in shape and contain microvesicles. The size of melanocytes in black skin is larger than the other races. Also, in blacks melanin is distributed in all levels of the epidermis, including the stratum corneum. In whites, melanin is found chiefly in the basal layer.

Environmental factors such as ultraviolet B (UVB) radiation increase the rate of melanocyte proliferation and increase melanocyte production of melanin. Keratinocytes in the stratum germinativum and stratum spinosum are stimulated to make more melanin migrate outward, carrying more melanin to the stratum corneum. Also, after two to three average sun exposures, ultraviolet radiation causes a thickening of the stratum corneum. The stratum corneum itself is a very effective screening layer for 280- to 300-nm radiation. Radiation of 299 to 320 nm is "sunburn radiation." Where the stratum corneum is very thick, such as the palm or sole of the foot, sunburn rarely occurs.

Merkel cells

Merkel cells are located in the basal stratum germinativum layer in areas highly sensitive to touch. They are found in hairy and glabrous skin of the fingers, outer root sheaths of hair follicles, and the lips and parts of the oral cavity. They serve as the skin touch receptors (slow-adapting type 1 mechanoreceptors). Merkel cells first appear in the fetus at 11 to 12 weeks. They contain keratin intermediate filaments, as do keratinocytes, but are thought to differentiate from keratinocytes rather than migrating from the neural crest. Merkel cells are rare and for the most part are seen only under electron microscopy. They attach to keratinocytes by desmosomes and are stimulated when external forces deform keratinocytes. Merkel cells may also be arranged in groups called *tactile disks* or *touch domes*. Microscopically, the Merkel cell has a lobulated nucleus, pale-staining cytoplasm, and spines on the cell surface projecting toward keratinocytes. The cytoplasm contains dense core granules that are found opposite a Golgi apparatus and adjacent to an unmyelinated extracellular neurite. The granules produced by the Golgi apparatus contain neurotransmitter-like substances and are analogous to neurosecretory granules in neurons.

Langerhans' cells

Langerhans' cells, comprising 2% to 8% of the epidermis, function as the macrophage of the epidermis. They react to contact antigens, may transport antigens to regional lymph nodes by dermal lymphatics, and present antigens to sensitized T lymphocytes. The activated T lymphocytes multiply in the regional lymph nodes and then are transported to the skin site where required. Langerhans' cells are dendritic and, like melanocytes, they do not form desmosomal junctions with keratinocytes. Langerhans' cells originate from bone marrow. They migrate to the epidermis via the blood stream early in embryonic development and continually replenish themselves as they process antigens and travel from the dermis to the regional lymph nodes via dermal lymphatics. They are found in the stratum germinativum, stratum spinosum, and stratum granulosum. Their largest concentration is external to the stratum germinativum. Microscopically, they have convoluted nuclei and are pale staining. Under electron microscopy, they have characteristic rod- or racquet-shaped Birbeck granules, also termed *Langerhans' cell granules*.

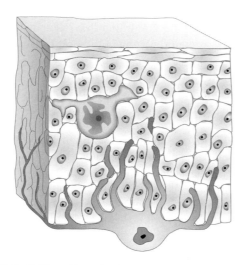

FIGURE 9–2 The epidermal melanin unit. (From Fitzpatrick TB, Eisen AZ, Wolff K, et al [eds]: Dermatology in General Medicine [4th ed], Vol 1. New York: McGraw-Hill, 1993:262. Reproduced with permission of the McGraw-Hill Companies, 1993.)

Birbeck granules are created when antigen bound on a cell membrane is engulfed by endocytosis. Langerhans' cells are responsible for contact sensitivity, rejection of skin allografts, and response against epithelial tumor antigens and infectious organisms such as herpesvirus and leishmanial organisms. Human immunodeficiency virus (HIV) is thought to infect Langerhans' cells, which may then serve as reservoirs of the disease. Langerhans' cells and keratinocytes act in concert, and Langerhans' cell activity is in part regulated by keratinocytes. Cytokines and other factors play a role in this interdependent regulation. Langerhans' cell effectiveness is diminished by ultraviolet radiation. UVB results in a decreased ability of Langerhans' cells to process antigen and a decreased production of cytokines by keratinocytes. Immune surveillance becomes less effective. Langerhans' cells are present in squamous epithelium outside the dermis, such as the oral cavity, esophagus, and vagina.

Dysmorphia

The normal differentiation of cells of the stratum germinativum to keratinized cells of the stratum corneum has been described above in detail. This differentiation proceeds with amazing regularity despite multiple environmental effects from radiation, chemicals, and organic compounds such as tobacco. However, basal cells of the stratum germinativum may be damaged over time, leading to the formation of actinic or solar keratoses on the skin and actinic cheilitis and leukoplakia of mucous membranes. These lesions are precancerous and they may evolve into a squamous cell cancer. The development of a keratosis from a single damaged cell of the stratum germinativum has been popularized by Pinkus. Dysplastic basal cells show increased mitosis, which leads to the formation of a scaly keratosis.

Basement Membrane Zone

Investigation of the basement membrane, or dermal-epidermal junction, has revealed a very complicated semipermeable barrier between epidermis and dermis. The dermal-epidermal junction is manufactured chiefly by basal keratinocytes with a small contribution from dermal fibroblasts. The outermost layer of the dermal-epidermal junction consists of the basal cell membranes and hemidesmosomes of the basal keratinocytes. Keratin intermediate filaments join the hemidesmosomes from the basal cell cytoplasm. The next layer, named the lamina lucida because it appears as a clear zone, begins just under the hemidesmosomes. It contains laminin, fibronectin, and entactin/nidogen (noncollagenous glycoproteins.) These molecules bind together and to cells and provide adherence between the epidermis and lamina densa.

The lamina lucida is the weakest part of the dermal-epidermal junction. It separates easily with heat and chemicals and in disease. The middle layer, the lamina densa, is composed mainly of type IV collagen produced by keratinocytes. Type V collagen is present in some but not all dermal-epidermal junctions. The lamina densa contains laminin and also contains sulfated proteoglycans, which impede the permeability of macromolecule cations. Thus the lamina densa has a significant barrier filter function. The deepest layer of the basement membrane zone, the sublamina densa, contains anchoring fibrils with type VII collagen, synthesized primarily by the keratinocyte. Anchoring fibrils originate in the lamina densa and insert into the dermis into anchoring plaques. Collagen types I, III, V, and VI and procollagens I and III are also present in the sublamina densa. For the first time in the structure of skin, elastic fibers are seen originating in the lamina densa. These fibers are part of an elastic fiber system holding the epidermis to the dermis. They apply tension to the epidermis, allowing deformation and recovery without loss of epidermal-dermal integrity.

Dermis

The majority of skin consists of dermis, which provides strength and elasticity. The outer layer of dermis, the papillary dermis, contains abundant ground substance and thin, randomly arranged elastic and collagen fibers. The reticular dermis, traversing from the papillary dermis to subcutaneous fat, consists of heavy elastin fibers and dense collagen bundles largely arranged in parallel to the skin surface. The dermis houses nerve and vascular systems, epidermal-derived skin appendages, fibroblastic macrophages, mast cells, plasma cells, and various white cells.

Collagen

Collagen makes up 70% to 75% of the human dermis by dry weight. Collagen types I (80% to 90%), III (8% to 12%), and V (≤5%) are in greatest abundance in human dermis. Collagen type V is incorporated into fibrils of type I and type III collagen and may play a role in determination of collagen fibril diameter. Fibroblasts synthesize procollagen, which consists of three polypeptide chains spiraled into a triple helix. Each polypeptide chain consists of approximately 1000 amino acids. Glycine repeats every third amino acid, with hydroxyproline and hydroxylysine also repeating frequently. The triple-helix assembly of procollagen occurs within the fibroblast endoplasmic reticulum. The procollagen molecules are secreted into the extracellular space, where cross-linking to form microfibrils and, finally, collagen fibers takes place. Cross-linking occurs side-to-side, not end-to-end.

Type I collagen fibrils are large-diameter fibrils (100 nm) arranged into thick bundles that stretch but give great tensile strength to dermis. A single fiber 1 mm in diameter can support a static load of 20 kg. Type III collagen fibrils are thinner and arranged in small bundles located around structures such as a blood vessel, where compliance is required. Type V collagen has been found surrounding nerves in epidermal appendages.

Elastin

Elastin fibers account only for 4% of dermal matrix by dry weight. However, they make up a continuous network from the lamina densa to the hypodermis. After deformation, the skin is returned to its normal shape by the action of elastin fibers. Elastic tissue is most dense in the ligamentum nuchae and in the wall of the aorta. Elastin fibers are produced by fibroblasts and are composed of 90% elastin. Elastin is assembled from a secreted precursor molecule, tropoelastin. Covalent bonding between four lysyl residues provides strength and stability.

Ground Substance

The ground substance is the amorphous substance that surrounds and supports the collagen and elastin fibers of the dermis. Proteoglycans and glycosaminoglycans (GAGs) are the primary molecules of ground substance. The most common of the proteoglycans and GAGs are hyaluronic acid, dermatan sulfate, and chondroitin sulfate G. The ground substance comprises only 0.2% of the dry weight of the dermis but is capable of binding water in a volume up to 1000 times its own weight. Ground substance determines water volume of the skin and skin turgor.

Cells of the Dermis

Fibroblasts, macrophages, dendrocytes, and mast cells commonly occupy the dermis. They are found in the greatest numbers in the papillary dermis and surrounding blood vessels of the subpapillary dermal plexus. In the reticular dermis, cells of the dermis are found between the dense collagen bundles.

Fibroblasts

Fibroblasts are derived from the mesenchyme. They synthesize collagen and elastin and ground substance proteins. They are found on the surface of structural fibers but not within. The same fibroblasts have the ability to synthesize more than one type of protein simultaneously.

Macrophages

Macrophages originate from bone marrow cells and migrate to the dermis. Macrophages are phagocytic and capable of processing and presenting antigen to lymph cells. Macrophages produce lysozyme, peroxide, and superoxides, which allow them to kill microbes. They also possess tumoricidal ability, are hematopoietic, and are involved in coagulation, atherogenesis, wound healing, and tissue remodeling. Macrophages also secrete growth factors, cytokines, and other immune regulatory molecules.

Dendrocytes

Dendrocytes are stellate or at times spindle-shaped dendritic cells that are very phagocytic. They are found chiefly in the papillary dermis and upper reticular dermis. They are frequently noted adjacent to blood vessels in the subpapillary plexus and reticular dermis and subcutaneous fat. The dermal dendrocyte, previously thought to be a fibroblast, also may function as a type of dermal stem cell that can turn into a fibroblast when needed in wounded skin.

Mast cells

Mast cells, originating in the bone marrow, are secretory cells present in connective tissues throughout the body. In the skin, mast cells are located in greatest concentration in the papillary dermis, in sheaths of epidermal appendages, and surrounding blood vessels and nerves in the subpapillary plexus. Mast cells are also found in fat of the hypodermis. Microscopically, mast cells have a round or oval nucleus and a large number of dark-staining granules in the cytoplasm. The granules are of two types, secretory and lysosomal. Secretory granules may contain histamine, heparin, tryptase, chymase, carboxypeptidase, neutrophil chemotactic factor, and eosinophil chemotactic factor. Mast cells are the primary cells involved in the onset of allergic reactions. Release of mast cell granules causes contraction of vascular smooth muscle, increase in vascular permeability, tissue edema, and influx of inflammatory cells.

Hypodermis

The dense fibrous tissue of the dermis ends abruptly as the subcutaneous layer of fat begins. However, these two very different layers have extremely important structural and functional relationships. Epidermal appendages such as hair follicles and apocrine and eccrine sweat glands extend into the hypodermis. Networks of blood vessels and nerves are organized in this layer into systems designed to supply the skin and epidermal appendages and to integrate functions of temperature regulation and protection. The hypodermis provides mobility of the skin, which protects against shearing of epidermis from dermis. The layer of fat supplies a reserve source of calories, insulates against heat loss, and cushions the skin, preventing pressure necrosis. The adipocyte of mesenchymal origin is the chief cell of the hypodermis. Adipose tissue is layered and subdivided into lobules. Connective tissue septae (e.g., Scarpa's fascia) separate fat into layers in various parts of the body and further organize layers into lobules. Blood vessels, nerves, and lymphatics run in these septi. Fat is first seen in the fetal hypodermis in the second trimester, and adipocytes continue to store fat throughout life. Depending on diet and metabolism, fat storage is accomplished by existing adipocytes, by adipocyte proliferation, and by the creation of new adipocytes from undifferentiated mesenchymal cells.

Blood Supply

The basic purpose of blood supply to an organ is to deliver nutrition and meet demands for repair and immunologic surveillance. The large number of blood vessels in the hypodermis and skin, however, exceed the requirements of most organs. This vascular network associated with the skin and hypodermis is complex because it is required to respond more frequently to injury and immunologic protection than most other organs. It is also involved in temperature regulation and blood pressure control. Because the skin is commonly subjected to shear forces, large arteries and veins in the skin, when compared to those in most other organs, are noted to have thicker walls containing smooth muscle and connective tissues.

The microcirculation to the skin consists of arterioles, terminal arterioles, precapillary sphincters, arterial and venous capillaries, postcapillary venules, and collecting venules. The macrocirculation, from deep to superficial, begins in the hypodermis with both horizontal vessels and vertical perforating vessels from underlying muscles. These small arteries pass through the hypodermis to the deep reticular dermis. At the level of the deep reticular dermis, arterioles are organized into a horizontal plexus. From this deep reticular plexus, arterioles pass vertically toward the epidermis. The ascending arterioles contain two layers of smooth muscle, a discontinuous elastic lamina, and another contractile cell, the pericyte. These ascending arterioles are thought to be the resistance vessels of the peripheral circulation. The vertical arterioles communicate with each other by forming vascular arcades. Where reticular dermis becomes papillary dermis, terminal arterioles form a second horizontally oriented subpapillary plexus. In the subpapillary plexus, the arterioles have one layer of smooth muscle and no elastic lamina. These vessels are thought to function as precapillary sphincters. Arterial capillary loops leave the terminal arterioles and extend into the papillary dermis, one or more loops per dermal papillae. The arterial capillaries have a continuous endothelium, basal lamina, and pericytes that form junctions with endothelial cells. Within the capillary loop, both the endothelium and basal lamina become very thin, allowing egress of intravascular contents.

The descending limb of the capillary loop becomes a venous capillary. The venous capillary empties into horizontally oriented postcapillary venules of the subpapillary plexus. Multiple postcapillary venules run with terminal arterioles in the subpapillary plexus. Both the venous capillary and postcapillary venule have a sheath of pericytes and veil cells. Veil cells encircle all segments of the microcirculation. They are not a component of the vessel wall but may support an open channel within the dermis for the delicate microcirculation. Postcapillary venules in the subpapillary plexus have an important function in the microcirculation. Histamine may act on the postcapillary venule to cause openings between endothelial cells. Postcapillary venules may be the site of the egress of fluid and inflammatory cells from the microcirculation. Actinic damage to skin and diabetes mellitus cause thickening of the postcapillary venule wall. Postcapillary venules flow into vertical venous channels that run along the ascending arterioles and empty into a deep horizontal venous plexus in the deep reticular dermis. Collecting venules carry blood from this deep reticular dermis venous plexus into the hypodermis. Valves are present in these collecting venules and are located to promote egress of blood from the skin.

Glomus bodies are special shunts typically found in the palms of the hand and soles of the feet that can bypass blood flow around congested capillary beds. The glomus body is a direct arteriovenous connection between an ascending arteriole and a venule. The ascending arteriole has three to six layers of smooth muscle and sympathetic innervation. Glomus bodies can close when blood pressure is low (Fig. 9–3).

Thermoregulatory Function of the Skin

The circulation of the skin also has an important thermoregulatory function. The skin has a large surface area and normally a blood flow of 450 mL/min (8.5% of total blood flow in the human body). Blood flow regulation can increase skin flow up to 10 times normal or almost totally shut down flow. The large subcutaneous venous plexus plays an important role. Arteriovenous anastomoses (AVAs) under sympathetic regulation connect arteries to veins in the subcutaneous venous plexus. At normal temperatures, the AVAs are essentially closed, but, when body temperature is increased, the AVAs open, shunting warm arterial blood directly to the subcutaneus venous plexus and allowing dissipation of heat. Also, to take advantage of the large surface area of the extremities, blood in the extremities can be regulated by sympathic nerves to run either in superficial veins or in the deep venae comitantes that run with the major arteries deep in the extremities.

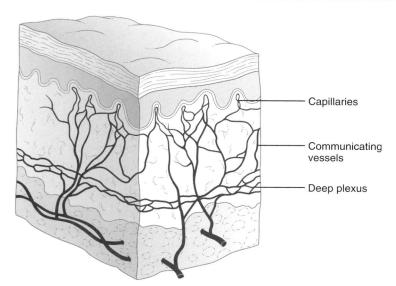

Capillaries

Communicating
vessels

Deep plexus

FIGURE 9–3 Circulation of the skin. (From Sams WM Jr, Lynch PJ [eds]: Principles and Practice of Dermatology [2nd ed]. London: Churchill Livingstone, 1996:8, with permission.)

Each arm represents 9% of the total body surface area, and each leg 18%, totaling 54% of body surface area. When body temperature is increased, blood flow is directed to the subcutaneous veins close to the surface to dissipate heat. When the body temperature drops, blood flow is directed to the venae comitantes both to prevent evaporative heat loss from the surface and to increase the venous return temperature by a heat exchange from the warmer deep arterial blood to the returning cooler blood in the venae comitantes.

Lymphatics

Lymphatic channels of the skin have an active and important role. The skin is often injured and frequently must process antigens, bacteria, and other organisms as it performs its protective function. Lymphatic channels must clear the skin of the discarded proteins and lipids, dead cells, and dead bacteria. Excess fluid released into the interstitium from the circulation under normal circumstances and after inflammatory processes also must be channeled away. Lymph flow is aided by deeper muscle contraction, adjacent arterial pulsations, and movement of the skin. Lymphatic vessels contain bicuspid-type valves to avoid backflow.

Lymph flow begins in blind-ending lymphatic channels called *lymphatic capillaries* or prelymphatic tubules in the papillary dermis. These lymphatics do not reach upward as close to the epidermis as do the vessel capillary loops and are not as numerous. The lymphatic capillaries empty into a horizontal subpapillary lymphatic plexus that is deep to the venous subpapillary plexus. Lymph vessels have a thinner wall and a larger diameter lumen than arteries or veins in this and other locations in the skin.

Their thin walls are composed of endothelial cells, a discontinuous basal lamina, and elastin fibers. The elastin fibers in the dermis may join the elastin fibers of the lymphatic vessel wall in a manner that promotes or "wicks" the passage of interstitial fluid into the lymphatic vessels. The subpapillary plexus lymphatic endothelium may abut or overlap, but gaps between cells are present. The gaps allow the influx of fluid and material from the interstitium. The subpapillary lymphatic plexus empties into larger vertical descending lymphatic channels that pass to the deep reticular dermis. At this level, there is a deep reticular plexus of lymphatics that empty into larger lymphatics that pass into the hypodermis. In the hypodermis, smooth muscle is first seen in the walls of lymph vessels.

Free Nerve Endings and Corpuscular Receptors

Touch, pain, pressure, temperature, and itch are mediated through free sensory nerve endings and specialized corpuscular receptors. Receptors are concentrated in hairless areas such as the palms, soles, labia, and glans penis. Both sensory somatic and sympathetic autonomic nerve fibers are found in the skin. Sympathetic motor fibers also run with sensory nerves into the dermis. Motor fibers branch off and terminate in vascular smooth muscle, arrector pili muscle, sweat glands, and sebaceous glands. The distribution of nerves through the skin follows a pattern similar to that of blood vessels and lymphatics. Dermatomes of skin are innervated by myelinated large cutaneous branches of musculocutaneous nerves. Small branches of these nerves pass through the hypodermis and enter the deep dermis. These branches possess epineurial, perineurial, and endoneurial seeds. Schwann cells encase bundles and individual fibers. A deep dermal plexus is formed by nerve fibers. Ascending fibers establish a superficial subpapillary plexus. Fibers branch from each plexus to innervate the skin, blood vessels, corpuscular receptors, and epidermal appendages.

Free nerve endings are the most significant and dominant sensory receptor in human skin. They consistently have a Schwann cell sheath and a basal lamina. Free nerve endings are widespread in the papillary dermis immediately below the epidermis. The basal lamina of these free nerve endings may fuse with the lamina densa of the dermal-epidermal junction. Fibers in this location have been categorized as penicillate and papillary. Penicillate fibers are the chief nerve fibers found just beneath the epidermis in hairy skin. They have an overlapping pattern and communicate pain, touch, temperature, and itch. On nonhairy ridged skin such as the palms and soles, they supply 60% of papillae, with a pattern of individual nerves supplying individual papillae. This nonoverlapping pattern provides fine discrimination. Corpuscular receptors provide the remaining sensibility in the skin of the palms and soles.

Papillary nerve endings are different from penicillate fibers. These nerve endings have vesicles and increased numbers of mitochondria. They are thought to be cold receptors. They are seen close to the orifices of hair follicles and arise from deeper nerves associated with hair follicles. The deep portion of a hair follicle is innervated by nerve fibers branching from myelinated axons in the plexus of nerves in the reticular dermis. These nerve fibers, covered by Schwann cells, are organized around the lower end of the hair follicle in both a longitudinal and a circular pattern to form a basket-like arrangement. They are stimulated by the motion of hair. These "basket" fibers contain cholinergic sympathetic nerves that branch to eccrine sweat glands and other fibers that go to the arrector pili muscle and sebaceous glands. The arrector pili muscle may contract in response to cold or fright, producing "goose bumps." These muscles are best developed in humans on the areolae and tunica dartos of the scrotum. Sebaceous glands found over most of the body empty into the outer portion of the hair follicle except in the labia minora, nipple areola, and inner aspect of the prepuce, where they empty directly onto the surface of the skin. They produce sebum, an oil that lubricates and protects skin and hair.

Additional free nerve endings lose their Schwann cell sheaths, penetrate the epidermis, and form touch domes. Touch domes, also known as Iggo's capsules, Pinkus corpuscles, and hederiform endings, may contain 50 Merkel cells associated with one branching nerve fiber in the epidermis. Touch domes are found in humans in hairy skin on the dorsal forearm and neck and in palmar and plantar skin.

Receptor Corpuscles: Meissner's Corpuscles and Pacinian Corpuscles

Receptor corpuscles in general consist of a capsule composed of perineurium and an inner structure of nerve fibers wrapped in Schwann cell lamellae. Meissner's corpuscles are elongated receptors in the palms and soles. They are vertically oriented in dermal papillae and mediate touch. Up to six myelinated fibers enter each Meissner's corpuscle and have bulbous endings. Specialized mucocutaneous end organs much like Meissner's corpuscles are found in the perianal canal, glans penis, labia minora, clitoris, and vermilion of the lips. They also mediate delicate touch.

The pacinian corpuscle is found in the deep dermis and hypodermis of the palms and the soles and responds to pressure and vibration. Its perineurium forms a complicated capsule of 30 or more layers of cells and connective tissue. The center consists of Schwann cell hemilamellae and nerve fibers and terminals. Pacinian corpuscles in the digit receive one myelinated branch from a digital nerve.

Epidermal Appendages

Eccrine Glands

Human skin houses 2 to 4 million sweat glands dispersed over the entire skin surface except for the vermilion of the lips, glans penis, inner prepuce, and labia minora. The greatest concentration of sweat glands is found in the axillae and in the palms and soles. The soles of the feet actually have the highest concentration at $620/cm^2$. An individual gland weighs 30 to 40 μg, but the total number found in human skin, which is between 2 and 4 million, weighs approximately 100 g, which is roughly equivalent to the weight of one kidney. As a functional unit, sweat glands can excrete as much as 10 L of fluid per day. Eccrine sweating is the most important method by which the human body controls temperature through evaporative heat loss, and this is an extremely important function of the human skin. Each gram of water lost through the skin dissipates 580 calories of heat.

The sweat glands consist of two parts: (1) the secretory coil situated deep in the dermis, and (2) a duct to transmit sweat directly to the skin surface. The secretory coil consists of clear secretory cells, dark mucoid cells, and myoepithelial cells. It produces an isotonic solution of sodium chloride when stimulated by acetylcholine release from sympathetic nerve endings. The duct, consisting of two layers of cuboidal cells, reabsorbs sodium chloride to preserve these electrolytes, yielding the final hypotonic solution. In addition to water and sodium chloride, sweat may contain heavy metals, lactate, urea, ammonia, amino acids, proteins, and certain drugs.

Apocrine Glands

Apocrine glands are located chiefly in the axillae and anogenital areas. Their major function is not to regulate heat but to act as scent glands. Every human has his or her own distinct "scent print" that can be recognized by dogs and other animals with an extremely well-developed sense of smell. Apocrine glands usually open not onto the skin surface but rather into the pilosebaceous hair follicle. Specialized apocrine glands are found in mammals. The mammary gland is an example of a specialized apocrine gland. Another example is the apocrine gland in the ear canal that makes cerumen.

Hair

The first hair follicles on the eyebrows, upper lip, and chin are seen in the 9-week fetus. The rest of the hair follicles develop at 4 to 5 months. Hair follicles are derived from both ectoderm and mesoderm. The hair follicle is a complicated epidermal appendage consisting of several concentric layers (Fig. 9–4). The follicle is surrounded by an outermost acellular basement membrane. The next layer is the cellular outer root sheath, followed by the inner root sheath, which is further subdivided into Henle's layer, Huxley's layer, and the cuticle of the hair follicle. The hair shaft consists of an outer cuticle, a cortex, and a central medulla. The hair shaft is attached to the follicular papilla, which is full of blood vessels that supply materials for hair production. Matrix cells lying above the basement membrane cap the follicular papilla and produce the

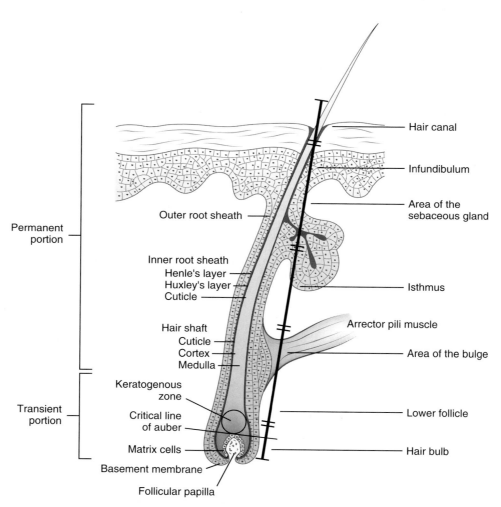

FIGURE 9–4 Anatomy of a hair follicle. (From Fitzpatrick TB, Eisen AZ, Wolff K, et al [eds]: Dermatology in General Medicine [4th ed], Vol 1. New York: McGraw-Hill, 1993:290. Reproduced with permission of the McGraw-Hill Companies, 1993.)

hair shaft. Hair color is determined by the type and amount of melanin. Darker hair has a large number of melanosomes of the eumelanin type. Lighter colored hair has fewer melanosomes that are of the pheomelanin type. Red hair displays erythromelanin. Each hair follicle has a smooth muscle, the arrector pilorum, attached. Contraction of this muscle when stimulated by cold or fright gives rise to "goose bumps" or hair standing up.

Sebaceous Glands

Sebaceous glands are epidermal skin appendages located on all parts of the body except the soles of the feet and palms of the hands. Sebaceous glands are structurally related to hair follicles and discharge into the outer portion of the hair follicle except on the nipple areolae, inner prepuce, and labia minora, where they empty directly onto the skin surface. In Montgomery's areolar tubercles of the female breast, sebaceous glands discharge directly into a lactiferous duct. The size and number of lobules in sebaceous glands vary. The main function of the sebaceous gland is to produce sebum. Sebum is oil consisting of triglycerides, phospholipids, and esterified cholesterol that provides both barrier protection and lubrication of the skin and hair.

Nails

Keratinized cells of the nail plate originate from the nail matrix. The nail plate is composed of two layers. The superficial layer is formed by the proximal nail matrix and the deep layer is formed by the distal nail matrix. The lunula denotes the distalmost portion of the proximal nail matrix. Fingernails grow at a rate of 0.1 mm/day, which is three times faster than the rate of toenail growth. Fingernails function as a protective covering of the fingertip and aid in picking up small objects (Fig. 9–5).

Langer's Lines

Elastic fibers in the dermis have special clinical significance. In 1861, Langer noted that a round puncture hole made into the skin assumes an elliptical shape as a result of innate skin tension. Elastic fibers in the dermis provide constant tension, so incisions in the skin spread open and skin grafts contract spontaneously following harvest. Innate tension in the skin is also determined by the motion of muscles and joints beneath the surface. The important concept of lines of minimal tension has developed from this knowledge. An incision made at 90 degrees to the lines of minimal tension will have a greater tendency to form a hypertrophic scar. Incisions made along the lines of minimal tension will be more likely to form a lesser scar.

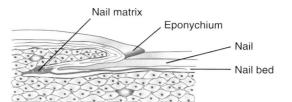

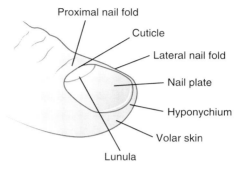

FIGURE 9–5 The nail. (From Sams WM Jr, Lynch PJ [eds]: Principles and Practice of Dermatology [2nd ed]. London: Churchill Livingstone, 1996:6, with permission.)

Skin Substitutes

The preceding detailed description of the structure and function of the skin illustrates how exceedingly difficult it is to engineer a skin substitute. Nevertheless, some real advancements have been made toward skin replacement.

Allograft (Cadaver Skin)

Reverdin is credited with the first skin graft using autograft in 1869. Soon thereafter, he applied allograft as a wound biologic dressing. James Barrett Brown popularized the use of allograft on burn wounds in the 20th century with his report in 1942. For more than 50 years now, allograft has been used extensively on burn wounds. Major burns cause significant immunosuppression, allowing allograft "take" historically to last for weeks or months. However, with early excision and grafting, better nutrition, and improved critical care over the last two decades, immune function has improved. Thus allograft may be rejected within 3 weeks.

Allograft take has significant beneficial effects on the burn wound. It first and foremost seals the wound to prevent the loss of fluids, electrolytes, and protein. Allograft prevents desiccation of healthy tissue to avoid further death of the wound surface. Nonviable surface tissue increases the depth of the burn and also provides a mechanism for bacterial growth. Placement of allograft on a viable wound surface promotes the ingrowth of blood vessels, which both prepares the wound for permanent grafting and reduces bacterial counts. Allograft take also diminishes pain, which may help decrease circulating catecholamines and decreases the associated burn hypermetabolic state. Pain reduction in the extremities also allows early range of motion and preservation of joint function.

Although fresh allograft stored at 4°C and used within several days of harvest may provide the best take, allograft bank skin may be more universally available. Both cryopreserved and lyophilized forms of allograft are available. Improvements in cryopreservation of allograft allow bank skin to remain viable for as long as 10 years. The risk of transmission of hepatitis B and C and HIV also has been reduced significantly.

Cadaver skin should be harvested from the cadaver donor and placed in standard cold storage within 18 hours to maintain two-thirds viability. In cases of a large third-degree surface burn, cadaver skin has been placed over widely meshed autograft. Cadaver skin has also been placed on large surface area full-thickness burn wounds following early excision. The cadaver skin has later been tangentially excised in preparation for the application of cultured keratinocytes.

Cultured Epithelium

Culturing of human keratinocytes has progressed to the point of allowing coverage of very large surface area burns in a relatively short time. A 10,000-fold expansion of a 2-cm^2 section of human skin has been achieved in 3 to 4 weeks. Epithelial cells mature in culture to show incomplete stratification but do form a keratinized layer. Significant contraction occurs in the burn wound treated with cultured epithelium. Reports of the durability of cultured keratinocyte grafts have varied from significantly less than to equal to that of meshed autografts. Cultured epithelial autograft (CEA) has been reported to show a more normal skin architecture at maturity, with rete ridges noted at 5 to 18 months. Conventional split-thickness skin graft controls showed no rete ridges at 5 years. At 1 to 2 years, an anchoring fibril system similar to that of normal skin was noted with CEA, and in 3 years elastin content approached that of age-matched normal skin. A neodermis was noted as well, with some improved degree of dermal organization under CEA compared to standard split-thickness autografts. However, contraction of CEA is a significant problem because of the lack of a functionally replaced dermis.

Biosynthetic Wound Coverings

When dermis is lost, it is not reproduced in adult mammals. Secondary healing, split-thickness skin grafts, and CEA coverage all provide an inelastic surface more like scar than normal skin because of the lack of a dermis. Thus attempts have been made to engineer a dermis. Integra, one of the first biosynthetic wound coverings, is sterilized and stored in 70% isopropyl alcohol or in a freeze-dried form. The product appears to be nonimmunogenic when placed on a wound, although immunoreaction to bovine injectable collagen (Zyderm) has been noted. Integra is a two-layer skin substitute with a dermal and an epidermal component. The dermal layer is bovine type I collagen cross-linked with a GAG chondrotin 6-sulfate. The mean pore size is 50 ± 20 μm. This replacement dermis, which is slowly biodegraded, provides a matrix for the ingrowth of fibroblasts and blood vessels. A clear Silastic epidermis allows passage of water vapor similar to normal skin. This clear layer allows inspection of the wound through the Integra to assess the take or lack of take of this product. Infection under the product is easily recognized. One to 4 weeks following placement, Integra "takes," the silicone layer is removed, and a split-thickness autograft of 2 to 8 one-thousandths of an inch or a CEA is applied. Clinical trials have demonstrated some advantages with the use of Integra. Less scar contracture occurred with Integra when compared to conventional split-thickness skin grafts or CEAs, and a better cosmetic appearance was provided in some cases. Also, there is no risk of transmission of hepatitis B or C or HIV as there is with the use of cadaver skin. Many other biosynthetic skin dressings or replacement products, such as Biobrane, Trancyte, and AlloDerm, have been developed. A functionally more complete skin substitute remains a difficult challenge, and research continues.

Bibliography

Fitzpatrick TB, Eisen AZ, Wolff K, et al (eds): Dermatology in General Medicine (4th ed), Vol 1. New York: McGraw-Hill, 1993.

Sams WM Jr, Lynch PJ (eds): Principles and Practice of Dermatology (2nd ed). London: Churchill Livingstone, 1996.

CHAPTER 10

Bone and Cartilage

Lawrence X. Webb, M.D. and Jeffrey S. Shilt, M.D.

Structure and Function

Bone and cartilage are tissues comprised of cells within an extracellular material whose composition determines the biomechanical behavior of the tissue. The composition of the extracellular material consists of collagen (90%) and protein polysaccharide macromolecules (10%). The polysaccharide molecules reside in the space between the collagen fibers as well as in the "hole zones" within the cross-linked portion of the collagen fibrils. These hole zones are thought to be the loci for the initiation of mineralization/hydroxyapatite crystallization. Functionally this composite of extracellular material is analogous to rods of rebar steel embedded in the concrete used in construction. Mechanically, the cement (hydroxyapatite crystal) provides a high resistance to compressive stress and the rebar steel rods (collagen fibers) provide a high resistance to tensile stress. The number and orientation of the collagen fibers determines the resistance of the bone to tensile load and accounts for the anisometric nature of the bone. For most situations, resistance to compressive stress is greater than it is for tensile stress for loads of the same magnitude, and therefore, when bone fails, it does so when loaded in tension.

This basic property of the matrix of bone explains its loading characteristics, as well as the pattern of its fracturing when loaded beyond capacity. In general, transverse fractures are produced by tensile loading along the axis of the bone, oblique fractures by axial loading in compression, and spiral fractures by torsional loading around the longitudinal axis. The loading characteristics of long bones and the correlation with fracture patterns is dictated by a complex mix of variables, including (1) the biomechanical properties of the heterogeneous extracellular material, as just discussed; (2) the distribution and orientation of that material in the bone; (3) the three-dimensional shape of the bone; (4) the magnitude, direction, and point of application of the load; and (5) the rate at which the load is applied.

Cartilage is a collection of cells (i.e., chondrocytes) whose extracellular gel is similarly characterized by collagen and ground substance consisting of proteoglycan macromolecules. Collagen is the major component of the matrix and is composed of three chains, which are wound around each other to form a triple helix. It is derived from its precursor, tropocollagen, which is elaborated by the chondrocyte in the case of cartilage or, in the case of bone, by the osteoblast/osteocyte, and in the case of fibrocartilage, by the fibroblast. The three chains that form the triple helix may differ in their amino acid sequence and biomechanical behavior. For example, type I collagen is found in tendon and bone, type II collagen is found in articular cartilage, type III collagen is found predominantly in early reparative tissue/fibrocartilage, and type IV is found in the basement membrane of blood vessels. Proteoglycan consists of a protein molecule backbone to which long-chain polysaccharides are attached. There are two main groups of such long-chain polysaccharide molecules: those whose constituent molecules are simple glycosaminoglycans, such as hyaluronic acid, and those whose constituent molecules are complex glycosaminoglycans, which are composed of sulfated molecules such as chondroitin sulfate and keratan sulfate. The sulfate groups on these constituent molecules are negatively charged and enable the complex glycosaminoglycans to function as a negatively charged colloid. The proportion of simple versus complex glycosaminoglycans can vary in different tissues as well as in the same tissue as the individual ages. It also varies in the stages of certain disease states. For example, in osteoarthritis, in early stages there is an increase in chondroitin sulfate, whereas in late stages there is a relative decrease in chondroitin sulfate compared to keratan sulfate.

In general, there are three types of cartilage: articular cartilage (which functions as the bearing surface in joints and acts as a precursor of bone in development, longitudinal growth, and fracture healing), elastic cartilage, and fibrocartilage. Articular (hyaline) cartilage is uniquely suited to allow a near-frictionless shearing on the opposing articular surface in a synovial fluid environment (coefficient of friction when lubricated with synovial fluid = 0.002, which is 15 times less friction than an ice skate on ice lubricated by water, whose coefficient of friction is 0.030!). Elastic cartilage contains many elastin fibers that have a high strain. This cartilage readily springs back to its original shape after deformation and is found in the nose and external ear. Fibrocartilage is the cartilage of repair tissue. It differs from articular cartilage in that it is stiffer and does not provide a near-frictionless bearing surface in a synovial fluid environment. However, this is the tissue that repairs injured specialized tissues such as articular cartilage, which helps to explain some of the deficient mechanics of the arthritic joint.

Bone

Formation and Cells

Bone is formed from the embryonic mesenchymal layer. It forms by one of two processes: endochondral ossification or intramembraneous ossification. Endochondral ossification is a process whereby a bone, which is preformed in cartilage, undergoes sequential focal degeneration and orderly replacement by osseous tissue. In long bones this process starts in the center of the bone at a site referred to as the primary center of ossification and later occurs at the ends of the bone (proximal and distal) at the secondary centers of ossification. (Some bones have more than two secondary centers.)

As time progresses, the ossification process fills the entirety of the cartilage precursor, and the residual "seam" of cartilage between the primary and secondary centers persists until the longitudinal growth of the bone is complete (at maturity). The cartilage seam between the two centers is the growth plate. The mitotic activity of the palisades of cartilage cells of the growth plate accounts for the growth in length of the bone and persists until maturity, at which point it is finally replaced by bone. The primary and secondary ossification centers appear and later fuse on a specific developmental timetable. For example, the distal femoral secondary epiphyseal center appears at 9 months' gestation and fuses with the primary center at age 14 to 16 years in females and 18 to 19 years in males.

Intramembranous ossification is also called "appositional growth," typified by the process that occurs at the outer surface of the long bone in the perichondrium (which later becomes the periosteum). This process accounts for the increase in the girth of the long bone. It also accounts for the growth of the flat bones, for example, those that comprise the cranium.

The cells of bone tissue are osteoblasts, osteocytes, and osteoclasts. Osteoblasts are cuboidal in shape and approximately 20 to 30 μm in average diameter. Osteoblast activity is controlled by parathyroid hormone (PTH) and the active metabolites of vitamin D. Products of their activity include carbohydrate-protein complexes as well as procollagen (tropocollagen), which is the precursor of collagen. Osteoblasts have alkaline phosphatase in their cytoplasm and nucleoplasm and elaborate the constituents of the extracellular matrix (ECM). The extracellular material is assimilated and undergoes calcification and matrix vesicle formation, histologic events that accompany the process of ossification.

The osteocyte is the cell that occupies the lacuna and is surrounded by ossified bone matrix (Fig. 10–1). Its cytoplasmic extensions occupy the canaliculi, and the cell is thought to play a primary role in mineral homeostasis.

Osteoclasts are multinucleated cells that resorb bone matrix. They have 15 to 20 nuclei and vary in size, ranging in diameter from 10 to 100 μm. The cytoplasm is rich in acid phosphatase. Osteoclasts occupy Howship's lacunae and possess an active brush border, which is rich in lysosomal enzymes and is thought to be the site on the surface of the cell where active bone matrix resorption occurs. Osteoclasts are essential for normal bone remodeling to occur. The disease process that occurs with osteoclast deficiency or malfunction is known as osteopetrosis or "marble bone disease." Patients with this disease have bones that, on radiographs, appear very dense with poorly formed marrow canals on the cross section of the long bones (cortical bone) (Fig. 10–2). Despite their density, these bones are prone to fracture because the stressed and theoretically partially fractured osteons are not cleared as a prelude to replacement, which occurs in normal bone. The process consisting of replacement and turnover of old osteons for new ones is called remodeling. The process occurs at an accelerated rate in growing bone and following a fracture and as an ongoing dynamic process

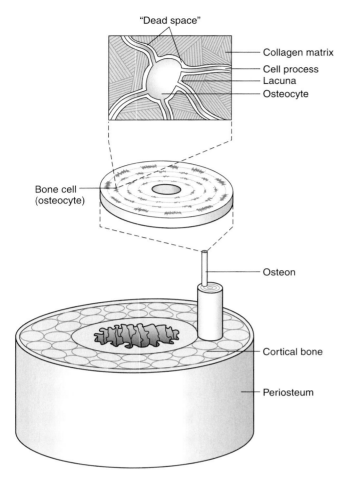

"Dead space"

Collagen matrix
Cell process
Lacuna
Osteocyte

Bone cell
(osteocyte)

Osteon

Cortical bone

Periosteum

FIGURE 10–1 An osteocyte in its lacuna with its cytoplasmic extensions in the canaliculi of the Haversian system of cortical bone.

in all living bone. It is this process that enables bone to be a self-replenishing, fatigue-resistant material.

Repair and Remodeling

Bone is unique in that it is the only specialized tissue in the body that repairs itself as itself (without a scar!). When a fracture of the bone occurs, the fracture zone is characterized by a tearing of the periosteum and by hematoma formation as well as local disruption of blood supply, which in turn results in a proportional amount of tissue anoxia and necrosis. The process of inflammation that follows the injury is characterized by the release of vasoactive substances and edema (sometimes manifesting as fracture blisters when this process affects the layers of the skin), white cell migration into the tissue space, and later proliferation of reparative tissues consisting of primitive mesenchymal cells, fibroblasts, chondrocytes, and osteoblasts.

Primitive mesenchymal cells can transform themselves into granulocytes, fibroblasts, chondroblasts, or osteoblasts, depending on the mechanical stability (and hence the strain)

imposed on the tissue at the fracture site. The correlation between cell/tissue types and the mechanical environmental of the fracture was initially proposed by Stephon Perren when research showed that the rupture strain for granulocytes is 100% of their resting length, while that for fibroblasts is 20%, that for chondroblasts is 10%, and that for osteocytes is 2%. Thus, if the relative motion between two bone fragments is 9%, fibroblasts and granulocytes can tolerate these strains but chondroblasts and osteoblasts cannot. Bone healing can only occur when mechanical conditions that permit bone formation exist (strains of 2% or less). Over the span of time, there is formation of increasing stiff tissue mass around the fracture.

In general, there are two types of bone healing. The first is adaptive bone healing, which is characterized by allowance for relative motion between bone fragments (e.g., a fracture treated by application of external or internal splints, which allow for some minor relative motion but negate excessive relative motion between the fracture fragments). Adaptive bone healing is characterized histologically by bone formation via a cartilage intermediary and radiographically by formation of "callus." Callus is an amalgamation of tissues the type of which change over time and whose mechanical characteristics change over time from elastic to rigid. The second type of bone healing is direct bone healing, which is characterized by absolute stability of the fracture fragments with the complete negation of all relative motion between the fractured bone ends. This type of healing is characterized histologically by direct haversian remodeling in areas of cortical contact and by intramembraneous bone formation in areas where there is a gap between the fragments. The bone that forms in the gap is woven bone, which is later remodeled into haversian bone. In conditions of absolute stability, bone forms in the gap without the need for a cartilage intermediary.

Clinically, the fulfillment of the condition of absolute stability between bone fragments is most reliably obtained by utilization of a properly applied lag screw(s) and/or compression plate in stabilizing the fracture. Examples of fractures and their modes of treatment that result in this type of healing are shown in Figure 10–3.

The type of fracture treatment chosen by the surgeon for a given fracture is determined by many factors and not primarily by the type of histologic or radiographic healing that occurs. Such factors as whether the fracture is open or closed, is associated with bone loss and/or overlying soft tissue loss, and is articular, periarticular, or diaphyseal all impact on this decision making, as does the patient's general medical condition, whether the patient has other injuries as well as the nature of the other injuries, the condition of the local soft tissue, and the quality of the bone.

On occasion, bone healing is delayed, incomplete, or no longer progressing. In a delayed union the process is

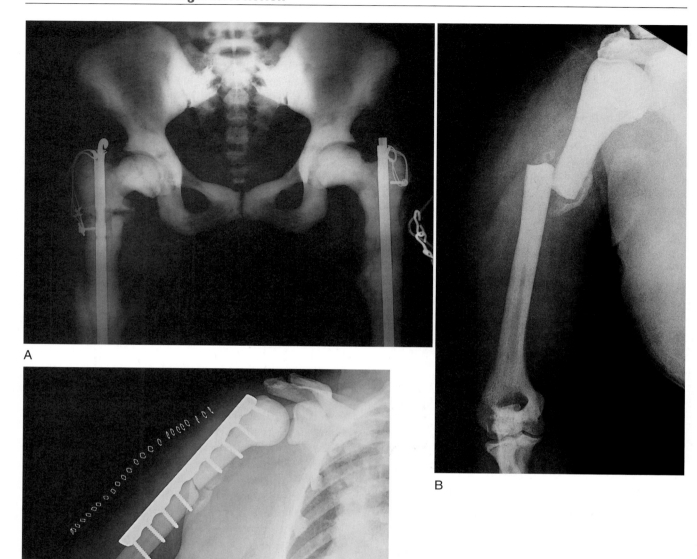

A

B

C

FIGURE 10–2 **A**, Anteroposterior radiograph of the pelvis and proximal femurs of a 30-year-old female with osteopetrosis. Note the increased density of the bones as well as the multiple fractures (in various stages of healing), which the intramedullary nails and wires address. **B**, Radiograph of this same patient's humerus, which failed to heal following a fracture. **C**, The delayed union was treated operatively with a plate fixation. Note the absence of an intramedullary canal in the proximal half of the bone.

prolonged beyond a normal timetable, and in nonunion the process of healing has reached a point of arrest with no further progression toward healing. Nonunions have been classified according to their biologic characteristics as (1) hypertrophic, (2) inert, and (3) atrophic (Fig. 10–4). The treatment chosen for delayed union or nonunion must take these biologic characteristics into account. For most atrophic and inert nonunions, stabilization (lowering fracture strain) and cancellous bone grafting are utilized. Stabilization utilizing compression without bone grafting will often suffice in the management of hypertrophic nonunions, whereas supplemental cancellous bone grafting is often advisable for atrophic or inert nonunions. For those nonunions whose biology includes active or indolent infection, the treatment algorithm becomes more complicated. One approach is to perform a radical débridement of all previously infected bone tissue followed by staged management as a gap (or defect) nonunion.

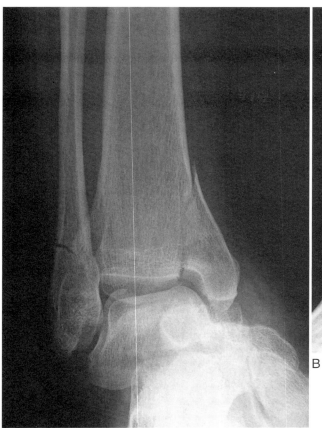

A

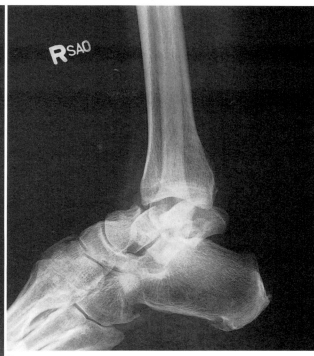

B

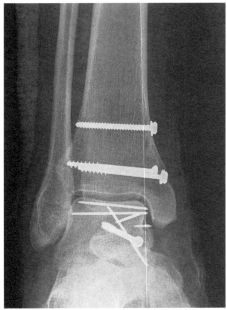

C

FIGURE 10–3 **A** and **B**, Preoperative radiographs of a foot/ankle in a patient with a fracture at the neck of the talus and tibial medial malleolus. **C** and **D**, This fracture has been managed with an open reduction and screws and pins, which negate all motion in the fracture, enabling it to heal without callus (by direct bone formation).

Figure continued on following page

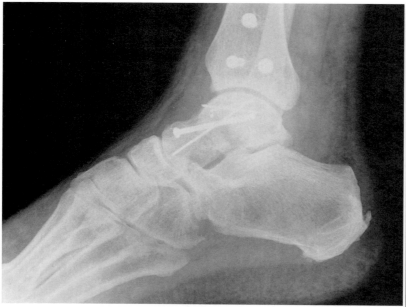

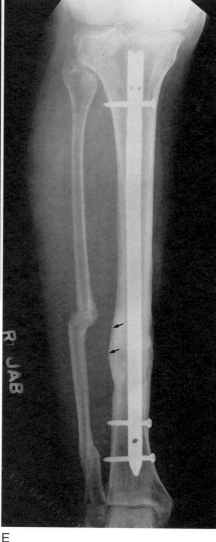

FIGURE 10–3 *Continued.* **E**, Anteroposterior radiograph of a fractured tibia and fibula that has been managed with a locked intramedullary nail. Some motion at the fracture site is permitted by the intramedullary nail, which functions as a plaint. Healing occurs by callus (with a cartilage intermediary), as evidenced by the slight bulge of the tibia at the fracture site *(arrows).*   E

Bone Grafts

Bone grafts are used to supplement and reinforce an area of bone deficiency or a zone of bone discontinuity for the purpose of correcting the deficiency/reestablishing bone continuity. Currently the gold standard material for bone grafting is autogenous bone, which is most commonly harvested from the iliac crest. Bone grafts may be structural as well as biologic. The former utilize cortical bone and the latter are derived from cancellous bone. Most commonly, however, autogenous cancellous bone is harvested from the iliac crest and directly implanted in the area of bone deficiency or as a supplement in the area of delayed union/nonunion. Another example of autogenous graft, which is both structural and biologic, would be a bicortical

or a tricortical graft from the iliac crest. When a living structural graft is required, it can be derived autogenously as a vascularized free fibular graft. This procedure entails the microsurgical transplantation of the fibular segment on its vascular pedicle.

The elements that comprise a fresh autogenous bone graft include cells, osteoconductive elements, and osteoinductive elements. For fresh autografts, it has been shown that significant proportions of bone cells survive the transplantation process. Osteoconductive elements act as a scaffold and provide a latticework upon which bone formation can occur. Osteoinductive elements provide the stimuli or chemical triggers to induce bone formation in the cells. Table 10–1 shows several different types of bone grafts/bone graft substitutes and lists their elements. Some substitutes

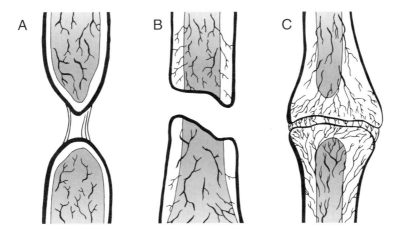

FIGURE 10–4 The types of nonunion as defined by Weber and Chech. **A**, Atrophic or "pencil-ended" nonunions are avascular. **B**, Inert or gap nonunions have either soft tissue interposition or an intercalary segment of bone loss resulting in a defect. The bones are otherwise normal, but the lack of bone contact or the position removes the stimulus to bone healing. **C**, Hypertrophic or "elephant foot" nonunions are vascular and characterized by hypertrophy of reparative tissues in the zone of healing. Usually, if appropriate mechanical conditions are established (strain <2%), bone healing will result.

act as space-occupying or filler material and are replaced over time (as they dissolve or resorb) within the host bone.

Although autogenous bone is currently the best bone graft material, there is the potential for donor site morbidity at the harvest site, and the amount of graft material is limited. Allograft bone, although less osteogenic, is not associated with any donor site morbidity. It does, however, have the potential (albeit extremely small) for disease transmission. Synthetic bone graft substitutes avoid the potential for disease transmission and donor site morbidity, but their osteogenic capacity is less than that of autogenous bone and their osteoconductive capacity has not been shown to be better than freeze-dried cancellous allograft bone.

Disease State: Osteoporosis

Osteoporosis is a skeletal disorder characterized by decreased bone strength and a predisposition to fracture. It is thought that 70% of bone strength is attributable to bone mineral density, a parameter considered to be an indirect measure of bone strength. Particularly affected are postmenopausal Caucasian females, whose bone mass is lost at an accelerated rate. Exercise, particularly impact exercise, as well as appropriate intake of vitamin D and calcium and measures taken to reduce the risk of falls, have been shown to lower the likelihood of osteoporosis-related fractures.

Table 10–1
Bone graft

Material	Trade Name	Biodegradeable	Cells	Donor Site Morbidity
Allograft bone (bone bank)		+	No	No
Autogenous bone graft		+	Yes	Yes
Demineralized bone matrix	Grafton Allomatrix (Wright Medical)	+	No	No
Collagen	Collografts (Zimmer)	+	No	No
65% Hydroxyapatite				
35% Collagen types I & III				
Coralline hydroxyapatite	Pro Osteon (Interpore)	±	No	No
Calcium sulfate	Osteo Set (Wright Medical)	+	No	No
Synthetic hydroxyapatite	Osteogen (Impladent, Holiswood, WY)	–	No	No

Hip fractures constitute about 20% of all osteoporosis-related fractures. They are associated with a 1-year mortality of 20%. Most of the survivors never regain their prefracture mobility. Nonoperative management is associated with unacceptably high rates of mortality and morbidity, hence surgical stabilization or prosthetic replacement is necessary. Adults with fractures of the vertebra, rib, hip, and wrist should be evaluated for osteoporosis and given appropriate counseling regarding intake of vitamin D and calcium as well as (when the patient is capable) impact-loading exercises.

Cartilage

Basic Composition

Cartilage consists of cells (chondrocytes) and the substance they secrete (ECM). The morphology and composition of the ECM determines the cartilage type and function. Many types of cartilage are described. Three commonly characterized cartilage subgroups include: articular or hyaline cartilage, fibrocartilage, and growth plate cartilage. These three types, with their subtypes, common locations, and unique characteristics of their respective ECMs, are presented in Table 10–2.

The ECM of all cartilage contains type II collagen. In minute amounts, proteoglycans and other proteins are present as well. However, water is the most prevalent ingredient, comprising approximately 75% of the wet weight of cartilage.

Several distinguishing characteristics are unique about cartilage. It is avascular and receives its nutrition from synovial fluid by diffusion. It maintains no lymphatic drainage system. Cartilage has no innervation and therefore does not communicate via neural impulses. However, it is believed that chondrocytes respond to their environment through integrins or molecules that are contained within the plasma membrane.

Cartilage Repair

Mature cartilage is metabolically active tissue. However, the cell-to-ECM ratio, mitotic activity, and turnover rate are significantly lower than those found in most other tissues of the body. These properties limit cartilage's ability to repair itself. This deficiency is primarily manifested in the mature chondrocytes' inability to proliferate and divide and neighboring chondrocytes' inability to migrate into the defect. The avascular nature of cartilage prevents effective systemic introduction of cells and growth factors to injured areas, further burdening the reparative process.

Simply stated, superficial lacerations in cartilage do not heal. Lack of hemorrhage following injury fails to initiate an inflammatory response. The scant matrix produced to fill an injured area by the chondrocytes does not adequately fill the defect or heal the lesion.

However, the limited reparative mechanisms maintained by cartilage can be utilized for repair. Full-thickness cartilage injuries that penetrate to subchondral bone does allow vascular invasion. Alternatively, superficial lesions can be artificially transformed into deeper lesions by drilling into the subchondral bone. In either case, a systemic inflammatory response occurs, resulting in the recruitment and proliferation of stem cells. These mesenchymal cells have the capability of differentiating into chondrocytes and filling the defect. By 6 months following injury, defects are commonly filled with a combination of bone, hyaline cartilage, and fibrous tissue. This latter tissue is inferior to normal articular cartilage, but provides some improvement to the lack of repair noted in superficial lacerations. This provides the clinical basis for drilling of cartilage defects.

Table 10–2
Cartilage types

Type	Location	Unique Characteristics
Articular or hyaline cartilage	Surfaces of synovial joints	Water comprises 75% of wet weight
Growth plate cartilage	Ossification centers of long bones	
Fibrocartilage	Interface between tendons/ligaments and bone	Strands of fibrous tissue intermixed throughout ECM
Elastic cartilage*	Auricles, nose, epiglottis, Eustachian tubes, trachea	Elastin fibers surrounding the chondrocytes
Fibroelastic cartilage*	Intervertebral disks, menisci	Fibers of elastin and fibrous tissue present

ECM, extracellular matrix.
*Subset of cartilage types.

This reparative process is much more notable and biomechanically sound in young individuals in comparison to the healing process that occurs in the elderly.

Disease States

▋*Osteoarthritis*

Osteoarthritis is a condition generally occurring later in life that affects load-bearing joints. Biochemically, osteoarthritic cartilage swells with water secondary to a loss of proteoglycans. Morphologically, this process results in fissuring and focal loss of the cartilage, subchondral bone sclerosis, and osteophyte and cyst formation. Clinically, patients present with pain, swelling, deformity, and limitation of motion that progress as the disease progresses. The etiology is unknown, but it appears that age-related changes in cartilage coupled with preceding trauma/abnormal joint loading and subsequent arrival of cartilage-derived chemical mediators likely play a significant role. Current treatment is aimed at symptomatic relief with nonsteroidal anti-inflammatory drugs. Intra-articular hyaluronates and "nutraceuticals" are becoming more popular as a form of conservative management. Finally, total joint arthroplasty is reserved as definitive management. Attempts at physiologic replacement with autograft and allograft cartilage are currently underway.

▋*Osteochondritis dissecans*

Osteochondritis dissecans is a focal fragmentation of subchondral bone with loss of the structural integrity of the overlying articular cartilage. This commonly occurs in children and adolescents, and the etiology is unknown. The knee, ankle, and elbow are the most common sites in decreasing order of incidence. Repetitive stress is thought to play some role in pathogenesis. Treatment is based on the stage of the disease. Observation and modification of weight bearing is the initial treatment for early disease. Arthroscopic débridement and drilling of the lesion is indicated for persistent lesions not amenable to the above treatment. The development of osteocartilaginous loose bodies created by separation of the articular cartilage from the underlying subchondral bone can occur, and arthroscopic removal of any loose chondral bodies is indicated. Osteochondral grafts are reserved for large lesions not responsive to débridement and drilling.

Mineral Homeostasis

Calcium, Phosphorus, and Magnesium Metabolism

Normal mineral homeostasis is responsible for all essential biochemical processes, skeletal growth during childhood, and maintenance of skeletal mass throughout adulthood. This delicate balance requires interaction between intestinal absorption, renal regulation, and bone remodeling to maintain the appropriate levels of calcium, phosphorus, and magnesium.

These minerals each play a unique role. Calcium and phosphorus help provide the structural integrity of the skeleton by combining to form hydroxyapatite $(Ca_{10}(PO_4)_6(OH)_2)$, a major constituent of the ECM of bone. Calcium is also critical for normal muscle contraction and cellular membrane permeability. Intracellular phosphorus, in the form of phosphate esters, is an integral component of cellular energy processes. Magnesium has no structural role but is an enzymatic cofactor needed in many chemical reactions.

Normal intestinal absorption of these minerals is dependent on adequate dietary intake and intact absorptive properties in the intestine. This latter process occurs primarily in the small intestine, but evidence exists that the colon maintains the ability to play a minor absorptive role. Two separate systems allow for such absorption: (1) *a nonsaturable, passive, paracellular absorption*, dependent only on each specific mineral concentration within the gut; and (2) *a saturable, active, transcellular absorption* that is physiologically regulated. The duodenum (20 cm length) is the location of the active transport system. The jejunum (100 cm length, 7- to 9-Å pore size) and ileum (150 cm length, 3- to 4-Å pore size) maintain the passive, paracellular system. Despite the location of the active system in the duodenum, the jejunum has the greatest absorptive potential because of its larger surface area and pore size, greater length, and relatively longer transit time.

The mineral load filtered by the kidneys is 40 times that absorbed by the intestine. Therefore, renal regulation has the capacity to play the dominant role in maintaining normal mineral homeostasis. The nephron acts as the functional unit of the kidney. Each nephron is composed of both vascular (glomeruli, afferent and efferent arterioles, and peritubular capillaries) and tubular (proximal and distal convoluted tubules connected by the loop of Henle) components. The peritubular capillaries are responsible for the majority of the nephrons' resorptive ability secondary to the high concentration of microvilli located there. Much of this resorption is through a passive system similar to that found in the intestine.

The skeleton serves as a large storage space for calcium and phosphate in the form of hydroxyapatite. Bone deposition by osteoblasts creates the crystalline hydroxyapatite, which creates a storage place for the minerals in the ECM. Bone resorption release these minerals back to the blood stream. This coupled interaction is a continual process that occurs throughout life. Under normal circumstances, bone remodeling plays a tertiary role in maintaining mineral homeostasis.

Normal calcium intake each day consists of approximately 1000 mg, of which 200 to 300 mg is absorbed. A similar amount is excreted in the kidneys to maintain normal plasma levels. Primary dietary intake is from dairy products. However, significant intake can also be obtained through broccoli, turnips, and collard and mustard greens. Spinach has a high calcium content, but is not readily absorbed secondary to the concomitant presence of a high oxalate concentration. Magnesium daily intake is approximately 300 mg, of which 100 mg is absorbed. It is widely distributed in all food types. Phosphorus intake varies from 800 to 2000 mg/day, with approximately 65% absorbed. It is also widely distributed throughout most food types.

Interaction of Parathyroid Hormone, Calcitonin, and Vitamin D

PTH regulates the calcium level in the blood stream through a complex feedback loop. Low serum calcium stimulates the parathyroid gland to increase secretion of PTH. This in turn leads to increased calcium serum levels from all sources: bone, intestine, and kidneys. Elevated PTH initiates resorption of bone. This hormonal effect on the osteoblast results in stimulation of the enzyme collagenase. Collagenase initiates osteoclast resorption in bone, releasing calcium and phosphate into the blood stream.

A second direct effect occurs through selective renal tubular resorption of calcium, while inhibiting the resorption of phosphate. This results in elevated serum calcium without stimulating calcium phosphate crystal deposition back into bone. It indirectly increases calcium levels through conversion of vitamin D to its active form, 1,25-dihydroxy vitamin D_3. This in turn increases the active, transcellular absorption of calcium and phosphate in both the intestine and kidney. The active resorption process is driven by an increase in the calcium-binding protein (calbindin) and by activating calcium pumps. Finally, bone resorption is stimulated through the induction of stem cells to differentiate into osteoclasts, resulting in release of calcium and phosphate similar to the method described above.

Once serum calcium levels have normalized, a negative feedback system is initiated. The increased calcium levels stimulate the parafollicular cells found in the thyroid to produce calcitonin. This results in renal excretion of calcium and phosphate, as well as inhibiting osteoclastic resorption of bone.

Disease States

Osteomalacia and rickets

Osteomalacia and rickets are considered the same disorder seen on either end of the age spectrum. These disorders are the result of impaired bone mineralization caused by a true or relative deficiency of calcium, phosphate, or both. This deficiency can be the result of poor nutrition, genetic insensitivity to vitamin D (vitamin D–resistant rickets), chronic renal disease, or a host of other problems. The age of disease onset produces different clinical manifestations because the effects of impaired bone mineralization on the developing skeleton are different from those on mature bones.

Rickets, the disorder present in children, produces a skeletal dysplasia signified by bowing of the extremities and dwarfism. These deformities are primarily present as a result of impaired mineral metabolism in the growth plate. Osteomalacia, the disorder present in adults, produces osteopenia and pathologic fractures. The symptoms are often much more subtle and can be difficult to diagnose.

Treatment of these disorders is aimed at correcting the underlying aberration in mineral metabolism. Nutritional rickets is corrected with dietary supplementation. Most genetic etiologies can be treated with physiologic doses of 1,25-dihydroxy vitamin D supplementation. The treatments of renal causes are more complex and require management of the underlying kidney disease, vitamin D and aluminum supplementation, and often parathyroidectomy to control tertiary hyperparathyroidism.

Bibliography

Athanasiou K, Shah AJ, LeBaron R: Basic science of articular cartilage repair. Clin Sports Med 2001;20:223.

Breslau NA: Calcium, magnesium, and phosphorus: renal handling and urinary excretion. In Favus MJ (ed): Primer on Metabolic Bone Diseases and Disorders of Mineral Metabolism. New York: Raven Press, 2001:50.

Bullough PG, Vigorita VJ: Injury and repair. In PG Bullough, Vigorita VJ (eds): Atlas of Orthopaedic Pathology: with Clinical and Radiologic Correlations. New York: Gower Medical Publishing, 1984:4.1.

Canalis E, Hock JM, Raisz LG: Parathyroid hormone: anabolic and catabolic effects on bone and interactions with growth factors. In Bilezikian JP, Marcus R, Levine MA (eds): The Parathyroids: Basic and Clinical Concepts. New York: Raven Press, 1994:65–82.

Cargo RD: Protein polysaccharides of cartilage and bone in health and disease. Clin Orthop 1970;68:182.

Chapay MC, Arlot ME: Vitamin D3 and calcium to prevent hip fractures in the elderly women. N Engl J Med 1992;327:1337.

Cummings RG, Nevitt MC: Calcium for the prevention of osteoporotic fractures in post menopausal women 65 years of age or older. J Bone Miner Res 1997;12:1321.

Gozna ER: Biomechanics of long bone injuries. In Gozna ER, Harrington IJ (eds): Biomechanics of Musculoskeletal Injury. Baltimore: Williams & Wilkins, 1982:1.

Gray JC, Elves MW: Early osteogenesis in compact bone isografts: a quantitative study of the contributions of the different graft cells. Calcif Tissue Int 1979;29:225.

Jackson DW, Scheer MJ, Simon TM: Cartilage substitutes: overview of basic science and treatment options. J Am Acad Orthop Surg 2001;9:37.

Manek NJ: Medical management of osteoarthritis. Mayo Clinic Proc 2001;76:533.

National Institutes of Health: Osteoporosis prevention, diagnosis and therapy. NIH Consens Statement 2000;17:145.

O'Driscoll S: The healing and regeneration of articular cartilage. J Bone Joint Surg Am 1998;80:1795.

Ogden JA: Femur. In Ogden JA (ed): Skeletal Injury in the Child. Philadelphia: WB Saunders, 1990:683.

Perren SM: Physical and biological aspects of fracture healing using prebending of compression plates. Clin Orthop 1979;138:175.

Perren SM: Fractures with absolute stability of surgical fixation. In Reudi T, Murphy WM (eds): AO Principles of Fracture Management. New York: Thieme Publishing, 2000:17.

Quinn CO, Scott DK, Brinckerhoff CE, et al: Rat collagenase: cloning, amino acid sequence comparison, and parathyroid regulation in osteoblastic cells. J Biol Chem 1990;265:22342.

Radin EL, Simon SR, Rose RM, Paul IL: Friction across joints. In Radin EL, Simon SR, Rose RM, Paul IL (eds): Practical Biomechanics for the Orthopaedic Surgeon. New York: John Wiley & Sons, 1979:124.

Robbins SL, Angell M: Inflammation and repair. In Robbins SL, Angell M (eds): Basic Pathology. Philadelphia: WB Saunders, 1971:28.

Rodrigo JJ: Physiology and biochemistry of the musculoskeletal system. In Rodrigo JJ (ed): Orthopaedic Surgery: Basic Science and Clinical Science. Boston: Little, Brown, 1986:177.

Schenck R, Goodnight J: Osteochondritis dissecans. J Bone Joint Surg Am 1996;78:439.

Gilbert SF: Collagen types. In Zygote: Cellular Approaches. Accessed 10 June, 2001. Available at *zygote.swarthmore.edu/cell6.html*

Weber BG, Chech O: Pseudarthrosis: Pathophysiology, Biomechanics, Therapy and Results. New York: Grune & Stratton, 1976.

Skeletal Muscle Physiology: Injury and Repair

Osvaldo Delbono, M.D., Ph.D.

A comprehensive approach to the structural and functional organization of skeletal muscle is needed to understand the primary role of skeletal muscle, which is the generation of force. A basic understanding of muscle structure and function also helps us understand muscle dysfunction in disease states and injury as well as the restorative capacity of muscle. Protein interactions at the external membrane (sarcolemma) and sarcoplasmic reticulum trigger a series of events leading to the generation of muscle force (excitation-contraction coupling). Alterations in molecular structure and/or interaction lead to impairment or failure of the primary function of muscle. Specific diseases and aging render the skeletal muscle more susceptible to injury. The ability of muscle tissue to recover from injury (plasticity) depends on the biologic conditions in which the injury occurs, the preservation of functional interaction with the nervous system, and the supply of trophic elements, among others factors.

This chapter is divided into seven sections. The first deals with basic embryology (myogenesis), the second with the structural and functional organization of skeletal muscle, and the third with mechanisms of muscle injury and repair. The last four sections are related to specific entities (malignant hyperthermia, tetanus, compartment syndromes, and hypoparathyroidism) that have skeletal muscle as their main target.

Basic Embryology (Myogenesis)

Myogenesis is a well-studied system because it became a preferred model system for the study of cell differentiation. Skeletal muscle derives from premyoblastic cells, which arise in the dermomyotome of the maturing somite and begin to differentiate into myoblasts at 4 to 5 weeks of gestation. By 6 weeks, cells have migrated from the dermomyotomal compartment to form the myotome in the center of the somite. Myotomal precursor cells are identified by the expression of myogenic determination factors such as Myf-5, myogenin, MyoD, and Myf-6. These factors have in common a 70-amino-acid, basic helix-loop-helix (bHLH) domain that is essential for protein-protein interactions and DNA binding. Myoblast migration to the prospective limb region follows a craniocaudal progression of growth, differentiation, and development. At various stages of myogenesis, myogenic bHLH factors activate transcription of a variety of muscle-specific genes by binding directly to conserved DNA sequence motifs (-CANNTG-, known as the E-box) in the promoter or 5′-flanking region of these genes. Myoblasts fuse to form myotubes with central alignment of their nuclei that evolve into mature muscle fiber after innervation and formation of neuromuscular junctions. This process is accompanied by development of transverse tubules (see Excitation-Contraction Coupling below), and changes from embryonic to mature myosin isoforms. Myotubes and myofibers are grouped into fascicles. Late during embryogenesis, a population of myoblasts destined to become the satellite cells of the adult muscle arises. These cells lie outside the sarcolemma but beneath the basement membrane and provide a reservoir of myoblasts capable of initiating regeneration in damaged adult muscle.

Structural Components and Function of Skeletal Muscle

Skeletal Muscle Structural Organization

Mature muscle fibers are long, multinucleated, cylindric units separated from other cells and surrounded by a membrane, the sarcolemma. Muscle fibers contain myofibrils made up of the contractile proteins myosin, actin, tropomyosin, and troponin and the structural supportive proteins actinin and titin. Myosin is an actin-binding protein provided with a catalytic site that hydrolyzes ATP, the source of energy for muscle contraction. Actin molecules polymerize in long, thin double helix filaments, forming a groove where tropomyosin molecules are located. Troponin molecules are located at regular intervals along the tropomyosin molecules. Troponin has three components: troponin T binds the other components to tropomyosin, troponin I inhibits the interaction of myosin with actin, and troponin C contains the binding sites for calcium, which initiates muscle contraction.

Muscle Fiber Subtypes and Types of Contraction

The most reliable method for differentiating fiber types is immunostaining of cross sections of cryopreserved muscles using specific antibodies to myosin isoforms (I, IIA, IIB, IIX-IID). However, ATPase staining based on the pH dependence of myosin ATPase activity, which relates closely to antigenic differences in myosin between fast- and slow-twitch muscle, also has been used for fiber classification. According to the histochemical classification, muscle fibers are divided into type I and type II (with subtypes IIA, IIB, and IIC). Human muscles fibers are classified into fast- and slow-twitch types based on their contractile properties in response to brief stimulation (an action potential). Fast-twitch fibers (type II, glycolytic, white) contract for less than 10 msec and are primarily concerned with fine, precise, and rapid movements. Slow-twitch fibers (type I,

oxidative, red) exhibit twitch durations up to 100 msec and are involved in strong, gross, and sustained movements.

Nerve-Muscle Functional Organization: The Motor Unit

Lower spinal cord motor neurons provide a common pathway for transmitting neural impulses from upper motor levels of the central nervous system to the skeletal muscles. This information is directed to skeletal muscles via the ventral roots, peripheral nerves, or cranial nerves. Each motor neuron innervates a number of muscle fibers within a single muscle; the various motor neurons innervating a single muscle are grouped in the spinal cord, forming the motor neuron pool for that muscle. During development, polyinnervated muscles become innervated by a single motor neuron. Axonal branches establish synapses with multiple muscle fibers of a single muscle. The activation of a motor neuron brings all the muscle fibers with which it establishes synapsis to the mechanical threshold; therefore, a single motor neuron and its associated muscle fibers constitute the motor unit, which is the smallest unit that can be activated to induce movement. On the basis of the speed of contraction, three types of motor units can be distinguished: fast-fatigable motor units, fatigue-resistant motor units, and slow-motor units that fall in between the first two subtypes in terms of time to fatigue onset. Differences in motor unit function depend on physiologic and biochemical characteristics of the constituent muscle fibers.

Excitation-Contraction Coupling

The motor neuron's generation and conduction of action potentials, release of acetylcholine at the motor end plate and its binding to nicotinic acetylcholine receptors, and increase in sodium and potassium conductance in the end plate membrane initiate skeletal muscle contraction. End plate potentials at the muscle membrane lead to generation of action potentials and their conduction to the sarcolemmal infoldings (T tubules). The transduction of changes in sarcolemmal potential into elevations in intracellular calcium concentration is a key event that precedes muscle contraction. Muscle electromechanical transduction requires the participation of a protein located at the sarcolemmal T tubule, the dihydropyridine receptor (DHPR), in the early steps of this signal transduction mechanism. The DHPR is a dihydropyridine-sensitive, voltage-gated, L-type Ca^{2+} channel, and its activation evokes Ca^{2+} release from the sarcoplasmic reticulum through ryanodine-sensitive calcium channels (RyR1) into the myoplasm. The functional consequence of alterations in the number, function, or interaction of these receptors is a reduction in the amount of intracellular calcium mobilization and in the development of force. Calcium is bound to troponin C, leading to formation of cross-linkages between actin and myosin and sliding of thin on thick filaments, producing shortening. Muscle relaxes as a result of calcium pumping back to the sarcoplasmic reticulum, release of calcium from troponin, and cessation of interaction between actin and myosin filaments.

Energy Metabolism

Energy metabolism is crucial for skeletal muscle contraction. The major fuels for muscle are glucose, fatty acids, and ketone bodies. Glucose is the preferred fuel for bursts of activity. In contracting skeletal muscle, the rate of glycolysis exceeds that of the citric acid cycle. Much of the pyruvate formed under these conditions is reduced to lactate, which flows to the liver, where it is converted into glucose. Muscle lacks glucose 6-phosphate, and so it does not export glucose. Three fourths of all the glycogen in the body (representing 1200 kcal) is stored in muscle. A large amount of alanine is formed in active muscle by the transamination of pyruvate, which in turn can be converted into glucose by the liver. In resting conditions, fatty acids are the major source of energy.

A group of neuromuscular disease entities are described in subsequent sections, with special emphasis on the molecular and cellular pathogenesis.

Muscle Injury and Repair: Role of Age

Age-related decreases in skeletal muscle mass and quality, termed *sarcopenia*, contribute to physical disability and loss of independence in the elderly. In addition to decreased muscle mass, sarcopenia is characterized by decreases in muscle contractile force or weakness that have been reported with age in several mammalian species, including humans. Sarcopenia is associated with limitations in activities of daily living, such as climbing stairs or rising from a chair, that lead to loss of independence. Statistical increases in frequency of falls, and in risk for fractures related to increased susceptibility to high-impact forces and accelerated bone loss, lead to periods of hospitalization with further decline in muscle strength. Reduced heat and cold tolerance, impaired glucose homeostasis, and obesity also have been related to sarcopenia. Decline in muscle performance with aging was quantitated in untrained and highly trained individuals more than two decades ago. These studies showed that, although the individuals with higher levels of physical activity were stronger, the rate of decrease in the level of muscle performance in both groups was similar. These results suggest that age-related deficits are independent of decreases in physical activity.

Despite the importance of muscle strength in preventing disability, the biologic mechanisms responsible for these phenomena are poorly understood. Some of the processes underlying sarcopenia have been investigated in human muscles, particularly the morphologic aspects. Cellular and molecular aspects have been explored both in human and more extensively in animal models of aging. Factors that determine sarcopenia with aging can be divided into three main groups: (1) neurogenic, (2) myogenic, and (3) a combination of both factors.

Neurogenic Mechanisms of Sarcopenia

The neurogenic mechanisms include alterations in muscle innervation and motor unit remodeling. Some elders present electromyographic evidence of muscle denervation suggestive of motor neuron alterations. These patients never develop classical amyotrophic diseases (e.g., amyotrophic lateral sclerosis). Muscle denervation is associated with reinnervation, as demonstrated by the presence of muscle fiber grouping in histologic sections. Cycles of muscle denervation associated with reinnervation lead to motor unit remodeling. The functional significance of motor unit remodeling still needs to be determined. The relative proportions of histologic area corresponding to fast- and slow-twitch muscle fibers change with aging, with slow-twitch muscle fibers becoming predominant. Age-related remodeling of motor units appears to involve denervation of fast muscle fibers with reinnervation by axonal sprouting from slow fibers. Therefore, motor unit remodeling leads to changes in fiber type distribution in mixed fiber-type muscles. Reinnervation of muscle fibers tends to compensate denervation; however, a net loss of fibers across age has been detected. This obviously occurs when the rate of muscle fiber denervation surpasses the rate of axonal sprouting and reinnervation. Indirect studies show a decrease in the total number of fast motor units and enlargement of the remaining motor units with age. Direct neuronal counting shows a reduction in the number and/or size of ventral spinal motor neurons at the cervical and lumbar regions with aging. Whether alterations in motor neuron, nerve terminal, or axonal transport account for muscle denervation is not clear. Studies on conduction velocity in peripheral nerves do not show significant changes with aging. This would suggest that alterations in myelin or severe reductions in nerve axonal composition do not occur with age. Although denervation has been suggested as a contributing factor to sarcopenia, the extent of denervation in individual muscles and its effect on human muscles remain to be determined. In addition, it is becoming apparent that denervation does not explain a significant deficit in specific maximum isometric tetanic force (muscle force normalized to cross-sectional area) recorded in aged skeletal muscles. Also, decreases in the number of spinal cord motor neurons occur after the eighth decade, when the loss in muscle mass and strength is already well established.

Myogenic Mechanisms of Sarcopenia

Primary muscular or myogenic factors in sarcopenia involve a group of alterations including (1) contraction-induced injury, (2) selective primary muscle fiber atrophy, and (3) alterations in muscle signal transduction. The phenomenon of contraction-induced injury has been related to increased mechanical frailty and decline in muscle restorative capacity with age that have not been well characterized. When muscles undergo lengthening contractions, the amount of injury to older animals is significantly greater. Also, older muscles recover slower and not as fully compared to muscles in younger controls. This suggested mechanism of sarcopenia has only been demonstrated in animal models of aging. Primary atrophy of type II fibers without alterations in fiber type distribution has been reported in aging muscles; however, it has been difficult to determine whether these changes result from aging or disuse. Alterations with age in muscle fiber signal transduction, such as sarcolemmal excitation–sarcoplasmic reticulum calcium release uncoupling and impaired insulin-like growth factor (IGF)-1–dependent modulation of muscle calcium channels, have been demonstrated.

Studies in muscle fibers deprived of sarcolemma (skinned muscle fibers) demonstrated that the force generated per unit of cross-sectional area does not differ in adult and old mice during isometric and shortening contractions. These results suggest that muscle atrophy does not explain entirely the age-related decline in muscle strength. They also suggest that other factors in addition to reductions in contractile proteins and in fiber number and size are contributing to age-related muscle weakness. Alterations with age in several mechanisms of signal transduction operate in skeletal muscles, and two of them in particular lead directly to development of muscle force. These are excitation-induced elevations in intracellular calcium and the mechanism of energy conversion from ATP into a mechanical response. It seems that changes in phosphorus metabolites involved in energy transduction (phosphocreatine, ADP, and ATP) and myosin isoforms do not change with aging. However, alterations in excitation-contraction coupling have been demonstrated in human quadriceps. Physiologic activation of the muscle membrane elicits elevations in intracellular Ca^{2+} that in turn induce muscle contraction by interaction with contractile proteins. Impairments in the mechanism of transduction of muscle activation into intracellular Ca^{2+} mobilization lead to decrease in muscle tension, with the clinical manifestation of muscle weakness. The basic mechanism underlying excitation-contraction uncoupling with aging is a molecular "unlinkage" between the two calcium channels, one that functions at the membrane voltage sensor and another that mediates

calcium release from intracellular stores. Alterations in excitation-contraction coupling result from significant changes in number and/or regulation of these molecules.

General mechanisms that may affect skeletal muscle directly or indirectly are oxidative DNA damage and mitochondrial DNA (mtDNA) mutations. Superoxide radicals and hydrogen peroxide, which are continuously produced in aerobic cells, undergo metal ion–catalyzed conversion into hydroxyl radicals. These hydroxyl radicals can cause oxidative damage, which in turn may be related to the development of mutations in mtDNA. Mutations in mtDNA have been associated with ischemic heart disease, late-onset diabetes, Parkinson's disease, Alzheimer's disease, and aging. The accumulation of damage to mtDNA by oxidation may be the basis for defects in oxidative phosphorylation capacity with age. It may be that a decline in oxidative phosphorylation capacity becomes symptomatic when tissue energetics fall below the threshold of an organ.

We are just beginning to identify the specific changes in muscle with age. A key question to be addressed at this moment is: Does cell signaling impairment with aging result from tissue resistance to trophic factors? There is increasing evidence supporting this concept. However, understanding this process requires further insight into a more general phenomenon, which is the role of trophic factors in mature tissue maintenance and restoration. In healthy individuals, deficiency with aging in spontaneous and stimulated growth hormone secretion, as well as circulating IGF-1 and IGF-binding protein-3 levels, is associated with decreased lean body mass, decreased protein synthesis, and increased percent body fat. Administration of recombinant human growth hormone improves nitrogen balance, increases lean body mass, and decreases body fat in older people with low IGF-1 levels. However, effects on muscle strength have not been measured in these studies.

Exercise interventions such as resistance training are being used in an attempt at least partially to restore muscle force in the elderly. Strength training in sedentary young and older individuals improves muscle force, improves metabolic capacities, and increases glycogen storage and oxidative enzyme activity. Aerobic training involving high-repetition, low-intensity muscle contractions leads to minimal strength gain when compared to the low-repetition, high-intensity stimulus of resistance training, in which both strengthening as well as endurance activities are included. Further studies on the use of trophic factors and specific exercise interventions are needed to determine the best means of preventing and/or reversing the decline in muscle function with age.

Malignant Hyperthermia

Malignant hyperthermia (MH) is an inherited autosomal dominant disease triggered by the administration of halothane and other inhalational anesthetics or succinylcholine. MH crisis develops most commonly in individuals between the ages of 3 and 30, with an incidence of 1 in 50,000 to 1 to 100,000 anesthetic administrations in adults. A high number of familial MH cases have been linked to point mutations in the ryanodine receptor. The analysis of the ryanodine receptor from probands from families with MH has associated MH with 17 mutations and 14 sites present in 40% of these families. Therefore, the causal MH mutations in 60% of families with MH have yet to be found. Mutation in the α_1-subunit of the L-type calcium channel has also been reported. MH episodes may occur in individuals who have inherited muscle diseases with deleterious phenotypes, such as central core disease, King-Denborough syndrome, Duchenne's muscular dystrophy, myotonia fluctuans, and possibly other myopathies. The main manifestations of MH are associated with rising end-tidal CO_2, tachycardia, unstable and rising blood pressure, hyperventilation, cyanosis, a falling arterial oxygen tension, an increasing arterial carbon dioxide tension, lactic acidosis, and eventually fever. Cellular damage results in elevation in serum levels of K^+, Mg^{2+}, and Ca^{2+} and a later rise in the serum and urine levels of muscle proteins such as creatine kinase and myoglobin (rhabdomyolysis). Different outcomes have been reported if therapy is not initiated immediately: the patient may die within minutes from ventricular fibrillation, within hours from pulmonary edema or coagulopathy, or within days from neurologic damage (postanoxic cerebral edema or encephalopathy) or obstructive renal failure. The in vitro caffeine/halothane contracture test was developed as a test for MH susceptibility and currently achieves 97% to 99% sensitivity and 78% to 92% specificity. A defect in the ryanodine receptor gives rise to abnormal chronic intracellular calcium regulation and accounts for all the clinical manifestations of MH.

MH should be treated with dantrolene at a dose of 1 to 2.5 mg/kg body weight per minute given intravenously until muscle tone softens, then 2.5 mg/kg IV every 6 hr for at least 24 to 48 hr until oral dantrolene can be administered. The patient is hyperventilated with 100% oxygen, and sodium bicarbonate is infused to correct metabolic acidosis. Furosemide and mannitol prevent acute renal failure. Procainamide should be administered because of the likelihood of ventricular fibrillation in patients with MH.

Tetanus

Tetanus is a neurologic disorder characterized by increased muscle tone and spasms produced by tetanospasmin, a powerful protein toxin elaborated by the anaerobic gram-positive organism *Clostridium tetani*. Waning immunity among the elderly contributes to tetanus being largely a geriatric disease in the United States. Only 27% of persons age 70 years or older have a protective level of antibody to *C. tetani*. Individuals aged 60 and older account for more than half of U.S. tetanus cases because routine immunization of infants since the 1940s has sharply decreased the incidence of tetanus in children and younger adults. *Clostridium tetani* is found worldwide in the soil and feces. The disease may complicate chronic conditions such as skin ulcers, gangrene, and abscesses. Tetanus also is associated with surgical procedures, burns, abortion, childbirth, drug abuse, and frostbite. The toxin is retrogradely transported from the wound to spinal cord or brainstem neurons through the axon. The toxin then crosses the central synapse, blocking the release of the inhibitory neurotransmitters glycine and γ-aminobutyric acid (GABA). The tetanic toxin cleaves protein(s) critical to proper function of the synaptic vesicle release apparatus. This results in increased alpha motor neuron resting firing rate, producing rigidity. Sympathetic hyperactivity and high circulating levels of catecholamines may result from loss of inhibition at the preganglionic sympathetic neurons in the lateral gray matter of the spinal cord. Similarly to the botulinum toxin, tetanospasmin may block neuromuscular transmission and produce weakness or paralysis. Recovery from paralysis requires sprouting of new nerve terminals.

Treatment is focused on the elimination of the toxin, neutralization of unbound toxin, muscle spasm prevention, and cardiorespiratory support until recovery. Diazepam or lorazepam, as benzodiazepine and GABA agonists, are widely used for the control of muscle spasms. Active immunization should be administered worldwide, including those persons recovering from tetanus, because immunity is not induced by the small amount of toxin that produces disease.

Compartment Syndromes

Acute compartment syndrome usually occurs with trauma, particularly long-bone fractures, crush injuries, burns, and vascular damage. In these injuries, bleeding and/or fluid accumulation within a muscular compartment containing one or more muscles leads to acute elevation of intracompartmental pressure. There are, however, a significant number of reports in the literature on acute exertional compartment syndrome, wherein unaccustomed exertion led to increases in intramuscular pressure sufficient to cause compromise of the arterial flow. Compartment syndrome is an increased pressure within a confined space that leads to microvascular compromise and ultimately to cell death. The microvasculature is affected, causing diffuse ischemia within the compartment. Pain is the hallmark sign. Fascia is the limiting entity that prevents "swelling out," so instead the compartment "swells in," decreasing blood flow in the small arteries and limiting venous return. It can affect any muscle compartment of the organism. It must be diagnosed immediately or irreversible neuromuscular and vascular damage occurs that can lead to renal failure (from myoglobinuria) and death (through arrhythmias).

The etiology of the compartment syndromes includes trauma, such as fractures, hematoma, gunshot/stab wounds, animal/insect bites, postischemic swelling, crush injuries, vascular damage, electrical injuries, frostbite, and burns; edema related to nephrotic syndrome; overuse injuries; prolonged use of tourniquets; genetic, iatrogenic, and acquired coagulopathies; external compression (i.e., cast, tight dressing); tight closure of fascial defects; hypo/hyperthermia; loss of consciousness; and *Clostridium perfringens* infection. Muscle injury leads to vascular compression, hypoxia, cell death, protein release, and edema. The increased intracompartmental pressure induces further vascular compression and cell damage, leading to muscle necrosis. Common clinical features are pain, paresthesias, passive stretch pain, pressure characterized by palpable tenseness in the affected compartment, and pulselessness. Consequences of this entity are irreversible tissue death (which determines the level of permanent disability), ischemic contractures, myoglobinuria, amputation, and death. The treatment is based on fasciotomy and urine alkalinization.

Hypoparathyroidism

A deficit of parathormone (PTH) causes hypocalcemia and hyperphosphatemia. PTH elicits a series of cellular events in response to interaction with the PTH receptor (PTHR) complex in target cells. Only two PTHR subtypes have been identified so far, one in bone and kidney and a different one in brain. The PTHR complex consists of a PTH receptor, an adenylate cyclase catalytic unit, and a guanyl nucleotide (GTP or GDP)–binding regulatory protein (G protein). Different G proteins (i.e., G_s, G_q) activate a cellular second messenger pathway involving either an effect on adenyl cyclase to enhance cyclic AMP or phospholipase C activation of diacylglycerol and inositol triphosphate. These second messengers then activate protein kinase A or protein kinase C, leading to protein phosphorylation and distal biologic responses. Neuromuscular symptoms usually are related to localized or generalized tetany. Hyporeflexia or areflexia is usually present. Elevated levels of serum creatine kinase may be secondary to muscle damage following tetany. Hereditary hypoparathyroidism occurs as an isolated entity or associated with other organ defects (DiGeorge syndrome, third and fourth branchial pouch syndrome, autoimmune polyglandular deficiency). Acquired hypoparathyroidism results from inadvertent surgical removal of all or part of the parathyroid glands. In this case, vascular compromise

of the remaining gland leads to fibrotic replacement and loss of function. Some cases of hypoparathyroidism result from radiation-induced damage subsequent to radioiodine therapy of hyperthyroidism. Transient hypoparathyroidism is frequent following surgery for hyperparathyroidism. The time to recover function varies from days to months. Oral calcium and vitamins restore the overall calcium-phosphate balance.

Bibliography

Bannister LH, Berry MM, Collins P, et al: Gray's Anatomy: The Anatomical Basis of Medicine and Surgery (38th ed). London: Churchill Livingstone, 1995.

Bogaerts Y, Lameire N, Ringoire S: The compartmental syndrome: a serious complication of acute rhabdomyolysis. Clin Nephrol 1982;17:206.

Buckingham M: Making muscle in mammals. Trends Genet 1992;8:144.

Buckingham M, Cossu G: Myogenesis in the Mouse Embryo. New York: Academic Press, 1998.

Burke RE, Levine DN, Tsairis P, Zajac FEI: Physiological types and histochemical profiles in motor units of the cat gastrocnemius. J Physiol (Lond) 1973;234:723.

Delbono O: Ca^{2+} modulation of sarcoplasmic reticulum Ca^{2+} release in rat skeletal muscle fibers. J Membr Biol 1995;146:91.

Delbono O: Regulation of excitation-contraction coupling by insulin-like growth factor-1 in aging skeletal muscle. Nutr Health Aging 2000;4:162.

Delbono O, Meissner G: Sarcoplasmic reticulum Ca^{2+} release in rat slow- and fast-twitch muscles. J Membr Biol 1996;151:123.

Delbono O, O'Rourke KS, Ettinger WH: Excitation-calcium release uncoupling in aged single human skeletal muscle fibers. J Membr Biol 1995;148:211.

Delbono O, Renganathan M, Messi ML: Excitation-Ca^{2+} release-contraction coupling in single aged human skeletal muscle fiber. Muscle Nerve Suppl 1997;5:S88.

Di Felice A, Seiler JG, Whitesides TE: The compartments of the hand: an anatomic study. J Hand Surg [Am] 1998;23:682.

Di Mauro A: Satellite cells of skeletal muscle fibers. J Biophys Biochem Cytol 1961;9:493.

Fitzpatrick LA, Arnold A: Hypoparathyroidism (3rd ed). Philadelphia: WB Saunders, 1995.

Fletcher JE, Tripolitis L, Rosenberg H, Beech J: Malignant hyperthermia: halothane- and calcium-induced calcium release in skeletal muscle. Biochem Mol Biol Int 1993;29:763.

Holloszy JO, Kohrt WM: Exercise. *In* Masoro EJ (ed): Handbook of Physiology. New York: Oxford University Press, 1995:633.

Jay CA: Infections of the Nervous System (4th ed). New York: McGraw-Hill, 1999.

Larsson L, Ansved T, Edstrom L, et al: Effects of age on physiological, immunohistochemical and biochemical properties of fast-twitch single motor units in the rat. J Physiol (Lond) 1991;443:257.

Loeser RF, Delbono O: The musculoskeletal and joint system. *In* Hazzard WR, Blass JP, Ettinger WH, et al (eds): Principles of Geriatric Medicine and Gerontology (4th ed). New York: McGraw-Hill, 1999:1097.

MacLennan DH, Britt BA: Malignant hyperthermia and central core disease. *In* Jameson JL (ed): Principles of Molecular Medicine. Totowa, NJ: Humana Press, 1998: 949.

MacLennan DH, Phillips MS: Malignant hyperthermia. Science 1992;256:789.

Marx SJ: Hyperparathyroid and hypoparathyroid disorders. N Engl J Med 2000;343:1115.

Melzer W, Herrmann-Frank A, Luttgau HC: The role of Ca^{2+} ions in excitation-contraction coupling of skeletal muscle fibres. Biochim Biophys Acta 1995;1241:59.

Orava S, Rantanen J, Kujala UM: Fasciotomy of the posterior femoral muscle compartment in athletes. Int J Sports Med 1998;19:71.

Pette D, Peuker H, Staron RS: The impact of biochemical methods for single muscle fibre analysis. Acta Physiol Scand 1999;166:261.

Phillips SK, Wiseman RW, Woledge RC, Kushmerick MJ: Neither changes in phosphorus metabolite levels nor myosin isoforms can explain the weakness in aged mouse muscle. J Physiol (Lond) 1993;463:157.

Renganathan M, Messi ML, Delbono O: Dihydropyridine receptor-ryanodine receptor uncoupling in aged skeletal muscle. J Membr Biol 1997;157:247.

Renganathan M, Sonntag WE, Delbono O: L-type Ca^{2+} channel-insulin-like growth factor-1 receptor signaling impairment in aging rat skeletal muscle. Biochem Biophys Res Commun 1997;235:784.

Wallace DC, Shoffner JM, Trounce I, et al: Mitochondrial DNA mutations in human degenerative diseases and aging. Biochim Biophys Acta 1995;1271:141.

Yu I, DeVita MV, Komisar A: Long-term follow-up after subtotal parathyroidectomy in patients with renal failure. Laryngoscope 1998;108:1824.

Zorzano A, Fandos C, Palacin M: Role of plasma membrane transporters in muscle metabolism. Biochem J 2000;349(Pt 3):667.

CHAPTER 12

Peripheral Nerve: Anatomy, Injury, and Repair

Linda Dvali, M.D., M.Sc., F.R.C.S.(C) and Susan E. Mackinnon, M.D.

For more than a century, the capacity of peripheral nerves to regenerate their axons and reinnervate distal targets after injury has been recognized. Despite this ability, poor functional results after peripheral nerve injury continue to be a frustrating problem. Dramatic advancements have been made in the techniques of microsurgical repair and in the understanding of the cellular and molecular basis of repair. Yet, complete functional recovery after a significant nerve injury is not guaranteed. The processes of nerve injury and regeneration are extremely complex. This chapter outlines the current knowledge of peripheral nerve anatomy, the cellular and molecular response to injury, and the mechanisms of repair. Having reviewed this complex subject, one can understand why functional improvement after nerve injury can be limited, and why continued research into this complex subject is warranted.

Anatomy of the Peripheral Nerves

Peripheral nerves have four basic components: neurons, Schwann cells, connective tissues, and end organs (motor end plates and sensory and autonomic receptors).

Neurons are the primary functional units of the peripheral nerve. They are composed of cell bodies and axons. Lower motor neuron cell bodies and presynaptic sympathetic ganglia reside in the ventral horn of the spinal cord. Lower motor neuron cell bodies send their axons through the ventral spinal root to join the spinal nerve that exits the vertebral foramen. The motor nerve fiber terminates at the neuromuscular junction in the muscle. Presynaptic sympathetic fibers send their axons to the sympathetic ganglia. Postsynaptic sympathetic neurons send axons to the periphery to innervate blood vessels, skin, and hair follicles. Sensory cell bodies reside in the dorsal root ganglia and send axons distally to join the spinal nerve and ultimately connect with sensory end organs.

Nerve fibers within motor and sensory nerves consist of unmyelinated and myelinated fibers in a ratio of 4:1. Unmyelinated fibers are composed of several axons, wrapped by a single Schwann cell. The axons of myelinated nerve fibers are each individually enveloped by a single Schwann cell (Fig. 12–1). Each Schwann cell has a double basement membrane that can only be identified on electron microscopy. The term *endoneurial sheath* refers to the basement membrane outside the Schwann cell. Myelinated axons are enveloped by a series of Schwann cells along the length of the axon. Between each Schwann cell is an interspace of unmyelinated axon known as the node of Ranvier. During development, the nerve is invested with a fixed number of Schwann cells. As growth occurs, the Schwann cells enlarge, increasing the internodal distance.

Unmyelinated axons conduct electrical impulses at speeds of 2 to 2.5 m/sec. Conduction begins with an action potential, which is propagated by voltage-gated channels as a depolarizing wave. Myelinated fibers, in contrast, are able to conduct impulses at speeds ranging from 3 to 150 m/sec. This is accomplished by saltatory conduction. A depolarization at one node of Ranvier is able to trigger a second depolarization at the next node without propagation of the depolarization in between the insulated axon segment. The greater the internodal distance, the faster the conduction.

Myelinated and unmyelinated axons combine into bundles known as fascicles. Within each fascicle is a loose collagen-containing connective tissue matrix known as the endoneurium. In surgical dissection, it is seen as a gelatinous material that partly extrudes from the sectioned ends of fascicles preceding repair. Surrounding each fascicle is a thicker, more substantial connective tissue layer known as the perineurium. Fascicles are arranged in various patterns within peripheral nerves from monofascicular, in which a single fascicle comprises the entire nerve, to oligofascicular and polyfascicular patterns, in which a few or many fascicles are contained within the nerve. Surrounding each fascicle is another connective tissue layer, the internal epineurium. The epineurium surrounding all of the fascicles of a nerve is known as the external epineurium. Surgically, the external epineurium is seen as a strong, loosely organized sheath around the nerve, which defines it anatomically and facilitates repair (Fig. 12–2). The mesoneurium makes up the loose areolar tissue around

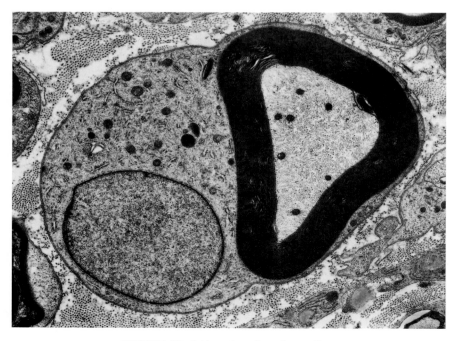

FIGURE 12–1 Normal myelinated nerve fiber.

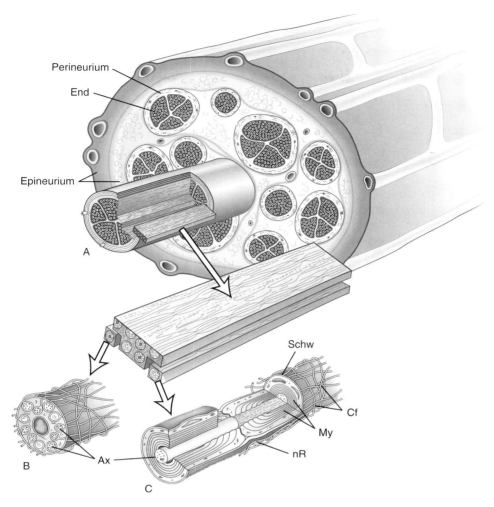

FIGURE 12–2 Microanatomy of a peripheral nerve trunk and its components. **A,** Fascicles surrounded by a multilaminated perineurium (*p*) are embedded in a loose connective tissue, the epineurium (*epi*). The outer layers of the epineurium are condensed into a sheath. **B** and **C,** The appearance of unmyelinated and myelinated fibers, respectively. *Schw,* Schwann cell; *my,* myelin sheath; *ax,* axon; *nR,* node of Ranvier. (From Lundborg G: Nerve Injury and Repair. Edinburgh: Churchill Livingstone, 1988, with permission.)

the outside of the nerve extending from the epineurium to the surrounding tissue. Segmental blood supply enters the nerve through the mesoneurium. Mesoneurium also permits longitudinal excursion of the nerve.

In addition to the mesoneurial function, the nerve itself has an internal architecture that allows for some degree of stretch. Healthy fascicles demonstrate transverse banding patterns along their length. These bands, known as the bands of Fontana, are often visible with loupe magnification in a normal nerve without removal of the epineurial layer. The bands of Fontana represent redundancy of nerve fibers within fascicles that allow for small changes in the length of the nerve. In areas of compression or stretch, these bands are absent. With relief of compression, such as with a successful neurolysis, the bands of Fontana will reappear. Similarly, if a normal nerve is pulled out to length with a pair of micropickups, the bands

will disappear. As the nerve is allowed to relax again, the bands will reappear.

Topography

Within the peripheral nerve, the relationship between the fascicles changes along its longitudinal course. Fascicular patterns in the proximal regions of peripheral nerves demonstrate little discernible organization relating to their more distal targets. Sunderland's work on the musculo-cutaneous nerve concluded that the maximum length of a nerve with a constant fascicular pattern was 15 mm. This study holds true for the proximal portion of peripheral nerves. However, other studies demonstrated that more distally in the extremity, nerve fascicles could be separated much more easily and that they demonstrated less branching over longer distances. The fact that these functionally distinct fascicles can be separated surgically has clinical application in traumatic and reconstructive peripheral nerve surgery and provides the anatomic basis for internal neurolysis.

Blood Supply

The peripheral nerve is supplied by a segmental, external blood supply as well as an intrinsic longitudinal blood supply. Blood flows from these vessels into the vasa nervorum, which enter the nerve from the mesoneurium and enter the epineurial space. From this point, there is considerable plexus formation in which nutrient vessels run longitudinally in the epineurium and perineurium. At the level of the endoneurium, only a fine network of capillaries is present. Venous drainage patterns parallel the arteriolar supply. The intrinsic blood flow is remarkable. Studies have shown that the internal blood supply of a nerve can support nerve viability over tremendous distances. Rabbit sciatic nerves can tolerate elevation and separation of a length 41 times their diameter when all extrinsic vessels except one are transected. This property allows for extensive mobilization of a peripheral nerve based on its intrinsic blood supply.

Physiology of the Peripheral Nerve

Blood-Nerve Barrier

Within each peripheral nerve there is a barrier that is a continuation of the blood-brain barrier. As the spinal nerves emerge from their foramina, they contain the pia-arachnoid layer of the meninges. This structure histologically is in continuity with the innermost layers of the perineurium and the endothelial cells of the endoneurium—the two sites of the blood-nerve barrier. These specialized endothelial cells contain tight junctions that maintain the internal environment of the peripheral nerve fibers. The blood-nerve barrier provides immunologic shielding to the endoneurial environment. Endoneurium and perineurium have no lymphatics and in cases of infection the perineurium provides a strong barrier to invasion. Disruption of the blood-nerve barrier by nerve compression, injection, or injury can result in loss of this homeostasis.

In compression neuropathies, leaking capillaries within the endoneurial space allow for the accumulation of proteins and fluid, with resultant endoneurial edema and nerve dysfunction. With an initial break in the barrier at the level of the tight junctions of the endothelial cells, pressures within the endoneurium will rise and produce subperineural edema and a mini–compartment syndrome within the endoneurium. In other nerve injuries and in repair, the blood-nerve barrier is directly disrupted by trauma. This triggers an inflammatory response directed toward previously protected antigens, and allows lymphocytes, macrophages, and fibroblasts to enter the perineural space and initiate further inflammation, injury, and, ultimately, scar.

Research has been directed toward modulating this inflammatory response with immunosuppressive therapy in the hope of alleviating its detrimental effects on nerve regeneration. Enhanced nerve regeneration has been demonstrated in animal models of nerve autografts when immunosuppressed with tacrolimus (FK506).

Axoplasmic Transport

Research in the 1940s demonstrated the accumulation of substances within a nerve after the application of a circumferential ligature, and it was postulated that this observation demonstrated axonal transport. Later, labeled amino acids were used to study the movement of neurotransmitter vesicles along the nerve, and the process of antegrade transport was calculated to occur at a rate of 1 to 1.5 mm/day. Today we know that neurotransmitters and structural elements are manufactured in the cell body and transported distally, and that recycled neurotransmitter vesicles are transmitted back to the cell body proximally. These processes consist of both a fast and a slow transport system in the antegrade direction and a fast system in the retrograde direction (Fig. 12–3).

Slow antegrade transport is used for major structural proteins such as tubulin, actin, and other components of microtubules, neurofilaments, and microfilaments. It occurs independently of ATPase and proceeds at a rate of 1 to 6 mm/day. Fast antegrade and retrograde transport are ATPase dependent and reach rates of 410 mm/day and 240 mm/day respectively. Distal neuromuscular junctions and Schwann cells also transport neurotrophic factors by this system in order to influence the neuronal cell body.

The Cellular Response to Nerve Injury

Peripheral nerves have the ability to regenerate and reinnervate distal targets. However, complete functional recovery is rarely achieved despite the considerable advances that have been made in our understanding of nerve regeneration and in our microsurgical techniques of repair. The process of nerve regeneration is complex and involves a multitude of factors. When a peripheral nerve is divided, complex changes occur in the nerve cell body, in

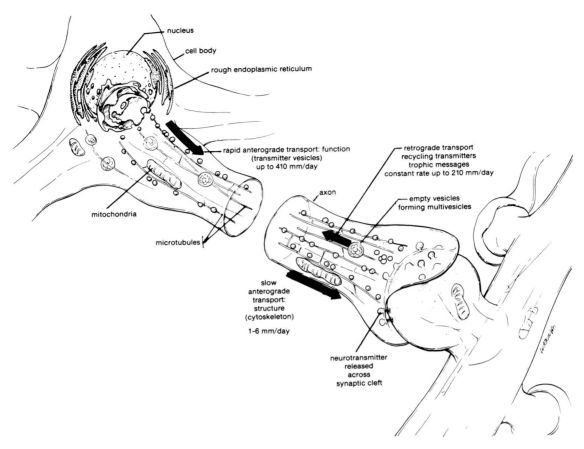

FIGURE 12–3 The axoplasmic transport system. Both fast and slow transport systems operate in an anterograde fashion. A fast transport system also works in a retrograde fashion. (From Mackinnon SE, Dellon AL: Surgery of the Peripheral Nerve [2nd ed]. New York: Thieme, 1998.)

the proximal and distal segment of the nerve, and at the end organs. First, the neuron must survive the injury and initiate regeneration. Second, the nerve stump distal to the injury must provide a growth environment that supports regeneration. Third, the regenerated axons must reinnervate the appropriate distal target. Lastly, the distal target must be able to recover from denervation.

The Nerve Cell

Following nerve transection, the cell body of the nerve will either undergo injury-induced cell death or transform from a cell that normally supports the production and turnover of neurotransmitters to one that is centered on repair. Survival depends on many factors, including age, neuron type, proximity of the injury to the cell body, and the degree of injury. In general, cranial motoneurons are more susceptible to death than spinal motoneurons, sensory neurons are more susceptible than motor neurons, developing neurons are more susceptible than mature neurons,

and proximal injuries are more susceptible than distal injuries.

The mechanisms involved in injury-induced neuronal death are only partially understood. It is accepted that axotomized neurons undergo apoptosis, and that this apoptosis is due in part, to the absence of neurotrophic factors. Neurotrophic factors are expressed and released by glial cells, fibroblasts, macrophages, target tissues, and the distal stump of the injured nerve. Experiments that prevent regenerating axons from accessing neurotrophic factors demonstrate increased evidence of nerve cell death.

Surviving neurons show significant morphologic and chromatolytic changes that demonstrate that the nerve cell has switched into repair mode. These changes include neuronal nuclear eccentricity, nucleolar enlargement, and Nissl body dissolution. Metabolic activities are now directed toward enhanced protein synthesis in order to replenish the cytoskeleton, and previous production of neurotransmitters is significantly downregulated. Some neurotransmitters that contribute to regeneration and survival of axotomized neurons are upregulated. The basis for this switch of gene expression in axotomized neurons remains unknown, but is likely secondary to reduced access of neurons to neurotrophic factors.

The Proximal Stump

Axonal degeneration in the proximal stump is more limited than degeneration distal to the injury. The proximal nerve axon usually will degenerate back to the first node of Ranvier if neuronal cell bodies survive the injury. More proximal degeneration can be seen in severe injuries. Swelling of the proximal nerve stump near the injury occurs and is likely due to an accumulation of transported material.

Within 24 hours of injury, regenerating axonal sprouts arise from the first node of Ranvier proximal to the injury site. Each injured proximal axon will produce numerous sprouts that resemble mini-axons. These sprouts form a growth cone that has an affinity for Schwann cell basal lamina. Without the proper distal environment, these branches will continue to grow and spiral around one another, forming a neuroma.

In the presence of a supportive distal environment, the axonal sprouts will advance more distally and comprise a "regenerating unit" (Fig. 12–4). The rate of axonal regeneration from the growth cone accelerates to a steady rate of 1 to 3 mm/day. The rate-limiting component of nerve regeneration is axonal transport of actin, tubulin, and neurofilaments.

Axons that proceed into the distal stump will subsequently undergo myelination. This myelination is initiated by contact between the axolemma and Schwann cells. However, conduction velocity will still be slower, despite this remyelination. This can be explained by the abnormally short internodal distances between the myelin sheaths secondary to an increase in Schwann cell number. Over time, remodeling occurs, resulting in increased internodal distances and improved conduction velocities.

Growth Environment of the Distal Stump

Complex changes occur in the distal nerve stump after injury in order to promote a favorable environment for axonal regeneration. These changes include wallerian degeneration, Schwann cell proliferation and alteration, and upregulation of regeneration-associated molecules.

Wallerian degeneration

The success of peripheral nerve regeneration depends on the growth environment of the distal nerve stump. After axotomy, the absence of a nucleus and other essential cellular synthetic subunits leads to wallerian degeneration. Through the process of wallerian degeneration, a series of changes take place that promote a favorable growth environment. Changes in the distal nerve stump are

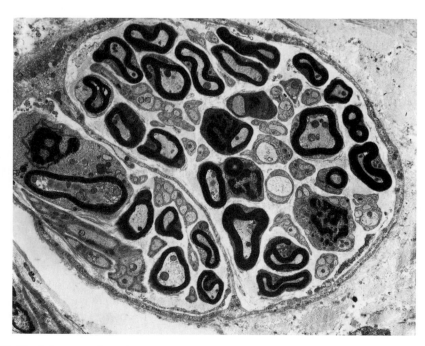

FIGURE 12–4 A regenerating unit containing myelinated and unmyelinated fibers surrounded by perineurium.

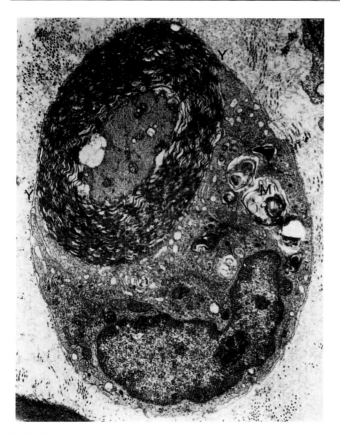

FIGURE 12–5 Changes in the distal nerve stump after injury: wallerian degeneration, Schwann cell proliferation, and myelin and axonal degeneration.

initially degenerative (Fig. 12–5). Axonal remnants and their myelin sheaths undergo degradation. Schwann cells initiate phagocytosis during the first 2 days, when macrophage invasion is minimal. This process is followed by the migration of macrophages through the disrupted blood-nerve barrier. These axonal remnants and myelin sheaths because they have been shown to inhibit axonal ingrowth from the proximal stump.

Schwann cell proliferation

Schwann cells, which were previously mitotically quiescent, begin to multiply under the influence of a multitude of factors. Macrophages release growth factors and cytokines that stimulate Schwann cell and fibroblast proliferation. The absence of axonal contact stimulates Schwann cell proliferation. Schwann cells alter their phenotype to become nonmyelinating; the presence of these nonmyelinating Schwann cells is essential for axonal growth in the distal nerve stump.

The Schwann cell also begins to elaborate growth factors. Several neurotrophic factors, including nerve

growth factor (NGF), neurotrophin (NT)-4/5, brain-derived neurotrophic factor (BDNF), epidermal growth factor, insulin-like growth factors I and II (IGF-I and -II), and glial-derived neurotrophic factor (GDNF) are produced by the Schwann cells, as well as several of the neurotrophin receptors. They continue to proliferate and form longitudinal columns known as "the bands of Büngner," which fill the endoneurial sheaths. These Schwann cell columns attract the proximal nerve growth cone through both contact guidance and the release of growth factors. Only after the completion of Schwann cell migration can nerve outgrowth occur. Cell adhesion molecules and basement membrane components are also upregulated by Schwann cells and aid in contact guidance of axonal growth cones.

These processes have relevance to current attempts to perfect nerve regeneration through various artificial conduits. The limitation in the length of regeneration that is currently achievable through an artificial or acellular conduit is likely representative of the limitation in the finite ability of the Schwann cell to migrate within the confines of the conduit and thus to provide an adequate gradient of trophic factors.

Regeneration-associated molecules

Many molecules participate in the regulation of axonal regeneration either directly or indirectly through their effects on non-neuronal cells. These factors include neurotrophic and neurotropic factors, cell adhesion molecules, and extracellular matrix proteins.

Neurotrophism is the process by which a native or regenerating neuron and its axonal projection are supported by factors that promote maturation and nutrition of regenerating axons. The neurotrophins include NGF, BDNF, NT-3, and NT-4/5. These factors bind to high-affinity tyrosine kinase receptors and to p75, a low-affinity NGF receptor. Their role in neural regeneration is likely mediated indirectly through their action on Schwann cells by encouraging Schwann cell migration and adhesion to axonal projections. Considerable research has been devoted to numerous other growth factors, including IGF-I and -II, the fibroblast growth factors, platelet-derived growth factor, and GDNF. Evidence suggests that these factors enhance axonal regeneration indirectly by mediating the growth environment rather than directly affecting neuronal activity.

Neurotropism is a related concept that refers to the process of directional guidance of regenerating axons, whether by diffusable or spatially fixed factors. The concept of guidance by chemotaxis was first suggested by Forssman in 1898. Support for the theory came from the work of Ramon y Cajal, who was able to demonstrate axons from the proximal ends of severed nerves traveling along convoluted paths toward distal nerve ends.

Through the decades, there has been debate regarding the control of motor/sensory nerve regeneration. Do motor axons regenerate preferentially toward a distal motor target, or do they just mature once they reach the motor end plate? Current research efforts have helped to clarify these issues. An injured motor axon will sprout into a regenerating unit containing many axons. Pioneer motor axons will initially regenerate randomly into sensory or motor Schwann cell tubes. Once the leading motor axon recognizes an environment of a motor Schwann cell tube, this *motor* axon will signal back to the cell body, allowing the other axons within that regenerating unit to *regenerate preferentially* within that motor Schwann cell tube. Once these motor axons reach the distal muscle environment, *preferential motor maturation* will occur so that the size of these motor axons increases. By contrast, a motor axon that randomly regenerates into the inappropriate sensory Schwann cell tube will not send information back to the cell body, and therefore other axons will not follow this errant axon. This axon, however, will not be pruned away, as previously thought.

Cellular adhesion molecules (CAMs) of the immunoglobulin superfamily (L1/Ng-CAM/NILE, N-CAM, and N-cadherin) and extracellular matrix molecules such as laminin, collagen, fibronectin, and tenascin-C are upregulated in the distal stump after axotomy. These molecules are involved in adhesion between axon and axon, axon and Schwann cells, and axon and basement membrane. These processes aid in the regulation of axonal growth in the distal nerve stump and enhance preferential growth of motor and sensory nerves toward their appropriate targets over longer distances.

Distal Receptors

Several factors account for poor functional recovery after delayed nerve repair. Prolonged denervation of the distal nerve stump itself can result in poor regeneration of axons through the distal segment. The reason for this finding is poorly understood; it is believed to be secondary to Schwann cell atrophy, disruption of the basal laminae, and progressive fibrosis. Other important factors are secondary to prolonged end-organ denervation. Irreversible changes are seen in motor end plates and muscle receptors with prolonged denervation that limits functional recovery.

Motor End Plates and Muscle Fibers

Following axotomy, changes occur in denervated muscle. Muscle fibers atrophy significantly, but the actual fiber number does not decrease. The type I fibers will undergo pathognomonic histologic changes in which "target cells"

become apparent. These are seen to be alternating zones of dark and light staining. In cross section, the normally eccentric nucleus migrates to a central position. Initially, the architecture of the neuromuscular junction remains unchanged, with synaptic folds being maintained for over a year.

However, significant changes occur in the distribution of acetylcholine receptors. Acetylcholine receptors normally are located in the midportion of the muscle fiber. Once denervated, acetylcholine receptors are present diffusely along the entire length of the muscle, creating supersensitivity to acetylcholine. This finding can be demonstrated on electromyography by the presence of fibrillations. With reinnervation, sprouting axons will follow their original path to reform the original neuromuscular junctions. In addition, collateral sprouting of axons close to the motor end plates will occur. This will create groups of muscle fibers that are of the same histologic staining type (i.e., all type I or type II). This is in contrast to normal muscle, which demonstrates a random mixture of type I and II fibers.

Within 3 months of injury, denervated muscles will demonstrate significant fibrosis, with deposition of connective tissue along the epimysium. This fibrosis continues to progress over time. In order for muscle to undergo meaningful recovery after denervation, reinnervation should occur within 12 to 18 months.

Sensory Receptors

The end organs of sensation found in the skin and soft tissue include Meissner's and pacinian corpuscles, Merkel cells, Ruffini's endings, and free nerve endings. Pacinian and Meissner's corpuscles are quickly adapting fiber receptors mediating moving touch and vibration. They differ in their sensitivities to vibration frequencies. The Merkel cell neurite complex is a slowly adapting fiber receptor mediating constant touch and pressure. Ruffini's endings transmit proprioception and vibration sense. The free nerve endings represent unmyelinated axons that are sensitive to pain, temperature, and touch.

Pacinian corpuscles receive only a single axon terminal and do not reinnervate. All other sensory receptors, however, are able to reinnervate. Sensory reinnervation is under fewer time constraints than motor reinnervation, and can occur many years after denervation. However, over time, the sensory organs may undergo changes that alter the ultimate quality of reinnervation. Therefore, the quality of reinnervation and sensory recovery may be enhanced by a more rapid reinnervation, but protective sensation may be achieved after much longer periods of time.

Clinical Classification of Nerve Injuries—Seddon and Sunderland Classifications and the Mackinnon Modification

In 1943, Sir Herbert Seddon reviewed 650 nerve injuries and presented a classification scheme consisting of three different types of injuries: neurapraxia, axonotmesis, and neurotmesis. In, 1951, Sir Sydney Sunderland expanded this classification system by emphasizing Seddon's division of the axonotmesis category into two separate degrees of injury based on the ability of the nerve to recover. He also added a neurotmesis category to include an incontinuity injury. Mackinnon further expanded this classification with the addition of a sixth-degree injury to emphasize mixed injuries (Table 12–1).

First-Degree Injury—Neurapraxia

This injury represents a localized conduction block at the site of trauma. Gross inspection reveals no obvious abnormalities. Histologically, demyelination of fibers may be present along with endoneurial and perineurial edema. Because there is no axonal discontinuity, no Tinel's sign is present. Recovery can vary from days to 12 weeks.

When the conduction block improves recovery is immediate, in contrast to the slower progression of neural recovery seen in more severe degrees of injury. Examples of neurapraxia include injuries induced by pressure (i.e., tourniquet palsy) and mild stretch injuries of nerves, often from surgical retraction. Complete recovery is the rule because the neural architecture has not been destroyed.

Second-Degree Injury—Axonotmesis

Second-degree injuries are the least serious of the degenerative injuries. It involves axonal disruption followed by wallerian degeneration, however, the endoneurial sheaths are completely preserved. The basal lamina of the Schwann cells within the endoneurium is intact, and axonal contact and guidance of the regenerating growth cones is unimpeded by the formation of scar or by topographic mismatch. A Tinel's sign will be present and will be noted to progress in accord with the regenerating axons at a rate of 1 to 3 mm/day. The axonotmetic injury will recover according to the sequential reinnervation of target sensory and motor end organs in a logical proximal-to-distal manner.

Third-Degree Injury—Axonotmesis

A third-degree injury is also axonotmetic, however, the architectural disturbances include the endoneurial sheath, the basal laminae of the Schwann cells, and other

Table 12–1
Classification of nerve injury

Seddon	Sunderland	Pathophysiology
Neurapraxia	1	Conduction block, focal demyelination at edges of nodes of Ranvier, or complete internode segments. No axonal abnormality, therefore no Tinel's sign. Full recovery with repair of conduction block or remyelination.
Axonotmesis	2	Axonal loss of continuity, intact endoneurium. Wallerian degeneration of distal nerve and myelin sheath. Axons will regenerate along their original endoneurial tubes to their original distal receptors. Full recovery expected.
	3	Loss of continuity of axons and endoneurium. Perineurium intact. Distal Wallerian degeneration. Endoneurial scarring, content of fascicle (pure vs. mixed) affect ultimate outcome. Recovery variable.
	4	Loss of continuity of axons, endoneurium, and perineurium. Epineurium intact. Nerve in continuity but complete scarring across it (i.e., neuroma in continuity). No regeneration or recovery without treatment.
Neurotmesis	5	Complete transection of nerve. No recovery without repair, grafting of nerve.
	6	Mixed neuroma in continuity.

connective tissue disruptions within the perineurium. The perineurial contents are no longer able to guide axonal regrowth, and mismatch of fibers from proximal to distal will occur. Some of the fibers will fail to progress from proximal to distal and may form scar tissue within the epineurial sheaths.

Clinically, the patient with a third-degree injury can demonstrate a wide range of outcomes depending on the extent of intrafascicular scarring and the fascicular topography at the level of the injury. Despite this variability, it is generally accepted that microsurgical repair with grafting is less successful than the results seen with spontaneous recovery of a third-degree lesion. Recovery of a third-degree injury may be improved with surgical decompression if the injury localizes to a known area of nerve compression (i.e., peroneal nerve at the fibular head). Similarly, a third-degree injury presenting with significant pain may be better treated with excision and nerve grafting.

Fourth-Degree Injury–Neuroma in Continuity

In a fourth-degree injury, the nerve is intact anatomically (i.e., the epineurium is intact) but all of the subepineurial layers have undergone complete disruption and replacement with scar. In this situation nerve regeneration is impossible and nerve growth cones, Schwann cells, and scar tissue combine to form a neuroma at the level of the injury. A Tinel's sign will be present, but it will fail to progress distally. This injury requires excision of the neuroma and microsurgical repair with grafting or conduit technique. Fourth-degree injuries require a period of observation for reliable diagnosis, although the absence of progression of a Tinel's sign can be an early sign of a significant injury.

Fifth-Degree Injury–Neurotmesis

A fifth-degree injury is defined as a complete anatomic division of the nerve. No recovery is possible without microsurgical repair. These injuries are usually associated with penetrating trauma, although severe avulsion injuries can also create fifth-degree injuries.

Sixth-Degree Injury

Mackinnon added this injury classification to Sunderland's original classification in order to address the problem of a mixed nerve injury. A nerve may undergo a combination of different degrees of injury. These are the most surgically challenging of injuries because of the possibility of downgrading function of the less severely injured portions of the nerve. In mixed nerve injuries it is important to try to differentiate fourth- and fifth-degree injured

fascicles from less severely injured or uninjured ones. A complete picture may only be accomplished with intraoperative electrodiagnostic studies.

Principles of Nerve Repair

The basic principles of nerve repair have remained unchanged for many years. These principles include accurate preoperative assessment, properly timed exploration and repair, microsurgical repair with magnification, tension-free coaptation, early protected movement to ensure nerve gliding, and postoperative sensory and motor rehabilitation.

Timing of Nerve Repair

From the previous discussion of the physiology and molecular biology of peripheral nerves and end organs, it is apparent that the timing of repair is critical in determining the eventual clinical outcome. As a general principle, nerve injuries should be repaired as soon as possible. The ideal timing, however, varies with the mechanism and type of injury.

Open Injuries

In general, nerve injuries associated with open wounds require early exploration. The injury is often a sharp laceration causing nerve injury that can be repaired immediately and primarily. However, it can be difficult to appreciate the proximal and distal extent of the zone of injury in anything other than a very clean injury from a knife or glass. With "messy" or contused injuries, if possible, the nerve should be approximated using fascicular patterns to help with topographic alignment. At 3 weeks, or when the wound permits, the nerve is reexplored and definitive repair or graft can be performed. By 3 weeks, the longitudinal extent of scar tissue will be apparent.

One exception to the general rule of exploring open injuries is the gunshot wound. Although these are open injuries, the mechanisms of nerve damage are predominately heat and shock effects. Gunshot wounds therefore are more appropriately treated as closed or blunt trauma.

Closed Injuries

In closed or blunt trauma, initial management is expectant. The clinical course is observed closely. If complete recovery is not observed within 6 weeks, nerve conduction studies should be obtained for baseline evaluation. At 12 weeks postinjury, further clinical and electrical assessment is performed. If motor unit potentials are seen on the electromyogram, then spontaneous reinnervation of that muscle should be anticipated, and these patients should be treated expectantly. Lack of clinical or electrical evidence of reinnervation at that time suggests that operative intervention is indicated. The type of surgical procedure performed is determined after exploration with intraoperative nerve conduction testing.

Epineurial Versus Fascicular Repair

Debate continues regarding the optimal technique of microsurgical neural repair. The pros and cons of epineurial versus fascicular (perineurial) repair have been the subject of much debate. The theoretical advantages of fascicular repair are obvious. Proper fascicle-to-fascicle repair should give superior results. However, accomplishing proper fascicular alignment can be quite difficult in clinical practice. The normal topography of the nerve can easily be distorted by trauma, edema, or scar. If fascicular mismatch occurs, then the coapted nerves may be excluded from the opportunity to find their own way to the proper target. As well, greater manipulation of the fascicles is required to accomplish a fascicular repair, and this may lead to increased fibrosis and scarring.

Comparisons of the various techniques have yielded conflicting results. However, in the only prospective comparison done in humans, no differences were seen between fascicular repair and epineurial repair.

Intraoperative Methods of Fascicular Identification

The task of matching fascicles in proximal and distal stumps remains a significant challenge. Currently there are three techniques available: anatomic, histochemical, and electrophysiologic.

Anatomic Techniques

Anatomic techniques consist of extending the dissection proximal and distal to the area of injury. Alignment is facilitated by identifying corresponding longitudinal vessels on both sides, or by using distal branches or fascicular groupings to determine topography. For some peripheral nerves, such as the median, radial, and ulnar nerves, specific studies have been performed to identify the motor and sensory topography. The motor/sensory topography within the peripheral nerve is very precise and can be identified in an intact, healthy nerve with a simple disposable nerve stimulator. A surgeon who has the incidental opportunity to stimulate a normal nerve will have a unique opportunity to identify the location within the nerve of motor/sensory fascicular groups for future reference.

Histochemical Techniques

Histochemical enzyme staining has been used to separate motor from sensory nerves. Karnovsky and Roots devised a thiocholine staining protocol that identifies the cholinesterases present in motor neurons. Carbonic anhydrase has been used to identify sensory fibers. These techniques are most useful for the proximal stump, where enzyme activity will be present indefinitely. In contrast, enzyme staining of the distal stump is limited to 5 days following the injury. Intraoperative histochemical staining requires particular attention to ensure that the specimens are properly oriented. Processing periods of about 1 hour are required, and not all surgical facilities are equipped to undertake these studies. Given these limitations, histochemical techniques are not used routinely in clinical practice.

Electrophysiologic Awake Stimulation

Awake stimulation of the patient with a nerve injury can provide useful information. The exposure of the nerve is accomplished with the patient under a short-acting anesthetic or intravenous regional anesthetic with sedation. Tourniquet time for the dissection is limited to 30 minutes to prevent transient neurapraxia. After a reperfusion period of 10 minutes, proximal stump fascicles are stimulated with a disposable nerve stimulator or a sterile nerve conduction stimulation electrode. Motor fascicle stimulation will yield a dull ache in the extremity. The same level of stimulation of a sensory fascicle will yield a more intense, sharp pain in a specific sensory territory.

The benefits of electrical mapping are limited to the proximal nerve stump. Electrical stimulation of the motor fascicles of the distal stump can elicit a motor contraction only in the initial 72 hours following a nerve injury. For injuries outside of the 72-hour window, anatomic techniques must be used.

Intraoperative Nerve Conduction Studies

Nerve conduction studies of surgically exposed nerves can provide direct evidence of the extent of neural injury. Electrodes are placed at least 5 cm apart and stimulating voltages of 1 to roughly 20 mV are applied until an action potential is observed. The proximal nerve, the injured segment, and the distal segment are all studied sequentially. Stimulation of the proximal nerve confirms that the equipment is functioning correctly. Lack of conduction across the injured segment or distally warrants excision and grafting of the injured segment. Conduction across the injured segment warrants neurolysis.

Nerve Gap Management

A *nerve gap* is defined as the distance between two ends of a severed nerve. It consists not only of the length of nerve tissue that has been lost to injury or to débridement of nonvital tissue by the surgeon but also of the distance that the nerve has retracted. A *nerve deficit*, in contrast, is the length of actual nerve tissue that has been lost to injury or to surgical débridement. Nerve gaps that are small and can be repaired with "minimal tension" may be repaired primarily. Any significant tension must be managed with another method. Excessive tension is any tension greater than that required to overcome an 8-0 nylon suture. Several methods of reconstruction exist for nerve injuries with a significant nerve gap. Nerve grafting, vascularized nerve grafting, conduit interposition, allografting, and distal nerve transfers are all options that are discussed below. Despite these options, the gold standard in nerve gap management continues to be autogenous nerve grafting.

Nerve Grafting

The surgical technique of nerve grafting is similar to primary repair. The proximal and distal ends of the nerve must be prepared by transversely sectioning the nerve in the injured segment until fascicles are visualized with visible herniation of endoneurium from the cut ends. The defect size is measured and the donor graft is obtained. The graft should be oriented in a reverse fashion from its native position so that regenerating fibers will not be diverted from the distal neurorrhaphy site and the distal stump. Graft neurorrhaphy may be performed in either an epineurial or a perineurial manner, depending on the goals of the particular repair. Care must be taken to place the grafts in the same sequence proximally and distally to avoid surgically created malalignment. Each graft requires only two or three sutures for neurorrhaphy.

Donor selection of nerve grafts is limited by the size of donor nerves and the functional and aesthetic deficits created by their harvest. The donor nerves available for grafting are typically the sural nerve, the lateral antebrachial cutaneous nerve, and the anterior division of the medial antebrachial cutaneous nerve (Table 12–2).

Specialized Nerve Grafts

Vascularized nerve grafts

The theoretical advantage of a vascularized nerve graft is the ability to provide immediate intraneural perfusion in a poorly vascularized bed, and to reconstruct large nerve gaps. Mixed results have been seen in experimental models. Clinically, favorable results have been reported; however, only one of these studies made a direct comparison between conventional nonvascularized and vascularized nerve grafts. Despite the introduction of this technique more than two decades ago, the role of vascularized nerve grafts in clinical practice has not yet been established.

Conduits

In 1880, Gluck first described the use of a non-neural tube to reconnect the proximal and distal ends of an injured nerve. Presently a tremendous amount of research energy is being devoted to the development of the ideal conduit. Nerve conduits have been constructed from bone, vein, artery, silicone, poly(glycolic acid), polyglactin, and collagen. The goals of current research are to maximize the principles of neurotropism, neurotrophism, and contact guidance to provide an ideal microenvironment for the regenerating nerve and to isolate the influence of the distal stump. To summarize these research efforts, it is well established that the influence of the distal stump can be exerted equally well through a conduit or a nerve graft over short distances. However, current research has met with tremendous difficulty when trying to develop a conduit that is successful for nerve gaps longer than 3 cm. Now, as our understanding of the neurobiology of nerve regeneration progresses, researchers are beginning to

Table 12–2		
Donor nerves available for grafting		
Donor Nerve	**Length (cm)**	**Deficit**
Sural	30–40	Lateral aspect of foot
Lateral antebrachial cutaneous nerve	5–8	Lateral forearm
Medial antebrachial cutaneous nerve (anterior branch)	10–20	Medial arm and elbow

report successes in advancing nerve regeneration beyond the critical 3-cm gap. Although the ideal conduit milieu has not yet been established, successful regeneration across larger gaps suggests an increased potential for the clinical utility of nerve conduits in the future.

The senior author's current practice includes the use of conduits only for gaps less than 3 cm in noncritical, small-diameter areas of sensation, in patients who decline autogenous nerve graft harvest.

Nerve allograft

The reconstruction of long nerve segments after trauma or tumor ablation continues to pose a considerable challenge. Traditionally an expendable sensory nerve is used as an interposition autograft. However, the use of nerve autografts is limited by the finite number of expendable donor nerves. This challenge has stimulated the search for alternatives for reconstruction. The earliest report of clinical nerve allografting was made by Albert in 1885. Since that time, many advances have been made: the advent of microsurgical techniques, the implementation of host immunosuppression, and an increased understanding of the neurobiology of peripheral nerve injuries. The last decade has seen a tremendous amount of research on host immunosuppression and cadaveric nerve allografts.

Investigators have studied a number of methods of graft pretreatment to prevent allograft rejection. As previously discussed, Schwann cell presence as well as intact basal laminae are critical to the support of neural regeneration. Schwann cells have been shown to survive cold storage in University of Wisconsin Cold Storage Solution for up to 3 weeks. One week of cold preservation in University of Wisconsin Cold Storage Solution is effective in reducing the expression of major histocompatability complex class II molecules but will not decrease the number of viable donor Schwann cells. Other pretreatments, including lyophilization and high-dose irradiation, can abolish immunogenicity of nerve allografts but are also toxic to Schwann cells.

Manipulation of the host's immune response is an important adjunctive strategy to pretreatment. A large body of evidence points to the donor Schwann cell as the primary target of nerve allograft rejection. This rejection, in the form of donor Schwann cell replacement with host Schwann cells, will proceed even in the presence of appropriate immunosuppression, however, it will occur without the destruction of the intraneural architecture. Nerve allografts function as biologic conduits for recipient nerve regeneration. Once that regeneration is complete, the neural elements within the graft are purely of host origin. Even in incomplete regeneration, reestablishment of the blood-nerve barrier results in significant shielding from the circulating elements of the immune system. These factors contribute to the gradual loss of nerve allograft antigenicity that enables immunosuppression to be discontinued without any deterioration of nerve function.

The clinical outcome of seven patients who had reconstruction of long peripheral nerve gaps with interposition peripheral nerve allografts has been reported recently by the senior author. Six of the seven patients demonstrated return of motor function or sensation in the affected limb. One patient experienced rejection secondary to subtherapeutic immunosuppression.

End-to-side neurorrhaphy

End-to-side neurorrhaphy is the technique of creating a neurorrhaphy between the distal end of an injured nerve and the side of an uninjured donor nerve, either by simple microsurgical attachment without alteration of the donor nerve or in conjunction with the creation of a surgical incision within the donor nerve. The earliest reports of end-to-side neurorrhaphy date back to the late 1800s. The technique, however, was lost until it was reintroduced in the early 1990s. Since then, numerous reports have been published.

Although our understanding of the cellular events following end-to-side neurorrhaphy is incomplete, several mechanisms have been studied. In the distal segment, the repair process is similar to that seen in end-to-end repair, with wallerian degeneration, proliferation of Schwann cells, and organization of Schwann cells into columns. Invasion of the Schwann cells from the distal segment into the epineurium of the donor nerve has been demonstrated to be critical in initiating collateral sprouting from intact axons. Normal, uninjured sensory axons will spontaneously sprout de novo, but motor axons may need to be injured in order to sprout. Collateral sprouting into the recipient nerve occurs from the nodes of Ranvier. The sprouting axons within the distal segment then become ensheathed by Schwann cells, forming regenerating units, and myelination of these axons occurs.

At this time, the use of end-to-side neurorrhaphy in the clinical setting for motor recovery remains controversial. We employ it in sensory nerve reconstruction in circumstances in which distal nerve ends would go without a source of proximal neurons. In the authors' anecdotal experience, this has met with reasonable success.

Summary

Advances in the field of peripheral nerve surgery have increased our understanding of the complex cellular and molecular events involved in nerve injury and repair. Innovative techniques utilizing microsurgical techniques, nerve conduits, growth factors, allografts, and end-to-side techniques are direct consequences of these advances. As we acquire more knowledge, it is hoped that many of the innovative techniques mentioned in this chapter may become the mainstays of treatment.

Bibliography

Albert E: Einige Operationen an Nerven. Wien Med Presse 1885;26:1285.

Al-Majed AA, Neumann CM, Brushart TM, Gordon T: Brief electrical stimulation promotes the speed and accuracy of motor axonal regeneration. J Neurosci 2000;20:2602.

Al-Qattan MM, Al-Thunayan A: Variables affecting axonal regeneration following end-to-side neurorrhaphy. Br J Plast Surg 1998;51:238.

Atchabahian A, Mackinnon SE, Doolabh VB, et al: Indefinite survival of peripheral nerve allografts after temporary cyclosporin A immunosuppression. Restor Neurol Neurosci 1998;13:129.

Atchabahian A, Mackinnon SE, Hunter DA: Cold preservation of nerve grafts decreases expression of ICAM-1 and class II MHC antigens. J Reconstr Microsurg 1999;15:307.

Bain JR, Mackinnon SE, Hudson AR, et al: The nerve allograft response in the rat immunosuppressed with cyclosporin A. Plast Reconstr Surg 1988;82:1052.

Bain JR, Mackinnon SE, Hudson AR, et al: The peripheral nerve allograft: a dose-response curve in the rat immunosuppressed with cyclosporin A. Plast Reconstr Surg 1988;82:447.

Bonney G, Birch R, Jamieson AM, Eames RA: Experience with vascularized nerve grafts. In Terzis JK (ed): Microreconstruction of Nerve Injuries. Philadelphia: WB Saunders, 1986:403.

Bora FW: A comparison of epineurial, perineurial and epiperineurial methods of nerve suture. Clin Orthop Rel Res 1978;133:91.

Bora FW, Pleasure DE, Didizian NA: A study of nerve regeneration and neuroma formation after nerve suture by various techniques. J Hand Surg 1976;1:138.

Brown MC, Lunn ER, Perry VH: Poor growth of mammalian motor and sensory axons into proximal nerve stumps. Eur J Neurosci 1991;3:1366.

Brushart TM, Gerber J, Kessens P, et al: Contributions of pathway and neuron to preferential motor reinnervation. J Neurosci 1998;18:8674.

Bunge RP: Tissue culture observations relevant to the study of axon-Schwann cell interactions during peripheral nerve development and repair. J Exp Biol 1987;132:21.

Chiu DTW, Janecka I, Krizek TJ, et al: Autogenous vein graft as a conduit for nerve regeneration. Surgery 1982;91:226.

Chiu DTW, Strauch B: A prospective clinical evaluation of autogenous vein grafts used as a nerve conduit for sensory nerve defects of 3 cm or less. Plast Reconstr Surg 1990;86:928.

Chow JA, Sunderland S, Van Beek AL: Surgical significance of the motor fascicular group of the ulnar nerve in the forearm. J Hand Surg [Am] 1985;9:605.

Cragg B: What is the signal for chromatolysis? Brain Res 1970;23:1.

Curtis R, Stewart HJS, Hall SM, et al: GAP-43 is expressed by non-myelin-forming Schwann cells of the peripheral nervous system. J Cell Biol 1992;116:1455.

Droz B, Leblond CP: Axonal migration of proteins in the central nervous system and peripheral nerves as shown by radio autography. J Comp Neurol 1963;121:325.

Droz B, Rambourg A, Koenig HL: The smooth endoplasmic reticulum: structure and role in the renewal of axonal membrane and synaptic vesicles by fast axonal transport. Brain Res 1975;93:1.

Evans PJ, Mackinnon SE, Levi AD, et al: Cold preserved nerve allografts: changes in basement membrane, viability, immunogenicity, and regeneration. Muscle Nerve 1998;21:1507.

Forssman J: Ueber de ursachen welche die waschstufstrichtung der peripheren nervenfasern vie der regeneration bestimmen. Beitr Pathol Anat 1898;24:55.

Fu SY, Gordon T: Contributing factors to poor functional recovery after delayed nerve repair: prolonged denervation. J Neurosci 1995;15:3886.

Fu SY, Gordon T: The cellular and molecular basis of peripheral nerve regeneration. Mol Neurobiol 1997;14:67.

Futenma C, Kanaya F: Evaluation of preferential motor reinnervation by measuring choline acetyltransferase (CAT) activity and by Karnovsky staining. (submitted for publication)

Gluck T: Ueber Neuroplastik auf dem Wege der Transplantation. Arch Klin Chir 1880;25:606.

Gorio A, Carmingnoto G: Reformation, maturation and stabilization of neuromuscular junctions in peripheral nerve regeneration. In Gorio A, Millesi H, Mingrino S (eds): Post-traumatic Peripheral Nerve Regeneration. New York: Raven Press, 1981:481.

Grabb WC, Bement SL, Koepke GH, et al: Comparison of methods of peripheral nerve suturing in monkeys. Plast Reconstr Surg 1970;46:31.

Greensmith L, Vrbova G: Motoneural survival: afunctional approach. Trends Neurosci 1996;19:450.

Gu Y, Zheng Y, Li H, Zu Y: Arterialized free sural nerve grafting. J Plast Surg 1985;15:332.

Hare GM, Mackinnon SE, Midha R, et al: Cyclosporin A inhibits lymphocyte migration into ovine peripheral nerve allografts. Microsurgery 1996;17:697.

Hildebrand C, Mystafa GY, Waxman SG: Remodelling of internodes in regenerating rat sciatic nerve: electron microscopic observations. J Neurocytol 1986;15:681.

Jabaley ME, Wallace WH, Heckler FR: Internal topography of major nerves of the forearm and hand: a current view. J Hand Surg [Br] 1980;51:1.

Korshing S: The neurotrophic factor concept: a reexamination. J Neurosci 1993;13:2739.

Lee M, Doolabh VB, Mackinnon SE, Jost S: FK506 promotes functional recovery in crushed rat sciatic nerve. Muscle Nerve 2000;23:633.

Levi AD, Evans PJ, Mackinnon SE, Bunge RP: Cold storage of peripheral nerves: an in vitro assay of cell viability and function. Glia 1994;10:121.

Levinthal R, Brown WJ, Rand RW: Comparison of fascicular, interfascicular, and epineurial suture techniques in the repair of simple nerve lacerations. J Neurosurg 1977; 47:744.

Lind R, Wood MB: Comparison of the patterns of early revascularization of conventional versus vascularized nerve grafts in the canine. J Reconstr Microsurg 1986;2:229.

Lo AC, Houenou LJ, Oppenheim RW: Apoptosis in the nervous system: morphological features, methods, pathology, and prevention. Arch Histol Cytol 1995;58:138.

Lubinska L, Niemierko S: Velocity and intensity of bidirectional migration of acetylcholinesterase in transected nerves. Brain Res 1971;27:329.

Mackinnon SE: New directions in peripheral nerve surgery. Ann Surg 1989;22:257.

Mackinnon SE, Doolabh VB, Novak CB, Trulock EP: Clinical outcome following nerve allograft transplantation. Plast Reconstr Surg 2001;107:1419.

Mackinnon SE, Hudson AR, Bain JR, et al: The peripheral nerve allograft: an assessment of regeneration in the immunosuppressed host. Plast Reconstr Surg 1987;79:436.

Mackinnon SE, Hunter D, Kelly L: A histological and functional comparison of regeneration across a vascularized and conventional nerve graft: a case report. J Microsurg 1988;9:226.

Mackinnon SE, Midha R, Bain J, et al: An assessment of regeneration across peripheral nerve allografts in rats receiving short courses of cyclosporin A immunosuppression. Neuroscience 1992;46:585.

Matsumoto K, Ohnishi K, Kiyotani T, et al: Peripheral nerve regeneration across an 80-mm gap bridged by polyglycolic acid (PGA)–collagen tube filled with laminin-coated collagen fibers: a histochemical and electrophysiological evaluation of regenerated nerves. Brain Research 2000; 868:315.

Matsumoto M, Irata H, Nishiyama M, et al: Schwann cells can induce collateral sprouting from intact axons: experimental study of end-to-side neurorrhaphy using a Y-chamber model. J Reconstr Microsurg 1999;15:281.

Mendell LM: Neurotrophic factors and the specification of neural function. Neuroscientist 1995;1:26.

Midha R, Mackinnon SE, Wade JA, et al: Chronic cyclosporin A therapy in rats. Microsurgery 1992;13:273.

Millesi H: The nerve gap: theory and clinical practice. Hand Clin 1987;2:651.

Morris JH, Hudson AR, Weddell GA: A study of degeneration and regeneration in the divided rat sciatic nerve based on electron microscopy. II. The development of the "regenerating unit." Z Zellforschung 1972;124:103.

Ramon y Cajal SR: Mechanismo de la degeneracion y regeneracion de nervos. Trab Lab Inbest Biol (Madrid) 1905;9:119.

Reichert F, Saada A, Rotshenker S: Peripheral nerve injury induces Schwann cells to express two macrophage phenotypes: phagocytosis and the galactose-specific lectin MAC-2. J Neurosci 1994;14:3231.

Rich KM, Disch SP, Eichiler ME: The influence of regeneration and nerve growth factor on neuronal cell body reaction to injury. J Neurocytol 1989;18:567.

Richardson PM: Neurotrophic factors in regeneration. Curr Opinion Neurobiol 1991;1:401.

Seckel BR, Ryan SE, Simons JE, et al: Vascularized versus nonvascularized nerve grafts: an experimental, structural comparison. Plast Reconstr Surg 1986;78:211.

Seddon HJ: Three types of nerve injury. Brain 1943;66:237.

Settergren CR, Wood MB: Comparison of blood flow in free vascularized versus non-vascularized nerve grafts. J Reconstr Microsurg 1984;1:95.

Sherren J: Some points in the surgery of the peripheral nerves. Edinburgh Med J 1906;20:297.

Shizhen Z, Xiangluo T, Muzhil L: The microsurgical anatomy of peripheral nerves. In Shizhen Z, Yongjian M, Wencyun Y (eds): Microsurgical Anatomy. Lancaster, UK: MTP Press, 1985:289.

Smith BH, Kornblith PL: Axoplasmic transport in neurological surgery. Neurosurgery 1982;10:268.

Snyder RE, Chen H, Smith RS: Structural and functional properties of the junction between the parent and regenerating portions of myelinated axons. In Gordon T, Stein RB, Smith PA (eds): Neurology and Neurobiology, Vol 38: The Current Status of Peripheral Nerve Regeneration. New York: Liss, 1988:84.

Stockel K, Schwab M, Thoenen H: Specificity of retrograde transport of nerve growth factor (NGF) and sensory neurons: a biochemical and morphological study. Brain Res 1975;89:1.

Strauch B, Rodriguez DM, Diaz J, et al: Autologous Schwann cells drive regeneration through a 6-cm autogenous venous nerve conduit. J Reconstr Microsurg 2001;17:589.

Strasberg SR, Mackinnon SE, Hare GM, et al: Reduction in peripheral nerve allograft antigenicity with warm and cold temperature preservation. Plast Reconstr Surg 1996; 97:152.

Suematsu N, Atsuta Y, Hirayama T: Vein graft for repair of peripheral nerve gap. J Reconstr Microsurg 1988;4:313.

Sunderland S: The intraneural topography of the radial, median and ulnar nerves. Brain 1945;68:243.

Sunderland S: A classification of peripheral nerve injuries producing loss of function. Brain 1951;74:491.

Tang JB, Shi D, Shou H: Vein conduits for repair of nerves with a prolonged gap or in unfavorable conditions: an analysis of three failed cases. Microsurgery 1995;16:133.

Viterbo F, Trindade JC, Hoshino K, Mazzoni A: Lateroterminal neurorrhaphy without removal of the epineurial sheath: experimental study in rats. Sao Paulo Med J 1992; 110:267.

Weiss P: Damming of axoplasm in constrictive nerve: a sign of perpetual nerve growth in the nerve fibers. Anat Rec 1944;88(Suppl):48.

Weiss P: Evidence of perpetual proximal-distal growth of the nerve fibers. Biol Bull 1944;87:160.

Williams HB, Jabaley ME: The importance of internal anatomy of the peripheral nerves to nerve repair in the forearm and hand. Hand Clin 1986;2:689.

Yan JG, Matloub HS, Sanger SR, Zhand LL: Nerve sprouting after termino-lateral neurorrhaphy [abstract]. J Reconstr Microsurg 1999;15:376.

Young L, Wray RC, Weeks PM: A randomized prospective comparison of fascicular and epineural digital nerve repairs. J Plast Reconstr Surg 1981;68:89.

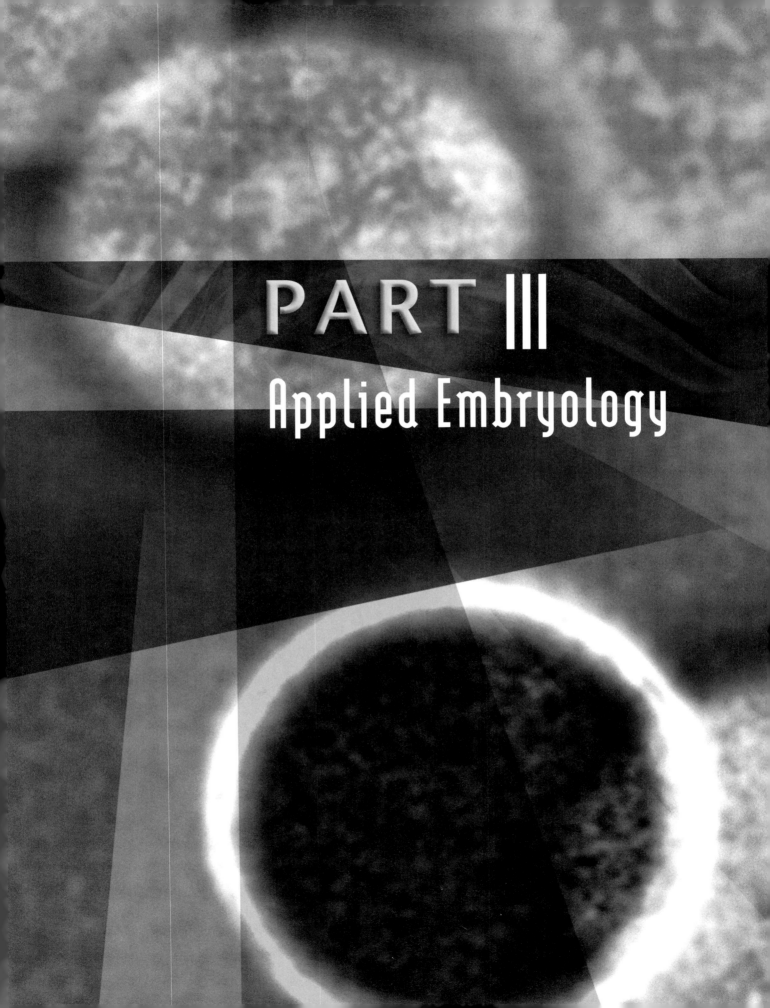

PART III
Applied Embryology

CHAPTER 13

Applied Neuroembryology

Alphonse R. Burdi, Ph.D.

Early Establishment of the Central Nervous Sytem

The human central nervous system is first apparent as a thickened plate (the neural plate) of neuroectoderm along the dorsal midline of the early third-week embryo. The formation of the thickened neural plate is associated with a group of signaling molecules in the transforming growth factor-β (TGF-β) family, which also includes fibroblast growth factors (FGFs). The lateral edges of the neural plate along the embryo's central axis elevate to form the neural folds. With continued elevation, the folds approach each other in the midline to begin forming the neural tube. Upon contacting each other, at day 22 the folds fuse together (almost zipper-like) beginning in the cervical region, and then proceeding toward the cephalic and proctodeal ends of the embryo. The tube's cephalic open end is the anterior neuropore, which closes at day 26, while its counterpart at the proctodeal end of the tube, the posterior neuropore, closes later at 28 days. Some cells from the neural folds give rise to pluripotent neural crest cells that migrate widely in the embryo, giving rise to a number of nervous system structures, including spinal cord dorsal root ganglia, autonomic ganglia, peripheral nerve sheaths, widely distributed pigment cells, the adrenal medulla, skeletal and muscular structures of the head and neck, and the brain and cord meninges. Although both the pia mater and arachnoid mater are neural crest derivatives, the dura mater arises from mesoderm surrounding the neural tube.

Morphogenesis and Growth of Brain and Ventricles

The cephalic end of the neural tube gives rise to the brain. As with the simpler picture of spinal cord morphogenesis (see Spinal Cord Morphogenesis and Growth below), the region of the neural tube giving rise to the brain also has identifiable basal and alar plates, representing motor and sensory functions, respectively. It progressively shows signs of segmentation, or selective regional growth, at approximately 27 days in the form of three dilatations, called the primary brain vesicles. Further differentiation and growth of these vesicles (at 32 days) give rise to the embryonic prosencephalon, mesencephalon, and rhombencephalon.

At day 35, the prosencephalon differentiates into the telencephalon and the diencephalon (future thalamus, epithalamus, hypothalamus, neurohypophysis, pineal gland, optic nerve, and retina). The telencephalon (future cerebral hemispheres, basal ganglia, lamina terminalis, hippocampus, corpus striatum, and olfactory system) is the most rostral of the brain vesicles. The bilateral outpocketings of the telencephalon become the prominent cerebral hemispheres, which contain cavities. The lateral ventricles are the largest of these cavities, all of which contain circulating cerebrospinal fluid. Cerebrospinal fluid in these lateral ventricles communicates with the lumen of the diencephalon through the interventricular foramina of Monro.

The mesencephalon (future midbrain) is separated from the neighboring rhombencephalon by a deep furrow, the rhombencephalic isthmus. It has efferent connections with the oculomotor and trochlear nerves that innervate eye musculature. The rhombencephalon (hindbrain region) is the most caudal of the brain vesicles, and subsequently gives rise to the metencephalon and the myelencephalon (future medulla oblongata). The metencephalon (future pons and cerebellum) has efferent connections with the abducens, trigeminal, and facial nerves. The myelencephalon tapers in diameter and becomes continuous with the spinal cord in the region of the foramen magnum. At about that time, the developing brain shows two major flexures, which are identified as the cervical flexure, located at the junction of the hindbrain and spinal cord, and the cephalic flexure, located in the midbrain region. The pontine flexure is the boundary between the metencephalon and rhombencephalon.

Molecular Regulation of Brain Morphogenesis

The brain is regionalized or patterned along its anteroposterior and dorsoventral axes. Once the neural plate is established, morphogenic signals unleash a pattern of brain segmentation into forebrain, midbrain, and hindbrain regions. Sonic hedgehog (SHH) proteins ventralize the brain's forebrain and midbrain regions, while bone morphogenetic proteins 4 and 7 from non-neural ectoderm induce and sustain the expression of dorsalizing genes. These proteins are important in the formation of craniofacial tissues and are under the direction of signaling genes, especially the *HOX* genes that are catalogued in the family of homeobox genes. Expressed as early the embryonic neural plate stage, these *HOX* genes have identifiable DNA sequences that pattern and control craniofacial morphogenesis. There is an overlapping expression of homeobox genes that specify the regionalization of brain regions (e.g., forebrain and midbrain). The exact mechanisms for such signaling are not yet fully understood, although retinoids (e.g., retinoic acid) have been linked with the regulation of *HOX* gene expression. Patterning, or the early specification, of forebrain and midbrain regions also is regulated by synergistic expressions of yet another family of genes, including *LIM1* and *OTX2*. Once the neural folds progressively engage in neural tube formation, additional homeobox genes are expressed. FGF-β is a key signaling molecule that induces and sustains subsequent gene expressions in craniofacial morphogenesis. In addition to their roles in brain segmentation, homeobox genes play an important role in the formation of rhombomeres (i.e., the building-block tissues for craniofacial structures).

Interface of Brain and Craniofacial Development

The size, shape, and proportionality of the craniofacial region are influenced by the development of the brain at key times during the prenatal and postnatal periods of life. As summarized in the previous section, there is increasing evidence to show that morphogenesis and growth of the head, face, jaws, and mouth is set in motion by molecular events that occur early in the formation of the embryonic brain. Morphogenesis and growth of the brain predominate in the embryonic and fetal periods. Much of this is reflected in the size and shape of the various components of the craniofacial skeleton. Although there are disproportionately large increases in the size of the cranium (brain case) during the second and third trimesters, there is even greater growth of the cranium during the first 2 years after birth, associated also with the rapid postnatal growth chiefly of the cerebral hemispheres.

The capacity of the cranium to accommodate to expanding brain size is linked to the sutures and synchondroses that join the bones of the two major skull regions. Such regions are the neurocranium (brain case or desmocranium, and cranial base or chondrocranium) and viscerocranium (nasomaxillary and mandibular skeletons). Sutures are five-layered fibrous joints (syndesmoses) that are limited to the skull and whose specific locations and types are genetically determined, as is the duration of their patency. At specific postnatal times, the closure of sutures by intramembranous ossification transforms the syndesmoses into synostoses. The timing and rate of fusion among calvarial sutures is sensitive to brain growth and overall size. In general, the metopic (interfrontal) suture, which allows the frontal bones to accommodate the increasing size of the brain's frontal lobes, begins to ossify after year 1 and typically is completely ossified by 4 to 6 years. The sagittal, coronal, and lambdoidal sutures fuse between 20 and 40 years of age, with the exact timing for each dependent upon the individual's population (i.e., population polymorphisms).

Sutures and synchondroses also play important roles in the downward and forward growth of the facial skeleton after birth, at least up to and through the period of mixed dentitions. The large flat bones of the brain case (frontal, parietal, temporal, occipital, and sphenoid) develop through intramembranous ossification within the soft tissue envelope (ectomeninx) covering the brain. A more localized region of the ectomeninx underlying the brain eventually chondrifies as the brain case floor (cartilaginous cranial base). The prenatal and postnatal shapes and sizes of the brain case have been associated with the arrangement of specific collagenous fiber tracts (dural stretch fields) within the soft tissue envelope observable as early as the second trimester of development. It has been suggested that missing or defective dural stretch fields can be associated with abnormal brain size and shape. Skull bones are separated by fibrous (syndesmotic) and cartilaginous (synchondrotic) joints throughout much of the prenatal period and into late adulthood. The syndesmoses separating the calvarial bones can be either narrow in width (i.e., sutures) or expansive in size (i.e., fontanelles). Sutures allow for normal enlargement of the brain by keeping the various calvarial bones connected (i.e., articulations). Fontanelles allow for the over-riding of calvarial bones to reduce the anteroposterior and bilateral dimensions of the calvarium during childbirth.

The rapid growth of the brain establishes an early predominance of neurocranium size over the size of the upper facial skeleton. In general, the growth predominance of the neurocranium over the facial regions is greatest in the fetal period, reducing to an 8:1 proportion at birth, to 6:1 in postnatal year 2, to 4:1 in the fifth year, and to 2.5:1 in the adult years. At birth, the neurocranium has attained 25% of its full adult growth; it attains 50% by age 6 months, and 75% by 2 years. By 10 years, the growth of the neurocranium is 95% complete, while the facial skeleton has achieved only about 65% of its anticipated adult size. Again, reflecting the precocious growth of the brain, the brain case in postnatal life increases 5 times in volume, whereas the facial skeleton increases to about 10 times its size at birth. The cranium typically increases in size and capacity until about 16 years of age. After that time, there is only a slight increase in size for the next 4 years, attributed less to brain growth and more to a progressive thickening of the cranial bones. The expansive brain displaces the individual calvarial bones laterally and upward from the brain itself, and, as the bones are displaced, there is a concomitant set of tension forces placed on the sutures themselves.

Because the rapidly enlarging brain has an effect on cranial form, in general, with increasing brain size there is a concomitant flattening of the developing cranial base and its cranial base angle (nasion-sella-basion angle). Progressive changes in the form (i.e., size and shape) of the cranial base are associated with changes in position of the optic fields and orbits and a forward displacement of the upper face. The intrauterine period showing the greatest forward displacement of the upper face is at approximately the second and third intrauterine months, at which time a disproportionate expansion of the brain's temporal lobes occurs. In anencephaly, the marked reduction in brain volume is associated with a flattened cranial base region and a concomitant retropositioning of the upper facial region. After birth, and more specifically after 4 years of age, there is a relative slowing of brain growth with increases in growth and repositioning of the facial regions. Differential growth of the mesenchymally derived brain meninges, especially that of the dural (collagenous) stretch fields, is associated with rapid brain growth in the first trimester. Such differential growth has known enlarging effects on the developing cranial base skeleton that eventually translate into the forward movement of the upper facial skeleton from beneath the anterior cranial base. As noted above, the skeletal elements of the cranium develop initially to support and protect the enlarging brain mass. Cartilages of the cranial base (chondrocranium) eventually transform into individual bones (ethmoid, sphenoid, and occipital) and intervening cartilaginous growth plates of the cranial base (spheno-occipital and sphenoethmoid synchondroses). These synchondroses are important to the growing face and pharyngeal regions beginning as early as 7 to 10 intrauterine weeks. Postnatally, proliferative growth in the anterior and downward extension of the chondrocranium (i.e., the nasal septum) plays a significant role in support and anterior and downward growth of the upper face throughout the adolescent years.

While the developing brain plays an important role in cranial form, extensions of the brain play an important role in the development of the face. Considering that the developing embryonic optic fields and future eyes (except for the lens) are extensions of the brain's diencephalon, it should be noted that the positions of the optic fields are associated with key states in facial development during the fifth to eighth embryonic weeks. To summarize, the face arises from the growth, migration, and consolidation of five major facial prominences, including the frontonasal (reflecting a forward extension of the brain) and paired maxillary and mandibular prominences. As noted earlier, neural crest cells surrounding the embryonic brain play an important role in formation of the face. Crest cells differentiating and migrating out from the developing midbrain and hindbrain regions eventually locate and further differentiate in the branchial arches, where they play key roles in formation of the face, jaws, tongue, palate, nasal cavities, mouth, and pharynx. A number of birth defects affecting the head and face (e.g., Treacher Collins syndrome, mandibulofacial dysostosis) arise from genetic errors in abnormal development of the brain and neural crest. The latter are referred to as *neurocristopathies.*

The pattern of normal repositioning of the embryonic optic fields between 5 and 8 intrauterine weeks has been linked to the migration and consolidation of the separate embryonic maxillary processes. At 5 weeks, the optic fields are situated on the sides of the embryonic head, at which time the frontonasal and the two maxillary prominences are typically separated blocks of tissue. Between 5 and 8 weeks (i.e., the peak period of facial morphogenesis), the maxillary prominences gradually are repositioned toward the midline, where each will contact and fuse with the frontonasal prominence, and the medionasal prominence in specific, to form the upper lip. The optic fields have a 180-degree angular relationship with each other at 5 weeks. By the eighth week, the angle between the right and left optic fields (formed by the intersecting optic nerves) becomes more acute, with a value of approximately 120 degrees, which is the value seen in the adult. In that this reduction in the optic field angle is associated temporally with the consolidation of the embryonic facial prominences, medial and forward movement of the eye fields has been theorized as bringing the face together. Significant interruptions of eye field migration have been associated with the conditions of cleft lip and hypertelorism. Overmigration of the embryonic optic fields has been associated with such conditions as hypotelorism, cyclopia, cebocephaly, and ethmocephaly.

Clinical Correlates of Brain and Skull Dysmorphogenesis

Dysmorphogenesis of the Brain

In general, dysmorphology is often a result of morphogenic disturbances or interruptions at critical periods of normal embryogenesis. A number of craniofacial phenotypes have been related to or implicated in abnormal morphogenesis and growth of the nervous system, especially that of the brain. *Holoprosencephaly* involves a loss of midline structures of the brain and face. In severe cases, lateral ventricles merge into a single telencephalic vesicle, in which the eyes may fuse, and there is a single nasal cavity along associated midline facial defects. Mutations in the *SHH* gene, which specifies the midline of the central nervous system at neural plate stages, have been linked causally to these conditions. Other causes have included defective cholesterol biosynthesis associated with the Smith-Lemli-Opitz syndrome, and fetal alcohol exposure, which can selectively destroy midline cells of the developing nervous system.

Meningocele, meningoencephalocele, and *meningohydroencephalocele* are related to ossification defects in skull bones (secondary to neural tube defects), which variously may involve both the herniating brain and meningeal coverings. *Exencephaly* is a condition characterized by a failure of the cephalic region of the neural tube to close, specifically in the region of the anterior neuropore, and is a condition in which the skull vault does not develop, leaving the malformed brain exposed. Later the rudimentary malformed brain degenerates, leaving a mass of necrotic cerebral tissue, as in anencephaly, although the brainstem

remains intact. *Anencephaly* (or meroanencephaly), a common lethal malformation readily imaged by ultrasonography, fetoscopy, and radiography, occurs at least once in every 1000 live births. A closure defect of the neural tube in the brain region (occurring typically in the fourth week) is generally called *cranioschisis*. *Schizencephaly* is a rare disorder showing as large clefts in the cerebral hemispheres, and etiologically linked with mutations within the homeobox gene family (e.g., the *EMX2* gene). The *Arnold-Chiari malformation* is a caudal displacement and herniation of cerebellar tissues through the foramen magnum. This malformation occurs in virtually every case of spinal bifida cystica and typically is accompanied by hydrocephalus.

Hydrocephaly involves the accumulation of abnormal levels of cerebrospinal fluid within the ventricular system, usually as a result of an obstruction of the aqueduct of Sylvius. This blockage prevents fluid of the lateral and third ventricles from passing into the fourth ventricle and on to the subarachnoid space, where the fluid can be resorbed. Buildup of fluid within the lateral ventricles in the prenatal and early childhood years can compress brain tissue against the calvarial bones and expand abnormally the calvarial sutures, producing an abnormal form (size and shape) of the brain case.

As compared to enlarged cranial sizes often seen in hydrocephaly, *microcephaly* is a condition in which the brain case is smaller than expected, which reflects a diminished growth and volume of the brain. Face size and form are usually within the normal range in microcephalic individuals. This condition may be genetic (chiefly but not entirely autosomal recessive inheritance) or due to prenatal insults such as infection or maternal exposure to drugs and teratogens (e.g., maternal alcohol abuse and fetal alcohol syndrome).

Dysmorphogenesis of the Skull

The skull, especially the calvarium, can be a dominant clinical feature in a number of birth defects. Premature fusion (*synostosis*) occurs chiefly in the calvarial sutures and less frequently among sutures of the facial skeleton. Reduced or excessive levels in TGF-β protein expression at developing suture sites have been linked with the early or delayed closure of sutures. As noted earlier, the timing and rate of fusion among calvarial sutures is sensitive to disturbances in brain growth. As examples, sutures and fontanelles fuse prematurely in microcephaly, whereas sutural fusion is delayed in hydrocephaly. Whether directly or indirectly associated with atypical growth of the brain, unilateral or bilateral premature closure of key calvarial sutures (e.g., coronal, sagittal, lambdoid) can be significant enough to result in a number of nonsyndromic calvarial distortions. Premature synostosis of the sagittal suture limits lateral growth of the skull. Bilateral synostosis of the coronal sutures limits anteroposterior growth of the skull, resulting in a "pointed" skull feature (*oxycephaly*) and reduced anteroposterior length (*brachycephaly*). Premature unilateral fusion of the coronal and lambdoid sutures causes an oblique calvarial distortion (*plagiocephaly*).

Premature calvarial fusions also can manifest as a family of syndromic cranial distortions called the *craniosynostoses*. In the craniosynostoses, the severity of calvarial distortion is related to the number and location of synostosed sutures and the onset of the premature fusions. These conditions invariably become more severe with increasing age. They include Crouzon's disease (craniofacial dysostosis) and the syndromes of Apert (acrocephalosyndactyly), Saethre-Chotzen, Carpenter, and Pfeiffer. In cases of cretinism, trisomy 21, and cleidocranial dysostosis, there is a delayed midline ossification of the frontal (metopic) and sagittal sutures of the calvarium that is associated with a delay or failure of ossification of the anterior fontanelle until adult life. The shape and size of the brain regions underlying these aberrant sutures and synchondroses also can be abnormal. Defects in ossification of the ethmoid-frontal suture are associated clinically with herniation of cranial contents (e.g., encephaloceles) into the nasal and facial regions. Occipital and basal encephaloceles may occur through the cranial base tissues. Premature ossification of the cranial base synchondroses, namely the spheno-occipital synchondrosis in the posterior cranial base and the sphenoethmoid synchondrosis in the anterior cranial base, can result in reduced lengths of those specific base segments and related structures (i.e., pharynx, facial skeleton). Although cranial base abnormalities, including those of the cranial base synchondroses, have been variously associated with orofacial clefting, such cranial base abnormalities may be only secondary disturbances, with the primary causal factors related to dysmorphogenesis of the brain and brainstem.

Spinal Cord Morphogenesis and Growth

Patterns of Cord Morphogenesis

The neural tube distal to the brain (i.e., below the fourth pair of somites) develops into the spinal cord. The neural canal of the neural tube within the spinal cord becomes the central canal of the spinal cord, which is gradually reduced in size (at 9 to 10 weeks) by continued thickening of the lateral neural tube walls surrounding the canal. Cells within the tube wall progressively differentiate into a variety of neuroepithelial cell types. One group constitutes the ventricular zone (ependymal layer), which gives rise

(at 6 to 9 weeks) to all neurons and macroglial cells (e.g., macroglial astrocytes and oligodendrocytes) of the spinal cord. Soon after, a marginal zone becomes recognizable that gradually becomes the spinal cord's white matter as axons grow into it from nerve cell bodies in the spinal cord, spinal ganglia, and brain. An intermediate zone (mantle layer) subsequently develops as neuroepithelial cells from the ventricular zone migrate into the zone between the ventricular and marginal zones. These migrating cells are neuroblasts and become neurons as they develop cytoplasmic processes. Following neuroblast formation, neuroepithelial cells differentiate into supporting glioblast cells (spongioblasts), which further differentiate into astroblasts (astrocytes) and oligodendroblasts (oligodendrocytes). When neuroepithelial cells stop producing neuroblasts and glioblasts, they differentiate into ependymal cells, which subsequently form the ependymal lining of the spinal cord's central canal. Small cells called microglia, thought to develop from mesenchyme, invade the central nervous system late in the fetal period and may be related to blood cells of the monocyte-macrophage lineage.

The continued thickening of the spinal cord wall is accompanied by the development of a longitudinal groove (at about 40 days) on each lateral wall. That groove is the sulcus limitans, which separates the tube's dorsal part, the alar plate, from its ventral part, the basal plate. This regional separation is of significance because the alar and basal plates eventually become associated with sensory and motor functions, respectively. Motor nerves first appear at about the fourth week, arising from nerve cells within the basal plate (ventral horns) of the spinal cord. Neuronal connections with unipolar neurons of the developing spinal (dorsal root) ganglia develop from neural crest cells. Much like the coverings of the brain, mesenchyme surrounding the spinal neural tube forms a trilaminar membrane (called the primordial meninx) from which arise the cord's dura mater, arachnoid mater, and pia mater layers. Embryonic cerebrospinal fluid begins to form and circulate within the subarachnoid space as early as the fifth intrauterine week.

Spinal Cord Growth

In the embryo, the spinal cord extends the entire length of the vertebral canal. Because the bony vertebral canal and dura mater grow in length more rapidly than the spinal cord, this relationship does not persist. At 6 months, the caudal end of the spinal cord is at the level of the first sacral vertebra. The caudal tip of the cord in newborns is found at the level of the second or third lumbar vertebra. Below those levels, a thread-like extension of the cord's pia mater forms the filum terminale that attaches to the first coccygeal vertebra. In the adult, the cord typically terminates at the level of the first lumbar vertebra. One outcome of this differential growth between cord and vertebral canal is that the spinal nerve roots, especially those in the lumbar and sacral cord segments, run obliquely from the spinal cord to the corresponding level of the vertebral column. These obliquely arranged nerves are collectively known as the cauda equina.

Myelin sheaths in the spinal cord begin to form during the late fetal period and continue to form during the first postnatal year. In general, fiber tracts become myelinated at about the same time they become functional. Oligodendrocytes form myelin sheaths surrounding nerve fibers within the spinal cord. Myelin sheaths around axons of peripheral nerves are formed by plasma membranes of neurolemmal cells (i.e., the neural crest–derived Schwann cells), which differentiate from neural crest cells. At about 20 prenatal weeks, peripheral nerve fibers begin to take on a whitish appearance, resulting from the deposition of myelin. In general, motor roots are myelinated before sensory roots, and tracts in the nervous system become myelinated at about the time function is established.

Molecular Regulation of Spinal Cord Morphogenesis

As with the molecular patterning of brain morphogenesis, the above picture of spinal cord morphogenesis is best understood on the basis of information coming from the world of developmental molecular biology. At the neural plate stage in spinal cord embryogenesis, the entire plate expresses the transcription factors PAX3, PAX7, MSX1, and MSX2. This expression pattern is linked with SHH protein expressed in the notochord and with bone morphogenetic proteins 4 and 7 (BMP4 and BMP7) as expressed in the non-neural ectoderm at the border of the neural plate. SHH represses expression of PAX3, PAX7, MSX1, and MSX2. Thus SHH positions the developing neural tube so that the ventral (motor/efferent) portion of the tube differentiates into the basal plate and motor neurons that subsequently grow out from the basal plate (i.e., ventral horns). BMP4 and BMP7 gene expression then upregulates PAX3 and PAX7 transcription factors in the tube's dorsal portions, giving rise to the alar (sensory/afferent) plate. PAX3 and PAX7 genes are required for formation of the neural crest cells along the tops of the neural folds, but their specific roles and those of the *MSX* genes in the differentiation of sensory and interneuron neurons is not clear. However, the expression of PAX3 and PAX7 genes throughout the neural tube in the earliest stages of tube morphogenesis is essential for the receptivity to *SHH* gene expression and for the formation of ventral horn cell types. While the PAX6 gene is expressed during and after neural fold elevation, its specific role is yet unidentified.

Clinical Correlates of Spinal Cord Dysmorphogenesis

Most congenital defects of the spinal cord and associated structures result from defective closure of the neural tube during the fourth intrauterine week. A closure defect of the neural tube and spinal cord is generally called *rachischisis*. Defects involving the vertebral arches are generally referred to as *spina bifida*. *Meningoceles* and *meningomyeloceles* may occur anywhere along the vertebral column, but are most common in the lumbar and sacral regions. Some cases of meningomyelocele can be associated with defective skull development, called *craniolacunia*, resulting in depressed, nonossified areas on the inner surfaces of calvarial flat bones.

Severe cases of spina bifida also involve the spinal cord and meninges. Usually present without clinical signs, *spina bifida occulta* occurs in the L5 or S1 vertebra in about 10% of otherwise clinically normal individuals, and has been linked with abnormal expression of the MSX2 gene. In a few instances, affected infants show functionally significant defects of the underlying spinal cord and attached dorsal roots. Severe types of spina bifida, collectively known as *spina bifida cystica*, can involve herniation of the spinal cord and/or meninges through the defect in the vertebral arches. Spina bifida cystica is often associated with the Arnold-Chiari malformation. Where the herniated sac contains meninges and cerebrospinal fluid, the malformation is called spina bifida with meningocele. Spina bifida with meningomyelocele is a more severe condition in which spinal cord and/or nerve roots also are included in the herniated sac. It is often marked by neurologic deficits. The incidence of meningoceles is rare compared with meningomyeloceles. Severe cases of spina bifida with meningomyelocele involving several vertebrae are often associated with partial absence of the brain (e.g., meroanencephaly or anencephaly).

Spina bifida with myeloschisis, the most severe kind of spina bifida, occurs when the spinal cord is open because the neural folds failed to fuse and form a tube (i.e., spinal cord). Spina bifida with myeloschisis may result from a neural tube defect caused by a significant overgrowth of the neural plate with a concomitant failure of closure (at about the fourth week) of the caudal neuropore. As a result, the spinal cord appears as a flattened mass of nerve tissue.

Spina bifida cystica and/or meroencephaly are strongly associated with high levels of α-fetoprotein in the amniotic fluid and, in some cases, in the maternal blood serum. Nutritional and environmental factors also have been assigned various roles in the etiology of neural tube defects. As examples, vitamins and folic acid supplements taken prior to or immediately after conception can reduce the incidence of tube defects in the offspring of some women. Certain drugs (such as the anticonvulsant valproic acid) increase the risk of meningomyeloceles, again in the offspring of some women. Hypothermia, hypervitaminosis A, and teratogens also can produce neural tube defects. The vertebral column and spina bifida cystica can be effectively imaged as early as the eighth postconceptional week.

Bibliography

Behrman RE, Kliegman RM, Arvin AM: Nelson Textbook of Pediatrics (15th ed). Philadelphia: WB Saunders, 1996.

Blechschmidt M: The biokinetics of the basicranium. *In* Bosma JF (ed): Symposium on the Development of the Basicranium (NIH/NIDR Publication No. 77-989). Bethesda, MD: National Institutes of Health, 1977.

Burdi AR: Early development of the basicranium: its morphogenic controls, growth patterns, and relations. *In* Bosma JF (ed): Symposium on the Development of the Basicranium (NIH/NIDR Publication No. 77-989). Bethesda, MD: National Institutes of Health, 1977.

Burdi AR, Lawton TJ, Grosslight J: Prenatal pattern emergence in early human facial development. Cleft Palate J 1988;25:8.

Cohen MM, MacLean RE: Craniosynostosis: Diagnosis, Evaluation and Management (2nd ed). Oxford: Oxford University Press, 2000.

David DJ, Poswillo D, Simpson D: The Craniosynostoses. Berlin: Springer-Verlag, 1982.

Dobbing J, Sands J: Head circumference, biparietal diameter and brain growth in fetal and postnatal life. Early Human Dev 1978;2:81.

Enlow DH, Hans MG: Essentials of Facial Growth. Philadelphia: WB Saunders, 1996.

Erickson CA: Control of pathfinding by the avian neural crest. Development 1988;103:63.

Eriksen E, Back-Petersen S, van den Eynde B, et al: Midsagittal dimensions of the prenatal human cranium. J Craniofac Genet Dev Biol 1995;15:44.

Farkas LG: Anthropometry of the Head and Face (2nd ed). New York: Raven Press, 1994.

Forman R, Chou S, Koren G: The role of folic acid in preventing neural tube defect. Contemp Ob/Gyn 1995;4:16.

Gorlin RJ, Cohen MM, Levin LS: Syndromes of the Head and Neck (3rd ed). London: Oxford University Press, 1990.

Jones KL: Smith's Recognizable Patterns of Human Malformations. Philadelphia: WB Saunders, 1988.

Kjaer I, Keeling JW, Graem N: Midline maxillofacial skeleton in human anencephalic fetuses. Cleft Palate Craniofac J 1994;31:250.

Kreiborg S, Cohen MM: Characteristics of the infant Apert skull and subsequent development. J Craniofac Genet Dev Biol 1990;10:399.

Laurence KM, Weeks R: Abnormalities of the central nervous system. *In* Norman AP (ed): Congenital Abnormalities in Infancy (2nd ed). Oxford: Blackwell Publications, 1971.

LeDouarin N, Smith J: Development of the peripheral nervous system from the neural crest. Annu Rev Cell Biol 1988;4:375.

LeDouarin NM, Catala M, Battini C: Embryonic neural chimera in the study of vertebrate head and brain development. Int Rev Cytol 1997;175:1109.

Lumsden A, Krumlauf R: Patterning the vertebrate neuraxis. Science 1996;274:1109.

Morriss-Kay G, Tan SS: Mapping cranial neural crest migration pathways in mammalian embryos. Trends Genet 1987;3:257.

Morriss-Kay G, Tuckett F: Early events in mammalian craniofacial morphogenesis. J Craniofac Genet Dev Biol 1991;11:181.

Moss ML: Malformations of the skull base associated with cleft palate deformity. Plast Reconstr Surg 1956;17:226.

Moss ML: The pathogenesis of premature cranial synostosis in man. Acta Anat 1959;37:351.

Moyers RM: Handbook of Orthodontics (4th ed). Chicago: Year Book Medical Publishers, 1988.

Noden DM: Origins and patterning of craniofacial mesenchymal tissues. J Craniofac Genet Dev Biol 1986;2:15.

Noden DM: Cell movements and control of patterned tissue assembly during craniofacial development. J Craniofac Genet Dev Biol 1991;11:192.

Opperman LA, Nolen AA, Ogle RC: TGF-beta 1, TGF-beta 2, and TGF-beta 3 exhibit distinct patterns of expression during cranial suture formation and obliteration in vivo and in vitro. J Bone Miner Res 1977;12:301.

Roessler E: Mutations in the human sonic hedgehog gene cause holoprosencephaly. Nat Genet 1996;14:357.

Sakai Y: Neurulation in the mouse: the ontogenesis of neural segments and the determination of topographical regions in a central nervous system. Anat Rec 1987;218:450.

Scott JH: The cartilage of the nasal septum. Br Dent J 1953;95:37.

Scott JH: Growth at facial sutures. Am J Orthod 1956;42:381.

Sperber GH: Craniofacial Development. Hamilton, Ontario: BC Decker, 2001.

Stewart RE, Prescott GH: Oral Facial Genetics. St. Louis: CV Mosby, 1976.

Sulik KK: Craniofacial development. *In* Turvey TA, Vig KWL, Fonseca RJ (eds): Facial Clefts and Craniosynostosis: Principles and Management. Philadelphia: WB Saunders, 1996.

Sutton JB: On the relation of the orbitosphenoid to the region pterion in the side wall of the skull. J Anat Physiol 1884;78:220.

Thompson MW, McInnes RR, Willard HF: Thompson and Thompson's Genetics in Medicine (5th ed): Philadelphia: WB Saunders, 1991.

Venes J, Burdi AR: Proposed role of the orbitosphenoid in cranial dysostosis. Concepts Pediatr Neurosurg 1985;5:126.

Warkany J: Congenital Malformations. Chicago: Year Book Medical Publishers, 1971.

CHAPTER 14

Applied Embryology of the Head and Neck

Lisa R. David, M.D.

As the Human Genome Project has become a reality, we have an increasing understanding of the etiology of errors that occur during development and their clinical consequences. This quantum leap has provided a better understanding of fetal development. For example, we now know the genes responsible for palatal development, including *MSX1* and *LHX8* (controlling palatal shelf growth and differentiation); *TGFA*, *EGFR*, and *HOXA2* (controlling elevation and depression of the tongue); *TGFB3* and *PVRL1* (controlling fusion of the midline palatal seam); and *TGFA* and *EGFR* (controlling the disappearance of the midline palatal seam). In the future this knowledge may allow earlier treatment or possible prevention of clinical malformations.

A basic understanding of embryology is necessary to adequately comprehend why certain developmental abnormalities occur. There is no area in the human body for which this is truer than for the head and neck region. This understanding not only will explain why these abnormalities produce the clinical manifestations we see, but also will facilitate the development of optimal treatment algorithms.

Overview of Normal Development

Embryo development begins with fertilization. Several cell divisions later, a fluid-filled cavity known as the blastocyst is formed. This blastocyst contributes only a portion of itself to the actual embryo (inner cell mass), but makes a significant contribution to what will become the placenta. The cells of the inner cell mass of the blastocyst separate into two layers called the epiblast and hypoblast. During a process known as gastrulation, some cells from the epiblast then migrate to form a middle germ layer. This migration is known as gastrulation. It is during this stage that three separate layers are formed in the developing embryo. The portion of the epiblast that does not migrate becomes the ectoderm, while the portion that migrates becomes the mesoderm. The endoderm is formed from the cells of the hypoblast. All adult structures can be traced to their origin in one of these three cell layers.

At this stage of development, the cells begin interacting and primary embryonic induction begins. This process results in a portion of the mesoderm inducing the formation of neural plate in the overlying ectoderm. The mesoderm is composed of three major components: notochord, paraxial mesoderm, and lateral plate. The induced neural plate then thickens and rolls up to form the neural tube. Simultaneously, the lateral part of the three germ layers folds under the embryo to form the gut. The forebrain then overgrows the regions that will become the face and cardiac structures. Tubulation, or the formation of two embryonic tubes (neural tube and gastrointestinal tube), has occurred. By this stage, much of the map of the head has been predetermined.

It is during this time that the complex migration of cells derived from the neural folds begins. Neural crest cells migrate over a long course, interacting with various other tissues along the pathway to their ultimate destination. It is this extended migratory pathway that explains how neural crest cells make contributions to a wide array of structures. Derivatives of neural crest cells include melanocytes and cells of the peripheral nervous system, cranial structures (Fig. 14–1), and the connective and skeletal tissue of the face and neck. Neural crest cells also play a dominant role in the development of the head and neck.

Neural crest cells reach the cranium after migrating under the ectoderm. Upon leaving the neural plate, they lose their close association with other cells. Ultimately these cells surround the mesoderm cores of the visceral arches and form all the mesenchyme of the rest of the face. Once their migration is completed, sites of rapid cell proliferation, known as growth centers, control head and neck development. Three growth centers, specifically the frontonasal, maxillary, and mandibular prominences, play a prominent role in development of the head.

The development of the lower face and neck is dominated by the development of visceral arches. Each arch has its own blood vessel, muscle, nerve, and skeletal elements. These pharyngeal (branchial) arches initially only contain mesoderm. Neural crest cells migrate and surround these arches. The mesoderm then becomes segmented by the ingrowth of ectoderm (cleft) and the outgrowth of endoderm (pouch). The pharyngeal apparatus plays a key role in the development of the head and neck.

The onset of skeletal formation usually is considered the end of the embryonic period and the beginning of the fetal period (Table 14–1).

The Skull

The skull can be divided into two components. The viscerocranium, which is derived from the pharyngeal apparatus, is discussed below. The neurocranium is the portion derived from neural crest cells, except for the basilar part of the occipital bone. This portion of the occipital bone is instead derived from mesoderm from the occipital somites.

The cranium is made up of the flat bones of the cranial vault and the base of the skull. During fetal life and infancy, these bones are separated by dense connective tissue known as sutures. There are five cranial sutures: the metopic, coronal, sagittal, lambdoid, and squamosal. These sutures allow the bones of the skull to move and permit deformation during the childbirth process as well as growth during childhood. The sutures come together in areas known as fontanelles. There are six of these: the anterior and posterior, two sphenoid, and two mastoid fontanelles. The posterior and sphenoid fontanelles are the first to close, at around 6 months after birth. The anterior and mastoid fontanelles can remain open up to 2 years of age, after the primary growth of the brain is completed. Failure of a fontanelle to close on time may be an indication of increased intracranial pressure.

Clinically Applied Embryology

Craniosynostosis, the premature fusion of cranial sutures, is most often responsible for abnormalities in skull shape. The major exception, positional or deformational plagiocephaly, is now known to be responsible for cranial asymmetry in 1 in 70 infants. Beginning in 1992, with the

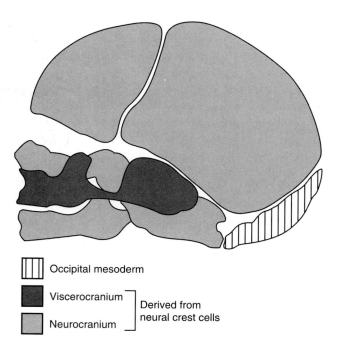

Occipital mesoderm

Viscerocranium ⎤
⎥ Derived from
⎦ neural crest cells
Neurocranium

FIGURE 14–1 Neural crest cell derivatives. (From Gordon ES: Collection of Images and Illustrations. Department of Plastic Surgery, Wake Forest University School of Medicine. January 2002. © 2001 WFUSM Plastic Surgery Collection.)

Table 14–1
Chronology of events during the embryonic period

Postconception Age (days)	Craniofacial Features
14	Primitive streak appears, oropharyngeal membrane forms
17	Neural plate forms
20	Cranial neural folds elevate, otic placode appears
21	Neural crest migration begins, fusion of neural folds, otic pits form
24	Frontonasal prominence swells, first arch forms, wide stomodeum, optic vesicles form, anterior neuropore closes, olfactory placode appears
26	Second arch forms, maxillary prominences appear, lens placodes commence, posterior neuropore closes
28	Third arch forms, dental lamina appears, fourth arch forms, oropharyngeal membrane ruptures
32	Otic and lens vesicles present, lateral nasal prominences appear
33	Medial nasal prominences appear, nasal pits form, widely separated face laterally
37	Nasal pits face ventrally, upper lip forms on lateral aspect of stomodeum, lower lip fuses in midline, retinal pigment forms, nasolacrimal groove appears and demarcates the nose
41	Contact between medial nasal and maxillary prominences, separating nasal pit from stomodeum, upper lip continuity is first established, vomeronasal organ appears
47–48	Nasal fin disintegrates, mouth width diminishes, mandibular ossification commences
50–51	Lidless eyes migrate medially, nasal pits approach each other, ear hillocks fuse
54	The eyelids thicken and encroach upon the eyes, the auricle forms and projects, the nostrils reach their definitive position
56–57	Eyes are wide apart but eyelid closure begins, nasal tip elevates, face assumes a human fetal appearance, mouth opens, palatal shelves elevate, maxillary ossification begins
60	Palatal shelves fuse, deciduous tooth buds form; embryo is now a fetus

American Academy of Pediatrics' recommendation to put children to sleep on their backs to prevent sudden infant death syndrome (SIDS), an increased incidence of children with posterior cranial asymmetry was seen. Initially this was misinterpreted by some as craniosynostosis; however, it is now clear that this is simply a result of the "Back to Sleep" campaign to decrease the incidence of SIDS. Since that time, many institutions have shown that this deformity can be managed conservatively with helmet therapy rather than the surgical intervention that is required for true craniosynostosis.

Craniosynostosis is the premature fusion of one or more cranial sutures that results in a restriction of head growth in a direction perpendicular to the involved suture. Specific types of craniosynostosis include (Fig. 14–2).

1. *Trigonocephaly*: premature fusion of the metopic suture, resulting in a triangulated forehead shape

2. *Scaphocephaly*: premature fusion of the sagittal suture, resulting in an elongated and narrow head

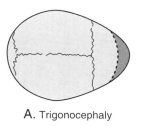
A. Trigonocephaly

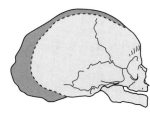
B. Scaphocephaly

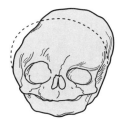
C. Plagiocephaly

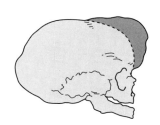
D. Brachycephaly

FIGURE 14–2 Types of craniosynostosis. (From Gordon ES: Collection of Images and Illustrations. Department of Plastic Surgery, Wake Forest University School of Medicine. January 2002. © 2001 WFUSM Plastic Surgery Collection.)

3. *Anterior plagiocephaly*: premature fusion of one of the coronal sutures, resulting in orbital dystopia and forehead asymmetry

4. *Posterior plagiocephaly*: premature fusion of one of the lambdoid sutures, resulting in occipital asymmetry

5. *Brachycephaly*: premature fusion of both of the coronal sutures, resulting in frontal bossing and a fetal appearance of the forehead

6. *Oxycephaly or turricephaly*: premature closure of both the lambdoid and coronal sutures, resulting in a tower-like skull shape

Craniosynostosis can have a sporadic or hereditary origin. The exact cellular mechanism that is responsible for this deformity is still under study. Current theories focus on changes in the concentration of growth factors at the site of the fused suture and the interaction of the suture with the underlying dura. Craniosynostosis requires surgical intervention, and the best results are obtained if this is done prior to 1 year of age. Surgical treatment usually involves the advancement and reshaping of the forehead and expansion of the cranial vault. Children with syndromic craniosynostosis, such as Crouzon's disease and Apert's syndrome, often require a series of operations to address both the fused suture and associated midface abnormalities.

The Pharyngeal Apparatus

The pharyngeal apparatus consists of arches, grooves, pouches, and membranes (Fig. 14–3). The pharyngeal arch begins to develop during week 4 when the neural crest cells migrate into the future head and neck regions. The first pair of arches is seen as surface elevations lateral to the developing pharynx. By the end of the fourth week, four pairs of arches are visible on the developing embryo. The fifth and sixth pairs are rudimentary and thus not visible on the surface of the embryo. During the fifth week, the second pharyngeal arch enlarges and overgrows the third and fourth arches, forming the cervical sinus. By the end of the seventh week, the second through fourth pharyngeal grooves and the cervical sinus have disappeared, giving rise to a smooth neck contour.

Pharyngeal Arches

Each pharyngeal arch is composed of a core of mesenchyme with an internal endodermal lining and an external cover of ectoderm. The mesenchyme that originates from migrating neural crest cells gives rise to the maxillary and mandibular prominences as well as many of the key derivatives of the arches. The original mesenchyme contributes to the skeletal muscle and vascular endothelium of the head and neck. Each pharyngeal arch contains an aortic arch, a cartilage rod that forms the skeleton of the arch, a muscular component that will contribute to the muscles of the head and neck, and a nerve (Table 14–2).

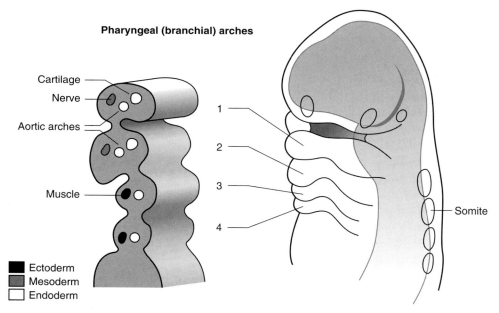

Pharyngeal (branchial) arches

Cartilage
Nerve
Aortic arches
Muscle

1
2
3
4

Somite

■ Ectoderm
■ Mesoderm
□ Endoderm

FIGURE 14–3 Pharyngeal apparatus derivatives. (From Gordon ES: Collection of Images and Illustrations. Department of Plastic Surgery, Wake Forest University School of Medicine. January 2002. © 2001 WFUSM Plastic Surgery Collection.)

Table 14–2
Adult derivatives of the pharyngeal arches

Arch	Cranial Nerve	Muscles	Skeletal Structures
First	V	Muscles of mastication, mylohyoid muscle, tensor veli palatini muscle, anterior belly of the digastric muscle	Maxilla, zygomatic bone, squamous temporal bone, palatine bone, vomer, mandible, incus, malleus, sphenomandibular ligament
Second	VII	Muscles of facial expression, posterior belly of the digastric muscle, stylohyoid muscle, stapedius muscle	Lesser horn and upper body of hyoid bone, stapes, styloid process, stylohyoid
Third	IX	Stylopharyngeal and upper pharyngeal muscles	Greater cornu of hyoid, lower part of body of hyoid bone
Fourth	X	Muscles of the soft palate (except tensor veli palatini), muscles of the pharynx (except stylopharyngeus), cricothyroid muscle, cricopharyngeus muscle, laryngeal cartilages	Thyroid, arytenoid, corniculate, and cuneiform cartilages
Fifth and sixth	X	Intrinsic muscles of the larynx (except cricothyroid), upper muscles of esophagus, laryngeal cartilages	Thyroid, arytenoid, corniculate, and cuneiform cartilages

From Johnston MC, Sulik KK: The neural crest. In Shields ED, Burzynsky NJ, Melnick M (eds): *Craniofacial Dysmorphology: Genetics, Etiology, Diagnosis and Treatment.* Littleton, MA: John Wright, PSG, 1983; and Dudek RW: High-Yield Embryology. Baltimore: Williams & Wilkins, 1996:30.

The first pharyngeal arch (mandibular) consists of a dorsal portion known as the maxillary process and a ventral portion known as the mandibular process. The first arch cartilage, Meckel's cartilage, regresses except for two small portions that persist to form the incus and malleus. The mesenchyme of the maxillary process ultimately gives rise to the premaxilla, maxilla, zygomatic bone, and part of the temporal bone through membranous ossification. The mandible also is formed by membranous ossification. The musculature of the first arch forms the muscles of mastication (temporalis, masseter, and pterygoids), anterior belly of the digastric, mylohyoid, tensor tympani, and tensor palatini. The embryonic origin of these muscles can be remembered because their nerve supply comes from the first arch. The mandibular branch of the trigeminal nerve provides the motor nerve supply to the muscles of the first arch. The mesenchyme of the first arch also contributes to the dermis of the face, so the sensory supply of this area is from all three branches of the trigeminal nerve (ophthalmic, maxillary, and mandibular).

The second pharyngeal arch, or hyoid arch cartilage, gives rise to the stapes, the styloid process of the temporal bone, the stylohyoid ligament, and, ventrally, the lesser horn and upper part of the body of the hyoid bone. The muscles derived from the second arch include the stapedius, stylohyoid, posterior belly of the digastric, and

auricular muscles and the muscles of facial expression. The facial nerve, derived from the second arch, supplies motor innervation to all of these muscles.

The third pharyngeal arch cartilage becomes the lower part of the body and the greater horn of the hyoid bone. The only known muscle to be derived from this arch is the stylopharyngeus. The glossopharyngeal nerve is derived from this arch and supplies the stylopharyngeus muscle. The third and fourth arch both contribute to the cartilage of the epiglottis.

The fifth arch completely regresses in humans, and the fourth and sixth arch cartilaginous components fuse to form the thyroid, cricoid, arytenoids, corniculate, and cuneiform cartilages of the larynx. The muscles of fourth arch origin include the cricothyroid, levator palatini, and pharyngeal constrictors. The nerve of the fourth arch, the superior laryngeal branch of the vagus nerve, innervates these muscles. The recurrent laryngeal branch of the vagus nerve, which is the nerve of the sixth arch, supplies the intrinsic muscles of the larynx.

Pharyngeal Pouches

The human embryo has five pharyngeal pouches that contribute to persistent structures in the head and neck. The endodermal lining of these pouches gives rise to a number of important structures in the head and neck. The first pharyngeal pouch makes contributions to the middle ear, providing epithelial lining to the middle ear and the eustachian tube. This lining also aids in the formation of the tympanic membrane. The second pharyngeal pouch epithelial lining proliferates and contributes to the formation of the palatine tonsil. As development progresses, the tonsil is infiltrated by lymphatic tissue, but part of the pouch will remain as the tonsillar fossa.

The third pharyngeal pouch develops a dorsal and ventral wing during the third week of development. The epithelium of the dorsal wing becomes the inferior parathyroid gland and the ventral part forms the thymus. As development progresses, both glands break their connection with the pharynx and migrate caudally, with the thymus pulling the inferior parathyroid gland along with it. The primary adult derivative of the fourth pharyngeal pouch is the superior parathyroid gland. The fifth pharyngeal pouch, often considered a part of the fourth, gives rise to the ultimobranchial body. This structure later is incorporated into the thyroid gland and gives rise to the parafollicular or C cells of the thyroid gland, which secrete calcitonin. Calcitonin plays an important role in the regulation of serum calcium levels.

Pharyngeal Grooves (Clefts)

At 5 weeks of age, the embryo contains four pharyngeal grooves. These grooves develop from invaginations of

ectoderm between the pharyngeal arches. Only one of these grooves contributes to a definitive adult structure. The first groove gives rise to the external auditory meatus. A portion of the epithelial lining of this structure contributes to the formation of the eardrum. The second, third, and fourth grooves make contributions to a cavity called the cervical sinus, but this ultimately disappears with growth of the embryo.

Pharyngeal Membranes

Pharyngeal membranes, consisting of ectoderm, intervening mesoderm, neural crest cells, and endoderm, are present between each pharyngeal arch. The only one with an adult derivative is the first one, which becomes the tympanic membrane. Pharyngeal membranes two, three, and four regress and form no definitive adult structure.

Clinically Applied Embryology

Errors in development during weeks 4 and 5, when the pharyngeal apparatus is forming, have described clinical correlations (Fig. 14–4). Persistence of the second pharyngeal pouch and groove can result in a pharyngeal fistula, usually identified along the anterior border of the sternocleidomastoid muscle. Treatment requires surgical excision of the entire tract. Failure of the second pharyngeal arch to overgrow the third and fourth arches results in remnants of the second, third, and fourth grooves

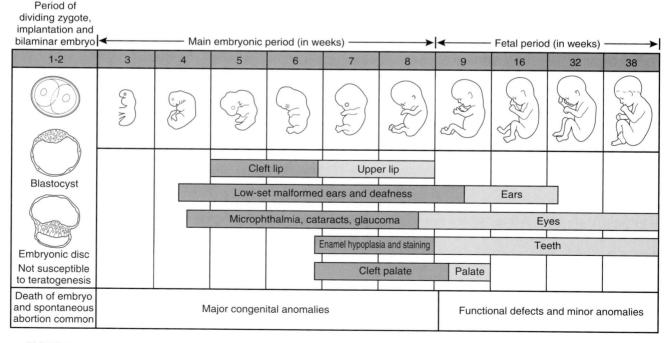

FIGURE 14–4 Correlation of timing of development and associated anomalies of the pharyngeal apparatus. (From Gordon ES: Collection of Images and Illustrations. Department of Plastic Surgery, Wake Forest University School of Medicine. January 2002. © 2001 WFUSM Plastic Surgery Collection.)

remaining in contact with the surface and can form a branchial fistula. These fistulas provide drainage for a lateral cervical cyst. These cysts are remnants of the cervical sinus and usually are located just below the angle of the jaw. Surgical treatment involves excision of the fistulous tract. This may require the injection of methylene blue into the tract to be sure it is excised in its entirety. An internal branchial fistula may occur if a rupture of the membrane between the second pharyngeal groove and pouch occurs sometime during development. As a result, the cervical sinus is connected to the lumen of the pharynx by a small patent canal.

The "first arch syndromes," including Treacher Collins syndrome and Pierre Robin syndrome, result from a lack of migration of neural crest cells into the first pharyngeal arch, or cell necrosis after migration, or decreased cell proliferation. Treacher Collins syndrome (mandibulofacial dysostosis) is caused by an autosomal dominant gene and consists of abnormalities of the external, middle, and inner ear; hypoplasia of the malar region and mandible; and defects of the lower eyelid. Treatment involves reconstruction of the ear and facial deformities. The facial reconstruction may require bone grafting and/or distraction osteogenesis of the underlying bony structures on the involved side of the face. Pierre Robin syndrome is characterized by a hypoplastic mandible, cleft palate, and eye and ear defects. Most of the time mandibular growth will catch up with the child; however, in severe cases early airway protection and jaw advancement/distraction may be needed.

Failure in the differentiation of the third and fourth pharyngeal pouches is responsible for DiGeorge syndrome. This syndrome is characterized by an absence of the thymus and parathyroids and a T-cell immunodeficiency. Other associated anomalies seen with this syndrome include facial (shortened philtrum, fish-mouth appearance, and nasal clefts) and cardiovascular anomalies. Treatment is individualized based on the clinical manifestations.

Failure of migration of the third and fourth pharyngeal pouches may result in ectopic parathyroid tissue. Variations in the number of parathyroid glands may result in too many, secondary to division of the parathyroid primordial, or too few, secondary to failure of the primordial to differentiate. This is clinically important in patients with hyperparathyroidism secondary to hyperplasia because treatment necessitates identification and removal of all involved glands. Failure to look for accessory glands can result in surgical failure.

The Tongue

The tongue is derived from parts of the first, second, third, and fourth pharyngeal arches. It arises in the ventral wall of the primitive oropharynx. At the same time as the pharyngeal apparatus is developing, two lateral lingual

swellings and one medial swelling originate from the first pharyngeal arch. The lateral swellings grow and ultimately fuse in the midline and provide the ectodermally derived mucosa of the anterior two thirds of the tongue. Laterally the epithelium proliferates into the underlying mesenchyme. The central cells of this lateral tissue then will degenerate and become the linguogingival groove. This groove frees the tongue from its attachment to the floor of the mouth except at the frenulum.

A second medial swelling, the copula, is formed by the mesoderm of the second, third, and fourth pharyngeal arches. A posterior part of the copula, the hypobranchial eminence, gives rise to the posterior one third of the tongue. This portion of the tongue is covered with mucosa derived from endoderm of the second, third, and fourth pharyngeal arches. The epiglottis, a third median swelling, is formed from the posterior part of the fourth arch.

Taste buds are induced by ectodermally and endodermally derived epithelial cells as well as by nerve cells derived from the chorda tympani, glossopharyngeal, and vagus nerves. Taste buds begin development around the 7th week of gestation but do not become functional until around the 15th week of development.

It is easy to remember that the mandibular branch of the trigeminal nerve provides the sensory innervation of the mucosa of the anterior two thirds of the tongue by recalling that this portion of the tongue is derived from the first pharyngeal arch. Although the third arch does not provide regular sensory innervation to the tongue, it does provide the special taste sensation to the anterior two thirds of the tongue via the chorda tympani branch of the facial nerve. The posterior one third of the tongue's sensory innervation is provided by the glossopharyngeal nerve, whose origin is the third pharyngeal arch. The very back of the tongue and epiglottis are innervated by the superior laryngeal nerve, thus indicating their primary site of origin as being the fourth pharyngeal arch. The motor supply to the intrinsic tongue muscles is the hypoglossal nerve, indicating their derivation from occipital somites.

The tonsils are derived from the endodermal lining of the second pharyngeal arch, which has invaded mesenchyme. Lymphoid tissue then becomes incorporated into these structures during the third through fifth months of development. The palatine tonsils reside at the site of the second pharyngeal arch. The pharyngeal and lingual tonsils develop in the posterior pharyngeal wall and tongue root, respectively.

Clinically Applied Embryology

Ankyloglossia, or being "tongue-tied," results from lack of degeneration of the tissue that connects the tongue to the floor of the mouth early in development. This anomaly occurs in 1 in 300 infants. The most common form of this abnormality is for the frenulum to extend to the tip of the tongue. Treatment involves releasing this persistent attachment if it fails to stretch with time.

Tongue cysts may occur secondary to remnants of the thyroglossal duct cyst. This can be problematic if they enlarge and produce dysphagia. Treatment involves surgical excision. Other abnormalities that are less common include underdevelopment (microglossia), overdevelopment (macroglossia), and failure of fusion (bifid or cleft tongue).

The Thyroid Gland

The thyroid gland makes its first appearance as an epithelial proliferation in the floor of the pharynx between the lateral and medial swellings of the developing tongue (tuberculum impar and copula, respectively). This site eventually will be the foramen cecum in the adult. As development progresses, the thyroid gland descends in front of the pharyngeal apparatus. It remains connected to its original location by the thyroglossal duct. Normally, this duct will eventually regress. The thyroid ultimately comes to rest in its final position in front of the trachea around week 7. By the time it reaches it final destination, it has become a structure with a central median isthmus and two lateral lobes. The thyroid gland becomes functional at the end of the third month of development.

Clinically Applied Embryology

If the thyroglossal duct does not obliterate, an external opening with a patent tract may be found anywhere along the pathway of migration from the foramen cecum to the adult location of the gland in the neck (Fig. 14–5). This cyst is almost always found in the midline of the neck. Approximately one half of such cysts are located around the hyoid bone. Surgical removal involves removing the entire tract, including a portion of the hyoid bone, to prevent recurrence. Methylene blue dye can be injected into the tract to better identify the wall and make sure it is completely excised. One must be judicious about this excision and be sure that this would not remove all of the thyroid gland in the patient. Thyroid visualization can be performed using preoperative nuclear scanning to localize all functioning thyroid tissue. Additionally, if the thyroid gland does not descend normally, there may be aberrant thyroid tissue along the pathway of descent. Again care must be taken prior to excising this ectopic thyroid tissue, to ensure that this is not the only thyroid tissue in the patient.

The Face

By the end of the fourth week of development, the facial prominences become distinguishable. These prominences are derived from mesenchyme containing neural crest

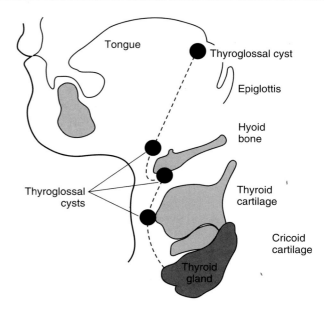

FIGURE 14–5 Pathway of descent of the thyroid. (From Gordon ES: Collection of Images and Illustrations. Department of Plastic Surgery, Wake Forest University School of Medicine. January 2002. © 2001 WFUSM Plastic Surgery Collection.)

cells and are formed by the time the first pair of pharyngeal arches appears. In relation to the stomodeum (ectodermal opening), the maxillary prominence is located laterally and the mandibular prominence is found in a caudal position. On the upper border of the stomodeum, the frontonasal prominence is identifiable. Local thickenings of surface ectoderm—the nasal placodes—develop on both sides of the frontonasal prominence. During the fifth week of development, the nasal placodes invaginate to form the nasal pits. After invagination, a ridge forms around the pit that has a distinct medial and lateral prominence. At first the nasal pit is separated from the underlying oral cavity by an oronasal membrane. This membrane eventually ruptures and the nasal cavity is connected with the oral cavity by foramina known as the primitive choanae. As the palate develops further, these structures become more definitive and reside at the junction of the nasal cavity and pharynx.

Over the next 2 weeks, maxillary prominence growth results in a compression of the medial nasal prominence toward the midline. Concomitantly, the separation between the maxillary prominence and the median nasal prominence is obliterated. The upper lip is formed as a result of the fusion of both the medial nasal prominence and the maxillary prominences. The lateral nasal prominence does not contribute to the upper lip, but rather contributes to the alae of the nose. Likewise, growth and fusion of the mandibular prominences in the midline give rise to the lower lip and jaw (Fig. 14–6).

Initially a furrow, the nasolacrimal groove, separates the maxillary and lateral nasal prominences. The ectoderm in the floor of this groove forms a solid cord that develops

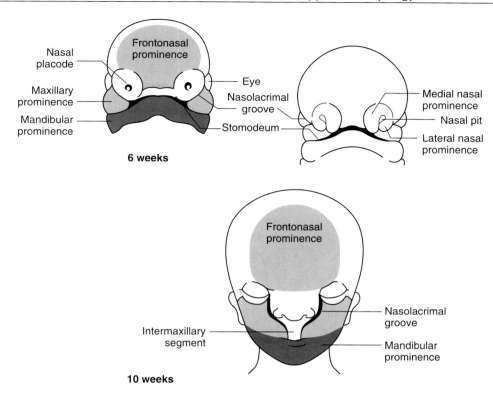

FIGURE 14–6 Facial prominences. (From Gordon ES: Collection of Images and Illustrations. Department of Plastic Surgery, Wake Forest University School of Medicine. January 2002. © 2001 WFUSM Plastic Surgery Collection.)

into a separate entity from the overlying ectoderm. This cord goes on to canalize and become the nasolacrimal duct. Once the cord has separated, the overlying maxillary prominence and the lateral nasal prominence fuse. This portion of the maxillary prominence develops into the upper cheek.

The frontonasal prominence contributes the forehead, bridge of the nose, and medial and lateral nasal prominences to the developing face. The external nose thus is formed by contributions from all five facial prominences (Table 14–3). The merged medial nasal prominences provide the crest and tip, and, as stated above, the lateral nasal prominences form the sides. Internally, the nasal pits have differentiated into nasal sacs. They are separated from the oral cavity by the oropharyngeal membrane. Once this connection is obliterated, the primordial choanae is formed. This eventually becomes the adult secondary choanae. At the same time, on the lateral nasal walls the superior, middle, and inferior conchae are developing. In the roof of nasal cavity, the ectoderm of the nasal placode forms the olfactory epithelium, which differentiates into neurons that contribute to the olfactory nerve.

The merger of the medial nasal prominences forms the intermaxillary segment. This is not simply a superficial merger, but includes all of the deeper layers as well. The intermaxillary segment is composed of a labial segment (philtrum of the lip), an upper jaw component containing four incisors, and the primary palate. Cranially, the intermaxillary segment is connected to the nasal septum, which is a derivative of the frontonasal prominence. The main part of the palate (secondary palate) is derived from outgrowths from the maxillary prominences. The palatine shelves appear in week 6 of development. They grow toward each other, fusing in the midline to form the secondary palate and fusing anteriorly with the primary palate. The incisive foramen is the landmark between the

Table 14–3	
Structures contributing to the formation of the face	
Prominence	**Structures Formed**
Frontonasal	Forehead, bridge of nose, medial and lateral nasal prominences
Maxillary	Cheeks, lateral portion of the upper lip
Medial nasal	Philtrum of the upper lip, crest and tip of the nose
Lateral nasal	Alae of the nose
Mandibular	Lower lip

primary and secondary palate. At the same time as palatal fusion is occurring, the nasal septum grows down to meet the palate.

Around the sixth week of development, the basal layer of the epithelial lining of the oral cavity forms a **C**-shaped structure. This structure contains the dental lamina, which gives rise to outbuddings that will become the ectodermal component of the teeth. Next, the deep surface of the bud will invaginate and produce the cap stage of tooth development. The cap is composed of an outer dental epithelium, an inner dental epithelium, and a central core of stellate reticulum. The dental papilla is formed from mesenchyme with neural crest cell origin. The developing tooth then undergoes a series of stages to become the deciduous tooth. The teeth therefore develop from an ectodermal and a mesodermal component. The buds for the permanent teeth are located on the lingual aspect of the deciduous teeth and are formed during the third month of development. The deciduous teeth erupt during the period from 6 to 24 months after birth. The permanent teeth buds remain dormant until approximately the sixth postnatal year and then begin to grow and push the deciduous teeth out of the way.

The mouth is formed from stomodeum (ectoderm) and the cephalic end of the foregut (endoderm), which provides a clue to the tissue of origin of most of the structures of the mouth. Ectoderm-derived structures include the oral part of the tongue, hard palate, sides of the mouth, lips, parotid gland and duct, Rathke's pouch, and tooth enamel. Endoderm-derived structures include the pharyngeal part of the tongue, floor of the mouth, palatoglossal fold, palatopharyngeal fold, soft palate, sublingual gland and ducts, and submandibular glands and ducts.

The three main salivary glands develop as an outgrowth from the stomodeal ectoderm during the sixth through eighth weeks of gestation. As previously mentioned, the parotid glands are derived from ectoderm, while the submandibular and sublingual glands are primarily derived from endoderm. The parotid glands are the first salivary glands to develop. They appear around 6 weeks of gestation and become functional around 18 weeks of gestation. The submandibular glands begin to develop at the end of the sixth week. Secretory activity begins around 16 weeks of gestation. The sublingual glands are the last to appear, at around 8 weeks of gestation. These glands develop as multiple buds and form ducts that open separately into the floor of the mouth.

Clinically Applied Embryology

There are multiple potential anomalous clinical outcomes from errors in this stage of development, including cleft lip, cleft palate, and choanal atresia (Fig. 14–7). Cleft lip and palate are thought to be multifactorial in etiology, with both genetic and environmental factors playing a role. The incidence of cleft lip and palate is approximately 1 in 1000, with males more commonly affected than females. Increased risk is associated with increasing maternal age and a positive family history.

Failure of fusion of the maxillary prominence with the medial nasal prominence can result in an incomplete or complete, unilateral or bilateral cleft lip. A cleft lip is the most common congenital malformation of the head and neck. If parents are not affected and have one child with a cleft lip, the risk for subsequent children is 4%. If they have two affected children, the risk for the next child

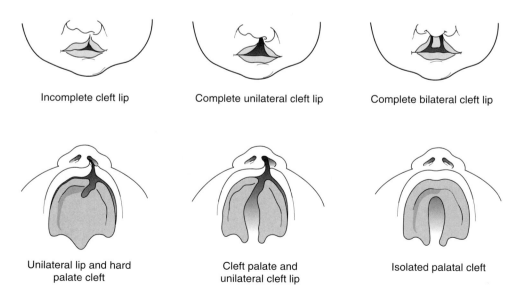

Incomplete cleft lip   Complete unilateral cleft lip   Complete bilateral cleft lip

Unilateral lip and hard palate cleft   Cleft palate and unilateral cleft lip   Isolated palatal cleft

FIGURE 14–7 Cleft lip and palate. (From Gordon ES: Collection of Images and Illustrations. Department of Plastic Surgery, Wake Forest University School of Medicine. January 2002. © 2001 WFUSM Plastic Surgery Collection.)

increases to 9%. If one of the parents is affected and they have an affected child, the risk for subsequent children increases to 17%. A cleft lip is surgically repaired when the child is around 3 months of age. The "rule of 10s" is the basis of the timing for repair; a weight of 10 pounds, 10 weeks of age, and a hemoglobin of at least 10 are required to minimize the operative risk. In patients with a very wide or a bilateral cleft lip, some institutions recommend early lip adhesion to help decrease the gap at the time of the definitive repair. The key components of a cleft lip repair are to increase the lip length on the cleft side and to restore the continuity of the orbicularis oris muscle.

Failure of the palatine shelves, which are derived from the maxillary prominence, to fuse will result in a cleft of the secondary palate with a cleft uvula. Isolated cleft palate is much less frequent than cleft lip and palate (1:2500) and is more common in females than males. It has been shown that the female palatal shelves fuse 1 week later than males, and this probably explains why an isolated cleft palate is more common in females. The risk for future children of a nonaffected parent is about 2%; this risk increases to 7% if the parent is affected. Treatment for a cleft palate involves fixing both the primary and secondary palate if involved. Ideally, the palatal cleft is repaired before 1 year of age to optimize long-term speech results. The key components of this procedure include the lengthening of the palate and the restoration of the connection of the levator palatini muscles in the midline.

Incomplete merging of the medial nasal prominences in the midline will result in a median or a Tessier type 0 cleft. This usually is accompanied by deep right and left grooves in the nose. Failure of the maxillary prominence to merge with the lateral nasal prominence will result in an oblique cleft (Tessier type 3, 4, 5, or 6) (Fig. 14–8). It is important to note that this is a cleft that occurs in both the

soft and underlying bony structures. The soft tissue cleft is repaired early on, while the bony cleft is repaired when the child gets a little older. Both problems must be addressed to achieve a good, long-lasting result. A type 7 Tessier cleft is a result of the failure of the maxillary and mandibular prominences to merge. If this occurs bilaterally, this is known as macrostomia. Macrostomia can be surgically repaired at an early age and involves closure of this soft tissue cleft and reapproximation of the orbicularis oris muscle at the oral commissure.

Choanal atresia is the failure of the oronasal membrane to rupture, resulting in an obstruction between the nasal and pharyngeal cavities. Treatment necessitates the re-creation of this connection, and adequate long-term patency is often difficult to achieve. A field defect affecting the frontonasal, medial, and lateral nasal prominence is most likely responsible for the development of proboscis lateralis and choanal atresia. A proboscis is a rudimentary tube-like structure composed of the deficient soft tissues of the nose that usually protrudes out from the level of the medial canthus (Fig. 14-9). The reported incidence is 0.06%, and the defect is even less frequent in live births. On a cellular level, this abnormality is likely to be secondary to an error in neural crest cell migration. Specifically, it has been postulated that imperfect mesodermal proliferation occurs during the formation of the frontonasal and maxillary process after the olfactory pits have been formed and that epidermal breakdown occurs, leaving the lateral nasal process sequestered as a tube in the frontonasal region. This epidermal breakdown causes failure of nasolacrimal duct formation. Treatment involves reconstructing the involved side of the nose both internally and externally. Additionally, the nasolacrimal system must be reconstructed. A staged surgical approach is used to treat this entity. If the nasal placodes do not form at all,

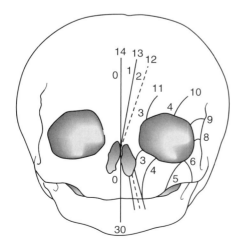
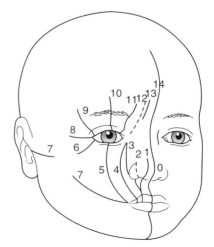

FIGURE 14–8 Tessier's cleft classification. (From Gordon ES: Collection of Images and Illustrations. Department of Plastic Surgery, Wake Forest University School of Medicine. January 2002. © 2001 WFUSM Plastic Surgery Collection.)

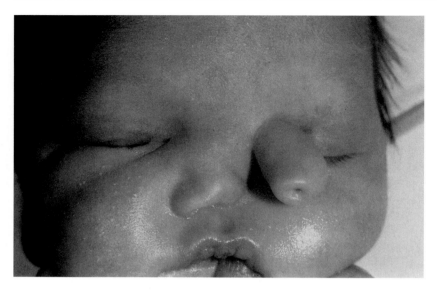

FIGURE 14–9 Child with untreated proboscis lateralis.

the nose will not develop. A single nasal placode will result in only one nostril. A bifid nose is a result of the medial nasal prominences not completely merging.

Failure of the mandibular prominences to merge completely results in a lower lip or jaw cleft (Tessier type 30 cleft). The lip can be repaired in the first few months of life. The bony defect is stabilized and then reconstructed using bone grafts when the child is a little older. Congenital microstomia is secondary to excessive merging of the mesenchymal masses of the maxillary and mandibular prominences of the first pharyngeal arch.

The Eye

The eye develops from three primordia. The retina is formed from an outgrowth of the brain. The skin ectoderm grows inward to form the lens. Local mesoderm is recruited to provide the fibrous and vascular coats.

The developing eye is first seen at around 3 weeks' gestation (day 22) as a groove on each side of the invaginating forebrain. Once the neural tube closes, these grooves form outpockets of the forebrain known as optic vesicles. The only connection with the forebrain from which they came is via the optic stalks. Each optic vesicle then invaginates and forms a double-layered optic cup still connected by an optic stalk. This double-layered cup is made up of an inner neural layer and an outer pigmented layer.

The optic cup gives rise to the retina. The outer layer of epithelium of the optic cup is invaded by pigment, which gives rise to the pigmented layer of the adult retina. The inner epithelial layer forms the neural portion of the retina, becoming photoreceptors, bipolar neurons, and ganglionic neurons. The central processes of the ganglionic neurons form the nerve fiber layer of the retina. These processes coalesce and enter the inner wall of the

optic fissure, forming the optic nerve. The fissure provides an exit for the axons of the ganglionic cells.

At the same time as the retina is developing, the optic vesicles stimulate thickening of the overlying ectoderm to form the lens placode. The placode then invaginates to form lens pits. The edges of the lens then come together, creating a spherical vesicle. The overlying ectoderm then reconnects and mesoderm migrates between it and the underlying lens. At the time of lens recession, the optic cup becomes concave to allow the lens to sit in the optic cup.

Linear grooves develop at this time on the ventral surface of the optic cup and along the optic stalk. These fissures (grooves) contain vascular mesenchyme that is responsible for the production of the hyaloid blood vessel development. Vascular mesenchyme infiltrates the optic fissure and migrates along the optic cup. Formation of this fissure thus allows the hyaloid artery to reach the inner chamber of the eye. The hyaloid vessels enter the fissure and traverse the vitreous humor to spread out on the lens. As the lens matures, the distal part of the hyaloid vessels regresses but the proximal part persists as the central retinal artery and vein.

Within the cup itself, the interstices of the mesenchyme become filled with gelatinous vitreous humor. The primary vitreous humor is derived from mesenchymal cells of neural crest origin. The primary vitreous humor does not increase but is surrounded by a gelatinous secondary vitreous humor of uncertain origin. After the lens vesicle is complete, a space (anterior chamber) develops in the mesoderm between the lens and the surface ectoderm (cornea). The cornea develops from surface ectoderm, mesoderm, and neural crest cells and lies anterior to the anterior chamber of the eye. The developing lens induces its formation.

A piece of ectoderm extends in front of the lens from the margin of the retina to form the iris. In the adult, the pigment-containing external layer and the unpigmented internal layer of the optic cup, as well as a layer of vascular connective tissue, forms the iris. Prior to birth, mesoderm stretches across the front of the lens, forming the papillary membrane. The portion of this mesoderm, which is not supported by ectoderm, breaks down to define the pupil structure. The area between the iris and the lens is the posterior chamber of the eye. The sphincter and dilator muscles develop at the free margin of the iris. These muscles are thought to be among the few that originate from neuroectoderm of the optic cup.

The mesoderm also forms a fibrous shell around the eye by the fifth week of gestation. This differentiates into an inner layer that forms the highly vascularized pigmented layer (the choroids) and an outer layer that becomes the sclera and gives rise to the dural sheath of the optic nerve. Vascular mesoderm forms the choroid coat of the eye between the sclera and retina. The ciliary muscle originates from mesoderm near the base of the iris. The ciliary body also develops from the pigmented and nonpigmented layers of the optic cup. It is an extension of the choroids. The ciliary body contains the processes that produce aqueous humor that circulates through the posterior and anterior chambers of the eye. It drains the venous circulation via the trabecular meshwork and the canal of Schlemm. The ciliary body also gives rise to the fibers that suspend the lens.

The extraocular muscles differentiate outside the sclera and then become attached. These muscles are thought to arise from mesoderm situated near the orbit. The eyelids are mesodermal folds with ectodermal lining that grow to meet each other anterior to the cornea during the sixth week of development. The eyelids adhere to each other by the beginning of the 10th week and remain adherent until around the 26th week of gestation. Under the developing eyelid is a conjunctival sac, which divides into two layers as the eyelids open. The eyelashes are derived from surface ectoderm and the tarsal plates come from mesenchyme in the eyelid. The orbicularis oculi muscle comes from the second pharyngeal pouch, and thus a branch of the facial nerve innervates it.

In summary, the origins of the adult components of the eye are derived from neuroectoderm (optic cup and optic stalk), surface ectoderm, and mesoderm. The optic cup gives rise to the retina, iris epithelium, dilator and sphincter muscles, and ciliary body epithelium. The optic stalk gives rise to the optic nerve, optic chiasm, and optic tract. The surface ectoderm gives rise to the lens and the anterior corneal epithelium. The mesoderm gives rise to the sclera, choroids, stroma of the iris, stoma of the ciliary body, ciliary muscle, substantia propria of the cornea, corneal endothelium, vitreous body, central retinal artery and vein, and extraocular muscles (Fig. 14–10).

Clinically Applied Embryology

The site of abnormal development dictates clinical anomalies. Failure of the inner and outer layers of the optic cup to fuse during the fetal period to form the retina and obliterate the intraretinal space results in congenital detachment of the retina. A defective closure of the optic fissure, characterized by a localized gap in the retina, results in a coloboma of the retina and/or iris and occurs during the sixth week of gestation. Abnormal elevation of intraocular pressure in newborns (congenital glaucoma) occurs secondary to an abnormal development of the

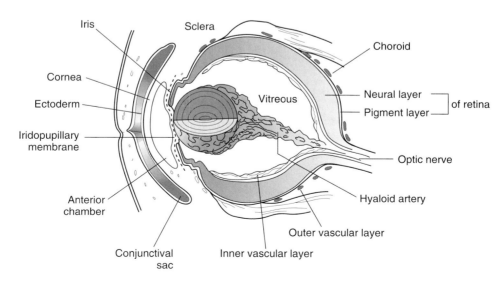

FIGURE 14–10 Fetal eye. (From Gordon ES: Collection of Images and Illustrations. Department of Plastic Surgery, Wake Forest University School of Medicine. January 2002. © 2001 WFUSM Plastic Surgery Collection.)

drainage mechanism of the aqueous humor during the fetal period. The etiology can be either genetic or environmental. A retinocele is a result of the failure of choroid fissure closure.

Failure of development of or injury to the levator palpebrae superioris muscle, or abnormal development of the superior division of the oculomotor nerve, may result in congenital ptosis (drooping) of the eyelid. Colobomas, or notching of the eyelid, are a result of local developmental disturbances in the formation of the eyelid. Failure of the optic vesicle to form is manifested by anophthalmia, or congenital absence of an eye. This can be a difficult problem because, without the eye as a stimulus for growth, the involved side of the face will not develop properly. Treatment involves serial tissue expansion and prosthetic replacement to both reconstruct the eye and maintain normal facial growth. Cyclopia (a single eye) is a direct result of a failure of the median cerebral structures to develop.

The Ear

The ear can be divided into three parts to understand its development more easily. A large part of the development of the middle ear was described in the discussion of the pharyngeal apparatus above and is reviewed here.

Inner Ear Development

Early in the fourth week of development, the otic placode appears as a surface ectodermal thickening on the caudal part of the hindbrain (myelencephalon). This thickening is induced by the notochord and paraxial mesoderm. The otic placode then invaginates into the underlying mesenchyme, and in doing so forms an otic pit. The edges of the otic pit come together to form the otic vesicle, which later will become the membranous labyrinth. The otic vesicle goes on to lose its ectodermal connection and develops an outgrowth that elongates and becomes the endolymphatic duct and sac. The otic vesicle now has two distinct components. The utricular part will give rise to the endolymphatic duct, utricle, and semicircular duct. The saccular part will give rise to the saccule and cochlear duct, where the organ of Corti is located.

The membranous labyrinth consists of all the structures derived from the otic vesicle. It is surrounded by mesoderm that becomes cartilaginous and then ossifies to become the bony labyrinth of the temporal bone. The mesoderm closest to the membranous labyrinth degenerates, forming the perilymphatic space containing the perilymph. The membranous labyrinth is suspended within the bony labyrinth by perilymph. The perilymph communicates with the subarachnoid space via the perilymphatic duct.

Middle Ear Development

The tympanic membrane develops from the first pharyngeal membrane. The proximal part forms the auditory tube and the distal part expands and becomes the tympanic cavity. This cavity gradually envelops the auditory ossicles. The ossicles are derived from the first pharyngeal arch (malleus and incus) and second pharyngeal arch (stapes). The trigeminal and facial nerves (respectively) are responsible for the innervation of the muscles controlling these ossicles.

External Ear Development

The external auditory meatus develops from the first pharyngeal groove. It becomes filled with ectodermal cells that form a temporary plug that disappears before birth. This meatus is fairly short at birth and does not reach adult length until around 9 years of age. The precursor of the tympanic membrane is the first pharyngeal membrane, as mentioned above. As development proceeds, mesenchyme grows between the two parts of the pharyngeal membrane and differentiates into the collagenic fibers of the tympanic membrane. The external covering of the tympanic membrane is derived from surface ectoderm, but the internal lining is derived from endoderm of the tubotympanic recess. As a result, the tympanic membrane receives contributions from all three germ cell layers.

The auricle (pinna) develops from six auricular hillocks that surround the first pharyngeal groove. The auricle begins to develop at the base of the neck, and, as the mandible develops, it moves to the adult position at the side of the head. The auricle continues to grow through puberty. The innervation of the ear is determined by its embryonic origin and includes the trigeminal, facial, glossopharyngeal, vagus, and second and third cervical nerves.

In summary, the adult derivatives of the otic vesicle are the components of the inner ear, including the utricle, semicircular ducts, vestibular ganglion, endolymphatic duct and sac, saccule, cochlear duct, organ of Corti, and spiral ganglion. The middle ear is derived primarily from pharyngeal arches one and two and the first pharyngeal pouch and membrane. The derivatives include the malleus, incus, tensor tympani, stapes, stapedius, auditory tube, tympanic membrane, and middle ear cavity. The external ear, which includes the auricle and external auditory meatus, is derived from the six auricular hillocks and the first pharyngeal groove (Fig. 14–11).

Clinically Applied Embryology

Clinical manifestations are dependent on site of aberrancy in ear development. Exposure of the organ of Corti to the

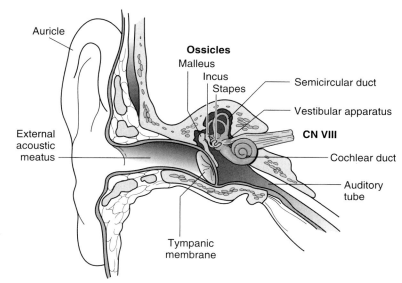

FIGURE 14–11 Anatomic divisions of the ear. (From Gordon ES: Collection of Images and Illustrations. Department of Plastic Surgery, Wake Forest University School of Medicine. January 2002. © 2001 WFUSM Plastic Surgery Collection.)

rubella virus during weeks 7 and 8 of development can result in congenital deafness. Failure of the meatal plug to canalize can result in conduction deafness and atresia of the external auditory meatus. This often is associated with first arch syndrome. Failure of inward expansion of the first pharyngeal groove and failure of the meatal plug to disappear may result in absence of the external auditory meatus entirely. This is a very rare entity. A congenital cholesteatoma is a result of an epidermoid thickening of the endodermal lining cells.

The external ear may develop accessory auricular hillocks that result in auricular appendages, or ear tags. Suppressed development of the auricular hillocks may result in microtia. This is often an indicator of associated internal anomalies such as middle ear anomalies. Depending on the amount of tissue that is absent, the ear will need to be reconstructed using autologous tissue. In children, this reconstruction is usually approached in two to three stages. Surgery is not started until the child is 6 to 7 years of age. This delay in surgical intervention is necessary to ensure adequate rib cartilage for the reconstruction and for the normal opposite ear, to which the reconstructed ear will be matched, to attain 90% of its final adult size. In the first stage, the cartilage framework is designed and put in proper position in the ear skin pocket. The next stages involve better defining the lobule and tragus as well as lifting the cartilage framework from the skull. Prosthetic reconstructions are used primarily for adult reconstructions after trauma or cancer. If there are inner ear problems as well, the external ear reconstruction should be completed prior to any surgical intervention for the inner ear.

Summary

A thorough understanding of the embryology of the head and neck gives a better appreciation of the mechanisms behind anomalies in this region. The next step to which we must now devote our attention is the prevention or correction of these errors in embryologic development. Genetically derived tools that are now being developed will enable us to do this in the future.

Bibliography

Albers GD: Branchial anomalies. JAMA 1963;183:399.

Anson BJ, Hanson JS, Richany SF: Early embryology of the auditory ossicles and associated structures in relation to certain anomalies observed clinically. Ann Otol 1960;69:427.

Argenta LC, David LR, Wilson JA, et al: An increase in infant cranial deformity with supine sleeping position. J Craniofac Surg 1996;1:5.

Bardi AR: Sexual differences in closure of the human palatal shelves. Cleft Palate J 1969;6:1.

Binns JH: Congenital tubular nostril (proboscis lateralis). Br J Plast Surg 1969;22:265.

Bottero L, LaJeunie E, Arnaud E, et al: Functional outcome after surgery for trigoncephaly. Plast Reconstr Surg 1998;102:952.

Carlson BM: Human Embryology and Developmental Biology. St. Louis: CV Mosby, 1994.

Diewert VM, Wang KY: Recent advances in primary palate and midface morphogenesis research. Crit Rev Oral Biol Med 1992;4:111.

Dudek R, Fix J: Embryology (2nd ed). Philadelphia: Lippincott Williams & Wilkins, 1998:149.

Dudek RW: High-Yield Embryology. Baltimore: Williams & Wilkins, 1996:30.

Fini ME, Strissel KJ, West-Mays JA: Perspectives on eye development. Dev Genet 1997;20:175.

Fraser FC: Genetics and congenital malformations. In Steinberg AG (ed): Progress in Medical Genetics. New York: Grune & Stratton, 1961:38.

Gorlin RJ, Cervenka J, Pruzansky S: Facial clefting and its syndromes. Birth Defects 1971;8:3.

Gorlin RJ, Cohen MM Jr, Levin LS: Syndromes of the Head and Neck (3rd ed). New York: Oxford University Press, 1990.

Hinrichsen K: The early development of morphology and patterns of the face in the human embryo. Adv Anat Embryol Cell Biol 1985;98:1.

Johnson MC, Bronsky PT: Prenatal craniofacial development: new insights on normal and abnormal mechanisms. Crit Rev Oral Biol Med 1995;6:368.

Johnston MC, Sulik KK: Embryology of the head and neck. In Serafin D, Georgiade NG (eds): Pediatric Plastic Surgery. St. Louis: CV Mosby, 1984:2451.

Johnston MC, Sulik KK: The neural crest. In Shields ED, Burzynsky NJ, Melnick M (eds): Craniofacial Dysmorphology: Genetics, Etiology, Diagnosis and Treatment. Littleton, MA: John Wright, PSG, 1983.

Jones KL: Smith's Recognizable Patterns of Human Malformation (5th ed). Philadelphia: WB Saunders, 1997.

Kapp-Simon KA, Figueroa A, Jocher CA, et al: Longitudinal assessment of mental development in infants with nonsyndromic craniosynostosis with and without cranial release and reconstruction. Plast Reconstr Surg 1993;92:831.

Karmody CS, Annino DJ Jr: Embryology and anomalies of the external ear. Facial Plast Surg 1995;11:251.

Khoo BC: The proboscis lateralis—a 14 year follow-up. Plast Reconstr Surg 1985;75:569.

Kjaer I, Keeling JW, Fischer-Hansen B: The Prenatal Human Cranium—Normal and Pathologic Development. Copenhagen: Munksgaard, 1999:65.

Kruchinskii GV: Classification of the syndromes of branchial arches 1 and 2. Acta Chir Plast 1990;32:178.

Mandarim-de-Lacerda CA, Alves MU: Growth of the cranial bones in human fetuses (2nd and 3rd trimesters). Surg Radiol Anat 1992;14:125.

Mann IC: Developmental Abnormalities of the Eye. Philadelphia: JB Lippincott, 1957.

Mann IC: The Development of the Human Eye (3rd ed; British Medical Association). New York: Grune & Stratton, 1974.

Marchac D, Renier D: Craniofacial Surgery for Craniosynostosis. Boston: Little, Brown, 1981.

Marchac D, Renier D, Broumand S: Timing of treatment for craniosynostosis and faciocraniosynostosis: a 20 year experience. Br J Plast Surg 1994;47:211.

Marshall SF, Becker WF: Thyroglossal cysts and sinuses. Ann Surg 1949;129:642

Martins AG: Lateral cervical sinus and preauricular sinuses. Br Med J 1961;5:255

Mathijssen IM, van Splunder J, Vermeij-Keer C, et al: Tracing craniosynostosis to its developmental stage through bone center displacement. J Craniofac Genet Dev Biol 1999;19:57.

Moore KL, Persaud TVN: The Developing Human: Clinically Oriented Embryology (6th ed). Philadelphia: WB Saunders, 1998.

Noden DM: Interactions and fates of avian craniofacial mesenchyme. Development 1998;103:121.

Noden DM, Van de Water TR: The developing ear: tissue origins and interactions. In Ruben RJ, van de Water TR (eds): The Biology of Change in Otolaryngology. Amsterdam: Elsevier/North Holland, 1986:15.

Patten BM: The normal development of the facial region. In Pruzansky S (ed): Congenital Anomalies of the Face and Associated Structures. Springfield, IL: Charles C Thomas, 1961:11.

Pearson AA, Jacobson AD: The Development of the Ear. Rochester, MN: American Academy of Ophthalmology and Otolaryngology, 1967.

Poswillo D: The pathogenesis of the first and second branchial arch syndrome. Oral Surg 1973;35:302.

Renier D, Marchac D: Craniofacial surgery for craniosynostosis: functional and morphological results. Ann Acad Med Singapore 1988;17:415.

Renier D, Sainte-Rose C, Marchac D, et al: Intracranial pressure in craniosynostosis. J Neurosurg 1982;57:370.

Scheuerle AE, Good RA, Habal MB: Involvement of the thymus and cellular immune system in craniofacial malformation syndromes. J Craniofac Surg 1990;1:88.

Shepard TH: Development of the thyroid gland. In Gardner LI (ed): Endocrine and Genetic Diseases of Childhood and Adolescence (2nd ed). Philadelphia: WB Saunders, 1975.

Tessier P: Anatomical classification of facial, craniofacial and latero-facial clefts. J Maxillofac Surg 1976;4:69.

Turk AE, McCarthy JG, Thorne CH, et al: The "Back to Sleep Campaign" and deformational plagiocephaly: is there cause for concern? J Craniofac Surg 1996;1:12.

Virtanen R, Korhonen T, Fagerholm J, et al: Neurocognitive sequelae of scaphocephaly. Pediatrics 1999;103:791.

Wright KW: Embryology and eye development. In Wright KW (ed): Textbook of Ophthalmology. Baltimore, Williams & Wilkins, 1997:57.

CHAPTER 15

Applied Cardiac Embryology

Michael H. Hines, M.D.

Development of the normal heart involves a series of complicated twists, turns, migrations, and dissolutions taking it from a simple tube to an intricate four-chambered pump. All this begins in about the third week of gestation as the fetus outgrows the ability to gain needed nutrition by diffusion alone, and it is essentially complete by the eighth week, except for the closures of the foramen ovale and ductus arteriosus, which normally occur soon after birth. The sequence of this embryology has been deduced over time from the examination of two-dimensional sections of embryos, and still involves several areas of controversy, including differences in nomenclature. However, the available information is more than sufficient for a clinician to obtain a clear understanding of the basic elements of the heart's formation and their relation to both the normal and the congenitally malformed heart. Because significant errors very early in gestation lead to fetal demise, this chapter concentrates on the later stages in the development of the cardiovascular system and describes the basic formation of the atria, ventricles, valves, and systemic and pulmonary venous return, as well as the arch and great vessels. It explains the relationship of the normal and abnormal development of these elements, and how interruptions or errors in these steps lead to the most commonly treated congenital cardiac defects.

Formation of the Cardiac Tube

Formation of the primitive heart tube occurs early in fetal development, with the tube lying along the ventral surface of the embryo. Four areas of constriction divide the tube into five general regions (Fig. 15–1A). Beginning at the venous pole at the inferior end of the tube, the sinus venosus accepts blood from the right and left sinus horns. Beyond the first constriction (the sinoatrial junction), the blood enters the primitive atrium. From here the blood traverses the next constriction, the atrioventricular (AV) canal, to enter the next two chambers that will together form the ventricles. These two chambers have been described most simply as the inlet and outlet portions of the developing ventricle, with the constriction between them called the inlet-outlet junction. A less descriptive nomenclature has labeled the two portions the ventricle and the bulbus cordis, separated by the bulboventricular sulcus. Beyond the two ventricular components lie the ventriculoarterial junction and the arterial segment or aortic roots. Bending of the primitive heart tube to about 90 degrees occurs at the AV canal, placing the venous and atrial components posteriorly. The ventricular portion bends to about 180 degrees at the inlet-outlet junction, placing the arterial tube or truncus in front of the AV canal. These two bends together leave the forming heart in its eventual "cardiac" position (Fig. 15–1B). The next few weeks of development involve septation of this single tube into two separate circulations. Anomalies at this level of formation involve major anomalies that frequently give rise to complex combinations of defects including atrioventricular discordance, valve and chamber underdevelopment or complete artesias, and multiple persistent septal defects. These more complex defects are beyond the scope of this chapter.

Systemic Venous Return

The embryologic sinus venosus is formed by the confluence of two superior cardinal veins (from the embryo), two inferior vitelline veins (from the yolk sac), and two inferior and more lateral umbilical veins (from the placenta)

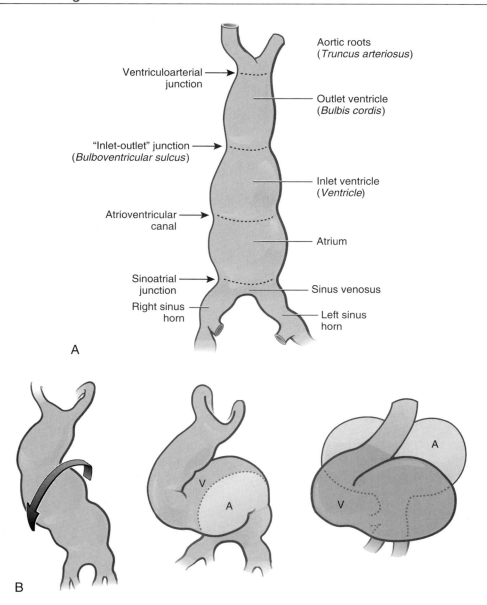

Ventriculoarterial junction

Aortic roots (*Truncus arteriosus*)

Outlet ventricle (*Bulbis cordis*)

"Inlet-outlet" junction (*Bulboventricular sulcus*)

Inlet ventricle (*Ventricle*)

Atrioventricular canal

Atrium

Sinoatrial junction

Sinus venosus

Right sinus horn

Left sinus horn

A

B

FIGURE 15–1 A, Primitive heart tube. **B,** Folding of heart tube.

(Fig. 15–2A). Formation of collateral connections superiorly and inferiorly allows direction of all systemic venous blood to the right side of the heart with regression of the left-sided structures. The superior connection will become the left brachiocephalic or innominate vein, directing left cranial and arm drainage to the right side. Inferiorly, the ductus venosus directs blood from the left umbilical vein into the right vitelline vein at the level of the liver. Both distal vitelline veins regress along with the left proximal vitelline vein. Therefore, the only remaining structures are right sided, and there is regression of the left horn of the sinus venosus, which remains to become the coronary sinus. The site of the previous left cardinal vein is marked by the ligament of Marshall near the origin of the coronary sinus, dividing the left atrial appendage of the primitive atrium from the posterior new left atrium formed by the pulmonary venous

component as described below. The remaining veins develop from the right cardinal vein (superior vena cava) and the right vitelline vein (inferior vena cava) (Fig. 15–2B).

Abnormal persistence of the left cardinal vein leads to a persistent left superior vena cava, and may be seen with or without a superior connection to the right-sided vena cava. Physiologically this creates no problem because the blood drains into the coronary sinus, emptying into the right atrium. Rarely, this may be associated with an unroofed coronary sinus, wherein the venous blood then drains directly into the left atrium, leading to a significant right-to-left shunt and mild to moderate cyanosis. Very rarely, there is persistence of the left vena cava with abnormal regression of the right vena cava, leaving a single left-sided vena cava draining into a very large coronary sinus. Abnormal regression of the right vitelline vein

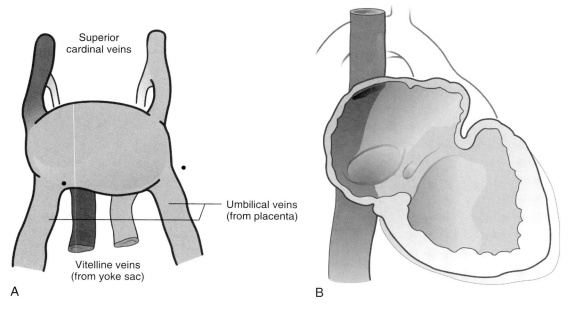

A

B

FIGURE 15–2 A, Embryonic systemic veins. **B,** Contribution of embryonic veins to systemic venous anatomy.

leads to an interrupted inferior vena cava. In this anomaly, the hepatic veins drain directly into the right atrium, but inferior truncal venous return ascends on the left, eventually draining into the hemiazygous system into the right atrium, or occasionally on the right via the azygous system. Rarely both vitelline veins persist, leading to duplicated inferior venae cavae. These venous anomalies are usually seen in association with various heterotaxy syndromes and other cardiac malformations. Very rarely, systemic veins drain into the left atrium; however, this is essentially a defect of atrial septation rather than a defect in vein formation.

Most of these anomalies are surgically significant with respect to proper cannulation for cardiopulmonary bypass, and in single-ventricle palliation such as cavoatrial anastomoses (bidirectional Glenn shunts) and Fontan procedures. At times abnormal connections also must be corrected as part of atrial septation procedures. As with most cardiac surgery, preoperative knowledge of the anatomy is helpful, if not essential.

Pulmonary Venous Return

The formation of the venous drainage of the lungs parallels the development of the lung itself as the trachea and lung buds form off the foregut. During this time, the primary pulmonary vein arises from the left posterior wall of the primitive atrium, eventually making contact with the venous plexus forming in the developing lung buds, and at the same time losing its connection with the splanchnic plexus of veins. The left atrium gradually absorbs the primary pulmonary vein and the first-level branches of the

newly formed pulmonary veins, thereby increasing the size of the new left atrium. The posterior wall of the left atrium therefore is formed primarily by the pulmonary vein contribution, with little residual from the primitive atrial portion of the heart tube, mainly the AV canal portion and the left atrial appendage.

Failure of the proper connection of the primary pulmonary vein to the pulmonary venous drainage leads to one of the many forms of total anomalous pulmonary venous connection (TAPVC) (Fig. 15–3). When the pulmonary venous confluence does not connect with the left atrium, there must be persistent connections to the systemic venous drainage or there will be fetal demise. The pulmonary confluence may drain into the left cardinal vein (persistent left vena cava) or directly into the right superior vena cava (TAPVC type I). It may enter into the coronary sinus or directly into the right atrium (TAPVC type II). It also may enter below the diaphragm into the left vitelline vein, entering the heart through the ductus venosus and the inferior vena cava (TAPVC type III). Rarely there is mixed drainage with right- and left-sided pulmonary venous drainage entering the systemic veins separately, without a central confluence. Most of the type III and some of the type I TAPVCs have obstruction to drainage leading to significant changes in the pulmonary vascular bed and pulmonary hypertension.

Another congenital anomaly is seen when the primary pulmonary vein connects properly with the posterior atrium, but there is incomplete absorption of the tissue between them, leading to a condition known as cor triatriatum. In this malformation, the pulmonary confluence is connected to the posterior left atrium, but there is a

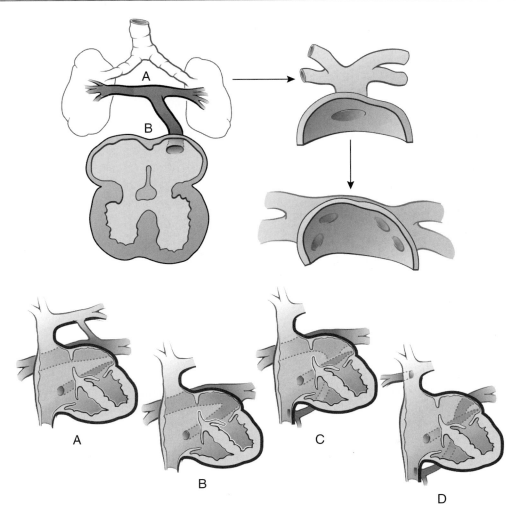

FIGURE 15–3 Formation of pulmonary venous confluence (**A**) and common pulmonary vein (**B**). Classification of TAPVC types I, II, III, and IV: supracardiac, intracardiac, infracardiac, and mixed. (Modified from Hines M, Hammon J: Anatomy of total anomalous pulmonary venous connection. *In* Cox J [ed]: Operative Techniques in Thoracic and Cardiovascular Surgery, Vol 6, No 1: Total Anomalous Pulmonary Veins. Philadelphia: WB Saunders, 2001:3–4, with permission.)

membrane-like structure between it and the left atrium proper, leading to a "three-atrium" heart. There is frequently a very small communication into the left atrium, leading to obstruction of flow and commonly some degree of pulmonary hypertension. Surgical correction involves removal of the membrane.

Atrial Septation

Reorganization of the venous channels allows direction of systemic venous blood toward the right side of the primitive atrium, and pulmonary venous flow to the left side. Simultaneously, many changes occur within the atrium to septate it into two chambers. At the junction of the primitive atrium and inlet portion of the ventricle, or the AV canal, two opposing masses of mesenchymal tissue called endocardial cushions grow toward each other,

working to septate the canal itself. These endocardial cushions will divide the inferior portion of the atrial chambers, as well as the inlet portion of the ventricles. Simultaneously, the AV valves form from the walls of the inlet portions of the ventricle and fusion of the endocardial cushions separates the common AV valve into two tricuspid valves. The rightward valve remains tricuspid, but the two adjacent leaflets of the leftward valve fuse to form a single leaflet, which will become the anterior leaflet of the bicuspid or mitral valve (Fig. 15–4).

Failure of proper fusion of these tissues leads to a spectrum of endocardial cushion defects, also known as AV canal defects. At the more minor end of the spectrum is a primum atrial septal defect (ASD). In this defect, only the inferior atrial wall component of the endocardial cushions has failed to fuse, leaving a communication between the left and right atria at the base of the atrial

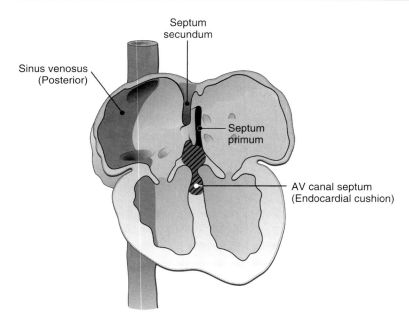

Septum
secundum

Sinus venosus
(Posterior)

Septum
primum

AV canal septum
(Endocardial cushion)

FIGURE 15–4 Atrial septation.

septum immediately over the AV valves. In almost all cases, although there are two distinct AV valves with separated fibrous rings or annuli, the two embryologic contributions to the anterior leaflet fail to fuse, leaving a central cleft within that leaflet. In rare circumstances a "cleft mitral valve" can be seen without the presence of an atrial communication. In some cases, the atrial septation is completed normally along with AV valve division; however, the inlet ventricular portions of the endocardial cushions fail to fuse, creating an "inlet" ventricular septal defect (VSD).

With increasing failure of fusion, a "transitional AV canal" defect is seen involving a single AV valve with a primum ASD, but with completed septation of the inlet ventricular septum. With total failure of the endocardial cushion masses to fuse, a complete AV canal defect or AV septal defect is created. There is a single AV valve with varying sizes of both the ASD and VSD. In the most severe forms of this defect, flow through an abnormally formed AV valve is disproportionate, with more flow directed into either the left or the right ventricle, leading to a hypoplastic ventricle on one side.

With other malformations of the valves, chordal structures may actually cross over from one side of the VSD to the opposite AV valve leaflets. In these more severe cases with an "unbalanced" AV canal, or with "straddling" AV valve leaflets, surgical correction with septation and valve reconstruction may not be possible. In severe forms of endocardial cushion malformation, either the left- or the right-sided AV valve may fail to form completely, leading to varying degrees of tricuspid or mitral stenosis or atresia. With underdevelopment of the AV valves, poor flow into the inlet ventricles leads to underdevelopment and

ventricular hypoplasia, seen clinically in syndromes such as tricuspid atresia and hypoplastic left heart syndrome.

While the endocardial cushions are fusing to divide the AV canal, an ingrowth appears on the internal superior wall of the primitive atrium, leftward of the sinus venosus contribution and rightward of the primary pulmonary vein outgrowth externally. This is the septum primum, which heads inferiorly toward the endocardial cushion tissue. The opening between the septum primum and the endocardial cushion tissue is called the ostium primum, or foramen primum. Gradually both superior and inferior endocardial cushions migrate to fuse with the approaching septum primum to obliterate the ostium primum. However, because there must be a pathway for blood to flow from the primitive right side to the left side, openings or fenestrations appear and then coalesce within the superior septum primum to form the ostium secundum, or foramen secundum. As the right sinus horn of the sinus venosus is incorporated into the right side of the primitive atrium, it enlarges, and another fold appears descending inferiorly toward the endocardial cushions. This septum secundum descends but never completely obliterates the interatrial communication. It moves inferiorly to form the superior limbus of the remaining communication, the foramen ovale, which is the residual of the ostium secundum. The remaining septum primum has two residual limbs from its descent from the roof of the atrium, and these sit on the leftward side of the newly formed septum secundum. This architecture allows flow from the right to the left atrium, but is structured such that, with the normal physiologic changes at birth, the septum primum is pushed rightward into the septum secundum, closing the communication.

Failure of septation of the atria is a relatively common occurrence and can range from a probe-patent foramen ovale (its most minor form) to complete absence of the atrial septum and a common atrium. It has been shown at autopsy that as many as 25% of hearts have a probe-patent foramen ovale at the superiormost aspect of the fossa ovale, which remains clinically insignificant except in very rare circumstances. More commonly, the presence of a patent foramen ovale (PFO) creates little problem with regard to significant left-to-right shunting, but may provide a scenario for paradoxical emboli in patients with systemic venous thrombi. A secundum ASD is a defect within the septum primum of the atria, resulting from failure in the descent or overlap of the septum secundum over the septum primum (essentially a large PFO), or from excessive disappearance of the septum primum during atrial development. This can involve a single defect within the septum, or several fenestrations. After birth, this leads to a left-to-right shunt across the defect because of the preferential flow into a thin-walled, very compliant right ventricle in comparison to the thicker walled, less compliant left ventricle.

Failure of proper fusion of the sinus horns of the sinus venosus to the right atrium leads to several sinus venosus types of ASD. The most common of these involves a defect in the posterosuperior right atrium over the insertion of the right superior pulmonary vein. This malformation of the right superior horn of the sinus venosus is often said to be accompanied by partial anomalous venous return, but in fact the pulmonary vein is coming into the left atrium correctly, but is "unroofed" into the right atrium because of the failed fusion of the sinus venosus. In this defect, the hole in the septum lies in the superior part of the right atrium at the insertion of the superior vena cava. The pulmonary veins are easily seen within this orifice and commonly are in close association with the superior vena cava. Occasionally the right upper lobe vein or an accessory pulmonary vein will enter the side of the superior vena cava. A less common sinus venosus defect involves failure in the right inferior horn, leaving a defect in the postero-inferior septum and similarly "unroofing" the right inferior pulmonary vein. A much less common defect involves the left inferior horn of the sinus venosus (which forms the coronary sinus), leading to an unroofing of the coronary sinus with drainage of the coronary venous flow directly into the left atrium. In the absence of an associated persistent left superior vena cava, this defect allows a right-to-left shunt that is not clinically significant.

Other unusual errors in septation have been reported, including left-sided inferior venae cavae and right-sided pulmonary venous connections, as well as complete absence of the atrial septum from lack of formation and descent of the septum primum and septum secundum. These defects usually are associated with very complex and multiple congenital cardiac malformations, and frequently are seen within the various heterotaxy syndromes.

Much confusion arises for students of embryology and clinical cardiology because of the somewhat unfortunate terminology used for the development of the heart and its specific defects. To briefly review and clarify, the embryologic ostium primum and ostium secundum are communications in the fetal heart during its formation. They occur sequentially, and normally both are closed at the end of gestation, except for the residual foramen ovale, which closes shortly after birth. The septum primum and septum secundum both arise from the superior atrium during septation, and both partially remain within the formed heart, contributing to the completed atrial septum. Clinically, a "secundum" ASD is one or more defects within or above the septum primum, and is in fact a residual of the embryologic ostium secundum, while a "primum" ASD is a defect in the endocardial cushion contribution of the atrial septum, immediately over the AV valves. The intact atrial septum therefore contains contributions from the sinus venosus (posteriorly near the venae cavae), the septum secundum (superiorly down to the limbus of the fossa ovale), the septum primum (from the fossa down to the endocardial cushions), and the endocardial cushions or AV canal septum (immediately above the AV valves). The primitive atrium contributes little more than the trabeculated portions of the right and left atrium, including the atrial appendages. The majority of the right atrium is formed by the right sinus horn of the sinus venosus, and the left atrium by the pulmonary venous confluence.

Ventricular Septation

The completely formed ventricular septum has four basic components, the formation of which is addressed separately. The closure of the inlet septum by the AV canal endocardial cushions was described above with the AV canal septation. The formation of the trabeculated septum and the membranous septum is described here, and that of the conotruncal or outlet septum is described later.

As the primitive heart loop forms into a U, the inlet and outlet portions have outgrowth of tissue at their bases on both sides of the foramen separating the two chambers. These pouches continue to expand and will form the trabeculated portions of the left and right ventricles, the left from the inlet portion and the right from the outlet portion. Next, though the precise mechanism is not clearly understood and is controversial even among experts, it is clear that there is a series of tissue reorganization, molding, and transfer movements to allow the two AV valves to overlie the appropriate ventricular inlet. That is, the left-sided AV orifice moves to position itself over the inlet ventricular trabeculated chamber that will be the left ventricle, and the right AV orifice transfers to a position over the outlet chamber, the future right ventricle. The actual primordial foramen between the original inlet and outlet chambers never actually closes, but instead is reoriented to become part of the junction of the inlet of the right ventricle and the outlet of the left ventricle. The aggregation of tissue between the two chambers below the original foramen enlarges to form the majority of the muscular septum and then migrates to fuse with the appropriate inlet septum formed from the AV canal endocardial cushion tissue. Until the completion of these complex reorganization movements, when each trabeculated pouch has its own inlet and outlet, there must remain some interventricular communication. After this, the final interventricular communication may fuse. This membranous septum is at the junction of the inlet septum of the AV canal endocardial cushion, the superior border of the muscular septum, and the inferior margin of the conotruncal septum below the semilunar valves, which is addressed in the next section along with the formation and septation of the conotruncus.

Failure of ventricular septation can involve failure at several of the levels described above. As previously mentioned, failure at the endocardial cushion level within the AV canal leaves an inlet VSD immediately below the septal leaflet of the tricuspid valve. This can also occur if the muscular septum fails to migrate up to fuse with the inlet septum. Muscular VSDs occur when the aggregation of tissue is insufficient to complete the septation between the two forming pouches of the original inlet and outlet chamber, or may involve abnormal resorption of septal tissue. They may be single or multiple and may occur at any site within the septum from the apex superiorly. Because the muscular septum continues to grow and thicken after birth, the majority of these VSDs close spontaneously over time unless they are initially large enough to cause significant heart failure and prevent normal growth. The most common VSD is found in the membranous septum, the last portion of the interventricular septum to close. Smaller membranous VSDs may close spontaneously in the first 6 months to 2 years of life, whereas others are sufficiently large to cause severe heart failure and require early surgical closure, particularly if they have extension into the inlet or muscular septum.

Conotruncal Formation

As the primitive heart tube bends into a U shape with the inlet portion of the ventricle connected to the AV canal segment of the tube, the outlet portion of the ventricle is similarly attached to the arterial segment. Just as the atrial-ventricular inlet connection is septated by the AV canal endocardial cushions, the outlet arterial segment has outlet cushions of mesenchymal tissue, also called bulbar

or conal cushions. These may be continuous with "truncal" cushions within the arterial segment, but, whether connected or separated, these tissues are responsible for the septation of the primordial truncus or arterial segment into aorta and pulmonary artery. These two ridges of tissue migrate distally in spiral fashion to divide the truncus into its two components, though actually forming only the most proximal portion of the two great vessels. As the arteries expand, the two opposing walls actually form the majority of the septum between them. Proximally, the right conal cushion terminates at the border of the tricuspid valve, and the left along the anterior rim of the muscular septum. As the aorta is transferred over the left ventricle, its fibrous annulus forms in continuity with the AV valves. The pulmonary artery, having formed from the original arterial trunk, maintains its position over the outlet pouch, which became the right ventricle, separated from the right AV valve and keeping its infundibulum within the outflow tract.

The most common congenital defect of conotruncal formation is tetralogy of Fallot, wherein anterior displacement of the conal septum creates outflow obstruction of the right ventricle and prevents normal closure of the ventricular septum, leaving a "malalignment" VSD. The associated aortic override is related to the malaligned septum, and the right ventricular hypertrophy is due to the right-sided outflow obstruction. Abnormal closure of the bulbar or conal septum creates a VSD that lies immediately below the aortic and pulmonary valves. The congenital defect of a persistent truncus arteriosus involves complete failure of septation of the arterial segment. There is a single outflow tract and single valve, which overrides both ventricles and a conal VSD, and gives rise to both the aorta and pulmonary arteries. Completed septation without the normal spiraling of the primordial truncus gives rise to transposition of the great arteries, with the aorta arising from the right ventricle and the pulmonary artery from the left ventricle. Another form of abnormal conotruncal development is double-outlet right ventricle, in which both great vessels arise from the right ventricle, with an associated VSD, frequently subarterial. An aortopulmonary window is a rare type of defect involving a localized failure of septation between the aorta and the pulmonary artery, above the level of two normally formed semilunar valves.

Semilunar and AV Valve Formation

The two semilunar valves are formed at the junction of the arterial segment with the outlet portion of the heart tube. As the septation of the truncus arteriosus is finishing, areas of mesenchymal tissue appear along the septating ridges and hollow out to form the trileaflet semilunar valves. The valve in persistent truncus arteriosus usually contains four, but occasionally has five or six leaflets, because it is by definition malformed and may be significantly insufficient. Congenital problems of the semilunar valves usually involve either complete atresia or stenosis from fusion of the leaflets. Malformed aortic valves are commonly bicuspid, with fusion of two of the three leaflets, but may be unicuspid with a small teardrop-shaped orifice. These malformed valves are rarely congenitally insufficient, but may begin to leak at an older age as the valve leaflets elongate and begin to prolapse. Complete atresia of the aortic valves is usually associated with ventricular and aortic hypoplasia. Pulmonary atresia, however, may be seen with a normally formed but thickened right ventricle in the presence of a VSD, or with an underdeveloped but potentially functional right ventricle when the septum is intact.

During septation of the AV canal as described above, the endocardial cushions may function as primordial valves, but actually have no part in the development of the valves themselves. Once the inlet portions of the two ventricles are in place, an undermining of tissue in the inlet chamber occurs to form the AV valve and the subvalvular apparatus. The tissue thins out to form the valve leaflets and the muscular connections are replaced by fibrous connective tissue to create the chordae tendineae, which are connected to the ventricular wall by the papillary muscles. The mitral apparatus involves chordae from each papillary muscle to both the anterior and posterior leaflets. The tricuspid valve has chordae to both its papillary muscle as well as from the interventricular septum. Abnormalities include failure of AV canal septation as previously described, as well as general malformation of the valve leaflets leading to either stenotic or incompetent valves. AV valve atresia is associated with underdevelopment of the involved ventricle, and it may be unclear whether the abnormal ventricle had insufficient inlet tissue to give rise to an AV valve, or the malformed valve created insufficient flow to allow complete ventricular development. Whatever the mechanism, the association of severe AV valve stenosis or atresia and ventricular underdevelopment is clear. Another specific congenital defect is Ebstein's anomaly, involving a malformation of the tricuspid valve with thinning or "atrialization" of various amounts of ventricular wall. The malformed valve has an inferiorly displaced annulus and may be stenotic or regurgitant depending on the amount of tethering of the anterior leaflet to the ventricular wall.

Coronary Arteries

The primordia of the coronary arteries exist as collections of tissue, or anlages, which lie within the primitive truncus and develop within its sinuses prior to septation. Abnormal fusion of the anlages leads to a single coronary artery, and abnormal migration leads to an anomalous origin of the circumflex artery off the right coronary artery. Very rarely, the anlages end up on the pulmonary side of the septation process, creating an anomalous origin of the coronary artery off the pulmonary artery. This usually involves the left coronary artery, but has also been reported with the right. In this circumstance, the flow of blood passes from the aorta, through collaterals, retrograde into the anomalous coronary artery, and into the low-pressure pulmonary artery. This "steal" of blood flow into the pulmonary artery leads to ischemia of the muscle in the distribution of the anomalous coronary artery. Another unusual but important anomaly of the coronary arteries involves passage of a major coronary artery between the aorta and the pulmonary artery. During increases in cardiac output, there may be compression of the anomalous coronary artery with resultant ischemia, arrhythmia, and even sudden death.

While the coronary arteries originate from the anlages above the truncal valve, the coronary arterial tree develops along with the myocardium. Occasionally fistulae may develop between the major branches of the coronary artery and one of the cardiac chambers, including the coronary sinus. While small fistulae are not infrequently noted at cardiac catheterization, larger fistulae can create left-to-right shunts sufficient to cause chamber enlargement and symptoms of heart failure, and require surgical repair. Because there is not really a "normal" distribution of coronary arteries, anomalies are very difficult to define. The majority of hearts develop with a "right-dominant" circulation wherein the posterior descending artery (PDA) is the terminal branch of the right coronary artery. The remaining 10% to 15% have left-dominant circulation, with the PDA as the terminal branch of the circumflex system. Less than 1% of patients have a true circumflex artery branch off the right coronary, although it is not unusual for a right-dominant system to wrap around the heart in the AV groove, well beyond the takeoff of the PDA, and give rise to numerous obtuse marginal branches normally from the circumflex artery. These hearts usually have a small residual circumflex artery, in contrast to the true anomalous circumflex artery, which is a distinct branch off the proximal right coronary artery. The most significant pattern from a surgical standpoint involves anomalous branches off the right coronary artery, including at times the true left anterior descending artery, that may cross directly over the right ventricular outflow tract in patients who require incisions into the infundibulum as part of a congenital repair, particularly for tetralogy of Fallot. This finding clearly will alter the surgical plan in order to avoid injury to important myocardial blood supply.

Aortic Arch Formation

Early in fetal life, several arches surround the tracheo-esophageal structures beyond the arterial end of the primitive heart tube. Classically six arches are described, although controversy exists as to whether the fifth arch is actually ever present in the human fetus; if it does exist, there are no known residual structures in the finally formed arterial tree (Fig. 15–5A). Regardless, the significant structures present in the newborn are primarily residuals of the fourth and sixth arches. Small vessels of the middle ear may be remnants of the first and second arches, while part of the third arch participates in common carotid artery formation. The fourth arch forms the majority of the true aortic arch and the proximal descending aorta. The sixth arch forms the proximal intrapericardial portions of the right and left pulmonary arteries. The connection between the left sixth arch (left pulmonary artery) and the fourth arch (proximal descending aorta) remains to become the specialized tissue of the ductus arteriosus (Fig. 15–5B).

The most common congenital anomaly of the aortic arches is a patent ductus arteriosus. Under normal circumstances, the ductus has specialized contractile elements within its walls that contract under the direction of chemical changes occurring at birth with initiation of respiration. The persistence of the ductus may be caused by abnormalities in chemical signaling, abnormal receptor responsiveness, or absence of normal contractile elements within its walls. The former is more likely in premature infants because the ductus frequently can be closed with intravenous indomethacin. In older children with a patent ductus, the reason the ductus fails to close remains unclear. Another common defect is coarctation of the aorta.

This defect involves a discrete narrowing in the periductal area. Although many authorities have distinguished between pre- and postductal coarctations, this discrimination has little clinical significance. The cause of the narrowing has been attributed to abnormalities within the media of the aorta with intimal proliferation. However, several pieces of evidence support the concept that this defect actually may be caused by abnormal infiltration of "ductal" elements into the aortic wall. First, newborns with critical coarctation who are treated with prostaglandins are noted by echocardiography to have not only opening of the ductus, but improvement of the narrowing at the level of the coarctation, implying that there is some ductal tissue involved within the coarctation segment. Whether classified as pre- or postductal in nature, essentially all coarctations are immediately adjacent to the ductus or ligamentum arteriosum. In addition, coarctation segments within the pulmonary artery adjacent to the ductus have been noted in complex lesions involving pulmonary atresia, wherein all flow across the ductus is from the aorta to the pulmonary artery, possibly carrying abnormal ductal cells further into the pulmonary artery. A similar mechanism may carry ductal cells abnormally further into the fourth arch of the proximal descending aorta, creating a coarctation of the aorta.

When abnormal resolution of the left fourth arch occurs, the aorta itself is interrupted along its path, with continuity to the descending aorta maintained by the ductus. There is usually complete absence of the missing segment, although occasionally an atretic band may connect the two ends. The three types of this defect involve interruption between the innominate and left common carotid arteries (type C), between the left common carotid and the left subclavian arteries (type B), and beyond the

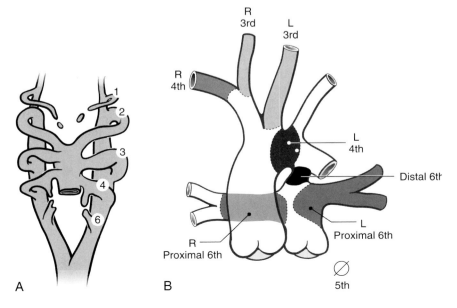

FIGURE 15–5 A, Embryologic aortic arches. **B,** Fate of the aortic arches.

left subclavian artery (type A). The more proximal the interruption, the less flow through the ascending aortic segment and the more hypoplastic the aortic valve and vessel and, at times, the left ventricle. Similarly, there may be atresia or malconnection of either branch pulmonary artery when there is abnormal resolution of the right or left sixth arch, or with misconnection of the arches, so that one or both of the branch pulmonary arteries arise from the aorta, the ductus, or a major arterial branch.

Vascular rings are formed when there is failure of regression of some component of the arches leading to a complete circular connection around the trachea and esophagus. The classic example is a true double aortic arch wherein the ascending aorta arises normally but then gives rise to two equally sized arches, right and left. Each of these then gives rise to a common carotid artery and then a subclavian artery, and then the two trunks fuse posteriorly. Other forms are asymmetrical, involve various patterns of branching, and usually have unequal size trunks. Frequently the completion of the ring is a small remnant of the contralateral arch and may even involve an atretic band only. One of the most common patterns of vascular rings is a persistence of a right aortic arch (right fourth arch) with resolution of the left. There is mirror image branching and an associated aberrant subclavian artery so that the sequence of branches off the rightward arch is left carotid artery, right carotid artery, right subclavian artery, and finally left subclavian artery, which arises posteriorly off Kommerell's diverticulum, a remnant "stump" of the left arch. The ring is actually completed by the ligamentum arteriosum, which extends on the leftward side from the diverticulum to the main pulmonary artery. Many other variations of rings have been reported but are less common.

Anatomic-Physiologic Changes at Birth

With the first few breaths at birth, the expanding lungs fill quickly with air and the blood flow through them rapidly increases. The pulmonary vascular resistance drops considerably over the next several days, and continues over weeks to months to reach a normal level. The dramatic rise in oxygenation over the fetal state leads to several physiologic and chemical changes that direct physical anatomic changes as well. With the increased oxygen

tension, smooth muscle contractions close the umbilical arteries, and shortly thereafter the umbilical veins close. Although they are physiologically closed in minutes after birth, clinically it is well known that these structures take days to weeks to form their final ligamentous configurations and can be cannulated in the newborn for venous and arterial access. With the change in oxygen tension along with chemical mediators such as bradykinin released from the newly inflated lung, the ductus arteriosus and ductus venosus close in the first minutes to hours after birth. The ductus arteriosus frequently can be manipulated pharmacologically within the first hours to days of life, either stimulating contraction and closure with indomethacin or maintaining ductal patency with prostaglandin infusions. As simple as the latter manipulation may seem, this discovery has had a tremendous impact on the survival of infants with "ductal-dependent" congenital heart lesions. These children, who previously were rushed to the operating room hypoxic and acidotic for lack of sufficient pulmonary blood flow for surgical palliation with a systemic-to-pulmonary shunt, now can be maintained on simple prostaglandin infusions, be resuscitated and stabilized, and undergo elective surgery with much less morbidity and mortality.

As the lungs expand, the pulmonary blood flow increases and the ductus arteriosus closes, the right-sided pressure drops, and the left-sided pressure rises with increasing pulmonary venous return. This forces the "trapdoor" of the foramen ovale to close, eliminating right-to-left communication. Some brief shunting may occur in the first few days of life with transient rises in pulmonary vascular resistance, such as with crying, or with sustained rises as with pulmonary hypertension of the newborn.

Bibliography

The literature is filled with a plethora of articles describing very specific and detailed information about cardiac development and classifications of defects, clearly too numerous to list or recommend, and which can be easily identified with detailed searches. However, for the student of embryology who wishes a more complete overall description of development of the heart, including excellent color illustrations, the author highly recommends Chapter 10 (pages 10.2–10.30) of *Cardiac Anatomy: An Integrated and Color Atlas* by Robert H. Anderson and Anton E. Becker, Gower Medical Publishing, London, England, 1980.

CHAPTER 16

Applied Urinary and Reproductive Embryology

John M. Park, M.D.

The study of embryology provides a useful basis for understanding definitive human anatomy and various congenital disease processes. During the last two decades, a torrent of molecular information and novel experimental techniques has revolutionized the field of embryology. From a surgeon's perspective, however, the classic, descriptive aspects of anatomic embryology continue to serve as an important reference point from which various congenital problems are solved. The aim of this chapter is to provide a concise presentation of the essential facts in urogenital system development, clarifying the important anatomic features and supplementing them with up-to-date molecular information.

Kidney Development

Development of Three Embryonic Kidneys

Mammals develop three kidneys in the course of intrauterine life. The embryonic kidneys are, in order of their appearance, the *pronephros*, the *mesonephros*, and the *metanephros*. The first two kidneys regress in utero, and the third becomes the permanent kidney. All three kidneys develop from the intermediate mesoderm. As the notochord and neural tube form, the mesoderm, located on either side of the midline, differentiates into three subdivisions: paraxial (somite), intermediate, and lateral mesoderm (Fig. 16–1). As the embryo undergoes transverse folding, the intermediate mesoderm separates away from the paraxial mesoderm and migrates toward the intraembryonic coelom (the future peritoneum). At this time, there is a progressive craniocaudal development of the bilateral longitudinal mesodermal masses, called *nephrogenic cords*. Each cord is seen bulging from the posterior wall of the coelomic cavity, producing the *urogenital ridge*.

The mammalian pronephros is a transitory nonfunctional kidney, analogous to that of primitive fish. In humans, the first evidence of pronephros is seen late in the third week, and it completely degenerates by the start of the fifth week (Fig. 16–2A). The second kidney, the mesonephros, is also transient, but in mammals it serves as an excretory organ for the embryo while the definitive kidney, the metanephros, begins its development. There is a gradual

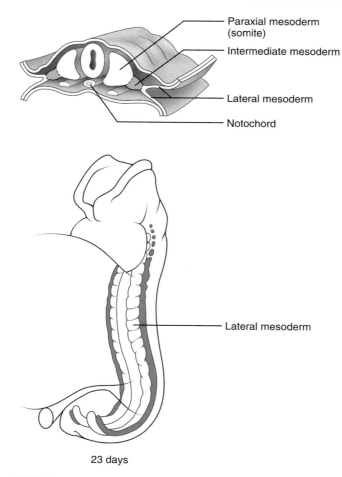

Paraxial mesoderm (somite)

Intermediate mesoderm

Lateral mesoderm

Notochord

Lateral mesoderm

23 days

FIGURE 16–1 The intermediate mesoderm gives rise to paired, segmentally organized nephrotomes from the cervical to the sacral region. Cervical nephrotomes are formed early during the fourth week and are collectively referred to as the pronephros. (Modified from Larsen WJ: Human Embryology [2nd ed]. New York: Churchill Livingstone, 1997.)

transition from the pronephros to the mesonephros at about the 9th and 10th somite levels. Development of the *mesonephric ducts* (also called *wolffian ducts*) precedes the development of the mesonephric tubules (Fig. 16–2B). The mesonephric ducts can be seen as a pair of solid longitudinal tissue condensations at about the 24th day, developing parallel to the nephrogenic cords in the dorsolateral aspect of the embryo. Their blind distal ends grow toward the primitive cloaca (see Bladder and Ureter Development below) and soon fuse with it at about the 28th day. This fused region later becomes a part of the posterior wall of the bladder. Soon after the appearance of the mesonephric ducts during the fourth week, mesonephric vesicles begin to form. Initially, several spherical masses of cells are found along the medial side of the nephrogenic cords at the cranial end. This differentiation progresses caudally and results in the formation of 40 to 42 pairs of

mesonephric tubules, but only about 30 pairs are seen at any one time because the cranially located tubules start to degenerate at about the fifth week (Fig. 16–2C). By the fourth month, the human mesonephros has almost completely disappeared, except for a few elements that persist into maturity. Certain elements of the mesonephros are retained in the mature urogenital system as part of the reproductive tract. In males, some of the cranially located mesonephric tubules become the *efferent ductules of the testis*. The *epididymis* and *vas deferens* are formed from the mesonephric (wolffian) ducts. In females, remnants of cranial and caudal mesonephric tubules form small, nonfunctional mesosalpingeal structures called the *epoophoron* and the *paroophoron*.

The definitive kidney, the metanephros, forms in the sacral region as a pair of new structures, called the *ureteric buds*, sprouts from the distal portion of the mesonephric ducts and comes in contact with the blastema of *metanephric mesenchyme* at about the 28th day (Fig. 16–3). The ureteric bud penetrates a condensing metanephric mesenchyme and begins to divide dichotomously. The tip of the dividing ureteric bud, called the *ampulla*, interacts with the metanephric mesenchyme to induce formation of future nephrons. As the ureteric bud divides and branches, each new ampulla acquires a caplike condensation of metanephric mesenchyme, thereby giving the metanephros a lobulated appearance.

The ureteric bud and metanephric mesenchyme exert reciprocal inductive effects toward each other, and the proper differentiation of these primordial structures depends on these inductive signals (see Molecular Mechanism of Kidney Development below). The metanephric mesenchyme induces the ureteric bud to branch, and in turn, the ureteric bud induces the metanephric mesenchyme to condense and undergo mesenchymal-epithelial conversion. The nephron, which consists of the glomerulus, proximal tubule, loop of Henle, and distal tubule, is thought to derive from the metanephric mesenchyme, while the collecting system, consisting of collecting ducts, calyces, pelvis, and ureter, is formed from the ureteric bud (Fig. 16–4).

In principle, all nephrons are formed in the same way and can be classified into fairly well-defined developmental stages. The first identifiable precursors of the nephron are cells of metanephric mesenchyme that have formed a vesicle completely separated from the ureteric bud ampulla (stage I). Cells of the stage I renal vesicle are tall and columnar in shape, and are stabilized by their attachments to the newly formed basement membrane (Fig. 16–5). It has not yet established a contact with the ampulla of the ureteric bud. The stage I renal vesicle then differentiates into an S-shaped stage II nephron that connects to the ureteric bud. At this stage, the cup-shaped glomerular capsule is recognized in the lowest limb of the S-shaped tubule.

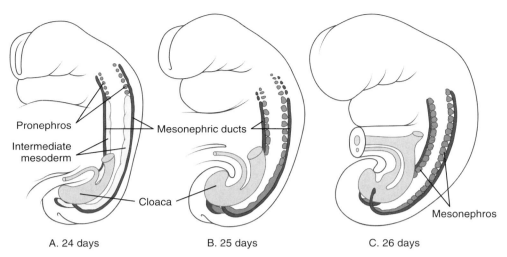

FIGURE 16-2 Development of pronephros and mesonephros. **A**, Pronephroi develop in each of five to seven cervical segments, but these primitive renal structures degenerate quickly during the fourth week. The mesonephric ducts first appear on day 24. **B** and **C**, Mesonephric vesicles and tubules form in a craniocaudal direction throughout the thoracic and lumbar regions. The cranial pairs degenerate as caudal pairs develop, and the definitive mesonephroi contain about 20 pairs confined to the first three lumbar segments. (Modified from Larsen WJ: Human Embryology [2nd ed]. New York: Churchill Livingstone, 1997.)

The rest of the **S**-shaped tubule develops into the proximal tubule, the loop of Henle, and the distal tubule. When the cup-shaped glomerular capsule matures into an oval structure, the nephron has now passed into stage III of development. Now the nephron can be divided into identifiable proximal and distal tubules. The stage IV nephron is characterized by a round glomerulus that closely resembles the mature renal corpuscle (Fig. 16–6).

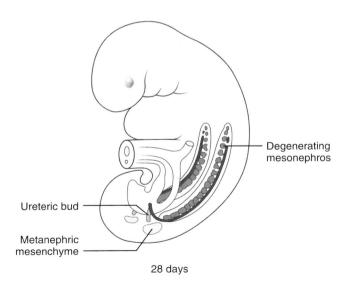

FIGURE 16-3 Metanephric mesenchyme condenses from the intermediate mesoderm during the early part of the fifth week and comes into contact with the ureteric bud, while the cranial mesonephroi continue to degenerate. (Modified from Larsen WJ: Human Embryology [2nd ed]. New York: Churchill Livingstone, 1997.)

The morphology of the proximal tubule resembles that of a mature nephron, whereas the distal segments are still primitive. In some species (e.g., the rodents), all stages of nephron development are present at birth, whereas in others (e.g., humans), all nephrons are in varying steps of stage IV at birth. Initially, vessels are seen in the cleft between the lower and middle portion of the **S**-shaped tubule, and they quickly branch into a portal system. Mesenchymal cells that do not become tubular epithelium either give rise to interstitial mesenchyme or undergo programmed cell death (apoptosis). Overall, these events are reiterated throughout the growing kidney, so that older, more differentiated nephrons are located in the inner part of the kidney near the juxtamedullary region and newer, less differentiated nephrons are found at the periphery (Fig. 16–7). In humans, although renal maturation continues to take place postnatally, nephrogenesis is completed before birth.

Development of the Collecting System

The bifurcation of the ureteric bud determines the eventual pelvicaliceal patterns and their corresponding renal lobules (Fig. 16–8). The first few divisions of the ureteric bud give rise to the renal pelvis, major and minor calyces, and collecting ducts. Thereafter, the first generations of collecting tubules are formed. When the ureteric bud first invades the metanephric mesenchyme, its tip expands to form an ampulla that will eventually give rise to the renal pelvis. By the sixth week, the ureteric bud has bifurcated at least four times, yielding 16 branches. These branches

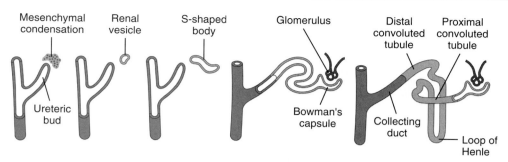

FIGURE 16–4 Development of the renal collecting ducts and nephrons. The tip of dividing ureteric bud induces the metanephric mesenchyme to condense, which then differentiates into a renal vesicle. This vesicle coils into an S-shaped tubule and ultimately forms a Bowman's capsule as well as the proximal convoluted tubules, distal convoluted tubules, and loops of Henle. The ureteric bud contributes to the formation of collecting ducts. (Modified from Larsen WJ: Human Embryology [2nd ed]. New York: Churchill Livingstone, 1997.)

then coalesce to form two to four major calyces extending from the renal pelvis. By the seventh week, the next four generations of branches also fuse, forming the minor calyces. By the 32nd week, approximately 11 additional generations of bifurcation have resulted in approximately 1 to 3 million branches, which will become the collecting duct tubules.

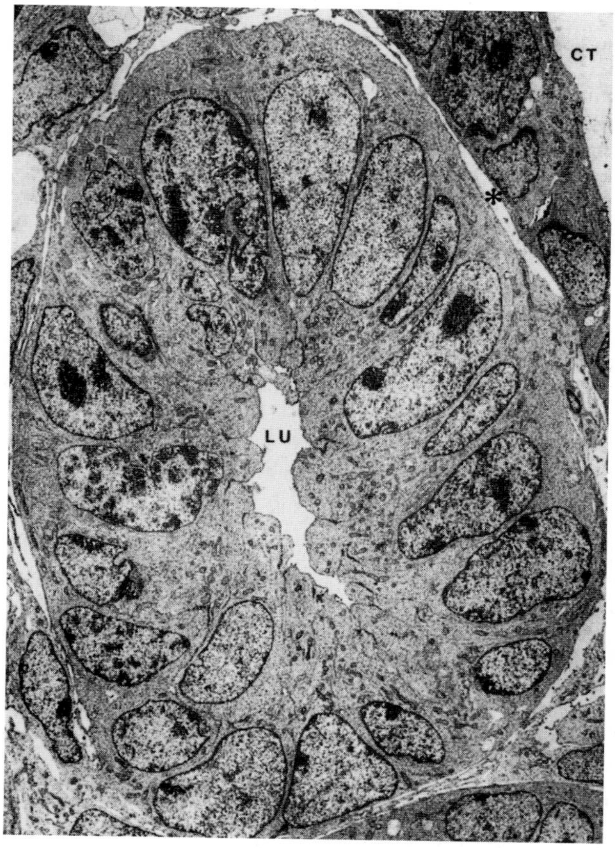

Renal Ascent

Between the sixth and ninth weeks, the kidneys ascend to a lumbar site just below the adrenal glands (Fig. 16–9). The precise mechanism responsible for renal ascent is not known, but it is speculated that the differential growth of the lumbar and sacral regions of the embryo plays a role. As the kidneys migrate, they are vascularized by a succession of transient aortic sprouts that arise at progressively higher levels. These arteries do not elongate to follow the ascending kidneys, but instead degenerate and are replaced by successive new arteries. The final pair of arteries forms in the upper lumbar region and becomes the definitive renal arteries. Occasionally, a more inferior pair of arteries persists as accessory lower pole arteries. When the kidney fails to ascend properly, its location becomes *ectopic*. If its ascent fails completely, it remains as a *pelvic* kidney. The inferior poles of the kidneys may also fuse, forming a *horseshoe* kidney that crosses over the ventral side of the aorta. During ascent, the fused lower pole becomes trapped under the inferior mesenteric artery and thus does not reach its normal site. Rarely, the kidney fuses to the contralateral one and ascends to the opposite side, resulting in a cross-fused ectopy.

Molecular Mechanism of Kidney Development

In mammalian embryos, the permanent kidney is derived from the reciprocal inductive interactions between two primordial mesodermal structures, the ureteric bud and the metanephric mesenchyme (Fig. 16–10A). Upon induction by the ureteric bud, the metanephric mesenchyme undergoes a series of morphogenetic events that converts the mesenchyme to an epithelium and eventually generates most of the renal tubules. In turn, the metanephric

FIGURE 16–5 Stage I nephron development. The cells are tall with large nuclei, and the renal vesicle is separated from the developing collecting tubule (CT) by a narrow zone of low electron density (*). (From Larsson L: The ultrastructure of the developing proximal tubule in the rat kidney. J Ultrastruct Res 1975;51:119, with permission from Elsevier.)

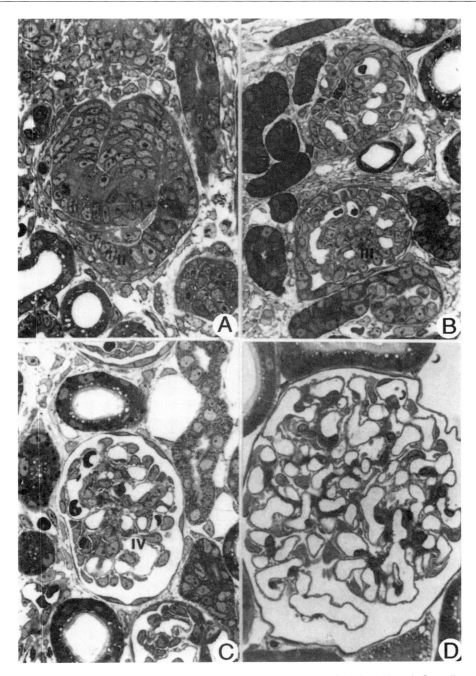

FIGURE 16–6 Stages II through IV nephron development as seen from a renal cortex of a 3-day-old rat. **A,** Stage II nephron with S-shaped body (II). **B,** Stage III nephron with oval-shaped glomeruli (III). **C,** Stage IV nephron resembles that of mature tubules and glomeruli (IV). **D,** Mature superficial glomerulus from adult rat kidney. (From Larsson L, Maunsbach AB: The ultrastructural development of the glomerular filtration barrier in the rat kidney: a morphometric analysis. J Ultrastruct Res 1980;72:392, with permission from Elsevier.)

mesenchyme provides a stimulus for continued growth and bifurcation of the ureteric bud, which eventually gives rise to the renal collecting ducts, calyces, renal pelvis, and ureter. Many of the early events in embryonic kidney development were first elucidated by manipulating lower vertebrate embryos and by utilizing a mammalian in vitro organ culture system. Clifford Grobstein's pioneering work

in the 1950s led to an organ culture technique whereby the metanephric mesenchyme is separated from the ureteric bud during the early part of kidney development and grown on a filter (Fig. 16–10B). This ingenious experimental approach has established the kidney as a model system for studying the role of epithelial-mesenchymal interaction in organ development. The development of

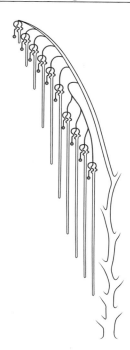

FIGURE 16–7 Schematic representation of progressive nephron differentiation. Older, more differentiated nephrons are located in the inner part of the kidney near the juxtamedullary region and newer, less differentiated nephrons are found at the periphery. (From Potter EL: Normal and Abnormal Development of the Kidney. Chicago: Year Book Medical Publishers, 1972, with permission.)

many other organs, including lung, salivary glands, gonads, prostate, and bladder, also requires epithelial-mesenchymal interaction for the controlled differentiation and proliferation of tissues.

Although much has been known about the morphologic events of kidney development, the molecular mechanisms involved in these processes have begun to be identified only during the last few years (Fig. 16–11). This is largely due to the identification of critical genes expressed during kidney development and the application of molecular recombinant techniques for single gene disruption (*gene knock out*). The advent of molecular biologic techniques has led to the identification of a large and growing number of genes expressed during kidney development. There are more than 200 genes and/or proteins currently listed in the Kidney Development Database, and a detailed, up-to-date summary can now be accessed on a website. However, to show that these genes are truly involved in kidney development, inactivation of these genes must demonstrate an abnormal kidney phenotype. There are now at least 11 genes that have been shown to play a critical role in kidney development via gene disruption studies (Table 16–1). Currently, studies using combinations of gene expression analyses, gene knockouts, and organ culture techniques are providing the most complete information. Several comprehensive reviews have been published on this topic.

The classic transfilter assay of Grobstein is carried out with a mesenchyme isolated from rodent embryos at 11 to 12 days of gestation. By this time, kidney morphogenesis is well under way, and the ureteric bud has come into full contact with the condensing metanephric mesenchyme. This early phase of kidney development has now come into focus in molecular genetic experiments that address the functions of various transcription factors, signaling molecules, and receptors. The results of these experiments suggest that formation of the ureteric bud is initiated by inductive signals from the metanephric mesenchyme. The first evidence for this paradigm came from the analysis of mice lacking the transcription factor WT-1, the product of

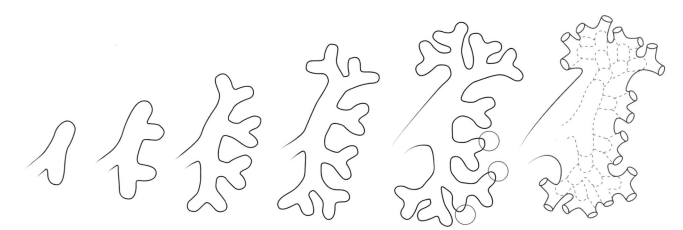

FIGURE 16–8 Dichotomous branching of the ureteric bud and subsequent fusion of the ampulla to form the renal pelvis and calyces. Circles indicate possible sites of infundibular development between the third, fourth, or fifth generations of branches and their subsequent expansions to give rise to the calyces. (From Potter EL: Normal and Abnormal Development of the Kidney. Chicago: Year Book Medical Publishers, 1972, with permission.)

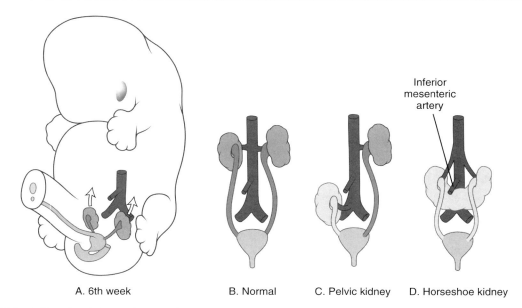

FIGURE 16–9 Normal and abnormal ascent of the kidneys. **A** and **B,** The metanephroi normally ascend from the sacral region to their definitive lumbar location between the sixth and ninth weeks. **C,** Rarely, a kidney may fail to ascend, resulting in a pelvic kidney. **D,** If the inferior poles of the metanephroi fuse before ascent, the resulting horseshoe kidney does not ascend to a normal position because of entrapment by the inferior mesenteric artery. (Modified from Larsen WJ: Human Embryology [2nd ed]. New York: Churchill Livingstone, 1997.)

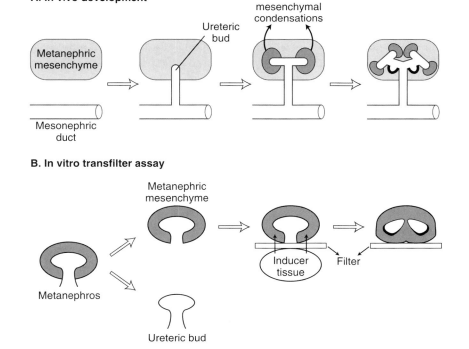

FIGURE 16–10 Schematic representation of in vivo kidney development (**A**) and an in vitro transfilter organ culture system of Grobstein (**B**). At an early stage of renal development, the metanephric mesenchyme is separated from the ureteric bud and cultured on a filter. If there is an inducer tissue grown on the opposite side of the filter, such as ureter and spinal cord, the metanephric mesenchyme will continue to differentiate into nephron structures. In the absence of inducer tissue, the metanephric mesenchyme will degenerate via apoptosis. (Modified from Vainio S, Muller U: Inductive tissue interactions, cell signaling, and the control of kidney organogenesis. Cell 1997;90:975, with permission from Elsevier.)

Table 16–1
Genes crucial for the development of functional kidneys*

Gene	Type	MM	UB	Defect
WT1	Transcription factor	Yes	No	Renal agenesis
PAX2	Transcription factor	Yes	Yes	Renal agenesis
GDNF	TGF-β family member/legand for c-Ret	Yes	No	Renal agenesis or severe dysgenesis
c-Ret	Receptor tyrosine kinase	No	Yes	Renal agenesis or severe dysgenesis
A8B1	Integrin	Yes	No	Renal agenesis or severe dysgenesis
Wnt4	Secreted glycoprotein	Yes	No	Renal dysgenesis
BF2	Transcription factor	Yes	No	Abnormal stromal cells leading to renal dysgenesis
BMP7	TGF-β family member	Yes	Yes	Renal dysgenesis
PDGFB	PDGF and ligand for PDGFR-β	Yes	No	Absence of mesangial cells
PDGFRB	Receptor tyrosine kinase	Yes	No	Absence of mesangial cells
A3B1	Integrin	Yes	Yes	Abnormal glomerular podocytes and basement membrane

MM, metanephric mesenchyme expression; UB, ureteric bud expression.
*The genes are listed in the order in which the developmental defects occur.
Adapted from Lipschutz JH: Molecular development of the kidney: a review of the results of gene disruption studies. Am J Kidney Dis 1998;31:383.

the Wilms' tumor suppressor gene. During embryonic kidney development, WT-1 is expressed in the metanephric mesenchyme, but not in the ureteric bud. Mutant WT-1 mice do not form ureteric buds, suggesting its involvement in the formation of ureteric bud. In organ culture, the WT-1–deficient metanephric mesenchyme does not respond to inducer tissues, indicating that it may also confer mesenchymal competence for induction. Other targeted mutations that cause defects in early kidney development include genes encoding the transcription factors Pax-2 and Lim-1. Pax-2 is expressed in the mesonephric ducts and the ureteric buds from the murine embryonic day 12 onward. In Pax-2 gene knockout mice, no mesonephric ducts, müllerian ducts, ureteric buds, or metanephric mesenchyme form, and the animals die within 1 day of birth as a result of renal failure. In humans, a Pax-2 gene mutation is related to a syndrome encompassing renal dysplasia, optic nerve colobomas, and vesicoureteral reflux. Further studies are required to establish their functions, but it seems likely that both Pax-2 and Lim-1 operate earlier than WT-1.

An important signaling molecule from the metanephric mesenchyme that regulates ureteric bud growth is glial cell line–derived neurotrophic factor (GDNF). In the mouse, targeted inactivation of c-Ret, a member of the receptor tyrosine kinase superfamily, results in renal agenesis and dysplasia. c-Ret is expressed in the ureteric bud as it invades the metanephric mesenchyme. Later, its expression is confined to the bifurcating ampulla of the ureteric bud. The primary defect in the homozygous c-Ret

gene knockout mice is a failure of the ureteric bud to emerge from the mesonephric duct and respond to signals from the metanephric mesenchyme. While the importance of c-Ret in kidney development was clearly demonstrated, it is only recently that its ligand, GDNF, has been identified. GDNF is a secreted glycoprotein that possesses a cystine-knot motif found in other growth factors such as platelet-derived growth factor, nerve growth factor, and transforming growth factor-β. GDNF is expressed within the metanephric mesenchyme prior to ureteric bud invasion, and later its expression is confined to the most peripheral mesenchyme of the developing kidney, where the induction of new nephrons occurs, complementing the expression pattern of c-Ret at the ureteric bud ampulla. GDNF can promote ureteric bud growth in vitro, but, more importantly, ureteric bud formation is impaired in GDNF knockout mice, a phenotype strikingly similar to the c-Ret knockout mice. There is now compelling evidence that GDNF and c-Ret are the elements of the same signaling pathway that regulates ureteric bud development.

Upon induction by mesenchymal signals, the growing ureteric bud reciprocates itself by expressing signal molecules that regulate the differentiation of the metanephric mesenchyme. This process is not well understood, but some candidate molecules such as FGF-2, BMP-7, and Wnt-11 have emerged. There is also evidence that expression of these signaling molecules by the ureteric bud is regulated by the homeobox transcription factor Emx-2. In Emx-2 gene knockout mice, the ureteric bud forms and invades the metanephric mesenchyme, but

A. Ureter induction

a. Initiation

b. Growth and differentiation

B. Tubule induction

a. Patterning

b. Tubulogenesis

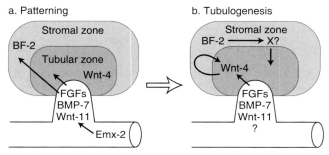

FIGURE 16–11 Molecular models for inductive interactions during early kidney development. **A,** Inductive signals that regulate the growth of the ureteric bud. *a,* Initiation: Glial cell line–derived neurotrophic factor (GDNF) is secreted from the metanephric mesenchyme and activates the c-Ret receptor tyrosine kinase in the presumptive ureteric bud epithelium. This leads to induction of downstream factors such as Wnt-11 and proteoglycans (PG). *b,* Growth and differentiation: multiple molecules contribute to continued ureteric bud formation and branching, including mesenchymal proteins, such as GDNF, and ureteric bud factors, such as Wnt-11, PG, BMP-7, and FGFs. Wnt-11 and PG might function as autocrine factors to maintain directional growth of the ureteric bud. Some of the ureteric bud signals may act on the mesenchyme as well. **B,** Signals involved in mesenchymal differentiation. *a,* Patterning: the transcription factor Emx-2 regulates the ureteric bud epithelium expression of yet-to-be identified signaling molecule(s). Candidates are Wnt-11, BMP-7, and FGFs, and these factors may be involved in patterning the mesenchyme into two zones, a tubular one (Wnt-4 positive) and a stromal one (BF-2 positive). *b,* Tubulogenesis: cells from the ureteric bud and the stromal zone provide inductive signals for cells in the tubular zone to become nephrons. Here Wnt-4 is induced by ureteric bud signal(s), which may then act as an autocrine factor in tubule development. (Modified from Vainio S, Muller U: Inductive tissue interactions, cell signaling, and the control of kidney organogenesis. Cell 1997;90:975, with permission from Elsevier.)

its development is arrested and the mesenchyme does not differentiate. It is not known whether the mesenchyme is a homogeneous cell population prior to interaction with the ureteric bud. It is clear, however, that the inductive signals from the ureteric bud pattern the mesenchyme into at least two different cell populations, a tubular one and a stromal one. The tubular cell population is thought to derive from mesenchymal cells in direct contact with the

ureteric bud ampulla, and they express Pax-2, Syndecan-1, and Wnt-4. The stromal cell population surrounds the tubular cells, and they express the transcription factor BF-2. Once the mesenchyme has been patterned, the cells in the tubular zone undergo morphogenesis to become renal tubular epithelial cells. There is recent evidence that this process is dependent not only upon signals from the ureteric bud but also upon signals from the mesenchyme itself. One of these autocrine signals may be Wnt-4, whose expression is induced in cells of the tubular zone upon interaction with the ureteric bud. In Wnt-4 gene knockout mice, the ureteric bud forms and invades the metanephric mesenchyme, but subsequent development of epithelial tubules is abolished. This suggests that two signals are essential for renal tubule formation: an initial ureteric bud–derived signal(s) activating Wnt-4 expression in the metanephric mesenchyme and Wnt-4 itself as a mesenchymal autocrine signal. Signals from the stromal cell population contribute to tubule formation as well, because tubulogenesis is perturbed in BF-2 gene knockout mice. The discovery that Wnt-4 acts as a downstream signal during the induction cascade leading to renal tubule formation leads to the question regarding the nature of the initial ureteric bud–derived signal. In vitro data suggest a role for FGF-2 and other uncharacterized factors secreted by the ureteric bud. Candidate molecules that may cooperate with FGF-2 are Wnt-11 and BMP-7.

Widespread apoptosis occurs in the metanephric mesenchyme in the absence of inductive signals. Thus it seems likely that induction of metanephric mesenchyme generates both survival and differentiation factors. Indeed, a number of growth factors, including epidermal growth factor and basic fibroblast growth factor, can prevent cell death in cultured metanephric mesenchyme and may function as survival factors. During renal development, apoptotic cells are characteristically found between maturing nephrons in the metanephric mesenchyme. Factors controlling apoptosis have been investigated, including Bcl-2, a form of cytoprotective protein. Bcl-2 gene knockout mice develop cystic kidneys that are hypoplastic and have fewer nephrons. In these mice, a dramatic increase in apoptosis within the metanephric mesenchyme was observed. These findings suggest that apoptotic regulation is required for normal renal development and that Bcl-2 may block apoptosis in many kidney cell types.

The renin-angiotensin system (RAS) is present and active during fetal life. It is generally thought that the major role of the RAS in the fetus is to maintain fetal glomerular filtration rate and ensure an adequate urine production. There is evidence that the RAS is also important for normal growth and development of the ureter and the metanephric kidney. The kidney is able to produce all components of the RAS, and thus the local (intrarenal) production of angiotensin II may play a critical role in this regard. Renin messenger RNA is detectable in the human mesonephros at about 30 days of gestation, and in the metanephros at about 56 days. A similar profile of expression is seen for angiotensinogen and angiotensin-converting enzyme (ACE). Both subtypes of angiotensin II receptors, AT_1 and AT_2, are expressed in the developing meso- and metanephros. AT_2 expression predominates in undifferentiated mesenchyme and declines with maturation, and this observation suggests AT_2's role in modulation of proliferation, apoptosis, and/or mesenchymal differentiation. AT_1 is expressed in more differentiated structures and may be involved in modulating later stages of renal vascular development and acquisition of classic angiotensin II–mediated effects of vasoconstriction and sodium reabsorption. The function of AT_2 receptor is not defined completely, but it appears to play an important role in ureteral development (see Role of Renin-Angiotensin System in Ureteral Differentiation below). AT_2 is highly expressed in undifferentiated periureteral and peripapillary mesenchymal cells. AT_2 gene knockout mice demonstrate a spectrum of congenital urinary tract abnormalities, including ureteropelvic junction obstruction, multicystic dysplastic kidney, megaureter, vesicoureteral reflux, and renal hypoplasia. Ten- to 12-month-old mutant mice lacking ACE are found to have abnormal renal vasculature and tubules as well as increased renin synthesis in intersitial and perivascular cells. Pharmacologic inhibition of ACE in the neonatal rat produces irreversible abnormalities in renal function and morphology, supporting that an intact RAS is crucial for normal kidney development and maturation. In addition to the high rate of fetal loss, infants born to mothers treated with ACE inhibitors during pregnancy have increased rates of oligohydramnios, hypotension, and anuria. Babies with high umbilical cord renin concentrations have significantly smaller kidneys, and infants with intrauterine growth retardation have high angiotensin II levels in the blood.

Bladder and Ureter Development

Formation of Urogenital Sinus

At the third week of gestation, the *cloacal membrane* remains a bilaminar structure composed of endoderm and ectoderm. During the fourth week, the neural tube and the tail grow dorsally and caudally, projecting themselves over the cloacal membrane, and this differential growth of the body results in embryo folding. The cloacal membrane is now turned to the ventral aspect of the embryo, and the terminal portion of the endoderm-lined yolk sac dilates and becomes the cloaca (Fig. 16–12). According to

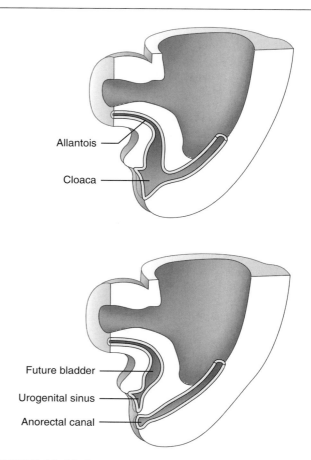

FIGURE 16–12 Development of the urogenital sinus. Between the fourth and sixth weeks, the cloaca is divided into an anterior urogenital sinus and a posterior anorectal canal. The superior part of the urogenital sinus, continuous with allantois, forms the bladder. The constricted narrowing at the base of the urogenital sinus forms the pelvic urethra. The distal expansion of the urogenital sinus forms the vestibule of the vagina in females and the penile urethra in males. (Modified from Larsen WJ: Human Embryology [2nd ed]. New York: Churchill Livingstone, 1997.)

the embryonic theories of Rathke and Tourneux, the partition of the cloaca into an anterior urogenital sinus and a posterior anorectal canal occurs by the fusion of two lateral ridges of the cloacal wall and by a descending urorectal septum. This process is thought to occur during the fifth and sixth weeks, and it is culminated by the fusion of this urorectal septum with the cloacal membrane. Recently, however, some investigators have challenged this classic view with evidence that there is neither a descending septum nor fusing lateral ridges of the cloacal wall. There is evidence that the urorectal septum never fuses with the cloacal membrane. According to these new observations, the congenital cloacal and anorectal malformations, which were previously thought to occur as a result of a failure of septum formation and its fusion with the cloacal membrane, may in fact occur from an abnormal development of the cloacal membrane itself (Fig. 16–13).

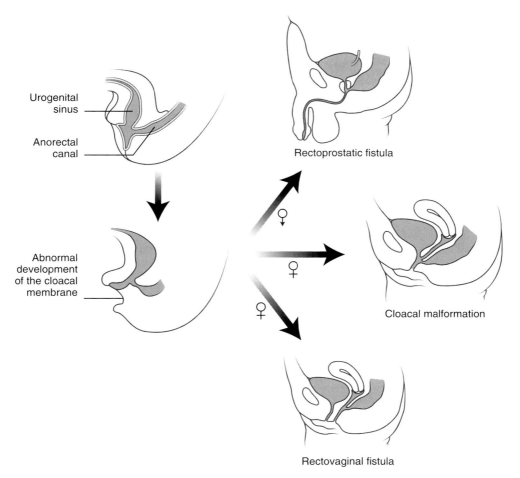

FIGURE 16–13 Abnormal development of cloacal membrane results in characteristic anomalies of the urogenital and lower gastrointestinal tract. (Modified from Larsen WJ: Human Embryology [2nd ed]. New York: Churchill Livingstone, 1997.)

The mesonephric (wolffian) duct fuses with the cloaca by the 24th day and remains with the urogenital sinus during the cloacal separation. The entrance of the mesonephric duct into the primitive urogenital sinus serves as a landmark distinguishing the cephalad *vesicourethral canal* from the caudad *urogenital sinus*. The vesicourethral canal gives rise to the bladder and pelvic urethra, while the caudal urogenital sinus forms the phallic urethra for males and distal vaginal vestibule for females.

Formation of Trigone

By day 33 of gestation, the common excretory ducts (the portion of the mesonephric ducts distal to the origin of the ureteric buds) dilate and become absorbed into the urogenital sinus (Fig. 16–14). The right and left common excretory ducts fuse in the midline as a triangular area, forming the primitive trigone. The ureteric orifice extrophies and evaginates into the bladder by day 37 and begins to migrate in a cranial and lateral direction within

the floor of the bladder. During this process, the mesonephric (wolffian) duct orifice diverges away from the ureteric orifice and migrates caudally, flanking the *paramesonephric (müllerian) duct* at the level of the urogenital sinus. This is the site of the future *verumontanum* in males and vaginal canal in females.

The mechanism of ureteric orifice incorporation into the developing bladder is inferred primarily from clinical observations of duplex kidneys. The upper pole ureteric orifice rotates posteriorly relative to the lower pole orifice and assumes a more caudal and medial position. Weigert and Meyer recognized the regularity of this relationship between upper and lower pole ureteric orifices, which has come to be known as the *Weigert-Meyer rule*. According to this concept, an abnormally lateral lower pole ureteric orifice may result from a ureteric bud arising too low on the mesonephric duct, therefore resulting in premature incorporation and migration within the developing bladder. In such a ureteric orifice, vesicoureteral reflux is more likely to occur as a result of an inadequate intramural tunnel.

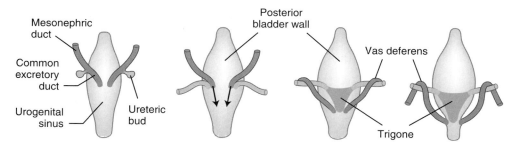

FIGURE 16–14 Incorporation of the mesonephric ducts and ureteric buds into the bladder wall. Between the fourth and sixth weeks, common excretory ducts, the terminal portion of the mesonephric ducts caudal to the ureteric bud formation, exstrophy into the posterior wall of the developing bladder. The triangular region of exstrophied mesonephric ducts forms the trigone of the bladder. This process brings the ureteric bud openings into the bladder wall, while the mesonephric duct openings are carried inferiorly to the level of pelvic urethra. (Modified from Langman J, Sadler TW: Langman's Medical Embryology [5th ed]. Baltimore: Williams & Wilkins, 1985.)

In contrast, an abnormally caudal upper pole ureteric orifice may result from a ureteric bud arising too high on the mesonephric duct. It may drain at the bladder neck and verumontanum, or remain connected to the mesonephric duct derivatives such as the vas deferens. In females, the ectopic upper pole ureter may insert into the remnants of the mesonephric (wolffian) ducts or vaginal vestibule (Fig. 16–15).

Anomalous development of the common excretory duct may lead to an ectopic vas deferens. In certain clinical situations, the vas deferens is connected to the ureter rather than the verumontanum, so that both the ureter and vas drain into a common duct. This situation may occur when the ureteric bud arises too high on the mesonephric duct, and the subsequent common excretory duct becomes too long, resulting in incomplete absorption

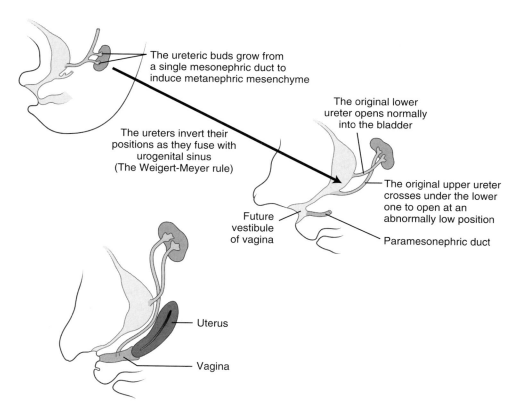

FIGURE 16–15 Development of an ectopic upper pole ureter draining into the vagina. (Modified from Larsen WJ: Human Embryology [2nd ed]. New York: Churchill Livingstone, 1997.)

into the developing bladder. This anomaly, although rare, should be kept in mind when evaluating males with epididymitis and ipsilateral hydronephrosis.

Development of Ureter

Only a small amount of descriptive information and speculative theories exist regarding the molecular mechanism of ureteral development. The ureter begins as a simple cuboidal epithelial tube surrounded by loose mesenchymal cells, and acquires a complete lumen at 28 days of gestation in human. It was suggested that the developing ureter undergoes a transient luminal obstruction between 37 and 40 days and subsequent recanalization. It appears that this recanalization process begins in the midureter and extends in a bidirectional manner both cranially and caudally. In addition, another source of physiologic ureteral obstruction may exist as Chwalla's membrane, a two-cell-thick layer over the ureteric orifice that is seen between 37 and 39 days of gestation. In humans, urine production is followed by proliferative changes in the ureteral epithelium. The epithelium attains a transitional configuration by 14 weeks. The first signs of ureteral muscularization and development of elastic fibers are seen at 12 weeks of gestation. In both rats and humans, the ureteral smooth muscle phenotype appears later than that of the bladder. Smooth muscle differentiation is first detected in the subserosal region of the bladder dome and extends toward the bladder neck and urethra, whereas smooth muscle differentiation of the ureter occurs later within the subepithelial region in the ureterovesical junction, ascending toward the intrarenal collecting system. In the embryonic ureter and bladder, it is likely that epithelial-mesenchymal interactions are also important in the development of urothelium, lamina propria, and muscular compartments, but the exact nature of this induction process is unknown at this time.

Role of Renin-Angiotensin System in Ureteral Differentiation

One of the best-investigated mechanisms of ureteral development at the present time involves the AT_2 gene. AT_1 was found to be expressed in mature glomeruli and developing S-shaped bodies throughout the various stages of nephrogenesis. Both the temporal and spatial expression of AT_1 coincided with the differentiation and proliferation of glomerular mesangial and tubular cells. In contrast, AT_2 was expressed only in the mesenchymal cells adjacent to the stalk of the ureteric bud at early developmental stages and decreased markedly after birth. The role of the AT_2 gene in ureteral development was further elucidated in AT_2 gene knockout mice. These mice demonstrated a high incidence of congenital anomalies of the kidney and urinary tract (CAKUT), including ureteropelvic junction (UPJ)

obstruction, vesicoureteral reflux, ureterovesical junction obstruction, multicystic dysplastic kidney, hypoplastic kidney, and megaureter. It was speculated that CAKUT phenotypes may have been caused by delayed apoptosis in the undifferentiated mesenchymal cells surrounding the ureteric bud. These findings in AT_2 gene knockout mice are especially fascinating in light of the fact that AT_2 gene mutations were also found in a selected cohort of patients with UPJ obstruction and megaureter.

Development of Bladder and Continence Mechanism

By the 10th week, the bladder is a cylindrical tube lined by a single layer of cuboidal cells surrounded by loose connective tissue. The apex tapers as the urachus, which is contiguous with the allantois. By the 12th week, the urachus involutes to become a fibrous cord, which becomes the *median umbilical ligament*. The bladder epithelium consists of bilayered cuboidal cells between the 7th and 12th weeks, and it begins to acquire mature urothelial characteristics between the 13th and 17th weeks. By the 21st week, it becomes four to five cell layers thick and demonstrates ultrastructural features similar to the fully differentiated urothelium. Between the 7th and 12th weeks, the surrounding connective tissues condense and smooth muscle fibers begin to appear, first at the region of the bladder dome and later proceeding toward the bladder neck. Collagen fibers first appear in the lamina propria and then later extend into the deeper wall between the muscle fibers. Embryologically speaking, the bladder is composed of two regions: the trigone and the bladder body. The bladder body is derived from the endoderm-lined vesicourethral canal and the surrounding mesenchyme. The trigone has a different embryologic origin in that it develops from the incorporation of the common excretory ducts (the portion of mesonephric ducts caudal to the origin of the ureteric bud) into the base of the developing bladder.

Bladder compliance is thought to change during gestation. When studied in a whole organ preparation using fetal sheep bladders, bladder compliance is very low during early gestation and increases gradually thereafter. The mechanism of these changes in bladder compliance is not known but may involve alterations in both smooth muscle tone and connective tissue composition. This phenomenon is also observed in developing human bladders. These changes in compliance seem to coincide with the time of fetal urine production, suggesting a possible role for mechanical distention. Using fetal mouse bladders as organ culture explants, bladder distention promoted a more orderly development of collagen fiber bundles within the lamina propria in comparison to decompressed bladder explants, suggesting that mechanical factors from accumulating urine may play a role during bladder development.

The epithelial-mesenchymal inductive interactions appear to be necessary for orderly differentiation and proper development of the bladder. A modified Grobstein technique was applied to study the mechanism of bladder smooth muscle cell differentiation. Undifferentiated rat bladder epithelial and mesenchymal rudiments were separated prior to bladder smooth muscle cell differentiation and then recombined to grow within the immunologically compromised host (athymic nude mouse). In the presence of epithelial cells, the mesenchymal cells differentiated into smooth muscle cells with sequential expression of appropriate muscle markers, whereas, in the absence of epithelial cells, they involuted with evidence of apoptosis. The signaling mechanism for this inductive interaction is not known at this time.

No functional study has been done to assess the fetal continence mechanism. Only a handful of ontogenic descriptions are available using human fetal specimens, but these provide a basis for speculative theories. A mesenchymal condensation forms around the caudal end of the urogenital sinus after the division of the cloaca and the rupture of the cloacal membrane. Striated muscle fibers can be seen clearly by the 15th week. At this time, the smooth muscle layer becomes thicker at the level of bladder neck and forms the inner part of the urethral musculature. The urethral sphincter, composed of central smooth muscle fibers and peripheral striated muscle fibers, develops in the anterior wall of the urethra. Beyond this point, sexual dimorphism develops in conjunction with the formation of the prostate in males and the vagina in females. The urethral sphincter muscle fibers extend to the posterior wall of the urethra. In males, these fibers project to the lateral wall of the prostate, whereas in females, the muscle fibers attach to the lateral wall of the vagina.

Genital Development

Formation of Genital Ridges and Paramesonephric Ducts

During the fifth week, primordial germ cells migrate from the yolk sac along the dorsal mesentery to populate the mesenchyme of the posterior body wall near the 10th thoracic level. In both sexes, the arrival of primordial germ cells in the area of future gonads serves as the signal for the existing cells of the mesonephros and the adjacent coelomic epithelium to proliferate and form a pair of *genital ridges* just medial to the developing mesonephros (Fig. 16–16). During the sixth week, the cells of the genital ridge invade the mesenchyme in the region of future gonads to form aggregates of supporting cells called the *primitive sex cords*. The primitive sex cords will subsequently invest the germ cells and support their development.

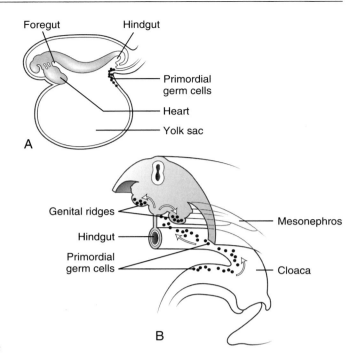

FIGURE 16–16 A, The site of the primordial germ cell origin in the wall of the yolk sac in a 3-week-old embryo. **B,** Migratory path of the primordial germ cells along the wall of the yolk sac and dorsal mesentery into the developing genital ridges. (Modified from Langman J, Sadler TW: Langman's Medical Embryology [5th ed]. Baltimore: Williams & Wilkins, 1985.)

The genital ridge mesenchyme containing the primitive sex cords is divided into the cortical and medullary regions. Both regions develop in all embryos, but, after the sixth week, they pursue different fates in the male and female.

During this time, a new pair of ducts, called the paramesonephric (müllerian) ducts, begins to form just lateral to the mesonephric ducts in both male and female embryos (Fig. 16–17). These ducts arise by the craniocaudal invagination of thickened coelomic epithelium, extending all the way from the third thoracic segment to the posterior wall of the developing urogenital sinus. The caudal tips of the paramesonephric ducts are adherent to each other as they connect with the urogenital sinus between the openings of the right and left mesonephric ducts. The cranial ends of the paramesonephric ducts form funnel-shaped openings into the coelomic cavity (the future peritoneum).

Development of Male Genital Structures

Under the influence of *SRY* (the sex-determining region of the Y chromosome; see Molecular Mechanism of Sexual Differentiation below), cells in the medullary region of the primitive sex cords begin to differentiate into *Sertoli cells*, while the cells of the cortical sex cords degenerate. Sex cord cells differentiate into Sertoli cells only if

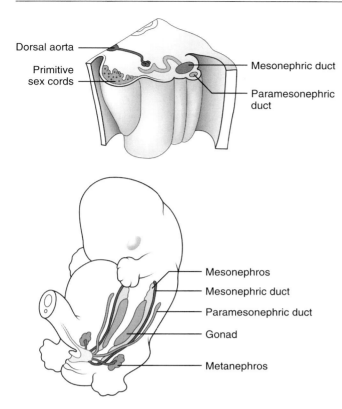

FIGURE 16–17 Formation of genital ridges and paramesonephric ducts. During the fifth and sixth weeks, the genital ridges form in the posterior abdominal wall just medial to the developing mesonephroi. The primordial germ cells induce the coelomic epithelial cells lining the peritoneal cavity and the cells of the mesonephros to proliferate and form the primitive sex cords. During the sixth week, the paramesonephric ducts develop lateral to the mesonephroi. The caudal tips of the paramesonephric ducts fuse with each other as they connect with the urogenital sinus. (Modified from Larsen WJ: Human Embryology [2nd ed]. New York: Churchill Livingstone, 1997.)

they contain the SRY protein; otherwise the sex cords differentiate into ovarian follicles. During the seventh week, the differentiating Sertoli cells organize to form the *testis cords*. These testis cords associated with germ cells eventually undergo canalization and differentiate into a system of seminiferous tubules. The testis cords distal to the presumptive seminiferous tubules also develop lumens and differentiate into a set of thin-walled ducts called the *rete testis*. Just medial to the developing gonad, the tubules of rete testis connect with 5 to 12 residual tubules of mesonephric ducts, called *efferent ductules*. The vas deferens develops from the mesonephric duct. At this time, the testicle begins to round up, and the degenerating cortical sex cords become separated from the coelomic (peritoneal) epithelium by an intervening layer of connective tissue called the *tunica albuginea* (Fig. 16–18).

As the developing Sertoli cells begin their differentiation in response to SRY, they begin to secrete a glycoprotein

hormone called *müllerian inhibiting substance* (MIS). MIS causes the paramesonephric (müllerian) ducts to regress rapidly between the 8th and 10th weeks. Small müllerian duct remnants can be detected in the developed male as a small tissue protrusion at the superior pole of the testicle, called the *appendix testis*, and as a posterior expansion of the prostatic urethra, called the *prostatic utricle*. MIS is absent in female embryos, so the müllerian ducts do not regress. Occasionally, genetic males have persistent müllerian duct structures (uterus and fallopian tubes), the condition known as *hernia uteri inguinale*. In these individuals, either MIS production by Sertoli cells is deficient or the müllerian ducts do not respond to normal MIS levels.

During the 9th and 10th weeks, Leydig cells differentiate from mesenchymal cells of the genital ridge in response to the SRY protein. These endocrine cells produce testosterone. At an early stage of development, testosterone secretion is regulated by placental chorionic gonadotropin, but eventually the pituitary gonadotropins assume control of androgen production. Between the 8th to 12th weeks, testosterone secretion by Leydig cells stimulates the mesonephric ducts to transform into the vas deferens. The cranial portions of the mesonephric ducts degenerate, leaving a small remnant of tissue protrusion called the *appendix epididymis*, and the region of mesonephric ducts adjacent to the presumptive testis differentiate into the epididymis. During the ninth week, 5 to 12 mesonephric ducts in the region of the epididymis make contact with the sex cords of the future rete testis. Meanwhile, the mesonephric tubules near the inferior pole of the developing testicle degenerate, sometimes leaving a remnant of tissue protrusion called the *paradidymis*.

The seminal vesicles sprout from the distal mesonephric ducts, whereas the prostate and bulbourethral glands develop from the urethra (Fig. 16–19). They therefore have different embryologic origins. The glandular seminal vesicles sprout from the mesonephric ducts near their attachment to the pelvic urethra during the 10th week. The portion of the vas deferens distal to the developing seminal vesicle is thereafter called the *ejaculatory duct*. The prostate gland also begins to develop during the 10th week as a cluster of endodermal evaginations budding from the pelvic urethra. These presumptive prostatic outgrowths are induced by the surrounding mesenchyme, and this process depends on the conversion of testosterone into dihydrotestosterone by 5α-reductase. The prostatic outgrowths initially form approximately five independent groups of solid prostatic cords. By the 11th week, these cords develop lumens and glandular acini, and by the 13th week, coincident with a rising testosterone level, the prostate begins its secretory activity. The mesenchyme surrounding the endoderm-derived prostatic acini differentiates into the smooth muscle and connective tissue of

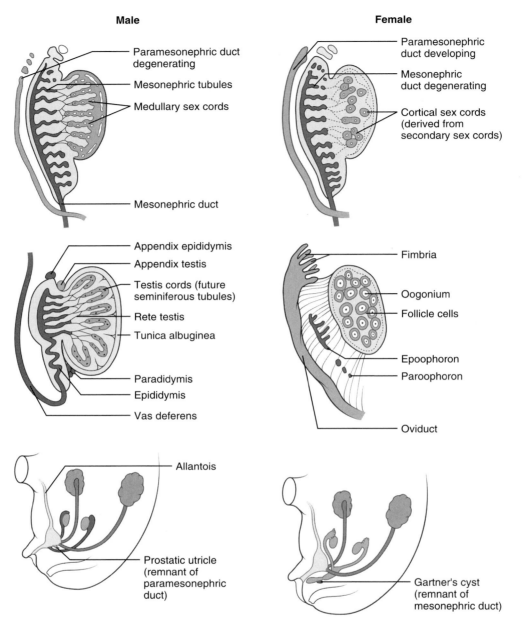

FIGURE 16–18 Male and female gonad and genital development. The male and female genital structures are virtually identical through the seventh week. In males, SRY protein produced by the Sertoli cells causes the medullary sex cords to become presumptive seminiferous tubules and causes the cortical sex cords to regress. Müllerian inhibiting substance (MIS) hormone produced by the Sertoli cells then causes the paramesonephric ducts to regress, leaving behind the appendix testis and prostatic utricle as remnants. The appendix epididymis and paradidymis arise from the mesonephric ducts. In females, cortical sex cords invest the primordial germ cells and become the ovarian follicles. In the absence of MIS hormone, the mesonephric ducts degenerate and the paramesonephric ducts give rise to the fallopian tubes, uterus, and upper vagina. The remnants of the mesonephric ducts are found in the ovarian mesentery as the epoophoron and paroophoron, and in the anterolateral vaginal wall as the Gartner's duct cysts. (Modified from Larsen WJ: Human Embryology [2nd ed]. New York: Churchill Livingstone, 1997.)

the prostate. As the prostate is developing, the paired bulbourethral glands sprout from the urethra just below the prostate.

Similar to renal and bladder development, prostatic development is dependent upon mesenchymal-epithelial interactions but under the influence of androgens. Studies using tissue recombination techniques have demonstrated that androgen receptor action in mesenchymal cells is essential for the induction of prostate and seminal vesicle development. This has led to the hypothesis that paracrine

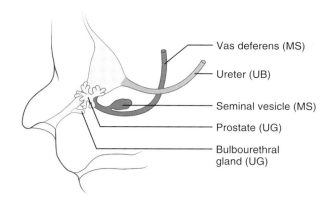

- Vas deferens (MS)
- Ureter (UB)
- Seminal vesicle (MS)
- Prostate (UG)
- Bulbourethral gland (UG)

FIGURE 16–19 Development of male accessory sex glands. During the 10th week, the seminal vesicles sprout from the distal mesonephric ducts in response to testosterone, whereas the prostate and bulbourethral glands develop from the urethra in response to dihydrotestosterone. Thus the vas deferens and seminal vesicle derive from the mesonephric ducts (MS), while the prostate and bulbourethral glands develop from the urogenital sinus (UG). *UB*, ureteric bud. (Modified from Larsen WJ: Human Embryology [2nd ed]. New York: Churchill Livingstone, 1997.)

factors, which are produced by the mesenchyme under the influence of androgens, may control the development of the male reproductive tract. The identity of these androgen-regulated paracrine factors, however, has not been elucidated. It was recently demonstrated using mutant mice that the Hox family of homeobox genes may be involved in the proper differentiation of male accessory sex glands. In particular, Hoxa-13 and Hoxd-13 transcription factors are expressed in both urogenital sinus and mesonephric ducts, and the loss-of-function mutation of these genes (knock out) results in agenesis of bulbourethral glands and defective morphogenesis of the prostate and seminal vesicles.

Development of Female Genital Structures

In female embryos, the primitive sex cords do not contain the Y chromosome, do not elaborate SRY protein, and therefore do not differentiate into Sertoli cells. In the absence of Sertoli cells and SRY protein, therefore, MIS synthesis, Leydig cell differentiation, and androgen production do not occur. Consequently, male development of the genital ducts and accessory glands is not stimulated, and female development ensues. In females, the primitive sex cords degenerate and the mesothelium of the genital ridge forms the secondary cortical sex cords. These secondary sex cords invest the primordial germ cells to form the ovarian follicles. The germ cells differentiate into oogonia and enter the first meiotic division as primary oocytes. The follicle cells then arrest further germ cell development until puberty, at which point individual oocytes resume gametogenesis in response to a monthly surge of gonadotropins (Fig. 16–18).

In the absence of MIS, the mesonephric (wolffian) ducts degenerate and the paramesonephric (müllerian) ducts give rise to the fallopian tubes, uterus, and upper two thirds of the vagina. The remnants of mesonephric ducts are found in the mesentery of the ovary as the epoophoron and paroophoron, and near the vaginal introitus and anterolateral vaginal wall as Gartner's duct cysts. The distal tips of the paramesonephric ducts adhere to each other just before they contact the posterior wall of the urogenital sinus. The wall of the urogenital sinus at this point forms a small thickening called the *sinusal tubercle*. As soon as the fused tips of the paramesonephric ducts connect with the sinusal tubercle, the paramesonephric ducts begin to fuse in a caudal-to-cranial direction, forming a tube with a single lumen. This tube, called the *uterovaginal canal*, becomes the superior portion of the vagina and the uterus. The unfused, superior portions of the paramesonephric ducts become the fallopian tubes (oviducts), and the funnel-shaped superior openings of the paramesonephric ducts become the infundibula.

While the uterovaginal canal is forming during the third month, the endodermal tissue of the sinusal tubercle in the posterior urogenital sinus continues to thicken, forming a pair of swellings called the *sinovaginal bulbs*. These structures give rise to the lower third of the vagina. The most inferior portion of the uterovaginal canal becomes occluded transiently by a block of tissue called the *vaginal plate*. The vaginal plate elongates between the third and fifth months and subsequently becomes canalized to form the inferior vaginal lumen.

As the vaginal plate forms, the lower end of the vagina lengthens, and its junction with the urogenital sinus migrates caudally until it comes to rest on the posterior wall of the definitive urogenital sinus (future vestibule of the vagina) during the fourth month. An endodermal membrane temporarily separates the vaginal lumen from the cavity of the definitive urogenital sinus. This barrier degenerates partially after the fifth month, but its remnant persists as the vaginal *hymen*. The mucous membrane that lines the vagina and cervix may also derive from the endodermal epithelium of the definitive urogenital sinus (Fig. 16–20).

Development of External Genitalia

The early development of the external genitalia is similar in both sexes. Early in the fifth week, a pair of swellings called *cloacal folds* develops on either side of the cloacal membrane. These folds meet just anterior to the cloacal membrane to form a midline swelling called the *genital tubercle*. During the cloacal division into the anterior urogenital sinus and the posterior anorectal canal, the portion of the cloacal folds flanking the opening of the urogenital

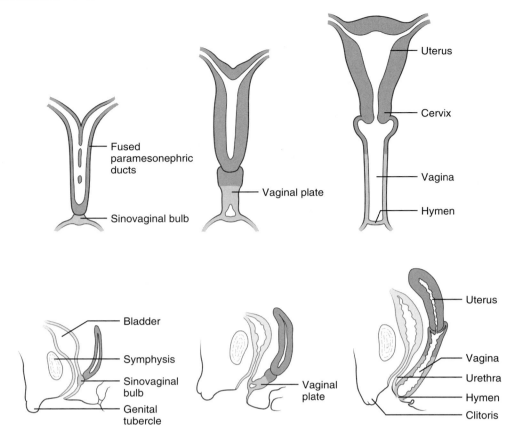

FIGURE 16–20 Development of uterus and vagina. During the 10th week, the paramesonephric ducts fuse at their caudal ends to establish a common channel and come into contact with a thickened portion of the posterior urogenital sinus called the sinovaginal bulb. This is followed by development of the vaginal plate, which elongates between the third and fifth month and becomes canalized to form the inferior vaginal lumen. (Modified from Langman J, Sadler TW: Langman's Medical Embryology [5th ed]. Baltimore: Williams & Wilkins, 1985.)

sinus becomes the *urogenital folds*, and the portion flanking the opening of the anorectal canal becomes the *anal folds*. A new pair of swellings, called the *labioscrotal folds*, then appears on either side of the urogenital folds (Fig. 16–21A).

The most popular hypothesis of external genital development is based upon work performed in the early part of this century. Inherent to this type of analysis is that many of the conclusions are speculative and unproven in terms of mechanistic validity. Most embryology texts today quote the mechanism of urethral development proposed by Glenister. The cavity of the urogenital sinus extends onto the surface of the enlarging genital tubercle in the form of an endoderm-lined *urethral groove* during the sixth week. This groove becomes temporarily filled by a solid endodermal structure called the *urethral plate*, but the urethral plate disintegrates and recanalizes to form an even deeper secondary groove. In males, this groove is relatively long and broad, whereas in females, it is shorter and more sharply tapered. In both sexes, an ectodermal *epithelial tag* is now present at the tip of the genital tubercle. The genital tubercle elongates to form the phallus, and a

primordium of the glans clitoris and glans penis is demarcated from the phallic shaft by a coronary sulcus. The appearance of the external genitalia is similar in male and female embryos until the 12th week.

Starting in the fourth month, the effects of dihydrotestosterone on the male external genitalia become readily apparent. The perineal region separating the urogenital sinus from the anorectal canal begins to lengthen. The labioscrotal folds fuse in the midline to form the scrotum, and the urethral folds fuse to enclose the penile urethra. The penile urethra is completely enclosed by the 14th week. However, because the urethral groove does not extend onto the glans of the penis, the penile urethra may exist transiently as a blind-ending tube. The formation of the distal glanular urethra may occur by a combination of two separate processes: the fusion of urethral folds proximally and the ingrowth of ectodermal cells distally (Fig. 16–21B). It is generally thought that the stratified squamous lining of the fossa navicularis results from an ingrowth of surface ectoderm as far proximally as the valve of Guérin. The lacuna magna (also known as the

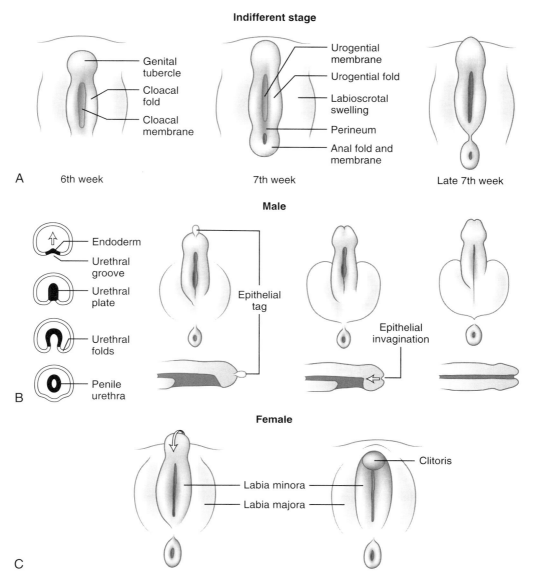

FIGURE 16–21 Development of external genitalia in male and female. **A,** The external genitalia derive from a pair of labioscrotal swellings, a pair of urogenital folds, and an anterior genital tubercle. Male and female genitalia are morphologically indistinguishable until the seventh week. **B,** In males, the urogenital folds fuse, and the genital tubercle elongates to form the penile shaft and glans. A small region of the distal urethra in the glans is formed by the invagination of surface epithelial tag. The fused labioscrotal folds give rise to the scrotum. **C,** In females, the genital tubercle bends inferiorly to form the clitoris, and the urogenital folds remain separate to become the labia minora. The unfused labioscrotal folds form the labia majora. (Modified from Larsen WJ: Human Embryology [2nd ed]. New York: Churchill Livingstone, 1997.)

sinus of Guérin), which can give symptoms of hematuria and dysuria in some boys, may form as a result of dorsal extension of this ectodermal ingrowth. It was suggested recently that the entire penile urethra might differentiate from the fusion of the urethral plate via the mechanism of epithelial-mesenchymal interactions.

In the absence of dihydrotestosterone, the primitive perineum does not lengthen, and the labioscrotal and urethral folds do not fuse across the midline in the female embryo. The phallus bends inferiorly, becoming the clitoris, and the definitive urogenital sinus becomes the vestibule of the vagina. The urethral folds become the labia minora, and the labioscrotal folds become the labia majora (Fig. 16–21C). The external genital develops in a similar manner in genetic males who are deficient in 5α-reductase and therefore lack dihydrotestosterone.

Gonadal Descent

During fetal development, the testes and the ovaries both descend from their original position near the 10th thoracic level. In both sexes, the initial descent of the gonads depends on a ligamentous cord structure called the *gubernaculum* (meaning "helm or rudder"). The testes complete their descent through the inguinal canal down to the scrotum, while the ovaries remain within the abdominal cavity. The mechanism of testicular descent is not known, but the most plausible theories of testicular descent in the human fetus are related to the development of the gubernaculum, processus vaginalis, inguinal canal, spermatic cord, and scrotum, because these structures differ substantially between male and female fetuses. Although it is not universally accepted that the gubernaculum "holds the key to the mystery of gonadal descent," the development of this structure in the male is unique in that it offers the most obvious explanation of why the fetal testicle descends to the scrotum while the ovary does not.

During the seventh week, the gubernaculum forms within the longitudinal peritoneal folds on either side of the vertebral column. The superior end of this cord is attached to the gonad, and its expanded inferior end, called the *gubernacular bulb*, is attached to the fascia between the developing external and internal oblique muscles in the region of the labioscrotal folds. At the same time, a slight evagination of the peritoneum, called the *processus vaginalis*, develops adjacent to the gubernacular bulb. The inguinal canal is a caudal evagination of the abdominal wall that forms when the processus vaginalis expands inferiorly, pushing out a "socklike" evagination through the abdominal wall layers. The first layer encountered by the processus vaginalis is the transversalis fascia, lying just deep to the transversus abdominis muscle. Next, the processus picks up the muscle fibers of the internal oblique muscle, which go on to become the cremasteric muscle of the spermatic cord. Finally, the processus picks up a thin layer of the external oblique muscle, which becomes the external spermatic fascia. In males, the inguinal canal extends down to the scrotum and allows the passage of the descending testicle. A complete inguinal canal also forms in females but appears to play no role in genital development. The processus vaginalis normally degenerates but occasionally remains patent, resulting in either a communicating hydrocele or indirect inguinal hernia. During the eighth week, the processus vaginalis begins to elongate caudally, carrying along the gubernacular bulb.

The testicles descend to the level of the internal inguinal ring by the third month and complete their descent into the scrotum between the seventh and ninth months. During the early period, the relative growth of the lumbar vertebral column is probably responsible for the intra-abdominal "descent" of the testicles, whose position is relatively fixed by the gubernacular anchoring near the inguinal canal. The testicles remain near the internal inguinal ring between the third and seventh months and later pass through the inguinal canal in response to the renewed "shortening" of the gubernaculum. This second phase of testicular descent appears to be a rapid process, probably occurring within a few days.

Once they pass through the inguinal canal, the testicles remain within the subserosal fascia of the processus vaginalis, through which they descend toward the scrotum. Further descent from the external inguinal ring to the dependent portion of the scrotum may take more than 4 to 6 weeks. By the ninth month, just before normal term delivery, most testicles have completely entered the scrotal sac, and the gubernaculum is reduced to a small ligamentous band attaching the inferior pole of the testis to the scrotal floor. The gonadotropins and androgens appear to have a role as well, although their target structures and mechanism of action remain undefined. It is generally accepted that the development of fetal spermatic vessels, vas deferens, and scrotum in regard to testicular descent is an androgen-dependent process, but this postulate has not been proven.

The ovaries also descend and become suspended within the broad ligaments of the uterus. As in males, the female embryo develops a gubernaculum-like structure extending initially from the inferior pole of the gonad to the subcutaneous fascia of the presumptive labioscrotal folds. This "female gubernaculum" later penetrates the abdominal wall as part of a fully formed inguinal canal and becomes the *round ligament*. In females, although the gubernaculum does not shorten as does that in males, it still causes the ovaries to descend during the third month (by anchoring the ovaries in the pelvis) and places them into a peritoneal fold (the *broad ligament of the uterus*). This translocation of ovaries appears to occur during the seventh week when the gubernaculum becomes attached to the developing paramesonephric (müllerian) ducts. As the paramesonephric ducts fuse together in their caudal ends, they sweep out the broad ligaments and simultaneously pull the ovaries into these peritoneal folds. In the absence of androgens, the female gubernaculum remains intact and grows in step with the rest of the body. The inferior gubernaculum becomes the round ligament of the uterus and attaches the fascia of the labia majora to the uterus, while the superior gubernaculum becomes the ligament of the ovary, connecting the uterus to the ovary. As in males, the processus vaginalis of the inguinal canal is normally obliterated, but occasionally it remains patent to become an indirect inguinal hernia.

Molecular Mechanism of Sexual Differentiation

Mammalian embryos remain sexually undifferentiated until the time of sex determination. When the Y-linked master regulatory gene, called *SRY*, is expressed in the male, the epithelial cells of the primitive sex cords differentiate into Sertoli cells, and this critical morphogenetic event triggers subsequent testicular development. Once the testicles are established, they produce androgens to give rise to the male phenotype. In the female gonads, no morphologic change is observable at the time of *SRY* expression. It follows from this general picture that, in mammals, sex determination is synonymous with testicle development, with the differentiation of Sertoli cells being the key event. It was thought that identification of the SRY

protein would rapidly lead to the identity of downstream elements regulating male sexual development. So far, however, the binding of SRY protein to other genes or factors has not been demonstrated, and the molecular mechanism by which genes interact to determine sex remains speculative (Fig. 16–22). It is now clear that only about 25% of sex reversals in humans can be attributed to disabling mutations of *SRY*. Indeed, chromosomal deletions of 9p and 10q as well as duplications of Xp can also lead to a female phenotype in XY individuals despite the intact *SRY*.

The activities of several new regulatory elements in male and female sexual differentiation have been described, including Wilms' tumor suppressor gene (*WT1*), steroidogenic factor-1 (*SF1*), SRY-related transcription factor-9

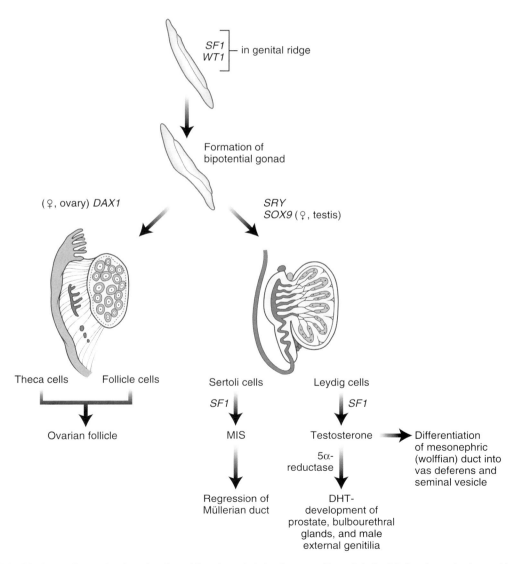

FIGURE 16–22 Molecular mechanism of male and female genital development. (From Schafer AJ: Sex determination and its pathology. Adv Genet 1995;33:275, with permission from Elsevier.)

(*SOX9*), and the *DAX1* gene. Humans heterozygous for mutations in the *WT1* gene exhibit abnormalities of the genital system in addition to abnormalities in renal development (see Molecular Mechanism of Kidney Development above) *WT1* is expressed within the genital ridges during the early gonad development in mouse and human embryos, prior to the expression of *SRY*. It has therefore been suggested that *WT1* directly or indirectly induced the expression of *SRY*. In females with *WT1* mutations, the gonads may consist of undifferentiated streaks of mesenchyme. In *Wt1* knockout mice, normal thickening of the genital ridge does not occur, even though primordial germ cells enter the presumptive gonadal tissue.

Translocation mapping of sex-reversed patients with camptomelic dysplasia (CD) led to the identification of the *SRY*-related gene SOX9. 46,XY individuals with heterozygous mutations in SOX9 show both CD and sex reversal, implicating SOX9 in both skeletal and sex determination. These individuals possess a normal *SRY* but may exhibit completely feminized genital structures. SOX9 is related to *SRY* and may be structurally similar. Its gene product therefore may bind to DNA in a manner similar to the SRY protein. SOX9 is expressed in differentiating Sertoli cells in male embryos of both mice and chickens.

SF-1 is an orphan nuclear receptor whose best known functions involve the regulation of steroid hydroxylase enzyme expression. This enzyme complex catalyzes multiple steps during the conversion of cholesterol to testosterone, and therefore SF-1 may play an important role in the steroidogenic function of the Leydig cells. *SF1* is expressed at an early stage of the genital ridge formation, and *SF1* gene knockout mice fail to develop gonads regardless of their genetic sex. These findings suggest that *SF1*, similar to *WT1*, shares a common pathway upstream of *SRY*, controlling the formation of the bipotential gonads. In addition, *SF1* is expressed in developing Sertoli cells, implying a male-specific role, and may be necessary in the activation of genes such as that for the MIS protein. As the bipotential gonad begins to differentiate, *SF1* expression is maintained in the testicles while it ceases in the ovaries.

The absence of functional *DAX1* gene induces adrenal hypoplasia congenita and hypogonadotrophic hypogonadism. *DAX1* maps to the human Xp21 region, which contains *DSS* (dosage-sensitive sex reversal), a locus that causes male-to-female sex reversal when duplicated. This situation occurs despite an intact, normal *SRY*. *DAX1* gene expression persists in the developing ovaries but rapidly decreases in the testicles. This implies a key role for *DAX1* in sex determination. Because this gene is not required for testicular development, it has been suggested that *DAX1* may function as an ovarian inducer. In fact,

SRY and *DAX1* may act antagonistically, and the precise degree and timing of their expression may be critical for the correct function of these genes during sex determination. According to this model, a single copy of *SRY* may be unable to counteract the effect of two active copies of *DAX1*, so that male-to-female sex reversal would occur, as observed in humans with a duplicate Xp21.

Bibliography

Alcaraz A, Vinaixa F, Tejedo-Mateu A, et al: Obstruction and recanalization of the ureter during embryonic development. J Urol 1991;145:410.

Baker LA, Gomez RA: Embryonic development of the ureter and bladder: acquisition of smooth muscle. J Urol 1998;160:545.

Bard JB, McConnell JE, Davies JA: Towards a genetic basis for kidney development. Mech Dev 1994;48:3.

Bardoni B, Zanaria E, Guioli S, et al: A dosage sensitive locus at chromosome Xp21 is involved in male to female sex reversal. Nat Genet 1994;7:497.

Baskin LS, Hayward SW, Young P, Cunha GR: Role of mesenchymal-epithelial interactions in normal bladder development. J Urol 1996;156:1820.

Baskin L, Meany D, Landsman A, et al: Bovine bladder compliance increases with normal fetal development. J Urol 1994;152(2 Pt 2):692; discussion 696.

Beauboeuf A, Ordille S, Erickson DR, Ehrlich HP: In vitro ligation of ureters and urethra modulates fetal mouse bladder explants development. Tissue Cell 1998;30:531.

Bourdelat D, Barbet JP, Butler-Browne GS: Fetal development of the urethral sphincter. Eur J Pediatr Surg 1992;2:35.

Chung LW, Cunha GR: Stromal-epithelial interactions: II. Regulation of prostatic growth by embryonic urogenital sinus mesenchyme. Prostate 1983;4:503.

Coplen DE, Macarak EJ, Levin RM: Developmental changes in normal fetal bovine whole bladder physiology. J Urol 1994;151:1391.

Cunha GR, Chung LW: Stromal-epithelial interactions—I. Induction of prostatic phenotype in urothelium of testicular feminized (Tfm/y) mice. J Steroid Biochem 1981;14:1317.

Davies JA, Bard JB: The development of the kidney. Curr Top Dev Biol 1998;39:245.

Davies JA, Brandli AW: The Kidney Development Database. Edinburgh, UK: University of Edinburgh, 1994. Available at *golgi.ana.ed.ac.uk/kidhome.html*

Foster JW, Dominguez-Steglich MA, Guioli S, et al: Camptomelic dysplasia and autosomal sex reversal caused by mutations in an SRY-related gene. Nature 1994;372:525.

Glenister TW: The origin and fate of the urethral plate in man. J Anat 1954;88:413.

Guron G, Adams MA, Sundelin B, Friberg P: Neonatal angiotensin-converting enzyme inhibition in the rat induces persistent abnormalities in renal function and histology. Hypertension 1997;29(1 Pt 1):91.

Hatini V, Huh SO, Harzlinger D, et al: Essential role of stromal mesenchyme in kidney morphogenesis revealed by targeted disruption of Winged Helix transcription factor BF-2. Genes Dev 1996;10:1467.

Hilgers KF, Reddi V, Krege JH, et al: Aberrant renal vascular morphology and renin expression in mutant mice lacking angiotensin-converting enzyme. Hypertension 1997; 29(1 Pt 2):216.

Hohenfellner K, Hunley TE, Schloemer C, et al: Angiotensin type 2 receptor is important in the normal development of the ureter. Pediatr Nephrol 1999;13:187.

Ikeda Y, Shen WH, Ingraham HA, Parker KL: Developmental expression of mouse steroidogenic factor-1, an essential regulator of the steroid hydroxylases. Mol Endocrinol 1994;8:654.

Kakuchi J, Ichicki T, Kiyama S, et al: Developmental expression of renal angiotensin II receptor genes in the mouse. Kidney Int 1995;47:140.

Karavanova ID, Dove LF, Resau JH, Perantoni AO: Conditioned medium from a rat ureteric bud cell line in combination with bFGF induces complete differentiation of isolated metanephric mesenchyme. Development 1996;122:4159.

Kim KM, Kogan BA, Massad CA, Huang YC: Collagen and elastin in the normal fetal bladder. J Urol 1991; 146(2 Pt 2):524.

Kispert A, Vainio S, Shen L, et al: Proteoglycans are required for maintenance of Wnt-11 expression in the ureter tips. Development 1996;122:3627.

Kluth D, Hillen M, Lambrecht W: The principles of normal and abnormal hindgut development. J Pediatr Surg 1995;30:1143.

Konje JC, Bell SC, Morton JJ, et al: Human fetal kidney morphometry during gestation and the relationship between weight, kidney morphometry and plasma active renin concentration at birth. Clin Sci 1996;91:169.

Koseki C, Herzlinger D, al-Awqati Q: Apoptosis in metanephric development. J Cell Biol 1992;119:1327.

Kreidberg JA, Sariola H, Loring JM, et al: WT-1 is required for early kidney development. Cell 1993;74:679.

Kurzrock EA, Baskin LS, Cunha GR: Ontogeny of the male urethra: theory of endodermal differentiation. Differentiation 1999;64:115.

Larsson L, Aperia A, Elinder G: Structural and functional development of the nephron. Acta Paediatr Scand Suppl 1983;305:56.

Lechner MS, Dressler GR: The molecular basis of embryonic kidney development. Mech Dev 1997;62:105.

Lipschutz JH: Molecular development of the kidney: a review of the results of gene disruption studies. Am J Kidney Dis 1998;31:383.

Lumbers ER: Functions of the renin-angiotensin system during development. Clin Exp Pharmacol Physiol 1995;22:499.

Luo X, Ikeda Y, Parker KL: A cell-specific nuclear receptor is essential for adrenal and gonadal development and sexual differentiation. Cell 1994;77:481.

Mackie GG, Stephens FD: Duplex kidneys: a correlation of renal dysplasia with position of the ureteric orifice. Birth Defects Orig Art Ser 1977;13:313.

McLaren A: Development of the mammalian gonad: the fate of the supporting cell lineage. Bioessays 1991;13:151.

Miyamoto N, Yoshida M, Kuratani S, et al: Defects of urogenital development in mice lacking Emx2. Development 1997;124:1653.

Moore MW, Klein RD, Farinas I, et al: Renal and neuronal abnormalities in mice lacking GDNF. Nature 1996; 382:76.

Morais da Silva S, Hacker A, Harley V, et al: Sox9 expression during gonadal development implies a conserved role for the gene in testis differentiation in mammals and birds. Nat Genet 1996;14:62.

Muscatelli F, Strom TM, Walker AP, et al: Mutations in the DAX-1 gene give rise to both X-linked adrenal hypoplasia congenita and hypogonadotropic hypogonadism. Nature 1994;372:672.

Nagata M, Nakauchi H, Nakayama K, et al: Apoptosis during an early stage of nephrogenesis induces renal hypoplasia in bcl-2-deficient mice. A J Pathol 1996;148:1601.

Newman J, Antonakopoulos GN: The fine structure of the human fetal urinary bladder. Development and maturation: a light, transmission and scanning electron microscopic study. J Anat 1989;166:135.

Nievelstein RA, van der Werff JF, Verbeek FJ, et al: Normal and abnormal embryonic development of the anorectum in human embryos. Teratology 1998;57:70.

Nishimura H, Yerkes E, Hohenfellner K, et al: Role of the angiotensin type 2 receptor gene in congenital anomalies of the kidney and urinary tract, CAKUT, of mice and men. Mol Cell 1999;3:1.

Patterson LT, Dressler GR: The regulation of kidney development: new insights from an old model. Curr Opin Genet Dev 1994;4:696.

Perantoni AO, Dove LF, Karavanova I: Basic fibroblast growth factor can mediate the early inductive events in renal development. Proc Natl Acad Sci U S A 1995;92:4696.

Pichel JG, Shen L, Sheng HZ, et al: Defects in enteric innervation and kidney development in mice lacking GDNF. Nature 1996;382:73.

Podlasek CA, Clemens JQ, Bushman W: Hoxa-13 gene mutation results in abnormal seminal vesicle and prostate development. J Urol 1999;161:1655.

Podlasek CA, Duboule D, Bushman W: Male accessory sex organ morphogenesis is altered by loss of function of Hoxd-13. Dev Dyn 1997;208:454.

Sanchez MP, Silos-Santiago I, Frisen J, et al: Renal agenesis and the absence of enteric neurons in mice lacking GDNF. Nature 1996;382:70.

Sanyanusin P, Schimmenti LA, McNoe TA, et al: Mutation of the gene in a family with optic nerve colobomas, renal anomalies and vesicoureteral reflux. Nat Genet 1996; 13:129.

Saxen L, Sariola H: Early organogenesis of the kidney. Pediatr Nephrol 1987;1:385.

Schuchardt A, D'Agati V, Larsson-Blomberg L, et al: Defects in the kidney and enteric nervous system of mice lacking the tyrosine kinase receptor Ret [see comments]. Nature 1994;367:380.

Schuchardt A, D'Agati V, Pachnis V, Costantini F: Renal agenesis and hypodysplasia in ret-k- mutant mice result from defects in ureteric bud development. Development 1996;122:1919.

Schutz S, Le Moullec JM, Corvol P, Gasc JM: Early expression of all the components of the renin-angiotensin system in human development [see comments]. Am J Pathol 1996;149:2067.

Schwarz R, Stephens FD: The persisting mesonephric duct: high junction of vas deferens and ureter. J Urol 1978;120:592.

Sedman AB, Kershaw DB, Bunchman TE: Recognition and management of angiotensin converting enzyme inhibitor fetopathy. Pediatr Nephrol 1995;9:382.

Shawlot W, Behringer RR: Requirement for Lim1 in head-organizer function [see comments]. Nature 1995; 374:425.

Shen WH, Moore CC, Ikeda Y, et al: Nuclear receptor steroidogenic factor 1 regulates the müllerian inhibiting substance gene: a link to the sex determination cascade. Cell 1994;77:651.

Shotan A, Widerhorn J, Hurst A, Elkayam U: Risks of angiotensin-converting enzyme inhibition during pregnancy: experimental and clinical evidence, potential mechanisms, and recommendations for use. Am J Med 1994;96:451.

Stark K, Vainio S, Vassileva G, McMahon AP: Epithelial transformation of metanephric mesenchyme in the developing kidney regulated by Wnt-4. Nature 1994;372:679.

Swain A, Narvaez V, Burgoyne P, et al: Dax1 antagonizes Sry action in mammalian sex determination. Nature 1998;391:761.

Tichy M: The morphogenesis of human sphincter urethrae muscle. Anat Embryol 1989;180:577.

Torres M, Gomez-Pardo E, Dressler GR, Gruss P: Pax-2 controls multiple steps of urogenital development. Development 1995;121:4057.

Vainio S, Lehtonen E, Jalkanen M, et al: Epithelial-mesenchymal interactions regulate the stage-specific expression of a cell surface proteoglycan, syndecan, in the developing kidney. Dev Biol 1989;134:382.

Vainio S, Muller U: Inductive tissue interactions, cell signaling, and the control of kidney organogenesis. Cell 1997;90:975.

van der Putte SC: Normal and abnormal development of the anorectum. J Pediatr Surg 1986;21:434.

Vukicevic S, Kopp JB, Luyten FP, Sampath TK: Induction of nephrogenic mesenchyme by osteogenic protein 1 (bone morphogenetic protein 7). Proc Natl Acad Sci U S A 1996;93:9021.

Weller A, Sorokin L, Illgen EM, Ekblom P: Development and growth of mouse embryonic kidney in organ culture and modulation of development by soluble growth factor. Dev Biol 1991;144:248.

CHAPTER 17

Applied Embryology of the Extremities

Loren J. Borud, M.D. and Joseph Upton, M.D.

Clinical Application

It is essential for a surgeon operating on the limbs to possess a thorough understanding of the functional anatomy of the extremities. Even if one does not specialize in surgical treatment of congenital disorders, a basic knowledge of fundamental embryology is useful to understand and remember the exquisitely complex anatomy of the adult extremity.

History

The history of embryology is no less than the history of the cultural, religious, and political philosophy of life itself. Although some records of embryologic history date as far back as the Assyrians and ancient Egyptians, the foundation of Western embryology is, not surprisingly, based on Aristotle, who wrote the first known text on the subject. *Embryology* is defined as the study of formation and development of organisms. Aristotle's theory crediting spontaneous generation of organisms was widely held until about 300 years ago—countered only by religious philosophy. The modern era of embryology was developed by Wolpert, who began asking basic questions about symmetry and pattern development and how they relate to events at the cellular and molecular level.

Development of the Limbs

Overview

Embryogenesis is defined as the period between fertilization and the completion of organogenesis. In the human, this encompasses the first 8 weeks following fertilization. Organogenesis occurs between the fourth and eighth weeks after conception. Most organs are completely developed by the time most pregnancies are first recognized. The organogenesis period is the time of greatest susceptibility to teratogenic agents. From the ninth week through the remainder of gestation, the "fetal period" is marked only by enlargement and differentiation of existing organ systems.

Limb formation begins with the activation of a group of mesenchymal cells in the somatic mesoderm of the lateral plate. Localization of fibroblast growth factor (FGF)-8 and retinoic acid in these cells is critical. Animal studies have demonstrated that, if this mesoderm is removed, a limb fails to form. If this mesoderm is transplanted to an ectopic location in the embryo, a supranumerary limb grows at that site. These animal experiments show that, at least in early limb development, the primary limb blueprint is in the mesoderm.

The first evidence of upper limb formation is the upper limb bud, which is evident at the fourth intrauterine week. This bud, known as "Wolff's crest," is apparent on the ventrolateral side of the embryo, extending from the 8th through the 12th myotomes, or the C6 through T2 vertebral levels. A thickened ridge of ectoderm (apical ectodermal ridge) forms along the anteroposterior plate of the apex of the limb. This ridge interacts with the underlying mesoderm to promote outgrowth of the developing limb. Injury to the apical ridge cells results in an arrest of limb development leading to distal truncation of the limb. As the limb bud begins to grow, the apical ridge produces FGF-2 and FGF-4. Abnormalities in local FGF have been recognized in mutations characterized by deficient or absent outgrowth of the limb.

The axillary fossa is seen as a small depression in the fifth week, accompanied by straightening and rotation in a supine direction. Apoptosis (programmed cell death) occurs in the portion of mesoderm destined to become the axillary fold. A flat, paddle-like structure known as the "hand plate" emerges by day 37. Vessels soon appear within the limb, supplying the ectodermal surface. Nerve trunks follow, and are in turn followed by muscle groups appearing around cartilage anlage. By about day 56, the pattern of the upper limb is complete in the 3-cm embryo (Fig. 17–1).

A well-developed vascular network supplies the mesoderm forming the early limb bud. There are no nerves in the early limb bud. These mesenchymal cells ultimately will give rise to the skeleton, connective tissue, and some small blood vessels. Mesenchymal cells that are derived from somites will migrate into the limb bud as precursors of muscle cells. Later, the neural crest contributes to migrating cells that form the Schwann cells of nerves and melanocytes.

Although the development of the upper and lower extremities involves similar mechanisms, the question of what determines the difference in form between arms and legs remains unanswered. Work with the homeobox (*HOX*)-containing gene reveals some difference of expression between arms and legs.

Development of Bones

Bone is the first major tissue to undergo specific differentiation in the limb. Bones of the extremity develop from cartilaginous precursors or anlage, which are initially clear, vascular "condensations" arising from mesenchymal cells during the fifth intrauterine week. These mesenchymal condensations begin in the central core of the proximal part of the limb bud. In comparison with the membranous bones of the cranial skeleton, the bones of the extremities are formed by replacing cartilage with bone in a process known as endochondral ossification. Of course, bone growth and remodeling continue—primarily at the growth plates—for some years following birth.

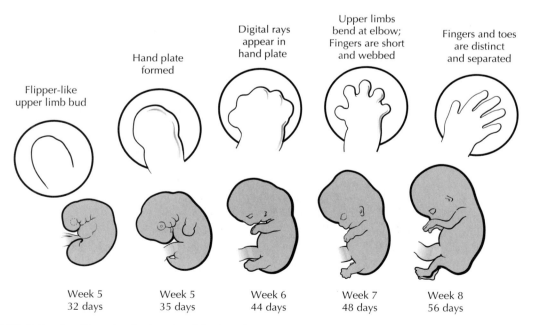

Flipper-like upper limb bud	Hand plate formed	Digital rays appear in hand plate	Upper limbs bend at elbow; Fingers are short and webbed	Fingers and toes are distinct and separated
Week 5 32 days	Week 5 35 days	Week 6 44 days	Week 7 48 days	Week 8 56 days

FIGURE 17–1 Drawings illustrating development of the limbs (32 to 56 days of gestation). (From Moore KL, Persaud TVN: The limbs. *In* Moore KL, Persaud TVN: The Developing Human: Clinically Oriented Embryology [6th ed]. Philadelphia: WB Saunders, 1998:436, with permission.)

The trapezium, trapezoid, and capitate are the only carpal bones that develop from analogous cartilaginous precursors, although none of the carpal bones begins to ossify until the postnatal period. The other bones of the carpus fuse in a complex process thoroughly described by meticulous dissections of aborted embryos in Prague in the late 1960s.

Joints are evident first as "interzones" or segmentations in the cartilaginous condensations. Transverse strips of dense cells grow across the cartilaginous condensations to split them. After the joint cavity forms, joint capsules and ligaments appear, followed by plates of hypertrophic chondrocytes that ultimately line the articular surfaces. Interestingly, in utero motion is required for normal joint development. Neurologic or mechanical restrictions in early development cause abnormal flat joints joined by stiff fibrous tissue.

The hand or foot "paddle" is a webbed structure that divides into the digits through a process of apoptosis that occurs in the "interzones" of the web spaces (Fig. 17–2). Recent work has implicated members of the bone morphogenic protein (BMP) family in this process.

The postaxial structures differentiate before the preaxial structures. Formation of the digits occurs first in the fifth and progresses to the first digit. The postaxial skeleton of the arm consists of the ulna digits 4 and 5 and the corresponding carpal elements. The preaxial skeleton includes the radius digits 1 through 3 and the corresponding carpal bones. Limb abnormalities known as hemimelias occur in which some or all of the preaxial or postaxial components of the limb may be missing.

The lower limb develops in an analogous manner, lagging the upper limb by about 2 to 3 days. Rotation of the lower limb is in the direction of pronation, allowing the plantar surface of the foot to be oriented posteriorly and inferiorly. The embryologic events of the first 8 weeks of life were classified by Streeter, who broke the process down into 23 stages of development. These range from stage 1 (fertilization) to stage 23, occurring at day 56 with a crown-rump length of 2.7 to 3.1 cm. This classic staging system is reproduced in Table 17–1.

Development of the Arterial System

The original vasculature of the limb bud originates from endothelial cells from several segmental branches of the aorta and cardinal vein. The original vasculature is only a fine capillary network, but rapidly some channels specifically enlarge to form the major vessels.

In the upper extremity, the subclavian artery can be seen entering the limb bud 3 weeks after conception (Fig. 17–3). A "median" artery continues down the midaxis of the limb. The ulnar artery can be identified by the sixth week, branching from the brachial artery. The radial artery develops later, and is therefore somewhat more variable in course. Ultimately, the median artery degenerates, only supplying vascularity to the median nerve in the adult.

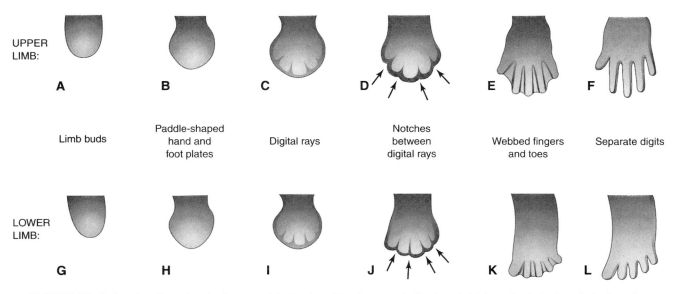

UPPER LIMB:

A   **B**   **C**   **D**   **E**   **F**

Limb buds   Paddle-shaped hand and foot plates   Digital rays   Notches between digital rays   Webbed fingers and toes   Separate digits

LOWER LIMB:

G   **H**   **I**   **J**   **K**   **L**

FIGURE 17–2 Drawings illustrating development of the hands and feet between the fourth and eighth weeks. **A,** 27 days. **B,** 32 days. **C,** 41 days. **D,** 46 days. **E,** 50 days. **F,** 52 days. **G,** 28 days. **H,** 36 days. **I,** 46 days. **J,** 49 days. **K,** 52 days. **L,** 56 days. (From Moore KL, Persaud TVN: The limbs. *In* Moore KL, Persaud TVN: The Developing Human: Clinically Oriented Embryology [6th ed]. Philadelphia: WB Saunders, 1998:437, with permission.)

Table 17-1
Streeter stages of human embryonic development

Stage	Age (days)	C-R Length*	Events
1			Fertilization
2			Zygote divides
3			Early blastocyte
4	6		Implantation begins
5	9–10		Complete blastocyte implantation
6	11–15		Primary villi
7	16–20		Notochord appears
8	20–21		Neural plate develops
9	21–22		Neural groove develops
10	23	2.0–3.5	Embryo straight; heart begins to beat
11	24–25	2.5–4.5	Embryo curved
12	26–27	3.0–5.0	Arm buds appear
13	28–31	4.0–6.0	Arm buds are flipper-like
14	32	5.0–7.0	Forelimbs are paddle shaped
15	33–36	7.0–9.0	Hand plates form
16	37–40	8.0–11.0	Foot plates form
17	41–43	11.0–14.0	Finger rays appear
18	44–46	13.0–17.0	Notches between finger rays
19	47–48	16.0–18.0	Fingers begin to separate
20	49–51	18.0–22.0	Fingers separate and elongate
21	52–53	22.0–24.0	
22	54–55	23.0–28.0	Toes separate and elongate
23	56	27.0–31.0	Head rounded

*Crown-rump length in millimeters.
Adapted from Upton J: Congenital anomalies of the hand and forearm. In McCarthy J, May JW, Littler JW (eds): Plastic Surgery, Vol VIII. Philadelphia: WB Saunders, 1990:5216.

From the original median artery, blood is distributed to the periphery via a capillary network. It then coalesces into a marginal sinus located beneath the apical ectodermal ridge. Later, the apical portions of the marginal sinus degenerate. The basilic and cephalic veins of the arm and the saphenous vein of the leg persist as the proximal channels of the remaining marginal sinus in adulthood.

Overall, the generalization can be made that arterial development occurs with significant access of vascular channels. These channels consistently change during limb development. Original channels may regress and new sprouts may come from previously existing channels. In addition, many sprouts may coalesce to form new vessels.

In the lower extremity, the primary axial artery evolves into the profundus femoris artery, which subsequently branches into the anterior and posterior tibial arteries (Fig. 17–4).

Development of the Peripheral Nerves

In lower vertebrates, there is a "one muscle–one nerve" correlation. In humans, however, spinal nerves intermingle in the brachial plexus, resulting in a complex pattern of innervation of the upper extremity. The brachial plexus, formed by the fourth week after conception, is exquisitely variable in humans, yet with certain consistent patterns. Sensory nerves derive from the neural tube, whereas motor neurons arise from neural crest tissue.

Motor axons from the spinal cord enter the limb bud at about the fifth week of development and preferentially

Development of the Arteries of the Upper Extremity

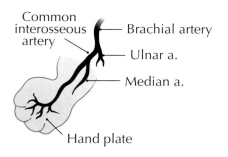

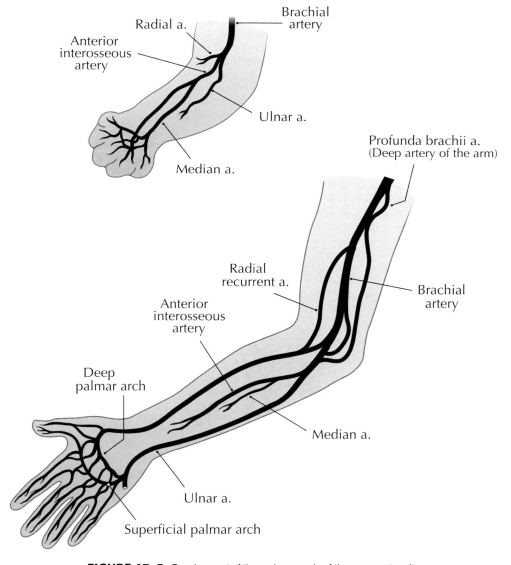

FIGURE 17–3 Development of the major vessels of the upper extremity.

Development of the Arteries of the Lower Extremity

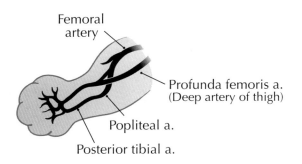

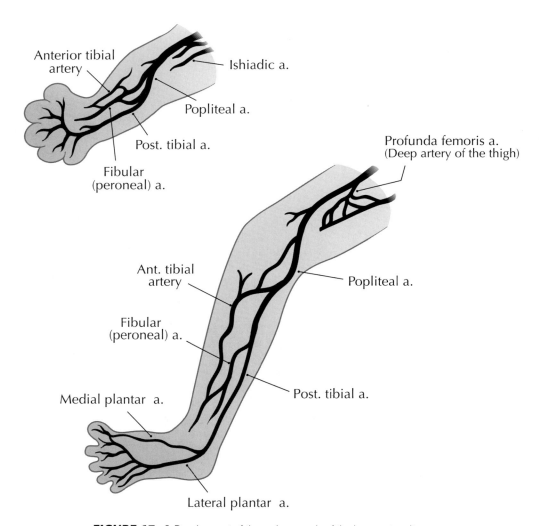

FIGURE 17–4 Development of the major vessels of the lower extremity.

grow into the dorsal and ventral muscle masses before individual muscle segmentation has occurred. Neurons located in the medial portions of the spinal cord send branches to the ventral muscle mass. Neurons located more laterally in the spinal cord supply the dorsal mass.

Mixed motor and sensory nerves enter the upper and lower limbs as "growth cones," following the path of major embryologic arteries. Once a branch of a nearby growing peripheral nerve innervates a muscle, the branch is then "pulled" and stretched distally by the growing muscle. However, muscles do not guide nerves to their destinations. Experiments in the avian limb bud show that destruction of somatic mesoderm, creating a muscleless limb, does not result in the absence of peripheral nerves. The major nerves develop normally, along the course of arteries, but simply lack branches to missing muscles.

Development of the sensory nerve axons occurs after the motor axons and appears to use them for directional guidance. Cells that are to become the Schwann cells (derived from the neural crest) that surround both the motor and sensory nerve fibers are added later. The growth pattern of the innervation of the adult limb has developed prior to formation of the digits.

Development of Muscles

Spinal segments known as somites split into three components: the sclerotome, which gives rise to vertebral segments and ribs; the dermatome, which provides for development of skin and fascia; and the myotome, which is responsible for muscle formation. In the developing limb, the dorsal "blastoma" ultimately forms the extensor muscles of the arm and the dorsiflexory muscles of the leg. The ventral "blastoma" forms the flexor muscles of the arm and the knee flexors and plantar flexors of the leg.

Proximal cells of the limb-forming area produce "scatter factor" (hepatic growth factor), which stimulates cells to leave the somite and migrate toward the limb. These migrating cells multiply to keep pace with the elongation of the limb bud. Division of the two common muscle masses, one the precursor of the flexor muscles and the other giving rise to the extensor muscles, is poorly understood. The division of muscles into anatomically recognizable precursors of the ultimate limb muscles occurs somewhere in the sixth and seventh week.

Tendons develop separately from their muscle bellies and ultimately fuse together in a poorly understood process. This explains why, in cases of some congenital disorders, distal tendons may adhere to the nearest bone, tendon, or fascial layer. Tendons that do not reach their muscle companions degenerate.

In the hand and foot, the intrinsic muscles have exceedingly complex origins and developmental patterns that are beyond the scope of this chapter. This is the most rich and interesting part of limb muscle development. Tissues from five embryonic muscle layers fuse in a logical but complex fashion to form the intrinsic muscles of the distal extremities.

Basic Events in Limb Development

Overview of Molecular Biology of Limb Development

Rapid advances in molecular biology have led to a number of incredible insights into the basic events that determine limb development. This work is based almost completely on animal models, starting from zebra fish, crickets, and newts, which are known to regenerate severed limbs or fins. The most widely used vertebrate models today are the mouse and the chick. Research using transgenic and knockout mouse has led to countless interesting strains of limb deformities, and these strains are ideal for creating "gain-of-function" and "loss-of-function" models for specific genes. Chick embryos are easy to manipulate in ovo, offering endless opportunities to study the developing limb.

The classic model of limb development, the so-called progress zone model, is a good starting point for understanding the developing limb. This model holds that there is a crucial, moving zone of action in the limb bud. The length of time a cell remains in this progress zone determines its differentiation and ultimate position. This accounts for patterning, segmentation, and differentiation of tissues from progenitor cells.

Limb bud–forming potential exists all along the lateral mesoderm of the embryo. Genes crucial in early limb bud formation include *FGF10*, *SNAIL*, and *TWIST*. The *PITX* and *TBX4* and *TBX5* genes seem to be involved in determination of upper versus lower limb morphology.

The terminal portion of the growing limb bud is covered by a tough cap of ectoderm known as the apical ectodermal ridge (AER). The total truncation of limb growth that results from removal of the AER can be rescued using a FGF-4 bead, although FGF-4 is now known not to be essential for development. There are currently over 24 known members in the *FGF* gene superfamily, many of which are known to act in complex interplay in the AER.

The Three Dimensions of Limb Development

Nature rigidly divides the genetic responsibility for the three spatial dimensions of limb development into three axes of genetic action. The *HOX* genes are a gene superfamily that, in large part, determines the proximal-distal limb pattern. For example, *HOXD13* is active in formation of the terminal digits. In the first published description of human mutation associated with a limb deformity, a *HOXD13* mutation was shown to be responsible for a large series of complex synpolydactyly in a Portuguese family settled in the Boston area.

The *anterior-posterior axis* of the extremities is the term biologists use to describe what surgeons might refer to as the radial-ulnar axis of the hand or the tibial-fibular axis of the foot. What determines a great toe or thumb versus a small toe or finger? The posterior zone of the limb bud (i.e., the ulnar or fibular side) was found in early transplant experiments to contain an area that, if transplanted to the anterior side, caused a posteriorizing influence such as a "mirror hand." This "zone of polarizing activity" works in this manner as a result of expression of a soluble protein known as "sonic hedgehog" (Shh). The gene for Shh is vital to pattern formation in almost all organisms, explaining its remarkable phylogenetic conservation in species from the zebra fish to the human.

Dorsal-ventral polarity is the last of the three spatial axes to note. In the hand, surgeons would refer to this as the dorsal-volar axis or the dorsal-palmar axis. In the foot, the term would be the dorsal-plantar axis. Cell labeling studies have shown that no cell in the developing embryo crosses the dorsal-ventral border. Molecular biologists have shown that the engrailed-1 gene (*En1*) is strictly expressed in the ventral compartment, and is controlled by members of the BMP superfamily. *En1* suppresses expression of *Wnt7a*. Unopposed *Wnt7a* activity results in a dorsalizing influence.

Anomalies of the Limb

Most anomalies of the limb are relatively minor and can be corrected surgically. These minor defects, however, should be considered as indicators of other coexisting anomalies that may be part of a recognizable syndrome.

Severe limb anomalies occur with the use of thalidomide, a drug commonly used by pregnant women as anti-nauseant in the late 1950s. Exposure to this drug before gestational day 32 caused severe anomalies such as the absence of limbs or the hands. Exposure to thalidomide at a later period resulted in absence or hypoplasia of the thumb. It should be noted that the most critical period for limb development is from the 24th to the 32nd days after fertilization, a period when most women are unaware they are pregnant.

Cutaneous syndactyly (simple webbing of digits) is a result of the failure of apoptosis to degenerate the tissue between digits. Osseous syndactyly, however, occurs when the notches between the digital rays fail to develop during the seventh week. Syndactyly is most frequently observed between the third and the fourth finger and between the second and third toe. Suppression of limb bud development in the early part of the fourth week results in absence of the limb (amelia). A disturbance of growth or differentiation

during the fifth week results in partial absence of a limb (meromelia). Cleft hand and cleft foot result when one or more digital rays fail to develop and a central cleft results. The remaining digits are usually partially or completely fused, resulting in a lobster-like clawhand. Failure of the mesenchymal primordium of the radius to form during the fifth week results in congenital absence of the radius. As the ulna (derived from a separate mesenchymal primordium) grows, it becomes bowed and a concavity develops on the lateral side of the forearm.

Conclusion

Knowledge of embryology of the limbs is vital to any surgeon operating on the extremities. In addition to understanding congenital disorders, it provides a road map to explain and organize the anatomy of these complex regions. Advances in molecular biology have shed light on the basic events controlling limb development. As time passes, more and more human deformities and syndromes of the limbs will be understood in molecular terms. This area of academic endeavor provides a new and fertile realm for surgical researchers and basic scientists.

Bibliography

Cihak R: Connections of the abductor pollicis longus and brevis in the ontogenesis of the human hand. Folia Morphol (Praha) 1972;20:102.

Cihak R: Differentiation and rejoining of muscular layers in the embryonic human hand. Birth Defects 1977;13:97.

Moore KL, Persaud TVN: The limbs. *In* Moore KL, Persaud TVN: The Developing Human: Clinically Oriented Embryology (6th ed). Philadelphia: WB Saunders, 1998:436.

Muragaki Y, Mundlos S, Upton J, Olsen BR: Altered growth and branching pattens in synpolydactyly caused by mutations in HOXD13. Science 1997;275:408.

Niswander L, Tickle C, Vogel A, et al: FGF-4 replaces the apical ectodermal ridge and directs outgrowth and patterning of the limb. Cell 1993;75:579.

Saunders JW: The experimental analysis of chick limb bud development. *In* Ede DA, Hinchliffe JR, Ballis M (eds): Vertebrate Limb and Somite Morphogenesis. Cambridge, UK: Cambridge University Press, 1977:23.

Summerbell D, Lewis JH, Wolpert L: Positional information in chick-limb morphogenesis. Nature 1973;244:492.

Upton J: Congenital anomalies of the hand and forearm. *In* McCarthy J, May JW, Littler JW (eds): Plastic Surgery, Vol VIII. Philadelphia: WB Saunders, 1990:5216.

Wolpert L: Positional information and the spatial pattern of cellular differentiation. J Theor Biol 1969;25:1.

Zou H, Niswander L: Requirement of BMP signaling in interdigital apoptosis and scale formation. Science 1996;272:738.

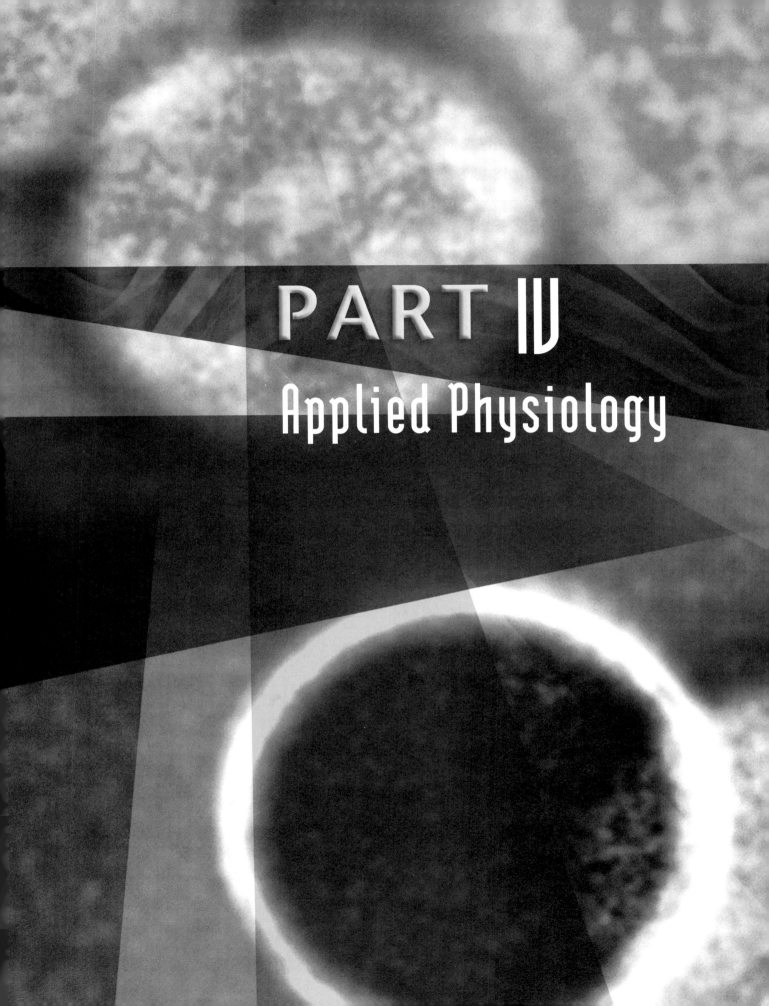

PART IV
Applied Physiology

CHAPTER 18

Fundamentals of Neurophysiology and Neurodysfunction

Rebekah C. Austin, M.D. and John A. Wilson, M.D.

▶ Electrical Signaling in the Nervous System
▶ Synapses and Neurotransmitters
▶ Cerebral Blood Flow
▶ Brain Metabolism
▶ The Blood-Brain Barrier
▶ Cerebrospinal Fluid System
▶ Brain Function and Integration
▶ Bibliography

Having a basic understanding of central nervous system physiology is an essential part of surgical training. Many disease processes can have neurologic signs or symptoms as part of their presentation or natural history, and it is important to identify these and determine what significance they have when deciding upon a course of treatment. The brain and spinal cord are unique because structure and function are so intimately related. Although computed tomography scans and magnetic resonance imaging are readily available, lesion localization may often be obvious based on history and physical examination. Global changes in cognition, however, may result from numerous disease processes, including infection, metabolic disturbances, hydrocephalus, psychosis, polypharmacy, and trauma.

This chapter serves to introduce general concepts of neurophysiology. It is not intended to be a comprehensive review. The goal is to provide a framework for understanding cerebral blood flow, cerebrospinal fluid (CSF) dynamics, neuronal conduction and synapses, metabolism, and the basic architecture and function of normal central nervous system components. This will provide the most utility in formulating broad differential diagnoses, choosing diagnostic modalities, and interpreting their results.

Electrical Signaling in the Nervous System

The function of the nervous system requires at its most basic level the initiation and conduction of electrical signals. These electrical signals are not conveyed by electrons traveling along wires, as is seen in electrical systems we encounter in our normal lives. The movement of inorganic ions across polarized cell membranes causes electrical signaling in the nervous system. Neurons are the basic cellular elements of the nervous system primarily concerned with electrical signaling. The membranes of all cells, including neurons, are structured such that there is an electrical potential across the cell membrane. Cells are polarized, with the interior of the cells being negatively charged. The potential that exists across the cell membrane when the cell is in its steady state is called the resting membrane potential.

The cell membrane is highly permeable to most inorganic ions but largely impermeable to most organic ions, such as proteins. There are two basic constraints affecting the distribution of ions across the cell membrane: (1) both the intracellular and extracellular matrix must be electrically neutral; and (2) the osmotic concentration within the cell must be equal to that of the extracellular fluid. The electrical potential of cells is the result of differential concentrations of ions on either side of the cell membrane. Inorganic ions will try to cross the cell membrane along a gradient from higher concentration to lower concentration. Given the high permeability of the cells to inorganic ions, the ionic gradient must be maintained by ionic pumps in the cellular membrane.

The equilibrium potential for an ion is the electrical potential at which the electrical force driving the ion in one direction across the cell membrane equals the

$$E_X = \frac{RT}{nF}\ \log_{10}\ \frac{[x]_0}{[x]_1}$$

E_X = Equilibrium potential for ion X
R = Gas constant
T = Absolute temperature
n = Ionic valance
F = Faraday constant (relates charge in coulombs to concentration in moles)
$[x]_0$ = Concentration of ion in cell
$[x]_1$ = Concentration of ion outside the cell

FIGURE 18–1 The Nernst equation.

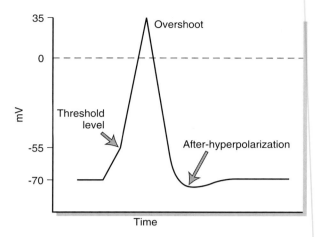

FIGURE 18–2 Action potential.

chemical force driving it in the opposite direction. The equilibrium potential for any given ion can be calculated by the Nernst equation (Fig. 18–1). The sum of the equilibrium potentials of all the ionic constituents of the cell is the resting membrane potential of the cell. This resting membrane potential is negative; the interior of the cell is negatively charged relative to the extracellular space. If the permeability of the cell membrane changes, there will be a resultant change in the resting membrane potential. This process is the basis for electrical signaling in the nervous system.

Two types of electrical signaling occur in the nervous system, localized potentials and action potentials. Localized potentials can occur as a response to a sensory receptor or as a result of synaptic transmission. Receptor potentials are localized potentials occurring at sensory receptors. These sensory receptors can transduce mechanical, thermal, or chemical stimulation into electrical signals. Localized potentials travel only over short distances, whereas action potentials can be conducted over much longer distances. Localized potentials are graded, meaning that the magnitude of the electrical potential is proportional to the magnitude of the stimulus. The effect of the stimulus is also additive, such that repeated stimuli over a short time span can result in a greater magnitude of the localized potential. If the magnitude of the localized potential reaches a certain threshold, an action potential is generated.

An action potential is a sequence of events that results in the propagation of an electrical impulse (Fig. 18–2). It is what allows the rapid transmission of electrical signals over long distances in the nervous system. The first phase of an action potential requires the depolarization of the cellular membrane. This depolarization occurs as a result of a localized graded potential as noted above. If the depolarization reaches a certain threshold (about 15 mV), the firing level is reached. When this firing level, also known as the threshold potential, is reached, there is a dramatic increase in the rate of depolarization related to a change in the membrane permeability. The generation of the action potential is an all-or-none phenomenon. Once the

threshold level is reached, the action potential will proceed to its completion. The rapid rate of depolarization results in an overshoot of the zero potential by about 35 mV. The process then reverses and the cell repolarizes. The rate of repolarization is initially quite rapid but then slows. During most of the depolarization and repolarization phases, the cell is refractory to the propagation of further action potentials. As the membrane potential returns towards its resting level, there is a variable period of hyperpolarization. During this period, a higher local potential is necessary to allow the cell to reach the threshold potential and trigger an action potential.

Action potentials can be conducted over relatively long distances in the nervous system by nerve fibers. There are three broad categories of nerve fibers, which can be further subdivided (Table 18–1). A fibers are large myelinated fibers with high conduction velocities. B fibers are smaller myelinated fibers that conduct signals relatively slowly.

Table 18–1
Nerve fiber types

Fiber Type	Function
Alpha	Motor, proprioception
Beta	Touch, pressure
Gamma	Motor to muscle spindles (intrafusal)
Delta	Pain and temperature, fine touch
B	Preganglionic autonomic
Sensory (dorsal root)	Pain, reflex
Motor (postganglionic autonomic)	Postganglionic autonomic

C fibers, the smallest fibers, are unmyelinated and have the slowest conduction velocities.

Myelinated fibers are able to conduct electrical signals at much higher speed than unmyelinated fibers. The process that allows myelinated axons to conduct impulses so much more rapidly is called saltatory conduction. The myelin sheath on an axon acts as an electrical insulator, permitting very little current flow. However, along the course of the axon there are periodic gaps in the myelin sheath called nodes of Ranvier. In saltatory conduction, the action potential jumps from node to node, resulting in a much higher conduction velocity.

Synapses and Neurotransmitters

Synapses, or functional connections between neurons, are a vital part of understanding neural conduction. These highly specialized clefts are responsible for conducting an impulse in a particular direction, blocking an impulse, or participating in impulse modulation based on the summation of information received in a temporal or spatial fashion. A typical synaptic cleft is 20 to 30 nm wide and separates a presynaptic terminal from a postsynaptic terminal. In the mammalian central nervous system, chemical synapses are predominant. Electrical synapses, which are formed by gap junctions in cardiac and smooth muscle, are rarely found in neural tissue.

Presynaptic terminals are the axonal end point for a propagated depolarization impulse. These areas are rich in mitochondria and contain synaptic vesicles, each filled with a quantum of specific neurotransmitter. Numerous voltage-gated calcium channels are opened by membrane depolarization at the axon terminus. This influx of calcium results in neurotransmitter vesicles fusing with the presynaptic membrane and releasing their quanta into the synaptic cleft. These molecules diffuse readily and bind receptors on the postsynaptic and presynaptic terminals to effect a response.

Postsynaptic terminals may be present on neuron cell bodies, axons, dendrites, or an effector organ such as a muscle cell or sweat gland. The membrane of postsynaptic terminals is studded with receptors that bind neurotransmitters in a reversible fashion. These receptors may be linked with intracellular second messengers such as cyclic AMP or G proteins. Both temporal and spatial summation may occur to increase or decrease a postsynaptic membrane potential relative to its threshold potential. When the postsynaptic membrane potential increases (hyperpolarization), a greater stimulation is required to reach threshold potential. This is called an inhibitory postsynaptic potential. This occurs when the localized membrane permeability is increased to potassium and chloride ions but not to

sodium ions. This results in an influx of negatively charged chloride ions and an efflux of positively charged potassium ions. The net result of these ionic shifts is to increase or hyperpolarize the negative resting membrane potential. An excitatory postsynaptic potential occurs when there is a decrease in the resting membrane potential of the postsynaptic cell membrane, bringing it closer to the threshold potential. This occurs when binding of the synaptic transmitter to receptors on the postsynaptic cell membrane opens gated channels locally within the membrane, which increases permeability to sodium, potassium, and chloride ions. With sodium having the highest concentration gradient, the net effect is that positive sodium ions move into the cell, resulting in depolarization of the cell. As more postsynaptic receptors are stimulated, more gated channels are opened in the cell membrane, and the resultant depolarization causes the cell membrane potential to approach the threshold potential. Once threshold is reached, depolarization occurs and an action potential is generated.

Over 40 neurotransmitters have been identified. They consist of small proteins, peptides, amines, and amino acids. Each axon terminus synthesizes only one type of neurotransmitter. Many antidepressant and antipsychotic medications have been developed that change the milieu of selected neurotransmitters such as serotonin or norepinephrine in brain tissue.

Acetylcholine is the most widely studied central nervous system neurotransmitter and is found in motor neurons, sympathetic and parasympathetic neurons, caudate nucleus, and adrenal medulla (Table 18–2). It is excitatory and acts on nicotinic and muscarinic receptors

Table 18–2 Common neurotransmitters	
Neurotransmitter	**Localization in Nervous System**
Acetylcholine (Ach)	Neuromuscular junction, caudate nucleus, putamen, limbic system, parasympathetic neurons, autonomic ganglia, motor ganglia of cranial nerves
Norepinephrine (NE)	Sympathetic nervous system, lateral tegmentum, locus ceruleus
Dopamine (DA)	Midbrain, nigrostriatal pathways, hypothalamus
Serotonin (5-HT)	Pineal gland, raphe nuclei of pons, parasympathetic neurons in gut
γ-Aminobutyric acid (GABA)	Cerebellum, hippocampus, cortex, nigrostriatal pathways

linked to G proteins. Excessive acetylcholine, as caused by exposure to organophosphates or black widow spider venom, results in profuse salivation, tearing, sweating, and urination. Functional acetylcholine deficiency has been associated with Alzheimer's disease, myasthenia gravis, and exposure to botulinum toxin.

Cerebral Blood Flow

The average brain constitutes 2% of the body's weight; however, it receives 17% to 20% of the cardiac output and utilizes 20% of the body's oxygen. The vessels responsible for maintaining cerebral blood flow are the paired carotid and vertebral arteries. The carotid system supplies the anterior circulation, including the majority of the cerebral hemispheres. The vertebral system supplies the posterior circulation, including the brainstem and cerebellum, but also contributes blood flow to the occipital and mesial temporal lobes. Multiple anastomoses are also present that provide retrograde flow in advanced disease states.

The common carotid arteries emerge in the thorax from the aortic arch on the left and the brachiocephalic (innominate) bifurcation on the right. These vessels continue a cephalad course under the sternocleidomastoid muscle toward the angle of the mandible. The common carotids divide into two terminal branches (internal and external carotids) at a variable level in the neck. The baroreceptive carotid body and chemoreceptive carotid sinus are found in the region of this bifurcation. The external carotid artery (ECA) has numerous branches supplying cervical and facial structures, whereas the larger internal carotid artery (ICA) ascends without branching until it enters the temporal bone at the base of the skull.

The ICA courses anteriorly through the cavernous sinus. Numerous named branches supply the pituitary, tentorium, anterior thalamus, and internal capsule. Terminal branches of the ICA are the anterior cerebral artery (ACA) and middle cerebral artery (MCA). The medial frontal and parietal lobes are supplied by the ACA, along with subcortical structures such as the hypothalamus, optic apparatus, fornix, and caudate nucleus. The MCA supplies the lateral frontal, temporal, and parietal lobes as well as the internal capsule, putamen, and globus pallidus. Branch points of the major intracranial arteries are the most common location of intracranial aneurysm formation.

Paired vertebral arteries arise from the subclavian arteries and ascend through the foramina transversarium of vertebral levels C6 through C2 before entering the skull base through the foramen magnum. The arteries join there, forming the basilar artery, which courses anteriorly along the clivus and supplies the pons, midbrain, and cerebellum. The basilar artery divides into two posterior cerebral arteries, which irrigate the posterior thalamus and occipital and mesial temporal lobes.

Normal cerebral blood flow is 50 mL/100 mg/min. Neurons will survive but not function at flows of 8 to 23 mL/100 mg/min. This is clinically relevant because the brain parenchyma adjacent to an area of infarct may be impaired but may potentially recover function if its vascular supply is promptly restored. This area is referred to as the "ischemic penumbra" during acute stroke states. At flow rates less than 8 mL/100 mg/min, neurons are irreparably injured, resulting in cell death and permanent neurologic deficits.

Numerous anastomotic channels provide some relief in ischemic states typically caused by advanced atherosclerotic disease. Examples include supply of the ophthalmic artery of the anterior circulation by way of the angular branch of the facial artery or middle meningeal artery, both of ECA derivation. Similarly, the vertebral arteries may augment flow from ECA branches such as the occipital or ascending pharyngeal artery. Persistent fetal-type connections between the carotid and vertebrobasilar systems are present in up to 20% of the population and may provide alternative sources of blood flow. The most common of these is the persistence of a large posterior communicating artery.

Brain Metabolism

Neural tissue is metabolically expensive to maintain. In addition to constitutive cellular proteins, neurons and glial tissue must vigilantly preserve chemical and electrical gradients essential for proper functioning. The synthesis, storage, release, and reuptake of neurotransmitters are also highly energy-dependent processes. Usable energy in the form of ATP is generated by oxidative metabolism of glucose supplied by the liver or muscle. The ultimate by-products of this metabolism are carbon dioxide and water.

Under normal physiologic conditions, consumption of oxygen may reach 35 to 70 mL/min. This is generally 20% of the entire body's utilization for an organ that comprises 2% of the body's mass. Although the brain may transiently increase oxygen extraction from the blood stream as a compensatory mechanism, this is a short-lived response, and oxygen deprivation for more than 3 to 8 minutes may result in permanent cell injury or death.

Regional cerebral blood flow is closely coupled to functional demand. As neuronal activity increases, the metabolic needs of that region of the brain are also increased. These increased metabolic demands are met by increasing regional blood flow. This can be demonstrated during functional positron emission tomography scanning when regional blood flow increases are consistently seen in areas of cerebral functional activity, representing an increased metabolic demand coupled with an instantaneous increase in substrate delivery.

Glucose enters the cells by facilitated carrier-mediated transport. Glycolysis takes place in the cell cytoplasm, forming the intermediate product pyruvate. Anaerobic conditions yield two ATP molecules per molecule of glucose, which is insufficient energy generation to meet the metabolic needs of a neuron. When oxygen is present, pyruvate enters the mitochondria and is completely oxidized to carbon dioxide and water, yielding 38 molecules of ATP per molecule of glucose.

Cerebral metabolic demand may be increased by mental or physical exercise, seizures, injury, or elevated core body temperature. Increased cerebral blood flow usually provides increased oxygen and glucose to meet this increased demand. In a similar way, phosphocreatine, ketone bodies, and dicarboxylic acids may be used during short periods of inadequate glucose supply. Reduced rates of metabolism are found in sleep or coma states, with hypothermia, and under barbiturate-induced coma.

As a conservation mechanism, a separation exists between functional and basal activity in the brain. Functional energy usage, reflected by electrical activity detectable by electroencephalography, represents 60% of total energy expenditure, whereas basal energy usage is roughly 40%. During times of short substrate supply, neurons may reduce their energy consumption by up to 60% by reducing or eliminating functional electrical activity in favor of maintaining cell integrity and survival. Clinicians may take advantage of this property by placing a severely head-injured patient under barbiturate-induced coma to reduce cerebral metabolism, subdue the increasing cerebral blood flow, and provide analgesia. These efforts aim to manage elevated intracranial pressure and preserve neuronal tissue to achieve the highest possible level of neurologic functional outcome.

The Blood-Brain Barrier

The brain requires highly selective substrates for growth and constitutive maintenance. A blood-brain barrier is formed from specialized cerebrovascular endothelial cells, which form tight junctions as well as astrocytic and pericytic foot processes that encircle the vessel walls. Molecular movement across this barrier occurs via diffusion, carrier-mediated (facilitated) transport, and active transport. A high permeability exists for H_2O, CO_2, O_2, and lipid-soluble substances such as alcohols. Protein-bound substances are impermeable. Selective permeability for ions such as Na^+, Cl^-, and K^+ exists. Enantiomer-specific transport proteins conduct only the D-glucose isomer for cerebral metabolic demands, excluding the L-glucose isomer. Similar specificity exists for L-dopamine, used in treating Parkinson's disease.

Fenestrated capillaries are present in the hypothalamus, pineal gland, and pituitary gland. These areas of the brain are responsible for sampling systemic blood and releasing hormones or other substances for regulation of growth, sexual function, and sleep-wake cycles. In addition to these natural breaches, the blood-brain barrier may be disrupted by blunt or surgical trauma, cytotoxic and vasogenic cerebral edema, sepsis/infections, and novel chemotherapeutic agents.

Drug manufacturers have had limited success in designing molecules capable of traversing the endothelial tight junctions of the central nervous system. Common delivery restrictions include molecular weight less than 500 Da, surface area less than 50 to 100 Å, and limited plasma protein binding. Few neuropharmaceuticals meet these criteria, and those that do have been limited largely to treatment of affective disorders, insomnia, epilepsy, and pain syndromes. Because of the difficulties that prevent drug distribution in the nervous tissue, alternative strategies have been considered, including craniotomy-based infusion, intracarotid hyperosmolar injections designed to disrupt the blood-brain barrier, and use of viruses as a vector for drug or gene delivery.

Cerebrospinal Fluid System

CSF is found in the ventricular system and subarachnoid space of the brain and spinal cord. It is produced by the choroid plexus, capillary ultrafiltrate, and metabolic water production. CSF is normally a clear, colorless fluid with a specific gravity of 1.007, a pH of 7.35, and an osmolarity that is similar to that of plasma (295 mOsm/L). There should be no more than five mononuclear white blood cells in CSF and no polymorphonuclear cells or red blood cells. The total protein content should be less than 40 mg/dL, and the normal glucose level should be approximately two thirds that of the serum. The electrolyte concentrations in CSF are similar to those in the serum with the exception of chloride, which is normally 116 to 120 mEq/L. CSF bathes the neural parenchyma and removes waste, regulates concentrations of neurotransmitters and hormones, and provides structural support. An average 70-kg adult produces 450 mL of CSF daily. CSF is absorbed in a pressure-dependent fashion into the venous system via the arachnoid granulations surrounding the sagittal sinus.

The ventricular system is composed of paired lateral ventricles found in the frontal, parietal, occipital, and temporal lobes; the midline third ventricle between the basal ganglia and thalami; the cerebral aqueduct (the smallest segment), which traverses the midbrain; the fourth ventricle found between the cerebellar hemispheres and adjacent to the pons and medulla; and the central canal of the spinal cord. Impedence of CSF outflow from the ventricles leads to noncommunicating or obstructive hydrocephalus. Commonly encountered etiologies include aqueductal stenosis or Chiari's malformation in children, cerebral edema, tumors, and intraventricular cysts. Communicating hydrocephalus occurs when CSF resorption is hindered or, rarely, when CSF is overproduced. Clinical examples include meningitis and subarachnoid or intraventricular hemorrhages (impeded resorption), and choroid plexus papillomas (overproduction). In infants prior to closure of the cranial sutures, hydrocephalus results in a disproportionate enlargement of the head circumference and developmental delays. Untreated obstructive hydrocephalus in adults results in elevated intracranial pressure and may rapidly lead to coma and death.

Treatment of hydrocephalus requires CSF diversion. This typically involves placement of a ventricular catheter into a lateral ventricle. This catheter may be tunneled and externalized for temporary drainage or internalized for permanent routing to the peritoneal cavity, pleural cavity, or atrium of the heart. A third ventriculostomy may also be performed by fenestrating the third ventricular floor, or lamina terminalis. This creates an alternate pathway for CSF flow to the subarachnoid space over the cerebral hemispheres and is most successful in cases of aqueductal stenosis. Administration of acetazolamide, a carbonic anhydrase inhibitor, has been shown to reduce CSF production but has limited clinical applications.

Brain Function and Integration

The cerebral cortex and spinal cord function as a set of complex integrated circuits with multiple levels of negative feedback. Each neuron acts as an information processor whose function depends on the summation of inputs it receives. There are discrete areas of cortex responsible for language expression, language reception, special and somatosensory perception, and motor generation. These areas are remarkably consistent in location as well as laterality throughout the human species. The ears, eyes, and nose are among the highly evolved special sensory receptors capable of transforming sound waves, light, and macromolecules from the environment into meaningful neuronal impulses in the brain. More diffuse functional connections of neurons are responsible for arousal, cognition, and learning.

Within the discrete areas of the brain corresponding to a specific function, there are somatotopically arranged areas of cortex. Somatotopy is a recurrent theme throughout organization of the brain and spinal cord. This refers to highly conserved arrays of neurons that correspond to specific locations within the body. In addition to detection

and recognition of a sensory stimulus, the brain must also locate where the stimulus occurred to prepare an appropriate response. The most straightforward example of this concept is the "homunculus," which allows visualization of this concept in the precentral gyrus or "motor strip" in humans. In this caricature, cortical surfaces responsible for initiating movement of the lower extremity are localized to the superior and interhemispheric portion of the gyrus, whereas those for the upper extremity and face are found in more inferior positions over the convexity. Larger areas are responsible for mouth and hand movements, commensurate with their more elaborate motor functions.

The two cerebral hemispheres are mirror images. For cortical functions such as sensory perception and movement, this corresponds to identical function in the contralateral (opposite) side of the body. For less tangible functions such as language and cognition, one hemisphere is referred to as "dominant." This asymmetry is apparent in early childhood. The left cerebral cortex is dominant with regard to language function in 99% of right-handed and over 80% of left-handed individuals. The remainder have right hemisphere dominance or no demonstrable dominance. This means that, for the majority, lesions involving the left frontotemporal lobes are expected to result in mutism. Lesions in the right hemisphere in this group will most likely result in more subtle deficits such as loss of emotional inflection in speech (prosody) but maintenance of the ability to express speech fluently.

Bibliography

Kuffler SW, Nicholls JG, Martin AR (eds): From Neuron to Brain: A Cellular Approach to the Function of the Nervous System (2nd ed). Sunderland, MA: Sinauer Associates, 1984.

Pardridge WM: Drug and gene delivery to the brain: the vascular route. Neuron 2002;36:555.

Pulvermuller F: A brain perspective on language mechanisms: from discrete neuronal ensembles to serial order. Prog Neurobiol 2002;67:85.

Renfro MB, Day AL, Rhoton AL: The extracranial and intracranial vessels: normal anatomy and variations. In Batjer HH (ed): Cerebrovascular Disease. Philadelphia: Lippincott–Raven, 1997:3.

Werner C, Kochs E, Hoffman WE: Cerebral blood flow and metabolism. In Albin MS (ed): Textbook of Neuroanesthesia with Neurosurgical and Neuroscience Perspectives. New York: McGraw-Hill, 1997:21.

CHAPTER 19

Physiology of Normal and Abnormal Respiration

Mark Knower, M.D. and David L. Bowton, M.D.

A basic understanding of respiratory physiology in both health and disease is essential to the optimal management of surgical patients. In addition to the obvious fact that surgical patients will be subject to the same chronic pulmonary diseases as the nonsurgical population, there are the considerations of changes in pulmonary function resulting from the surgical procedure itself and from the anesthesia provided for the surgery. This accounts for the finding that perioperative pulmonary complications are the most frequent severe complication in postoperative patients and the most costly. In this chapter, we review normal pulmonary physiology and the impact of surgery and anesthesia on this physiology. Although the relevance of this to specific complications is discussed, the diagnosis and treatment of these disorders are the subjects of other chapters.

Pulmonary Mechanics

The lungs are responsible for providing adequate oxygen to permit ongoing metabolic activity in tissues and excreting carbon dioxide produced during tissue metabolic processes in varying environments and under widely varying loads and demands. This requires the cooperative function of the pulmonary circulation and the gas-exchanging components of the lung. This section first examines gas exchange and then the pulmonary circulation. Because analysis of arterial blood gases is so commonly performed, it is tempting to relate changes in physiology to changes to blood gases. A reasonable guide is that changes in partial pressure of arterial carbon dioxide ($PaCO_2$) are linearly and inversely related to changes in minute alveolar ventilation (V_A), while changes in partial pressure of arterial oxygen (PaO_2) are related to changes in ventilation/perfusion (V/Q) ratios:

$$PaCO_2 \propto 1/V_A$$

$$PaO_2 \propto V/Q$$

In the discussion below, we refer back to these concepts to review the mechanisms by which common disease processes alter gas exchange. The process of delivering oxygen to hemoglobin and removal of carbon dioxide from blood can be divided into the individual components of (1) bulk gas flow (moving air from the environment to the alveolus), (2) blood flow to the alveolus, (3) the transfer of gases at the alveolar interface, and (4) the integration and matching of gas movement and blood flow, matching gas transfer to cellular needs.

Bulk Gas Movement

The gas exchange functions of the lung require bulk gas flow, moving air in and out of the alveoli, and transfer of gas across alveoli. Bulk gas flow results from changes in pressure and volume of the alveoli caused by the changes in the volume of the thoracic cage consequent to activation of the respiratory muscles, predominantly the diaphragm and intercostal muscles. The primary muscle of ventilation is the diaphragm, contraction of which increases the intrathoracic volume, resulting in a reduction in pleural pressure. This drop in pleural pressure is then transmitted to the alveoli, resulting in gas flow from the mouth to the alveolus. Exhalation results from relaxation of the diaphragm, a reduction in intrathoracic volume, and an increase in pleural pressure causing an increase in alveolar pressure, with gas again flowing down the pressure gradient.

The volumes of gas that can be inhaled and exhaled by the patient can be measured by spirometry. However, not all the gas in the lungs can be exhaled. This gas, the residual volume (RV), and those volumes and capacities that contain or include the RV (e.g., total lung capacity and functional residual capacity [FRC]), can only be measured by more specialized measurements involving helium dilution, nitrogen washout, or body plethysmography. Figure 19–1 illustrates commonly measured lung volumes and capacities.

Ventilation is not homogeneously distributed even in the healthy lung. There is more lung tissue in the lung bases, but also the lung units that are gravity-dependent (the bases in an upright individual) are better ventilated than are nondependent (apical) units. This is due in part to gradients in pleural pressure that are generated by gravitational forces on the lung. The effect is to reduce the pleural pressure (more negative) in the nondependent lung regions and to increase pleural pressure (less negative) in the dependent regions. This places these lung units along different portions of the lung's pressure-volume

curve (Fig. 19–2). The fall in pleural pressure consequent to inspiratory effort (typically 5 cm H$_2$O during quiet breathing) is fairly uniformly distributed throughout the pleural space. However, because at the onset of inspiration from FRC, the dependent units lie on the steeper, more compliant, portion of the curve and the nondependent units are on the upper, flatter, less compliant part of the curve, more ventilation occurs in the dependent than nondependent lung units. Hence, changes in posture affect regional ventilation. In the supine position, the dorsal lung units tend to be best ventilated, while in the right lateral decubitus position, the right (dependent) lung is better ventilated than the left. The difference in ventilation between dependent and nondependent lung units tends to be less in recumbent positions than when upright because the gravitational moment arm (the distance through which gravity is acting) is less in the anteroposterior than in the cephalocaudad direction. That is, because the lungs are taller than they are wide, gravitational effects are more noticeable when acting along the length of the lung than its breadth.

The FRC is the resting volume of the lung, that is, the volume the chest and lungs assume when a subject is told to "relax." This is the volume at the end of a normal exhalation or the volume the lungs return to without additional expenditure of energy. It is determined by the opposing tendencies of the lungs to shrink or recoil (lung elastic recoil), and of the chest wall to expand. Lung elastic recoil acts like a stretched spring and is due to tension in the

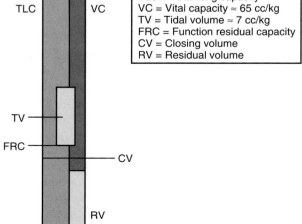

FIGURE 19–1 Lung volumes.

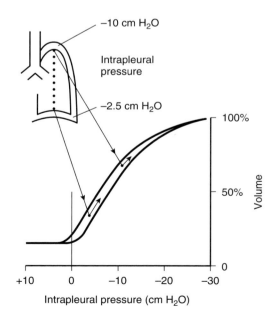

FIGURE 19–2 Explanation of the regional differences of ventilation down the lung. (From West JB: Respiratory Physiology: The Essentials [6th ed]. Philadelphia: Lippincott Williams & Wilkins, 2000:87, with permission.)

parenchymal architecture of the lung and to surface tension at the alveolar air-liquid interface. A host of disease processes can alter lung elastic recoil: pulmonary edema (cardiogenic or noncardiogenic) and lung inflammation (chronic, as with fibrosing alveolitis, or acute, as in pneumonia) typically increase lung elastic recoil, whereas processes that destroy alveolar septa, such as emphysema, decrease lung recoil. Increased lung elastic recoil results in a lower FRC, whereas decreases will cause an increase in FRC. These concepts are important because of their relationship with yet another volume, the closing volume (CV) (and its congener, closing capacity). The CV is the volume at which previously patent airways begin to close. In healthy individuals, the CV is below the FRC (see Fig. 19–1) so that, during normal breathing, there is little airway closure. The CV can be increased in many diseases processes (emphysema, pulmonary edema), which can result in airway closure during the normal breathing cycle. Hence, a variety of lung diseases can reduce FRC, increase CV, or both. The net effect of these processes then will be to increase the amount of airway closure during normal breathing cycles (tidal breathing), with resultant decreased ventilation to these closed units. This will commonly have the effect of reducing V/Q ratios and, accordingly, the PaO_2.

The characteristics of gas flow in and out of the lung are dependent on lung resistance and compliance. Resistance is the pressure required to push air through a hollow tube. Resistance increases as an exponential function of the radius of the tube (r^4); much more force or pressure is required to blow a given volume within a fixed time frame (flow in liters/second) through a narrow tube than a wider one. Lung compliance is the pressure (force) required to inflate the lungs to a given volume. Inflating lungs that are highly compliant is like inflating a thin, floppy balloon, whereas, with lungs that are noncompliant, it is more like blowing up a thick, stiff balloon. The conducting airways are the airways not involved in gas exchange (i.e., proximal to the respiratory bronchioles); they extend from the nose to the terminal bronchioles and account for the majority of the resistive properties of the lung. The distal airways, the site of gas exchange, include the respiratory bronchioles, alveolar ducts, and alveoli, and it is the properties of these distal airways that, in large measure, determine lung compliance. Though varying with lung volume and other factors, normal resistance in the lungs is quite low, generally approximately 2 cm H_2O/L/sec. In other words, generating a flow of 1 L/sec into the lungs will require a pressure of only 2 cm H_2O. The normal lung and chest wall are also quite easily distensible, with the total thoracic (i.e., chest wall and lung together) compliance typically 90 to 100 mL/cm H_2O. Hence a distending pressure or drop in pleural pressure of 5 cm H_2O will result in a volume change of

approximately 500 mL—just what is normally observed during quiet tidal breathing.

Pulmonary Circulation

The pulmonary circulation behaves much differently than its systematic analog. It includes the huge alveolar capillary network, whose surface area is over 50 m². Under normal circumstances, it operates at much lower pressure because of the very low resistance of the pulmonary vascular bed. Normal pulmonary artery pressures are in the range of 25/8 mm Hg, with mean pressure of 15 mm Hg. This is a consequence of both the large cross-sectional area of the pulmonary vascular bed (again, resistance is inversely proportional to r^4) and its distensibility. The pulmonary vascular bed is far more distensible than the systemic circulation because it is thin walled and, at the alveolar level, is separated from atmospheric pressure only by the attenuated epithelial and endothelial cells of the alveolar septa. Furthermore, not all pulmonary capillaries are open all the time. A certain amount of pressure is required to maintain the patency of small vessels—the so-called critical opening pressure. Because of the low pressures in the pulmonary circulation, many capillaries remain collapsed or closed until increases in pressure (e.g., caused by increased cardiac output) increase the pressure in the pulmonary circulation to above the critical opening pressure of these capillaries. This phenomenon of increasing the number of perfused or open capillaries is called *recruitment* (Fig. 19–3). Increasing cross sectional area through distension and recruitment accounts for the finding that, under normal circumstances, pressures in the pulmonary circulation do not increase very much even with maximal increases in cardiac output (Fig. 19–4). Patients with a reduced pulmonary vascular bed (e.g., those with emphysema), however, will elevate their pulmonary artery pressures with only modest increases in cardiac output.

Just as with ventilation, pulmonary blood flow is not uniformly distributed (Fig. 19–5). If the normal lung is 24 cm tall, and the mean pulmonary artery pressure is 20 cm H_2O (15 mm Hg) at midlung (midchest), then the perfusion pressure 12 cm higher in the apex (in the upright person) will be, very approximately, 8 cm H_2O, while

COMPLIANT AND RECRUITABLE VASCULATURE

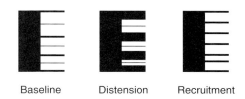

Baseline   Distension   Recruitment

FIGURE 19–3 Compliant and recruitable vasculature.

PRESSURE FLOW RELATIONSHIPS

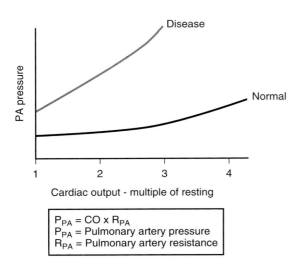

$$P_{PA} = CO \times R_{PA}$$
$$P_{PA} = \text{Pulmonary artery pressure}$$
$$R_{PA} = \text{Pulmonary artery resistance}$$

FIGURE 19–4 Pressure-flow relationships.

in the bases (12 cm lower) it will be about 32 cm H_2O. Hence, when upright, the lung bases are better perfused than the apices. The gravity-dependent changes in perfusion are, however, greater than those for ventilation. The decrement in perfusion going from base to apex (again in an upright subject) is greater than the decrement in ventilation. This is why V/Q ratios are higher in the lung apex than the lung base.

Gravity-dependent changes in perfusion can lead to significant impairment in gas exchange. Perhaps the most

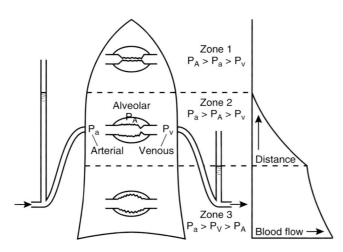

FIGURE 19–5 Three-zone model designed to account for the uneven topographic distribution of blood flow in the lung. P_a, pulmonary arterial pressure; P_A, pulmonary alveolar pressure; P_v, pulmonary venous pressure. (From West JB, Dollery CT, Naimark A: Distribution of blood flow in isolated lung: relation to vascular and alveolar pressures. J Appl Physiol 1964;19:713, with permission.)

common clinical scenario is the patient with asymmetrical lung disease, for example, with a pneumonia involving the right lung. The pneumonia, by flooding alveoli and small airways with secretions and inflammatory debris, will result in decreased ventilation to the affected lung. If this lung is then made dependent, by turning the patient with his or her right side down, perfusion to the right lung will be increased. This increase in perfusion to poorly ventilated alveoli will have the net effect of increasing the number of lung units with low V/Q ratios, and, as noted above, this will result in hypoxemia.

Hypoxic pulmonary vasoconstriction (HPV) helps to minimize the impact of lung disease on V/Q ratios and oxygenation. HPV is the response to a reduction in alveolar oxygen tension producing vasoconstriction in the small precapillary arterioles, thereby reducing blood flow to these alveoli and preserving V/Q ratios. Arterial and mixed-venous hypoxemia are much less important in causing pulmonary arteriolar vasoconstriction. HPV is rapid in onset and offset, and, though the response is a focal one (in the small arterioles supplying the hypoxic alveolus), generalized HPV can be seen when there is widespread alveolar hypoxia, as when environmental oxygen tension is reduced, as is seen at high altitude, or when there is diffuse lung disease. HPV can be augmented by acidemia (increased $[H^+]$) or increases in partial pressure of carbon dioxide (PCO_2). The response to hypoxia is also modulated by genetic factors. The mediator of HPV remains unknown, however. HPV can be antagonized by a variety of vasodilators, including nitrates and the calcium channel blockers. By virtue of increasing perfusion to poorly ventilated alveoli, hence increasing the number of lung units with low V/Q ratios, vasodilator agents can reduce the PaO_2 in subjects with underlying lung disease.

Gas Transfer and O_2 and CO_2 Transport

Gas transfer across the alveolar epithelium and capillary endothelium is by passive diffusion. The rate of gas transfer across the alveolar-capillary membrane is therefore dependent upon the difference in partial pressure of the gas across the membrane, the surface area of the membrane, and its thickness. It is also proportional to the solubility of the gas and the molecular weight of the gas traversing the membrane. Because CO_2 is much more soluble than O_2, it traverses the alveolar-capillary membrane about 20 times faster than oxygen.

Oxygen is transported in the blood in two forms: bound to hemoglobin and dissolved. The dissolved fraction represents much less than 5% of the oxygen content of blood under usual conditions. The amounts of oxygen carried in the blood are noted in Figure 19–6. The shape

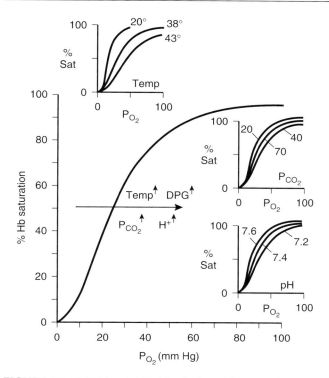

FIGURE 19–6 Rightward shift of the O_2 dissociation curve by increase of H^+, P_{CO_2}, temperature, and 2,3-diphosphoglycerate (DPG). (From West JB: Respiratory Physiology: The Essentials [6th ed]. Philadelphia: Lippincott Williams & Wilkins, 2000:67, with permission.)

of the oxyhemoglobin dissociation curve and the low solubility of oxygen in blood result in the observation that little additional oxygen can be carried in the blood as PaO_2 is increased above 70 mm Hg. The shape of the oxyhemoglobin dissociation curve ensures, however, that oxygen can be effectively "offloaded" to the tissues, where the partial pressure of oxygen (PO_2) is typically 40 mm Hg or less. Facilitating the offloading of oxygen is the rightward shift in the oxyhemoglobin dissociation curve with acidosis (i.e., increasing $[H^+]$), the so-called Bohr effect. This is most commonly a result of increasing PCO_2 in the capillaries, which serves to increase oxygen release to the tissues as carbon dioxide is loaded into the blood in the tissue capillary. As noted in Figure 19–6, enhancement of release of oxygen to the tissues by rightward shifting of the curve is also observed with increases in temperature and increased red blood cell levels of 2,3-diphosphoglycerate.

Carbon dioxide is transported in the blood in three forms: dissolved, as bicarbonate, and attached to proteins, especially the globin moiety of hemoglobin. Again, as for oxygen, the majority of CO_2 is transported bound to hemoglobin. Dissolved CO_2 accounts for approximately 10% of the CO_2 transported in blood. The dissolved CO_2 is in equilibrium with bicarbonate by the reaction

$$CO_2 + H_2O \xrightarrow{\text{carbonic anhydrase}} H_2CO_3 \leftrightarrow H^+ + HCO_3^-$$

This reaction is catalyzed by carbonic anhydrase, which, while absent from plasma, is present within red blood cells. Some of the hydrogen ion produced by this reaction is bound to hemoglobin. Reduced hemoglobin carries more CO_2 than oxidized hemoglobin at any given $PaCO_2$ (the Haldane effect). Therefore, as CO_2 diffuses from the tissues to the blood, its major transport protein becomes even more efficient.

Control of Respiration

The respiratory system has an extensive control system to facilitate its response to changing metabolic demands, changing characteristics of the mechanical properties of the system, and its involvement in volitional activities such as speech. These control mechanisms endeavor to maintain constancy of $PaCO_2$ and acid-base status, as well as adequacy of blood oxygen content, and to do this with the least amount of respiratory system work possible. These control mechanisms integrate signals from the central nervous system, lung and airway receptors, and peripheral and central chemoreceptors.

Areas of high concentrations of neurons responsible for respiratory activity are localized to the dorsal respiratory group (DRG) and the larger ventral respiratory group (VRG), both located in the medulla, and the pontine respiratory group (PRG) in the dorsal pons. The precise centers in the midbrain responsible for the generation of rhythmic respiration are not well defined, though generation of the respiratory rhythm itself may be due to collections of neurons just rostral to the VRG. The VRG, DRG, and PRG are each involved in coordinating respiratory rate and depth and duration of inspiration, and initiation of exhalation using input from the myelinated vagal fibers within the airway, unmyelinated vagal fibers within the lung interstitium and adjacent to pulmonary capillaries, and mechanoreceptors within the muscle spindles and Golgi tendon organs of the respiratory muscles. The integration is complex, and the stimuli can be mechanical (such as lung inflation) or chemical (either endogenous such as bradykinin, or exogenous such as capsaicin). Both mechanical and chemical stimulation of the nasal upper airway receptors can initiate a sneeze, while stimulating laryngeal receptors often results in cough, and lower airway stimuli commonly cause cough and mucus secretion as well as bronchospasm. Furthermore, steady lung inflation will usually result in slowing of the respiratory rate by prolonging the exhalation time—the classic Hering-Breuer inflation reflex.

Chemical modulation of respiratory drive can be effected by changes in PaO_2, $PaCO_2$, or pH acting on the peripheral or central chemoreceptors. The central chemoreceptors appear to be the primary sensors and response generator for changes in $PaCO_2$ and arterial pH. The sensors are located in the ventrolateral superficial medulla adjacent to the fourth ventricle. Ventilation increases in experimental animals when the surface of the medulla is bathed with mock cerebrospinal fluid made acidotic either by increasing the carbon dioxide level or by decreasing the bicarbonate. Peripheral chemoreceptors are located in the carotid and aortic bodies. They are sensitive to changes in pH, PO_2, and PCO_2. In humans, the carotid bodies play the dominant role. The carotid bodies are located at the bifurcation of the common carotid arteries and are intensely vascular. Reductions of PaO_2 or increases in $PaCO_2$ or $[H^+]$ result in an increase in the discharge of sensory nerve fibers of the carotid bodies. The response to changes in $PaCO_2$ and $[H^+]$ is nearly linear (Fig. 19–7). Although the response to changes in PaO_2 is nonlinear, the response is almost linear when examined as a function of hemoglobin oxygen saturation (Fig. 19–8). Hence, large changes in ventilation do not occur in response to reduction in PaO_2 until the PaO_2 falls below approximately 70 mm Hg (nearing the steep portion of the oxyhemoglobin dissociation curve). Furthermore, the response to individual stimuli is additive to the others so that, if PaO_2 falls simultaneously with an increase in $PaCO_2$ (or fall in pH), the ventilatory response will be greater than the response to any of the individual changes. Figure 19–8 illustrates that reductions in PaO_2 alter the ventilatory response to changes in $PaCO_2$. Ventilatory responsiveness to changes in $PaCO_2$ and PaO_2 vary greatly among individuals and can be reduced by a variety of factors, including age, drugs, and level of consciousness.

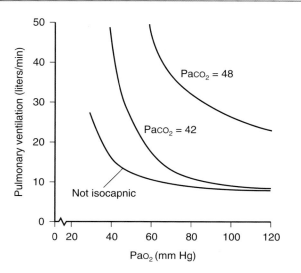

FIGURE 19–8 Ventilatory responses to alterations in partial pressure of alveolar oxygen (PaO_2) under both nonisocapnic and two levels of isocapnic (alveolar carbon dioxide partial pressure [$PaCO_2$]) conditions are depicted. (From Loeschcke HH, Gertz KH: Einfluss des O_2-Druckes in der Einatmugsluft auf die Atemtotigkeit des Menschen, gepruft unter Konstanthaltung des alveolaren CO_2-Druckes. Pflugers Arch Ges Physiol 1958;267:460, with permission.)

Effects of Surgery and Anesthesia

General anesthesia is associated with changes in lung mechanics, ventilatory drive, and gas exchange. These effects must be borne in mind when caring for the patient intraoperatively, but may also have an impact on postoperative care. Furthermore, surgery itself, independent of anesthesia, further impairs lung function in many situations. These effects are reviewed briefly, followed by a discussion of selected perioperative concerns in common disease states.

General anesthesia causes a widening of the alveolar-arterial oxygen tension gradient. The cause is multifactorial and appears to be due to increases in V/Q mismatch and in intrapulmonary shunt. Inhalation anesthetic agents can inhibit hypoxic pulmonary vasoconstriction, increasing perfusion of poorly ventilated lung units (increased V/Q mismatch) and of completely unventilated lung units (increased shunt). Additionally, the FRC decreases appreciably during general anesthesia. This is independent of use of neuromuscular blockade and is largely independent of the duration of anesthesia. It may be due, in part, to alteration of the mechanical properties of the chest wall and to cephalad shift in the position of the diaphragm with anesthesia. This may result in the FRC falling below the closing capacity, again

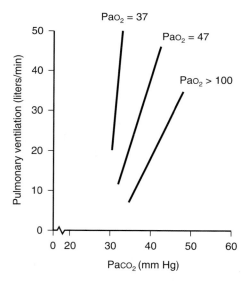

FIGURE 19–7 Ventilatory responses to alterations in partial pressure of alveolar carbon dioxide ($PaCO_2$) are shown at different levels of alveolar oxygen partial pressure (PaO_2). (From Nielson M, Smith H: Studies on the regulation of respiration in acute hypoxia. Acta Physiol Scand 1952;24:293, with permission.)

producing lung units that are poorly ventilated and contributing to V/Q mismatch.

Surgical factors also have an impact on lung mechanics. The vital capacity and FRC both fall 30% to 50% after upper abdominal incisions. Similar changes are observed after posterolateral thoracotomy incisions, with smaller, though significant, changes after lower abdominal surgery. Clearly, if preoperative lung function is impaired, changes in lung function of this magnitude may have major consequences for postoperative morbidity and recovery. These changes are not, primarily, related to pain, because animal studies suggest that most of the decrement in function persists even when pain is completely relieved. Similarly, in humans, epidural anesthetics may alleviate postoperative pain, but lung function remains significantly compromised. These lung function abnormalities are maximal approximately 72 hours postoperatively, and require 7 to 10 days to fully resolve. These observations underlie the observation that perioperative pulmonary complications are maximal about 3 days after surgery.

Dysfunction

Chronic Obstructive Pulmonary Disease

The chronic obstructive pulmonary diseases (COPDs) include emphysema, chronic bronchitis, and asthma. While the underlying pathology differs, they are each characterized by narrowing and increased resistance in the conducting airways. In asthma and chronic bronchitis, the airway walls are narrowed by inflammatory edema and the airways are plugged by excessive secretions. Though increased reactivity or "twitchiness" of the airways can be seen in patients with chronic bronchitis, it is ubiquitous and generally more severe in asthma. In emphysema, the widespread destruction of alveolar septa results in a loss of airway support, resulting in the narrowing and collapse of airways during exhalation. In most patients with COPD caused by cigarette abuse, emphysema and chronic bronchitis will coexist, though features of one or the other commonly predominate. Nonspecific bronchial hyperresponsiveness, or airway twitchiness, is a sine qua non of asthma, but is also commonly observed in patients with emphysema and chronic bronchitis (henceforth termed COPD). Hence, a variety of stimuli, including airway instrumentation, coughing, and excessive airway secretions, can result in bronchospasm and increased airflow resistance. In addition to the increased work of breathing and impaired gas exchange, increased resistance can markedly impair the ability to clear secretions by cough. This, in turn, can lead to atelectasis, pneumonia, and respiratory failure.

Prevention of perioperative complications in patients with obstructive lung diseases has been surprisingly poorly studied. Bronchodilator therapy will improve lung mechanics and therefore assist with secretion removal. The most effective bronchodilators are generally β_2-agonists such as albuterol. Anticholinergic agents are longer acting, and their combination with β_2-agonists in patients with COPD may decrease the frequency of treatments needed. These agents are almost always administered via inhalation, and it has been well demonstrated that administration by metered-dose inhaler (MDI) is equivalent to administration by wet nebulizer in patients who are able to use a MDI with a spacer device. A dose of albuterol by MDI of approximately 6 to 10 puffs (0.54 to 0.9 mg) is equipotent to the usual nebulizer dose of 2.5 mg.

Early ambulation, deep breathing, and coughing are important to reduce the impact of reduced lung volumes on cough efficiency and the development of atelectasis. Incentive spirometry may serve to create a protocol for deep breathing, or provide a means of reminding patients to breath deeply and cough. As such, it is inexpensive and safe; however, it is no more efficacious than frequent (hourly) encouragement to breath deeply and cough. Despite its widespread use, there are few data supporting the utility of chest physiotherapy (CPT) in the perioperative period. Indeed, in patients with obstructive lung diseases, increased bronchospasm and worsening oxygenation had been observed, without evidence for counterbalancing benefit. Hence, the use of CPT in this setting cannot be recommended unless there is evidence of lobar atelectasis (see below) or the patient has significant bronchiectasis, as seen, for example, in patients with cystic fibrosis.

Pulmonary Edema–Cardiogenic and Noncardiogenic (Acute Respiratory Distress Syndrome)

Pulmonary edema is characterized by diffuse increases in lung water both in the interstitial spaces and ultimately in the alveolar spaces. Lung compliance is reduced; that is, the lungs are stiffer or more difficult to inflate. This leads to a reduction in FRC to a level that is less than closing capacity and results in airway closure, which increases the number of lung units with low V/Q ratios and results in hypoxemia. The application of positive airway pressure (continuous positive airway pressure or positive end-expiratory pressure [PEEP]) recruits lung units, increases the FRC, and decreases the venous admixture and improves oxygenation.

The differentiation of cardiogenic from noncardiogenic pulmonary edema can often be done on the basis of history, physical examination, and the radiographic appearance. A history of congestive heart failure, acute myocardial infarction, or acute coronary syndromes increases the likelihood of a cardiac etiology for diffuse infiltrates, as does an S_3 heart sound on physical examination, pleural effusions or evidence of venous engorgement (azygos vein enlargement or redistribution of pulmonary blood flow) on chest radiography, or echocardiographic evidence of left ventricular dysfunction. In the setting of severe sepsis, trauma, or multisystem organ failure, or with aspiration syndromes, noncardiogenic pulmonary edema is more likely. When the clinical picture is confusing, a pulmonary artery catheter (PAC) may be useful to establish a diagnosis.

Acute coronary syndromes should be treated with aspirin and anticoagulation, with β-blockade and urgent coronary angiography considered in selected patients. While the use of a PAC has not been shown to improve outcomes in well-designed trials, it can certainly support the use of vigorous afterload reduction and diuresis when a cardiac etiology is present. In noncardiogenic pulmonary edema, the use of low tidal volume ventilation has been shown to decrease mortality, and its use in all cases of pulmonary edema can likely be justified. A recent randomized, controlled trial demonstrated a reduction in mortality from 39% to 31% with the use of small tidal volumes (6 mL/kg or less based on ideal body weight) in comparison to using larger tidal volumes (10 mL/kg). Careful attention to tidal volumes and plateau pressures (maintaining the latter less than 35 cm H_2O) should be paid in all these patients. PEEP should be applied to enable decreasing the fraction of inspired oxygen (FiO_2) to less than 60% whenever feasible. The Acute Respiratory Distress Syndrome (ARDS) Network trial utilized PEEP levels of 15 cm H_2O or less, and controlled trials examining PEEP levels above this are few. Treating underlying disease processes such as sepsis is essential to improving the outcomes in these patients. With current therapy, the mortality of ARDS has been reduced from 65% to 70% to approximately 40%.

Atelectasis

Atelectasis (pulmonary collapse) occurs when a portion of the lung parenchyma is rendered airless. Atelectasis is caused by either obstruction of airways at normal lung volumes or by airway closure as a result of elevation of closing capacity above the FRC. Obstruction of airways can result from inspissated secretions or other obstructing material in the airways, including inflammatory exudates, blood, edema, foreign body, or intraluminal mass lesions. As described above, in healthy young adults, closing capacity is below FRC and airway closure does not occur during tidal breathing. A variety of pathologic processes may cause atelectasis via the loss of opposing forces to lung elastic recoil. Compression of lung by the heart or diaphragm, chest wall trauma (rib fractures or flail chest), intrathoracic abdominal herniation, pneumothorax, hemothorax, pleural effusion, or empyema all may result in atelectasis by diminishing normal opposing forces to lung elastic recoil. Similarly, after cardiac surgery,

phrenic nerve paralysis or surfactant dysfunction may also contribute to postoperative lung collapse. Alternatively, the closing capacity may be increased above a relatively normal FRC and result in airway closure during tidal breathing. This can occur as a normal part of aging, in which the closing capacity increases with resultant airway closure at up to 40% of the vital capacity above residual volume. Therefore, airway closure and atelectasis in dependent lung segments may be present during tidal breathing of patients in their seventh or eighth decades, especially when high concentrations of oxygen are inspired. A similar mechanism accounts for atelectasis during anesthesia in healthy patients, with diaphragmatic paralysis and the supine position both resulting in a reduction in FRC leading to tidal breathing at or below closing capacity and consequent airway closure. The resorption of alveolar gas distal to airway closure is hastened with the use of higher FiO_2, which can further promote alveolar collapse.

Atelectasis with or without effusion is one of the most common chest radiograph abnormalities seen in hospitalized patients, especially those in the intensive care unit. Because FRC will inevitably fall after all cardiac, thoracic, or upper abdominal procedures, measures to prevent atelectasis are especially important in the early postoperative period. Prevention of pulmonary collapse can be achieved with several interventions, including encouragement of cough or deep breathing, routing incentive spirometry, and intermittent positive pressure ventilation. All appear to be equally efficacious, with coughing and deep breathing clearly the easiest and least expensive. Pain control in the postoperative patient permits early ambulation and deep breathing maneuvers. Although routine CPT has never been shown to assist in prevention of pulmonary collapse, CPT combined with tracheobronchial toilet is as efficacious as fiberoptic bronchoscopy in the treatment of established lobar atelectasis and should be the first intervention attempted once atelectasis has been documented. CPT with nasotracheal or tracheobronchial suctioning should be performed with the patient in decubitus positioning and the atelectatic lung superior. Resolution of the chest radiograph after CPT or bronchoscopy can be delayed for up to 24 hours after intervention. In mechanically ventilated patients, intermittent sighs as well as low levels of PEEP will assist in preventing or clearing areas of collapse. Frequent (every 2 hours) position changes or a rotating bed is a useful adjunct to other noninvasive preventative measures in the intubated patient. Of course, any other mechanical cause of atelectasis (effusion, pneumothorax, flail chest, etc.) must be corrected for maximal benefit.

Contusion

Pulmonary contusion is a relatively common injury after blunt trauma to the thorax or upper abdomen. Often rib fractures or overt flail chest will coexist; however, the absence of rib fracture does not rule out the possibility of contusion. The typical appearance on chest radiograph is a localized area of increasing alveolar opacification, which is greatest at 24 to 48 hours after injury and may resolve over the following week. In some patients, the initial chest radiograph will be normal, and chest wall contusion with worsening hypoxia is the only clue to the diagnosis. In cases of severe trauma, a more generalized pulmonary injury can result in a syndrome of noncardiogenic pulmonary edema (ARDS) secondary to massive release of inflammatory mediators from the injured lung. As blood fills the interstitial and alveolar spaces, lung compliance and FRC are both reduced, leading to tidal breathing near closing capacity and promoting airway collapse in areas adjacent to the injury. Capillary disruption in injured lung parenchyma essentially stops blood flow to these affected areas. Therefore, the hypoxemia that follows is a result not of intrapulmonary shunt (i.e., lung units with V/Q = 0) through the most contused lung, but rather of the contribution of low V/Q ratios in adjacent areas with compromised gas exchange. Management of simple pulmonary contusion involves pain control, oxygen supplementation, adequate pulmonary toilet, and other measures to prevent atelectasis.

Pneumonia

Invasion of the lower respiratory tract by microorganisms is a potent stimulus for the migration of neutrophils into the lung parenchyma. Neutrophils and alveolar macrophages then produce a cascade of inflammatory mediators that result in a cellular alveolar inflammatory exudate, seen as an infiltrate on chest radiography. A localized severe inflammatory process can cause a more generalized injury to the lung parenchyma through the release of inflammatory mediators, resulting in ARDS and/or the sepsis syndrome. Lung consolidation causes a decrease in compliance and FRC, thereby decreasing lung volumes to below closing capacity in adjacent airways, and promoting airway closure. Unlike the case for pulmonary contusion, intrapulmonary shunt through areas of consolidation is a major cause of hypoxemia in pneumonia. This hypoxemia is worse than that seen with atelectasis alone, in part because of antagonism of hypoxic pulmonary vasoconstriction by the inflammatory mediators associated with the pneumonia. This increases the percentage of lung units with low V/Q ratios.

Hospital-acquired pneumonia (HAP) occurs at a rate of 5 to 10 cases per 1000 hospital admissions, and ventilator-associated pneumonia (VAP) may occur in up to 20% to 30% of patients ventilated for over 48 hours. Crude mortality of HAP and VAP may be as high as 50% to 70%, with a highly variable attributable mortality ranging from 0 to 30%. The risk for HAP increases in patients with severe chronic illness and comorbidities such as coma, prolonged malnutrition, and advanced age. Poor infection control practices, corticosteroids, sedatives, cytotoxic agents, prolonged surgery, inappropriate antibiotic use, and intubation also play a role. Factors that impart a high risk for VAP include an admission diagnosis of burns or trauma, central nervous system disease, previous underlying respiratory disease, paralytic agents, ventilation for greater than 48 hours, and witnessed aspiration. The initial bacterial inoculum reaches the lung primarily via inhalation (including aspiration), though hematogenous spread from a distant site or via translocation of bacteria from the gastrointestinal tract has been implicated in some series.

Diagnosis of HAP or VAP is clinically challenging. Fever, purulent sputum, hypotension, worsening hypoxemia, and new infiltrates suggest the diagnosis, but these clinical findings are nonspecific and their use can lead to the overdiagnosis of pneumonia. Culture of normally sterile material from blood or pleura may produce an etiologic organism, but the yield is low. Quantitative culture of tracheal aspirates or bronchoscopically obtained material is more specific, though potentially less sensitive. Gram-negative enterics, *Staphylococcus aureus*, and *Pseudomonas* are among the most frequently isolated organisms, though in HAP or VAP occurring within the first 5 days of hospitalization, *Haemophilus influenzae* and pneumococcus can be seen. At least two recent studies have demonstrated a survival advantage with the use of bronchoscopically obtained quantitative cultures to guide antibiotic prescription. Several protocols exist for treatment of HAP and VAP, but modulation of risk factors, proper infection control practices, and the early use of empiric antibiotic coverage are important to prevent unnecessary morbidity or mortality. In addition, emerging evidence suggests that prolonged antibiotic usage in patients with infiltrates but little other clinical or culture evidence of pneumonia may worsen outcome. A high index of suspicion is necessary to avoid misdiagnosis of patients with HAP, and treatment must be tailored not only to the individual patient but also to the microbial prevalence and resistance profiles of individual institutions.

Aspiration

Aspiration can be defined as the inhalation of either oropharyngeal or gastric secretions into the respiratory tract. Two distinct syndromes will result depending on the type of aspirated material and frequency of aspiration. Aspiration pneumonitis is a chemical inflammation that typically occurs after the inhalation of sterile gastric secretions, while aspiration pneumonia is an infection resulting from inhalation of secretions containing a high load of microorganisms, typically from the oropharynx.

Aspiration of acidic gastric contents causes a chemical burn with a subsequent intense inflammatory response by the lung parenchyma. The pattern of injury in the lung is biphasic. The first, early inflammatory injury is likely secondary to the direct effects of acid inhalation, while the second injury occurs as a result of infiltration of neutrophils 4 to 6 hours later. Because gastric secretions are normally sterile, direct bacterial invasion into the lung after aspiration does not play a significant role in early inflammatory responses. However, the lung injury induced by acid aspiration may predispose patients to late bacterial colonization and secondary infection. Hypoxemia is multifactorial: alveolar/interstitial inflammatory exudates and pulmonary edema increase shunt fraction while decreased lung compliance and FRC promote adjacent airway closure and V/Q mismatch. The pathophysiology of aspiration pneumonia is similar to that described for pneumonia above.

Aspiration is a known complication after anesthesia, and may occur in 1 in 3000 operative procedures, accounting for up to one third of anesthesia-related deaths. Risk factors for aspiration include advanced age, dysphagia, stroke, anatomic abnormalities of the upper aerodigestive tract, gastric dysmotility, and depressed level of consciousness. The risk is further increased in critically ill patients as a result of supine position, sedatives, paralytics, intubation, and gastroparesis. Controversy exists in the literature as to whether prophylaxis with H_2 antagonists increases the risk for aspiration pneumonia or VAP, with at least one large study showing no difference in pneumonia incidence between ranitidine and sucralfate treatment. A high risk for aspiration exists immediately after extubation, especially if residual sedative effects, nasogastric intubation, or swallowing dysfunction is present. As stated above, not all patients who aspirate will develop pneumonia. The majority of otherwise healthy adults will demonstrate aspiration of small amounts of oral secretions during sleep without sequelae. However, the low bacterial load and the presence of intact defense mechanisms prevent the development of overt pneumonia. If immune function is impaired or the aspiration is large or frequent, pneumonia can result. Poor oral hygiene also increases the risk for pneumonia after inhalation of oropharyngeal contents by increasing the burden of pathogenic organisms, and gastroparesis or small bowel obstruction increases the risk after gastric aspiration by increasing bacterial colonization of gastric secretions. Although it is common practice in critically ill patients to place postpyloric tubes for feeding, the efficacy of this approach in protecting against aspiration is not clear. Furthermore, postpyloric placement of a feeding tube does not protect against aspiration of oral secretions, which are "milked" around the balloon of the endotracheal tube and into the airway. Aspiration of pharyngeal contents from above the balloon of an endotracheal tube may decrease aspiration of oropharyngeal contents and reduce the incidence of pneumonia.

Bibliography

Acute Respiratory Distress Syndrome Network: Ventilation with lower tidal volumes as compared with traditional tidal volumes for acute lung injury and the acute respiratory distress syndrome. N Engl J Med 2000;342:1301.

Berger AJ: Control of breathing. *In* Murray JF, Nadel JA (eds): Textbook of Respiratory Medicine. Philadelphia: WB Saunders, 1994:199.

Bowton DL: Nosocomial pneumonia in the ICU—year 2000 and beyond. Chest 1999;115:28S.

Bryan AC, Bentivoglio LG, Beerel F, et al: Factors affecting regional distribution of ventilation and perfusion in the lung. J Appl Physiol 1964;19:395.

Carrillo EH, Williams MJ: Thoracic surgery. *In* Civetta JM, Taylor RW, Kirby RR (eds): Critical Care. Philadelphia: Lippincott Williams & Wilkins, 1997:1131.

Cook D, Guyatt G, Marshall J, et al: A comparison of sucralfate and ranitidine for the prevention of upper gastrointestinal bleeding in patients requiring mechanical ventilation. N Engl J Med 1998;338:791.

Cook DJ, Kollef MH: Risk factors for ICU-acquired pneumonia. JAMA 1998;279:1605.

D'Oliveira M, Sykes MK, Chakrabarti MK, et al: Depression of hypoxic pulmonary vasoconstriction by sodium nitroprusside and nitroglycerine. Br J Anaesth 1981;53:11.

Esparza J, Boivin MA, Hartshorne MF, Levy H: Equal aspiration rates in gastrically and transpylorically fed critically ill patients. Intensive Care Med 2001;27:660.

Fagon JY, Chastre J, Vuagnat A, et al: Nosocomial pneumonia and mortality among patients in intensive care units. JAMA 1996;275:866.

Fagon JY, Chastre J, Wolff M, et al: Invasive and noninvasive strategies for management of suspected ventilator-associated pneumonia: randomized trial. Ann Intern Med 2000;132:621.

Grippi MA: Distribution of ventilation. *In* Grippi MA (ed): Pulmonary Pathophysiology. Philadelphia: Lippincott Williams & Wilkins, 1995:41.

Hakim TS, Lisbona R, Dean GW: Effect of cardiac output on gravity-dependent and nondependent inequality in pulmonary blood flow. J Appl Physiol 1989;66:1570.

Hall JB, Schmidt GA, Wood LDH: Acute hypoxemic respiratory failure. *In* Murray JF, Nadel JA (eds): Textbook of Respiratory Medicine. Philadelphia: WB Saunders, 1994:2589.

Hall JC, Tarala R, Harris J, et al: Incentive spirometry versus routine chest physiotherapy for prevention of pulmonary complications after abdominal surgery [see comments]. Lancet 1991;337:953.

Hendolin H, Lahtinen J, Lansimies E, et al: The effect of thoracic epidural analgesia on respiratory function after cholecystectomy. Acta Anaesthesiol Scand 1987;31:645.

Heyland DK, Cook DJ, Griffith L, et al: The attributable morbidity and mortality of ventilator-associated pneumonia in the critically ill patient. Am J Respir Crit Care Med 1999;159:1249.

Heyland DK, Drover JW, MacDonald S, et al: Effect of postpyloric feeding on gastroesophageal regurgitation and pulmonary microaspiration: results of a randomized controlled trial. Crit Care Med 2001;29:1495.

Ibrahim EH, Ward S, Sherman G, Kollef MH: A comparative analysis of patients with early-onset vs late-onset nosocomial pneumonia in the ICU setting. Chest 2000;117:1434.

Kearns PJ, Chin D, Mueller L, et al: The incidence of ventilator-associated pneumonia and success in nutrient delivery with gastric versus small intestinal feeding: a randomized clinical trial. Crit Care Med 2000;28:1742.

Kollef MH: The prevention of ventilator-associated pneumonia. N Engl J Med 1999;340:627.

Kollef MH, Sherman G, Ward S, Fraser VJ: Inadequate antimicrobial treatment of infections: a risk factor for hospital mortality among critically ill patients. Chest 1999;115:462.

Lumb AB: Parenchymal lung disease. In Lumb AB (ed): Nunn's Applied Respiratory Physiology. Oxford: Butterworth Heinemann, 2000:559.

Lykens MG, Bowton DL: Aspiration and acute lung injury. Int J Obstet Anesth 1993;2:236.

Marik PE: Aspiration pneumonitis and aspiration pneumonia. N Engl J Med 2001;344:665.

Marini JJ, Pierson DJ, Hudson LD: Acute lobar atelectasis: a prospective comparison of fiberoptic bronchoscopy and respiratory therapy. Am Rev Respir Dis 1979;119:971.

Merhav H, Rothstein H, Eliraz A, et al: A comparison of pulmonary functions and oxygenation following local, spinal or general anaesthesia in patients undergoing inguinal hernia repair. Int Surg 1993;78:257.

Murray JF: The Normal Lung (2nd ed). Philadelphia: WB Saunders, 1986.

Rehder K, Sessler AD, Marsh HM: General anesthesia and the lung. Am Rev Respir Dis 1975;112:541.

Ruiz M, Torres A, Ewig S, et al: Noninvasive versus invasive microbial investigation in ventilator-associated pneumonia: evaluation of outcome. Am J Respir Crit Care Med 2000;162:119.

Santos C, Ferrer M, Roca J, et al: Pulmonary gas exchange in response to oxygen breathing in acute lung injury. Am J Respir Crit Care Med 2000;161:26.

Sleszynski SL, Kelso AF: Comparison of thoracic manipulation with incentive spirometry in preventing postoperative atelectasis. J Am Osteopath Assoc 1993;93:834, 843.

Tenling A, Joachimsson P-O, Tyden H, Hedenstierna G: Thoracic epidural analgesia as an adjunct to general anaesthesia for cardiac surgery: effects on pulmonary mechanics. Acta Anaesthesiol Scand 2000;44:1071.

Truedson H, Stjernberg N: Postoperative pulmonary ventilation after cholecystectomy with and without peritoneal drain. Acta Chir Scand 1983;149:401.

Valles J, Artigas A, Rello J, et al: Continuous aspiration of subglottic secretions in preventing ventilator-associated pneumonia. Ann Intern Med 1995;122:179.

Voelkel NF: Mechanisms of hypoxic pulmonary vasoconstriction. Am Rev Respir Dis 1986;133:1186.

Wagner WW: Pulmonary circulatory control through hypoxic vasoconstriction. Semin Respir Med 1985;7:124.

Warner MA, Warner ME, Weber JG: Clinical significance of pulmonary aspiration during the perioperative period. Anesthesiology 1993;78:56.

CHAPTER 20

Renal Physiology and Dysfunction

Jack W. Strandhoy, Ph.D.

The kidney is an organ of excretion, metabolism, and homeostasis of the body's fluids. By exquisite coupling between intake and output, variations in the urinary excretion of solutes and water maintain extracellular fluid balance, osmolality, pH, and electrolyte concentration. The urine serves as the primary excretory route for urea, other products of metabolism such as ammonia, many drugs, and some toxins. The kidney is also critically necessary for the production and release of several hormones. Renin is an enzyme synthesized and released primarily into the renal circulation to cleave a peptide from its globulin precursor. Angiotensin II, and likely other members of this peptide family, regulate blood pressure through vasoconstriction and sodium transport. Erythropoietin secretion stimulates red blood cell synthesis, and its deficiency contributes to the anemia of end-stage renal disease (ESRD). The kidney is also responsible for the final hydroxylation of vitamin D, so that damage to the tubules explains the osteodystrophy of renal failure. The kidney responds to many hormones as well. Parathormone and calcitonin regulate phosphate and calcium metabolism; aldosterone influences sodium, potassium, and pH balance; and vasopressin is critical for osmotic regulation by influencing water permeability.

Structure of the Kidney and Lower Urinary Tract

Each of the two kidneys in humans weighs about 150 g. The organs lie in the retroperitoneal space and are perfused through renal arteries branching off the aorta. While most renal arteries bifurcate within the kidney, extrarenal bifurcation or multiple renal arteries are not uncommon. The renal vessels and parenchyma are innervated with sympathetic nerves. Fluids exit the kidney through the renal vein into the vena cava or the lymphatics or as urine into the ureter. If the kidney is bisected, two zones are clearly apparent from their color differences. The outer layer is the cortex, and microscopic examination of this tissue shows that it contains all of the glomeruli along with segments of proximal tubules, distal tubules, and portions of the collecting ducts. The medulla is the inner portion of the kidney and it contains the loops of Henle along with the more inner portions of the collecting ducts. These structures are critical for the regulation of urine concentration and dilution. In the human kidney, the medulla is organized into pyramidal regions that extend to the papilla, the innermost tissue. The papilla hangs freely in the pelvis of the kidney and is bathed by the final urine.

The main renal artery branches to form interlobar arteries. They branch at right angles to form arcuate arteries that course along the corticomedullary junction. The arcuates in turn form interlobular arteries that head toward the surface of the cortex and arborize into afferent arterioles. The glomeruli are clustered like grapes at the ends of the afferent arterioles, branching off intralobular arteries in the cortex. The afferent arteriole that enters Bowman's capsule forms a glomerular capillary tuft, so that many vessels in parallel expand the filtration surface area. These vessels then coalesce to form the efferent arteriole and eventually the peritubular capillary network and the renal venous circulation. This very unusual arrangement of glomerular capillaries juxtaposed between two arterioles permits the high hemodynamic pressures that account for such large amounts of fluid ultrafiltration.

Renal sympathetic nerves originate mainly in the celiac plexus. Although there are muscarinic receptors in the kidney, there is no parasympathetic innervation. The renal nerves help regulate renal blood flow (RBF), glomerular filtration rate (GFR), and salt and water reabsorption by the nephron. The smooth muscle of the major blood vessels and even the periglomerular arterioles is innervated. Moreover, sympathetic discharge acting through β adrenoceptors stimulates renin secretion from cells lining the afferent arteriole. Nerve fibers also directly innervate the proximal tubule, Henle's loop, the distal tubule, and the collecting duct. Stimulation of adrenoceptors can directly modulate sodium transport. The activation of renal sympathetic nerves to change these processes is frequency dependent. Increasing strength of nerve activity affects sodium transport first, then renin secretion, and finally vasoconstriction.

The anatomic and functional unit of the kidney is the nephron. In each kidney there are approximately 1 million nephrons. Each one begins with a glomerulus and continues with a tubule composed of one layer of epithelial cells. The tubule take a torturous path from the cortex into the medulla, back into the cortex, and finally into the medulla again. This seemingly inefficient anatomic arrangement is, in fact, critical to the kidney's extremely efficient regulation of urine composition and osmolality. The various portions of the nephron are derived from two embryologic sources. Nephrogenesis proceeds in a centrifugal fashion and is not complete at birth in humans.

Along the nephron, the fluid that is filtered at the glomerulus is continuously modified as it passes through successive epithelial segments with different transport functions. In fact, at least 13 distinct epithelia can be categorized, although the main anatomic and physiologic divisions of the kidney can be limited to the glomerulus, proximal tubule, loop of Henle, distal tubule, and collecting duct.

Once the urine leaves the kidney, it flows down the ureters to the bladder. The ureters have both spiral and longitudinal smooth muscle, so that peristaltic waves help propel the urine downward. The ureters and bladder are lined with transitional epithelium in several layers. The ureters enter the bladder on the posterior side near the base and just above the bladder neck. This area of the bladder is known as the trigone. The bladder is composed of the main body or fundus. The neck, also called the posterior urethra, is funnel shaped and is the end of the urinary tract in females. In males, an additional anterior urethra extends through the penis. Contractile detrusor smooth muscle surrounds the bladder and extends to the neck. At the neck, the muscle fibers thicken to form the internal sphincter, which is not under conscious control. The urethra finally passes through a urogenital diaphragm

that contains the external sphincter. This sphincter is under voluntary control, especially in males, so that urination can be voluntarily started or stopped.

The innervation of the lower urinary tract is critical to the normal physiology of urination and is subject to interruption by trauma, surgery, or drugs. The bladder neck at the trigone region receives sympathetic innervation from the hypogastric nerves emanating from L1 to L3. Stimulation of α_1-adrenergic receptors constricts the urethra to help urinary storage. However, hyperplastic prostatic tissue can further impinge upon the ureter and contribute to difficult urination. The α_1-antagonists, such as terazosin, reduce sympathetically mediated constriction so that urination is easier in these patients. Sacral (S2 to S4) parasympathetic efferent and visceral afferent nerves are also present. The muscarinic efferent fibers innervate the body of the bladder and cause contraction. Sensory fibers of the pelvic nerves emanate from the fundus to detect bladder fullness, pain, and temperature. Sacral pudendal efferent nerves innervate the skeletal muscle of the external sphincter, where excitation causes sphincter contraction.

The process of micturition is an autonomic spinal cord reflex that can be modulated by centers in the brainstem and cerebral cortex. Progressive filling of the bladder initiates reflex muscle contraction through stretch receptors. At the same time, sensory signals from the fundus travel to the spinal cord via the pelvic nerves. Efferent parasympathetic nerves cause the detrusor muscle and bladder neck to contract. Because of the orientation of the muscle fibers, contraction opens the bladder neck and allows urine to flow through the posterior urethra. Voluntary relaxation of the external sphincter initiates urination. Damage to bladder innervation has varying consequences. Interruption of the lumbar sympathetic (hypogastric) nerves or the sacral parasympathetic pudendal nerves to the lower urinary tract does not interrupt the micturition reflex. In contrast, interruption of the parasympathetic nerves to the fundus and neck of the bladder results in bladder dysfunction. Pharmacologic modulation of muscarinic receptors can affect micturition as well. Anticholinergic drugs such as atropine or its derivatives can cause urinary retention, and stimulation of bladder muscarinic receptors with an agonist such as bethanecol increases bladder contractions.

Measurement of Renal Function

The kidneys are responsible for the exquisite control of extracellular volume and composition. This involves close coupling between intake and excretion of solutes and water. In order to quantitate the processes involved, it is necessary to be able to measure them. Measuring the urinary excretion of a substance is relatively straightforward. One needs a measured, timed collection of urine in which concentration of the substance is determined. Because amount = volume × concentration, the amount excreted per unit time can be calculated. Determining the intrarenal handling of this substance requires knowing how much went in to the kidney at the glomerulus, and how the tubules reabsorbed or secreted this filtered amount. Thus the amount filtered at the glomerulus (filtered load) is equal to the GFR (mL/min) times the plasma concentration (mg/mL). This requires measurement of the most useful general index of renal function—the GFR.

Because there are no easy direct measurements of the balance of Starling forces resulting in fluid filtration in microscopic glomeruli, indirect measurements are used. A marker such as inulin or creatinine can be used because it has been shown that these substances are inert, easily filtered at the renal glomerulus, not transported in or out of the tubule once filtered, and excreted unchanged in the urine. Thus the clearance of such marker substances can be determined. The clearance represents a volume of plasma from which all the substance has been removed and excreted in the urine per unit time. In the case of an endogenous marker such as creatinine, we know that muscle metabolism produces it at a relatively constant rate. We also know that the amount that is excreted is precisely the amount that was filtered at the glomerulus. If this is the case, and if amount = volume × concentration, then amount filtered = amount excreted, so that

$$GFR \times P_{cr} = U_{cr} \times V$$

where P_{cr} is the plasma creatinine level, U_{cr} is the urine creatinine level, and V is the urine flow rate (mL/min). When solved for GFR, it is equal to ($U_{cr}V/P_{cr}$), or the familiar clearance of creatinine. This now allows us to determine the amount of any other substance that is filtered because all that is additionally required is to measure the plasma concentration of that substance and multiply it by the GFR. Furthermore, if the amount of the substance excreted per unit time is less than the calculated filtered load, then net reabsorption has occurred. An example of this process is glucose in normal patients. Glucose is easily filtered but so extensively reabsorbed that its excretion is normally zero. Patients with uncontrolled diabetes exceed the transport capacity of the tubules and excrete glucose. Its osmotic effect in the tubule results in polyuria. Conversely, an excreted amount of a substance can be larger than its filtered load if net secretion occurs. Drugs such as penicillin are avidly secreted and quickly cleared by the kidney. Some substances, such as urate, undergo filtration, secretion, and reabsorption, so that the net excretion is the sum of all of the processes.

As useful and fundamental as the clearance relationship is, it may still be too cumbersome for routine clinical assessment of kidney function. If creatinine is produced endogenously at a relatively constant rate and only cleared by the kidney, then, as renal function declines, the blood concentration of creatinine rises. Thus a simple, but relatively crude, index of renal function is the serum creatinine concentration (S_{cr}). Its drawback is that a small amount of creatinine secretion makes the measurement less precise and that increases in the blood follow a hyperbolic rise. This means that GFR must decrease substantially before large increases in S_{cr} occur. Nevertheless, it is a commonly used index of renal function. The S_{cr} can be used in the Cockcroft-Gault formula, along with age, gender, and weight, to give an estimation of GFR. An index of the rate of change of GFR in chronic renal disease is $1/S_{cr}$. The straight-line decreasing slope allows one to determine if renal function is deteriorating at a set rate, if interventions slow or accelerate the rate, and at what future time renal function can be predicted to require renal replacement therapy, such as dialysis.

Physiologic Control of Renal Function

GFR and RBF are buffered by minute-to-minute changes in renal perfusion pressure. The process is known as autoregulation and prevents large swings in filtered load of solutes and fluid. If RBF and GFR are measured over a normal range of renal perfusion pressures, these variables remain relatively constant between a mean blood pressure of around 80 and 180 mm Hg. Both RBF and GFR remain relatively constant by changing afferent arteriolar resistance. In this manner, increased afferent resistance drops glomerular capillary pressure to buffer increases in GFR and at the same time increases overall renal vascular resistance, so that RBF does not rise with increased pressure.

The autoregulatory modulation of afferent arteriolar resistance has two components. The first, myogenic component relates to the ability of the vascular smooth muscle to increase tension in response to the change in transmural pressure produced from stretching the vessel at a higher perfusion pressure. This is now known to involve a stretch-activated calcium channel such that increased tension in the wall minimizes dilatation. This mechanism likely participates in other vascular beds that also show autoregulation of flow in response to changing pressure. The second mechanism is unique to the kidney and serves to minimize changes in filtration. It is known as tubuloglomerular feedback. For example, if a sudden increase in renal perfusion pressure were to be transmitted to the glomerular capillaries, this would result in increased filtration of salt and water. Some of the increased filtrate is reabsorbed by the proximal tubule, but some increased delivery occurs through the loop of Henle to the level of the macula densa cells at the start of the distal tubule. At this location, the distal tubule, glomerulus, and afferent arteriole are in close anatomic proximity. Transport of this increased salt load by the cells of the distal tubule releases mediators that constrict the afferent arteriole. This completes a feedback loop to keep renal perfusion and glomerular filtration relatively constant.

The nature of the afferent vasoconstrictor substance(s) is still controversial. Leading candidates include adenosine as a by-product of ATP breakdown involved in transport, one or more prostanoid metabolites, and perhaps other compounds such as nitric oxide or endothelin. Changes in renin and angiotensin production occur through signals coupled to transport at the macula densa as well, but the renin-angiotensin system cannot explain all of tubuloglomerular feedback. Angiotensin preferentially constricts the efferent rather than the afferent arteriole, and changes in salt transport across macula densa cells have effects on renin secretion that are opposite from the effects on the mediators of feedback. Nevertheless, the systems appear loosely coupled because interference with renin production modulates the efficiency of feedback control of GFR.

The reabsorption of NaCl and water quantitatively represents the greatest function of the kidney. Over 25 mol/day of sodium and 180 L/day of water are reabsorbed. Many other solutes are coupled directly or indirectly to the reabsorptive transport of sodium. Obviously, with such a huge filtered load compared to the daily excretion, reabsorption must be extensive and tightly regulated. Sodium reabsorption by the nephron can be divided into two main processes. The first half of the nephron, through the loop of Henle, is responsible for bulk reabsorption of large quantities of solute. The last half of the nephron is an area of fine-tuning of the final urine composition. This can be best appreciated by considering that, on average, perhaps 99% of the sodium originally filtered at the glomerulus is reabsorbed by the time urine exits the collecting duct. If the final portion of the nephron reduces sodium reabsorption to only 98%, this means that sodium excretion has doubled. The ability to sense and adjust to changes in volume and composition of the extracellular fluid is a critical function of the kidney (Fig. 20–1).

The proximal tubules in the cortex reabsorb about two thirds of the glomerular filtrate. This consists of Na^+, Cl^-, K^+, and water and virtually all of the filtered glucose, amino acids, and bicarbonate. The primary driving force for transport is the Na^+,K^+-ATPase in the basolateral membrane. This primary active transport keeps intracellular Na^+ low and K^+ high to provide the driving gradient for Na^+-coupled transporters on the luminal membrane. One of the most quantitatively important steps for Na^+ influx into the proximal tubule cells is an exchange transporter (antiporter) with H^+ on the luminal membrane. The proton that is extruded from cells into the lumen combines with HCO_3^- with the help of carbonic anhydrase that is on the surface of the microvilli of the luminal membrane.

The resulting CO_2 and H_2O easily diffuse into the cell, where they are resynthesized under the influence of intracellular carbonic anhydrase, and the bicarbonate ion is transported across the outside, basolateral membrane back to the blood. This area of the nephron is very efficient at reclaiming almost all of the filtered bicarbonate, and any that remains is reabsorbed by similar mechanisms in the loop. The solutes that are reabsorbed in the proximal tubule carry with them an equivalent amount of water, so that the reabsorbate is isotonic. The main driving force for water to follow solute comes from an area of hypertonicity in the space between cells. Thus the proximal tubule accounts for a large reabsorption of both solutes and water in equivalent proportions.

Beyond the proximal tubule, solute and water reabsorption can be regulated independently. This gives the kidney the ability to create a final urine with an osmolality that is as low as 50 and as high as 1200 mOsm/kg H_2O. This process requires the coordinated efforts of the loop of Henle, the distal tubule, and the collecting ducts. The reduced volume of isotonic tubule fluid that enters the descending thin limb of Henle's loop becomes more concentrated as it reaches the tip of the loop. This is primarily because water permeability is high and the solute gradient of the medullary interstitium provides the driving force. As fluid turns the bend at the tip of the loop, water permeability suddenly decreases and salt and urea permeability comparatively increase. The tubule fluid is now flowing into tissues that are increasingly less concentrated in solutes, so that sodium diffuses passively out of the tubule and some urea enters. The thick limb of Henle's loop is an area of a large amount of active transport of NaCl. The main carrier in this epithelium is a Na^+, K^+, $2Cl^-$ cotransporter on the luminal membrane. This transporter is inhibited by diuretics such as furosemide (Lasix). Approximately another 25% of the NaCl from the original glomerular filtrate is reabsorbed in this portion of the nephron and helps generate the high solute gradient in the medullary interstitium. Water permeability is nil, so that the fluid is actually hypotonic. Tubule fluid now enters the distal tubule, where additional salt is reabsorbed.

As this epithelium transitions into the collecting duct, additional NaCl is reabsorbed and K^+ secretion occurs under the influence of aldosterone. The collecting duct also depends upon vasopressin (antidiuretic hormone) for its water permeability. If the hormone is released from the posterior pituitary in response to volume or osmotic stimuli, it binds to the outside of the tubule, increases cyclic AMP, and imbeds water channels into the luminal membrane. This family of water channels is known as aquaporins. Some are constitutive and account for water movement across lipid membranes throughout the body, but aquaporin-2 requires vasopressin in order to be translocated to the renal collecting duct membrane.

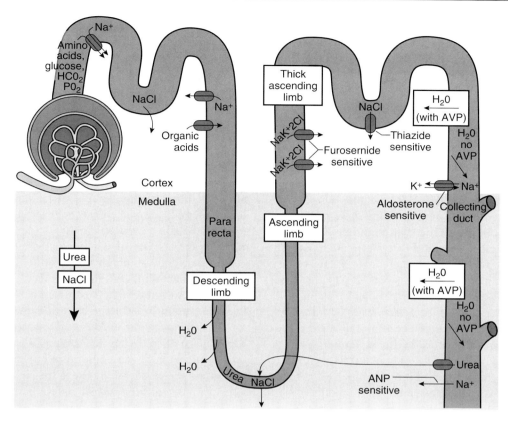

FIGURE 20–1 Major sites of transport and diuretic action along the nephron. The processes involved are described in the text. (From Lingappa VR, Farey K: Physiological Medicine: A Clinical Approach to Basic Medical Physiology. New York: McGraw-Hill, 2000:438. Reproduced with permission of The McGraw-Hill Companies.)

The last component needed for regulation of urine osmolality is urea in the medullary interstitium. Vasopressin-regulated urea channels in the innermost areas of the collecting duct permit its recycling in order to contribute to the hyperosmolality of the gradient. With all of the components now assembled, the kidney can quickly change from making a concentrated urine to a dilute urine simply in response to vasopressin levels. If vasopressin is high, solute gradients, including urea, are maximal in the medullary interstitium. The permeability to water is high as the tubule fluid passes through the collecting duct and equilibrates quickly with the hypertonic tissue. If vasopressin is low, urea contributes little to the medullary gradient, water reabsorption is reduced from the descending limb, and thick limb transport still produces a hypotonic tubule fluid, but now the distal tubule and collecting duct cannot remove the water because permeability is low. Large amounts of dilute urine are excreted. The clinical importance of transport at the loop of Henle can also be appreciated from this mechanism. This area of the tubule is responsible for much of the salt transport that provides the hypertonic medullary interstitium. If a patient is given enough loop diuretic to inhibit these transporters, then the interstitial solute gradient will approach isotonicity rather

than be hypertonic. Water reabsorption and passive salt transport in the thin limbs will be reduced and water removal from the collecting duct will be minimal regardless of the presence of vasopressin, because the driving gradient is dissipated. Therefore, the urine osmolality will approach isotonic. If this patient is administered free water through intravenous or oral routes, hyponatremia may result because the ability of the kidney to excrete the extra free water is compromised.

Although the kidney strives to maintain homeostasis of the extracellular fluid volume, the cardiovascular sensors may misinterpret the fullness of the vasculature if fluid is sequestered as edema or ascites, or if cardiac output is reduced secondary to heart disease. Thus an effective circulating volume (ECV) is actually sensed by low-pressure stretch receptors in the atria and pulmonary vasculature and by high-pressure receptors in the carotid sinus, aortic arch, and juxtaglomerular cells of the renal afferent arteriole. The response of integrated central nervous system afferent and efferent neural pathways to a perceived decrease in ECV involves (1) an increase in renal sympathetic nerve activity to decrease GFR, increase renin secretion, and increase tubular NaCl reabsorption; and (2) activation of the renin-angiotensin-aldosterone system to increase angiotensin II–mediated proximal NaCl transport, increase aldosterone-mediated loop and distal nephron NaCl reabsorption, and increase vasopressin secretion; so that (3) vasopressin increases water reabsorption from the collecting duct. These factors operate in reverse as well to help correct a sensed volume overload. In this case, additional natriuretic substances such as atrial natriuretic peptide augment NaCl loss through the kidney along with reducing the secretion of antinatriuretic hormones.

Potassium excretion is regulated in the kidney by secretion into the distal nephron fluid. Filtered K^+ is extensively reabsorbed in the proximal tubule and loop of Henle, so that the luminal concentration of K^+ is very low by the time the fluid enters the late distal tubule and early collecting duct. In this area of the nephron, Na^+ channels permit Na^+ entry into the cells, where it is pumped out across the basolateral membrane by Na^+,K^+-ATPase. This brings K^+ into the cells so that intracellular K^+ is high. Potassium is diffused out of the cells toward the lumen because the concentration gradient is favorable and the negative lumen provides a further driving force. Aldosterone regulates Na^+ reabsorption and K^+ secretion by stimulating the expression of more luminal Na^+ channels, more Na^+,K^+-ATPase pumps, and more ATP synthesis. Spironolactone is an aldosterone receptor blocker that prevents these changes, so that it is a K^+-sparing diuretic. Amiloride and triamterene provide the same pharmacologic changes in kidney function but do so by blocking the Na^+ channel entry step.

The kidney works in concert with the lungs and the liver to regulate extracellular pH. Under normal physiologic conditions, the kidney efficiently reabsorbs virtually all of the filtered bicarbonate. The pH of the urine is, in most individuals, acidic because the kidney excretes approximately 80 mmol of fixed acid each day. This consists mainly of sulfates and phosphates derived from ingested proteins. However, most of the protons secreted by the nephron into the urine need to be buffered or the tubule fluid pH would be much too low. Buffering is achieved by fixing a proton onto HPO_4^{2-} to form $H_2PO_4^-$ (titratable acid) and onto NH_4^+. The latter is a very important sink for protons because, in metabolic acidosis, the liver increases glutamine synthesis and the kidney increases glutamine breakdown. In the process, bicarbonate is generated and helps replenish the body stores, and NH_4^+ is formed to help excrete the proton excess. The hepatic and renal enzymes involved take some time to be induced, so that renal compensation for an acid-base imbalance takes several days to correct yet is very efficient.

Acute Renal Failure

Acute renal failure (ARF) can occur in almost any medical setting but is most common in hospitalized or postsurgical patients. It develops in 5% of hospitalized patients and has significant morbidity and mortality. The family of syndromes categorized as ARF can logically be subdivided into three etiologies: prerenal, intrinsic (intrarenal), and postrenal. In all types of ARF, the glomerular filtration rate decreases rapidly, in days to weeks. As a result, the kidney poorly filters fluids, electrolytes, and waste products. The filtrate that is produced may have exaggerated or decreased reabsorption depending upon the integrity of the nephrons. The condition is often diagnosed by measuring elevated levels of blood urea nitrogen (BUN) and creatinine. Because of the elevation in nitrogenous wastes, the condition is correctly referred to as azotemia, since the kidney may or may not have failed early in the disease. Acute azotemia or ARF may be defined as an acute increase of the serum creatinine of at least 0.5 mg/dL (44 μmol/L) over baseline. Oliguric renal failure, or renal shutdown, is present when the serum creatinine increases at least 0.5 mg/dL/day and the urine output is less than 400 mL/day (Fig. 20–2).

Prerenal azotemia, or ARF, is due to impaired RBF. This is most often due to true extracellular volume depletion but may also involve other reasons that renal perfusion is compromised. While the kidney normally has a large percentage of the cardiac output perfusing it, the distribution of RBF is heterogeneous. Under normal conditions, the outer medulla extra extracts 80% to 90% of the oxygen from the blood perfusing it, so that it borders on hypoxia. This layer of the kidney contains metabolically active nephron segments such as the thick ascending limb of Henle's loop and the pars recta of the proximal tubule. Because of this, the outer medulla is at risk of ischemia when total RBF is diminished. Unless prerenal causes of

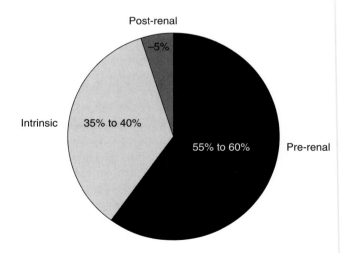

FIGURE 20–2 Types of acute renal failure. (Data from Brady HR, Brenner BM, Clarkson MR, Lieberthal W: Acute renal failure. *In* Brenner BM [ed]: Brenner & Rector's the Kidney [6th ed, vol I]. Philadelphia: WB Saunders, 2000:1201; and Agrawal M, Swartz R: Acute renal failure. Am Fam Physician 2000;61:2078.)

renal ischemia are recognized and corrected quickly, acute tubular necrosis can result. True intravascular volume depletion can result from hemorrhage, poor fluid intake, sepsis or other third-space losses, diarrhea, or vomiting. Decreased ECV perfusing the kidney can be a consequence of congestive heart failure, hepatorenal syndrome, or loss of oncotic retention of fluid in the vasculature from the nephrotic syndrome. Additionally, perfusion of the kidney can be compromised by stenoses or by some drugs. The most important culprits are angiotensin-converting enzyme (ACE) inhibitors or angiotensin receptor blockers, and nonsteroidal anti-inflammatory drugs (NSAIDs). In the former case, glomerular filtration in some patients, especially those with bilateral renal artery stenosis or hypovolemia, may depend upon angiotensin to maintain GFR. This is because it preferentially constricts the postglomerular efferent arteriole, which raises intraglomerular filtration pressure. Blocking the formation or action of angiotensin reduces GFR, and ARF can develop. These consequences can be avoided by ensuring adequate hydration of patients and by monitoring potassium, BUN, and creatinine soon after starting these drugs. In like manner, GFR is maintained in some patients by preglomerular dilatation from intrarenal prostaglandins. Prerenal ARF can result from inhibition of their synthesis with NSAIDs. Newer cyclooxygenase-2 inhibitors still share in this concern. Finally, some drugs that directly constrict the kidney, such as cyclosporine and tacrolimus (FK506), can complicate the management of renal transplantation.

Intrinsic ARF involves damage to the renal parenchyma. Because the acute azotemia is due to problems within the kidney, altering factors extrinsic to the kidney, such as improving hydration, cannot change it. The term *acute tubular necrosis* is often used as a synonym for intrarenal ARF. However, proximal tubular necrosis is not always present, so the terms are not strictly interchangeable. There are four main causes of intrinsic ARF: tubular disease, glomerular disease, vascular disease, and interstitial disease. Tubular diseases most often result from ischemic or toxic insults to the kidney. Acute tubular necrosis from ischemia may be reversible, but, if longer standing cortical necrosis occurs, the failure may be irreversible. Ischemia may follow surgery or trauma where redistribution of blood flow results in poor renal perfusion. Rhabdomyolysis with myoglobinuria or hemolysis with hemoglobinuria are important causes and are now known to contribute to renal vasoconstriction by antagonizing nitric oxide vasodilatation. Nephrotoxicity may result from some anti-infective agents such as aminoglycosides, cancer drugs such as cisplatin, contrast media, heavy metals, and ethylene glycol antifreeze. Because the nephrons are damaged, the abilities to transport electrolytes and urea and to generate a high urine osmolality are compromised.

Table 20–1

Distinguishing prerenal from intrinsic acute renal failure (ARF)

Type	BUN/Creatinine Ratio	Urine Osmolality	Fractional Excretion of Na[+]*
Prerenal ARF	>20:1	>500 mOsm	<1%
Intrinsic ARF	<20:1	250–300 mOsm	>3%

BUN, blood urea nitrogen; cr, creatinine; s, serum; u, urine.
*The fractional excretion of Na[+] (percentage of the filtered sodium remaining in the urine) is calculated by $(U_{Na}/S_{Na}) \div (U_{cr}/S_{cr}) \times 100$.

This compares to poor prerenal perfusion of an otherwise normal kidney (Table 20–1)

Acute tubular necrosis evolves from an initiation phase, which may last hours to days, to an oliguric phase with maximally decreased GFR and poor urine output. This may be followed by a polyuric recovery phase in which volume, electrolyte, and pH homeostasis may still be unbalanced because of damaged nephrons. Glomerular disease or glomerulonephritis can be characterized by hypertension, proteinuria, and hematuria. Although there are many types, the rapidly progressive and acute proliferative glomerulonephritides may lead to ARF. Microvascular or macrovascular disease can also cause ARF. Examples are thrombocytopenic purpura, hemolytic uremic syndrome, and the hemolysis, elevated liver enzymes, and low platelet count in association with preeclampsia (HELLP) syndrome of pregnancy. Atheroembolic events following surgery or invasive procedures risk irreversible ARF. The evidence may manifest in the skin and other organs as well as in reduced renal function. Acute interstitial nephritis can present as fever, rash, and eosinophilia. It may be due to an allergic reaction to drugs such as NSAIDs, penicillins, sulfonamides, cephalosporins, diuretics, and allopurinol. The suspected drug should be withdrawn, and treatment with corticosteroids may be helpful. Interstitial nephritis may also be an autoimmune disease or due to an infection.

Differentiating between prerenal and intrarenal causes of failure is a common clinical problem. An analysis of urine and serum reflects the pathophysiology and helps determine the cause. In the case of prerenal azotemia, perfusion and delivery to the nephrons is decreased but the tubules are intact and functioning. Therefore, urea, sodium, and water have extended transit time through the nephron and are extensively reabsorbed. Creatinine undergoes some secretion but not reabsorption. The ratio of BUN to creatinine rises, and sodium and water are conserved. When tubular epithelium is damaged in intrinsic ARF, the ability to efficiently conserve urea, water, and sodium is compromised. Postrenal ARF occurs if the urinary outflow tracts are obstructed at the level of the kidney, ureter, or bladder. This usually results in severe oliguria or anuria and may be due to crystals, tumors, or myeloma light chains. The back pressure on the kidney may produce hydronephrosis that is detectable by ultrasound. Treatment of postrenal failure is aimed at relieving the obstruction.

Treatment of the major types of ARF begins with eliminating the cause if possible and correcting the extracellular volume. Prerenal failure requires adequate volume correction. Patients who are oliguric from intrinsic ARF may be volume overloaded. Urine flow can be increased with diuretics such as furosemide, but disturbances in potassium and acid-base balance require correction. In many cases hypovolemia may outweigh any benefit. Mannitol may have benefit in rhabdomyolysis but may be deleterious in other situations. Dopamine, atrial natriuretic peptide, and calcium antagonists have equivocal benefit and should not substitute for adequate volume restoration.

Evaluation of Renal Function in the Surgical Patient

As discussed above, most situations of azotemia result from prerenal causes. Therefore, careful perioperative attention to adequate hydration and factors that may compromise RBF can prevent compromised renal function. Gastrointestinal fluid loss or third-space sequestration in burn or trauma patients must also be considered. Initial preoperative measurements of serum creatinine and BUN and urinalysis are appropriate. This permits estimation of the GFR, suggests euvolemia if the BUN and creatinine serum concentrations are not elevated and their ratio is about 10:1, and excludes proteinuria, hematuria, hyaline casts, or incipient stone disease. Postrenal consideration for urinary obstruction should be considered in older men with prostatic hyperplasia, in other causes of lower urinary tract obstruction, and in patients receiving adrenergic or anticholinergic drugs. Hypovolemia compromises renal function more than hypervolemia, but the latter is also of concern in the surgical patient. It will be manifested in elevated venous pressures measured directly or estimated by jugular venous distention. Too-vigorous fluid replacement can result in cardiopulmonary congestion. Creatinine is a product of muscle catabolism. Therefore, transient increases with trauma or surgery may not accurately reflect a decrease in GFR. Urine flow appropriate to the amount of fluid being administered is consistent with adequate renal perfusion and function.

Chronic Renal Insufficiency and End-Stage Renal Disease

Chronic renal insufficiency, or chronic renal failure (CRF), manifests a decrease in GFR and a reduction in nephron number. The course is typically progressive, with continued loss of functioning nephrons, eventually leading to ESRD. Renal disease is classified in general terms by the rate at which the GFR falls. This fall occurs over days in ARF, over months in subacute failure, and over years in CRF. This time between initial onset of disease and ESRD varies considerably between patients and with various renal diseases. When patients present with already decreased GFR, the differentiation becomes more complex but important because ARF is potentially reversible, whereas reversal of CRF is unlikely.

The etiology of CRF guides treatment. Diabetes and hypertension are responsible for over 60% of ESRD patients, but genetic factors such as race and human leukocyte antigen (HLA) haplotype play a role in addition to disease severity in the individual. Patients with type 1 diabetes mellitus (DM) have a higher prevalence of ESRD, but the incidence is higher in type 2 patients because the patient population is so much greater. In other patients, congenital kidney diseases, glomerulonephritis, obstructive uropathy, and interstitial nephritis are common causes of CRF.

Hypertension and DM damage glomerular membranes in part because high pressure is transmitted to the glomerular capillaries. Blood pressure may be lowered by a variety of mechanisms, but ACE inhibitors and angiotensin receptor blockers relax the efferent arteriole to lower intraglomerular pressure. Proteinuria, an index of glomerular capillary damage and nephrotoxicity per se, can be reduced when the capillary pressure is lowered. This approach has become a mainstay of protecting the kidneys in diabetic nephropathy and is increasingly applicable to other forms of chronic renal disease.

CRF progresses to a constellation of abnormalities. Fluid and electrolyte balance may be relatively well maintained until GFR is reduced to nearly 10 mL/min. The remaining nephrons then become overloaded, which eventually destroys them, but in the interim each nephron excretes a greater fraction of the filtrate. The ability to regulate high amounts of sodium or potassium in the diet becomes reduced as function deteriorates. With nephron damage, calcium and phosphate regulation is disturbed. Patients have decreased 1,25-dihydroxy vitamin D_3 and decreased phosphate excretion. This results in a secondary hyperparathyroidism, renal osteodystrophy, and extraskeletal calcification if not corrected. Therapy rationally reduces dietary phosphate by binding it in the gut, increases calcium, and provides an active analog of vitamin D. Anemia results from the kidney's inability to produce erythropoietin. The anemia is usually not severe until later in the disease, and treatment may be withheld until ESRD stage. Although a potential complication of erythropoietin is hypertension, patients' physiologic and psychological function often improves considerably with therapy. Because of the expense, the timing and dose of the drug are the subjects of many pharmacoeconomics analyses. Edema is a frequent complication and results from decreased albumin synthesis as well as salt and water ingestion beyond the excretory ability of the remnant kidneys.

When residual renal function can no longer cope with the metabolic demands, ESRD ensues. Symptomatic uremia ("uremic syndrome") occurs when the creatinine reaches 8 to 10 mg/dL and the BUN is greater than 100 mg/dL. The first symptoms may be subtle, such as lethargy, malaise, and weakness. Gastrointestinal symptoms of nausea, vomiting, and anorexia are common. With further progression, motor neuropathy, malnutrition, volume overload, impaired cognition, and intractable itching are seen. Endogenous renal function is no longer adequate, and renal replacement therapy is required.

Renal Replacement Therapy

Most patients with acute renal insufficiency can be managed without dialysis, although short-term hemodialysis (HD) may be useful for drug or toxin overdose or for brief support of renal function. Patients with CRF who progress to ESRD may be candidates for forms of renal replacement therapy depending upon comorbid conditions and patient preferences. Therapy for ESRD involves three main approaches: (1) HD, usually at a dialysis center but sometimes at home; (2) automated peritoneal dialysis (PD); or (3) renal transplantation from a living-related, living-unrelated, or cadaveric donor. The presence of uremic syndrome accelerates the need for dialysis.

Hemodialysis involves the simple principles of solute-gradient and pressure-gradient movement of fluids across a semipermeable membrane. These simple principles have evolved into highly complex technology to accurately control each patient's ion, pH, glucose, and water balance while simultaneously removing urea, creatinine, and other waste products. This is accomplished by adjusting the concentration, osmolality, flow rate, and pressure gradient of the dialysate across the dialysis membrane. Most patients require HD three times a week for several hours. The high flux rate (porosity) of modern dialysis cartridges permits rapid exchange of solutes and water for more rapid and efficient dialysis. If net removal of water from the patient is to be accomplished for fluid and blood pressure control, the dialysate is made hypertonic with a relatively poorly permeant solute, so that net flux is from blood to dialysate.

Vascular access remains a limiting factor in dialysis. Direct vessel cannulation is quickly limiting and painful, so a more permanent surgical solution is sought. An arteriovenous fistula, most commonly from the radial artery to the cephalic vein, can last for years with native vessels. If these vessels are inadequate, synthetic grafts are a common solution, but thrombosis, infection, and aneurysms require constant vigilance and occasional replacement. Graft material composition, design, intervention and repair techniques, and salvage protocols continue to extend arteriovenous graft life span.

The adequacy of a dialysis treatment remains a clinical judgment. However, one important clinical reason for administering dialysis is to reduce complications of the uremic syndrome. Many endogenous toxins likely participate, but clinical severity also correlates well with urea concentration, measured as the BUN. Because urea is a small molecule that is easily dialyzed, its blood concentration becomes a useful marker of dialysis adequacy. However, simply measuring BUN does not give an adequate picture because dialysis occurs over short intervals three times weekly. In the interim, protein catabolism and volume changes contribute to a constantly changing BUN. A time-averaged urea concentration gives a more integrated picture, but modeling urea kinetics gives the most currently reproducible guidelines. Just as first-order pharmacokinetics describes the elimination of drugs from the body, similar exponential kinetics describes urea fluxes. When BUN is measured at several time intervals, a slope of its reduction can be generated. The efficiency of dialysis is expressed as Kt/V. The K, a clearance term, represents dialyzer urea clearance, and t is the time on dialysis. This product represents the volume of dialysis delivered. This is normalized for the patient's size by dividing by the volume of distribution of urea (V) in the patient. The dimensionless quotient is a useful index of time-integrated dialysis efficiency. Experience has determined that Kt/V needs to be over 1.0. Although higher values, often in the 1.6 to 1.8 range, are desirable, the efficiency is limited by time, equipment, complications of fluid shifts, and hypotension. Another way of representing dialysis efficiency is by simply describing a linear decrease in urea between two time points. This urea reduction ratio (URR) of about 60% corresponds to a Kt/V of 1.0 and therefore represents a minimum for dialysis adequacy. These factors are related by the expression

$$Kt/V = \ln[1 - (URR/100)]$$

PD is technically much less complex than HD. A warmed, sterile electrolyte and dextrose (or other osmolyte) dialysate is infused into the peritoneum. Typically, 2 L is infused. After a dwell time of several hours or overnight, the fluid is allowed to drain and is replaced by fresh dialysate. The peritoneum becomes the semipermeable membrane across which diffusion occurs. The fluid exchange can be done manually, which is called continuous ambulatory PD, or can be done by an automated machine, which is called continuous cycling PD. Although the process may be simple, it involves the same principles and some of the same problems associated with HD.

Access to the peritoneum requires silicone rubber or polyurethane catheter placement. A double-cuffed Tenckhoff catheter or a variation, such as a swan-neck design, is placed through the rectus muscle and tunneled subcutaneously. A goal of PD is to remove waste product molecules such as urea and creatinine, as well as many larger "middle molecules" of undetermined composition. Larger molecular weight molecules diffuse slower across the peritoneal membranes, so that a longer dwell time more efficiently removes them. This must be balanced by the clinical practicality of the patient's lifestyle to encourage compliance. Unlike HD, the adequacy of dialysis in PD is less clearly defined by clinical trials. However, it is known that maintaining BUN at 70 mg/dL or less will prevent uremic symptoms, and that an average patient needs to remove about 10 L of dialysate per week to maintain this. Because the hypertonicity of the dialysate is designed for a net removal of fluid in order to control blood volume and pressure, this means that approximately four 2-L dialysis exchanges per week are needed to remove this much urea. If urea reduction is calculated in a fashion similar to that for HD, this results in a weekly Kt/V of 1.7 to 2.1, or a creatinine clearance of about 50 L/wk. Important complications of PD include peritonitis and catheter infections, peritoneal fibrosis, anemia (corrected with supplemental erythropoietin), malnutrition resulting from protein loss, and hypertriglyceridemia.

Renal transplantation has allowed a major improvement in quality of life of ESRD patients. Kidneys can be obtained from cadavers, living-related donors, or living-unrelated donors. In general, 1-year graft survival rates for living-related and cadaveric donors are 90% and 80%, respectively. Potential kidney recipients are evaluated for concurrent life-limiting diseases and comorbid conditions that complicate management, such as obesity, diabetes, cardiovascular diseases, infections, and metabolic bone disease. Recipients and donor tissues are blood group and HLA crossmatched and screened for blood-borne infectious diseases, including human immunodeficiency virus and hepatitis B and C.

Renal transplant surgery has not changed much since its advent and is relatively straightforward. The donor kidney is placed in the retroperitoneal iliac fossa, and the renal artery and vein are anastomosed to the iliac vessels. If possible, the cadaveric kidney is obtained with a cuff of donor aorta. This reduces the chance of vascular stenosis at the anastomotic site. The ureter is implanted into the bladder with an antireflux technique in the area of the trigone. Lymphatic vessels in the vicinity of the transplant are ligated to prevent leakage and lymphocele formation. Careful attention to detail is critical because the patient risks infections as a result of immunosuppressive agents and poor healing from malnutrition associated with ESRD and dialysis.

Post-transplant immunosuppression varies widely but generally starts with an aggressive induction phase for the first 5 to 14 days, a more moderate maintenance phase with lifetime immunosuppression, and acute treatment with higher doses or different drugs for rejection episodes. Current drugs target interleukin production or affect cytokine and T cell production. A current review of immunosuppression in a general renal medicine text can provide further details. Most transplant centers use corticosteroids, cyclosporine, tacrolimus, mycophenolate mofetil, and sirolimus. Patient groups expected to mount a strong immune response such as children, African-Americans, and repeat transplant recipients receive additional induction therapy with anti-thymocyte globulin. Antibodies to lymphocytes and to CD3$^+$ T cells (OKT3) are added to combat rejection episodes. Long-term management of these patients involves recognition and treatment of acute and chronic rejection episodes, minimizing infections (especially of cytomegalovirus), and minimizing coronary artery disease risk factors such as hypercholesterolemia and hypertension. Immunosuppressed patients are more susceptible to skin cancers, lymphomas, and some other cancers, so patient counseling and surveillance are warranted.

Bibliography

Agrawal M, Swartz R: Acute renal failure. Am Fam Physician 2000;61:2077.

Brenner BM (ed): Brenner & Rector's the Kidney (6th ed), Vols I and II. Philadelphia: WB Saunders, 2000.

Crowley S: Slowing the progression of chronic renal insufficiency. N C Med J 2000;61:80.

Koeppen BM, Stanton BA: Renal Physiology (3rd ed). St. Louis: Mosby, 2000.

Kriz W, Bankir L: A standard nomenclature for structures of the kidney. Am J Physiol 1988;254:F1.

Lingappa VR, Farey K: Physiological Medicine: A Clinical Approach to Basic Medical Physiology. New York: McGraw-Hill, 2000.

Schrier RW (ed): Manual of Nephrology (4th ed). Boston: Little, Brown, 1995.

CHAPTER 21

Reproductive Physiology and Dysfunction

Peter A. Argenta, M.D.

Human reproduction is the culmination of physiologic processes beginning with sex determination and proceeding through phases of organogenesis, endocrine maturation, and secondary structural development. Departure from normal clinical development in any stage may signify underlying pathology and result in failure to achieve or maintain reproductive capacity.

Sex Determination

Assignment of sex can be based on genotype, gonad type, or physical appearance. Genotypic sex is determined at conception when an oocyte, which always carries 22 autosomes and an X sex chromosome, is fertilized by a spermatid carrying a complementary 22 autosomes and either an X chromosome (yielding 46,XX, the female genotype) or a Y chromosome (yielding 46,XY, the male genotype). Only one X chromosome will remain viable in each cell. In females, one of the sex chromosomes is randomly selected to undergo condensation and inactivation. The condensed chromatin remains in the nucleus, forming a microscopically visible Barr body, but is not functional for protein production. Because the inactivation process is random, half of all cells will have an active maternal X chromosome, and half a paternal X. Gonadal and phenotypic determination depend on the chromosomal complement, intact endocrine axes, functional cellular receptors, and hormonal environment.

Development of Gonads and Genitalia

All embryos remain identical with regard to phenotypic differentiation in early gestation. Each maintains both a müllerian duct system, capable of becoming a uterus and oviducts, and a wolffian duct system, capable of becoming the epididymis, vas deferens, and seminal vesicles. Each embryo also contains two undifferentiated gonads, which originate in the genital ridge and migrate caudally. The gonads remain bipotential, that is, capable of becoming ovaries or testes, for the first 6 weeks of gestation.

Testicular development begins during the sixth and seventh weeks after conception in the presence of a Y sex chromosome. Specifically, the sex-determining region of the Y chromosome, or SRY locus, is required. The SRY locus encodes a protein transcription factor that binds to DNA and increases the production of testicular proteins, including anti-müllerian hormone (AMH). The SRY locus is generally considered "both necessary and sufficient" for male gonadal determination because, in its absence, regardless of the other chromosomal compliment, female determination proceeds. Thus female determination is often referred to as the "default pathway."

The gonads begin to differentiate in males during the seventh week of gestation. The cortex regresses and the medulla develops, becoming populated with spermatogonia, which will be responsible for gamete production, and Sertoli and Leydig cells. Leydig cells secrete testosterone, which supports development of the wolffian ducts. Some testosterone is converted to dihydrotestosterone (DHT) in the end organ by the cytosolic enzyme 5α-reductase. Dihydrotestosterone induces formation of the external genitalia and later some of the male secondary characteristics. Simultaneously, Sertoli cells secrete AMH, a member of the transforming growth factor-β superfamily, which stimulates apoptosis in the cells of the müllerian system. AMH has been thought to play a role in the descent of the testes, but recent evidence has called this into question.

Ovarian differentiation is detectable by the eighth to ninth week after conception. Contrary to the sequence of development of the testis, the medulla of the undifferentiated gonad regresses and the cortex develops, becoming populated with germ cells called oogonia, and supporting theca and granulosa cells. There is little or no hormone production in the immature ovary. Without AMH, the müllerian system develops into the uterus, fallopian tubes, and upper vagina by the 10th week of gestation. Conversely, the wolffian ducts regress in the absence of testosterone. Occasionally regression of the wolffian system is incomplete, and remnants, also called Gartner's duct cysts, can be detected as cystic masses in the lateral vagina of otherwise normal females.

Either the wolffian or müllerian system is established internally by the end of the eighth week in normal embryonic development. External differentiation is usually evident by 10 weeks and complete by 14 weeks, when the urogenital slit closes in males but remains open in females, creating the vaginal introitus. Further development of the external genitalia will come primarily through growth.

Abnormal Sexual Differentiation

Errors of sex chromosome assortment are not uniformly lethal. The most common mechanism is a nondisjunction event in which the sex chromosomes fail to split evenly during meiosis. The result is one gamete with no sex chromosomes, and one gamete with two. Fertilization with a normal gamete results in embryos with either 45 or 47 chromosomes (Table 21–1). Assortment defects need not involve an entire chromosome. For instance, the *SRY* gene may be absent from the Y chromosome as a result of deletion or translocation; in this case the phenotype is female while the genotype remains 46,XY. Conversely, phenotypically normal 46,XX males have been observed when the *SRY* locus has migrated to the X sex chromosome.

Phenotypic variation of the external genitalia from that predicted by the gonadal type is usually due to abnormal androgen effect: too little in males or too much in females. The exception is true hermaphroditism, in which both ovarian and testicular tissue can be found in the same individual, usually in the same gonad (an ovotestis). True hermaphroditism is usually the result of XX/XY mosaicism. The term *pseudohermaphrodite*, indicating that there is a partial discordance between the gonad type and the clinical phenotype, is more appropriate in most cases of sexual ambiguity. A female pseudohermaphrodite has ovaries but displays masculine characteristics, most commonly clitoromegaly. Almost 50% of such cases are caused by congenital adrenal hyperplasia, with cholesterol metabolites being shunted inappropriately from cortisol production to sex hormone production. Male pseudohermaphrodites have testes but are incompletely masculinized. The spectrum of phenotypes extends from normal-appearing, infertile females (complete testicular feminization) to normal-appearing, fertile males. The common causes of pseudohermaphroditism are listed in Box 21–1.

Table 21–1
Common disorders of sex chromosome assortment

Genotype	Viable	Fertile	Phenotype
45,XO (Turner's syndrome)	Yes*	Rarely	Short stature, mental retardation, absent or rudimentary gonads, webbed neck, cardiac anomalies
45,YO	No	No	Lethal in utero
47,XXX ("super female")	Yes	Yes	Normal female, Barr bodies visible microscopically
47,XXY (Kleinfelter's syndrome)	Yes	Rarely	Tall stature, normal male genitalia with small testes, mental retardation, gynecomasia
47,XYY	Yes	Yes	Usually normal male, tall stature, subfertility, and aggressive behavior seen occasionally

*While many of these embryos survive to birth, 45,XO is the single most common karyotype in first-trimester spontaneous abortions (miscarriages).

Box 21-1
Causes of Pseudohermaphroditism

Female
Congenital adrenal hyperplasia
  21β-Hydroxylase deficiency
  11β-Hydroxylase deficiency
  3β-Hydroxysteroid dehydrogenase deficiency
Maternal ingestion of androgenic substance, progestational agents
Maternal androgen overproduction
Placental aromatase deficiency

Male
Defective hormone production
  AMH synthesis defect
  Testosterone synthesis defect
  5α-Reductase deficiency
  $P450_{scc}$ deficiency
  3β-Hydroxysteroid dehydrogenase deficiency
  17β-Hydroxylase deficiency
  17β-Hydroxysteroid dehydrogenase deficiency
Abnormal receptor response
  Androgen insensitivity (testosterone receptor defect)
  Gonadotropin-resistant testes
Gonadal degeneration or dysgenesis

AMH, anti-müllerian hormone.

Failure of the testis to complete migration to the scrotum is called cryptorchidism. Migration to the scrotum, however, is influenced by multiple factors. Cryptorchidism is present in up to 10% of newborn males. Most of these (80%) will spontaneously resolve within the first year of life, and only 0.3% persist into puberty. Despite this, prompt surgical correction of cryptorchidism is now standard because undescended testes have a higher risk of tumor development and because prolonged exposure to the core body temperature can cause permanent decreases in sperm production.

Adolescence/Puberty

Both sexes go through a period of quiescence from birth through adolescence, during which both gonadal secretion of steroids and pituitary secretion of gonadotropins is relatively low. Hypothalamic production of gonadotropin-releasing hormone (GnRH) begins to increase between the age of 7 and 10. Gonadal estrogen or testosterone production increases shortly thereafter, effecting development of the secondary sexual characteristics. In females these changes include breast development (thelarche), followed by the appearance of pubic and axillary hair growth (pubarche), and finally the onset of menstrual cycles (menarche). Male secondary sexual changes include deepening of the voice, enlargement of the penis and testicles, acne, and male pattern facial, axillary, and pubic hair growth. Pubarche in both sexes is augmented by spontaneous increases in adrenal production of the androgen dehydroepiandrosterone sulfate.

The term *adolescence* describes this final period of structural maturation, and should be distinguished from the term *puberty*, which connotes attainment of reproductive capacity. Sufficient characterization of the physical and hormonal changes exists to identify pathologically premature or delayed maturation. Standard clinical milestones are listed in Table 21–2.

The average age of puberty varies regionally, but in general has been steadily decreasing at a rate of 1 to 3 months per decade in industrialized nations for over 150 years. Pubertal ages have stabilized in the United States during the last half-century, with males reaching puberty between the ages of 9 and 14 and females between 8 and 13. Improved nutrition, increased adiposity, and reduction of environmental stresses all have been implicated in decreasing the age of puberty.

Precocious and Delayed Puberty

True precocious puberty is the early but otherwise normal activation of the hypothalamic-pituitary-gonadal axis, with resultant appearance of the secondary sexual characteristics and gametogenesis before the age of 8. Precocious pseudopuberty implies that the secondary sexual characteristics have developed in the absence of gametogenesis. Pseudopuberty arises from abnormal exposure in immature males to androgens or in immature females to estrogens. For this reason, true precocious puberty is sometimes called GnRH dependent to distinguish it from pseudopuberty, which is GnRH independent. Precocity is five times more common in females than males and, though most often constitutional, it may indicate significant underlying pathology. Complete physical and endocrinologic evaluation is mandated in all cases. Causes for precocious sexual development are listed in Table 21–3.

Puberty is not considered pathologically delayed unless menstruation has failed to occur by age 17 or testicular development by age 20. Delay can result from disruption at any point along the hypothalamic-pituitary-gonadal axis, but ultimately results from functional hypogonadism. It can occur in the setting of overproduction (hypergonadotropic) or underproduction (hypogonadotropic) of GnRH. Hypergonadotropic hypogonadism implies a deficient gonadal response to luteinizing hormone (LH) and follicle-stimulating hormone (FSH). In males, this can occur in the absence of Leydig cells, as seen in some

Table 21–2
Clinical stages of pubertal development

Stage	Average Age	Findings
Males		
I (preadolescent)	0–7.5	Genitalia small
II	12	Enlargement of the testes
III	13.7	Penile enlargement
IV	15.7	Glans penis enlargement
V (adult)		Adult genitalia
Females		
I	0–7.0	Undeveloped breast, areola; no pubic hair
II	9.8	Breast budding; sparse hair extends to mons
III	11.2	Elevation, enlargement of breast, hair covers mons
IV	12.1	Projection of areolas, adult hair on mons only
V	14.6	Adult breast, female escutcheon

dysgenetic gonads, in the absence of functional LH receptors, or following castration. Clinically, eunuchoidism develops when the deficit is intrinsic to the testes. Eunuchoid individuals are tall, as a result of delayed epiphysial plate closure, but have typically female morphology, with narrow shoulders, widened hips, small muscles, and female pattern escutcheon (maintained through the production of adrenal-cortical androgen production), though secondary hair in general is sparse. Their genitalia are small and they have high-pitched voices.

Hypogonadotropic hypogonadism describes normal gonads that remain unstimulated by the upper endocrine axis. In some families there is a constitutional delay in maturation of the endocrine axis; however, this accounts for less than 10% of patients with delayed pubertal anomalies. Other causes are listed in Table 21–4.

Once established, the secondary male sexual characteristics require minimal testosterone for maintenance. Thus hypogonadism that follows puberty (usually after trauma, infection, or castration) results in few if any physical changes. Psychosocially, castrated patients may experience decreased libido, irritability, and depression. In females, the onset of menopausal symptoms usually follows castration, but, as in males, the secondary sexual characteristics regress slowly or not at all.

Male Reproductive Physiology

The mature testis is composed largely of the seminiferous tubules and interstitium. Leydig cells populate the interstitial spaces of the testis and provide testosterone to the developing spermatozoa. Sertoli cells line the inner surface of the

Table 21–3
Causes of sexual precocity

Cause	Females	Males
GnRH Dependent		
Constitutional	74%	41%
CNS/hypothalamic disorder (tumor, infection, developmental anomaly)	7%	26%
GnRH Independent		
Ovarian origin (functional cyst, granulosa cell tumor, polyostotic fibrous dysplasia)	16%	
Testicular origin (Leydig cell tumor)		10%
Adrenal origin	2%	22%
Ectopic gonadotropin production	1%	1%

CNS, central nervous system; GnRH, gonadotropin-releasing hormone.

Table 21-4
Causes of hypogonadotropic hypogonadism

Reversible	Nonreversible
Physiologic delay	GnRH deficiency
Weight loss/anorexia	Pituitary disease
Poor nutrition (malabsorption, ileitis, renal disease)	Craniopharyngioma
Congenital adrenal hyperplasia	Kallmann's syndrome (congenital anosmia and GnRH deficiency)
Prolactinoma	
Drug abuse—notably marijuana	

GnRH, gonadotropin-releasing hormone.

seminiferous tubules, forming bedding for the primitive germ cells. Sertoli cells are closely apposed to one another through tight junctions, creating a blood-testis barrier (BTB) that separates the dividing germ cells from the circulation. The BTB impedes the flow of large molecules between the circulation and the tubular lumen, allowing the tubular lumen to maintain a milieu relatively low in glucose and protein but high in potassium, androgens, estrogens, inositol, and amino acids. The BTB may also limit exposure of the developing gametes to the immune system. Disruption of the BTB, as seen in testicular trauma, is associated with formation of autoantibodies to sperm and subsequent infertility.

The seminiferous tubules coalesce in the rete testis and drain into the epididymis, where the sperm mature await ejaculation. During the process of emission, sperm are mobilized from the epididymis by smooth muscle contractions. They pass through the vas deferens, the ejaculatory ducts in the prostate, and finally the urethra.

Spermatogenesis

Spermatogenesis occurs from puberty through senescence in normal males. Primitive germ cells, called spermatogonia, populate the basal layer of the seminiferous tubules couched in a bed of Sertoli cells. Spermatogonia are present in the fetal testis but remain quiescent until puberty. Mitotic division of the spermatogonium yields two diploid (2n) primary spermatocytes. These remain linked through cytoplasmic bridges, which are thought to contribute to the synchronization of sperm development. Each primary spermatocyte undergoes meiotic division, yielding secondary spermatocytes and finally haploid (n) spermatids. Spermatids will lose most of their cytoplasm and develop flagella during the later stages of spermiogenesis, taking on the appearance of mature spermatozoa. The mature spermatid has three parts: the head, the middle or neck, and the tail. The head is composed almost entirely of the nucleus and the acrosome, a lysosome-like organelle containing the

enzymes necessary for penetration of the ovary. The middle portion contains a mitochondria-rich sheath and provides the energy that drives the tail portion. The tail portion is composed of a complex system of actin and tubulin. The whipping motion of the tail provides motility to the spermatozoa.

It has been noted that "[c]reation of functional sperm requires an optimal endocrine and paracrine milieu. Development from spermatogonia to spermatid is androgen independent, but further differentiation requires elevated local testosterone levels." Local testosterone levels are modulated by the gonadotropins FSH and LH, secreted by the anterior pituitary. Clinical evidence for their importance comes from the fact that infertility inevitably develops after hypophysectomy or pituitary infarct. Injections of LH can reverse infertility in these patients by increasing the activity of cholesterol desmolase, which in turn increases testosterone production. In addition to enveloping the developing spermatids, Sertoli cells secrete androgen-binding protein (ABP). The function of ABP is to maintain elevated levels of androgens within the tubular lumen.

Spermatids are not motile on delivery to the lumen of the seminiferous tubules, though they are capable of fertilizing the ovum if injected intracytoplasmically. Instead, they leave the testes through the rete and complete their maturation in the epididymis, where they are stored until ejaculation. Sperm concentration occurs during passage through the rete by reabsorption of the tubular fluid. Once in the epididymis, the sperm remain viable for months.

Spermatogenesis takes between 64 and 74 days, with about 125,000 sperm produced daily under normal conditions.

Male Fertility

Male fertility depends on both the quantity and quality of the sperm. Normal semen contains about 100 million sperm/mL, with 2.5 to 3.5 mL in an average ejaculate. Though ultimately only one sperm will fertilize the ovum, men with 20 to 40 million sperm/mL have a 50% reduction in fertility, and those with less than 20 million/mL are usually sterile. Temperature regulation is critical for normal sperm production. Normal testicular temperature is 1° to 2°C below core temperature. Homeostasis is regulated by a vascular countercurrent exchange and air exposure through contraction or relaxation of the cremaster muscles. Prolonged exposure to heat greater than 43° to 45°C for more than 30 minutes, as seen with hot tub usage and some insulated athletic wear, may decrease both sperm production and fertility by up to 90%.

Sperm quality is defined clinically by motility and morphology. The World Health Organization defines normal as at least 50% of sperm with forward mobility and 30% with normal form. These measurements are decidedly subjective, however, and many authors agree that normal fertility can be seen with much lower measurements.

Even optimally motile spermatozoa, which travel about 3 mm/min, must undergo a process called capacitation in the female reproductive tract before they can fertilize the ovum. During the 4- to 6-hour capacitation process, surface membrane proteins are redistributed, leading to an influx of calcium that increases sperm motility. Simultaneously, the acrosomal membrane fuses with the cellular membrane, allowing the egress of the proteolytic enzymes required for penetration of the ovum.

Endocrine Function of the Testes

The second broad function of the testes is to secrete testosterone and other hormones systemically. Testosterone is a C19 steroid with a hydroxyl group in the 17 position. It is synthesized from cholesterol in the Leydig cells in response to LH, and from androstenedione in the adrenal cortex. Leydig cells contain 17β-hydroxylase but lack both 11- and 21-hydroxylase activity; thus pregnenolone is shunted from the production of cortisol, as in the adrenals, to dehydroepiandrosterone and androstenedione, which are both converted into testosterone (Fig. 21–1). Normal adult males produce 4 to 9 mg of testosterone per day, resulting in blood levels of 300 to 1000 ng/dL. In general, production decreases slowly with advancing age. Females produce testosterone in the adrenal gland at a lower rate, with normal serum levels between 30 and 70 ng/dL. About 98% of circulating testosterone is in the bound form, with two thirds bound to gonadal steroid–binding globulin and one third to albumin. The remaining 2% is in the active, unbound form.

Testosterone suppresses the secretion of both GnRH from the hypothalamus and LH from the anterior pituitary. This mechanism has been examined as a potential means for male contraception.

Both testosterone and DHT act as transcription promoters when complexed to receptors in the cytoplasm. Both are androgens, but their effects are not identical, and both are necessary for normal male development. The differential effects of testosterone and DHT are listed in Box 21–2. Congenital absence of the 5α-reductase enzyme prohibits conversion of testosterone to DHT and results in male pseudohermaphroditism. Phenotypically these children have normal male internal genitalia, owing to normal testosterone and AMH production, but female-appearing external genitalia. They are usually raised as females and remain undiagnosed until puberty, when testosterone-dependent male secondary sexual characteristics appear. Drugs that inhibit 5α-reductase, such as finasteride, are used therapeutically to mitigate the negative effects of DHT seen in prostate hypertrophy.

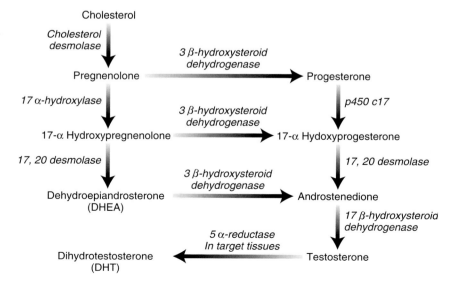

FIGURE 21–1 Biosynthesis pathway for testicular testosterone.

Box 21–2

Differential Effects of Testosterone and Dihydrotestosterone

Effects of testosterone

Differentiation of internal genitalia (epididymis, vas deferens, seminal vesicles)

Pubertal growth changes

    Initiation of growth spurt

    Epiphyseal plate closure

    Voice deepening

    Male bone and muscle development

    Hypertrophy of penis

Spermiogenesis

Psychic influences (libido/aggression)

Negative influence on gonadotropin production

Effects of dihydrotestosterone

Differentiation of external genitalia (penis, scrotum)

Adolescent sebaceous gland hyperactivity

Male hair and baldness pattern

Prostate hypertrophy

Most testosterone is excreted in the urine after it is converted to 17-ketosteroids, which are weak androgens. A smaller amount is converted into estrogens.

Female Reproductive Physiology

The müllerian ducts give rise to the uterus, cervix, fallopian tubes, and upper vagina. Unlike the testis, the ovary ceases migration in the pelvis near the fimbriated end of the fallopian tube. All reproductive organs are present at birth but remain essentially dormant until puberty.

Oocyte Development

Oocyte development begins early in utero. Primordial germ cells undergo constant mitotic divisions, reaching a maximum of about 7 million oogonia during midgestation. At this point mitosis stops, and the total number of oocytes will only decrease thereafter. Between 8 weeks gestation and 6 months of life, the oogonia enter meiosis. The first meiotic division is arrested in prophase, forming a primary oocyte. Primary oocytes remain in arrested prophase until ovulation, which begins around age 10 and ends around age 50. Most oocytes, however, will not reach ovulation but instead will undergo atresia and be resorbed. The steepest decline in oocyte number occurs in utero, such that at birth less than 2 million oocytes remain, of which half are already atretic. By puberty, less than 400,000 remain. The population continues to dwindle until, at menopause, there are few or no oocytes left. In all, about 500 oocytes will reach ovulation.

Each oocyte develops in a primordial ovarian follicle, composed of a single germ cell and its accompanying granulosa and theca cells. During the first phase of follicular development, the primary oocyte grows in size and the surrounding granulosa and theca cells undergo a proliferative spurt. The granulosa cells produce little estrogen at this time, maintaining instead an androgen-laden environment. The resulting primary follicle remains suspended in this condition until recruited for ovulation.

A cohort of primary oocytes/follicles is recruited to mature during each menstrual cycle, marking the onset of the second phase of follicular development. Granulosa and theca cells proliferate. In the theca cells, expression of the LH receptor is upregulated, as is production of the cytochromes $P450_{scc}$ and $P450_{c17}$ and 3β-hydroxysteroid dehydrogenase, which control rate-limiting steps in the metabolism of cholesterol to androgens. Each follicle develops a central fluid collection that bathes the oocyte in steroid hormones, proteins, and mucopolysaccharides. The second stage takes 10 to 12 weeks and results in the production of multiple graafian follicles, which are between 2 and 5 mm in diameter.

During the final stage, a single graafian follicle becomes dominant, and the other follicles regress. Selection is achieved by modulation of estrogen, FSH, and inhibin levels. Pituitary FSH secretion stimulates production of inhibin and cytochrome $P450_{arom}$, the aromatase enzyme for converting androgens to estrogens in the granulosa cells. Systemic estrogen and inhibin, in turn, suppress FSH secretion. Locally, however, estrogen augments the effects of FSH, including the elaboration of FSH receptors and hyperplasia of the granulosa cells. Suppression of FSH secretion affects less dominant follicles disproportionally, and the relative withdrawal induces apoptosis, or programmed cell death. Selection begins in the midfollicular phase, and within 48 hours a single dominant follicle swells to 20 mm in diameter. At ovulation, the follicle ruptures, releasing the oocyte into the peritoneal cavity.

Multifetal gestations occur when two or more of the recruited follicles survive to ovulation. This occurs spontaneously at a rate of about 1 in 90 births in the United States, but can be made to occur with hormonal manipulation. Clomiphene citrate is an orally active, nonsteroidal agent that increases GnRH secretion by binding hypothalamic estrogen receptors without suppressing GnRH. Without negative feedback, GnRH is constitutively pulsed, causing overexpression of gonadotropins. Gonadotropins in excess support the development of nondominant follicles. Likewise, human gonadotropins, isolated from the urine of postmenopausal women, are used to overcome the selection process in women undergoing in vitro fertilization.

The Reproductive Cycle

Unlike lower mammals, which go through periods of estrous, humans and other primates undergo regular cyclic reproductive cycles. The overt manifestation of the reproductive cycle is menstruation. Thus the term *menstrual cycle* is used interchangeably. Cycle length in normal females ranges from 21 to 35 days, but once established is usually consistent within a single woman. The reproductive cycle can most easily be described in terms of ovarian and uterine physiology, with each end organ having a pre- and postovulation component.

The ovarian cycle

The follicular phase begins with menstruation and concludes at ovulation. During the follicular phase, primary follicles are recruited for possible ovulation. The primary function of the follicle bed during the luteal phase, which extends from ovulation to menses, is to prepare the uterine lining for possible implantation.

Ovulation is ultimately under the control of the hypothalamus. Hypothalamic GnRH is secreted into the portal circulation in a pulsatile fashion. The pituitary is responsive to both the amplitude and interval of the pulses; it becomes sensitized with decreasing interval between pulses. Frequency of pulses is augmented by estrogen and diminished by progesterone, accounting for the LH surge that occurs midcycle, following the estradiol peak (Fig. 21–2). Continuous infusion of GnRH or long-acting GnRH analogs actually have the reverse effect, decreasing gonadotropin production by downregulating GnRH receptor expression. This strategy has been used therapeutically to suppress gonadal hormone production in the treatment of precocious puberty, uterine fibroids, and prostate cancer.

Ovulation occurs reliably 36 to 38 hours after the LH surge, usually on day 15 of a 28-day cycle. The ovum remains viable up to 72 hours after ovulation. Conception has been documented to follow intercourse on virtually every day of the cycle, but is most effective (up to 33%) on the day of or immediately prior to ovulation. Conception rates decrease dramatically if copulation is delayed as few as 24 to 48 hours after ovulation. Clinical signs that ovulation has occurred result from progesterone production and include an elevation in morning basal body temperature, thickening of the cervical mucus, and maturation of the endometrial lining.

The follicular bed fills with blood after ovulation, forming the corpus hemorrhagicum. Granulosa and theca cells again proliferate, filling the defect and forming a corpus luteum. The corpus luteum produces both

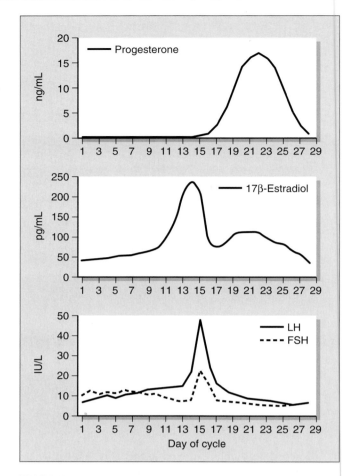

FIGURE 21–2 Serum hormone levels during menstrual cycle.

progesterone and estrogens, giving it a yellow color. If implantation occurs, β-human chorionic gonadotropin (hCG) is elaborated from the syncytiotrophoblasts of the forming placenta. Placental β-hCG maintains the corpus luteum, and thus its own progesterone supply, until the placental production of progesterone is adequate to maintain the pregnancy independently. Surgical or other disruption of the corpus luteum during early pregnancy results in miscarriage. If implantation does not occur, the corpus luteum involutes, and eventually becomes the white, scar-laden corpus albicans.

The uterine cycle

The uterine cycle is divided into three components called the proliferative, secretory, and menstrual phases. Cycle length averages 28 days, but lengths between 21 and 35 days are considered normal. By clinical convention, the first day of the menstrual cycle is marked by the onset of vaginal bleeding. It is easiest, however, to imagine each reproductive cycle beginning with the proliferative phase, which lasts from the conclusion of menses to ovulation. During the proliferative phase, follicular estrogen stimulates rapid expansion of the endometrial glands from the thin stratum basalis that is left after menstruation. This growth gives rise to the stratum functionale, a thick, more superficial layer supported by new coil-shaped spiral arteries. Despite hyperplasia and hypertrophy of the endometrial lining, the glands remain linear and nonproductive during the proliferative phase.

The secretory phase follows ovulation and is marked by edema and increased vascularity in the stratum functionale resulting from the combined influence of progesterone and estrogen. The glands begin to secrete a clear, mucin-rich fluid, and later detectable levels of prolactin. The secretory phase is fixed in length at 14 days and is remarkably consistent both within and between individuals. Therefore, differences in menstrual cycle length between individuals result from baseline differences in the preovulatory portion of the cycle.

Progesterone support decreases precipitously if implantation does not occur. The stratum functionale becomes thinner, resulting in increased coiling and spasm of the spiral arteries. These conformational changes compromise blood flow, causing focal necrosis and sloughing of the stratum functionale. Vasospasm is further augmented by local production of prostaglandins. The stratum basalis, which is supplied by the short, straight basilar arteries, is less affected by fluctuations in progesterone, and is thus immune from the cyclic sloughing process.

Normal menses may last from 1 to 8 days but is usually 3 to 5 days in length, and produces between 5 and 80 mL

of blood and necrotic endometrium. Prolonged bleeding is among the most common presenting complaints in gynecology and may be a sign of underlying structural, endocrine, or hematologic pathology.

Other end organs are influenced by the cyclic hormonal changes of the reproductive cycle. In the cervix, estrogen makes the mucus thin and alkaline, with the thinnest composition at the time of ovulation, which optimizes sperm motility. Progesterone, in contrast, causes the mucus to thicken, making sperm progress difficult and accounting in part for the poor conception rates seen when intercourse follows ovulation. Progesterone also causes the vaginal epithelium to increase mucus production. Mammary ducts in the breast proliferate during the follicular phase. Progesterone causes growth of the lobules and alveoli, which become edematous and hyperemic, causing tenderness prior to menses in some women.

Estrogen is the predominant hormone produced by the ovary. Naturally occurring estrogens, in order of decreasing potency, are 17β-estradiol, estrone, and estriol. All are C18 steroids, derived from androgens and differing only in the number of hydroxyl groups. Estrogens are synthesized from cholesterol through the combined interaction of the theca interna and granulosa cells of ovarian follicles (Fig. 21–3). Less than 2% of circulating estrogen is in the unbound, free form. About 60% is bound to albumin and 38% is bound to sex steroid–binding globulin.

Estrogen production is under variable feedback regulation at the level of the pituitary gland. In the early follicular phase, estradiol exerts a repressive effect on FSH secretion. This relationship reverses during the midcycle

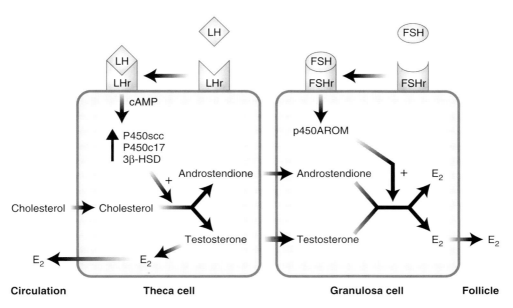

FIGURE 21–3 Granulosa and theca cell interaction. Follicular estrogen production: E_2, estradiol; E_1, estrone; FSH, follicle stimulating hormone; FSHr, FSH receptor; LH, luteinizing hormone; LHr, LH receptor; HSD, hydroxysteroid dehydrogenase.

and estradiol and FSH begin to form a positive feedback loop, which results in rapidly rising levels of both hormones immediately prior to ovulation. The positive feedback loop is broken after ovulation by the elaboration of progesterone, which downregulates FSH secretion.

Like most steroid hormones, estrogen exerts its effects by complexing with a receptor in the cell nucleus to promote the transcription. There are two prominent estrogen receptors, ER-α and ER-β, which appear to have different distributions and conflicting actions. The α receptor is widely distributed in men and women, and is implicated in the development of secondary sexual characteristics and bone density maintenance. ER-β is found throughout the genitourinary system, but also in the vasculature and prostate. Other receptors, including cytoplasmic membrane receptors, probably exist, accounting for some of estrogen's most rapid effects, which appear too rapid in onset to be genomically mediated.

The end-organ effects of estrogens, in concert with progesterone, support the reproductive potential of the female from development of oocytes through pregnancy. These are summarized in Box 21–3.

Estrogens are metabolized by conjugation to glucuronide or sulfate in the liver and are excreted either in the urine or bile. Some synthetic estrogens, such as ethinyl estradiol (used in oral contraceptive pills), are resistant to conjugation and are thus immune to first-pass effect making them ideally suited for oral formulations. Naturally occurring plant and animal hormones are easily conjugated and thus have decreased efficacy in the oral form.

Progesterone is secreted primarily by the corpus luteum and placenta, but smaller amounts are made by the remainder of the ovary, the adrenal cortex, and the testes. The production of progesterone is driven by LH through activation of adenylate cyclase, and follows a bimodal baseline, with serum levels up to 20-fold higher during the luteal phase than in the follicular phase (see Fig. 21–2). Progesterone is largely protein bound, with less than 2% in the free form. The end-organ effects of progesterone are listed in Box 21–4. Progesterone is metabolized in the liver; it is converted to pregnanediol, conjugated to glucuronic acid, and excreted in the urine.

The progesterone receptor (PR) is complexed to a heat shock protein (HSP), which obstructs the DNA-binding domain. Interaction with progesterone causes a

---

Box 21–3
End-Organ Effects of Estrogens

Reproduction
- Facilitates growth of ovarian follicle
- Enhances tubal motility
- Increases thickness of endometrial lining
- Decreases viscosity of cervical mucus
- Increases uterine blood flow

Growth and morphology
- Increases uterine muscle mass and contractility
- Contributes to epiphyseal plate closure
- Increases ductal growth, breast enlargement, and areolar pigmentation at puberty

Endocrine regulation
- Decreases FSH secretion
- Increases anabolic steroid metabolism
- Increases pituitary size
- Increases secretion of angiotensin and thyroid-binding globulin
- May increase salt and water retention premenstrually

Other
- Decreases serum cholesterol levels
- Stimulates production of nitric oxide, decreasing vascular smooth muscle proliferation and increasing vasodilatation
- Increases clotting factor production in liver

FSH, follicle-stimulating hormone.

Box 21–4
End-Organ Effects of Progesterone

Uterus
- Increases endometrial gland production/secretion
- Decreases myometrial excitability and spontaneous electric activity
- Downregulates estrogen receptor concentration
- Increases estrogen metabolism to inactive forms

Breast
- Stimulates differentiation and development of lobules and alveoli
- Supports lactation

Brain
- Inhibits, in large doses, LH production, thus inhibiting ovulation
- Increases basal body temperature
- Stimulates respiration ($Paco_2$ decreases in luteal phase and pregnancy)

LH, luteinizing hormone; $Paco_2$, carbon dioxide tension.

conformational change, releasing the HSP and freeing the binding site. Mifepristone (RU-486), a synthetic steroid, binds the PR-HSP complex intact, blocking the DNA-binding site. Mifepristone has been used to interrupt pregnancy in the first trimester.

Relaxin is a polypeptide hormone secreted by the corpus luteum, uterus, placenta, mammary glands, and prostate. Relaxin produces some of the physiologic changes that facilitate delivery of a baby, including relaxation of the pubic symphysis and pelvic joints, and softening and dilatation of the cervix. Its function in nonpregnant women and men is unclear, but some authors suggest that prostatic relaxin may augment sperm motility.

Fertilization and Implantation

The first meiotic division is completed at ovulation. The oocyte splits unevenly into a diploid secondary oocyte, which contains most of the cytoplasm, and a smaller polar body, which dissolves spontaneously. The second meiotic division begins immediately, but is arrested in metaphase until the oocyte is fertilized. At fertilization, a second polar body is ejected, leaving a diploid single-cell embryo.

Fertilization usually takes place in the distal fallopian tube shortly after ovulation. The fertilized ovum begins to divide immediately and forms a blastocyst of about 100 cells by the fourth day after ovulation. Implantation occurs between 5 and 7 days after ovulation, by which time the dividing blastocyst has developed an embryonic and placental component. Syncytiotrophoblastic tissue invades the endometrium and elaborates hCG, which rescues the corpus luteum from involution. A positive feedback loop is thus established. The corpus luteum maintains an optimal environment for the embryo, and the viable embryo secretes hCG, which prevents destruction of the corpus luteum.

Anovulation

An anovulatory cycle is one in which no oocyte is released from the ovary. Follicular estrogen exerts its proliferative effects unopposed by progesterone in anovulatory cycles because no corpus luteum is formed. Eventually the unchecked growth of the endometrial lining causes it to outstrip its own blood supply, resulting in asynchronous areas of focal necrosis. A single anovulatory cycle will most often spontaneously correct with the next ovulation. Repetitive anovulatory cycles result in prolonged exposure to unopposed estrogen and increase the risk of malignancy and premalignant conditions of the uterus and breast. Anovulation results from dysregulation of the feedback signals in the hypothalamic-pituitary-ovarian axis. Extragonadal estrogen production, as seen in obesity and polycystic ovaries, is seen commonly in these patients.

Coitus

Arousal in both sexes may result from both tactile and psychic stimulus. Physiologically, either stimulus results in activation of the efferent pelvic splanchnic nerves (nervi erigentes), which effect vasodilatation of the genitalia through the release of norepinephrine, vasoactive intestinal polypeptide, and nitric oxide. Increased blood flow in the erectile tissue in the penis compresses the venous return and causes erection. The same mechanism contributes to clitoral swelling. Drugs that block the degradation of these agents and their metabolites, such as sildenafil (Viagra), have been used to treat impotence.

Emission, the process of sperm mobilization before ejaculation, is integrated into the arousal response by nerves in the upper lumbar region of the spinal cord and mediated through stimulation of the hypogastric nerve trunk. Semen is formed by combining the sperm with secretions from the vas deferens, seminal vesicles, and prostate. The secretions, which ultimately make up 90% of the ejaculate, contain fructose and citrate, which provide energy to the sperm. Prostaglandins in the semen thin the cervical mucus, facilitating sperm motility. In some mammals, prostaglandins increase motility further by causing rhythmic contractions in the uterus and fallopian tubes; however, evidence for this activity in humans is lacking. The prostate secretions are highly alkaline, which neutralizes the acidity of both the vas deferens and the vaginal secretions. At orgasm, the semen is ejaculated through contraction of the bulbocavernosus muscle. The ejaculation reflex is coordinated in the lower lumbar spine and mediated by the first three sacral roots and the pudendal nerves.

In females, the vaginal epithelium and vestibular gland begin to secrete lubricating fluid and mucus during arousal. Tactile stimulation of the vaginal apex, clitoris, labia minora, and breasts as well as visual, auditory, and olfactory sensation increase excitement, which may culminate in orgasm. At orgasm, autonomic and pudendal nerve activation results in rhythmic contractions of the vaginal walls and the extravaginal bulbocavernosus and ischiocavernosus muscles. Whether this assists in mobilizing sperm is unclear; however, orgasm is not required for fertility.

Menopause/Senescence

The female reproductive capacity is finite. Between ages 45 and 55, the ovaries of most women undergo a precipitous oocyte atresia, which may predate menopause by 2 to 8 years. FSH production rises and inhibin production falls during this period. Estradiol, progesterone, and LH production remain stable until ovulation ceases, and then fall precipitously.

During the perimenopause, or climacteric, menstrual cycles become lighter, less frequent, and less predictable. Ultimately both ovulation and menses cease altogether, marking the onset of menopause. The entire process takes an average of 4 years, and the current average age of menopause in the United States is 52.

Concomitant with the decrease in ovarian function, there is an increase in vasomotor and often psychophysiologic symptoms. Hot flushes are the most frequent complaint and often among the earliest symptoms, occurring sometimes within 24 to 48 hours after surgical castration. The cause of hot flushes is unknown. Onset of symptoms correlates with the pulsatile LH surges, but can occur in patients who have undergone hypophysectomy, indicating that an upstream event in the hypothalamus is likely responsible for both the LH surges and the hot flushes. Hormone replacement ameliorates these symptoms, usually within a few days, probably through a negative feedback mechanism.

Overall estrogen production decreases at menopause from 350 to about 45 μg/day. What estrogen is produced comes almost entirely through the aromatization of androstenedione to estrone in the peripheral circulation, specifically in adipose tissue. Estrone, a relatively weak estrogen, is the most prevalent female hormone after menopause. These weaker estrogens do not support the long-term benefits of stronger estrogens on bone density and lipid profiles. Bone density loss occurs more rapidly during the perimenopause than at any other time.

Though the level of testosterone in men decreases steadily after puberty, there is little appreciable decrease in fertility potential during the later years. Nor are there acute episodes of vasomotor instability, which would correspond to those of the female climacteric.

Bibliography

Allan GF, Leng X, Tsai SY, et al: Hormone and antihormone induce distinct conformational changes which are central to steroid receptor activation. J Biol Chem 1992;267:19513–19520.

Amann RP, Howards SS: Daily spermatozoal production and epididymal spermatozoal reserves of the human male. J Urol 1980;124:211–215.

Anderson DJ, Alexander NJ: Consequences of autoimmunity to sperm antigens in vasectomized men. Clin Obstet Gynaecol 1979;6:425–442.

Barratt CL, Naeeni M, Clements S, Cooke ID: Clinical value of sperm morphology for in-vivo fertility: comparison between World Health Organization criteria of 1987 and 1992. Hum Reprod 1995;10:587–593.

Bedford JM: Effects of elevated temperature on the epididymis and testis: experimental studies. Adv Exp Med Biol 1991;286:19–32.

Berkowitz GS, Lapinski RH, Dolgin SE, et al: Prevalence and natural history of cryptorchidism. Pediatrics 1993;92:44–49.

Bryant-Greenwood GD, Schwabe C: Human relaxins: chemistry and biology. Endocr Rev 1994;15:5–26.

Caldwell BV, Behrman HR: Prostaglandins in reproductive processes. Med Clin North Am 1981;65:927–936.

Chikasawa K, Araki S, Tameda T: Morphological and endocrinological studies on follicular development during the human menstrual cycle. J Clin Endocrinol Metab 1986;62:305.

Dechering K, Boersma C, Mosselman S: Estrogen receptors alpha and beta: two receptors of a kind? Curr Med Chem 2000;7:561–576.

de Ridder CM, Thijssen JH, Bruning PF, et al: Body fat mass, body fat distribution, and pubertal development: a longitudinal study of physical and hormonal sexual maturation of girls. J Clin Endocrinol Metab 1992;75:442–446.

Devaja O, King RJ, Papadopoulos A, Raju KS: Heat-shock protein 27 (HSP27) and its role in female reproductive organs. Eur J Gynaecol Oncol 1997;18:16–22.

Emmen JM, McLuskey A, Adham IM, et al: Hormonal control of gubernaculum development during testis descent: gubernaculum outgrowth in vitro requires both insulin-like factor and androgen. Endocrinology 2000;141:4720–4727.

Enmark E, Gustafsson JA: Oestrogen receptors - an overview. J Intern Med 1999;246:133–138.

Federman DD, Donahoe PK: Ambiguous genitalia—etiology, diagnosis, and therapy. Adv Endocrinol Metab 1995;6:91–116.

Fink HA, Mac Donald R, Rutks IR, et al: Sildenafil for male erectile dysfunction: a systematic review and meta-analysis. Arch Intern Med 2002;162:1349–1360.

Ganong WF: The gonads: development and function of the reproductive system. In Review of Medical Physiology (15th ed) London: Appleton and Lange, 1991:403–406.

Gipson IK: Mucins of the human endocervix. Front Biosci 2001;6:D1245–D1255.

Gordon N: Undescended testes: screening and early operation. Br J Clin Pract 1995;49:318–320.

Griswold MD, Morales C, Sylvester SR: Molecular biology of the Sertoli cell. Oxf Rev Reprod Biol 1988;10:124–161.

Harlan WR, Harlan EA, Grillo GP: Secondary sex characteristics of girls 12-17 years of age: the U.S. Health Examination Survey. J Pediatr 1980;96:1074–1078.

Huirne JA, Lambalk CB: Gonadotropin-releasing-hormone-receptor antagonists. Lancet 2001;8:1793–1803.

Hutson JM, Baker M, Terada M, et al: Hormonal control of testicular descent and the cause of cryptorchidism. Reprod Fertil Dev 1994;6:151–156.

Jost A, Vigier B, Prepin J, Perchellet JP: Studies on sex differentiation in mammals. Rec Prog Horm Res 1973;29:1–41.

Koskimies AI, Kormano M, Alfthan O: Proteins of the seminiferous tubule fluid in man—evidence for a blood-testis barrier. J Reprod Fertil 1973;32:79–86.

Laven JS, Haverkorn MJ, Bots RS: Influence of occupation and living habits on semen quality in men (scrotal insulation and semen quality). Eur J Obstet Gynecol Reprod Biol 1988;29: 137–141.

Lobl TJ: Androgen transport proteins: physical properties, hormonal regulation, and possible mechanism of TeBG and ABP action. Arch Androl 1981;7:133–151.

Lyon MF: Gene action in the X-chromosome of the mouse (Mus musculus L). Nature 1961;190:372–373.

MacLeod J, Pazianos A, Ray B: The restoration of human spermatogenesis and of the reproductive tract with urinary gonadotropins following hypophysectomy. Fertil Steril 1966;17:7–23.

Magoffin DA: Regulation of differentiated functions in ovarian theca cells. Semin Reprod Endocrinol 1991;9:321–327.

Maslar IA, Ansbacher R: Effects of progesterone on decidual prolactin production by organ cultures of human endometrium. Endocrinology 1986;118:2102–2108.

McDaniel EC, Nadel M, Woolverton WC: True hermaphrodite with bilaterally descended ovotestes. J Urol 1968;100:77–81.

Meriggiola MC, Costantino A, Cerpolini S: Recent advances in hormonal male contraception. Contraception 2002;65: 269–272.

Meyer F, Moisan J, Marcoux D, Bouchard C: Dietary and physical determinants of menarche. Epidemiology 1990;1:377–381.

Obeid ML, Corkery JJ: Wolffian duct cyst. J Urol 1975;114: 946–947.

Pettersson K, Gustafsson JA: Role of estrogen receptor beta in estrogen action. Annu Rev Physiol 2001;63:165–192.

Rigola MA, Carrera M, Ribas I, et al: A comparative genomic hybridization study in a 46,XX male. Fertil Steril 2002;78:186–188.

Rock J, Robinson D: Effect of induced intrascrotal hyperthermia on testicular function in man. Am J Obstet Gynecol 1965;93:793–801.

Sinclair AH, Berta P, Palmer MS, et al: A gene from the human sex-determining region encodes a protein with homology to a conserved DNA-binding motif. Nature 1990;346: 240–244.

Speroff L: The ovary–embryology and development. In Speroff L, Glass RH, Kase NG (eds): Clinical Gynecologic Endocrinology and Infertility (5th ed). Baltimore, Williams and Wilkens, 1994:95–96.

Speroff L: The uterus. In Speroff L, Glass RH, Kase NG (eds): Clinical Gynecologic Endocrinology and Infertility (5th ed). Baltimore, Williams and Wilkens, 1994:118–119.

Speroff L: Regulation of the menstural cycle. In Speroff L, Glass RH, Kase NG (eds): Clinical Gynecologic Endocrinology and Infertility (5th ed). Baltimore, Williams and Wilkens, 1994:183–185.

Tanner JM: Growth at Adolescence (2nd ed). Oxford: Blackwell Scientific Publications, 1962.

Tho SP, Layman LC, Lanclos DK, et al: Absence of the testicular determining factor gene SRY in XX true hermaphrodites and the presence of this locus in most subjects will gonadal dysgenesis caused by Y aneuploidy. Am J Obstet Gynecol 1992;167:1794–1802.

Thomas F, Renaud F, Benefice E, et al: International variability of ages at menarche and menopause: patterns and main determinants. Hum Biol 2001;73:271–290.

Tilly JL, Kowalski KI, Schomberg DW, Hsueh AJ: Apoptosis in atretic ovarian follicles is associated with selective decreases in messenger ribonucleic acid transcripts for gonadotropin receptors and cytochrome P450 aromatase. Endocrinology 1992;131:1670–1676.

Uruena M, Pantsiotou S, Preece MA, Stanhope R: Is testosterone therapy for boys with constitutional delay of growth and puberty associated with impaired final height and suppression of the hypothalamo-pituitary-gonadal axis?. Eur J Pediatr 1992;151:15–18.

Waites GM, Gladwell RT: Physiological significance of fluid secretion in the testis and blood-testis barrier. Physiol Rev 1982;62:624–671.

Weiss G: Relaxin in the male. Biol Reprod 1989;40:197–200.

Wilcox AJ, Dunson DB, Weinberg CR, et al: Likelihood of conception with a single act of intercourse: providing benchmark rates for assessment of post-coital contraceptives. Contraception 2001;63:211–215.

Wise GJ: Hormonal treatment of patients with benign prostatic hyperplasia: pros and cons. Curr Urol Rep 2001;2:285–291.

CHAPTER 22

Cardiac Physiology and Dysfunction

Jakob Vinten-Johansen, M.S., Ph.D., Lawrence J. Mulligan, M.S., Ph.D., Jason M. Budde, M.D., and Cullen D. Morris, M.D.

Electrical Activity of the Heart

Constituent cells of the myocardium (myocytes, pacemaker and conduction tissue) have the property of electrical excitability. This electrical excitability is responsible for the rhythmic origin of the electrical signal in pacemaker cells, the propagation of the electrical depolarization in an orderly fashion from atria to ventricles, and synchrony in muscular contraction. The property of electrical excitability is conferred by the presence of differential concentrations of select ions, most notably Na^+, K^+, Ca^{2+}, and Cl^-, across the sarcolemma, and a selectively permeable membrane with voltage-gated channels for K^+, Na^+, and Ca^{2+}. The concentrations of ions involved in electrical activity of the heart are summarized in Table 22–1. Note that, at rest, the intracellular concentrations of Na^+ and Ca^{2+} are lower, and that of K^+ is higher, than in the extracellular compartment. During rest (diastole), the cardiac cell has a membrane potential (difference between charges across the sarcolemma) created by the higher concentration of K^+ intracellularly versus extracellularly, and a selective permeability to K^+. This selective permeability to K^+ allows this cation to diffuse out of the cell, leaving behind a relative overabundance of negative charges, contributed mostly by amino groups on proteins. Hence the intracellular environment is electronegative with respect to the extracellular environment. This intracellular electronegativity tends to attract K^+ back into the cytoplasm, but at some point the electrical and chemical forces come into balance, creating an equilibrium potential for K^+ of about −90 mV (inside of the cell more negative than outside). Therefore, K^+ ions determine the resting transmembrane potential of the cell.

Table 22-1
Intracellular and extracellular ion concentrations and equilibrium potentials in cardiac muscle cells

Ion	Extracellular Concentrations (mM)	Intracellular Concentrations (mM)*	Equilibrium Potential (mV)[†]
Na^+	145	10	81
K^+	4	135	−94
Ca^{2+}	2	10^{-4}	132
Cl^-	114	4	−90

*Estimates of free calcium concentration in cytoplasm.
[†]Calculated from the NERNST equation at 37°C body temperature.

The cardiac action potential is caused by changes in the membrane's selective permeability properties and, hence, the transmembrane movement of ions in response to their respective electrochemical gradients. Action potentials for fast fibers (ventricular myocytes) and slow fibers (nodal tissue and conduction tissue) are shown in Figure 22–1A and B, respectively. The following description relates to action potentials developed specifically in fast fibers. An electrical current externally applied to the cell (in the intact heart this is provided by the pacemaker

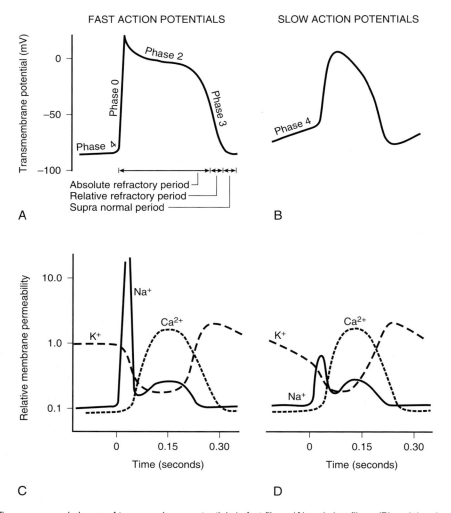

FIGURE 22–1 Time course and phases of transmembrane potentials in fast fibers (**A**) and slow fibers (**B**) and the changes in membrane permeability to Na+, K+, and Ca2+ in the respective fiber types (**C** and **D**, respectively) during development of the action potential. (From Mohrman DE, Heller LJ: Cardiovascular Physiology [4th ed]. New York: McGraw-Hill, 1997:23 with permission.)

tissues) decreases the conductance for K^+ (gK^+) through the selective K^+ channels while simultaneously increasing the conductance for Na^+ (gNa^+) (Fig. 22–1C). Activation gates in the membrane Na^+ channels open at approximately −70 to −50 mV, thereby increasing permeability to this cation, causing a fast inward current of Na^+ in response to the greater concentration of Na^+ in the extracellular space (chemical gradient) and the intracellular negative charge (electrical gradient), moving the membrane potential toward the Na^+ equilibrium potential. This fast inward Na^+ current depolarizes the cell, corresponding to phase 0 of the action potential (Fig. 22–1A). The duration of the open state of the Na^+ channels is very short, and Na^+ permeability rapidly decreases by the rapid closing of the inactivation gates of the cation channel. However, there is a slight overshoot of the depolarization such that the transmembrane potential becomes slightly positive (phase 1). The Na^+ channel remains relatively closed (impermeable) until the end of the action potential and the resting membrane potential is again reached (phase 4).

Phase 2 of the action potential follows the closing of the fast Na^+ channels. This phase, in which the action potential is prolonged, is very abbreviated in neural tissue, and is due largely to an opening of Ca^{2+} channels and subsequent calcium inward currents. The initial inward Ca^{2+} current is through T (transient) channels that open nearly simultaneously with the fast Na^+ channels, but then quickly close. These fast Ca^{2+} channels may be more important in nodal tissue. However, a slow inward current subsequently develops with the influx of Ca^{2+} through L-type channels, which open approximately at −30 to −20 mV and are inactivated relatively slowly, thereby producing a prolonged plateau phase 2 of the fast fiber action potential. The inward Ca^{2+} current increases the intracellular calcium concentration by about 2 orders of magnitude, and provides the initial calcium current that stimulates the greater release of calcium from the sarcoplasmic reticulum necessary to trigger muscle contraction. Repolarization of the cell (phase 3) results from both the delayed closing of the Ca^{2+} channels and an opening of the K^+ channels with K^+ efflux, which restores intracellular electronegativity to the resting state (phase 4). In summary, the action potential of the fast cardiac fibers is characterized by a rapid upstroke related to Na^+ influx (phase 0), an overshoot (phase 1) resulting from an overshoot in the inward Na^+ movement, a prolonged plateau (phase 2) related to the slow inward Ca^{2+} current, repolarization (phase 3) during which Ca^{2+} influx stops and K^+ efflux begins, and a relatively stable resting potential (phase 4). The imbalance of ions (intracellular loss of K^+, accumulation of both Na^+ and Ca^{2+}) that the action potential produces is corrected by the Na^+,K^+-ATPase and Ca^{2+}-ATPase pumps.

During the first two thirds of the repolarization phase, the cell is *absolutely refractory* to any depolarizing electrical current regardless of strength (Fig. 22–1A). Following

this period and lasting to the beginning of phase 4 is the *relative refractory period*, during which the cell can be excited by a stronger depolarizing current. Following the relative refractory period is the supranormal excitability period, in which weaker depolarizing currents than those normally necessary to activate the cell will elicit another action potential. The refractoriness of cardiac cells prevents premature re-excitation of cells that have just completed activation, thereby facilitating an orderly and unidirectional movement of excitation.

The action potential of the slow fibers of the nodal tissue (sinoatrial [S-A] node and atrioventricular [A-V] node) differs from that in the fast fibers in a number of ways (Fig. 22–1B). First, the rapid upstroke and overshoot are less prominent or even absent because of a smaller population of fast Na^+ channels. Second, the plateau phase is shorter and less stable because of the lack of a lingering active Na^+ inward current. Third, the repolarization phase leads to a resting phase that begins to slowly depolarize again. This automatically depolarizing resting potential is called the *diastolic depolarization*, or *pacemaker potential*. Ultimately the diastolic potential reaches threshold potential, which stimulates another action potential in an all-or-none fashion. The diastolic depolarization potential is the hallmark of pacemaker tissue, and is the mechanism underlying the property of *automaticity* in cardiac cells. This diastolic depolarization is due to the concerted actions of (1) a decrease in the outward K^+ current during early diastole (phase 4), (2) a persistence of the slow inward Ca^{2+} current, and (3) gradually increasing inward Na^+ current. The increasing Na^+ inward current most likely predominates in nodal and conduction tissue, causing a slow depolarization of the cell to its threshold potential and automatic triggering of another action potential. The slope of the diastolic depolarization, or the rate of diastolic depolarization, determines the rate of pacemaker activity, and hence is a primary mechanism determining heart rate. The slope of the diastolic depolarization is decreased by acetylcholine (parasympathetic action), thereby slowing heart rate. Hyperpolarization (more negative resting potential) or raising the threshold potential will also increase the time necessary to reach threshold potential, and thereby decreases the heart rate. Conversely, β-adrenergic agonists such as epinephrine and norepinephrine will accelerate the rate of depolarization, which will cause heart rate to increase. In the intact normal heart, the intrinsic rate of diastolic depolarization is faster, and the number of action potentials triggered is greater, in the S-A node (70 to 80/min), followed by the A-V node (40 to 60/min), and then by the ventricular myocytes (30 to 40/min). Once a depolarization is initiated in a pacemaker cell and propagated to other cells, it will depolarize the remainder of the heart in a synchronized and well-choreographed manner. Hence, there is a hierarchy of pacemaker activity, normally originating first in the S-A node.

If this node fails to initiate a depolarization, then pacemaker activity will be assumed by the A-V node with a characteristic slower heart rate (and absent P wave). If both the S-A node and the A-V node are dysfunctional, then pacemaker activity is taken over by the conduction tissue or, lastly, by the ventricular myocytes at a markedly slower rate.

Afterdepolarizations

Afterdepolarizations are spontaneous variations or oscillations in the postrepolarization potential that achieve threshold and elicit premature or triggered depolarizations. Afterdepolarizations can occur early after repolarization, and may be due to abnormalities in the outward K^+ or inward Na^+ current. They can be triggered by hypoxia, hypokalemia, ischemia, β-adrenergic agents, and some classes of antiarrhythmic drugs. Late or delayed afterdepolarizations occur later after repolarization has been completed, and occur primarily in calcium-overloaded hearts.

Myocardial Contraction and the Cardiac Cycle

Molecular Basis of Cardiac Contraction

The functional unit of the heart is the *sarcomere*. Sarcomeres are arranged longitudinally (end to end) to compose myofibrils; groups of myofibrils are surrounded by a cell membrane (the *sarcolemma*), forming the cardiac cell (the *cardiomyocyte*) (Fig. 22–2). The sarcolemma periodically invaginates to form transverse tubules, or T tubules, which increase the proximity of the sarcolemmal membrane to intracellular structures important to contraction. The sarcoplasmic reticulum (SR) is an intracellular membranous tube system with projections or feet that abut closely to the T tubules. Myocytes are connected longitudinally with attachments to adjacent cells to form a branched network, or *syncytium*. However, each myocyte is separated anatomically from the others by intercalated disks, which are specialized intercellular junctions that provide a low-resistance pathway for the rapid conduction of electrical impulses longitudinally between cells.

Each sarcomere is made up of specific proteins that are important in producing or regulating cardiac contraction. The major proteins are *myosin*, comprising the thick filament of the sarcomere, and *actin*, making up the thin filament of the sarcomere. Myosin is an elongated molecule forming a tail consisting of two "heavy" chains intertwined to form a helix, which serves as the rigid structural backbone of the thick filament (Fig. 22–3A). A globular head is attached to each of the heavy chains by

a mobile hinge molecule. Two pairs of light chains are associated with the hinged portion of the myosin molecule. The globular myosin head has two important biologic functions: (1) binding to actin to form actomyosin "cross-bridges"; and (2) binding and hydrolyzing ATP, with a resultant release of energy for contraction. In the sarcomere, the heavy myosin tails are connected to each other tail to tail, with the globular heads projecting outward.

Actin is the protein forming the thin filament of the sarcomere (see Fig. 22–2). It is a globular monomeric protein (G-actin) that is polymerized into filaments (F-actin; Fig. 22–3B); two filaments intertwine to form a double-stranded helix with a groove running the length of the filament. Actin has two important biologic functions: (1) it binds to the myosin globular head to form the actomyosin complex; and (2) it activates the myosin ATPase to hydrolyze ATP to ADP and inorganic phosphate (P_i).

There are two primary regulatory proteins or protein complexes that modulate the activity of actin and myosin in the process leading to contraction. Tropomyosin is a filamentous protein composed of two tightly coiled helical peptide chains. Tropomyosin lays in the groove formed by the two intertwined filaments of actin, and it binds a second complex of regulatory proteins, the *troponins* (Fig. 22–3B). The troponin complex consists of three components:

1. Troponin I—this is the inhibitory component that cloaks the myosin-binding site on actin and prevents interaction with myosin to form the actin-myosin cross-bridge.

2. Troponin T—this component anchors the three-unit complex to tropomyosin and is therefore primarily a structural component.

3. Troponin C—this component contains a calcium-binding site that is involved in the initiation of contraction.

The binding of calcium to troponin C removes the inhibitory effect of troponin I on the myosin-binding site of actin, thereby exposing the binding site on actin to the reciprocal site on myosin, allowing the formation of the cross-bridge.

In the relaxed heart, calcium is not bound to troponin C, and the myosin-binding site on actin is covered, which prevents formation of the actin-myosin complex necessary for contraction. However, during the depolarization process, calcium enters the intracellular space through the L-type calcium channels which are in close proximity to the SR. This calcium stimulates a

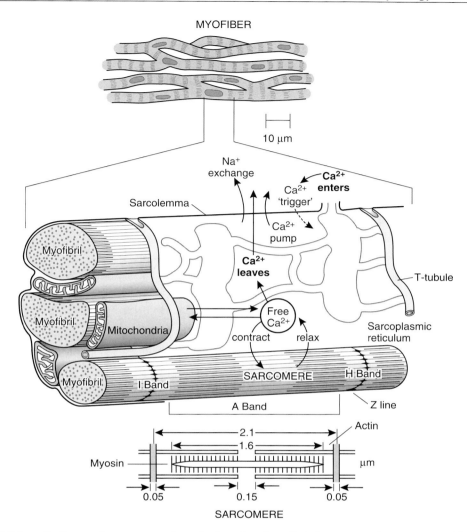

MYOFIBER

10 μm

FIGURE 22–2 Schematic diagram of sarcomere anatomy, the formation of myofibrils from groups of sarcomeres, and the formation of myocytes by groups of myofibrils. Shown also is the invagination of the sarcolemma to form T tubules, to which abut appendages of the sarcoplasmic reticulum (SR). This close proximity between the T tubules and the SR facilitates the calcium-induced calcium release into the cytosol, thereby increasing free cytosolic calcium (Ca^{2+}) levels after electrical depolarization. This increased intracellular calcium then binds to the troponin complex, allowing the formation of the actin-myosin complex and mechanical contraction of the sarcomeres by drawing the Z lines toward the center of the sarcomere. Calcium is therefore the excitation-contraction coupling agent that links electrical depolarization to mechanical contraction. (From Opie LH: The Heart: Physiology, Metabolism, Pharmacology and Therapy. New York: Grune & Stratton, with permission.)

sudden release of additional calcium from the SR, thereby raising intracellular Ca^{2+} from 10^{-7} M (in diastole) to 10^{-5} M (in systole). It is this additional calcium-induced calcium release from the SR that provides sufficient calcium to bind to troponin, which in turn initiates the contractile sequence. With Ca^{2+} binding to troponin C, the inhibitory effect of troponin I is lifted, allowing the association between actin and myosin to form the actomyosin complex (Fig. 22–3C). This association activates the ATPase on myosin and hydrolyzes ATP to ADP and P_i, which is followed by release of these products and a movement in the myosin "hinge" at the globular head. The movement of the myosin globular head slides the actin filament forward into a contraction, thereby moving the Z lines closer together. At the end of the hinge movement, the contractile proteins are reenergized when ATP reassociates with the myosin globular head and "cocks" the hinge, making it ready for another contraction. Simultaneously, calcium is removed from troponin C, which restores the inhibition of the myosin-binding site on actin, and the actin and myosin disengage from one another. The process then repeats itself until the end of muscular contraction is signaled, perhaps by the removal of intracellular calcium by sequestration into the sarcoplasmic reticulum, via

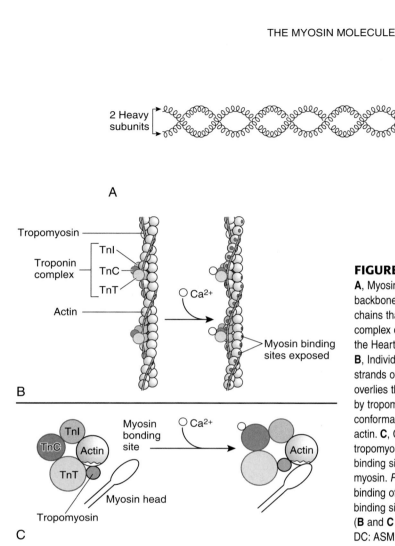

THE MYOSIN MOLECULE

FIGURE 22–3 The cardiac proteins important in contraction. **A**, Myosin molecule showing the two heavy chains that make up the backbone of myosin thick filament, the dual globular heads, and the light chains that act like hinges, allowing movement of the actin-myosin complex during the contraction process. (From Katz AM: Physiology of the Heart [2nd Ed]. New York, Raven Press, 1992:153, with permission.) **B**, Individual globular units of G-actin polymerize to form F-actin, two strands of which intertwine to form the actin thin filament. Tropomyosin overlies the groove of actin. The troponin complex is anchored to actin by tropomyosin. The binding of calcium (Ca^{2+}) to troponin C produces a conformational change in tropomyosin that exposes the binding site of actin. **C**, Close-up of the troponin complex tethered to actin and tropomyosin. *Left*, The troponin complex allowing inhibition of the myosin-binding site on actin, preventing the interaction between actin and myosin. *Right*, The conformational change in troponin associated with the binding of molecular calcium that disinhibits the cloaking of the actin-binding site, thereby allowing the interaction between actin and myosin. (**B** and **C** from Cooper GM: The Cell: A Molecular Approach. Washington, DC: ASM Press, 1977:439, with permission.)

SERCA2, the protein responsible for calcium uptake in the SR, and by other energy-dependent pump systems. Both contraction (systole) and relaxation (diastole) are ATP-requiring steps.

The strength of sarcomere contraction (i.e., inotropy) is increased by any intervention or event that increases intracellular calcium and its binding to the contractile apparatus. In addition, the rate of reassociation between myosin and ATP can lead to an increase in strength of contraction. For example, β-adrenergic stimulation increases reassociation of actin-myosin complexes by phosphorylation of the myosin, resulting in a contraction with more force and a greater degree of shortening.

Regulation of the SR calcium uptake, and hence relaxation, is under the control of phospholamban. This protein acts in an inhibitory manner in the unphosphorylated state and, when phosphorylated, stimulates the rapid uptake of calcium into the SR by Ca^{2+}-ATPase. This sequestration increases the calcium available in the SR for

release during the next cardiac cycle. During β-adrenergic stimulation, uptake of calcium by the SR is increased as a result of a loss of this inhibition. Conversely, heart failure is associated with a hyperphosphorylation of phospholamban and a small loss in SERCA2 function. Accordingly, less calcium is released into the proximity of the contractile apparatus, and less calcium is resequestered during diastole. This results in impairment in both diastolic and systolic function.

Attempts to restore contractile function in hearts exposed to ischemia-reperfusion or in failing hearts have recently focused on the SERCA2 pump as a therapeutic target. Complete reversal of systolic and diastolic dysfunction has been observed in rats receiving functional SERCA2. The role of calcium release (i.e., calcium-induced calcium release) via the ryanodine receptor on the SR in pathophysiologic states is less understood, but recent studies suggest that this site of calcium release may also be impaired in the diseased state.

The Cardiac Cycle

The cumulative and synchronized contraction of individual sarcomeres and myofibrils drives the contraction and relaxation actions of the four chambers of the heart: the right atrium, left atrium, right ventricle, and left ventricle. Moreover, synchronized contraction of the atria followed by the respective ventricles constitutes the cardiac cycle, which is shown for the left side (i.e., left atrium, left ventricle) relative to time in Figure 22–4. Similar events occur on the right side (i.e., right atrium, right ventricle). The rapid conduction of depolarization to the atria via specialized conduction fibers in Bachman's bundle (coincident with the P wave on the electrocardiogram), and the deceleration of conduction through the A-V node coincident with the PQ interval, allows contraction of the atrium before activation and contraction of the ventricle. Although the majority of ventricular filling is passive, atrial contraction fills the ventricle by an additional 10% before ventricular systole takes place, which maximizes loading and strength of ventricular contraction (discussed below). The introduction of this additional aliquot of blood with atrial contraction causes an "a wave" impulse, or "atrial kick," in the ventricular pressure tracing immediately before the onset of systole.

The onset of mechanical systole of the ventricle is preceded by electrical activation, the time delay being related to the trans-sarcolemmal influx of calcium and the calcium-triggered calcium release (i.e., excitation-contraction coupling), which is necessary for mechanical contraction to proceed. The initiation of ventricular systole raises intracavitary pressure without a change in ventricular volume (i.e., isovolumically; see the ventricular volume tracing in Fig. 22–4) because both the mitral and aortic valves are shut. However, when intraventricular pressure exceeds aortic pressure, the aortic valve opens, and ejection of blood proceeds with a reduction in ventricular volume, causing a comparable increase in aortic pressure (ejection phase; phases II through IV in Fig. 22–4). Ejection first occurs in a rapid phase, followed by a slower phase as the end-systolic volume is approached. At the end of ejection of blood into the aorta (i.e., end-systole), the ventricular pressure rapidly decreases below that in the aorta; the snapping shut and rebounding of the fibrous aortic valves creates the dicrotic notch or "incisura" that clinically heralds the end of systole. Ventricular relaxation begins first isovolumically (phases V and VI) without volume change, since both the aortic and mitral valves are closed, followed by opening of the mitral valve and a rapid filling phase (phases VI and VII), and then by a slower filling phase, or diastasis (phases VII and VIII).

On average, the duration of systole is 0.27 seconds. The duration of systole remains relatively constant over a range of heart rates, whereas the duration of diastole

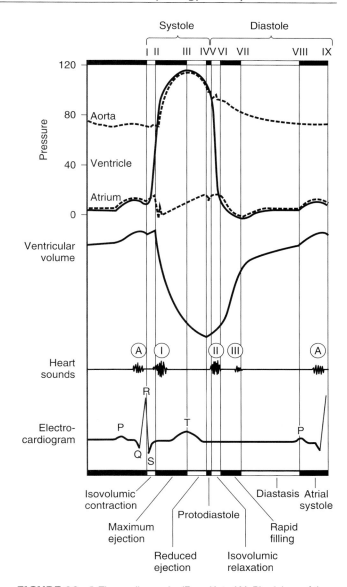

FIGURE 22–4 The cardiac cycle. (From Katz AM: Physiology of the Heart [2nd ed]. New York: Raven Press, 1992:362, with permission.)

changes inversely with heart rate. That is, as heart rate increases, the duration of diastole decreases, and as heart rate decreases, the duration of diastole increases. Clinically useful data derived from the cardiac cycle include (1) the stroke volume, which is the difference between the end-diastolic volume (EDV) and end-systolic volume (ESV), or the ejected volume; and (2) the ejection fraction, which is the stroke volume divided by the end-diastolic volume.

The pressure-volume loop

The function of the heart is to develop sufficient blood pressure and stroke volume to adequately perfuse all tissues of the body under all conditions. Accordingly, it is natural to view the cardiac cycle described in Figure 22–4 in terms of ventricular pressure and volume. In this view, the cardiac cycle generates a characteristic pressure-volume "loop." Referring to Figure 22–5A, the end-diastolic point is a convenient and conventional starting point. With electrical activation and excitation-contraction coupling, tension (pressure) develops isovolumically in the left ventricle, against closed aortic and mitral valves without ejection of volume. When left ventricular pressure exceeds aortic pressure, the aortic valve opens, and ejection of blood into the aorta is accompanied by a corresponding decrease in ventricular volume (ejection phase). At the end of systole and ejection, left ventricular pressure decreases rapidly; the aortic valve closes, and relaxation proceeds first isovolumically, and then with filling of the chamber after the mitral valve opens (diastolic filling phase). The most important points of the pressure-volume loop are the *end-systolic pressure-volume* (ESPV) point, located in the upper left corner of the loop, and the *end-diastolic pressure-volume* (EDPV) point, located in the lower right corner of the loop. Integration of the individual pressure-volume loops represents the *internal work* of the chamber, as opposed to the *external work*, determined by the product of stroke volume and aortic pressure measured externally to the heart. The rate of filling gives information on the compliance of the ventricle. The effects of increasing filling (preload) and arterial pressure (afterload) on the pressure-volume loop at a constant inotropic state are shown in Figure 22–5B. Pressure-volume loops may be visualized clinically during left heart catheterization and when echocardiography is performed, but this requires that high-fidelity measurements of left ventricular pressure be made.

Cardiac Function

The Frank-Starling Response

The resting length of the cardiac sarcomere or of a segment of myocardium determines the extent of contraction of the subsequent beat. As the resting length of the muscle increases, the force of contraction, or developed tension, increases without application of any other external influences, such as positive inotropic agents. This intrinsic response describes the length-tension relationship of cardiac muscle, shown in Figure 22–6. Peak contractile force can be achieved by optimally stretching the myocardium, after which a decline in function is observed (the descending portion of the length-tension relationship). In the intact heart, stretching the left ventricular muscle is achieved by increasing the EDV, as by increasing the venous return, decreasing the heart rate with a constant venous return, or reducing the efficiency of contraction (decreasing ejected volume while venous return remains constant). The end-diastolic muscle length or ventricular

volume is termed the *preload* of the myocardium; hence an increase in preload is associated with an increase in tension developed during systole or, speaking more physiologically, an increase in the stroke volume and/or pressure generated.

The length-tension relationship was determined in the intact heart by Frank in 1895 and later by Starling in 1914. For the intact heart, the length-tension relationship, or *Frank-Starling law*, states that an increase in the EDV (stretching sarcomeres or increasing preload) of the ventricular chamber increases the ejection volume (i.e., the stroke volume). Conversely, decreasing the EDV of the left ventricle is associated with a decrease in stroke volume with all other factors, such as inotropic state, heart rate, and arterial pressure, being unchanged. The Frank-Starling relationship is extremely important in the beat-to-beat regulation of cardiac performance. For example, right and left ventricular outputs are matched largely through the Frank-Starling relationship. In addition, the variation in cardiac filling accompanying respiratory efforts is based largely on the Frank-Starling relationship. In cardiac tamponade, the decreased stroke volume is due to a constraint on left ventricular filling and consequently on stroke volume. Importantly, the effect of preload on cardiac performance as described by the Frank-Starling relationship is an *intrinsic* property of cardiac muscle, independent of external forces such as alterations in inotropic state induced by sympathetic activity; these external forces superimpose upon the Frank-Starling curve (see Fig. 22–6). The curve shifts upward with positive inotropic forces and downward with negative inotropic forces. Hence a family of curves is described, each having the intrinsic Frank-Starling effect superimposed on other external forces.

Frank-Starling curves have often been used as measures or indices of cardiac function. The advantage of these curves is that they describe cardiac function in physiologic terms, that is stroke volume or, more appropriately, cardiac output. In addition, the curves are sensitive to externally applied changes in inotropic state. However, quantifying and describing cardiac function by the Frank-Starling curves requires a fairly wide range of preload achieved by either volume loading or volume depleting the subject. In addition, changes in afterload (i.e., aortic pressure) will profoundly change the nature of the curves. Increased afterload shifts the Frank-Starling curve down and to the right (i.e., increased afterload reduces stroke volume), or requires greater ventricular filling to achieve comparable stroke volumes. Hence the curves are afterload sensitive, and may be different in patients with hypertension compared to patients with normal pressures. In addition, the stretch response of sarcomeres to increasing preloads is influenced by compliance of the cardiac tissue. While the Frank-Starling curve is descriptive of cardiac

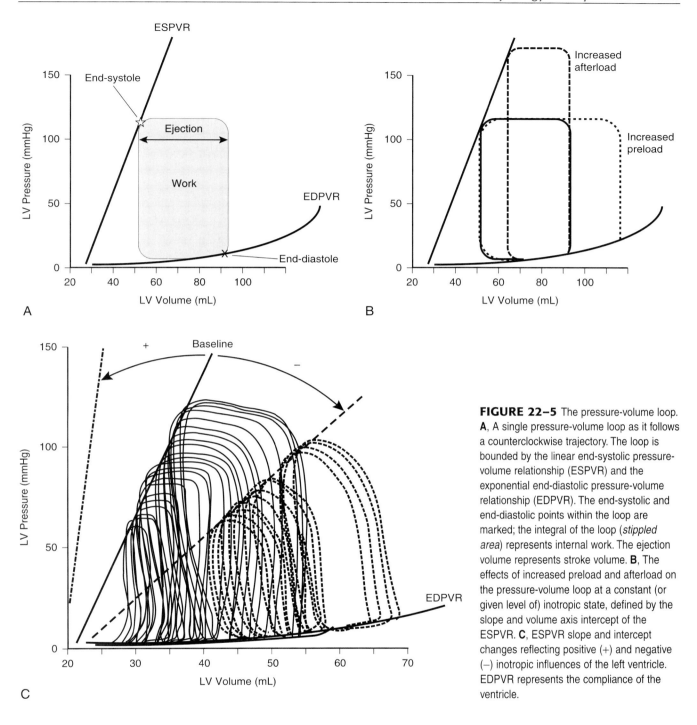

FIGURE 22–5 The pressure-volume loop. **A,** A single pressure-volume loop as it follows a counterclockwise trajectory. The loop is bounded by the linear end-systolic pressure-volume relationship (ESPVR) and the exponential end-diastolic pressure-volume relationship (EDPVR). The end-systolic and end-diastolic points within the loop are marked; the integral of the loop (*stippled area*) represents internal work. The ejection volume represents stroke volume. **B,** The effects of increased preload and afterload on the pressure-volume loop at a constant (or given level of) inotropic state, defined by the slope and volume axis intercept of the ESPVR. **C,** ESPVR slope and intercept changes reflecting positive (+) and negative (−) inotropic influences of the left ventricle. EDPVR represents the compliance of the ventricle.

function, comparing an earlier versus a later series of Frank-Starling curves in the same patient may produce erroneous conclusions if there are changes in ventricular compliance induced by hypertrophy (thickening of the chamber walls), scarring, cardiac edema, or diastolic dysfunction. Practically, volume loading of patients is cumbersome, and is not without its problems (e.g., hemodilution). In addition, volume loading often increases afterload, while volume reduction decreases afterload, thereby influencing the trajectory of the Frank-Starling curve. Hence, the methods used to inscribe Frank-Starling curves impose physiologic changes that alter the very nature of the curves themselves, introducing confounding factors that make diagnostic accuracy very difficult. Therefore, indices have been devised that indirectly measure cardiac performance.

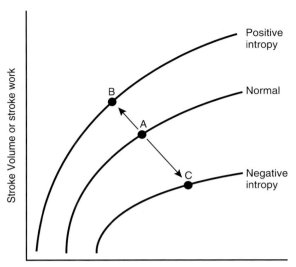

FIGURE 22–6 The Frank-Starling relationship of the left ventricle. A positive inotropic influence shifts the curve upward, resulting in an increase in stroke volume. However, physiologically, a positive inotropic influence will also decrease left ventricular (LV) end-diastolic volume or left atrial (LA) filling pressure, represented as a shift from point A to point B. Similarly, a decrease in inotropic state not only decreases stroke volume, but is associated with an increase in LV end-diastolic volume and LA filling pressure (point A to point C).

Pressure-Volume Relations for Assessment of Cardiac Function

The inotropic state (contractility) of the left ventricular chamber relates to the strength of contraction, expressed physiologically in terms of force, velocity, and extent of muscle shortening and clinically in terms of stroke volume, cardiac output, and EDV and end-diastolic pressure. Contractility of the whole heart can best be described physiologically by the slope (end-systolic ventricular elastance [E_{es}]) and volume axis intercept (left ventricular volume at zero pressure [V_0]) of the end-systolic pressure-volume relationship (ESPVR) (see Fig. 22–5C) generated by a series of loops developed during a preload reduction maneuver, increased preload, or a change in arterial pressure caused by vasoactive drugs. The end-systolic points in the series of declining loops conform to a linear relationship, forming the ESPVR, which is largely linear in the physiologic range of ventricular pressures (from 120 to 50 mm Hg), and has asymptotes horizontally at higher pressures and vertically at lower pressures.

A positive inotropic influence such as administration of catecholamines is associated with an increase in the slope of the ESPVR and/or a decrease in the V_0 (Fig. 22–5C). This shift in the ESPVR is in agreement with an increase

in the ejection fraction in which there is a generalized decrease in both systolic and diastolic dimensions but maintained or increased stroke volume. Conversely, a decrease in inotropic state with heart failure, ischemia, myocardial infarction, and β-adrenergic antagonists is associated with a decrease in the slope and/or an increase in V_0 (Fig. 22–5C), which is consistent with a decrease in the ejection fraction secondary to a decrease in stroke volume and/or an increase in EDV.

Evaluation of the inotropic state through the use of slope of the ESPVR requires control of heart rate. The early studies evaluating the responses of ESPVR over wide ranges in heart rates demonstrated that increases of 20 beats/min in heart rate resulted in significant increases in E_{es}, while later studies suggested that larger increases in heart rate (40 beats/min) were required for significant increases in E_{es} (Fig. 22–7). The impact of inotropic agents on the contractile function were then evaluated at specific heart rates. The results demonstrate that β-adrenergic stimulation results in greater increases in E_{es} compared with chronotropic stimulation. However, with the recent introduction of chronic β blockade as a therapy in patients suffering from heart failure, the use of inotropic stimulation to assess contractile function is less likely to be successful, whereas increases in heart rate may be the more effective means of altering inotropic state.

Accurate assessment of the inotropic state in patients undergoing coronary artery bypass grafting or valve surgery

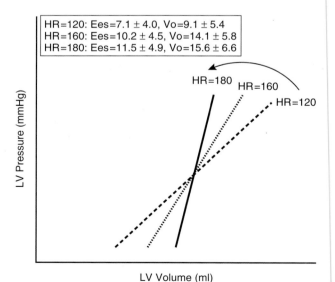

FIGURE 22–7 The progressive increase in the slope of the ESPVR with increasing heart rate, representing an intrinsic positive inotropic effect of heart rate. *Inset* shows the values for the ESPVR slope (E_{es}) and volume axis intercept (V_0) at each heart rate. (Data from Freeman GL, Little WC, O'Rourke RA: Influence of heart rate on left ventricular performance in conscious dogs. Circ Res 1987;61:455.)

is difficult because of the instability of the patient's hemodynamic state. Assessing the E_{es} provides unique information regarding ventricular function not available through assessment of the stroke volume or cardiac index, such as diastolic mechanics and systolic function independent of preload and afterload.

Diastolic Properties of the Heart

The exponential curve that describes the EDPV relationship, derived from the series of EDPV loops, represents diastolic properties of the left ventricle (see Fig. 22–5A and C), or its ability to fill during diastole. The end-diastolic points of the declining loops conform to a curvilinear relationship that is largely exponential, and reflects the *lusitropic* (i.e., compliance) properties of the left ventricular chamber. The EDPV curve shifts upward when compliance is lost, as with edema, scarring, or fibrosis of the chamber, or other abnormalities that reduce the rate and extent of chamber relaxation. The diastolic relationship also shifts upward when external forces such as tamponade, pericardial effusion, or fibrosis of the pericardium constrain the filling of the left ventricle. Reduced filling caused by such filling defects is associated with decreases in stroke volume via the Frank-Starling mechanism.

Hence the pressure-volume relationship is a very useful tool by which to understand and describe the systolic and diastolic properties of the heart. The advantage of the pressure-volume platform of analyzing systolic and diastolic properties of the heart is that it is relatively uninfluenced by hemodynamics. The disadvantage is that quantitative measurements of left ventricular volume are difficult to obtain clinically using surface or trans-esophageal echocardiography, ventriculography, or nuclear scans.

Clinical Indices of Cardiac Performance

Stroke Volume and Cardiac Index

Stroke volume shows considerable variation in humans depending on body size and weight, metabolic state, and the performance characteristics of the heart. The cardiac index, which is the cardiac output corrected for body surface area, expressed in liters per minute per meter squared, suffers from these same variations and has only limited usefulness as an accurate index of cardiac performance. At rest, the cardiac index averages approximately 3 L/min/m². A summary of the factors regulating stroke volume is shown in Figure 22–8.

dP/dt_{max}

The first derivative of the upstroke of the left ventricular pressure waveform has been used as an index of cardiac inotropic state and functional status. However, the reliability of this parameter from one time to another is dependent on stable filling pressures at the time of measurement. For example, an increase in dP/dt_{max} from 1000 to 1500 mm Hg/sec with an increase in left ventricular end-diastolic pressure (LVEDP) of 10 mm Hg between the two measurement time points makes the 33% increase in dP/dt_{max} suspicious of being due to an increase in preload rather than changes in inotropic state. However, numerous studies have demonstrated that dP/dt_{max} increases with positive inotropic influences without changes in LVEDP, providing strong evidence for the sensitivity and accuracy of the parameter as an index of contractile performance.

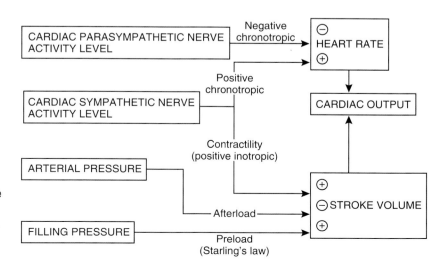

FIGURE 22–8 A summary of factors that influence cardiac output. (+) indicates a stimulatory effect, and (–) indicates an inhibitory effect. (From Mohrman DE, Heller LJ: Cardiovascular Physiology [2nd ed]. New York: McGraw-Hill, :66 with permission.)

Because dP/dt_{max} is dependent on the left ventricular pressure, and hence on afterload, changes in afterload will invariably alter the dP/dt_{max} independent of inotropic state. For example, an increase in afterload will increase the dP/dt_{max} independent of inotropic state because a greater pressure is achieved roughly during the same duration of systole, necessitating an increase in the rate of pressure development. Therefore, vasoconstrictors could possibly increase both aortic pressure and dP/dt_{max} in the absence of changes in inotropic state. The converse is observed for vasodilators and venodilators, which can decrease dP/dt_{max} in the absence of changes in inotropic state.

Ejection Fraction

The ejection fraction is most frequently used as a clinical index of global cardiac function. The ejection fraction is calculated as (EDV − ESV)/EDV. Ejection fraction is simply the percent of the EDV that is ejected as the stroke volume. These coefficients are obtained with fairly good accuracy by readily available clinical tools, such as ventriculography, cineangiography, echocardiography, and positron emission tomography. Normal values for ejection fraction range between 55% and 75%. In patients with heart failure or large myocardial infarctions, the ejection fraction can decrease to as low as 15% to 20%. The ejection fraction can give a fairly accurate indication of the contractile state of the heart, but has the disadvantages of being sensitive to preload, afterload, and heart rate and being influenced by ventricular compliance by its effect on filling. In addition, ejection fraction can be inaccurate in patients with valve abnormalities. For example, in patients with mitral insufficiency, a portion of the stroke volume regurgitates into the atrium, and ejection fraction is overestimated unless this regurgitant volume is taken into account. Despite these disadvantages, ejection fraction is a standard method used for clinical diagnosis of global cardiac performance.

Coronary Blood Flow

Coronary blood flow (CBF) is under mechanical, neural, and local control. The impact of ventricular contraction (mechanical effect) and relaxation on CBF was a fertile area of research in the late 1960s and the 1970s. The cyclical contraction and relaxation of the left ventricle produces obvious phases in the blood flow pattern in the left coronary artery and its main tributaries, the left anterior descending and left circumflex coronary arteries. These phasic blood flow patterns in a left coronary artery are shown in Figure 22–9. Note that blood flow during systole is low relative to that occurring during diastole. In Figure 22–9, coronary blood is rapidly decreasing at point

a during the isovolumic phase of systole, as a result of increasing resistance from extravascular compression produced by the pressure generated in the myocardial wall and the squeeze of cardiac muscle around the intramyocardial arterial vessels during systole. CBF may actually reverse and become retrograde during this phase as a result of pressure generation in the midmyocardial and endocardial layers squeezing blood back into the epicardial arteries. Point *c* represents the increase in coronary blood flow occurring in diastole, when the extravascular compression forces surrounding the intramyocardial vessels release, thereby decreasing the resistance and impedance to blood flow. Because the myocardial contraction and mural pressure are greater in subendocardial tissue than subepicardial tissue, vascular resistance during systole is greatest in this inner layer of myocardium. Hence, during systole, primarily the subepicardial tissue (where extravascular compressive forces are less) is perfused, whereas in diastole, both subepicardial and subendocardial tissues are perfused; subendocardial tissue is perfused primarily during diastole (i.e., during half the cardiac cycle). While pressure generation by the left ventricle has a significant impact on the impediment to CBF, contractile state, defined by E_{es}, appears to have a greater influence.

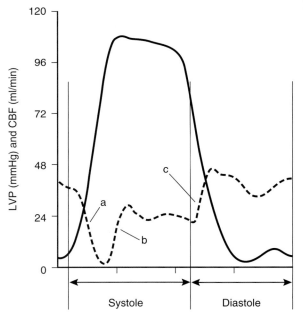

FIGURE 22–9 Phasic blood flow patterns in the left coronary artery (*dashed line*) with respect to left ventricular pressure tracings (*solid line*). Heavy vertical lines mark the phasic blood flow patterns in systole and diastole. Coronary blood flow during systole is markedly decreased compared to that in diastole, and perfuses primarily subepicardial tissue. Subendocardial tissue is perfused primarily during diastole. Therefore, subendocardial tissue receives blood flow during only half of the cardiac cycle, whereas subepicardial myocardium receives blood flow throughout the entire cardiac cycle. *a*, onset of systole; *b*, during systolic ejection; *c*, diastolic perfusion.

The restoration of blood flow occurs after the maximal pressure-volume relationship occurs, at the ESPV point.

In contrast to the phasic nature of blood flow in the left coronary artery, blood flow in the right coronary artery is relatively constant during the cardiac cycle. The constancy of blood flow is related to the lower mural pressures and extravascular compressive forces in the right ventricle compared to the left ventricle, and the thinner wall over which such forces are distributed. The lower extravascular compressive forces generated in the myocardial wall of the right ventricle does not impede blood flow to the same degree as in the left ventricle.

Myocardial perfusion is also controlled by local metabolic need and neural control mechanisms (the sympathetic-parasympathetic balance). The local control mechanisms include the release of adenosine in the local area surrounding arterioles, local tissue partial pressure of oxygen, and local pH. This local control tightly couples metabolic needs to CBF so that increasing needs are met precisely by appropriate increases in CBF—that is, metabolic or oxygen supply meets demand. Local control mechanisms can dominate, resulting in up to a fourfold increase in CBF following a brief (20-second) period of coronary occlusion (reactive hyperemia), which causes the involved coronary vasculature to dilate near-maximally. These local control mechanisms are responsible for autoregulation of blood flow to meet ambient energy demands. The extraction of oxygen from the arterial blood is normally high, averaging approximately 60% to 75% under normal conditions. The physiologic limit of extraction is approximately 90% to 95%, which leaves a limited oxygen extraction reserve to call on when oxygen delivery becomes inadequate for any number of reasons (e.g., ischemia, hypoxia). Under these conditions, increases in CBF are the primary mechanism of increasing oxygen delivery.

If perfusion pressure (arterial pressure − coronary sinus pressure) decreases, coronary arteries adjust by vasodilating in response to the buildup of local vasodilating factors until blood flow again meets demands. Because the extraction of oxygen carried in coronary arterial blood is very high, large increases in oxygen supply cannot be met by increasing extraction, but rather are met by increasing blood flow rate. A significant coronary reserve (up to four-fold increases in blood flow) exists in the healthy heart to accommodate a wide range in metabolic needs dictated by cardiac workloads. However, in the diseased heart, a loss of dilator capacity as a result of, for example, a coronary stenosis may compromise function through the presence of a mismatch between coronary artery blood flow and oxygen needs (i.e., a perfusion-function mismatch). As mentioned previously, mechanical contraction is dependent on oxidative metabolism. The loss of coronary artery dilatation and autoregulation is associated with coronary artery disease and hypertension, both commonly found in patients with heart failure. Under conditions of a compromised vasodilator reserve, the heart (teleologically speaking) will attempt to increase oxygen availability by increasing extraction. Increased extraction and decreased coronary sinus oxygen content are the hallmarks of coronary artery insufficiency.

Myocardial Energetics

The heart is, loosely speaking, a metabolic omnivore; that is, it will metabolize whatever substrate is available in greatest abundance. The chief myocardial fuels are non-esterified free fatty acids and carbohydrates (glucose and lactate). Under fasting conditions, when the blood levels of free fatty acids are relatively high, these lipids may account for up to 60% to 70% of the fuel metabolized, with carbohydrates accounting for the remaining 40%. However, when carbohydrate levels increase postprandially, myocardial metabolism will shift to utilize this source predominantly. Under resting conditions, or during exercise when blood lactate levels rise, the heart will use lactate as a metabolic fuel. Measurement of coronary sinus blood shows an extraction of lactate relative to arterial blood. Although the heart can utilize a wide range of substrates, it is largely an aerobic organ. It has a very limited anaerobic reserve; that is, it cannot undergo glycolysis to a great extent when there is insufficient oxygen to fully support oxidative phosphorylation.

Myocardial Oxygen Consumption

In the normal myocardium in the presence of oxygen, nearly all chemical energy used by the heart is generated by oxidative phosphorylation, regardless of the substrate used. As discussed previously, anaerobiosis accounts for very little of the total high-energy phosphates used by the myocardium. Therefore, the rate of minute volume of myocardial oxygen consumption ($M\dot{v}O_2$) is roughly indicative of the metabolic rate of the heart. Oxygen consumption is measured by the product of the arterial-venous oxygen content difference and CBF, optionally indexed to heart weight in one fashion or another. Therefore, $M\dot{v}O_2 = [(CaO_2 − C\dot{v}O_2)/CBF]/$heart weight, where CaO_2 is arterial oxygen content, measured in milliliters of O_2 per 100 mL blood; $C\dot{v}O_2$ is coronary venous (i.e., coronary sinus) oxygen content, measured in milliliters of O_2 per 100 mL blood; and CBF is measured in milliliters per minute.

The major determinants of $M\dot{v}O_2$ are wall stress, heart rate, and inotropic state. Minor determinants of $M\dot{v}O_2$ include energy used in maintenance of cell viability and to drive ATP-dependent ionic pumps. A large percentage of ATP hydrolysis (therefore energy expenditure) is involved in the liberation of heat, rather than in the process of generating mechanical work. Work per se is not a determinant of $M\dot{V}O_2$, in that two forms of work (pressure work and volume work) are considered. The development of pressure by the left ventricle (i.e., "pressure work") is somewhat more expensive in terms of $M\dot{V}O_2$ than the generation of stroke volume per se (i.e., "volume work"), even though the amount of external work is the same. More recent studies have shown that the $M\dot{V}O_2$ differences between pressure work and volume work at equivalent levels of external work are actually relatively small. Hence patients with hypertension may have a slightly greater oxygen demand than patients with volume-loading conditions resulting from aortic insufficiency (described above) for a given value of external work. One reason for this small difference in oxygen demand between pressure work and volume work is that the process of myocardial fiber shortening is relatively inexpensive in terms of $M\dot{V}O_2$ in comparison to the development of pressure during isovolumic systole.

Wall stress is a primary determinant of $M\dot{V}O_2$, and conceptually integrates both pressure and volume (vis-à-vis chamber diameter or radius) into one platform by including these terms as coefficients in the calculation, as discussed below. By the law of Laplace, wall stress is the product of pressure (P) and internal chamber radius (R_i), divided by wall thickness (h) (i.e., $[P \times R_i]/2h$), whereas wall tension is represented as the product of P and R_i. This equation is for a sphere, which is an oversimplification of the geometry of the heart, which more nearly approximates that of an ellipsoid or truncated ellipse. It is the static wall stress at peak or at systole that correlates with $M\dot{V}O_2$, and not specifically the integral of dynamic changes in wall stress during the cardiac cycle. Studies have shown that wall stress more accurately correlates with measured $M\dot{V}O_2$ under many conditions than does measuring either the pressure or volume coefficient alone or deriving some index based on these coefficients. Increased wall stress is associated with higher levels of $M\dot{V}O_2$, and lower wall stress with lower levels of $M\dot{V}O_2$. Clinically, $M\dot{V}O_2$ is greater in dilated left ventricles than in ventricles with smaller radii at a given left ventricular pressure, which is one reason why it is important to reduce ventricular geometry in the clinical treatment of heart failure. Heart rate determines $M\dot{V}O_2$ by the number of times wall stress (or tension) is generated per minute. An intrinsic positive inotropic effect of heart rate may also contribute to the increase in $M\dot{V}O_2$ of higher heart rates. Inotropic state determines $M\dot{V}O_2$ principally through its effect on velocity and extent of contraction. However, increases in the $M\dot{V}O_2$ by positive inotropic agents may be counterbalanced by a concomitant decrease in left ventricular size, and hence in wall stress.

Several indices of oxygen consumption have been developed to avoid directly measuring $M\dot{V}O_2$ from arterial and coronary sinus oxygen content differences and myocardial blood flow, parameters that are not always available to the clinician. Numerous basic and clinical studies assessing the strengths and weaknesses of these indices have been conducted. These indices are essentially based on the major determinants of $M\dot{V}O_2$ (i.e., wall stress and its coefficients, pressure and heart rate), and largely omit ventricular volume (dimension). The pressure-rate product is calculated as the product of peak systolic or mean arterial (or peak ventricular) pressure and heart rate. The integral of left ventricular pressure over the duration of systole, known as the tension-time index or the pressure-time index, has also been used as an index of $M\dot{V}O_2$. Although these indices are relatively easy to obtain by methods that are readily available in the cardiac catheterization laboratory, they have significant limitations in that none of the indices considers inotropic state or the volume component of wall stress. The product of pressure, heart rate, and systolic ejection time partially takes inotropic state into consideration because positive inotropic influences increase the velocity of contraction. The most recently developed index is the "pressure work index," which takes into account both pressure work and volume work. The $M\dot{V}O_2$ estimated with this index was well correlated with actual $M\dot{V}O_2$ measured experimentally.

Cardiac Efficiency

Cardiac efficiency relates the energy equivalent of the oxygen consumed and the work performed by the heart. Hence, cardiac efficiency = work/$M\dot{V}O_2$. The overall efficiency of the heart ranges from 5% to 40% depending on the type of work (pressure versus volume versus velocity) performed. Recent studies conducted in chronically instrumented animals provide additional in vivo data to support the original hypotheses regarding cardiac efficiency. One reason for the low efficiency of the heart is that a predominant portion of the oxygen consumed is expended in generating pressure and stretching internal elastic components of the myocardium during isovolumic systole (a form of internal work), which does not contribute to stroke volume and external work.

Following cardiac surgery, efficiency generally decreases as a result of the increase in $M\dot{V}O_2$ relative to cardiac work performed. The additional consumption of oxygen by the postsurgical heart may be due to an increase in basal metabolism, an increase in the cost of the excitation-contraction process, or left ventricular dilatation secondary to transient dysfunction, which would increase wall stress. These changes can only be assessed using the pressure-volume approach, which limits their clinical applicability because of the problems associated with attaining ventricular volume measurements as discussed above.

The Cardiac Valves

The heart has four valves. On the right side, the *tricuspid valve* lies between the right atrium and right ventricle, and the *pulmonary valve* lies between the right ventricle and the pulmonary artery. On the left side, the *mitral valve* lies between the left atrium and left ventricle, and the *aortic valve* lies between the left ventricular chamber and the aorta. The valves are fibrous structures without muscular components. Movement of the valves is governed by pressure gradients; the valves will open in response to, and blood will flow in the direction of, lower pressure. For example, when left atrial pressure exceeds that in the ventricle, the mitral valve opens to initiate ventricular filling. Conversely, the mitral valve shuts when pressure in the left ventricle exceeds that in the respective atrium during systole. The valves ensure the effective unidirectional flow of blood from atrium to ventricle to great vessel.

For the heart to function effectively as a pump, all four valves must properly open and close to propel the blood volume in a unidirectional manner. The common end point for all forms of untreated valvular dysfunction is heart failure, yet each form of valve dysfunction produces its own unique hemodynamic burden. Because valve surgery has been the major therapeutic advance in treating patients with severe heart valve disease, it is imperative for the physician to understand the pathophysiology of valve dysfunction.

Aortic Valve

Aortic stenosis

Aortic stenosis (AS) is the most common valvular lesion, and it is primarily the result of degenerative calcium deposition on the collagen framework of the valve leaflets, especially in adults older than 70 years of age. AS secondary to calcific degeneration in the older patient is the most common valve lesion presenting for valve replacement.

As the aortic valve narrows to 1 cm^2 from its normal diameter of 2.6 to 3.5 cm^2, a fixed resistance to left ventricular filling occurs. This increased resistance to ejection causes a greater pressure to be generated in the left ventricle (pressure loading) that exceeds aortic pressure, which presents clinically as a ventricular-aortic gradient. This gradual pressure loading causes myocardial sarcomere replication in parallel, with a resulting left ventricular concentric hypertrophy. Such hypertrophy results in decreased compliance. Hypertrophy in AS may also result in inadequate perfusion of the subendocardium with resultant ischemia, which occurs in 50% of AS patients in addition to significant coronary disease. By the Frank-Starling relationship, a higher LVEDP is needed to maintain the same stroke volume and cardiac output. Diastolic dysfunction ensues, and the patient with AS becomes more dependent on the "atrial kick" to generate adequate left ventricular filling to achieve appropriate stroke volume. Generally, systolic function remains normal, even during exercise, until late in the disease.

Aortic regurgitation

Aortic regurgitation (AR) is the fourth most common isolated valvular lesion. Aortic root and/or annular dilatation secondary to medial disease of the arterial wall is the usual cause of chronic isolated AR in North America. Regurgitant flow from the aortic root during diastole secondary to an incompetent valve or enlarged annulus produces a volume-loading strain on the left ventricle, similar to that produced by mitral regurgitation (MR), causing increases in end-diastolic pressure, left ventricular work, M$\dot{v}$O$_2$, and hypertrophy. The regurgitation of blood during diastole causes an increase or widening in the aortic pulse pressure. The left ventricular chamber enlargement is proportional to the amount of regurgitant flow, and the increase in diastolic stress results in parallel replication of myofibrils that extend the full length of each myocyte. In addition, the law of Laplace predicts that left ventricular wall tension increases proportionately with the increase in chamber radius. Early on in chronic AR, wall stress and oxygen demand are minimized by the resultant increase in wall thickness, which compensates for the increase in wall tension. In the compensated state, the left ventricular pressure-volume curve in AR is moved to the right of normal, with maintenance of ventricular diastolic pressure. The adaptive process of chamber enlargement and increasing wall thickness creates the greatest augmentation in ventricular mass of all valve lesions. However, as the process continues, myocardial fibrosis ensues, and the left ventricular pressure-volume relationship moves farther to the right. Left ventricular diastolic pressure increases, and heart failure results as the forward stroke volume declines (i.e., the descending portion of the Frank-Sterling carve).

Mitral Valve

Mitral stenosis

Mitral stenosis (MS) is the second most frequent valvular anomaly. Worldwide, rheumatic heart disease is the most common cause of MS, and it is usually associated with group A streptococcal pharyngitis. The acute inflammatory infiltrate forms on the valve leaflets, which then heal by fibrosis with fusion of the commissures and chordae, and calcification of the leaflets and subvalvular apparatus.

The pathophysiologic features of MS result from the obstruction of flow from the left atrium to the left ventricle caused by the stenotic valve. The normal adult mitral valve has an area of 4 to 6 cm^2, and an increased transvalvular gradient begins at 2 cm^2. The transvalvular pressure gradient is a function of the square of the transvalvular flow rate: doubling the flow quadruples the gradient. This increased pressure gradient is manifest as increased left atrial pressure, and if severe enough is reflected back to the pulmonary circulation and right ventricle, causing pulmonary venous hypertension. The chronically elevated left atrial pressure causes dilatation of that structure. Left atrial dilatation contributes to the development of atrial fibrillation, as the atrial fibers become disorganized and fibrotic. Eighty percent of patients older than 40 with MS and left atrial diameter greater than 45 cm develop atrial fibrillation. In MS, atrial fibrillation and the loss of the left atrial kick may cause a 20% decrease in stroke volume by the Frank-Starling relationship. Cardiac output will fall in severe cases of MS as a result of inadequate filling of the left ventricle and right ventricular failure. The increased transmitral gradient in MS can produce irreversible pulmonary arteriosclerosis with right ventricular failure. With pulmonary artery pressures greater than 70 mm Hg, right heart output is generally impeded.

Mitral regurgitation

MR is the third most common isolated valve lesion. The most common causes of MR are myxomatous changes of the valve, rheumatic disease, chordal rupture, bacterial endocarditis, and ischemia. With MR, the mitral valve fails to close sufficiently during systole, thereby allowing blood to "regurgitate" back into the left ventricle during diastole. As much as one half of the left ventricular volume regurgitates into the left atrium in patients with MR. Accordingly, the primary pathologic feature is the systolic unloading of the left ventricle into the low-pressure atrium, and a backup of pressure into the atrium and low-resistance pulmonary system. The reflow of this regurgitant volume from the left atrium to the left ventricle during subsequent diastolic intervals is essentially additive to the normal ventricular filling volume, and hence produces a volume-loaded state with falsely elevated stroke volume, and eccentric hypertrophy.

Tricuspid Valve

Diseases causing tricuspid regurgitation (TR) are more numerous than those causing tricuspid stenosis (TS). The most common cause of TS is rheumatic fever. The hemodynamic burden in TS is most often exacerbated by the presence of coexisting MS. When rheumatic disease affects the tricuspid valve, it usually creates a fibrotic lesion with commissural fusion that results in regurgitation and stenosis. The most common type of TR is secondary to enlargement of the orifice and annulus secondary to congestive heart failure with right ventricular dilatation

caused by disease of the left ventricle. The most common cause of pathologic isolated TR is infective endocarditis in drug addicts. In TR, a portion of the systolic blood flow from the right ventricle regurgitates into the right atrium, thereby elevating the right atrial pressure, which reflects back into the systemic venous system, producing a visible jugular venous distention, hepatic congestion, and pedal edema in severe circumstances. Diastolic volume overload of the right ventricle causes chamber dilatation, and the interventricular septum may protrude into the left ventricle during diastole, displacing left ventricular volume (preload) and subsequently reducing stroke volume by the Frank-Starling response. TS with a tricuspid gradient as small as 5 mm Hg can increase right atrial pressure and cause systemic congestion. Cardiac output is decreased as the normal tricuspid valve area of 7 cm^2 is reduced to less than 1.5 cm^2.

Pulmonary Valve

Acquired lesions of the pulmonary valve typically lead to pulmonary regurgitation (PR) more than pulmonary stenosis (PS). Pulmonary hypertension from any cause (MS, chronic obstructive pulmonary disease, or pulmonary emboli) can create PR. Severe PR may result in volume overload of the right ventricle, producing signs and symptoms of right-sided failure such as right ventricular dilatation, high right ventricular end-diastolic pressures, and high venous pressures. If pulmonary hypertension exists simultaneously with PR, the volume overload is superimposed on a hypertrophied myocardium. Severe hemodynamic changes resulting from injury to the pulmonary valve are unusual. In fact, isolated PR may be tolerated for years without decompensation.

PS is most commonly the result of a congenital defect. However, carcinoid syndrome with cardiac involvement can produce mild PS along with PR. Patients with severe stenosis may develop right-sided failure with syncope. PS may be treated with balloon valvotomy in the cardiac catheterization laboratory.

Myocardial Ischemia

Ischemic heart disease is the primary cause of death in this country. The central cause of cardiac ischemia is a mismatch between myocardial energy supply and demand, that is, a situation in which energy supply is inadequate to fully meet normal energy demands of the heart to support function. A decrease in delivery of blood flow, oxygen, and nutrients to the myocardium is called "supply ischemia." The chief cause of this type of ischemia is severe obstruction to CBF to the myocardium, caused by atherosclerotic heart disease, that is beyond the ability of the arteries to vasodilate in compensation. The second type of ischemia is caused by an increase in myocardial energy demands that exceeds the delivery of CBF, termed "demand ischemia." In the normal state, the heart consumes approximately 9 mL of oxygen per 100 g of muscle per minute, and extracts 70% to 80% of the arterial oxygen delivered, which is much higher than most other organs. During heavy exercise, the oxygen consumption may triple in the left ventricle. Under normal conditions, the vasodilatory capacity of normal coronary arteries will adjust blood flow to meet increased myocardial oxygen and nutrient demand during periods of increased cardiac work, primarily by local mechanisms as discussed above. However, partial occlusion of the coronary arteries by a stenosis that limits the vasodilator reserve prevents increases in blood flow during conditions of increased work and metabolic demand, producing a supply-demand mismatch. Factors contributing to excessive cardiac demand include states of increased sympathetic discharge (e.g., stress, exercise), cardiac hypertrophy, or states of aortic outflow obstruction (e.g., aortic valve stenosis, subvalvular stenosis, or aortic coarctation). Demand ischemia may occur more frequently in patients who have coronary lesions because of the combination of impaired CBF reserve and increased energy demands.

Ischemia occurs first and is more severe in the subendocardium than in the subepicardial myocardium. The proclivity of ischemia to affect the subendocardium is due to a number of factors. The contractile effort of subendocardial fibers is greater in this region, and hence the corresponding energy demands are greater in this region specifically. In addition, the extravascular compressive forces are greater in this layer. Hence, the vasodilatory reserve is expended in the subendocardial region first, thereby limiting blood flow to that region to a greater extent. Myocardial necrosis occurs if blood flow is not restored within a number of hours. Accordingly, with the greater severity of ischemia occurring in the subendocardial tissue, necrosis occurs first in this region and progresses toward the subepicardial region in a "wavefront" pattern. Necrosis begins in the subendocardium after approximately 40 to 60 minutes of severe ischemia, and migrates in a wavefront pattern to envelop the subepicardial tissue within the area at risk after approximately 6 hours. The progression of this wavefront, and the amount of at-risk myocardium that succumbs to infarction, depends on the degree of collateral blood flow that offsets blood flow deficits, as well as on the ambient myocardial oxygen requirements. The lower the collateral blood flow, the more severe the ischemia and the faster the progression of the necrotic wavefront.

Effects of Ischemia on Myocardial Contraction

The heart involved in a severe or total occlusion of a coronary artery may exhibit contractile dysfunction, which

may progress to failure if a sufficient amount (>35% to 40%) of the myocardium is involved. The affected region of myocardium may demonstrate a depressed systolic contraction and a delayed and incomplete diastolic relaxation, secondary to insufficient CBF and oxygen supply to support contractile efforts. In severe myocardial ischemia-reperfusion leading to necrosis, the loss of function is undoubtedly due to death of the myocytes. However, with short periods of ischemia, such as transient vasospasm or the short periods of occlusion involved in angioplasty procedures, some degree of contractile dysfunction in the area of at-risk myocardium affected by the involved coronary arteries is observed in the absence of infarction. This myocardium appears to be "stunned" because there is absence of obvious morphologic injury, and contractile activity can be recruited over time or with either inotropic interventions or postsystolic potentiation. On a subcellular level, the cause of myocardial stunning may be explained by lack of available ATP for muscle contraction. However, more likely explanations are temporary calcium dyshomeostasis, cytoskeletal disruption, and abnormalities in the contractile elements of the cardiac muscle resulting from the ischemic episode. Stunning is temporary; it is a self-reversing process with no known pattern related to restoration of perfusion, pharmacologic intervention, or any other therapeutic regimen.

Interestingly enough, short episodes of ischemia—up to 20 minutes—may both damage and protect the myocardium: Stunning occurs after as little as 5 minutes of ischemia, and yet brief episodes of total ischemia may induce an adaptive response in the myocardium that protects the tissue from lethal ischemia causing necrosis. This adaptive response may be triggered by the release of endogenous substances such as adenosine, nitric oxide, low levels of inactive oxygen spacies, and bradykinin, which are known to protect the heart from ischemia-reperfusion. This cardioprotective phenomenon is known as *ischemic preconditioning* and may also be induced pharmacologically, without the use of ischemia, by adenosine and other substances.

In cases of partial coronary artery occlusion that does not cause necrosis of the myocardium, there is evidence that the heart downregulates its level of activity during this incomplete ischemia. This phenomenon is known as "hibernation," and may be an adaptive response to limitations in CBF to save the myocardium from fully depleting its high-energy phosphate stores. The control mechanism may be that of the limited energy supply, limiting contractile effort to a level supported by the available oxygen supply during hypoperfusion. This hibernation may be fully reversible upon restoration of blood flow.

Clinically, the patient with an ischemic event or acute heart attack may present with increased EDVs and end-diastolic pressures, and reduced end-systolic pressures commensurate with the degree of ischemia (total versus subtotal) and the amount of left ventricular myocardium involved. When small regions of the left ventricle are affected, no compromise in global ventricular function may be expressed, and regional wall motion abnormalities may only be evident on echocardiographic or angiographic examination. However, with prolonged dysfunction involving 35% to 40% of the left ventricle, heart failure or cardiogenic shock may occur. The development of cardiogenic shock itself becomes a vicious cycle: loss of myocardial function reduces aortic pressure, further limiting coronary perfusion pressure and exacerbating ischemia by further limiting supply. Furthermore, decreased ejection increases EDV and end-diastolic pressure (preload), thereby increasing the ventricular wall tension and oxygen demand. These contractile abnormalities of the ischemic heart may be further exacerbated by accompanying disorders of rate and rhythm, which may contribute to half of the postischemic deaths that occur.

Timely restoration of flow will salvage myocardium and limit the size of the infarct. However, reperfusion may also paradoxically lead to more myocardial damage, a process called *ischemia-reperfusion injury*. The process of reperfusion injury is complex and multifactorial. The severity of reperfusion injury is predicated on the severity and duration of ischemia, which in effect sets the stage for reperfusion injury. Other studies indicate that the sudden normalization of extracellular pH precipitates an influx of calcium, which poisons the mitochondrial apparatus, leading to metabolic derangements, and precipitates a contracture of the myocardium (so-called stone heart). The process of contracture can lead to membrane damage and exacerbate the influx of calcium. Other studies suggest that the phenomenon of reperfusion injury is partially inflammatory in nature, mediated acutely primarily by neutrophils and their interaction with and adherence to vascular endothelium at the site of ischemia-reperfusion during the early moments of reflow. The process of reperfusion injury triggers cell death by both necrosis and apoptosis, or programmed cell death.

Bibliography

Alkhulaifi AM, Yellon DM, Pugsley WB: Preconditioning the human heart during aorto-coronary bypass surgery. Eur J Cardiothorac Surg 1994;8:270; discussion 276.

Amsterdam EA, Stahl GL, Pan HL: Limitation of reperfusion injury by a monoclonal antibody to C5a during myocardial infarction in pigs. Am J Physiol 1995;268:H448.

Anderson JR, Hossein-Nia M, Kallis P: Comparison of two strategies for myocardial management during coronary artery operations [see comments]. Ann Thorac Surg 1994;58:768; discussion 772.

Anderson PAW, Rankin JS, Arentzen CE: Evaluation of the force-frequency relationship as a descriptor of the inotropic state of canine left ventricular myocardium. Circ Res 1976;39:832.

Arentzen CE, Rankin JS, Anderson PAW: Force-frequency characteristics of the left ventricle in the conscious dog. Circ Res 1978;42:64.

Barnes CS, Coker SJ: Failure of nitric oxide donors to alter arrhythmias induced by acute myocardial ischaemia or reperfusion in anaesthetized rats. Br J Pharmacol 1995;114:349.

Berne RM, Levy MN: Special circulations. *In*: Physiology (2nd ed). St. Louis: Mosby, 1988:540.

Bohn H, Schonafinger K: Oxygen and oxidation promote the release of nitric oxide from sydnonimines. J Cardiovasc Pharmacol 1989;14(Suppl 11):S6.

Braunwald E: Control of myocardial oxygen consumption: physiologic and clinical considerations. Am J Cardiol 1971;27:416.

Braunwald E: 50th Anniversary Historical Article. Myocardial oxygen consumption: the quest for its determinants and some clinical fallout. J Am Coll Cardiol 2000;35:45B.

Braunwald E, Ross J Jr: Control of cardiac performance. *In* Berne RM (ed): Handbook of Physiology, Vol 1. Bethesda, MD: American Physiological Society, 1979:533.

Brillantes AM, Allen P, Takahashi T: Differences in cardiac calcium release channel (ryanodine receptor) expression in myocardium from patients with end-stage heart failure caused by ischemic versus dilated cardiomyopathy. Circ Res 1992;71:18.

Canty JM, Klocke FJ: Reductions in regional myocardial function at rest in conscious dogs with chronically reduced regional coronary artery pressure. Circ Res 1987;61:II-107.

Chilian WM: Microvascular pressures and resistances in the left ventricular subepicardium and subendocardium. Circ Res 1991;69:561.

Collis MG, Hourain SMO: Adenosine receptor subtypes. TiPS 1993;1:360.

Davia K, Bernobich E, Ranu HK: SERCA2A over expression decreases the incidence of aftercontractions in adult rabbit ventricular myocytes. J Mol Cell Cardiol 2001;33:1005.

del Monte F, Hajjar RJ, Harding SE: Overwhelming evidence of the beneficial effects of SERCA gene transfer in heart failure. Circ Res 2001;88:E66.

del Monte F, Williams E, Lebeche D: Improvement in survival and cardiac metabolism after gene transfer of sarcoplasmic reticulum Ca(2+)-ATPase in a rat model of heart failure. Circulation 2001;104:1424.

Downey JM, Downey HF, Kirk ES: Effects of myocardial strains on coronary blood flow. Circ Res 1974;34:286.

Downey JM, Kirk ES: Inhibition of coronary blood flow by a vascular waterfall mechanism. Circ Res 1975;36:753.

Factor SM: Pathophysiology of myocardial ischemia. *In* Hurst JW (ed): The Heart (7th ed). New York: McGraw-Hill, 1990:940.

Feigl EO: Physiological Review: Coronary Physiology. Bethesda, MD: American Physiological Society, 1983:63.

Freeman GL, Colston JT: Role of ventriculovascular coupling in cardiac response to increased contractility in closed-chest dogs. J Clin Invest 1990;86:1278.

Freeman GL, Little WC, O'Rourke RA: Influence of heart rate on left ventricular performance in conscious dogs. Circ Res 1987;61:455.

Gibbs CL, Chapman JB: Cardiac energetics. *In* Berne RM (ed): Handbook of Physiology, Vol 1. Bethesda, MD: American Physiological Society, 1979:775.

Glower DD, Spratt JA, Snow ND: Linearity of the Frank-Starling relationship in the intact heart: the concept of preload recruitable stroke work. Circulation 1985;71:994.

Gorlach G, Podzuweit T, Dapper F: Einfluss der Reperfusionsdauer auf die metabolische Erholung wahrend Entlastung des hypertrophen Herzens nach induziertem Herzstillstand [Effect of the duration of reperfusion on metabolic recovery during unloading of the hypertrophic heart following induced heart arrest]. Z Kardiol 1990;79:28.

Goto M, Flynn AE, Doucette JW: Cardiac contraction affects deep myocardial vessels predominantly. Am J Physiol (Heart Circ Physiol) 1991;261:H1417.

Goto M, Tsujioka K, Ogasawara Y: Effect of blood filling in intramyocardial vessels on coronary arterial inflow. Am J Physiol (Heart Circ Physiol) 1990;258:H1042.

Guyton AC: Muscle blood flow and cardiac output during exercise; the coronary circulation; and ischemic heart disease. *In*: Textbook of Medical Physiology (8th ed). Philadelphia: WB Saunders, 1991: 234.

Headrick JP, Northington FJ, Hynes MR: Relative responses to luminal and adventitial adenosine in perfused arteries. Am J Physiol 1992;263:H1437.

Heineman FW, Balaban RS: Control of mitochondrial respiration in the heart in vivo. Annu Rev Physiol 1990;52:523.

Hendry PJ, Anstadt MP, Plunkett MD: Improved donor myocardial recovery with a new lazaroid lipid antiperoxidant in the isolated canine heart. J Heart Lung Transplant 1992;11:636.

Heyndrickx GR, Vatner SF: Stunned myocardium: historical perspective. *In* Kloner RA, Przyklenk K (eds): Stunned Myocardium: Properties, Mechanisms, and Clinical Manifestations. New York: Marcel Dekker, 1993.

Jones CJ, Kuo L, Davis MJ: Role of nitric oxide in the coronary microvascular responses to adenosine and increased metabolic demand. Circulation 1995;91:1807.

Jordan JE, Zhao Z-Q, Vinten-Johansen J: The role of neutrophils in myocardial ischemia-reperfusion injury. Cardiovasc Res 1999;43:860.

Kass DA, Yamazaki T, Burkhoff D: Determination of left ventricular end-systolic pressure-volume relationships by the conductance (volume) catheter technique. Circulation 1986;73:586.

Katz AM: The ischemic heart. *In*: Physiology of the Heart (2nd ed). New York: Raven Press, 1992:609.

Kawabata K, Netticadan T, Osada M: Mechanisms of ischemic preconditioning affects Ca^{2+} paradox-induced changes in heart. Am J Physiol (Heart Circ Physiol) 2000;278:H1008.

Kirklin JW, Barratt-Boyes B: Stenotic arteriosclerotic coronary artery disease. *In* Kirklin JW, Barratt-Boyes B (eds): Cardiac Surgery (2nd ed), Vol 1. New York: Churchill Livingstone, 1993:28.

Kloner RA, Przyklenk K: First evidence: postischemic dysfunction of viable myocardium. *In* Kloner RA, Przyklenk K (eds): Stunned Myocardium: Properties, Mechanisms, and Clinical Manifestations. New York: Marcel Dekker, 1993:17.

Kohin S, Stary CM, Howlett RA: Preconditioning improves function and recovery of single muscle fibers during severe hypoxia and reoxygenation. Am J Physiol 2001;281:C142.

Koss KL, Grupp IL, Kranias EG: The relative phospholamban and SERCA2 ratio: a critical determinant of myocardial contractility. Basic Res Cardiol 1997;92:17.

Koss KL, Kranias EG: Phospholamban: a prominent regulator of myocardial contractility. Circ Res 1996;79:1059.

Landzberg J, Parker JD, Gauthier DF: Effects of intracoronary acetylcholine and atropine on basal and dobutamine-stimulated left ventricular contractility. Circulation 1994;89:164.

Lee J, Chambers DE, Akizuki S: The role of vascular capacitance in the coronary arteries. Circ Res 1984;55:751.

Luscinskas FW, Brock AF, Arnaout MA, Gimbrone MA: Endothelial-leukocyte adhesion molecule-1-dependent and leukocyte (CD11/CD18)-dependent mechanisms contribute to polymorphonuclear leukocyte adhesion to cytokine-activated human vascular endothelium. J Immunol 1989;142:2257.

Mann J, Renwick AG, Holgate S: Release of adenosine and its metabolites from activated human leukocytes. Clin Sci 1986;70:461.

Mohrman DE, Feigl EO: Competition between sympathetic vasoconstriction and metabolic vasodilation in the canine coronary circulation. Circ Res 1978;42:79.

Mulligan LJ, Escebedo D, Freeman GL: Mechanical determinants of coronary blood flow during dynamic alterations in contractility. Am J Physiol (Heart Circ Physiol) 1993;34:H1112.

Nanoff C, Jacobson KA, Stiles GL: The A_2 adenosine receptor: guanine nucleotide modulation of agonist binding is enhanced by proteolysis. Mol Pharmacol 1990;39:130.

Newton GE, Azevedo ER, Parker JD: Inotropic and sympathetic responses to the intracoronary infusion of a beta2-receptor agonist: a human in vivo study. Circulation 1999;99:2402.

Nishida K, Harrison DG, Navas JP: Molecular cloning and characterization of the constitutive bovine aortic endothelial cell nitric oxide synthase. J Clin Invest 1992;90:2092.

Noack E, Feelisch M: Molecular aspects underlying the vasodilator action of molsidomine. J Cardiovasc Pharmacol 1989;11:S1.

Odiet JA, Boerrigter ME, Wei JY: Carnitine palmitoyl transferase-I activity in the aging mouse heart. Mech Ageing Dev 1995;79:127.

Parent R, Lavallee M: Contribution of nitric oxide to dilation of resistance coronary vessels in conscious dogs. Am J Physiol 1992;262:H10.

Phillips RM, Narayan P, Gomez AM: Sarcoplasmic reticulum in heart failure: central player or bystander? Cardiovasc Res 1998;37:346.

Prabhu SD, Freeman GL: Left ventricular energetics in closed-chest dogs. Am J Physiol 1993;265:H1048.

Prasad MR, Jones RM: Enhanced membrane protein kinase C activity in myocardial ischemia. Basic Res Cardiol 1992;87:19.

Rees DD, Palmer RMJ, Moncada S: Role of endothelium-derived nitric oxide in the regulation of blood pressure. Proc Natl Acad Sci U S A 1989;86:3375.

Reiken S, Gaburjakova M, Gaburjakova J: Beta-adrenergic receptor blockers restore cardiac calcium release channel (ryanodine receptor) structure and function in heart failure. Circulation 2001;104:2843.

Restoration of contractile function in isolated cardiomyocytes from failing human hearts by gene transfer of SERCA2a. Circulation 1999;100:2308.

Rooke GA, Feigl EO: Work as a correlate of canine left ventricular oxygen consumption, and the problem of catecholamine oxygen wasting. Circ Res 1982;50:273.

Schipke JD: Cardiac efficiency. Basic Res Cardiol 1994;89:207.

Shen JG, Zhou DY: Efficiency of Ginkgo biloba extract (EGb 761) in antioxidant protection against myocardial ischemia and reperfusion injury. Biochem Mol Biol Int 1995;35:125.

Simmerman HK, Jones LR: Phospholamban: protein structure, mechanism of action, and role in cardiac function. Physiol Rev 1998;78:921.

Sisto T, Paajanen H, Metsa-Ketela T: Pretreatment with antioxidants and allopurinol diminishes cardiac onset events in coronary artery bypass grafting. Ann Thorac Surg 1995;59:1519.

Snyder R, Downey JM, Kirk ES: The active and passive components of extravascular coronary resistance. Cardiovasc Res 1975;9:161.

Steingart RM, Scheuer J: Assessment of myocardial ischemia. In Hurst JW (ed): The Heart (7th ed). New York: McGraw-Hill, 1990:351.

Suarez J, Rubio R: Regulation of glycolytic flux by coronary flow in guinea pig heart: role of vascular endothelial cell glycocalyx. Am J Physiol 1993;261:H1994.

Suga H: Ventricular energetics. Physiol Rev 1990;70:247.

Suga H, Hisano R, Hirata S: Mechanism of higher oxygen consumption rate: pressure-loaded vs. volume-loaded heart. Am J Physiol 1982;242:H942.

Takaoka H, Takeuchi M, Odake M: Comparison of hemodynamic determinants for myocardial oxygen consumption under different contractile states in human ventricle. Circulation 1993;87:59.

Tao S, Calza G, Lerzo F: Activation of the intracellular glutathione system by oxidative stress during cardiopulmonary bypass and myocardial perfusion. Perfusion 1995;10:45.

Van Winkle DM, Swafford AN, Downey JM: Subendocardial coronary compression in beating dog hearts is independent of pressure in the ventricular lumen. Am J Physiol (Heart Circ Physiol) 1991;261:H500.

Vinten-Johansen J, Barnard RJ, Buckberg GD: Left ventricular O$_2$ requirements of pressure and volume loading in the normal canine heart and inaccuracy of pressure-derived indices of O$_2$ demand. Cardiovasc Res 1982;16:439.

Vinten-Johansen J, Duncan HW, Finkenberg JG: Prediction of myocardial O$_2$ requirements by indirect indices. Am J Physiol 1982;243:H862.

Vinten-Johansen J, Johnston WE, Mills SA: Reperfusion injury after temporary coronary occlusion. J Thorac Cardiovasc Surg 1988;95:960.

Vinten-Johansen J, Weiss HR: Oxygen consumption in subepicardial and subendocardial regions of the canine left ventricle: the effect of experimental acute valvular aortic stenosis. Circ Res 1980;46:139.

Yamada H, Yoneyama F, Satoh K: Comparison of the effects of the novel vasodilator FK409 with those of nitroglycerin in isolated coronary artery of the dog. Br J Pharmacol 1991;103:1713.

Zhao Z-Q, Nakamura M, Wang N-P: Administration of adenosine during reperfusion reduces injury of vascular endothelium and death of myocytes. Coron Artery Dis 1999;10:617.

CHAPTER 23

Physiology of Arterial Venous and Lymphatic Systems

Sheila M. Coogan, M.D. and Christopher K. Zarins, M.D.

Normal Arterial Structure and Function

Layers of the Arterial Wall

The arterial wall is organized into three layers: the intima, the media, and the adventitia. The innermost layer of an artery is the intima. The intima is composed of an endothelial layer, a basal lamina that bonds the endothelium to the subendothelial layer, and the internal elastic lamina. The media, made up of smooth muscle cells oriented circumferentially in a collagen and elastin matrix, carries most of the tensile load of the arterial system and contains the vasa vasorum (Fig. 23–1). In some arteries, there is an external elastic lamina that separates the media from the outer adventitia. The adventitia provides a support function to the artery. The adventitia consists of fibrous connective tissue (the vasa vasorum) that provides nutrients to the outer layers of the artery, and nerve fibers that help regulate the smooth muscle tone of the media.

Vessel Diameter

The arterial tree originates at the aortic root. The aorta and its primary branch vessels are called elastic arteries. *Elastic arteries* are large in diameter and have a large elastin component in the media that accommodates the significant pressure changes of the cardiac cycle. In systole, vessels undergo significant distention, momentarily pooling blood and thus storing potential energy. In diastole, the elastic recoil of these arteries continues to propagate flow and release this potential energy (called the Windkessel effect). *Muscular arteries* are slightly smaller in diameter and have less elastin than elastic arteries. The media in these arteries has a thick layer of smooth muscle that reflects the primary function of the muscular arteries. These vessels regulate the distribution of blood throughout the body, shifting it into different vascular beds as needed. The microcirculation consists of *arterioles* and *capillaries*. Arterioles and capillaries are much smaller in diameter but greater in number than muscular or elastic arteries. The total cross-sectional area of arterioles is 50 times that of the aorta and capillaries, and 800 times that of the aorta. Arterioles, whose media has a large percentage of smooth muscle, act as control valves of the arterial system. Arterioles can severely constrict or become dilated severalfold to accommodate the needs of a particular vascular bed. Capillaries are thin walled and provide the site of nutrient exchange at the cellular level.

Blood Pressure

Blood pressure, obtained indirectly using a sphygmomanometer or directly using an intra-arterial pressure catheter, is expressed as a ratio of the systolic pressure (SBP), or the peak intra-arterial pressure during each pulse generated by systolic contraction, over the

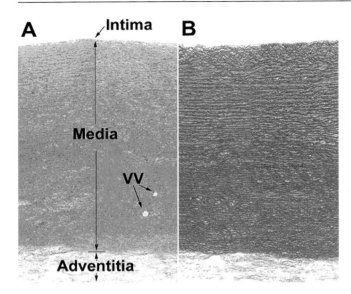

FIGURE 23–1 Histologic features of a normal thoracic aorta. **A**, Hematoxylin and eosin–stained cross section of the aorta shows three layers of the aorta: the intima, the media, and the adventitia. Vasa vasorum (VV) can be seen in the one-third zone of the outer media. **B**, Mason trichrome staining of the section depicts the rich component of elastic lamellae (purple stained). Original magnification: 50X for **A** and **B**.

diastolic pressure (DBP), or the basal intra-arterial pressure during cardiac relaxation. The pulse pressure wave that is generated by each systolic contraction of the left ventricle is dependent on not only the stroke volume but also the compliance (distensibility) of the aortic arch and proximal aorta, as well as the peripheral resistance. This maintains the diastolic pressure. The elastic nature of the major proximal arteries allows them to expand during systole and recoil during diastole, creating a more constant intra-aortic pressure as well as propagating the pulse distally. During exercise, sympathetic-mediated smooth muscle contraction results in reduced aortic expansion, which produces a higher systolic pressure, and peripheral vasodilatation, resulting in reduced peripheral resistance. The net result is an increase in pulse pressure (pulse pressure = SBP – DBP). In older patients with calcified, noncompliant vessels, systolic hypertension with increased pulse pressure is noted because of the increased stiffness of the aorta.

The arterial pressure waveform changes along the course of the aorta and peripheral arteries. In the aortic arch and descending thoracic aorta, the pressure waveform is rounded with a dicrotic notch during the systolic downslope as a result of closure of the aortic valve. There is a gradual increase in the peak systolic pressure wave amplitude in the descending thoracic and abdominal aorta. Reflection of the pulse wave at the bifurcation of the abdominal aorta into the

iliac arteries results in pulse amplification and a higher systolic pressure as the pulse proceeds peripherally. Diastolic pressure decreases slightly, with mean aortic pressure remaining the same throughout the aorta.

Blood Pressure and Energy

The total energy of a system is the sum of the kinetic energy (KE) and the potential energy (PE). The PE of the arterial system is the sum of the intra-arterial pressure and gravitational energy. Intra-arterial pressure is derived from the cardiac pump (Pc). Gravitational pressure (P_H) is the pressure from the hydrostatic column of blood:

$$P_H = -\rho gh$$

where ρ is the density of blood (1.056 g/cm^3), g is the acceleration of gravity (980 cm/s^2), and h is the height (cm) above a fixed reference point (the right atrium). Thus

$$PE\ [\text{erg/cm}^2] = Pc + P_H + \rho gh$$

In an ideal system, $KE = \frac{1}{2}\rho v^2$ where ρ is the density of fluid and v is the mean velocity. This equation is only applicable in a nonpulsatile, laminar flow scenario of Newtonian fluids and therefore cannot be applied to the arterial tree. It is useful, however, in reminding us that the KE of flowing blood is derived primarily from velocity or flow rate.

Blood Flow and Peripheral Resistance

Blood flow (Q) is influenced by pressure gradient (ΔP), radius (r), viscosity (η), and conduit length (L). The interrelationship of these variables is reflected in *Poiseuille's law*:

$$Q = \frac{\pi \Delta P r^4}{8 \eta L}$$

where Q is the flow (cm^3/sec), ΔP is the pressure gradient (dynes/cm^2), r is the radius (cm), η is the viscosity (dynes/sec/cm^2), and L is the length (cm). From this equation, one can see that small changes in radius will greatly affect flow because flow is proportional to the fourth power of the radius.

Ohm's law of electrical circuits can be borrowed to help define the relationship between flow, pressure gradient, and resistance in the arterial tree. Ohm's law is

$$Q = \frac{\Delta P}{R}$$

where Q is the flow (cm^3/sec), ΔP is the pressure gradient (mm Hg), and R is the resistance (mm Hg/min/cm^3). Thus peripheral arterial resistance is $R = \Delta P Q$. Using a pulmonary artery catheter to measure, one can obtain the pressure gradient and cardiac output and indirectly determine the systemic vascular resistance:

$$SVR = \frac{MAP - CVP}{CO} \times 80$$

where SVR is the systemic vascular resistance (dynes/sec/cm^{-5}), MAP is the mean arterial pressure (mm Hg), CVP is the central venous pressure (mm Hg), CO is the cardiac output (mL/min), and 80 is a constant to convert SVR into dynes/sec/cm^{-5}.

Systemic vascular resistance is a major determinant of cardiac output and hemodynamic forces.

Hemodynamic Forces

Flow in the human arterial tree is generally laminar, with fluid displacements following predictable and stable linear paths. Blood generally flows in smooth layers, with cells and particles tending to stay in ordered layers. If blood velocity exceeds a critical level, which may occur in areas of critical lumen stenosis, flow can be disordered or turbulent.

In turbulent flow, particles in the blood disperse and follow an erratic and unpredictable pathway. There are random movements of elements in the flow field. Whether or not flow will be turbulent depends on viscosity, mean velocity, and the diameter of the vessel. The *Reynold's number* (R$_e$) takes these into account and is given by

$$R_e = \frac{pVd}{\mu}$$

where p is the density, V is the mean velocity (m/sec), d is the diameter of the vessel lumen, and μ is the absolute viscosity (Nsec/m^2). A Reynolds number exceeding a critical value for a given situation predicts the occurrence of turbulent flow. Abrupt changes in geometry distal to a stenosis, or other obstacles in the flow stream, may cause focal turbulence.

In straight vessels, blood flow is typically laminar and parabolic. Velocity is greatest in the center of the vessel and declines symmetrically toward the endothelial surface of the arterial wall, where there is frictional resistance at the blood-endothelium interface. The distribution of velocities in the arterial lumen is displaced if there is an eccentric lesion in the vessel, or if the vessel curves. The velocity profile returns to a symmetrical parabolic state when the vessel is again straight. The curvature of a vessel, its branchings and bifurcations, and the angle of the branches all affect the velocity profile and can cause local flow disturbances. For example, the downstream edge of a branch vessel intercepts and divides the flow stream, and is exposed to higher flow velocities and shear stress than the upstream rim of the branch. Flow separation occurs when the flow velocity profile has been displaced away from the vessel wall. The flow velocity gradient is steeper on the inside of a flow divider, or on the convex or outer aspect of a curved vessel. These variations in hemodynamic forces and their effects on the blood-endothelium interface are thought to play a role in the development and localization of artery wall pathologies such as atherosclerosis.

Local Effects of Turbulent Flow

Shear stress has received much attention in the literature with respect to endothelial function and atherosclerotic plaque formation. Wall shear stress is defined as the tangential drag force per unit area produced by blood moving along the endothelial surface. This force tends to displace the endothelium and inner layers of the artery wall in the direction of flow. The expression for wall shear stress for parabolic flow in a cylindrical vessel is

$$\tau_w = \frac{4\mu Q}{\pi r^3}$$

where τ_w is the wall shear stress (N/m^2), μ is the viscosity of blood, Q is the blood flow rate (L/sec), and r is the vessel radius. Because shear stress is inversely related to the cube of the radius, small changes in the radius can have a significant impact on wall shear stress. Wall shear stress is also defined as the product of the viscosity and the velocity gradient of the fluid in the direction parallel to the blood endothelial surface.

Intraluminal blood pressure exerts a distending and compressive force on the artery wall, with a circumferential stretching force exerted in a direction tangential to the artery wall (Fig. 23–2). This force is known as *wall tension* and is described by the law of Laplace ($T = Pr$), where T is tension (N/m), P is pressure (N/m^2), and r is the lumen radius. This equation is accurate if the thickness of the arterial wall is small compared to the diameter. Increasing wall tension is counterbalanced by increases in wall thickness to maintain a constant wall *tensile stress*.

Pathologic Conditions of Arteries

Pathologic conditions of arteries include processes that obstruct blood flow, such as stenoses and occlusions, and processes that result in weakening of the artery wall with dilatation, aneurysm formation, and rupture.

Arterial Stenosis

Atherosclerotic disease primarily affects the circulation through energy loss at arterial stenoses, where the velocity must increase to maintain constant flow:

$$Q = vA = v\pi r^2$$

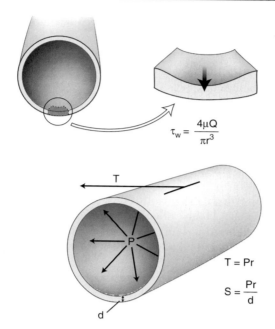

$$\tau_w = \frac{4\mu Q}{\pi r^3}$$

$$T = Pr$$

$$S = \frac{Pr}{d}$$

FIGURE 23–2 Schematic depiction of wall shear stress and wall tension.

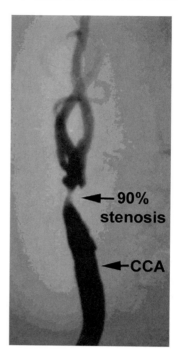

FIGURE 23–3 Angiogram of carotid artery showing critical stenosis.

where Q is the flow, v is the velocity, A is the area, and r is the tube radius. Upon entering and exiting an arterial stenosis, there are considerable inertial energy losses in the form of viscous energy loss resulting from turbulent flow.

The loss of kinetic energy as a result of turbulence has been estimated as follows:

$$\Delta P = k\rho(v_s - v_e)^2/2$$

where k is dependent on the geometric configuration, v_s is the velocity in the stenosis, v_e is the velocity after the exit of the stenosis, and ρ is the fluid density; or

$$\Delta P = kv^2[(r/r_s)^2 - 1]^2$$

where v is the velocity after stenosis, r is the radius of the uninvolved artery, and r_s is the radius of the stenosis. Hence energy lost at an arterial stenosis is proportional to the *fourth power of the change in radius* and the *second power of the velocity within the normal artery*.

Critical and subcritical stenoses

In experimental studies, a pressure gradient or flow reduction does not occur until there is a 75% to 90% reduction in cross-sectional area at the site of arterial stenosis. The reduction in cross-sectional area corresponds to a 50% to 75% reduction in diameter. Figure 23–3 represents a high-grade carotid artery stenosis.

A stenosis is *critical* when there is a pressure gradient or a reduction in pressure distal to the stenosis and a reduction in blood flow caused by the stenosis. A flow-limiting stenosis generally occurs at a 50% to 75% diameter

reduction of the artery. The degree of stenosis required to become "critical" is dependent on the volume and velocity of blood flow within the artery. At low flow, a stenosis may not be critical; however, at a higher flow rate (i.e., exercise), a stenosis may become critical. When this is the case, it is called *subcritical stenosis*.

Arterial stenoses become more significant in high-flow states. During resting states, a setting of low blood flow exists; however, with exercise, blood flow substantially increases and a stenosis may become critical. Using the formula $P = QR$, where Q is the flow, P is the pressure, and R is the resistance, one can determine the effect of exercise in the setting of a fixed stenosis.

In this setting, flow (Q) increases in response to the increased heart rate resulting from exercise. Resistance (R) must remain constant because of the fixed stenosis. Using $P = QR$, the pressure gradient must increase in response to increased flow across a fixed stenosis. This results in a decreased distal blood pressure, whereas distal blood pressure would normally increase in individuals with compliant blood vessels. In this setting, the increased metabolic demands of exercise are not met, leading to metabolite accumulation and pain (claudication). After a period of rest, the metabolites are cleared and pain subsides.

Multiple stenoses

Atherosclerosis is a systemic disease. Rarely does a patient have a single focal stenosis. More commonly, one finds that a patient will have multiple sequential stenoses. Resistances in series are additive:

$$R_T = R_1 + R_2 + R_3 \ldots$$

where R_T is the total resistance. Although sequential stenoses are additive, the single most critical stenosis determines the limitation of blood flow.

Collateral circulation

Proliferation of collateral arteries occurs as a compensatory mechanism to improve the delivery of blood around a fixed stenosis. Collateral arteries are smaller than the primary diseased vessel. Therefore, to compensate for a stenosis in the primary vessel, a much larger number of collaterals must develop. Resistance is an inverse function of the fourth power of the radius. Thus, for a 50% stenosis of a 0.5-cm artery, 625 1-mm collaterals would be needed to compensate for the stenosis.

Arterial Aneurysms

Aneurysms are focal arterial dilatations more than twice the normal artery diameter. Figure 23–4 represents an infrarenal abdominal aortic aneurysm.

The pathophysiology of aneurysm enlargement is still not well understood, but there is a well-defined hemodynamic contribution to aneurysm expansion and rupture. Aneurysms are believed to expand as a result of tangential stress (τ) within the wall of the aneurysm. Rupture occurs when τ exceeds the wall tensile strength. In an idealized cylinder, circumferential wall stress (τ_c) is defined by

$$\tau_c = P \cdot r / \delta$$

where P is the pressure, r is the internal radius, and δ = wall thickness.

This is a modification of Laplace's law for cylinders with negligible thickness:

$$T = P \cdot r$$

Based on these formulas, risk of aneurysm expansion and rupture is linearly proportional to arterial pressure and aneurysm size and inversely proportional to wall thickness. More recently, an alternative method using computer modeling has been proposed to determine peak wall stress that appears to be more sensitive than the above modification of Laplace's law in predicting potential aneurysm rupture.

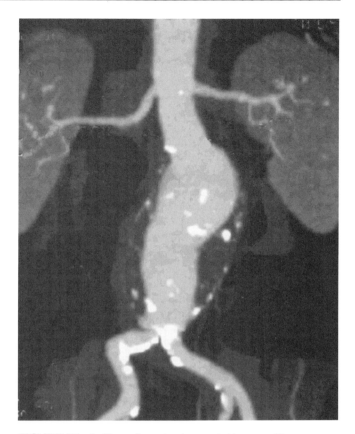

FIGURE 23–4 Three-dimensional computed tomographic reconstruction of an infrarenal abdominal aortic aneurysm.

Bibliography

Fillinger MF, Raghavan ML, Marra SP, et al: In vivo analysis of mechanical wall stress and abdominal aortic aneurysm rupture risk. J Vasc Surg 2002;36:589.

Glagov S, Zarins C, Giddens DP, Ku DN: Hemodynamics and atherosclerosis: insights and perspectives gained from studies of human arteries. Arch Pathol Lab Med 1988;112:1018.

Guyton AC: Textbook of Medical Physiology (7th ed). Philadelphia, WB Saunders, 1986.

Strandness DE, Sumner DS: Hemodynamics for Surgeons. New York: Grune & Stratton, 1975.

Sumner DS: Essential hemodynamic principles. In Rutherford RB (ed): Vascular Surgery (3rd ed). Philadelphia: WB Saunders, 1989:18.

Tropea BI, Zarins CK: Hemodynamics and atherosclerosis. In Sidawy AN (ed): The Basic Science of Vascular Disease. Armonk, NY: Futura, 1997:107.

CHAPTER 24

Gastrointestinal and Hepatic Physiology and Dysfunction

Gordon L. Kauffman, Jr., M.D.

Stomach

The stomach is divided into two functionally distinct organs. The fundus is the portion of the stomach that secretes acid and intrinsic factor from parietal cells and pepsinogen from chief cells. In contrast, the distal portion of the stomach, the antrum, is devoid of parietal and chief cells but contains G cells that secrete gastrin, which is the primary endocrine agent for parietal cell stimulation. Both the fundus and the antrum contain surface epithelial cells that line the luminal surface. Their primary products are mucus and bicarbonate, which provides some measure of defense against secreted protons in the gastric lumen.

Hydrochloric acid converts pepsinogen to the active form of the enzyme, pepsin, which denatures proteins and provides a bacteriocidal effect. In normal humans, the stomach is usually sterile. Pepsin begins the process of proteolysis when proteins are in the lumen of the stomach. Circulating gastrin from the antrum has an effect on the enterochromaffin-like (ECL) cell and the parietal cell to stimulate hydrochloric acid secretion, in addition to which it regulates mucosal growth and has a stimulatory effect on the chief cell to release pepsinogen. The appearance of the gastric mucosa macroscopically is velvety, and microscopically it is lined with surface epithelial cells between gastric pits and glands. The parietal cell and chief cell of the fundus are found deep in the glands, as are the G cells in the antrum (Fig. 24–1).

Parietal Cell Secretion

The secretory surface of the parietal cells is lined with a number of H^+,K^+-ATPase units. This is the final transport mechanism for the release of protons into the lumen, which occurs in exchange for potassium. It is thought that the parietal cell is the only cell in the body that contains this H^+,K^+-ATPase. It is 1000 amino acids in length and has eight transmembrane domains. During stimulation, the parietal cell increases its secretory surface several hundred fold, thus exposing more of the H^+,K^+-ATPase to the lumen, dramatically increasing the rate of proton secretion. The protons are generated primarily from the metabolism of glucose and fatty acids, which yields carbon dioxide, OH^-, and H^+. Carbonic anhydrase catalyzes the conversion of water and carbon dioxide to carbonic acid, which then dissociates, leaving a free proton to be exchanged for potassium by H^+,K^+-ATPase. The bicarbonate moiety diffuses down the concentration gradient on the nutrient side, a process that is referred to as the "alkaline tide."

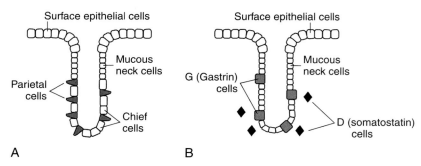

FIGURE 24–1 Histologic structure of the gastric fundic (**A**) and antral (**B**) mucosa. The fundus contains parietal and chief cells deep in the gastric glands, above which are mucus neck cells that differentiate primarily into surface epithelial cells but can differentiate into parietal or chief cells. Similarly, in the gastric antrum, the G cells that contain gastrin and the D cells that release somatostatin as a paracrine agent are found deep in the glands of the gastric antral mucosa, above which are also mucus neck cells, the majority of which differentiate into surface epithelial cells but can also differentiate to become G cells.

Chloride enters the lumen via active transport from the cytosol. Potassium leaves the cytosol via active transport across the nutrient membrane (Fig. 24–2).

The parietal cell has three primary receptors that, when activated, result in stimulation of H^+,K^+-ATPase units through either the protein kinase A or protein kinase C pathways. Ligand binding to the gastrin receptor, also referred to as the cholecystokinin B (CCKB) receptor, and the cholinergic (M_3) receptor activates H^+,K^+-ATPase through an increase in cytosolic protein kinase C. Ligand binding to the histamine₂ (H_2) receptor activates H^+,K^+-ATPase through activation of adenylate cyclase and an increase in cytosolic cyclic AMP (cAMP) protein kinase A. Recently, it has been found that a primary effector cell for stimulation of acid secretion is the ECL cell, which resides in close proximity to the parietal cells. It also contains the gastrin/CCKB receptor, as well as the cholinergic muscarinic M_1 receptor, both of which, when activated, cause the ECL cell to release histamine. Histamine acts as a paracrine agent to activate the H_2 receptor on the parietal cell. Thus the integrated acid secretory response to a meal is a result of a neurocrine component, acetylcholine acting on the M_3 receptor of the parietal cell and the M_1 receptor of the ECL cell; an endocrine component, gastrin acting on the CCKB receptor of both the ECL cell and the parietal cell; and a paracrine component, histamine released from the ECL cells, diffusing to the parietal cell on which it activates the H_2 receptor (Fig. 24–3).

Pharmacologically, the parietal cell can be inhibited by two classes of compounds. The H_2 receptor antagonists have been developed to block the H_2 receptor on the parietal cell. These are compounds that are similar in structure to histamine, allowing them to bind to the H_2 receptor without activating the cell. A second group of compounds, the substituted benzimidazoles, are direct inhibitors of H^+,K^+-ATPase. They are weak bases that enter the lumen, where they are acidified. The acidified form of the substituted benzimidazole then binds irreversibly to a portion of H^+,K^+-ATPase, thus inhibiting all forms of stimulated acid secretion. Some specific muscarinic M_1 receptor antagonists have been developed, but are not in clinical use in the United States.

The parietal cell also synthesizes and releases intrinsic factor, which combines with two vitamin B_{12} moieties and, as a complex, moves down the gastrointestinal tract where, in the terminal ilium, the components are dissociated and there is active transport of vitamin B_{12} across the enterocyte, into the portal circulation. Thus patients who have had a near-total gastrectomy or have had resection of

PARIETAL CELL

$$CO_2 + H_2O$$
$$\downarrow$$
$$H_2CO_3$$
$$\downarrow$$
$$HCO_3^- + H^+$$

FIGURE 24–2 Proposed mechanism of parietal cell secretion of HCl. Protons and bicarbonate are made available in the cytosol by the dissociation of carbonic acid. The protons leave the cytosol in exchange for potassium by means of the H^+,K^+-ATPase located on the luminal membrane of the parietal cell. There is also a chloride channel through which chloride traverses from the cytosol into the gastric lumen. Potassium leaves the cell through a similar channel on the nutrient membrane. Bicarbonate leaves the cell, moving down its concentration gradient into the submucosa in a process referred to as the "alkaline tide." The H^+,K^+-ATPase requires the energy derived from ATP.

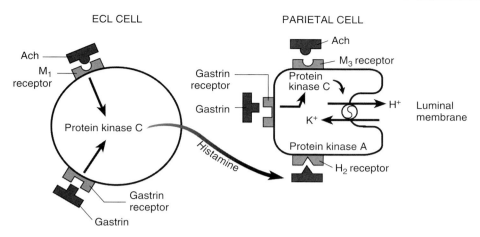

FIGURE 24-3 Proposed mechanism of interactions between the enterochromaffin-like (ECL) cell and the parietal cell, including signal transduction pathways. Following the ingestion of a meal, circulating gastrin has a primary effect on the gastrin/CCKB receptor of the ECL cell, activating protein kinase C and the subsequent release of histamine from the ECL cell that acts on the H_2 receptor of the parietal cell. When this receptor is activated, the parietal cell, through adenylate cyclase, realizes an increase in cAMP, protein kinase A, and the activation of H^+,K^+-ATPase. The effect of gastrin on a human parietal cell is thought to stimulate H^+,K^+-ATPase through activation of inositol triphosphate (IP_3) and protein kinase C. Acetylcholine released by cholinergic neurons near the ECL causes activation of the M_1 receptor on the ECL cell, which results in an increase in protein kinase C on the ECL cell, causing the release of histamine, which acts on the H_2 receptor of the parietal cell. In addition, the direct effect of acetylcholine on the parietal cell acts through the M_3 receptor, activating IP_3, protein kinase C, and H^+,K^+-ATPase. Thus there are endocrine, neurocrine, and paracrine mechanisms involved in postprandial gastric acid secretion.

their terminal ilium are likely to require parenteral vitamin B_{12} administration on a routine basis, to prevent the development of a macrocytic anemia.

Chief Cell Secretion

The chief cell of the gastric fundus synthesizes pepsinogen, of which there are seven isozymes. The chief cell can be stimulated by vasoactive intestinal polypeptide (VIP)/secretin, epinephrine, acetylcholine, and gastrin. Activation by VIP/secretin and epinephrine affects the adenylate cyclase, cAMP, and protein kinase A cytosolic pathway, whereas activation of the acetylcholine muscarinic receptor and the gastrin/CCKB receptor activates the cell through the inositol triphosphate, calcium-dependent protein kinase C pathway. In addition to activation of any of these receptors, acid bathing the lumen also stimulates the release of pepsinogen, which, on entering the acidic milieu of lumen of the stomach, is converted to the active form of the proteolytic enzyme, pepsin.

Antral Gastrin Release

The G cells in the antrum synthesize the peptide gastrin. The 17-amino-acid form is the most abundant and is the primary circulating form of the peptide. Stimulants for the release of gastrin include intraluminal amino acids as well

as di- and tripeptides. The most potent amino acids are aromatic: tryptophane and phenylalanine. Antral distention also causes the release of gastrin into the blood stream through intramural cholinergic mechanisms. During the cephalic phase of acid secretion, stimulated by the senses (sight, smell, and taste), gastrin is released into the systemic circulation through a long neural network involving the vagal nucleus in the thalamus. The neural transmitter for this is gastrin-releasing peptide (GRP), released from the postganglionic neurons terminating on the G cell. There are also D cells in the antrum, in close proximity to the G cells, that contain somatostatin. Somatostatin acts as a paracrine agent to inhibit the release of gastrin, primarily when the antral lumen is acidified, serving as a negative feedback mechanism to inhibit the release of gastrin. There are some data suggesting that the colonization of the antrum by *Helicobacter pylori* is associated with increased rates of acid section in some patients. One of the mechanisms seems to be related to the ability of *H. pylori* to interfere with this negative feedback mechanism, inhibiting the release of somatostatin from the D cell. These patients also have mild hypergastrinemia. In addition to stimulation of acid secretion by its effect on both the parietal cell and the ECL cell, gastrin is trophic to the mucosa. Patients with gastrin-secreting pancreatic or duodenal tumors, called gastrinomas, often have very high rates of acid secretion and hypertrophic gastric mucosa.

Surface Epithelial Cell Secretion

The surface epithelial cells lining both the fundus and the antrum produce mucus and a bicarbonate-rich fluid that is continually secreted into the lumen. Bicarbonate is actively secreted, stimulated by cholinergic agents and intraluminal acidification and inhibited by anticholinergic agents. Mucus is a complex glycoprotein that is secreted in the form of a gel. It has no proton-neutralizing capabilities. This layer of bicarbonate-rich mucus overlying the entire gastric mucosa does possess a pH profile such that, when the luminal fluid pH is 3, the pH at the apical membrane of the surface epithelial cell is much closer to neutral pH. If the pH is lower than 3, however, this gradient dissipates. One of the mechanisms by which nonsteroidal anti-inflammatory compounds have deleterious effects on the gastric mucosa has to do with their ability to inhibit the release of both bicarbonate and mucus from the surface epithelial cell through inhibition of cyclooxygenase.

Phases of Acid Secretion

Acid secretion is divided into four phases; cephalic, gastric, intestinal, and interdigestive. The cephalic phase is stimulated by activation of the senses; smell, taste, and sight. It is centrally mediated through the dorsal complex of the thalamus, resulting in parasympathetic outflow. Release of acetylcholine at the neural-ECL and neural-parietal cell interfaces activates the ECL cells to release histamine and the parietal cells to increase the rate of acid secretion. Neural release of the neurotransmitter GRP results in the release of gastrin from the D cell in the antrum. The cephalic phase represents approximately 30% of the total response to a meal.

The gastric phase of acid secretion represents 50% of the total response to a meal. The stimuli for the gastric phase of acid secretion, when ingested food is in the stomach, are gastric distention and the presence of intraluminal proteins. Not only are there intramural cholinergic reflexes that respond to stretch, causing the activation of both ECL and parietal cells, but also distention causes the release of gastrin. Thus all of these stimulants of acid secretion—paracrine, endocrine, and neurocrine—are activated during this phase of the acid secretory response to a meal. Once food has left the stomach and entered the duodenum and small bowel, a number of mechanisms come into play to shut down the acid secretory mechanism.

The intestinal phase of acid secretion represents only 5% of the total response to a meal. The duodenum does contain G cells that respond to proteins and amino acids by releasing gastrin, primarily the 34-amino-acid peptide. There also are humoral agents, termed *enterogastrones*, that stimulate acid secretion by some unknown mechanism(s).

As food moves down the gastrointestinal tract, the distal small bowel releases a yet to be identified peptide called enterogastrone into the systemic circulation, which inhibits acid secretion. The presence of protein in the stomach actually buffers the protons that have been secreted. Thus the highest concentration of free protons in the stomach usually occurs 2 to 3 hours after a meal, because that is the time when there is still mild activation of the parietal cells but no protein in the stomach to neutralize the free protons. For this reason, if antacids are recommended for a patient with acid-peptic symptoms, they should be taken approximately 2 to 3 hours after a meal. This also accounts for the symptoms found in patients with peptic ulcer disease, in which the epigastric pain is usually worse before a meal and sometimes awakens them at night. Eating often relieves the pain. When the luminal pH of the antrum falls to 4.5 or less, the antral D cells release somatostatin, causing inhibition of gastrin release through a paracrine mechanism, resulting in acid secretory inhibition.

Motor Activity

From a motor standpoint, the stomach has three anatomically contiguous but functionally distinct units. The proximal stomach, or fundus, functions are designed for accommodation and receptor relaxation. The distal portion of the stomach, or gastric antrum, does the grinding and sieving. The pylorus, at the outlet of the stomach, allows for the emptying of particles of food less than or equal to 2 mm in size. The proximum gastric muscular tone has no spontaneous contractions. It serves a reservoir function, and accommodates the intraluminal contents that pulsed retrograde during antral contraction. The tone of the proximal stomach seems to increase after ingestion of a meal. The relaxation of tone is neurogenic and mediated through nonadrenergic inhibitory nerves whose cell bodies lie in the myenteric plexus. These nerves are stimulated in response to gastric distention.

The antral musculature exhibits rhythmic peristalsis at the rate of approximately 3 waves per minute. There is a gastric pacesetter, located on the greater curvature of the stomach, that generates these slow-wave contractions, which accelerate and thicken as they move toward the pylorus. This peristaltic activity in the antrum, with retropulsion of ingested food, and the activity of free protons and pepsin allows the food to be broken down into particles less than or equal to 2 mm, a process referred to as sieving. The pylorus controls the release of intraluminal contents into the duodenum, and it is rare for particles greater than 2 mm in size to transit the pylorus. The antral-pyloric mechanism tightly controls the size of the particles that leave the stomach (Fig. 24–4).

Gastric emptying can be inhibited by neural and hormonal mechanisms related to the activation of

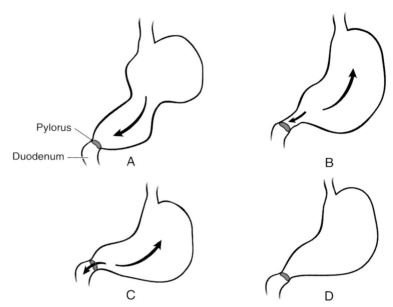

FIGURE 24-4 A, Gastric peristaltic contractions begin in the midregion of the stomach, forcing the movement of intragastric contents toward the duodenum. **B,** As the peristaltic wave moves toward the pylorus, small particles (≤2 mm) pass through the pylorus, whereas larger particulate intragastric contents are retropulsed back into the body of the stomach, where receptor relaxation accommodates them. **C,** When contraction force of velocity causes near-complete closure of the gastric antrum, small particles (≤2 mm) again pass through the pylorus, and the remainder of the gastric contents are retropulsed into the gastric body. **D,** Between contractions, there is no evidence of movement of the gastric contents.

chemoreceptors in the duodenum by protons, fats, and changes in osmolarity. Acid bathing the duodenum causes the release of secretin, fats bathing the duodenum cause the release of cholecystokinin (CCK), and gastrointestinal polypeptide and hypertonic solutions cause the release of an as yet unidentified hormone, all of which cause a decrease in gastric emptying.

Approximately 4 to 6 hours after a meal, the motility pattern changes from no contractions to very strong contractions; this has been termed the migrating myoelectric complex (MMC). There are three phases of the MMC: phase I is associated with no contractions, lasting about 70 minutes; phase II is associated with contractions every 5 minutes, lasting about 10 to 20 minutes; and phase III is associated with contractions every 1 to 5 minutes, lasting about 10 to 20 minutes. The MMC effectively evacuates the stomach and small intestine into the colon and may play a role in proximal flow of colonic bacteria.

Clinical disorders may be associated with gastric motor dysfunction, such as pyloric stenosis, as a result of long-standing peptic ulcer disease. Patients with long-standing diabetes can develop a neuropathy producing gastroparesis that can be diagnosed by doing an electrogastrogram, allowing the gastroenterologist to determine whether there is an abnormality of the gastric pacing system.

Small Intestine and Colon

Digestion and Absorption

Digestion refers to the process by which ingested foodstuffs are cleaved into smaller particles, catalyzed by enzymes on the luminal surface of the small intestine. As a result of the digestion, ingested foodstuffs are converted to absorbable forms of carbohydrates, proteins, and fat. *Absorption* refers to the process by which molecules are transported into epithelial cells that line the small bowel, referred to as enterocytes, from which the molecules enter the portal venous circulation or lymphatic drainage system. Absorption occurs as a result of concentration gradients and the large surface area of the small bowel, as defined by Fick's first law of diffusion. The absorbing surface of the small bowel is over 200 m² as a result of folds, villi, and microvilli. Absorption can occur either actively or passively. The active form is transcellular, carrier mediated, and energy dependent. Passive absorption can occur through the tight junctions between cells, a process referred to as paracellular diffusion. Passive diffusion also can occur transcellularly by diffusion, concentration gradient, or convection.

Digestion and absorption of carbohydrates

Amylopectin is a very-high-molecular-weight branched-chain molecule of glucose. The linear changes are 1,4α, linkages and the branch points are 1,6α linkages. The majority of dietary plant starch consists of amylopectin. Amylose makes up the remainder of dietary plant starch, and its composition is similar to amylopectin, but its molecular weight is usually less than 100,000, compared to that of amylopectin, which is greater than 1 million. Cellulose is a 1,4β-linked glucose polymer. Humans do not have appropriate enzymes to hydrolyze these linkages. Glycogen is a glucose polymer like amylopectin but with more branching, and is the form of stored starch in humans. Sucrose is a disaccharide composed of glucose and fructose, while lactose is composed of galactose and glucose.

Animal and plant starches are broken down by salivary and pancreatic amylase. The breakdown products include dextrins and maltoligosaccharides (maltase and maltotriose). Pancreatic amylase is released from the stimulated pancreas, as a result of both neural and humoral mechanisms, and enters the gastrointestinal tract in the duodenum, through the papillae of Vater. Further digestion of oligosaccharides is accomplished by intestinal brush border–bound enzymes in the duodenum and jejunum: α-dextranase, which breaks down the 1,6α linkages; glucoamylase, which breaks down the maltoligosaccharides; lactase, which breaks down lactose into its constituents, galactose and glucose; and sucrase, which breaks down sucrose into its components, fructose and glucose.

The absorption of carbohydrates occurs primarily in the duodenum and proximal jejunum. The only dietary sugars that are well absorbed are glucose, galactose, and fructose. Glucose and galactose are transported by the same carrier-mediated mechanism, requiring a Na$^+$-dependent symport (SLGT-1) that simultaneously moves sodium with galactose or glucose into the enterocyte, across its apical membrane. The sodium then leaves the cytosol and moves into the interstitial space between the enterocytes as a result of the energy derived from Na$^+$,K$^+$-ATPase. Glucose and galactose exit the cytosol on the nutrient side of the cell, presumably by another carrier-mediated mechanism employing the GLUT-2 transporter. These sugars then diffuse into capillaries, where they enter the blood stream, moving down a concentration gradient. Fructose does not compete with glucose and galactose for the same transporter and does not require sodium to be transported across the apical membrane into the enterocyte. The fructose transporter referred to as GLUT-5 is carrier mediated. This transporter of fructose is not energy requiring, and therefore transport of fructose is considered to occur by facilitated diffusion. Fructose also exits the cell on the interstitial membrane of the enterocyte, using the GLUT-2 transporter as well (Fig. 24–5).

Digestion and absorption of proteins

Approximately 0.5 to 0.8 g of protein per day per kilogram of body weight is required to maintain nitrogen homeostasis. The gastrointestinal tract digests 10 to 30 g of protein per day that are secreted into the lumen, as well as mucus, desquamated cells, and secreted enzymes. Approximately 50% of protein entering the gastrointestinal tract is dietary, 25% is derived from digestive juices, and 25% from desquamated cells. Nearly all of this protein is digested and absorbed.

The digestion of proteins begins in the stomach when pepsinogen, released from the chief cell, is converted to the active form of the enzyme (pepsin) by protons and pepsin in the lumen of the stomach. Pepsin cleaves peptides primarily at aromatic amino acids. The majority of the digestion of proteins occurs in the small bowel. The pancreas produces proenzymes designed to digest proteins and fats. These proenzymes are activated by the active form of the enzyme in the lumen and by interaction with enterokinase, an enzyme found on the brush border of the proximal small bowel enterocytes. For example, trypsinogen is activated to trypsin, chymotrypsinogen is activated to chymotrypsin, proelastase is activated to elastase, procarboxypeptidase A is converted to carboxypeptidase A, and procarboxypeptidase B is converted to carboxypeptidase B. Insoluble exopeptidases that include aminopeptidases and carboxypeptidases are also found in the brush border of enterocytes.

The final product of digestion of protein is primarily di- and tripeptides and individual amino acids. The rate of absorption of di- and tripeptides exceeds that of amino acids. There appears to be a single peptide carrier present on the apical membrane of the enterocyte that has a higher affinity for di- and tripeptides than for larger peptides. Transport of di- and tripeptides is sodium dependent and requires active transport of sodium into the intracellular space, as a result of a Na$^+$,K$^+$-ATPase. Some amino acids in the lumen of the small bowel move through the tight junctions and into capillaries by simple diffusion.

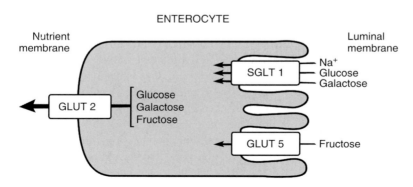

ENTEROCYTE

Nutrient membrane

Luminal membrane

SGLT 1 — Na$^+$ / Glucose / Galactose

GLUT 2 — Glucose / Galactose / Fructose

GLUT 5 — Fructose

FIGURE 24–5 Absorption of glucose, galactose, and fructose occurs on the luminal membrane of the enterocyte. Glucose and galactose enter the epithelial cell against the concentration gradient using the SGLT-1 transport protein. The sodium gradient provides energy for monosaccharide entry. Facilitated transport of fructose across the brush border membrane is mediated through the GLUT-5 transporter. All three sugars leave the cytoplasm of the enterocyte by facilitated transport via a common transporter, GLUT-2.

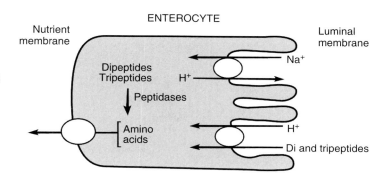

FIGURE 24–6 Protein in the form of dipeptides and tripeptides is taken up across the luminal membrane of the enterocyte by a single H^+-powered secondary active transport protein. The proton gradient is created by Na^+, H^+ exchangers in the brush border membrane. Peptidases break down the dipeptides and tripeptides into amino acids, which then leave the cytosol through the nutrient basolateral membrane by facilitated transport.

There are some specific transporters on the apical membrane of the enterocyte for the transport of amino acids into the cytosol of the enterocyte, from which they are transported across the nutrient membrane by a different type of transporter. There are specific transporters that have preferred substrates, such as neutral amino acids, basic amino acids, imino acids, acidic amino acids, and β-amino acids. There are also different transporters on the basolateral membrane of the enterocyte that have preference for these types of amino acids (Fig. 24–6).

Digestion and absorption of fats

The primary form of ingested fat is the triglyceride. The length of saturation of fatty acids on the triglyceride determines whether it is liquid or solid. Other than triglycerides, phospholipids, sterol esters, the fat-soluble vitamins (D, E, and K), cholesterol, and fatty acid esters are also ingested. Lingual lipase begins the process of fat digestion. There is also a gastric lipase that further breaks down lipids; however, the majority of lipids are broken down in the small bowel. The primary pancreatic enzymes required are a lipase that cleaves 1- and 3-fatty acid groups, leaving the 2-monoglyceride, and a lipase that digests triglycerides, found in fat droplets. Cholesterol esterase cleaves fatty acids of sterol esters, and phospholipase A_2 cleaves the ester bond at the 2 position of glycerophosphate. These enzymes, too, are secreted from the pancreas. Because the luminal contents are primarily an aqueous medium, the solubility of fats requires that micelles be formed to emulsify bile salts, phospholipids, and cholesterol. These cylindrical micelles allow for the solubility of the lipid moieties as emulsified lipids rather than large fat droplets. Lipids are delivered to the enterocyte by the micelles.

Because the apical membrane of the enterocyte is composed of lipids, it does not pose a significant barrier to the movement of lipids from the micelles into the cytosol. There is no known specific transport mechanism for uncharged lipids to cross this membrane. Triglycerides are digested by lipases into monoglycerides and fatty acids, which diffuse from micelles across the apical membrane

into the enterocyte cytosol, where they are resynthesized into triglycerides. Cholesterol and cholesterol esters are hydrolyzed to cholesterol and fatty acids. How cholesterol is transported into the enterocyte cytosol is not well understood. Long-chain fatty acids may be transported by a Na^+-dependent symport. Short-chain (C2 to C6) and medium-chain (C8 to C12) fatty acids are more water soluble and do not require the presence of micelles for absorption. This is why many enteral feeding supplements contain short- and medium-chain fatty acids.

The fat-soluble vitamins require micelles for solubilization and absorption into the enterocyte. Vitamin A is ingested as keratin, that is, two molecules of retinol. Retinol is absorbed by diffusion from the mixed micelle, re-esterified in the enterocyte cytosol, and packaged into chylomicrons for transport across the basolateral membrane and into the lymphatics. Vitamin E absorption also requires the presence of micelles and is handled by the enterocyte in fashion similar to that for vitamin A. Vitamin K requires micellar solubilization and is absorbed by diffusion. Vitamin D is also absorbed into the enterocyte cytosol; however, it is packaged into chylomicrons without being esterified.

In the enterocyte, these fats are resynthesized as triglyceride droplets and are coated with a stabilizing layer of polar lipids, resulting in the formation of a chylomicron. The actual exocytosis of chylomicrons occurs across the basolateral membrane of the enterocyte, where they enter central lacteals of the villus. From there, they pass into larger lymphatic channels draining the intestine, into the thoracic duct, and finally into the left subclavian vein (Fig. 24–7).

Patients with pancreatic insufficiency may have difficulty digesting any of these primary foodstuffs. Steatorrhea occurs when fats are not appropriately broken down and absorbed. Bile acid deficiency caused by hepatic dysfunction or extrahepatic biliary obstruction may also result in steatorrhea.

Absorption of water and salts

Nearly 99% of the water ingested into the gastrointestinal tract is absorbed. *Efflux* refers to the movement of water

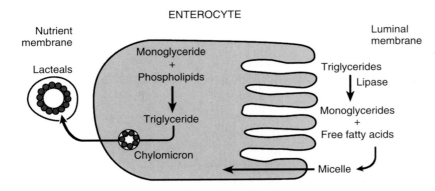

FIGURE 24–7 In the enteric lumen, triglycerides are broken down by lipase into monoglycerides and free fatty acids. These are presented to the luminal membrane of the enterocyte in micelles. Within the enterocytes, triglycerides are reformed by the synthesis of monoglycerides and phospholipids. They are packaged into chylomicrons and leave the cytosol by exocytosis through the nutrient membrane, whereupon they are taken up by lymphatics called lacteals.

and ions from the lumen into the blood, and *influx* refers to the movement of water and ions from the blood to the lumen. Secretion occurs when influx predominates, and absorption occurs when efflux predominates. Sodium is absorbed along the entire length of the intestine. Sodium crosses the brush border membrane, moves down an electrochemical gradient, and is actively extruded by the basolateral membrane of the enterocyte, requiring the presence of a Na^+,K^+-ATPase. Because the luminal contents of the small bowel and the blood have similar sodium concentrations, sodium absorption is normally not diffusional but rather active by a transcellular route. The presence of glucose, galactose, small peptides, neutral amino acids, and imino acids in the lumen enhances the absorption of sodium, particularly in the jejunum.

Given the ingestion of approximately 2 L of water per day and the production of nearly 7 L of saliva, gastric juice, bile, pancreatic juice, and intestinal secretions, combined with the fact that only about 100 mL of water is found in the stool, there is a huge absorption of water volume throughout the gastrointestinal tract. The majority of water absorption occurs in the small bowel and the colon. Transmucosal water movement occurs via the paracellular pathway by a mechanism referred to as the "standing gradient osmosis." There is a Na^+,K^+-ATPase that mediates the transport of sodium into the lateral intracellular space. Chloride enters this same space by flow from the lumen through tight junctions or by facilitated transport from adjacent epithelial cells. This creates a hypertonic solution of sodium chloride near the luminal portion of the lateral intracellular space. Water then flows by osmosis into the lateral intracellular spaces, raising hydrostatic pressure. This hydrostatic flow of water and ions down the lateral intracellular space and across the epithelial basement membrane allows the water to enter the blood stream.

Calcium ions are actively absorbed throughout the small intestine, but particularly in the duodenum and proximal jejunum. Calcium is absorbed as a divalent ion, and its absorption is stimulated by vitamin D. Calcium moves down an electrochemical gradient across the apical membrane. An intestinal brush border membrane protein, IMCal, may be the transporter for calcium. There also are thought to be calcium channels through which calcium moves down a concentration gradient from lumen to enterocyte cytosol. In the cytosol, calcium is chelated by calbindin, which binds two calcium ions per calbindin molecule. Calbindin prevents precipitation with cytosolic anions that would form insoluble calcium salts and prevents appropriate activation of calcium-sensitive enzymes. Calbindin transports calcium from the apical membrane to the basolateral membrane, where it is then transported out the cytosol in exchange for sodium as well as by a specific Ca^{2+}-ATPase. Vitamin D is essential for the absorption of calcium because it stimulates each phase of calcium transport by the epithelial cells. Vitamin D_3 also induces the synthesis of calbindin and increases the level of Ca^{2+}-ATPase activity on the nutrient membrane (Fig. 24–8).

Absorption of iron

Although normal iron intake is 15 to 20 mg/day, only about 0.5 to 1 mg is absorbed. Iron absorption occurs primarily in the duodenum and proximal jejunum. Dietary iron is in the ferric (Fe^{3+}) form as a water-insoluble salt, when combined with phosphate, hydroxide, or bicarbonate. In the gastric lumen, Fe^{3+} is solubilized by protons and reduced by ascorbate to the ferrous (Fe^{2+}) form, which is much less likely to form insoluble complexes. Heme iron is relatively well absorbed, because proteolytic enzymes release heme from proteins that is then taken into the enterocyte by facilitated diffusion. In the enterocyte, heme is split from iron, a process requiring the enzyme xanthine oxidase. Ferrous ions in the cytosol are bound to transferrin and transported in the cytosol to the basolateral plasma membrane, where they bind to transferrin receptors on the basolateral membrane. Ferritin in the cytosol prevents excess absorption of iron by irreversibly binding iron. It remains in this form until the enterocyte is desquamated. Ferritin-bound iron is then excreted in the stool. Patients with iron deficiency anemia respond with

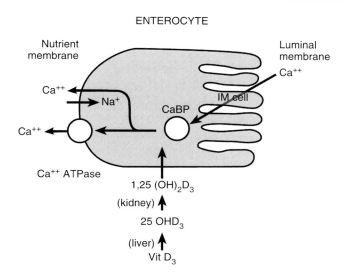

ENTEROCYTE

FIGURE 24–8 Calcium crosses the luminal membrane through calcium channels. A membrane-bound calcium-binding protein, calbindin (CAL), may assist in this process. In the cytosol, calcium is bound to calbindin and leaves the cytosol at the basolateral membrane by an active transport mechanism requiring a calcium-dependent ATPase. Some calcium also leaves the cytosol across the basolateral membrane in exchange for sodium.

an increase in iron absorption. Iron deficiency anemia is reflected in microcytic and hypochromic indices.

Absorption of vitamin B_{12}

Vitamin B_{12} is required for the maturation of red blood cells. Ingested vitamin B_{12} is bound to intrinsic factor, a product of the gastric parietal cells, and other cobalamin-binding glycoproteins present in saliva and gastric secretions. Intrinsic factor binds vitamin B_{12} with a lower affinity than the other proteins; thus, in the gastric lumen, most of the vitamin B_{12} present in food is bound to other proteins. Intrinsic factor secretion parallels vitamin B_{12} intake and need. Vitamin B_{12} and intrinsic factor form a complex (a dimer of intrinsic factor and two vitamin B_{12} molecules) that is resistant to proteases throughout the gastrointestinal tract. In the terminal ilium, the vitamin B_{12}–intrinsic factor dimer is recognized by a brush border receptor that does not recognize intrinsic factor alone. The binding of the vitamin B_{12}–intrinsic factor complex to this receptor is followed by active transport of vitamin B_{12} across the luminal membrane of the terminal ileal enterocytes. Intrinsic factor is probably not transported into the cytosol. How vitamin B_{12} is transported through the enterocyte cytosol is not well understood. When the vitamin B_{12} is transported across the nutrient membrane, however, it binds to a globin known as transcobalamin II, which is synthesized by the liver, and the complex enters the portal venous circulation.

Patients who have pernicious anemia, have had significant gastric or terminal ileal resections, or are on a strong

antisecretory medication may develop megaloblastic anemia because of inadequate intrinsic factor synthesis and secretion. These patients require the administration of parenteral vitamin B_{12} to ensure normal red cell maturation.

Small Intestinal Motility

The small intestine contains both circular and longitudinal smooth muscle. The muscularis mucosa is thin and gives off small bundles that extend into the villi. The myenteric plexus of the submucosa has regularly spaced ganglia and prominent secondary and tertiary plexuses. The ganglia lie on two planes, one closer to the mucosa and the other closer to the circular muscle. This neural network that produces peristaltic and segmentation motility is referred to as the enteric nervous system. The movements of the small intestine are important to mix chyme with digestive secretions, allowing the various nutrients to come into contact with the absorptive surface of the small intestine. Intestinal smooth muscle contraction is rhythmic, with contraction of the circular muscle beginning at any point and moving caudad over variable distances at velocities up to 3 cm/sec. Longitudinal muscles also take part in this motor activity, known as propulsive peristalsis. Segmentation is the most frequent type of movement, in which tonic contraction of rings of circular muscle develop at uniform distances. Rhythmic contractions occur at a rate of approximately 12 per minute in the duodenum, 9 per minute in the jejunum, and 7 per minute in the ileum. These rhythmic contractions are controlled by slow waves from the gastric antrum.

In general, ingested food traverses the small intestine within 2 to 4 hours, ultimately arriving at the terminal ileum and passing through the ileocecal valve into the colon. The ileocecal valve, when competent, prevents colonic bacteria from refluxing into the ileum. Relaxation or contraction of the ileocecal center is coordinated primarily by neurons of the interneural plexus. Distention and peristalsis in the terminal ileum trigger the ileocecal valve to relax so that chyme is allowed to enter the cecum.

Colonic Motility

The colon receives between 500 and 1500 mL of chyme from the ileum per day. It absorbs water to the point that daily feces contain only 50 to 100 mL of water. Colonic contractions mix the chyme and circulate it across the mucosal absorbing surface. Localized segmental contractions divide the colon into neighboring ovoid segments called haustra. There is some anatomic thickening of the circular smooth muscle that is a component of the haustra. Antipropulsive movements occur primarily in the right colon, where the peristalsis moves from the hepatic flexure toward the cecum. These movements help retain chyme in the proximal colon to facilitate water absorption. The remainder of the colon exhibits rhythmic contraction that moves the chyme short distances caudad. From time to time the proximal and midportion of the colon contract simultaneously, referred to as mass movements. When this occurs, the chyme moves within the colon both cephalad and caudad. This allows the chyme to come into contact with more of the absorbing surface.

Pancreatic Exocrine Secretion

The exocrine function of the pancreas represents the secretion of proteins or proenzymes required for the digestion of carbohydrates, proteins, and fats as well as the secretion of bicarbonate, causing the duodenal luminal fluid to have a pH near 8.0, which, for most of the activated enzymes, is the optimum pH for their activity (Fig. 24–9). Anatomically, there are pancreatic lobules that contain clusters of acini. Protein secretion is a product of the acinar cell. Bicarbonate and water secretion is a product of the centroacinar or duct cell. The secreted protein and fluid move through the intercalated ducts into the interlobar ducts, terminating in the main pacreatic duct, from which they enter the duodenum along with biliary secretion through the papillae of Vater. The proteolytic, amylolytic, lipolytic, and mucolytic enzymes are secreted from the pancreas as proenzymes. They are activated in the lumen, duodenum, and jejunum by the active form of the enzyme itself as well by enterokinase, a component of the brush border membrane of the duodenal and jejunal enterocytes. Enzymes or proteins are secretory products of the acinar cell.

The volume of pancreatic secretion approaches 1 L/day. The primary anions are bicarbonate and chloride, whereas the primary cations are sodium and potassium. Pancreatic juice is isotonic with plasma at all rates of

secretion, because water is able to move freely across the duct epithelium. As the rates of secretion increase, however, there is an exponential increase in bicarbonate concentration with a reciprocal decrease in chloride concentration. This allows the pH of the fluid, at high rates of secretion, to be approximately 8 to 8.2. Water and bicarbonate are secretory products of the centroacinar cells that line the proximal pancreatic ducts.

The acinar cell has receptors for several secretagogue agonists: acetylcholine, gastrin, CCKB, substance P, and secretin/VIP (Fig. 24–10). Occupation of receptors for gastrin/CCKB, acetylcholine, and substance P activate the inositol triphosphate, protein kinase C pathway, resulting in an increase in enzyme formation, packaging, and exocytosis from the acinar cell into the lumen. In contrast, occupation of the secretin/VIP receptor is associated with increases in membrane-bound adenylate cyclase activity, activation of protein kinase A and cytosolic cAMP, and stimulation of protein synthesis, packaging, and exocytosis into the lumen. Thus the acinar cell can release its proenzymes as a result of both neural and humoral activation.

The cellular mechanism associated with bicarbonate and water production from the centroacinar cells lining the proximal pancreatic ducts is thought to be related to the availability of chloride within the lumen of the duct. Carbon dioxide that has diffused into the centroacinar cell is hydrated to H_2CO_3 and catalyzed by carbonic anhydrase to dissociate into H^+ and HCO_3^-. The H^+ is extruded across the basal lateral membrane in exchange for potassium. The bicarbonate moiety is then secreted into the lumen in exchange for chloride. The rate of bicarbonate secretion is directly related to the luminal chloride concentration, which is dependent upon opening of a calcium channel that is cAMP dependent, representing the cystic fibrosis transmembrane conducting regulator. Hence patients with cystic fibrosis do not have aqueous pancreatic exocrine

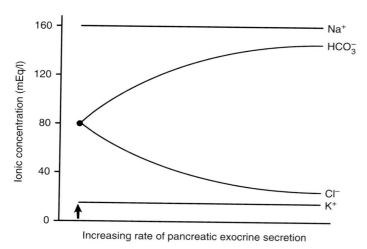

FIGURE 24–9 With increasing rates of pancreatic protein and bicarbonate secretion, the composition of the duodenal luminal fluid changes. An exponential fall in [Cl⁻] and a similar exponential rise in bicarbonate yields a secretory product with a pH greater than 8.0.

ACINAR CELL OF PANCREAS

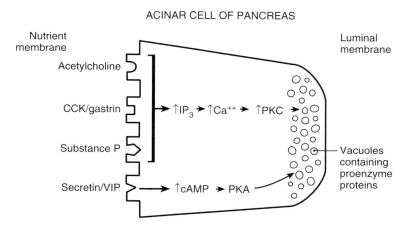

FIGURE 24–10 The pacreatic acinar cell has receptors for acetylcholine, gastrin/CCKB, substance P, and secretin (VIP). Activation of the secretin/VIP receptor results in an increase in membrane-bound adenylate cyclase, cytosolic cAMP, and protein kinase A, causing the vacuoles containing the proenzymes to be released into the secretory ducts by exocytosis. Activation of the acetylcholine receptor, the CCK/gastrin receptor, or the substance P receptor results in a cytosolic increase in inositol triphosphate, cytosolic [Ca^{2+}], and protein kinase C, which also stimulates the exocytosis of prepackaged proenzymes in the vacuoles.

secretion because of the defect in this chloride channel resulting from a mutation in the gene that encodes it (Fig. 24–11).

Secretin

Secretin is the hormone that is the primary stimulant of bicarbonate and water secretion from the centroacinar cells lining the proximal pancreatic ducts. The secretin family of peptides includes VIP, gastric inhibitory polypeptide, glucagon, and enterogon. Secretin is a 27-amino-acid peptide, and the entire molecule is required for full biologic activity. Secretin is synthesized by the S cell in the duodenum and jejunum. The primary stimulant of the release of secretin is a luminal pH of 4.5 or less. Circulating secretin stimulates bicarbonate-rich fluid from the centroacinar cells of the pancreas and from Brunner's glands in the duodenum.

Cholecystokinin

Cholecystokinin is the hormone that is the primary stimulant of protein secretion from the acinar cell. It is in

the gastrin/CCKB family of peptides. The predominant circulating forms of CCK are the octapeptide (CCK8) and CCK33. Cholecystokinin is synthesized in the I cells of the duodenum and jejunum. The primary stimulant of CCK release is the presence of interluminal proteins, particularly aromatic amino acids, and intraluminal fats. The biologic action of circulating CCK is primarily to activate the acinar cells to synthesize and release proenzymes. In addition, it has a strong contractile effect on the smooth muscles of the gallbladder and causes the sphincter of Oddi to relax, allowing bile stored in the gallbladder to flow down the biliary tract to enter the duodenal lumen through the papillae of Vater.

Following a meal, as gastric emptying occurs, acid will cause the S cell to release secretin, which then circulates in the vascular system, causing the centroacinar cells to release bicarbonate and water. Similarly, when proteins and fats enter the duodenum, they activate the I cell to release CCK. Circulating CCK has a direct effect on the acinar cell, stimulating it to synthesize and release proteins or prohormones. There also are cholinergic neural pathways between the duodenum and acinar and centroacinar cells that respond to stretch. As the duodenal wall is

CENTROACINAR CELL OF PANCREAS

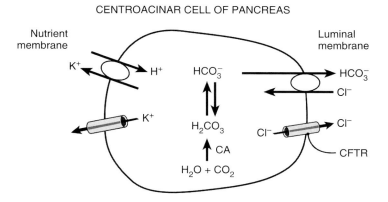

FIGURE 24–11 Proposed mechanism of bicarbonate secretion into the secretory ducts by the centroacinar cells. In the cytosol, dissociation of carbonic acid leaves a free proton and free bicarbonate anion. The proton is actively transported across the nutrient membrane in exchange for potassium. There is also a nutrient membrane potassium channel. On the secretory surface, the bicarbonate enters the lumen in exchange for chloride. The chloride available within the lumen is dependent upon the chloride channel on the luminal or apical membrane, which is the cystic fibrosis transmembrane conducting regulator (CFTR).

distended by the intraluminal contents, cholinergic nerves are activated that also have direct effects on both the acinar and centroacinar cells. Thus, following a meal, full protein and bicarbonate secretion response to a meal occurs by both neural and humoral mechanisms.

Biliary Secretion

Anatomically, the biliary tree consists of bile canaliculi within the liver, hepatic ducts, the common hepatic duct, the cystic duct and gallbladder, the common bile duct, and the sphincter of Oddi. Lobules of the hepatocytes are the source of hepatic bile secretion. Blood flow to the hepatocytes comes from branches of both the portal vein and the hepatic artery. Blood from the portal vein flows through sinusoids past the hepatocyte to the central vein, where it drains into the hepatic veins and inferior vena cava. Only one layer of hepatocytes separates the sinusoids. Kupffer's cells are anchored to the sinusoidal epithelium. The microscopic architecture of the liver shows portal triads consisting of bile ducts, branches of the hepatic artery, and branches of the portal vein.

Bile is a solution of both organic and inorganic compounds. The electrolyte composition of bile is similar to that of plasma with the exception of the bicarbonate concentration, which is twice as high in bile as it is in plasma. The hepatocyte secretes two primary bile acids, cholic acid and chenodeoxycholic acid. These are synthesized in the hepatocyte from cholesterol and recycled through the enterohepatic circulation to conserve bile salts. Primary bile acids, when in the lower gastrointestinal tract, are converted to secondary bile acids (deoxycholic acid and lithocholic acid) by 7α-dehydroxylation when in contact with bacteria. In order to make bile salts more soluble, they are conjugated with either glycine or taurine in the cytosol of the hepatocyte before being secreted.

The primary purpose of secretion of bile acids is to allow for the formation of micelles, as noted in the earlier section Digestion and Absorption of Fats. Micelles are cylindrical moieties that contain bile acids, phospholipids, and cholesterol. All of these compounds are amphipathic, because they have both hydrophilic and hydrophobic aspects to their structure. As the micelles are formed, bile acids form the outer layer and their hydrophilic portions are oriented toward the aqueous environment. Phospholipids are also positioned within the micelle so that their hydrophilic portions are oriented to the aqueous medium. Cholesterol, too, is oriented in the center of the micelle so that it will be more soluble in the aqueous medium. The emulsions then move down the gastrointestinal tract and allow lipids that are ingested to freely move in and out of the micelles so that they can be presented to the enterocytes for absorption (Fig. 24–12).

The primary pigment of bile, which gives it its yellow color, is bilirubin. Bilirubin is derived from the degradation of hemoglobin in the reticuloendothelial system. Because bilirubin itself is not soluble in an aqueous medium, it is conjugated primarily with glucuronide and occasionally with sulfate. Circulating bilirubin is bound to albumen, from which it dissociates at the hepatocyte on the portal venous membrane. Bilirubin is conjugated in the cytosol of the hepatocytes, primarily catalyzed by glucuronosyl-transferase. It enters the bile canaliculus as bilirubin diglucuronide. In this way, the body removes the breakdown products of red blood cells. Bilirubin is also the pigment that gives stool its color.

Patients who have had hepatocellular dysfunction may become hyperbilirubinemic, primarily with unconjugated or indirect bilirubin. In contrast, when there is extrahepatic biliary obstruction, the hyperbilirubinemia is caused by excessive circulating conjugated or direct bilirubin. Both may be associated with tea-colored urine and

MICELLE COMPOSITION

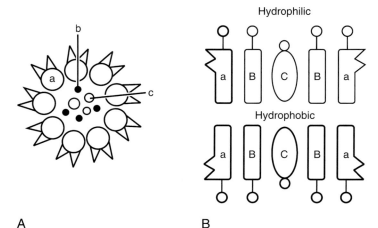

A   B

FIGURE 24–12 The cylindrical micelle is depicted, viewed from the top (**A**) and from the side (**B**). The hydrophilic portions of bile acids, phospholipids, and cholesterol are exposed to the aqueous solution, which is the primary component of bile, whereas the hydrophobic portions of bile acids, phospholipids, and cholesterol are found within the center of the micelle. Lipids freely move in and out of the micelle, which allows ingested fats to be emulsified and delivered to the enterocytes for absorption.

clay-colored stools, related to an excess of urobilinogen entering the urine and a paucity of bilirubin in the stool. Fractionating the bilirubin in this way may allow for the distinction between hepatocellular dysfunction and extrahepatic obstruction as the cause of hyperbilirubinemia.

The primary component of bile, the bile acids, are synthesized or reused by the hepatocytes as they are presented as conjugated and unconjugated bile acids from the portal circulation. The liver produces approximately 500 to 1000 mL of bile per day. Most of the bile acids secreted by the hepatocyte are recirculated through the enterohepatic circulation. The bile acids in the small intestine are passively absorbed throughout its entire length, and those in the terminal ileum are actively absorbed. These bile acids are then presented to the hepatocyte through the portal circulation, where they are taken up by an active cotransport mechanism that requires sodium. The unconjugated bile acids are then conjugated with glycine or taurine in the cytosol of the hepatocyte and attached to a specific bile acid–binding protein that moves them from the sinusoidal membrane to the secretory membrane. On the secretory or canalicular membrane of the hepatocyte, there is a specific ATP-dependent bile acid transporter that moves the conjugated bile acids from the cytosol into the lumen of the bile canaliculus. Water and electrolytes enter the canalicular bile by diffusion through the transcellular route. The liver also synthesizes cholesterol and phospholipids. They are transported across the canalicular membrane into the lumen of the bile canaliculus as a nonmicellar vesicle. When all three components enter the canaliculus, micelles are formed (Fig. 24–13). Thus the final product is a yellow fluid that contains micelles consisting of bile acids, phospholipids, and cholesterol. These flow down the biliary tree and join with the secretions from the pancreas before entering the duodenum through the sphincter of Oddi. Together, hepatic and pancreatic exocrine secretion allows for the breakdown of carbohydrates, proteins, and fats. The micelles allow intraluminal fats to emulsify. Thus all three nutrients can then be presented to the enterocytes along the small intestine for absorption.

Hepatic Metabolism

The liver synthesizes proteins, stores vitamins and iron, degrades hormones, and inactivates or excretes certain drugs and toxins. Carbohydrate, lipid, and protein metabolism is regulated by the liver. Skeletal muscle and liver are the two primary sites of glycogen storage in the body. When serum glucose levels are high, there is conversion of glucose to glycogen, which is deposited within the liver. As blood glucose levels fall, glycogen is then broken down to glucose by a process called glycogenolysis. Thus the liver is key to the relatively constant level of circulating glucose in the blood. The liver also has the capability of converting amino acids, lipids, and simple carbohydrates into glucose by a process known as gluconeogenesis. This carbohydrate metabolism is regulated by insulin and glucagon. The liver is also involved in lipid metabolism. Many of the absorbed lipids leave the

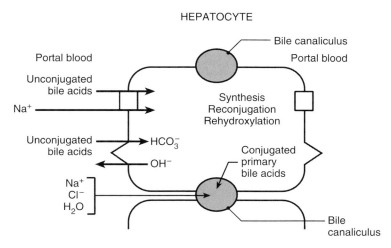

FIGURE 24–13 Unconjugated bile acids are presented to the hepatocyte through the sinusoidal capillaries of the portal venous system after they have been absorbed in the jejunum or actively transformed in the terminal ileum. Conjugated bile acids are taken up by the hepatocyte with sodium, by a mechanism of facilitated diffusion. Unconjugated bile acids are taken up in exchange for bicarbonate or hydroxyl anions. Within the cytosol, the unconjugated bile acids are conjugated. Conjugated bile acids are transported to the secretory membrane by specific transport-binding proteins. Secondary bile acids are converted to primary bile acids by rehydroxylation. The conjugated bile acids are then transported across the secretory membrane into the bile canaliculus by a yet to be described mechanism. Water, Na^+, and Cl^- move down a concentration gradient from the portal venous blood through a paracellular pathway into the bile canaliculus.

GALLBLADDER EPITHELIAL CELLS

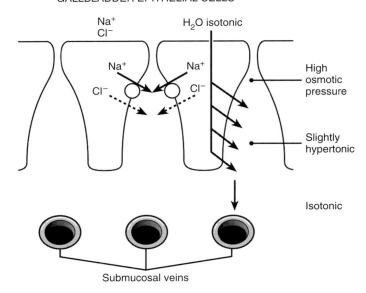

FIGURE 24–14 Water is constantly being removed from the gallbladder luminal fluid because of a standing osmotic gradient within the lateral intracellular space between the epithelial cells. There is active Na$^+$ transport across the apical portion of the basolateral membrane that continually pumps sodium and chloride into the lateral intracellular space. The apical portion of the lateral intracellular space is hypertonic, and there is a gradient toward the basal membrane. Water then flows into the lateral intracellular space, transcellularly, down a concentration gradient and into the submucosa, where it is removed by venous drainage.

enterocytes in the form of chylomicrons that are taken out by the lacteals and lymphatic channels, traveling through the cisterna chyli and the thoracic duct and into the left subclavian vein. Lipoprotein lipase is found on the surface of the endothelial cells of blood vessels, causing the hydrolysis of triglycerides into chylomicrons, releasing glycerol and fatty acids. Adipocytes take up cholesterol and fatty acids, leaving chylomicron remnants that are rich in cholesterol. These remnants are taken up by the hepatocytes and degraded. The hepatocytes also synthesize very-low-density lipoproteins, which are then converted to high-density and low-density lipoproteins. These lipoproteins are the major source of circulating cholesterol and triglycerides. Hepatocytes play a major role in lipid metabolism, being the primary source of cholesterol in the body and forming bile, which is the only route of excretion for cholesterol, thus regulating the serum cholesterol level.

Gallbladder

The gallbladder functions primarily as a reservoir for secreted bile during the interdigestive period. Not only does it store bile, but also it concentrates bile. The concentrating ability of the gallbladder is based on the presence of active sodium transport at the basolateral membrane, which is active continually, causing a standing osmotic gradient in the lateral intercellular space, with the portion closest to the lumen being hypertonic. Thus water moves both trans- and paracellularly down a concentration gradient, leaving the lumen and entering the interstitial fluid and blood stream (Fig. 24–14). Following a meal, the primary

humoral mechanism causing gallbladder contraction is circulating CCK from the S cells of the duodenum and proximal jejunum, as discussed earlier. Cholecystokinin has a direct effect on the gallbladder smooth muscle cells, causing them to contract while simultaneously causing relaxation of the sphincter of Oddi. This allows the gallbladder to empty its contents into the common hepatic duct, hence flowing into the duodenum. The normal ejection fraction of the gallbladder should exceed 40%. Some patients have a low ejection fraction, called biliary dyskinesia, which may be associated with intermittent abdominal discomfort and a chronic feeling of nausea. The gallbladder appears to be relatively superfluous given the number of cholecystectomies that are performed annually and the relative lack of any significant postoperative gastrointestinal sequelae.

Bibliography

Brandt SJ, Schmidt WE: Gastrointestinal hormones. *In* Yamada T, Alpers DW, Owyang C, et al (eds): Textbook of Gastroenterology (2nd ed). Philadelphia: JB Lippincott, 1995:25.

Caspary WF: Physiology and pathophysiology of intestinal absorption. Am J Clin Nutr 1992;55:299S.

Chen D, Monstein HJ, Nylander AG, et al: Acute responses of rat stomach enterochromaffinlike cells to gastrin: secretory activation and adaptation. Gastroenterology 1994;107:18.

Civitelli R, Avioli LV: Calcium, phosphate, and magnesium absorption. *In* Johnson LR, Alpers DH, Christensen J, et al (eds): Physiology of the Gastrointestinal Tract (3rd ed). New York: Raven Press, 1994:2173.

Davenport HW: Secretion of bile. *In* Physiology of the Digestive Tract: An Introductory Text (4th ed). Chicago: Year Book Medical Publishers, 1977:141.

Flemstrom G: Gastric and duodenum mucosal secretion of bicarbonate. *In* Johnson LR, Alpers DH, Christensen J, et al (eds): Physiology of the Gastrointestinal Tract. New York: Raven Press, 1987:1285.

Ganapathy V, Brandsch M, Leibach FH: Intestinal transport of amino acids and peptides. *In* Johnson LR, Alpers DH, Christensen J, et al (eds): Physiology of the Gastrointestinal Tract (3rd ed). New York: Raven Press, 1994:1773.

Hasler WL: Motility of the small intestine. *In* Yamada T, Alpers DH, Owyang C, et al (eds): Textbook of Gastroenterology (2nd ed). Philadelphia: JB Lippincott, 1995:207.

Hersey SJ: Pepsin secretion. *In* Johnson LR, Alpers DH, Jackson MJ, et al (eds): Physiology of the Gastrointestinal Tract (3rd ed). New York: Raven Press, 1994:1227.

Hersey SJ, Sachs G: Gastric acid secretion. Physiol Rev 1995;75:155.

Hofmann AF: Bile secretion and the enterohepatic circulation of bile acids. *In* Feldmann F, Scharschmidt BF, Sleisenger MH (eds): Gastrointestinal and Liver Disease: Pathophysiology, Diagnosis, Management (6th ed). Philadelphia: WB Saunders, 1997:937.

Kidd M, Modlin IM, Tang LH: Gastrin and the enterochromaffin-like cell: an acid update. Dig Surg 1998;15:209.

Phillips SF: The growth of knowledge in human digestion and absorption. Gastroenterology 1997;112:1404.

Quigley EM: Gastric and small intestinal motility in health and disease. Gastroenterol Clin North Am 1996;25:113.

Raeder M: The origin and subcellular mechanism causing pacreatic bicarbonate secretion. Gastroenterology 1992;103:1674.

Samloff IM: Pepsins, peptic activity, and peptic inhibitors. J Clin Gastroenterol 1981;3:91.

Sarna SK: Cyclic motor activity: migrating motor complex. Gastroenterology 1985;89:894.

Schubert ML, Makhlouf GM: Neural, hormonal, and paracrine regulation of gastrin and acid secretion. Yale J Biol Med 1992;65:553.

Schubert ML, Makhlouf GM: Gastrin secretion induced by distention is mediated by gastric cholinergic and vasoactive intestinal peptide neurons in rats. Gastroenterology 1993;104:834.

Seetharam B, Alpers DH: Absorption and transport of cobalamin (vitamin B_{12}). Annu Rev Nutr 1982;2:343.

Soll AH, Berglindh T: Receptors regulating acid secretory function. *In* Johnson LR, Alpers DH, Christensen J, et al (eds): Physiology of the Gastrointestinal Tract (3rd ed). New York: Raven Press, 1994:1139.

Teichmann R, Stremmel W: Iron uptake by human upper small intestine microvillous membrane vesicles: indications for a facilitated transport mechanism mediate by a membrane iron-binding protein. J Clin Invest 1990;86:2145.

Tso P: Intestinal lipid absorption. *In* Johnson LR, Alpers DH, Christensen J, et al (eds): Physiology of the Gastrointestinal Tract (3rd ed). New York: Raven Press, 1994:1867.

Williams JA: Regulatory mechanism in pancreas and salivary acini. Annu Rev Physiol 1984;46:361.

Wright EM, Hirayama BA, Loo DDF, et al: Intestinal sugar transport. *In* Johnson LR, Alpers DH, Christensen J, et al (eds): Physiology of the Gastrointestinal Tract (3rd ed). New York: Raven Press, 1994:1751.

CHAPTER 25

Endocrine Physiology and Dysfunction

Maria D. Allo, M.D.

This chapter describes the general physiologic and regulatory functions of the endocrine system as related to surgically treated endocrine disease. The chapter is divided into five parts: (1) common features, which describe aspects of the endocrine system that are not organ specific; (2) pituitary; (3) thyroid; (4) parathyroid; and (5) adrenal. Although one normally thinks of the endocrine system as including reproductive function, that area is covered in Chapter 21 and is not included here. Similarly, diabetes and morbid obesity are covered in Chapters 30 and 29, respectively.

Common Features of the Endocrine System

The endocrine system is the control center for the body, and performs complex regulatory functions necessary for growth and development, response to acute needs, and maintenance of homeostasis. These functions are accomplished by a wide variety of hormones. Chemically, hormones are either peptides, iodothyronines, steroid derivatives, or catecholamines. Knowing the chemical structure of a hormone provides clues as to how the hormone works at a cellular and molecular level.

Functionally, steroid hormones, 1,25-dihydroxyvitamin D [1,25-$(OH_2)D$], and thyroid hormone act similarly and can be classified as steroid-type hormones. These hormones usually diffuse into cells (with some exceptions) and bind to receptor proteins, forming complexes that have high affinity for DNA-binding sites. Subsequently the steroid dissociates from the receptor and diffuses from the cells. The receptor is used again and again to bind new steroid. Because these hormones are protein bound, they tend to have relatively longer half-lives than do the peptide hormones. Once they are unbound, they can be transformed peripherally in ways that can alter their activity. The steroid hormones generally affect regulatory body functions that help maintain homeostasis.

Peptide hormones, which include growth factors, neurotransmitter hormones, and the prostaglandins, generally act at the cell surface. Their receptors are on the plasma membranes of target cells. The specific, high-affinity binding of the hormone to the plasma cell receptor results in the generation of a "second messenger" that affects intracellular function. Because these hormones are unbound, they arrive in "active form." Consequently, they have very short biologic half-lives and their activity cannot be increased peripherally. These hormones generally help the body adjust to episodic conditions.

Independent of their chemical structure, hormones have some universal features that are summarized in Box 25–1. The reactions that result in hormone synthesis are very nonspecific and can occur in tissues that are not the target organ. In some cases, hormone that cannot be synthesized in an organ can be made by transformation of a precursor substance in the target organ.

Feedback mechanisms are another important feature of endocrine systems, and several types of systems are operative. The simplest of these systems is the negative feedback loop, in which the rate of hormone release is regulated by the blood concentration of either the hormone or a chemical controlled by the hormone. For example, corticotropin (adrenocorticotropic hormone [ACTH]) acts on the adrenal gland to regulate cortisol release. Release of cortisol acts on the pituitary to regulate corticotropin-releasing factor, which in turn affects release of ACTH. Understanding of feedback loops is essential to understanding and interpreting many of the tests used to measure endocrine function. When there is a functional abnormality associated with a hormone system, it is important to identify where in the feedback loop the abnormality is occurring, because ablation of the end organ may not correct the abnormality (Box 25–2).

Abnormalities of endocrine function are first evaluated by screening tests that answer the question, is there an endocrine abnormality? Once it is established that an abnormality is present, diagnostic tests can help determine where in the complex process of hormone production and secretion the abnormality arises.

Most endocrine diseases fall into one of the categories listed in Box 25–3. In addition, the endocrine system is closely linked to the nervous system and the immune system, and consequently aberrations in either of these systems

can result in endocrine dysfunction. Most endocrine diseases that can be treated surgically present as a mass, a functional abnormality, or both. When a mass is present, it is important to determine whether it is associated with malignancy, with inappropriate hormone production, or both. The determination of malignancy frequently falls on the surgeon rather than on the pathologist. The finding of a mass that attaches to or erodes into surrounding structures, or of metastases distant from the organ from which the mass originates, may be the sole feature suggesting malignancy. Benign endocrine tissue often exhibits cellular pleomorphism, mitoses, and other histologic characteristics suggestive of malignancy; at the same time, malignant endocrine neoplasms may be so well differentiated as to be microscopically indistinguishable from their benign counterparts.

Box 25–2

Important Negative Feedback Loops

Aldosterone System
1. Renal potassium excretion → aldosterone release
   ↑ potassium balance ↓
2. ↑ Aldosterone → sodium retention (kidney) → renin release
   ↑ angiotensin activation ↓

Cortisol
CRF (hypothalamus) → ACTH (pituitary) → cortisol (adrenal)
   ↑ high cortisol inhibits CRF ↓

Thyroid
TRH (hypothalamus) → TSH (pituitary) → T_3 and T_4
   T_3 suppresses stimulation of TSH release by TRH

Prolactin Secretion
Prolactin (pituitary) ↔ dopamine (hypothalamus)

Box 25–1

Universal Features of Hormones

1. All have mechanisms to direct them to their target site:
   - Receptors in target tissues
   - Delivery via portal or other restricted circulatory systems
   - Local formation of active hormone from inactive precursors
2. Plasma concentrations are very small (picomoles to micromoles per liter).
3. All have target tissues on which they have major actions.
4. Rate of hormone release is limited by rate of synthesis.
5. There is feedback control of hormone production.

Box 25–3

Mechanisms of Endocrine Disease

1. Disruption of a feedback system
2. Disruption in the cyclic pattern of hormone release
3. Abnormal amounts of hormone production
4. Normal amounts of production of abnormal hormone
5. Abnormal transport of hormones
6. Abnormal hormone metabolism

Pituitary and Hypothalamus

Anatomy

The hypothalamus has efferent and afferent fibers connecting it to the rest of the nervous system, and is located below the thalamus and surrounding the third ventricle of the brain. Although its primary blood supply comes from the circle of Willis and its primary drainage system is via the vein of Galen, a secondary, but important, part of its venous drainage flows from the median eminence as a capillary plexus into a sinusoidal network in the adenohypophysis (anterior pituitary gland) to form the hypothalamo-hypophysial portal system.

The pituitary gland is located in the hypophysial fossa of the skull, also known as the sella turcica. The sphenoid bone lies lateral and inferior to the gland. Superiorly it is covered by the diaphragmatic sella. Both the diaphragmatic sella and the sphenoid bone are lined with dura. The adenohypophysis, or anterior pituitary, represents about 80% of the pituitary gland and is composed of three parts: the pars distalis, which is the site of hormone-producing cells; the pars intermedia, which has little significance in humans; and the pars tuberalis, which produces some glycoprotein hormones. The posterior pituitary is part of the neurohypophysis, which consists of the supraoptic and paraventricular nuclei in the hypothalamus, and nerve fibers from the cell bodies of the hypothalamic nuclei as well as the posterior lobe of the pituitary. Unlike the adenohypophysis, the neurohypophysis gets its blood supply from the superior and the inferior hypophysial arteries, which form a capillary plexus throughout the gland and which ultimately drain into the jugular veins.

Physiology

Box 25–4 lists common features of the six major hormones produced in the adenohypophysis. The six hormones are corticotropin (ACTH), prolactin, pituitary growth hormone, thyrotropin (thyroid-stimulating hormone [TSH]), and the two gonadotrophins: luteinizing hormone (LH) in females/interstitial-cell stimulating hormone in males and follicle-stimulating hormone (FSH). These hormones can be thought of in three groups: corticotropin; prolactin and growth hormone; and the glycoprotein hormones (TSH, LH, and FSH).

Corticotropin binds to cell membrane receptors in the presence of extracellular calcium. Its second messenger is cyclic AMP, generated by activation of adenyl cyclase. Its chief function is to stimulate the synthesis and secretion of cortisol in the adrenal cortex.

Prolactin and pituitary growth hormone are structurally similar, and have receptors that are similar. It is

> **Box 25–4**
> ### Common Features of Anterior Pituitary Hormones
>
> 1. They are regulated by hormones made in the hypothalamus via the hypothalamo-hypophysial portal system
> 2. Most are under feedback regulation with hormones secreted by the target organ (EXCEPTION: prolactin).
> 3. The hypothalamic hormones bind to high-affinity receptors in individual pituitary cells and regulate secretion at the cell level.
> 4. There is "short-loop" feedback whereby hormones from the pituitary are transported back to the hypothalamus to reduce hypothalamic secretion.
> 5. Secretion of anterior pituitary hormones is discontinuous.

thought that their genes may have a common origin. However, they are distinct hormones with distinct functions. Although there are prolactin receptors in many tissues, the main site of action of prolactin is in the breast, where it initiates and maintains lactation. Its secretion is controlled by substances made in the hypothalamus, including dopamine, which has an inhibitory effect; and thyrotropin-releasing hormone (TRH), vasoactive intestinal peptide, and other similar substances, which have a stimulatory effect. Pituitary growth hormone acts on multiple sites, including the liver, muscle, bones, and soft tissue. The exact mechanism of action and specific effects are still under investigation; however, it does regulate insulin metabolism in muscle, growth in growth plates, and lipolysis in adipose tissues. Its secretion is regulated at the level of the hypothalamus by somatostatin and growth hormone–releasing hormone.

Thyrotropin binds to cell membrane receptors in the thyroid gland to activate adenyl cyclase. It indirectly regulates synthesis and secretion of thyroid hormones by stimulating blood flow to the thyroid, decreasing the amount of colloid and increasing the height of the follicular cells. These changes result in formation of iodothyronine and iodotyrosine, release of triiodothyronine (T_3) and thyroxine (T_4), synthesis of thyroglobulins, and increased iodide transport.

Clinical Correlation

Most operations performed in the pituitary gland are for removal of pituitary tumors. Pituitary tumors are divided into two major groups: hormone secreting versus non–hormone secreting, and macroadenomas (≥ 1 cm) versus microadenomas (< 1 cm). The most common hormone-secreting tumor of the pituitary secretes prolactin, and this is the one pituitary tumor that often can be successfully managed medically using bromocriptine. For most other pituitary tumors, surgical treatment is the mainstay of therapy. Most pituitary tumors present either with symptoms referable to hormone excess or with visual symptoms, particularly bitemporal hemianopsia.

Thyroid

Anatomy

The thyroid gland lies in the anterior neck between the sternal notch and the thyroid cartilage. It consists of two lobes, connected by an isthmus, that originate from the fusion of the fourth and fifth branchial pouches. Two functional cell groups can be identified histologically: follicular cells, which line the edges of the colloid-containing follicles; and parafollicular cells, also known as C cells, which secrete calcitonin, a hormone that lowers calcium levels. The thyroid receives its blood supply from the superior thyroid artery, which is a branch of the external carotid artery, and the inferior thyroid artery, which is a branch of the subclavian artery. A third unpaired artery, the thyroidea ima, occurs in about 30% of patients. The venous drainage of the thyroid is via the superior thyroid veins, the middle thyroid vein, and the inferior thyroid veins. Nervous innervation is via both adrenergic fibers from the cervical ganglia and cholinergic fibers from the vagus. These nerves are important because they regulate blood flow to the thyroid, which in turn influences the delivery of trophic substances, iodine and TSH, to the thyroid gland.

Physiology

Thyroid hormone is important for maintenance of homeostasis. In particular, it helps in the maintenance of body temperature and body weight; supports nutrition by stimulating protein synthesis, and the synthesis and degradation of cholesterol and triglycerides; and stimulates heart contraction. As mentioned earlier, thyroid hormones, like steroid hormones, function as ligand-dependent transcription factors. Thyroid hormones diffuse through cell membranes and enter the nuclei of cells. Once in the nuclei, they bind to hormone-specific intranuclear receptors to form hormone-receptor complexes that interact with specific DNA sequences of promoter genes to stimulate or inhibit transcription. In this way, they modulate gene expression.

Thyroid hormone is made within the thyroid cell as follows. Iodine is trapped when it is actively transported into the thyroid cell. Once in the cell, an oxidation reaction occurs that results in iodination of tyrosyl in thyroglobulin.

Iodotyrosine then is coupled in thyroglobulin to form T_3 and T_4. Free iodotyrosine and iodothyronine are released from the thyroglobulin by proteolysis; then the iodine is recycled as the iodotyrosines are deiodinated.

Secretion of thyroid hormone is regulated by the hypothalamic-pituitary axis. The feedback loop is as follows: TRH stimulates secretion of TSH, which in turn controls the synthesis and release of T_3 and T_4. TRH is made in the hypothalamus. Its secretion is influenced by many external factors, including changes in temperature. TSH is the most important regulator of thyroid synthesis. TSH binds to receptors found on thyroid epithelial cells. TSH in high concentration increases the rate of endocytosis of colloid, which, in turn, causes thyroid hormone to be released into the circulation.

Clinical Correlation

Thyroid surgery is done for solitary thyroid nodules suspicious for, or proven to be, malignant; for large symptomatic goiters; and, rarely, for hyperthyroidism or thyroiditis.

Solitary thyroid nodules

Solitary thyroid nodules usually are found on routine physical examination. If there is a question as to whether the nodule is actually solitary, thyroid scanning may be helpful. However, thyroid scanning is rarely helpful in the preoperative evaluation of thyroid lesions. The primary modality for evaluating thyroid nodules is fine-needle aspiration cytology. Where this is not available, core needle biopsy will provide histologic diagnosis. Colloid nodules do not require operation, thus eliminating need for surgical treatment in about 75% of palpable nodules. Many medullary and papillary carcinomas can be diagnosed preoperatively. Follicular cancers, because the criterion for malignancy is capsular or vascular invasion, cannot be definitively diagnosed preoperatively. Consequently, a cellular aspirate with predominance of follicular cells is an indication for surgical intervention. Of note, most patients with thyroid cancer are clinically and chemically euthyroid. The minimal operation for a thyroid nodule suspected to be malignant is hemithyroidectomy and isthmusectomy. There is controversy as to whether well-differentiated thyroid cancers (papillary and follicular carcinomas) should all be treated with total thyroidectomy, or whether lesser resection is adequate treatment. Total thyroidectomy makes it easier to follow patients for recurrence because any rise in serum thyroglobulin, which generally becomes undetectable after total thyroid ablation, heralds recurrence. It also simplifies treatment of metastases with radioactive iodine because uptake following ablation likely represents tumor, and the scanning dose of radioactive iodine is not taken up by the residual thyroid tissue.

Medullary thyroid carcinoma arises from the parafollicular cells of the thyroid that produce calcitonin. Elevation of serum calcitonin levels confirms the diagnosis, and is also an important marker for recurrent or metastatic disease after surgical treatment. Treatment is total thyroidectomy with central compartment lymph node dissection. Medullary thyroid carcinoma can be associated with familial cancer syndromes associated with mutation of the *ret* oncogene. These include familial medullary thyroid carcinoma, multiple endocrine neoplasia (MEN) type IIa, and MEN type IIb. It is important to screen family members for *ret* mutations when familial disease is suspected. In addition, when MEN IIa or IIB is suspected, pheochromocytoma (which occurs as often as 40% of the time) must be ruled out before proceeding with thyroidectomy.

Anaplastic thyroid carcinoma, the rarest form of thyroid carcinoma, has the worst overall prognosis. It presents with a rapidly enlarging neck mass, dysphagia, and/or airway compromise. Surgery plays only a palliative role, and generally is indicated primarily as a means of securing an airway.

Hyperthyroidism

It is uncommon to treat hyperthyroidism surgically. Graves' disease, the most common form of hyperthyroidism, usually is managed medically, then definitively treated with radioactive iodine. When surgical treatment is used, subtotal thyroidectomy is the operation of choice.

It is important that surgeons be aware of thyrotoxic storm, one of the serious complications of hyperthyroidism. This can occur when patients with untreated or inadequately treated hyperthyroidism undergo stress, including the stress of surgery. Patients with hyperthyroidism should be made euthyroid with antithyroid drugs or radiotherapy prior to undergoing elective operation. When urgent or emergent surgical situations force operation before the patient can be made euthyroid, treatment with propylthiouracil or methimazole, followed by treatment with potassium iodide and hydrocortisone, should be initiated prior to operation and continued perioperatively.

Large goiters

Very large goiters can cause symptoms of dysphagia or respiratory compromise. Some will extend substernally. Malignancy can be found within the gland about 8% of the time. When large goiters fail to suppress with levothyroxine, cause obstructive symptoms, or extend substernally, surgical intervention is indicated. Subtotal thyroidectomy is the treatment of choice.

Thyroiditis

Subacute thyroiditis, also known as de Quervain's disease, is an inflammatory disorder likely caused by a viral infection. Patients present with soreness over the thyroid, fever, malaise, and signs of hyperthyroidism without ophthalmopathy. Like Graves' disease, there is elevation of T_3 and T_4 and suppression of TSH; unlike Graves' disease, there is low uptake of radioiodine and absence of thyroid antibodies. Treatment is nonsurgical and consists of anti-inflammatory drugs, and occasionally steroids and thyroid suppression. Chronic thyroiditis, or Hashimoto's disease, is the most common cause of goiter in the United States. It is an autoimmune disease that results in lymphocytes becoming sensitized to thyroid antigens, which in turn results in production of autoantibodies. The end result is hypothyroidism. Fine-needle aspiration biopsy showing predominance of lymphocytes and Hürthle cells, and the presence of thyroglobin antibody and thyroid peroxidase antibody, establish the diagnosis. Rarely, surgical intervention is indicated to relieve tracheal compression associated with the fibrotic variant of this disease, also known as Riedel's struma.

Parathyroid

Anatomy

As the name implies, the parathyroid glands are located adjacent to the thyroid gland in the neck. They are four small structures that arise embryologically from the third and fourth branchial pouches. The superior glands arise from the fourth branchial pouch and migrate with the thyroid anlage; the lower glands arise from the third branchial pouch and descend with the thymic remnant. The embryologic relationship between the lower parathyroids and the thymus explains why lower parathyroid glands may be located anywhere from as cephalad as the hyoid to as caudad as the mediastinum.

The parathyroids are made up of two predominant cell types: chief cells and oxyphilic cells. Both cell types secrete parathyroid hormone (PTH), and it is not known if or how their functions differ.

Physiology

The primary function of the parathyroid gland is calcium regulation. It does this by its actions on bone, kidney, and, indirectly, intestinal mucosa. PTH is an 84-amino-acid, single-chain polypeptide that is synthesized within the parathyroid glands. The amino-terminal sequence (amino acids 1 to 27) is responsible for binding the hormone to receptor sites, for activating adenyl cyclase, and for biologic activity.

Control of PTH secretion is by negative feedback with the serum calcium concentration. Parathyroid cells "sense" extracellular calcium concentration by means of a G protein–coupled receptor, which appears to be the same receptor that regulates calcium in the C cells of the thyroid and the distal tubule of the kidney. Extracellular calcium inhibits the secretion of PTH when there is an increase in calcium ion concentration. Conversely, high extracellular calcium levels inhibit the secretion of preformed PTH.

PTH has a circulating half-life of 2 to 4 minutes, which is why intraoperative assays for PTH have been used to document successful parathyroidectomy. The active hormone is rapidly cleared by the liver and kidney and cleaved into amino-terminal and carboxy-terminal moieties. Early PTH assays measured the carboxy-terminal moiety. These have been replaced by the much more sensitive intact PTH assays, such as immunoradiometric assay, which detect both high levels of PTH, diagnostic of hyperparathyroidism, and suppressed levels of PTH, which occur in cases of hypercalcemia from causes other than hyperparathyroidism.

Clinical Correlation

Primary hyperparathyroidism

Hyperparathyroidism often is first detected by finding elevated serum calcium on a screening blood panel. However, with increasing measurement of bone densities as part of osteoporosis screening in women and less use of blood screening panels as a cost-saving measure, decreased bone density may become the most common presentation. It is not unusual for patients with hyperparathyroidism to have nonspecific symptoms of lethargy, constipation, and aches and pains, which miraculously go away once their hyperparathyroidism has been treated. There are many causes of hypercalcemia; however, primary hyperparathyroidism is the most frequent cause in the ambulatory population. Most adult patients presenting with primary hyperparathyroidism will have a single adenoma. Surgical resection of the adenoma is generally curative. There is no curative medical treatment. About 3% of patients will have a second adenoma, and about 3% will have their adenoma in the chest rather than in the neck.

The finding of hypercalcemia and elevated PTH is virtually diagnostic for primary hyperparathyroidism. That said, two important variants need be considered: familial hypocalciuric hypercalcemia (FHH) and MEN-related hyperparathyroidism. FHH is an autosomal dominant trait that represents a mutation in the parathyroid calcium receptor. It should be suspected when both the hypercalcemia and the elevation in PTH are mild. Like primary hyperparathyroidism, it is associated with hypophosphatemia and hypermagnesemia; unlike primary hyperparathyroidism, there is hypocalciuria. The clinical significance in identifying patients with this variant is that they are actually harmed by parathyroidectomy: serum calcium levels do not fall, and patients become hypoparathyroid.

MEN-related hyperparathyroidism occurs in both MEN type I and MEN type II, but the etiology and penetrance are different. MEN I has a penetrance of 90%; MEN II, about 25% to 30%. MEN I–related hyperparathyroidism is thought to be caused by a mutation on the tumor suppressor gene of chromosome 11q12-13, similar to what is thought to occur with parathyroid adenomas, whereas MEN II–related hyperparathyroidism is due to a mutation of the *ret* oncogene. Both are treated with subtotal parathyroidectomy, although it is relatively uncommon for patients with MEN II to develop hypercalcemia requiring operation. Finally, primary hyperparathyroidism is extremely rare before puberty. Children presenting with hyperparathyroidism must be evaluated for MEN or other familial disease.

Secondary Hyperparathyroidism

Secondary hyperparathyroidism is a form of renal osteodystrophy that occurs when the kidney cannot synthesize adequate amounts of 1,25-$(OH)_2$D, and cannot maintain phosphate balance. Decreased formation of 1,25-$(OH)_2$D means that there is less calcium absorbed from the gut. Phosphate retention drives the serum phosphate up. Each of these in turn results in decreased serum calcium that results in increased PTH. Increased PTH results in increased bone resorption, which in turn causes phosphate to be released into the serum. Ideally this condition can be treated medically with a low-phosphate diet, phosphate binders, and calcitriol. However, when these measures are inadequate, operation is sometimes necessary. The usual indications for operation include any of the following: serum calcium:phosphorus ratio of greater than 70; pathologic fractures; and severe symptoms such as pruritus, calciphylaxis, soft tissue deposition of calcium, or bone pain. The usual operation is either subtotal parathyroidectomy (excision of three and one-half glands) or total parathyroidectomy with implantation of parathyroid tissue in forearm or neck muscle.

Adrenal

Anatomy

The adrenal glands are located in the retroperitoneum superomedially to the upper poles of the kidney. Ninety percent of the gland is composed of cortical tissue, which surrounds the remaining 10%, which is the medulla. The blood supply to the adrenal consists of a series of arterial twigs deriving from the inferior phrenic arteries, the renal arteries, and the aorta. The right adrenal venous drainage is to the vena cava; the left adrenal vein drains into the left renal vein. About 30% of the time there is a prominent accessory renal vein that on the right drains into the right renal vein and on the left into the inferior phrenic vein.

The cortex is the color of gold leaf and derives from mesoderm, whereas the medulla is brown and derives from neuroectoderm. The cortex is further subdivided into three layers: the outermost layer (zona glomerulosa), which makes aldosterone; and the middle and thickest layer (zona fasciculata) and the innermost layer (zona reticularis), which make cortisol and androgens. The medulla is made of chromaffin cells, which contain large numbers of storage vesicles for catecholamines. The cells of the medulla are nested among blood vessels and sympathetic ganglia.

Physiology of the Adrenal Cortex

The primary function of the adrenal cortex is steroid production. Cholesterol is cleaved by the action of ACTH on the enzyme cholesterol mono-oxygenase (side chain cleaving), or $P450_{scc}$, to produce pregnenolone. This reaction, like most of the steroidogenic reactions, is cytochrome P-450 dependent. Because of enzymatic differences in the different zones of the adrenal cortex, different reactions can occur, and consequently different products are synthesized. In the zona glomerulosa, for example, the enzyme aldosterone synthetase, or $P450_{aldo}$, mediates the conversion of 11-deoxycorticosterone to aldosterone by catalyzing 11β-hydroxylation, 18-hydroxylation, and 18-oxidation. Because 17-hydroxylase is not found in the zona glomerulosa, cortisol and androgens cannot be produced. Conversely, aldosterone synthetase is not found in either the zona reticularis or the zona fasciculata, but 17-hydoxylase is present there, allowing production of cortisol and androgens but not aldosterone.

Aldosterone

Although both cortisol and aldosterone have mineralocorticoid activity, cortisol undergoes local degradation, and in fact has relatively little actual mineralocorticoid effect, nor is it under control of the renin-angiotensin system, as is aldosterone. Unlike cortisol and the androgens, aldosterone is only weakly bound to cortisol-binding globulins, so that about one third to one half of all aldosterone is free in plasma, as opposed to the other corticosteroids, which are about 90% to 95% bound. Both deoxycorticosterone and aldosterone compete for mineralocorticoid receptors, but, because more aldosterone is free in plasma, it is functionally more important. The high amount of free aldosterone in plasma accounts for its relatively short half-life (15 to 20 minutes).

Glucocorticoids

The glucocorticoids regulate glucose metabolism in the liver, osteoclast activity in bone, lipolysis in adipose tissue,

lactate release in muscle, catecholamine synthesis, and production of factors important to immune response. Glucocorticoids are made in the adrenal and secreted into the circulation, where about 95% are bound to plasma protein. The unbound 5% diffuse into target cells and become bound to proteins in the cells' cytosol. Then the hormone-receptor complexes enter the nucleus and react with acceptor sites in the nuclear chromatin, influencing the expression of specific genes.

Physiology of the Adrenal Medulla

Catecholamines are made in the adrenal medulla by a four-step reaction: (1) tyrosine is hydroxylated to form dihydroxyphenylalanine (DOPA), (2) DOPA is decarboxylated to form dopamine, (3) dopamine undergoes β-hydroxylation to norepinephrine, and (4) norepinephrine undergoes N-methylation to epinephrine. Catecholamine biosynthesis is coupled to secretion so that the amount of norepinephrine stored at nerve endings is constant. However, in times of prolonged hypoglycemia, catecholamine stores in the adrenal medulla can be depleted. Catecholamines are stored within storage granules in the adrenal medulla and sympathetically innervated organs. Secretion of the catecholamines is mediated by the release of acetylcholine from preganglionic fibers, which in turn causes calcium flux, which initiates exocytosis that releases contents of the storage vesicles. Once in the circulation, the catecholamines are bound to albumin.

Clinical Correlation

Surgical diseases of the adrenal present clinically as (1) incidental adrenal masses found on imaging studies; (2) hypertension and its surgically treatable causes, primary hyperaldosteronism, Cushing's syndrome, and pheochromocytoma; or (3) symptoms directly related to hyperfunction, such as physical stigmata of Cushing's syndrome, or Cushing-related amenorrhea.

Incidental adrenal masses

The evaluation of the incidental adrenal mass begins with an exhaustive history and physical exam directed at eliciting any signs or symptoms of a functioning adrenal tumor. Blood pressure is carefully checked. Screening is done for primary hyperaldosteronism (serum potassium level), Cushing's syndrome (low-dose overnight dexamethasone suppression test), and pheochromocytoma (urinary vanillylmandelic acid, norepinephrine, epinephrine, nor-metanephrine, and metanephrine levels). If any of these screens are positive, surgical excision is indicated. If not, if the lesion is 4 cm or larger, it should be excised; if smaller, serial re-evaluations should be done.

Hypertension

Primary hyperaldosteronism, Cushing's syndrome, and pheochromocytoma are three surgically amenable causes of hypertension. Most patients with primary hyperaldosteronism come to medical attention because of hypokalemia, or are incidentally found to be hypertensive on routine medical exam. Clinically significant hypertension is more common in patients with Cushing's disease than in those with Cushing's syndrome, which is caused by an adrenal adenoma; however, even though as many as 80% of patients with Cushing's syndrome have hypertension, it is usually not the presenting complaint. Pheochromocytoma has both sustained and paroxysmal hypertension, which can be very severe and associated with dramatic symptoms of chest pain, sweating, severe headache, anxiety, and visual disturbances. Hypertensive crises during times of stress can occur, especially in patients with occult pheochromocytoma undergoing surgery. Screening is recommended for patients with hypertension who are young, who have associated symptoms suggestive of pheochromocytoma, who have mucosal neuromas or body habitus suggestive of MEN type IIb, or who have a family history of pheochromocytoma or neurofibromatosis or of unusual pressor response during surgery.

Primary hyperaldosteronism

Excessive levels of aldosterone cause increased sodium retention and increased extracellular volume. Stretch receptors at the juxtaglomerular apparatus and sodium ion flux at the macula densa cause renin suppression. The concomitant potassium depletion results in hypokalemia. The constellation of hypokalemia, high plasma aldosterone level, and decreased plasma renin are the hallmarks of this disorder. Primary aldosteronism is caused by a solitary aldosterone-producing adenoma of the adrenal cortex about 70% of the time. Five percent of these tumors are renin-responsive adenomas that are biochemically more similar to changes seen with hyperplasia; however, these adenomas are responsive to surgical resection and therefore are treated the same way as the solitary adenomas. Diagnosis is made by demonstrating elevations in plasma aldosterone levels and decreased plasma renin. Localization is best done using computed tomography (CT) scanning or magnetic resonance imaging (MRI) to demonstrate a unilateral adrenal mass.

The important cause of primary hyperaldosterone to be differentiated from the adenomas is idiopathic hyperaldosteronism with bilateral hyperplasia, which occurs in about 15% of patients presenting with signs and symptoms of primary hyperaldosteronism. It is usually treated with spironolactone rather than operation. Localization studies and measurement of plasma aldosterone levels after postural stimulation help to differentiate the two. Very rarely, primary hyperaldosteronism can be associated with adrenal cortical carcinoma or with a rare genetic disorder, glucocorticoid-remediable aldosteronism.

Secondary hyperaldosteronism

This entity usually results from excessive renin secretion resulting from a low effective blood volume. Management of secondary hyperaldosteronism depends on the underlying factor that causes the low effective blood volume.

Hypercortisolism (Cushing's syndrome)

Hypercortisolism can result from excessive stimulation by ACTH to produce cortisol, from a cortisol-secreting adrenal adenoma, or from an ectopic source of ACTH. The evaluation of a patient with suspected Cushing's disease first requires establishing that there is hypercortisolism, then determining its etiology. The simplest and best screening test is the low-dose (1 mg) overnight dexamethasone suppression test. The patient takes a single 1-mg dose of dexamethasone at 11 PM, and the following morning a plasma cortisol level is determined. If the plasma cortisol level is less than 3 μg/dL, Cushing's disease is excluded; if the level is greater than 10 μg/dL, further work-up is indicated. Measurement of plasma ACTH will determine whether an adrenal adenoma is the cause or whether an ACTH-dependent tumor (pituitary adenoma, or other tumor producing ectopic ACTH) is the cause. A low ACTH level indicates adrenal adenoma, and CT scanning or MRI should be obtained to localize the lesion. Unilateral adrenalectomy is the treatment of choice, and has a very good success rate. If the ACTH level is high, other tests such as an overnight high-dose dexamethasone suppression test or the metyrapone test can be done to determine whether the elevated ACTH is of pituitary or ectopic origin. Imaging with MRI sometimes will visualize a pituitary adenoma. Inferior petrosal sinus sampling also is sometimes used to detect a gradient of ACTH levels.

Perioperatively and following operation for Cushing's adenomas, it is very important to give the patient steroid supplements with the assumption that the contralateral adrenal is suppressed.

Pheochromocytoma

Pheochromocytomas are catecholamine-secreting tumors. They may arise from the adrenal medulla or from the organs of Zuckerkandl. Symptoms are described above in the section on Hypertension. The "rule of 10s" applies: 10% of pheochromocytomas are extra-adrenal, 10% bilateral, 10% familial, and 10% malignant. In the absence of an obvious adrenal mass, localization studies, including MRI, should be done. In selected cases, scanning with [^{131}I]-metaiodobenzylguanidine may help to localize extra-adrenal or metastatic tumors that elude detection by MRI.

Bilateral pheochromocytomas should raise suspicion for MEN type II, and an appropriate family history should be taken. As is the case with many endocrine tumors, malignant tumors are well differentiated and malignancy often is determined at the time of operation. Diagnosis is made by demonstrating elevated urinary catecholamine levels. Treatment is surgical removal; however, it is very important to give patients preoperative blockade with α-adrenergic agents, and to closely monitor blood pressure and the electrocardiogram intraoperatively. Intraoperative availability of agents to treat both hyper- and hypotension is very important.

Adrenal insufficiency

Adrenal insufficiency, though not a surgically treated disease, is one that all surgeons must be aware of and know how to manage. Although there are many causes, the single most frequent cause is the use of exogenous corticosteroids. Whenever a patient on chronic steroid treatment is to undergo a surgical intervention, physiologic doses of steroid (300 mg of hydrocortisone per day in divided doses) should be administered perioperatively.

Bibliography

Endocrine system in general

Clark OH, Duh QY (eds): Textbook of Endocrine Surgery. Philadelphia: WB Saunders, 1997.

Greenspan FS, Strewler GJ: Basic and Clinical Endocrinology. Stamford, CT: Appleton & Lange, 1994.

Thyroid

Allo MD, Thompson NW: Rationale for the operative management of substernal goiters. Surgery 1983;94:969.

DeGroot LJ, Kaplan EL, McCormick M, Straus FH: Natural history, treatment and course of papillary thyroid carcinoma. J Clin Endocrinol Metab 1990;71:414.

Farid NR, Shi Y, Zou M: Molecular basis of thyroid cancer. Endocr Rev 1994;15:202.

Grebe SKG, Hay ID: Follicular thyroid cancer. Endocrinol Metab Clin North Am 1995;24:761.

Mazzaferri EL: Management of a solitary thyroid nodule. N Engl J Med 1993;328:553.

Moley JF: Medullary thyroid cancer. Surg Clin North Am 1995; 75:405.

Singer PA, Cooper DS, Daniels GH, et al: Treatment guidelines for patients with thyroid nodules and well-differentiated thyroid cancers. Arch Intern Med 1996;156:2165.

Soh EY, Clark OH: Surgical considerations and approach to thyroid cancer. Endocrinol Metab Clin North Am 1996; 25:115.

Parathyroid

Bilezikian JP: Management of acute hypercalcemia. N Engl J Med 1992;326:1196.

Carney JA, Roth SI, Heath H III, et al: The parathyroid glands in multiple endocrine neoplasia type 2b. Am J Pathol 1980;99:387.

Marx SJ, Spiegel AM, Levine MA, et al: Primary hyperparathyroidism in familial multiple endocrine neoplasia type I: long term follow-up of serum calcium after parathyroidectomy. Am J Med 1982;307:416.

Maselly MJ, Lawrence AM, Brooks M, et al: Hyperparathyroid crisis. Surgery 1981;90:741.

Rothmund M, Wagner PK, Schark C: Subtotal parathyroidectomy versus total parathyroidectomy and autotransplantation in secondary hyperparathyroidism: a randomized trial. World J Surg 1991;15:745.

Saxe AW, Brennan MF: Reoperative parathyroid surgery for primary hyperparathyroidism caused by multiple gland disease: total parathyroidectomy and autotransplantation with cryopreserved tissue. Surgery 1982;91:616.

Wells SA, Leight GF, Ross A: Primary hyperparathyroidism. Curr Probl Surg 1980;17:398.

Adrenal

Conn JW: Primary aldosteronism: a new clinical syndrome. J Lab Clin Med 1955;45:3.

Curry DB, Tuck ML: Secondary aldosteronism. Endocrinol Metab Clin North Am 1995;24:511.

Gifford RW Jr, Manger WM, Bravo EL: Pheochromocytoma. Endocrinol Metab Clin North Am 1994;23:387.

Kloss RT, Gross MD, Francis IR, et al: Incidentally discovered adrenal masses. Endocr Rev 1995;16:460.

Samuels MH, Loriaux DL: Cushings's syndrome and the nodular adrenal gland. Endocrinol Metab Clin North Am 1994;23:555.

Udelsman R, Holbrook NJ: Endocrine and molecular responses to surgical stress. Curr Probl Surg 1994;31:653.

Young WF Jr, Hogan MJ, Klee GG, et al: Primary aldosteronism: diagnosis and treatment. Mayo Clin Proc 1990;65:96.

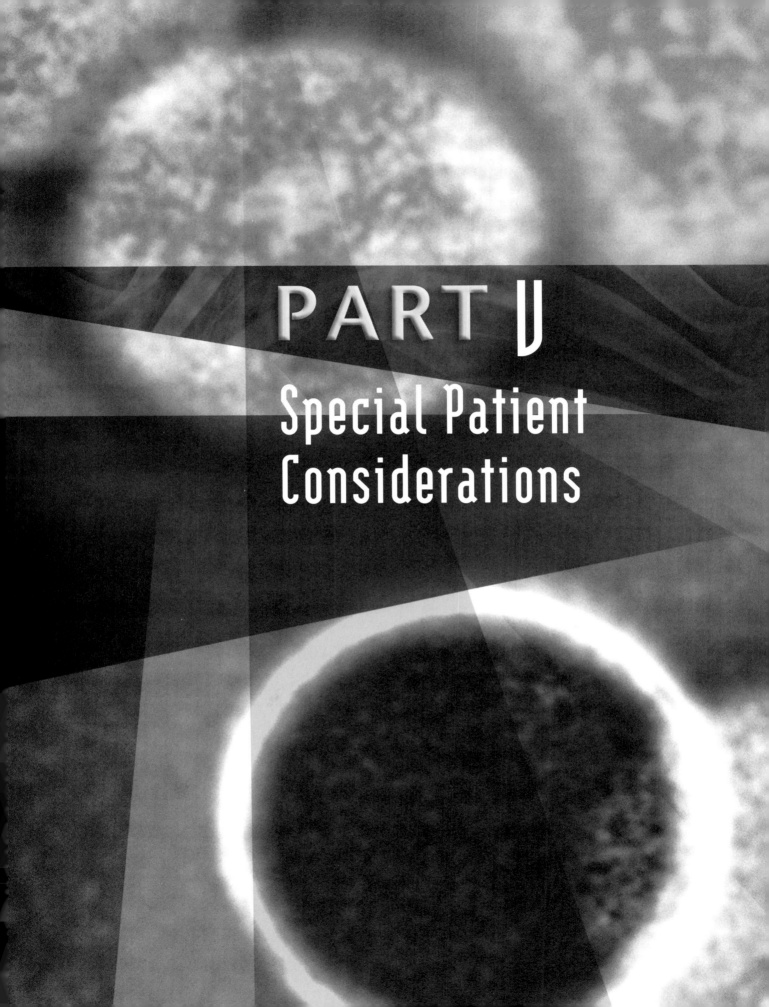

PART V
Special Patient Considerations

CHAPTER 26

The Pregnant Surgical Patient

Bonnie J. Dattel, M.D. and Marya Zlatnik, M.D.

Pregnancy is a time of unique physical and physiologic changes. These changes can pose challenges in the management of otherwise seemingly straightforward medical and surgical concerns. The presence of a pregnancy does not preclude the usual necessary interventions for disease treatment. Rather, it is a time when the surgeon and the obstetrician can work together to assure the best possible outcome for both mother and child.

Physiologic Changes of Pregnancy: Mechanical and Hormonal

An understanding of the basic physiologic changes of pregnancy is important for every practitioner caring for the gravida. Pregnancy has diverse effects on physiology, and these changes influence both the course of medical treatment and the woman's response to medical intervention. The physiologic changes of pregnancy can be conceptually divided into those related to the increased metabolic needs of the pregnancy, those that result from the hormonal milieu of pregnancy, and those that arise from the mechanical changes of the enlarging uterus.

The increased metabolic needs of pregnancy arise from the metabolism of the developing fetus, the hormonal and synthetic functions of the placenta, and the increase in maternal metabolism and fat deposition. In order to meet these increased metabolic needs, the pregnant woman undergoes a vast array of changes in her cardiovascular and respiratory systems. Cardiac output increases by 30% to 50% in pregnancy, and this increase begins early in gestation. This increase is accomplished by a 15% increase in heart rate and a 30% increase in stroke volume. Blood volume also increases in pregnancy, with the increase in plasma volume relatively greater than the increase in red cell mass.

Accompanying these changes is a decrease in peripheral vascular resistance and an increase in renal blood flow and glomerular filtration rate. Additionally, there is a decrease in vascular impedance in the uterine arteries and an increase in uterine blood flow from early in pregnancy. Uterine blood flow is approximately 0.5 L/min at term, accounting for approximately 10% of maternal cardiac output. This increase in blood flow is used for the metabolic needs of the uterine muscle as well as the placenta and fetus. The term fetus consumes 7.4 mL/min/kg of oxygen and benefits from this hyperdynamic circulation.

In addition to the cardiovascular changes, the respiratory system is also in overdrive. Minute oxygen uptake is increased by 30% in pregnancy. The gravida has a 40% increase in minute ventilation, mostly accomplished by an increase in tidal volume, with not much change in respiratory rate. The increase in tidal volume comes at the expense of decreased residual volume. Functional residual capacity (FRC) is reduced by approximately 20%. Vital capacity is essentially unchanged. The increase in minute ventilation results in a decreased carbon dioxide tension (PCO_2) and a partially compensated respiratory alkalosis. It is thought that progesterone is the hormone responsible for the increased respiratory drive that results in these changes. The oxygen dissociation curve is shifted to the left, resulting in less oxygen release to maternal tissues.

The hormonal changes of pregnancy affect many other systems. The predominant hormones of pregnancy are estrogen and progesterone. Levels of relaxin, plasma renin, angiotensin II, and aldosterone increase as well. Estrogen has been shown to cause vasodilatation. This results in a small decrease in systemic blood pressure and in a significant decrease in peripheral vascular resistance. The increase in circulating estrogen levels is thought to result in an increase in clotting factor, including fibrinogen and factors VII, VIII, IX, and X. Free protein S levels decrease in pregnancy, also increasing coagulability. Although plasminogen levels increase, fibrinolytic activity is prolonged in pregnancy.

In addition to its effects on respiration, progesterone is implicated in the relaxation of smooth muscle throughout the body. Progesterone influence is believed to be responsible for the slowing of intestinal transit times and the delay of gastric emptying, which is especially pronounced in labor, making aspiration of increased concern. Gastroesophageal reflux is common in pregnancy. The combination of decreased tone in the lower esophageal sphincter and increased pressure in the stomach is the likely cause.

Progesterone is also thought to be partially responsible for dilatation of the urinary tract based on animal studies. The gallbladder is also affected by pregnancy. Increased distention and hypotonia of the gallbladder are typical. Progesterone is thought to be responsible for this change, via inhibition of cholecystokinin-mediated smooth muscle contraction. Estrogen also affects the biliary tract. Estrogen increases serum cholesterol levels, predisposing to cholesterol gallstones. Estrogen can also inhibit intraductal transport of bile acids, increasing the risk of cholestasis. These changes lead to an increase in cholesterol stone formation in pregnant women. Asymptomatic gallstones are seen in 2% to 10% of pregnant women, and almost one third have sludge. The diameter of the common bile duct is also increased.

The uterus increases dramatically in size and weight during the course of pregnancy, increasing its capacity by 500 to 1000 times. The growing mass of the uterus displaces other organs in the abdomen. It is important to understand how this can change maternal physiology and affect diagnosis and treatment of common illnesses.

Prior to 6 weeks, the enlargement of the uterus has little impact on surrounding structures. By 12 weeks, the uterus is globular and arises out of the true pelvis, becoming an abdominal organ. By 18 to 20 weeks, the weight of the uterus is enough to affect blood flow in the great vessels when the gravida is in the supine position. Compression of the inferior vena cava impedes venous return to the heart, decreasing preload and decreasing blood pressure. Additionally, compression of the descending aorta also occurs, increasing afterload to the heart and decreasing blood pressure. The hypotension resulting from the effect of the uterus can cause maternal hypotensive symptoms and can decrease uterine blood flow, resulting

in fetal distress. Supine hypotension can be avoided by simple displacement of the uterus to the left or right using a hip wedge. Displacement can be accomplished in a patient restrained on a backboard by tilting the entire board with a wedge.

As the uterus grows, the stomach and large and small intestines are displaced laterally and superiorly. The appendix also moves over the course of pregnancy, ending up near the right flank at term. Although traditional teaching has suggested that the pain of appendicitis moves upward as well over the course of pregnancy, two recent studies of appendicitis in pregnancy suggest that right lower quadrant pain is the most common finding, regardless of gestational age. Hemorrhoids are common in pregnancy, a result of frequent constipation, obstruction of venous return, and increased venous pressure.

Pregnancy-associated changes in the urinary tract may be a result of both hormonal influence and mechanical obstruction. As the uterus rises out of the pelvis, its weight rests on the ureters, resulting in partial obstruction at the pelvic brim. The extent of hydronephrosis and hydroureter is often greater on the right. This may be due to dextrorotation of the uterus.

Biochemical and Hematologic Status

The biochemical and hematologic changes in pregnancy reflect the basic physiologic changes. The normal values of the arterial blood gases and basic electrolytes differ from those in the nonpregnant state. The increased respiratory drive of pregnancy results in a lower PCO_2 (Table 26–1). The relative increase in plasma volume over red blood cell mass results in the physiologic anemia of pregnancy. Iron deficiency may exacerbate the anemia. Plasma oncotic pressure and osmolality decrease, along with the concentrations of ions such as sodium, potassium, magnesium, and chloride.

Production of clotting factors increases in pregnancy. Plasma levels of factors I (fibrinogen), VII, VIII, IX, X, and XII increase. Factor II (prothrombin) levels increase only slightly. Fibrinolytic activity is decreased, and levels of free protein S decline. The increase in circulating clotting factors, in addition to venous statis secondary to obstruction of venous return by the gravid uterus, increases the likelihood of thromboembolic phenomena during pregnancy. Postoperative obstetric patients confined to bed rest are also at increased risk of thrombosis. Furthermore, pregnancy can be associated with the release of tissue thromboplastin secondary to placental abruption/separation, amniotic fluid embolism, fetal demise, or vascular injury during delivery. Women with inherited or acquired thrombophilic states are at increased risk for thromboembolic complications.

Table 26–1
Normal laboratory values in pregnancy

Analyte	Normal Pregnancy Range
Sodium	130–140 mg/dL
pH	7.44
P_{CO_2}	30 mm Hg
P_{O_2}	Slight increase
Bicarbonate	18–25 mEq/L
Creatinine	<1.0 mg/dL
Hemoglobin	10.5–14 g/dL
Hematocrit	33–44%
Fibrinogen	300–600 mg/dL
Alkaline phosphatase	Activity increases 3–5 times
Triglycerides	2–3 g/L

P_{CO_2}, carbon dioxide tension; P_{O_2}, oxygen tension.

Table 26–2
Estimated frequency of surgical disease in pregnancy per 1000 births

General Conditions	
Major abdominal trauma	1.53
Other major trauma	1.47
Cholecystitis	1.18
Appendicitis	1.05
Breast cancer	0.3
Bowel obstruction	0.3
Intracranial hemorrhage	0.2
Negative laparotomy	0.3
Gynecologic Conditions	
Adnexal mass	10–50
Ectopic pregnancy	10–15
Cervical neoplasia requiring biopsy	1.25

From Newton ER: Surgical problems in pregnancy. Clin Obstet 1996;35:2, with permission.

Thromboembolic events account for up to 25% of direct maternal mortality.

Evaluation of Fetal Risk

The need for surgical therapy can occur at any time during pregnancy (Table 26–2). Certain times in pregnancy, however, are more likely to be associated with the need for surgery. For example, during the first trimester, ovarian cysts associated with the corpus luteum may result in adnexal torsion, rupture, and possible hemorrhage. This particular risk factor usually disappears as the pregnancy progresses. However, appendicitis, the most common cause for surgery during pregnancy, can occur during any time in gestation.

Regardless of when the need for surgery arises, surgical intervention carries with it some element of fetal risk. This is especially dependent on gestational age. In the first trimester, the risk to pregnancy is related to medications used before, during, or after surgical procedures. These include anesthetic agents, pain medications, antimicrobials, muscle relaxants, and vascular agents. Most medications that are in general use can be safely used in pregnancy. The Food and Drug Administration (FDA) has classified drugs into different categories depending on their potential fetal effect (Table 26–3). Clearly, agents that have been shown to be safe for use during pregnancy and lactation should be chosen whenever possible.

In general, the first trimester is the one that has the greatest or the least potential for fetal harm because it is subject to an "all or nothing" phenomenon. Data gathered from cases in which surgery was performed without prior knowledge of a current pregnancy suggest that surgical procedures, anesthesia, and recovery are well tolerated in the first trimester of pregnancy, but may carry a small increased risk of miscarriage. Clearly, knowledge of pregnancy prior to anesthesia and surgery offers the greatest protection to the fetus because the least potentially harmful agents can be chosen for use.

In addition to potentially harmful agents, the maintenance of uterine perfusion through minimizing blood loss during surgical procedures is of utmost importance. Clearly, the further the gestational age, the more critical is uterine perfusion. However, significant blood loss, even in the first trimester, may carry an increased risk of spontaneous fetal loss (miscarriage).

Historically, the second trimester of pregnancy is the preferred time for performance of nonemergent, but needed, surgical procedures. Examples of such instances include symptomatic gallbladder disease, cancer surgery, and gynecologic procedures. The second trimester of pregnancy affords protection to the fetus in terms of malformations that could result from exposure to potential teratogens while reducing the risk of preterm labor and delivery because the uterus is still small enough to avoid excessive manipulation during surgical procedures. Similarly, risks of supine hypotension are also minimized because of smaller uterine size. The third trimester of pregnancy is perhaps the riskiest time to the fetus depending on the gestational age. Usually, nonemergent surgical procedures should be delayed until after 34 weeks'

Table 26–3
U.S. Food and Drug Administration pregnancy risk categories

Category A	Controlled studies in women fail to demonstrate a risk to the fetus in the first trimester (and there is no evidence of a risk in later trimesters), and the possibility of fetal harm appears remote.
Category B	Either animal reproduction studies have not demonstrated a fetal risk but there are no controlled studies in pregnant women or animal reproduction studies have shown an adverse effect (other than a decrease in fertility) that was not confirmed in controlled studies in women in the first trimester (and there is no evidence of a risk in later trimesters).
Category C	Either studies in animals have revealed adverse effects on the fetus (teratogenic or embryocidal or other) and there are no controlled studies in women or studies in women and animals are not available. Drugs should be given only if the potential benefit justifies the potential risk to the fetus.
Category D	There is positive evidence of human fetal risk, but the benefits from use in pregnant women may be acceptable despite the risk (e.g., if the drug is needed in a life-threatening situation or for a serious disease for which safer drugs cannot be used or are ineffective).
Category X	Studies in animals or human beings have demonstrated fetal abnormalities or there is evidence of fetal risk based on human experience or both, and the risk of the use of the drug in pregnant women clearly outweighs any possible benefit. The drug is contraindicated in women who are or may become pregnant.

gestational age. At this point, should delivery occur or be necessary for the surgery to take place, the risk is significantly reduced, and the long-term outcome for children delivered after 34 weeks is excellent. The highest risk period is between 26 and 34 weeks' estimated gestational age. Surgery performed during this time in pregnancy is associated with an increased risk of preterm labor and preterm delivery. The neonatal outcome is directly associated with the exact gestational age at delivery. Naturally the later in the third trimester the delivery, the better the outcome (Table 26–4).

Other risks associated with surgical procedures during pregnancy include blood loss and infection. Clearly, minimal blood loss is the goal in all surgical procedures, but during pregnancy, especially in the latter stages, this is essential to fetal well-being. Uterine perfusion is the only source for fetal oxygenation. Cases of significant blood loss (>50% decrease in maternal hematocrit and 50% decrease in maternal blood pressure, or a maternal $PaO_2 < 60$ mm Hg or O_2 saturation < 90%) result in fetal compromise. Blood flow to the uterus is shunted to other more vital maternal organs. This can result in fetal hypoxia. During early pregnancy, significant blood loss followed by restoration of blood flow to the uterus can be associated with pregnancy loss.

Intrauterine fetal demise can occur later in pregnancy, as can the long-term sequelae of fetal hypoxia, such as cerebral palsy, vital organ infarct, and even placental abruption. Another potential risk of surgical procedures is infection. Depending on the particular procedure, infection risk can be quite high. Infection is injurious to the fetus either by direct extension (intra-amniotic infection) or via sepsis, which can result in preterm labor. For procedures that carry a high risk of infectious morbidity, such as

appendicitis, antibiotic therapy should be instituted. In other instances, as soon as infection is suspected, antimicrobial agents should be initiated. The choice of the particular antimicrobial agent should be directed at the most likely source of infection. Avoidance of broad-spectrum antibiotics is preferable because of the risk of resistant organisms. This avoids reduction in available therapeutic modalities later in pregnancy or for the newborn. Certain antibiotics should be avoided during pregnancy because of their teratogenic potential. These include quinolones and tetracycline derivatives. Most other antibiotic therapies can be safely used (Box 26–1). However, even with drugs such as aminoglycosides, it is important to be sure that serum levels are both efficacious and safe by following peak and trough drug levels at intervals during treatment. This avoids ototoxicity and renal toxicity in the fetus, potential drug side effects.

Although there is certainly an appreciable risk to the fetus, when surgery occurs during pregnancy, it is usually well tolerated and can be safely performed. The outcome is most dependent on the gestational age at the time of the surgery and the ability to choose therapeutic agents and techniques that pose the least fetal harm.

Indications and Contraindications

Generally speaking, there are no absolute contraindications to surgery during pregnancy. The basic tenet of obstetrics is that maternal well-being comes first. Therefore, when surgery is absolutely indicated, it should be performed and not delayed because of pregnancy. Elective procedures, however, should be delayed until some time postpartum.

Table 26–4
Neonatal morbidity rate (percent) by gestational age at birth

	Gestational Age													
	24	25	26	27	28	29	30	31	32	33	34	35	36	37–38
Respiratory distress syndrome	66.7	87.0	92.6	83.9	64.3	52.8	54.7	37.3	28.0	33.9	13.5	6.4	3.3	4
Intraventricular hemorrhage, grades III and IV	25.0	30.4	29.6	16.1	3.6	2.8	1.9	2.0	.9	.0	.0	.0	.0	.0
Sepsis	25.0	8.7	33.3	35.5	25.0	25.0	11.3	13.7	2.8	5.4	3.5	2.3	1.3	.3
Necrotizing enterocolitis	8.3	17.4	11.1	9.7	25.0	13.9	15.1	7.8	5.6	1.8	3.1	.3	.9	.0
Patent ductus arteriosus	33.3	60.9	48.1	38.7	42.9	44.4	22.6	15.7	9.3	1.8	1.7	1.3	.4	.3
Phototherapy for hyperbilirubinemia	66.7	43.5	9.26	80.6	67.9	75.0	73.6	58.8	63.6	43.8	29.3	16.4	9.0	3.5
Exchange transfusion for hyperbilirubinemia	.0	4.3	3.7	6.5	.0	2.8	.0	.0	.9	.0	.9	.3	.4	.2
Hypoglycemia	8.3	17.4	14.8	9.7	7.1	8.3	5.7	3.9	4.7	3.6	4.4	4.4	1.1	.9
None of the above	16.7	4.3	.0	.0	7.1	5.6	9.4	21.6	28.0	40.2	58.5	74.8	86.6	94.8
Admission to neonatal intensive care unit	100.0	100.0	100.0	100.0	100.0	100.0	94.3	96.1	98.1	83.9	70.3	41.6	24.1	10.2
N	12	23	27	31	28	36	53	51	107.0	112	229	298	544	4803

From Robertson PA, Sniderman SH, Laros RK Jr, et al: Neonatal morbidity according to gestational age and birth weight from five tertiary centers in the United States, 1983 through 1986. Am J Obstet Gynecol 1992; 166:1629, with permission.

Box 26-1
Pregnancy Risk Categories of Available Antibiotics*

Aminoglycosides
Amikacin (C)
Gentamicin (C)
Kanamycin (D)
Neomycin (C)
Paromomycin (C)
Streptomycin (D)
Tobramycin (C/D$_M$)[†]

Antibiotics/Anti-infectives
Azithromycin (B$_M$)
Aztreonam (B$_M$)
Bacitracin (C)
Chloramphenicol (C)
Chlorhexidine (B)
Clarithromycin (C$_M$)
Clavulanate Potassium (B$_M$)
Clindamycin (B)
Colistimethate (B)
Dirithromycin (C$_M$)
Erythromycin (B)
Fosfomycin (B$_M$)
Furazolidone (C)
Hexachlorophene (C$_M$)
Imipenem-cilastatin
    sodium (C$_M$)
Lincomycin (B)
Meropenem (B$_M$)
Metronidozole (B$_M$)
Novobiocin (C)
Oleandomycin (C)
Pentamidine (C$_M$)
Polymyxin B (B)
Spectinomycin (B)
Spiramycin (C)

Trimethoprim (C$_M$)
Troleandomycin (C)
Vancomycin (C$_M$)

Antifungals
Amphotericin B (B)
Butoconazole (C$_M$)
Clotrimazole (B)
Fluconazole (C$_M$)
Ketoconazole (C$_M$)
Nystatin (B)
Terconazole (C$_M$)

Antivirals
Acyclovir (C$_M$)
Amantadine (C$_M$)
Didanosine (B$_M$)
Ganciclovir (C$_M$)
Indinavir (C$_M$)
Lamivudine (C$_M$)
Nevirapine (C$_M$)
Ribavirin (X$_M$)
Saquinavir (B$_M$)
Valacyclovir (B$_M$)
Zalcitabine (C$_M$)
Zidovudine (C$_M$)

Cephalosporins
Cefaclor (B$_M$)
Cefadroxil (B$_M$)
Cefamandole (B$_M$)
Cefatrizine (B$_M$)
Cefazolin (B$_M$)
Cefepime (B$_M$)
Cefixime (B$_M$)
Cefonicid (B$_M$)

Cefoperazone (B$_M$)
Ceforanide (B$_M$)
Cefotaxime (B$_M$)
Cefotetan (B$_M$)
Cefoxitin (B$_M$)
Cefpodoxime (B$_M$)
Cefprozil (B$_M$)
Ceftazidime (B$_M$)
Ceftibuten (B$_M$)
Ceftizoxime (B$_M$)
Ceftriaxone (B$_M$)
Cefuroxime (B$_M$)
Cephalexin (B$_M$)
Cephalothin (B$_M$)
Cephapirin (B$_M$)
Cephradine (B$_M$)
Loracarbef (B$_M$)
Moxalactam (C$_M$)

Iodine
Iodine (D)
Providone-iodine (D)

Leprostatics
Dapsone (C$_M$)

Penicillins
Amoxicillin (B)
Ampicillin (B)
Bacampicillin (B$_M$)
Carbenicillin (B)
Cloxacillin (B$_M$)
Cyclacillin (B$_M$)
Dicloxacillin (B$_M$)
Hetacillin (B)
Methicillin (B$_M$)

Nafcillin (B)
Oxacillin (B$_M$)
Penicillin G (B)
Penicillin G, benzathine (B)
Penicillin G, procaine (B)
Penicillin V (B)
Piperacillin (B$_M$)
Ticarcillin (B)

Quinolones
Ciprofloxacin (C$_M$)
Enoxacin (C$_M$)
Levofloxacin (C$_M$)
Lomefloxacin (C$_M$)
Nalidixic Acid (C$_M$)
Norfloxacin (C$_M$)
Ofloxacin (C$_M$)
Sparfloxacin (C$_M$)

Sulfonamides[‡]
Sulfasalazine (B/D)
Sulfonamides (B/D)

Tetracyclines
Chlortetracycline (D)
Clomocycline (D)
Demeclocycline (D)
Doxycycline (D)
Methacycline (D)
Minocycline (D)
Oxytetracycline (D)
Tetracycline (D)

Trichomonacide
Metronidazole (B$_M$)

Urinary Germicides
Nitrofurantoin (B)

Subscript M indicates manufacturer rating of risk.

[†]*Generally risk category C; risk category D if administered near term.*

[‡]*Generally risk category B; risk category D if administered near term.*

This is not only because of the pregnancy, but also because surgical outcome will be optimized for most elective procedures once the physiologic and hormonal changes of pregnancy are gone. What constitutes "elective" versus "nonelective" procedures can differ among providers.

A good rule of thumb is that any procedure whose delay would result in maternal morbidity or mortality can and should be performed during pregnancy. Those procedures that do not directly affect the mother medically should be delayed until a safer time during the mother's life (Table 26–5). Any emergency/ life-threatening condition that requires surgery should *not* be delayed because of pregnancy. This is not only because of the potential risk to the mother's life but also because of the direct relationship between maternal and fetal well-being. Cases such as this include trauma and any hemorrhagic or infectious condition that cannot be managed medically.

In other cases in which the maternal condition is best treated by surgery, it may be in the best interest of the fetus to delay the procedure. These procedures often include treatment for cancer, gallbladder disease, or other chronic conditions that become worse or exacerbated during pregnancy. In these instances, it is the gestational age that will determine the timing for surgery. A team of high-risk obstetricians, anesthesiologists, neonatologists, and surgeons best addresses the timing and approach for the procedure needed.

Pain Management in the Pregnant Patient

Although pregnancy and steroid hormones are believed to influence the expression of opioid receptors, basic pain management in the perioperative period is unchanged in the pregnant patient. The only significant difference is the avoidance of nonsteroidal anti-inflammatory medications unless indicated for tocolysis. Prostaglandin synthase inhibitors such as indomethacin and ibuprofen influence uterine contractility. This property makes them useful as tocolytics, but in doses smaller than commonly used for pain control. Patients undergoing tocolysis should be monitored for contractions, fetal heart rate abnormalities, and cervical change. Nonsteroidal anti-inflammatory medications can also cause oligohydramnios and premature closure of the fetal ductus arteriosus. Therefore, nonsteroidal anti-inflammatory medications should not be used for postoperative pain control without consultation with an obstetrician.

Acetaminophen is considered safe in pregnancy, unless the gravida has liver disease. Plain acetaminophen or combinations with narcotics are acceptable medications for mild postoperative pain. For moderate to severe postoperative pain, narcotics are the medications of choice in pregnancy. Although a fetus can develop narcotic dependence from long-term use of narcotics, this is not a concern in the perioperative period. An infant born shortly after maternal administration of narcotics with display respiratory depression, but this can be treated with naloxone and/or mechanical ventilation. If a postoperative pregnant woman goes into labor, she may be treated with narcotic pain medication until delivery is thought to be imminent. The neonatologist should be notified of recent narcotic administration. Narcotic medications may be administered by intravenous, intramuscular, and epidural routes. Patient-controlled analgesia via an intravenous route is also appropriate.

Although teratogenicity is of general concern in the first trimester, it should not affect postoperative pain management. Acetaminophen (FDA pregnancy risk category B) and narcotic pain medications (oxycodone, morphine, and fentanyl; FDA pregnancy risk category B) are not thought to cause birth defects.

It is important to treat pain appropriately in the postoperative gravida. Adequate pain control is as important during pregnancy as it is outside of pregnancy. It is unethical to deny pain control because of unfounded concerns for harm to the fetus. Furthermore, biochemical studies suggest that pain and stress can adversely influence uterine blood flow.

Table 26–5

Elective and nonelective surgery in pregnancy

Elective	Nonelective
Plastic and reconstructive surgery	Hemorrhage/trauma
Nonemergent cholecystectomy	Acute appendicitis
Nonemergent orthopedic procedures	Acute cholecystitis
Urinary stress incontinence repair	Suspected liver rupture
	Cancer resection
	Biopsy
	Abscess drainage
	Dental procedure (noncosmetic)
	Adnexal torsion/rupture

Anesthetic Considerations

Anesthetic management of the gravida is influenced by the physiologic changes of pregnancy. Management of general anesthesia must include consideration of an increased difficulty of intubation as a result of airway edema and increased vascularity of the nasal, oropharyngeal, and laryngeal mucosal linings. Furthermore, the decrease in FRC and increase in oxygen utilization result in a smaller window for safe intubation after induction of anesthesia. Because of increased gastroesophageal reflux and delayed gastric emptying, pregnant women are always treated as having "full stomachs," even if they have had nothing by mouth for several hours.

Nonparticulate antacids and β receptor antagonists are given preoperatively to neutralize the pH of gastric secretions in case of aspiration. Rapid-sequence induction is preferred, after adequate preoxygenation (because pregnant women desaturate more quickly). If a difficult airway is a concern, alternatives such as awake intubation should be considered. Continuous pulse oximetry is important in monitoring of anesthetized gravidas. Additionally, pregnant women should be wide awake for extubation to decrease the risk of aspiration.

The commonly used anesthetic agents are considered to be safe in pregnancy. Pregnant women are more sensitive to these agents, and the minimum alveolar concentration is decreased by 20% to 40%.

Regional anesthetics are considered safe in pregnancy. Preloading with intravenous crystalloid is used to prevent hypotension from vasodilatation. Ephedrine is considered the agent of choice for treating hypotension because of its beneficial effect on uterine blood flow. A hip wedge is used or the operating room table is tilted to prevent supine hypotension during both regional and general anesthesia.

Fetal Maturity and Elective Delivery

The second trimester of pregnancy, estimated to be between 13 and 23 weeks gestational age, is usually considered the safest time to perform surgery of any kind during pregnancy. This is because the fetus at this time is fully "formed" and therefore at a much reduced risk for any possible teratogenic or other harmful effects of medications that may be used. In the second trimester, the uterus is also not so large as to obstruct surgical procedures, and therefore less manipulation of the uterus is needed for visualization during surgery. This results in a reduced risk of premature labor and delivery as well as improved visualization for the surgery performed. At times, surgery must be scheduled to occur during pregnancy because of the nature of the condition.

Classically, cancer surgery, gallbladder surgery, necessary repairs of orthopedic conditions, and other surgeries may be delayed because of pregnancy, to be performed at a time when delivery of the fetus would be safe.

One consideration is scheduling of surgery to coincide with fetal lung maturity (FLM). FLM occurs at relatively predictable times in pregnancy. The risk of severe respiratory distress syndrome diminishes as pregnancy progresses toward term. This is directly related to the development of the fetal lung during pregnancy. Fetal lung development is divided into three stages: pseudoglandular, canalicular, and terminal sac. The pseudoglandular stage (7 to 17 weeks' gestation) is the progressive division of airways from terminal bronchioles to respiratory bronchioles. Simultaneously, arterial and venous pathways also develop. The venous pathways demarcate lung segments and subsegments. At this stage of development the distal tubules are lined with undifferentiated epithelial cells. The canalicular stage (16 to 25 weeks' gestation) represents the previable human lung. The importance of this stage is characterized by the development of type II alveolar cells necessary to assure gas exchange by maintaining open alveoli through the production of surfactant. Finally, the terminal sac stage (25 weeks' gestation to term) is characterized by alveolarization. At term, the human lung has 10 to 150 million alveoli (the adult lung has 300 million alveoli).

The major physiologic importance of these events is the rapid increase in potential lung gas volumes and surface area after about 25 weeks of gestation. At this time, there is potential for neonatal survival. It is important to recognize that the fetal lung is not filled with air, but rather with fluid. Lung fluid production is an intrinsic mechanism of the fetal lung. This fluid mixes with the amniotic fluid and is swallowed as well as mobilized in and out of the fetal lung. This process allows sampling of amniotic fluid around the fetus to provide indicators of FLM that are key features in decision making for elective delivery. Available methods for the evaluation of fetal pulmonary maturity involve measurements of surfactant (lecithin/sphingomyelin [L/S] ratio) and phosphatidylglycerol (PG).

The L/S ratio is perhaps the most important of the amniotic indices for the prediction of fetal lung maturity (Table 26–6). Developed by Gluck and associates, it was based upon the fact that the amniotic fluid concentration of lecithin increases by 35 weeks of gestation, while sphingomyelin levels remain the same or decrease. Amniotic fluid lecithin exceeds sphingomyelin until about 31 to 32 weeks' gestation, when the ratio of the two becomes 1. Lecithin then rises rapidly, and an L/S ratio of 2 is observed at approximately 35 weeks (Fig. 26–1). There is wide variation in the timing of the appearance of an L/S ratio of 2. It is usually associated with lung maturity (98%) and the absence of severe respiratory distress

Table 26–6
Tests of fetal lung maturity

Test	Principle	Mature Level	Advantages	Disadvantages
L/S ratio	Quantity of surfactant lecithin compared with sphingomyelin	≥ 2.0 (method dependent)	Few falsely mature values; not altered by changes in amniotic fluid volume	Many falsely immature values, long turnaround time, special laboratory equipment required
Lung profile	Includes determination of L/S ratio, percentage precipitable lecithin, PG, and PI	L/S ratio ≥ 2.0; >50% acetone-precipitable lecithin, 15–20% PI, 2–10% PG	Reduces falsely immature L/S ratios; PG not altered by blood, meconium	Requires more time and equipment than L/S ratio
Amniostat-FLM*	Immunologic test with agglutination in presence of PG	Test positive with PG ≥ 0.5 µg/mL amniotic fluid	Rapid, few falsely mature tests; can be used with contaminated specimens	Many falsely immature results
Disaturated phosphatidylcholine	Direct measure of primary phospholipid in surfactant	≥ 500 µg/dL	Few falsely mature tests; may reduce falsely immature tests	May be altered by changes in amniotic fluid volume
Microviscosimeter*	Fluorescence depolarization used to determine phospholipid membrane content	p < 0.310–0.336	Few falsely mature tests; fast, easily performed	Requires expensive equipment
Shake test*	Generation of stable foam by pulmonary surfactant in presence of ethanol	Complete ring of bubbles 15 min after shaking at 1:2 diluation	Few falsely mature tests; fast, easily performed	Concentration of reagents critical; many falsely immature results
Lumadex-FSI*	Modification of manual foam stability index; stable foam in presence of increasing concentration of ethanol	≥ 47	Few falsely mature tests; fast, easily performed	Concentration of reagents critical; some falsely immature results
Optical density*	Evaluates turbidity changes dependent on total phospholipid concentration	At 650 nm, ≥ 0.15	Few falsely mature tests; fast, easily performed	Many falsely immature results; need clear amniotic fluid

L/S, lecithin/sphingomyelin ratio; PG, phosphatidylglycerol; PI, phosphatidylinositol.

*Screening test.

Adapted from Gabbe S: Recent advances in the assessment of fetal lung maturity. J Reprod Med 1979;23:277.

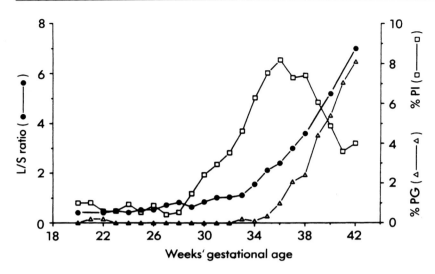

FIGURE 26–1 Lecithin/sphingomyelin (L/S) ratio, percentage phosphatidylglycerol (PG), and percentage phosphatidylinositol (PI) in amniotic fluid from normal pregnancies as a function of gestational age. (Data from Jobe A: Fetal lung development, test for maturation, induction of maturation and treatment. *In* Creasy RK, Resnik R [eds]: Maternal-Fetal Medicine. Philadelphia: Saunders, 1999:404.)

syndrome. Another test that can be performed on amniotic fluid is the slide agglutination test for PG. This test is a rapid, semiquantitative test that can detect PG in as little as 1.5 mL of amniotic fluid. Test results take approximately 20 to 30 minutes. The sensitivity is extremely high, and in studies no cases of respiratory distress syndrome occurred in the presence of a positive Amniostat-FLM.

A variety of other tests on amniotic fluid can be used to assess FLM; however, most of these are not in common usage. All of these tests are based upon the same chemical indicators of FLM that require either the presence of PG or an L/S ratio greater than 2. All of these tests also require the ability to do ultrasound-guided amniocentesis. While the risk of amniocentesis is low (<0.5%), it carries with it a risk of preterm premature rupture of the membranes, premature contractions/labor, puncture of placental or umbilical cord vasculature, or puncture of fetal parts. Fetal distress requiring cesarean section has also been reported from third-trimester amniocentesis. However, in general, when all the risks of the pregnancy, the medical condition, and the risks to the fetus are taken into consideration, the risk of amniocentesis is indeed low.

Once fetal lung maturity is assured, delivery can be accomplished. Vaginal delivery is the optimal method if at all possible. This can be accomplished with the assistance of cervical ripening agents and induction of labor.

There are very few contraindications to vaginal delivery (Table 26–7). However, there are fetal and other obstetric conditions that may preclude induction of labor and a trial for vaginal delivery. The most common indication for cesarean delivery in the premature infant is malpresentation. At term, less than 3% of fetuses are in the nonvertex position. As gestational age decreases, the likelihood of a nonvertex position increases (Table 26–8). Current obstetric management does not include induction of labor for breech or other malpresentations, especially in premature

infants, because of the likelihood for both mechanical and asphyxial trauma. Therefore, cesarean section may be indicated for optimal fetal outcome. Similarly, other obstetric indications, such as placenta previa, nonreassuring fetal status, or fetal anomalies, may make cesarean delivery preferable. The risk of cesarean delivery after induction of labor, especially at a premature gestational age, may also be increased. Finally, the nature of the surgical procedure may make cesarean delivery the preferred option so that both procedures can be combined and the patient may have a single recovery period (Box 26–2).

Table 26–7
Indications for cesarean section

Maternal	Fetal
Placenta previa	*Malpresentation
Prior classic cesarean section	*Hydrocephalus
*Prior uterine surgery	Certain fetal anomalies
*Pulmonary hypertension	Omphalocele
*IHSS	Bladder exstrophy
*Prior MI	Open neural tube defects
Alloimmune thrombocytopenia	Nonreassuring fetal testing
Obstructive uterine myomas	Fetal arrhythmia
*Cervical cancer	
*Multiple cesarean sections (>2)	

IHSS, idiopathic hypertrophic subacute stenosis; MI, myocardial infarction.
Relative indication.

Table 26–8	
Percent breech with advancing gestational age	
Gestational Age (wk)	**% Nonvertex**
18–24	24
28–30	7
38–40	2.8

Box 26–2

Common Surgical Procedures Performed at the Time of Cesarean Section

Cervical cancer
Adnexal pathology/malignancy
Bowel resection/repair
Bladder resection/repair

Complications of Pregnancy

Pregnancy itself may present complications that require surgical intervention. Clearly, cesarean section is one of the most commonly performed surgical procedures in the United States. Cesarean section delivery rates range from 10% to 25% depending upon the health center studied. Four indications have been found to account for most cesarean section deliveries: dystocia (30%), repeat cesarean (25% to 30%), breech presentation (10% to 15%), and "fetal distress" (10% to 15%). In general, delivery by cesarean section is a safe procedure, with mortality and morbidity rates directly related to underlying maternal medical conditions. There are conditions that arise as a result of cesarean section that may require further surgical intervention. These include hemorrhage, bowel obstruction, endometriosis in the wound site, and repeat cesarean delivery. For many years, there has been a national emphasis on vaginal birth after cesarean section. This had been based on many studies that showed a very high rate of successful vaginal delivery (up to 60%) and a very low rate of maternal and fetal complications (<1%) in the presence of a single prior low uterine segment transverse cesarean section. The major complication suffered was catastrophic uterine rupture, which could result in maternal and fetal death. Recent data suggest that there may be higher complication rates to both the mother and especially the fetus than have previously been suggested. Therefore, although vaginal birth after cesarean is still considered safe, the number of repeat cesarean deliveries is anticipated to increase.

Other complications relating to pregnancy that may require surgical intervention include ectopic pregnancy and severe preeclampsia/hemolysis, elevated liver enzymes, and low platelet count in association with preeclampsia (HELLP) syndrome. Ectopic pregnancy rates have been rising in the United States. This is in some part due to technological advances in therapies for disease states that may affect tubal function. It may also be due to sociological changes affecting sexual activity. Despite the increase in the absolute number of ectopic pregnancies in the United States, surgical therapy as a primary modality has declined. This is because of early diagnosis via quantitation of pregnancy hormones (human chorionic gonadotropin) as well as the advancements in ultrasound diagnostic capabilities (Fig. 26–2). Many women with the diagnosis of early ectopic pregnancy can be adequately treated with the chemotherapeutic agent methotrexate and avoid surgical intervention (Fig. 26–3).

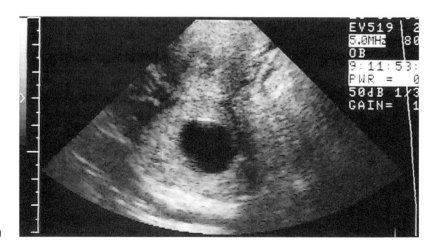

FIGURE 26–2 Ultrasound image of ectopic pregnancy. (Courtesy of the Division of Maternal-Fetal Medicine, Eastern Virginia Medical School, Norfolk, VA.)

Methotrexate Therapy for Ectopic Pregnancies

Criteria for Eligibility

1. Hemodynamically stable
2. Stable living situation
3. Availability of responsible adult for 24 to 48 hr
4. Fetal heart tones is a "relative" contraindication

Lab and Diagnostic Criteria

1. CBC, Type and Screen
2. SMA-18
3. Quantitative β-HCG < 15,000
4. Gestational sac size < 4 cm
5. No chronic hepatic or renal disease

Treatment

1. Document discussion of risks, benefits, alternatives, and consent in chart
2. Consider 23 hr admission for significant discomfort
3. Methotrexate (MTX) dose = 50 mg/M^2 on day 1. Calculate and recheck with 3rd or 4th yr resident, attending or pharmacy before writing order.
4. Advise patient that to call for ↑ pain, orthostatic sx, heavy vaginal bleeding, F/C/N/V
5. Advise patient she may experience increased pain on days 3 to 5

Follow-up

1. β-HCG levels on day 4 and 7. (Day 4 = baseline after 1st MTX R$_x$)
2. Day 7 expect decrease ≥15% of baseline—if not repeat MTX dose as above
3. Repeat β-HCG levels q wk until negative

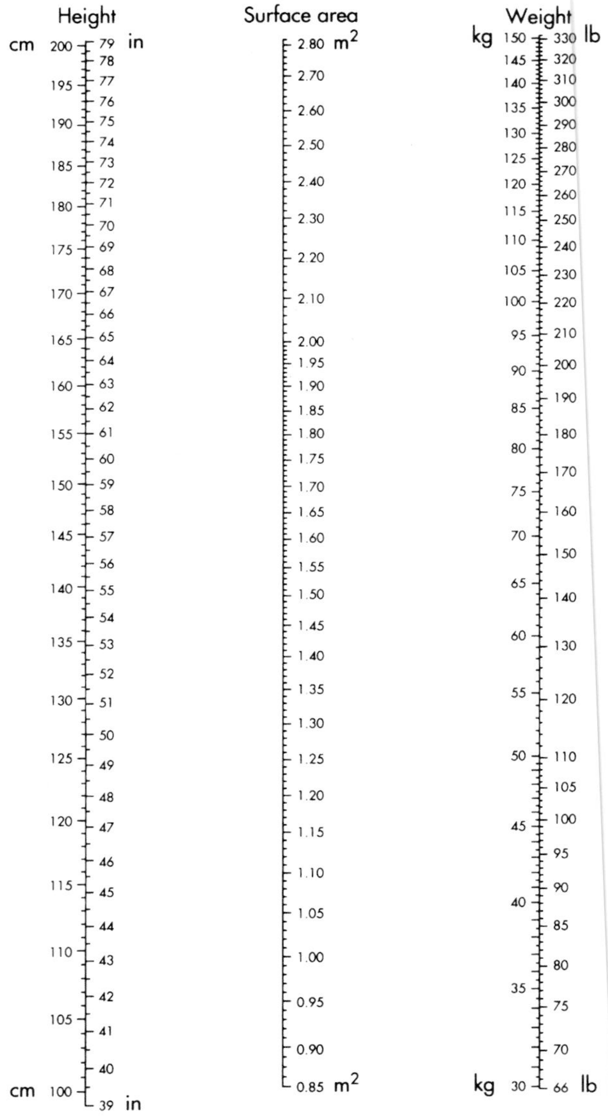

FIGURE 26–3 Data on methotrexate therapy for ectopic pregnancies. (From DiSasa PJ, Creasman WT: Epithelial ovarian cancer. *In* Clinical Gynecologic Oncology [4th ed]. St. Louis: Mosby–Year Book, 1993, with permission.)

An additional group of women can be treated for more advanced ectopic pregnancy via laparoscopic surgery to avoid complications of other more invasive surgical procedures. This leaves only a small percentage of women who require exploratory laparotomy for the treatment of ectopic gestation. In most of these cases, the laparotomy is reserved for emergent, large, or complicated cases.

One of the most catastrophic indications for extensive surgery during pregnancy is liver rupture as a consequence of preeclampsia/HELLP syndrome. Although a rare complication (1 in 45,000 live births), until recently maternal mortality rates exceeded 60%. Most of this mortality has been due to delayed diagnosis. In the setting of preeclampsia, shock, and right upper quadrant pain, the obstetrician and the surgeon should proceed to the operating room together. The advent of advances in imaging techniques has improved the prognosis of liver rupture. Similarly, less invasive surgical techniques such as packing and embolization rather than hepatic resection have lessened both the morbidity and mortality.

Summary

Pregnancy does not afford protection from other medical conditions and indeed may pose maternal risk. Therefore, surgical intervention may be necessary during pregnancy for many indications. Pregnancy poses a unique clinical circumstance wherein management decisions affect not just one, but two separate individuals. It must be remembered that fetal health and well-being are directly related to that of the mother. Surgical procedures for life-threatening events should never be delayed because of pregnancy. Similarly, purely elective procedures that can best be performed outside of pregnancy should be postponed. In other cases, where surgery provides the optimal therapy for a maternal condition, every consideration to assure fetal well-being should be entertained. In such instances, awaiting an optimal time in pregnancy and documenting FLM followed by delivery will not only allow for the best possible pregnancy outcome, but in most circumstances will facilitate the surgical procedure as well. In all cases, communication between surgeons, obstetricians, anesthesiologists, and neonatologists will assure that every aspect of maternal and child health is well attended.

Bibliography

Ashwood ER: Standards of laboratory practice: evaluation of fetal lung maturity. Clin Chem 1997;43:211.

Chan MTV, Mainland P, Gin T: Minimum alveolar concentration of halothane and enflurane are decreased in early pregnancy. Anesthesiology 1996;85:782.

Cugell DW, Frank NR, Gaensler ER, et al: Pulmonary function in pregnancy: serial observations in normal women. Am Rev Tuberc 1953;67:568.

Duncan PG, Pope WEB, Cohen MM, Greer N: Fetal risk of anesthesia and surgery during pregnancy. Anesthesiology 1986;64:790.

Gabbe S: Recent advances in the assessment of fetal lung maturity. J Reprod Med 1979;23:277.

Galle PC, Meis PG: Complications of amniocentesis: a review. J Reprod Med 1982;27:149.

Gluck L, Kulovich M, Borer R, et al: The interpretation and significance of the lecithin/sphingomyelin ratio in amniotic fluid. Am J Obstet Gynecol 1974;120:142.

Greiss FC: Uterine vascular response to hemorrhage during pregnancy. Obstet Gynecol 1966;27:549.

Jobe AH: Fetal lung development, tests for maturation, induction of maturation and treatment. In Creasy RK, Resnik R (eds): Maternal-Fetal Medicine. Philadelphia: WB Saunders, 1999:404.

Lederman RP, Lederman E, Work BA, et al: The relationship of maternal anxiety, plasma catecholamines, and plasma cortisol to progress in labor. Am J Obstet Gynecol 1978;132:495.

Mabie WC, DiSessa TG, Crocker LG, et al: A longitudinal study of cardiac output in normal human pregnancy. Am J Obstet Gynecol 1994;170:849.

Mazze RI, Kallen B: Reproductive outcome after anesthesia and operation during pregnancy: a registry of 5404 cases. Am J Obstet Gynecol 1989;161:1178.

McGrath JM, Chestnut DH, Vincent RD, et al: Ephedrine remains the vasopressor of choice for treatment of hypotension during ritodrine infusion and epidural anesthesia. Anesthesiology 1994;80:1073.

McMahon MJ, Luther ER, Bowes WA Jr, et al: Comparison of a trial of labor with an elective second cesarean section. N Engl J Med 1996;335:689.

Mourad J, Elliott JP, Erickson L, et al: Appendicitis in pregnancy: new information that contradicts long-held clinical beliefs. Am J Obstet Gynecol 2000;182:1027.

Newton ER: Surgical problems in pregnancy. Clin Obstet 1996;35:1.

Niermeyer S, Kattwinkel J, Van Reempts P, et al: International Guidelines for Neonatal Resuscitation: An excerpt from the Guidelines 2000 for Cardiopulmonary Resuscitation and Emergency Cardiovascular Care: International Consensus on Science. Contributors and Reviewers for the Neonatal Resuscitation Guidelines. Pediatrics 2000;106:E29.

Pereira AP, O'Donohue J, Wendon J, et al: Hepatic rupture: maternal and perinatal outcome in severe pregnancy-related liver disease. Hepatology 1997;26:1258.

Pritchard JA: Changes in the blood volume during pregnancy and delivery. Anesthesiology 1965;26:393.

Rosen MG (Chairman): Cesarean section rates: Consensus Task Force on Cesarean Childbirth (NIH Publication No 82-2022). Bethesda, MD: National Institutes of Health, 1981.

Rosen MG, Dickinson JC, Westhoft CL: Vaginal birth after cesarean: a meta-analysis of morbidity and mortality. Obstet Gynecol 1991;77:465.

Scott JR: Mandatory trial of labor after cesarean delivery: an alternative viewpoint. Obstet Gynecol 1991;77:811.

Smith LG, Moise KJ, Dildy GA, et al: Spontaneous rupture of the liver during pregnancy: current therapy. Obstet Gynecol 1991;77:171.

Wittich AC, DeSantis RA, Lockrow EG: Appendectomy during pregnancy: a survey of two army medical activities. Mil Med 1999;164:671.

Young BK: Report on third trimester amniocentesis at New York University Medical Center, New York. In Antenatal Diagnosis: Report of a Consensus Development Conference, March 5–7. Bethesda, MD: National Institutes of Health, 1979:II-61.

Yudkin P, Frumar AM, Anderson ABM, et al: Increased risk of cesarean section with induction: a retrospective study in induction of labor. Br J Obstet Gynaecol 1979;86:257.

Zhu Y, Pintar JE: Expression of opioid receptors and ligands in pregnant mouse uterus and placenta. Biol Reprod 1998;59:925.

CHAPTER 27

The Elderly Surgical Patient

Lisa S. Dresner, M.D., F.A.C.S. and Michael E. Zenilman, M.D., F.A.C.S.

As the population of the United States ages more and more, elderly patients become candidates for major elective and emergency surgical procedures. Elderly patients benefit from a variety of elective and emergency surgical procedures because *average* life expectancy for elderly patients is often underestimated. In fact, statistically the average life expectancy of a person who has reached the age of 65 is 17.5 years, and that for a 75-year-old is 11 years. Surgeons of all types must understand the changes in physiology that occur with aging, how to assess risk of surgery, and how to minimize comorbidity in their elderly patients. The goal of this chapter is to provide a foundation for the practicing surgeon for evaluation and management of the elderly patient.

The Problem

It should be no surprise that increased age adversely affects operative mortality and morbidity. In one study, mortality risk was 0.8% for patients 21 to 30 years of age, 3.1% for those 51 to 60 years of age, 6.8% for those 71 to 80 years of age, and 8.2% for those greater than 80. Mortality is similarly stratified for the oldest of the old, with mortality for patients greater than 100 reported as high as 15%. Several factors other than age contribute to the complexity of assessment of perioperative risk. The incidence of concurrent disease rises significantly with age to as much as 90% of 71- to 80-year-olds. In addition, the elderly population is a very heterogeneous one. Some have multiple medical ailments and limited cardiovascular reserve, while others of the same age are generally healthy and live an active, independent life. Although gradual and progressive loss of organ function is inevitable, the rate of decline varies widely across the population. Therefore, the ability to recover from stress of surgery varies across the population of elderly.

Physiologic Changes That Occur with Aging

Aging is accompanied by predictable declines in organ systems as well as a decrease in physiologic reserve that is manifest as a decreased ability to maintain homeostasis. Mortality from surgery, trauma, and systemic infection increases consistently with age, but physiologic status seems to be a more important determinant of outcome. Some elderly persons live independently and continue moderate physical activity, with preserved muscle mass and cardiovascular reserve, and therefore their responses to stress are similar to those of younger patients. In contrast, other elderly patients require care for their daily activities, and have multiple chronic medical conditions that include cardiovascular and pulmonary disease. This cohort of patients has much more substantial surgery-associated risks. Knowing the physiologic changes that occur with aging is important to assessing and managing risk.

Body Composition

Aging causes substantial changes in body composition. With advancing age there is a substantial decline in muscle mass, with up to 40% loss by age 80. This loss of lean body mass is balanced by a proportional increase in body fat. Therefore, an overall decrease in intracellular water and thus total body water occurs. Plasma volume is *unchanged* in physically active and healthy patients but may be substantially reduced in those who are bedridden, deconditioned, chronically ill, hypertensive, or on chronic diuretics.

Metabolic Activity

Basal resting metabolic activity decreases with aging as well. Metabolic activity decreases in direct proportion to the age-related loss of lean body mass. This loss of muscle mass results in a 30% to 50% decrease in maximal and resting oxygen consumption. In clinical practice, this is manifest as decreased resting cardiac output and a relatively diminished rise in cardiac output with stress. This may impair response to stress and illness, and also impairs the ability to maintain body temperature. Therefore, it is important to avoid the increase in morbidity associated with hypothermia by using a variety of clinical methods to prevent and treat hypothermia. Ambient temperature should be increased, intravenous fluids infused at body temperature, and air-warming blankets routinely used.

Renal Function

With advancing age, total kidney glomerular mass and renal cortical blood flow are decreased. Decreased glomerular filtration rate and measured creatinine clearance may not be reflected as an increase in serum creatinine above normal until renal function is severely impaired. This is due to loss of muscle mass and decreased muscle turnover and may be more pronounced in chronically ill and deconditioned patients. Any small rise in serum creatinine, therefore, signals a significant change in renal function. Thus nephrotoxic drugs and dehydration should be avoided in elderly patients, and renal function carefully monitored when nephrotoxic drugs are given.

Glucose Physiology

As humans age, there is a progressive decrease in the ability to handle a glucose load. It takes 50% longer for elderly adults without clinically diagnosed diabetes to return to fasting glucose levels compared to young adults. This change occurs in all patients, including those who have normal fasting glucose levels. This is likely due to impaired insulin function and secretion and insulin antagonism. Furthermore, decreased lean body mass results in diminished capacity to store carbohydrates. These changes result in increased risk for hyperglycemia and hypoglycemia in the perioperative period, and during other treatments where fasting is required. Poor glucose control during critical illness seems to impair immune function and increases risk of infection and death.

Immune Function

The decline in immune function that occurs with advancing age leads to increased risk of infection and cancer rates. Measurable changes in immune function occur gradually with advancing age. T-cell function specifically declines; this may be due to loss of thymus function and total lifetime exposure to antigens. In contrast, humoral immunity and macrophage function generally are preserved. Cytokine production, responsible for differentiation, proliferation, and survival of lymphoid cells, undergoes complex changes, with increased production of proinflammatory cytokines with aging. The impact of this change is important. The risk of acquiring a nosocomial infection is three times greater in the elderly, with hospital-acquired pneumonia occurring in about 15% of elderly surgical patients and increasing mortality by 20% to 50%. Risk factors for nosocomial pneumonia include aspiration, chronic lung disease, mechanical ventilation, pre-existing or acquired malnutrition, thoracoabdominal surgery, altered consciousness, and immunosuppression.

Nutritional Status

The risk and morbidity of infection specifically depend on immune responses and on nutritional status before the onset of illness in aged subjects. Protein-energy malnutrition is found in more than 50% of hospitalized elderly patients and in most with chronic diseases. In addition, micronutrient deficit appears to be common in independent-living, otherwise apparently healthy elderly subjects. Micronutrient deficits are now thought to be partly responsible for the decreased immune responses observed in the healthy elderly. Nutritional support in the elderly therefore may improve metabolic processes as well as maintain body reserves and should be considered as a necessary adjuvant therapy in the treatment of elderly patients.

Nutritional depletion has been documented frequently in adult surgical patients. In the elderly in particular, this has serious implications for health and for recovery from illness or surgery. Furthermore, among those whose nutritional status is borderline, the stress of illness may bring about deficiency. In addition, failure to correct malnutrition contributes to delayed recovery and prolonged hospital stay.

A careful examination and history are important in order to identify patients with nutritional risks. Several methods should be used to increase diagnostic accuracy in suspected malnutrition. For example, calculation of weight loss over time, muscle mass–height comparisons, and biochemical and hematologic measurements are important. Enteral feeding with supplementation as needed is the best first choice because it sustains the integrity of the gastrointestinal tract. Nutritional goals for the elderly patients are not significantly different from those for other adults, which generally are 30 to 35 kcal/kg/day, including 0.7 to 1 g/kg/day of protein. Parenteral nutrition is used to fill the gap between intake and needs. Vitamin and mineral supplementation should be remembered. It also is important to remember to continue supplementation throughout the postoperative period because energy, protein, and vitamin needs are increased from baseline as a result of stress of surgery and wound healing.

Respiratory Function

A significant contribution to excess operative risk in the elderly is respiratory complications that are in part due to age-related changes. Aging is accompanied by readily measurable changes in respiratory system mechanics, gas exchange, ventilatory control, and respiratory muscle strength (Table 27–1). Specifically, forced vital capacity decreases with age while total lung capacity is unchanged. With loss of elasticity, closing volume increases over the lifetime from 5% to 10% of total lung capacity at age 20 to 30% at age 70. These changes are not generally evident in the lives of healthy elderly individuals because of the substantial functional reserve of the respiratory system. The most consistent age-related change can be measured as an increase in residual volume and a decrease in ventilatory capacity. This loss of reserve may be exacerbated by a lifetime of tobacco use, environmental and occupational exposures, and other illnesses. In the perioperative period, the loss of excess capacity becomes important. Operative stresses, pain, and bed rest are always less tolerated by the respiratory system of elderly patients. Changes in chemoreceptor and respiratory center function result in impaired responses to hypoxemia and hypercapnia. Therefore, an elderly patient with impending respiratory failure may appear comfortable and without tachypnea. Overall outcome may depend on prevention and early recognition of and early intervention for respiratory dysfunction.

Cardiovascular Function

Cardiovascular illness is increasingly the most common cause of death with advanced age (Table 27–2). Anatomically, the cardiovascular system demonstrates aging long before middle age. Fibrous plaque is present in large blood vessels in as many as 30% of persons ages 15 to 24, and in 85% of persons ages 35 to 44. With aging, there is an overall increase in arterial stiffness of large vessels, which results in left ventricular hypertrophy. Atherosclerosis during aging also affects the coronary artery system, with stenoses (i.e., more than 50% decrease in luminal diameter) documented in half of those ages 55 to 64. Advanced large and small vessel disease leads to myocardial ischemia and excess cardiac work, ultimately leading to diastolic dysfunction and heart failure. The incidence of coronary artery disease also increases markedly with advanced age; however, it may not be evident until perioperative stress. This is particularly true in disabled patients with limited exercise in their day-to-day life.

Cardiac output at rest and with exercise declines with age. Diastolic dysfunction occurs commonly, and causes an increased dependence of ventricular filling (preload) on atrial contraction (the atrial kick). Myocardial infarction and myocardial ischemia cause global myocardial dysfunction and contribute to decreased cardiac output. Maximal heart rate in response to stress is decreased as well. Older individuals often exhibit little change in heart

Table 27–1
Changes in the respiratory system with aging

Airways	Calcification, disease-related changes
Lung parenchyma	Enlarged alveoli, loss of elasticity, ventilation-perfusion mismatch
Respiratory muscles and diaphragm	Decrease in respiratory muscle strength; increased chest wall rigidity
Control of ventilation	Decreased responses to hypoxemia and hypercapnia

Table 27–2
Causes of death in people age 65 and older, United States, 1999

Diseases of the heart	35.05%
Malignant neoplasm	22.15%
Cerebrovascular disease	8.10%
Chronic obstructive pulmonary disease	5.44%
Pneumonia and influenza	4.40%
Diabetes	2.72%
Unintentional injury	1.79%
Alzheimer's disease	1.28%
Renal disease	1.26%
Sepsis	1.05%

Data from Kramarow E, et al: Health and Aging Chartbook: Health, United States 1999. Hyattsville, MD: National Center for Health Statistics, 1999.

rate with exercise or stress. They increase cardiac output less efficiently by increasing stroke volume via raised end-diastolic volume. This occurs in patients with or without β-blocker treatment.

Congestive heart failure (CHF) is the end result of abnormal hypertrophy of the left ventricle, and is typically associated with long-standing significant hypertension or coronary artery disease. The incidence of CHF is six times higher in patients ages 65 to 74 years when compared to those 45 to 54 years. The renin-angiotensin-aldosterone system is activated during CHF, which promotes fluid retention and worsened CHF. Angiotensin II is the main target for drug therapy today for CHF. Blocking its action will reduce fluid overload, cardiac afterload, and the innate cardiac hypertrophy seen in CHF. Angiotensin-converting enzyme inhibitors are first-line therapy for CHF. Preserving cardiac function by treatment of hypertension and hyperlipidemia are important and life-extending therapies. Furthermore, there is evidence that perioperative treatment with β-blockers decreases mortality.

Risk Assessment

Assessment of risk will assist patients and their surgeons with decision making in planning surgical therapy. History and physical examination remain essential in preoperative assessment and are the first screen of cardiac risk of surgery. Medical history, medication use, and exercise tolerance will give clues to a patient's cardiac reserve. Careful examination for evidence of heart failure, S_3 gallop, murmurs, and arrhythmias will provide other important information.

A classical strategy to assess cardiac risk of patients undergoing noncardiac surgery was outlined by Goldman in 1977 and has been refined subsequently by Goldman and others. Goldman used history, physical exam, and type of surgery planned, among other factors, to identify criteria that increased the risk of cardiac complications, such as infarction, arrhythmia, and death. Goldman's multifactorial cardiac risk index is shown in Box 27–1. In Goldman's study, age greater than 70 was not as important as cardiac disease in determining risk of death. Goldman's analysis identifies patients for whom there is a significant risk of mortality and morbidity so that medical and cardiovascular intervention can be attempted to decrease risk or planned surgery can be altered. Control of blood pressure, treatment with β-blockers, and correction of critical coronary artery stenosis with angioplasty have been shown to decrease perioperative risk of cardiovascular morbidity and mortality.

The American Society of Anesthesiologists (ASA) physical status classification is another important tool that has been validated for assessment of perioperative

---

Box 27–1

Goldman Cardiac Risk Classification Variables

History: age >70, myocardinal infraction within 6 mo

Physical exam: S_3 gallop or jugular venous distention or aortic valvular disease

Electrocardiogram: rhythm other than sinus or atrial premature contraction

General status

- Po_2 <60 mm Hg, Pco_2 >50 mm Hg
- Serum potassium <3 mEg/L
- BUN >50 mg/dL, or creatinine >3 mg/dL
- Serum bicarbonate <20
- Liver disease/abnormal aspartate transaminase value
- Bedridden from noncardiac cause

Operation

- Intrathoracic, intraperitoneal, aortic
- Emergency

Adapted from Goldman L, Caldera DL, Nussbaum SR, et al: Multifactorial index of cardiac risk in noncardiac surgical procedures. N Engl J Med 1977;297:845, with permission. Copyright 1977 Massachusetts Medical Society. All rights reserved.

---

risk (Table 27–3). This scale divides patients into five groups based on general clinical criteria and gross severity of coexisting medical disease. Class I indicates a healthy patient undergoing elective surgery and class V is a moribund patient unlikely to survive 24 hours with or without surgery. ASA classification has been shown to accurately predict postoperative mortality even in patients older than 80 years.

Table 27–3

American Society of Anesthesiologists physical status classification

Class I	A normal, healthy patient
Class II	A patient with mild systemic disease
Class III	A patient with severe systemic disease that limits activity but is not incapacitating
Class IV	A patient with an incapacitating systemic disease that is a constant threat to life
Class V	A moribund patient not expected to survive 24 hr with or without an operation
Prefix E	In the event of an emergency operation, precede the number with an "E"

History of exercise tolerance and even the ability to perform activities of daily living may be the most sensitive predictor of perioperative complications in the elderly. A study that compared predictive tests, including the Goldman clinical criteria and ASA physical status criteria, demonstrated that the inability to increase heart rate to 99 while doing 2 minutes of exercise was the most sensitive predictor of perioperative morbidity and mortality. Other measures of functional capacity, such as the ability to perform activities of daily living, also have been correlated with postoperative mortality and morbidity. Preoperative functional deficits also contribute to postoperative immobility and its associated complications, such as atelectasis and pneumonia, venous stasis and pulmonary embolism, and multisystem deconditioning.

Evaluation of all elderly patients should begin with a careful medical history and review of symptoms and lifestyle. Additional tests to assess cardiovascular risk should be undertaken as appropriate. Healthy, active patients without chronic disease undergoing a relatively low- or moderate-risk surgical procedure do not need any perioperative cardiovascular or pulmonary testing other than an electrocardiogram. Others, such as patients with physical disabilities, deconditioning, or chronic medical disease or those undergoing high-risk surgery, should undergo additional testing. Echocardiography, for example, will identify global cardiac myocardial and valvular function as well as demonstrate any wall motion abnormalities. Stress testing may be especially important in patients who are physically disabled or deconditioned, those with diabetes, or patients undergoing higher risk elective procedures. Baseline arterial blood gas determination or oximetry may identify patients with significant pulmonary risk. Wherever possible, patients with chronic medical conditions such as hypertension, CHF, diabetes, and chronic lung disease should have their medical therapies optimized before surgery to ensure optimal outcome.

Bibliography

Chakravarti B, Abraham GN: Aging and T-cell-mediated immunity. Mech Ageing Dev 1999;108:183.

Chung OY, Beattie C, Friesinger GC: Cardiovascular disease in the elderly: assessment of overall risks for noncardiac surgery. Cardiol Clin 1999;17:197.

Gerson MC, Hurst JM, Hertzberg VS, et al: Prediction of cardiac and pulmonary complications related to elective abdominal and noncardiac thoracic surgery in geriatric patients. Am J Med 1990;88:101.

Hosking MP, Warner MA, Lobdell CM, et al: Outcomes of surgery in patients over 90 years of age. JAMA 1989;261:1909.

Josephson RA, Lakatta EG: Cardiovascular changes in the elderly. *In* Katlic MR (ed): Geriatric Surgery. Baltimore: Urban & Schwarzenburg, 1990:63.

Khuri SF, Daley J, Henderson W, et al: Risk adjustment of the postoperative mortality rate for the comparative assessment of the quality of surgical care: results of the National Veterans Affairs Surgical Risk Study. J Am Coll Surg 1997;185:315.

Kramarow E, et al: Health and Aging Chartbook: Health, United States 1999. Hyattsville, MD: National Center for Health Statistics, 1999.

Lesourd B: Immune response during disease and recover in the elderly. Proc Nutr Soc 1999;58:85.

Lesourd B, Mazari L: Nutrition and immunity in the elderly. Proc Nutr Soc 1999;58:685.

Poldermans D, Boersma E, Bax JJ, et al: The effect of bisoprolol on perioperative mortality and myocardial infarction in high-risk patients undergoing vascular surgery. N Engl J Med 1999;341:1789.

Van den Berghe G, Wouters P, Weekers F, et al: Intensive insulin therapy in critically ill patients. N Engl J Med 2001;345:1359.

Wei JY: Age and the cardiovascular system. N Engl J Med 1992;327:1735.

Zenilman ME (ed): Gastrointestinal Surgery in the Elderly. Probl Gen Surg 1997:13.

CHAPTER 28

The Pediatric Surgical Patient

Robert W. Letton, Jr., M.D., F.A.C.S., F.A.A.P. and
Walter J. Chwals, M.D., F.A.C.S., F.A.A.P.

The perioperative care of infants and children presents many differences in management compared to the perioperative adult patient. Even within the pediatric population itself, there is a tremendous amount of variation depending on the age, maturity, and weight of the patient. This chapter is intended to touch on some of these differences and provide a framework upon which to base decisions regarding perioperative fluids, electrolytes, and nutrition in the pediatric surgical patient. In addition, a brief discussion of the important metabolic differences encountered in infants and children is provided.

Critical Parameters

Temperature

Temperature regulation is critical in infants and neonates. Because of their large body surface area in relation to body weight and their decreased subcutaneous fat, infants lose significant amounts of heat when exposed to ambient atmosphere. In addition, there is a reduced lean body mass for generating heat compared with older children and adults. Hypothermia can be a significant problem in the operating room or emergency department if one does not actively attempt to keep the child warm. Most of the heat loss occurs as loss to the atmosphere through convection and evaporation. In the nursery setting, premature infants are kept in covered incubators to decrease loss through convection and evaporation. In the operating room, the room temperature must be raised and warming lights utilized to prevent hypothermia in infants and children. Furthermore, rapid infusion of cold crystalloid or colloid will further aggravate heat loss, and all measures for warming the fluids used to resuscitate the patient, as well as those used for irrigation, skin prep, and the like, should be employed. A more complete discussion of evaporative losses is included in the Fluid and Electrolytes section below.

Temperature can be monitored by measuring skin temperature or rectal temperature. In the operating room, esophageal temperature probes are utilized as well. Skin temperature is usually 1°C less than oral temperature, and rectal temperature is approximately 1°C more than oral temperature. Skin temperature should not be allowed to drop below 35°C, nor rectal temperature below 36°C. Active rewarming must be considered when temperatures drop below these levels.

Body Weight

Serial body weight measurements, in addition to measurement of urine output, are the easiest and most reliable monitors for volume status in infants and children. Most acute changes in body weight occur as a result of changes in body water, and serial measurement allows the physician to accurately monitor fluid losses and helps determine the volume of fluid replacement. It must be kept in mind that infants go through a normal diuresis period the first 24 to 48 hours of life to reduce extracellular fluid volume and total body water (TBW), and therefore body weight will decrease in the first few days of life.

Oxygenation and Ventilation

The umbilical artery can be easily cannulated in the critically ill newborn infant for arterial blood gas monitoring. In the infant with persistent fetal circulation, one must keep in mind that this line will be postductal in position. Mixing of unoxygenated blood as it bypasses the lungs through the patent ductus arteriosus with oxygenated blood from the left ventricle just past the left subclavian takeoff will result in a lower oxygen tension. Arterial partial pressure of oxygen and carbon dioxide ($PaCO_2$) can be readily determined. Capillary or venous aspiration can be used to determine pH and partial pressure of carbon dioxide (PCO_2) relatively accurately as long as the infant is perfusing well. Capillary PCO_2 tends to run approximately 5 mm Hg higher than $PaCO_2$ and capillary pH approximately 0.05 units lower.

Pulse oximetry is now standard in all nurseries and pediatric wards. It is based on the light absorption properties of oxygenated and unoxygenated hemoglobin. It is readily available and provides accurate monitoring of pulse rate and oxygen saturation, and the probe can remain in place for days. Monitoring of the concentration of carbon dioxide at the end of expiration, or end-tidal CO_2 ($ETCO_2$), is also available in most pediatric intensive care units and nurseries. A monitor can be placed in line with the endotracheal tube on ventilated children, and $ETCO_2$ continuously monitored. $ETCO_2$ runs approximately 5 mm Hg higher than $PaCO_2$, similar to a capillary blood gas value.

Cardiac Function

Continual monitoring of heart rate with electrocardiography and of arterial blood pressure with an automatic blood pressure cuff or arterial line is mandatory in critically ill infants and children. One must take care when monitoring blood pressure to choose an appropriate-sized cuff. A cuff that is too large for the patient tends to overestimate the blood pressure, whereas one that is too small will underestimate it. Another disadvantage of blood pressure monitoring with a cuff is the difficulty of detecting the pulse with palpation or auscultation in infants and children. Automatic cuffs, which utilize Doppler to detect the loss

and return of pulse, are more accurate. However, they still do not allow for continuous monitoring of pressure, and, in situations where minute-to-minute pressure changes must be monitored, an arterial line is appropriate. Even in the smallest of children, most arterial lines can be established via percutaneous technique. The radial artery is used most commonly, but the posterior tibial artery can be used as well. In neonates, the umbilical artery can be used sometimes for as long as 2 to 3 days after conception.

Very rarely are Swan-Ganz catheters used in the management of critically ill infants and children. Some postoperative cardiac patients may benefit from them, as well as some older, severely injured trauma patients with closed head injury or cardiac dysfunction. In children with an otherwise healthy heart, central venous pressure correlates well with blood volume, and is utilized frequently for managing children in the intensive care unit. Central venous catheters can be placed safely in the internal jugular, subclavian, or even femoral position in children as small as 1000 g by a physician accustomed to this. Cutdown and placement via the external jugular, facial vein, or internal jugular is possible as well. There are some data to suggest that lines placed by a cutdown approach tend to have a higher rate of infection. The external jugular is a readily available vein, but, in our experience, it can be difficult to direct the tip of the catheter into the vena cava without the use of fluoroscopy.

Shock

Shock is the inadequate delivery of oxygen and substrate to the tissues to meet demand. It is not a state that can be easily detected just by evaluating the vital signs. There is no particular blood pressure or pulse rate that defines it. Obviously vital signs are useful tools in assessing whether or not a child is in shock, but children have such physiologic reserve that waiting for a change in vital signs will often dangerously delay the child's resuscitation. Normal pediatric vital signs are listed in Table 28–1. Most children respond to shock with an increase in pulse rate, although neonates and children with profound shock will often become bradycardic. Because the child's blood pressure is already lower than that in an adult, the change that may occur is very small and difficult to distinguish. Waiting for hypotension to occur before diagnosing shock is inappropriate, and other clinical variables should be monitored to detect it sooner.

Mental status changes and lethargy may be the earliest warning signs. Decreased skin perfusion with increased capillary refill time and cool extremities soon follow. The skin may appear mottled, the child does not respond to painful stimuli appropriately, and slight tachycardia occurs. Urine output should be accurately monitored with a Foley catheter in any individual suspected of being in shock, and

Table 28-1
Normal age-adjusted vital signs

Age (yr)	Pulse Rate (beats/min)	Blood Pressure (mm Hg)	Respirations (breaths/min)
0–1	120	80/40	40
1–5	100	100/60	30
5–10	80	120/80	20

output of at least 1 mL/kg/hr should be maintained. As shock progresses, cardiac dysfunction and hypotension may occur, and the child starts becoming acidotic secondary to poor perfusion of the tissues. If the process is not addressed at this point, further decline and potential cardiac arrest can occur. Resuscitation from shock is discussed in the next section.

Fluid and Electrolytes

Despite the advances that have been made in caring for critically ill infants, the mismanagement of fluid and electrolyte therapy remains a potential cause of morbidity and mortality in this patient population. Managing fluids in the critically ill pediatric population requires dynamic monitoring and frequent adjustment of fluids and electrolytes. Subtle differences in the perioperative management of these patients can be amplified more than in the adult population. Fluid and electrolyte balance should be viewed from the three perspectives of total amount of water and solute in the body, distribution of water and solute in the various body compartments, and the osmolar concentration of each in these various compartments.

Fluid Compartments

The most abundant component of the human body is water. Liters of TBW can be calculated from the patient's body weight in kilograms, with adults having 0.6 times body weight, infants 0.7 times body weight, and neonates 0.8 times body weight. TBW can be divided into extracellular fluid (ECF) and intracellular fluid (ICF) compartments. The major components of the ECF compartment are an intravascular component (plasma volume) and an interstitial component. The principal cation of the ECF compartment is sodium; the principal anions are chloride and bicarbonate. In the ICF compartment, potassium is the principal cation while phosphates and nondiffusible proteins are the principal anions. The ICF compartment consists of the fluid found inside the cells of the body. It is separated from the ECF compartment by the cell membrane. ICF volume is estimated as the difference between

TBW and ECF volumes. Because cell membranes are freely permeable to water, the osmolality values of the ICF and ECF are always equal.

During the course of gestation, there is a decrease in the percentage of body weight represented by TBW and a relative decrease in the ECF-to-ICF compartment ratio. At 20 weeks' gestation, TBW accounts for 85% of total weight, three fourths of which is in the ECF (60% of body weight) versus only one fourth in the ICF (25% of body weight). At term, TBW is equal to roughly 80% of total body weight, with near-equal distribution between the ECF and ICF compartments (45% and 35% of body weight, respectively). By 18 months of age, fluid and electrolyte distribution reaches adult proportions, with the TBW compartment representing 60% of total body weight, two thirds of which is now intracellular (40% body weight), and one third extracellular (20% body weight). These changes are demonstrated graphically in Figure 28–1. The plasma compartment in newborn infants represents approximately 8% of total body weight and decreases to the adult volume of 6% of total body weight by 12 to 18 months of age.

Insensible Water Loss

Water expenditure in the neonatal and infant populations can be divided into insensible water loss, excretion of renal solute, water loss in stool, and water and electrolytes lost during normal homeostasis. Insensible losses are free water losses that occur through the skin and respiratory tract. The rate of loss via the respiratory tract is dependent on tidal volume, respiratory rate, temperature, and the humidity of inspired/expired air. In all infants, regardless of age, transepithelial water loss (TEWL) makes up the majority of insensible losses. The degree of TEWL varies inversely with body weight and age because younger infants have a higher ratio of body surface area to body weight. Using radiant warmers and phototherapy can increase temperature and decrease humidity, exacerbating evaporative losses. TEWL can be reduced significantly during transport by the use of an impermeable plastic cover. Fever can increase insensible losses by approximately

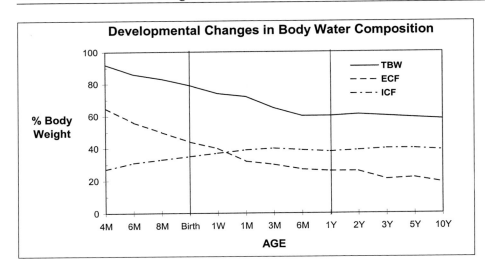

FIGURE 28–1 Developmental changes in body water composition.

7 mL/kg/day for each degree above 99°F. Because hyper-osmolality can lead to an increased risk of intracerebral hemorrhage, free water should be used to replace insensible losses. The simplest estimate of TEWL is 30 to 60 mL/kg/day for neonates less than 1500 g and 15 to 35 mL/kg/day in neonates greater than 1500 g.

Fluid Resuscitation

Any infant or child who is believed to exhibit clinical signs of shock should receive an isotonic fluid bolus of 20 mL/kg over no more than 30 to 60 minutes. Either normal saline or lactated Ringer's solution is adequate. The bolus should be given in addition to normal maintenance fluids. Samples for electrolytes and a blood count should be sent as early as possible to guide fluid therapy after the initial bolus. The child should be reassessed frequently for clinical response to the fluid challenge. A Foley catheter should be placed in order to accurately monitor the quantity of urine output as well as concentration of the urine, and capillary refill and peripheral pulses should be checked, as well as warmth of the extremity. An arterial or capillary blood gas measurement may be useful to check for acidosis and to monitor the response to resuscitation.

Fluid replacement postoperatively should be based on both a maintenance fluid component and a component that accounts for losses. Maintenance fluid requirements are listed in Table 28–2. For children less than 1 year of age, 5% dextrose (D_5) in 0.25% saline is an appropriate choice under normal circumstances. For older children, D_5 in 0.5% saline is an appropriate choice for most postoperative circumstances to replace maintenance fluids. In addition to maintenance fluids, another component should account for ongoing losses. This may be gastric output in a nasogastric tube, or pancreatic drainage from a drain, or third-space fluid shifts after an abdominal exploration for a perforated appendix. Fluids that can be measured and monitored are preferable. The electrolyte content of most gastrointestinal fluids can be found in Table 28–3. Knowing the volume and concentration of electrolytes allows one to choose the best replacement fluid.

For large abdominal operations we use the "quadrant" rule. For every quadrant of the abdomen involved in the process, we give an additional 25% of fluid volume in the form of lactated Ringer's solution to account for third-space losses. A patient with an inflamed appendix would thus get "maintenance and a quarter," whereas a sick child with a perforated appendix with severe inflammation involving the majority of the abdominal cavity would receive twice the amount of normal maintenance fluids for the first 12 to 24 hours postoperatively. For example, a

Table 28–2
Estimation of maintenance fluid requirements

Body Weight	Fluid (mL/kg/day)	Fluid (mL/kg/hr)
750–1000 g	80*	3
1000–1500 g	70*	3
First 10 kg	100	4
Second 10 kg	50	2
Each additional kg	20	1

* Maintenance rate for first 2 to 5 postnatal days; then increase to 100 mL/kg/day.

Table 28–3

Electrolyte composition of gastrointestinal fluids

Fluid	Na+ (mEg/L)	K+ (mEg/L)	Cl- (mEg/L)	HCO3- (mEg/L)
Salivary gland	10	26	10	30
Stomach	60	10	130	0
Duodenum	140	5	80	0
Bile	145	5	100	35
Pancreas	140	5	75	115
Ileum	140	5	104	30
Colon	60	30	40	0

3-year-old, 20-kg child with a perforated appendix localized to the lower abdomen and pelvis would receive D_5 in 0.5 N saline + 20 mEq/L KCl at 60 mL/hr. In addition, he or she should receive 30 mL/hr of lactated Ringer's solution to account for third-space losses, and, if a nasogastric tube was present with 40 mL/hr of bilious drainage, another 40 mL/hr of lactated Ringer's in addition to the other fluids. Total fluids initially would equal 130 mL/hr in this patient. As soon as urine output was established and stable, this would be titrated back to maintenance only plus ongoing losses. For severe electrolyte abnormalities, deficits should be calculated as discussed in the next sections on electrolyte abnormalities. Common formulas are found in Table 28–4.

Sodium

Sodium balance plays a major role in the maintenance of the ECF volume. It is the total amount of sodium present in the whole body, not just the serum concentration of sodium, that determines the ECF volume. A decrease, an increase, or no change in the sodium concentration can accompany changes in the ECF volume. The total amount of sodium in an adult is approximately 60 mEq/kg. The sodium content of the fetus is much higher, approximately 85 to 90 mEq/kg, because of the proportionally increased ECF compartment as compared to that in the adult. Serum osmolality is in large part (approximately 80%) dependent on the sodium concentration, but also

Table 28–4

Common equations to calculate fluid and electrolyte deficits and excesses

Serum osmolality	$2[Na^+] + (BUN/2.8) + (glucose/18)$	
Total body water (TBW)	Neonate:	$0.8 \times kg$
	Infant:	$0.7 \times kg$
	Adult:	$0.6 \times kg$
Electrolyte deficit	$d \times kg \times (desired\ [mEq/L] - actual\ [mEq/L])$	
	Sodium	$d = 0.6$
	Bicarbonate	$d = 0.4$
	Chloride	$d = 0.2$
Free water deficit	$TBW \times ([Na^+]/140 - 1)$	
Free water excess	$TBW \times (1 - [Na^+]/140)$	
Corrected calcium (hypoalbuminemia)	$[Ca^{2+}] + [0.8 \times (normal - current\ albumin)]$	
Corrected sodium (hyperglycemia)	$Serum\ [Na^+] + [1.8 \times (glucose - 100)]$	

BUN, blood urea nitrogen; [Ca2+], concentration of calcium; d, xxxx; kg, weight in kilograms; [Na+], concentration of sodium.

depends on blood urea nitrogen (BUN) and glucose concentrations, and can be estimated with the following formula:

$$2[Na^+] + (BUN/2.8) + (glucose/18)$$

Hyponatremia

Hyponatremia is defined as a serum concentration of sodium less than 135 mEq/L and may occur with hypovolemia, euvolemia, or hypervolemia. Symptoms usually do not become apparent until the level drops to below 120 mEq/L. Because water can easily cross the blood-brain barrier into the central nervous system, symptoms arise as a result of cerebral overhydration and include apathy, nausea, vomiting, headache, seizures, and coma. The rate and magnitude of the shift determine the degree of symptoms. Acute hyponatremia, which occurs over a period of 24 hours or less, is associated with the most rapid onset of symptoms. Rapid movement of water into the brain initiates protective mechanisms in the central nervous system, and intracellular amino acids and potassium are lost in order to reduce cellular swelling. Because of these changes, the brain is particularly susceptible to dehydration during the fluid and electrolyte correction phase. Rapid correction of the low plasma sodium will increase the plasma osmolality in advance of correction in the cerebral intracellular compartment, and a net shift of fluid out of the brain may occur, leading to central pontine myelinolysis. Therapeutic correction of hyponatremia should occur over 24 to 48 hours in order to avoid secondary injury from this mechanism.

The renal response to hyponatremia is to produce dilute urine; however, this can be complicated by release of antidiuretic hormone (ADH). Urine sodium concentration is a useful measure because it may provide clues to the underlying condition causing the hyponatremia. Urine sodium concentrations less than 10 mEq/L indicate that renal sodium handling is intact and that effective blood volume is decreased. A sodium concentration greater than 20 mEq/L indicates intrinsic renal tubular damage or a natriuretic response to a state of hypervolemia.

Hypovolemic hyponatremia occurs with excess loss of sodium relative to loss of water and is associated with total body sodium depletion and ECF volume contraction. It most commonly occurs secondary to increased gastrointestinal losses from vomiting (especially in cases of pyloric stenosis), diarrhea, or fistula output. Increased losses through perspiration can occur, especially in infants with cystic fibrosis and adrenal insufficiency. Intake of hypotonic solutions then leads to a hyponatremic, hypovolemic ECF volume, and the hyponatremia is maintained by the kidney's inability to excrete free water. The excessive renal loss of sodium induced by diuretics can lead to a hypovolemic hyponatremia. Adrenal insufficiency should

be suspected when hypovolemic hyponatremia exists in conjunction with hyperkalemia and renal sodium wasting (urinary sodium greater than 20 mEq/L) despite normal renal function. Intrinsic renal disease can lead to an impaired ability to conserve sodium, resulting in hyponatremia.

Euvolemic hyponatremia is rare and usually exists in a state of increased ECF volume, often associated with a normal amount of total body sodium. The syndrome of inappropriate secretion of ADH (SIADH) is the most common cause in children. It is diagnosed by exclusion and is found in certain malignancies, pulmonary diseases, and disorders of the central nervous system. SIADH is a problem of water retention, not decreased sodium, and should be managed with fluid restriction. Attempts to correct this condition with the administration of saline solutions usually cause an increase in renal sodium excretion with little change in serum sodium. Increased levels of ADH postoperatively, combined with the infusion of hypotonic fluids, can place the infant at risk of iatrogenic hyponatremia. Acute water intoxication is rare but can occur in infants as a result of their inability to effectively excrete a water load.

Cerebral salt-wasting syndrome is another cause of hyponatremia associated with central nervous system injury in children that is similar to SIADH. Rather than euvolemic or hypervolemic hyponatremia, this syndrome results in a hypovolemic hyponatremia, and is best treated by hydration and salt replacement, not fluid restriction. It is most likely secondary to increased levels of atrial natriuretic factor, and clinically is distinguished from SIADH by the fact that the patients have urine salt wasting and volume depletion.

Patients with *hypervolemic hyponatremia* present with peripheral and pulmonary edema. Despite the low serum concentration of sodium, they usually have elevated total body sodium and TBW. This condition can occur in infants with congestive heart failure, cirrhosis of the liver, nephrotic syndrome, and renal failure. The hyponatremia is a result of a decreased effective blood volume, which leads to an increased release of ADH resulting in water retention. A decreased glomerular filtration rate leads to increased water reabsorption, and, with active sodium reabsorption, urine sodium is usually less than 20 mEq/L.

Any patient with significant symptoms of hyponatremia and a serum sodium less than 120 mEq/L should receive hypertonic saline in order to rapidly (within more than 4 hours) increase the sodium to 125 mEq/L. Further correction toward normal should occur more slowly over the next 24 to 48 hours, and subsequent therapy will be based on the patient's volume status. Hypovolemic patients should receive isotonic saline or iso-oncotic colloid solutions. An estimate of the amount of sodium necessary for adequate correction can be obtained with the following formula:

$$Na\ required\ (mEq) = (desired\ [Na^+] - actual\ [Na^+]) \times 0.6 \times body\ weight\ (kg)$$

Euvolemic patients with SIADH require fluid restriction, and, if symptoms persist with little change in serum sodium, furosemide followed by hypertonic saline may be effective. In chronic SIADH, lithium and demeclocycline can inhibit the renal response to ADH. Hypervolemic patients require both salt and water restriction. The amount of fluid excess can be calculated from the following formula:

$$H_2O\ excess\ (L) = TBW \times (1 - [Na^+]/140)$$

Acute hyponatremia can be corrected at a rate of 12 to 14 mEq/L/day, and chronic hyponatremia should be corrected no faster than 12 mEq/L/day. In instances of renal failure, diuretics and dialysis also will help correct the hyponatremia.

Hypernatremia

Hypernatremia is defined as a serum sodium concentration greater than 145 mEq/L, with severe symptoms occurring at levels above 160 mEq/L. This condition is most often a disorder of water balance as opposed to sodium balance. Total body sodium content may be high, normal, or low in relation to TBW content, depending on the cause of the hypernatremia. The most common cause of hypernatremia in the pediatric population is the loss of hypotonic fluid without adequate water intake. Though diarrhea most often leads to isonatremic or hyponatremic dehydration, when it is additionally associated with decreased fluid intake or prolonged vomiting, hypernatremic dehydration may occur. Excess sodium intake is unusual but can occur iatrogenically if infants are fed an inappropriately concentrated formula. The loss of pure water, which occurs in diabetes insipidus, is characterized by decreased secretion of ADH (primary) or end-organ unresponsiveness (secondary). Excessive sweating or increased insensible losses, especially in the premature infant, result in increased free water loss.

Hypernatremic dehydration is associated with extremely dry mucous membranes and "doughy" skin. Periods of lethargy and irritability, increased muscle tone, seizures, and coma also can occur. In the central nervous system, the shrinkage of brain matter associated with ICF losses can result in intracerebral hemorrhage from the tearing of cerebral vessels. In response to persistent hypernatremia, the accumulation of intracellular taurine occurs in an attempt to increase the osmotic gradient for the intracellular return of water. Hypernatremic dehydration should first be treated with volume expansion using isotonic crystalloid solutions to promote volume expansion.

When urine output has been re-established, hypotonic solutions should be used to correct the hypernatremia in no less than 48 hours. Free water deficit can be calculated from the following formula:

$$Free\ H_2O\ deficit = TBW \times ([Na^+]/140 - 1)$$

Rapid rehydration will lead to cellular swelling and cerebral edema, thus increasing the likelihood of permanent neurologic deficit. Hypocalcemia commonly is associated with hypernatremia and also may require correction. In cases of central diabetes insipidus, the administration of vasopressin can be used cautiously as an adjunct to volume expansion to help correct the hypernatremia.

Potassium

The most important function of the potassium ion is the role it plays in regulating the electrical activity of biologic systems. Disorders of potassium homeostasis occur frequently in the hospitalized pediatric population and can lead to signs and symptoms ranging from muscle weakness to cardiac arrhythmias. Potassium is the principal intracellular cation, remaining primarily unbound and osmotically active. Although it is not freely diffusible through the cytoplasmic membrane, it is more easily diffusible than sodium or calcium.

Hypokalemia

Hypokalemic states are relatively common in the pediatric surgical population. Often, these are iatrogenic, most frequently associated with the use of diuretics without appropriate potassium replacement. Loop diuretics promote potassium secretion and trigger the release of aldosterone, which further aggravates the hypokalemia. In addition to renal loss, extrarenal potassium losses are common in the pediatric population, and the urine concentration of potassium can be helpful in distinguishing between the two. A urine concentration of potassium that is less than 15 mEq/L indicates renal conservation of potassium, suggesting loss from an extrarenal source. Increased gastrointestinal losses through vomiting and diarrhea lead to a dehydrated, contracted physiologic state, which can be associated with significant potassium losses. Increased levels of hormones, such as insulin and catecholamines, cause a significant shift of potassium into the cells, leading to a loss of extracellular potassium even though total body potassium remains constant.

Treatment of mild hypokalemia in asymptomatic patients may not be necessary, except in patients receiving digitalis preparations (to whom supplements should be given). In severe depletion, potassium replacement should be given parenterally. Potassium chloride doses of 0.5 to 1 mEq/kg are given with frequent electrocardiographic monitoring and measurement of serum values.

Concentrations of 40 to 60 mEq/L can be tolerated in peripheral veins, but concentrations of 1 mEq/3 mL can be given via central access with continuous heart monitoring required. Because potassium is located intracellularly, it is difficult to calculate the exact deficit and, therefore, frequent monitoring of the plasma potassium level should be performed as repletion is continued. Generally, a 1-mEq/L decrease in serum potassium (as a result of an actual decrease in total body potassium) represents a loss of approximately 5% to 10% of total body potassium. In patients with a significant hypochloremic alkalosis, such as infants with pyloric stenosis, potassium will be difficult to replace until the chloride is corrected. This is also true for patients who have a significant hypomagnesemia.

Hyperkalemia

Hyperkalemia is most often present in patients who have impaired renal excretion. Children with congenital urologic abnormalities, such as reflux nephropathy and prune-belly syndrome associated with bilateral hydronephrosis, have an associated dysfunction of the tubular epithelium. If this involves the epithelium responsible for potassium secretion, an associated hyperkalemic, hyperchloremic metabolic acidosis may ensue. Adrenal insufficiency causes hyperkalemia as a result of impaired secretion of potassium in the kidney and colon (secondary to decreased mineralocorticoid production). Insulin-dependent diabetes mellitus limits the ability of muscle and liver to take up potassium. Severe crush injuries associated with trauma or the lysis of tumor cells associated with chemotherapy can lead to acute, life-threatening hyperkalemia. Excess hydrogen ion decreases the membrane electrical gradient, allowing potassium to follow its chemical gradient out of the cell into the ECF. In adults, for every decrease in pH of 0.1 unit, a shift of 1.5 mEq of potassium occurs.

Hyperkalemia causes clinical sequelae by depolarizing electrically excitable cells. Early electrocardiograms show peaked T waves, which progress to a lengthening of the P-R interval and a widening of the QRS complex. If hyperkalemia persists, the infant is at risk for life-threatening arrhythmias, including asystole. When the QRS complex is widened or asystole is present, immediate intravenous infusion of 10% calcium gluconate (1 mL/kg per dose) increases the threshold potential, allowing cells to repolarize and once again generate action potentials. The hyperkalemia itself should be treated with an infusion of insulin (0.1 U/kg) and glucose (D_{50} in water, 1 mL/kg), which will transiently shift potassium into the intracellular compartment. If a metabolic acidosis also exists, the administration of sodium bicarbonate (1 mEq/kg) will shift potassium into the intracellular compartment. These maneuvers will transiently lower the extracellular potassium concentration for a few hours, allowing time to more definitively reduce total body potassium. Loop diuretics

are effective at removing potassium in patients with adequate renal function. In those without adequate renal function and with severe hyperkalemia, the administration of sodium polystyrene sulfonate (Kayexalate; 1 g/kg PO q6h), a cation-exchange resin, into the gastrointestinal tract will bond potassium and remove it from the system. Kayexalate is usually administered with sorbitol to enhance its removal from the gastrointestinal tract and avoid obstruction resulting from concretion formation. Hemodialysis or peritoneal dialysis is effective at correcting the hyperkalemia as well as the associated metabolic acidosis.

Other Electrolytes

Hypocalcemia is relatively common in the neonate. An exaggerated primary parathyroid response often persists into adulthood, but with a relatively benign course. The immunologic compromise associated with DiGeorge syndrome results in a hypoparathyroid hypocalcemia that requires aggressive management. A decreased parathyroid hormone response leads to neonatal hypocalcemia in infants of mothers with maternal diabetes, and may be related to hypomagnesemia. In this condition, a postprandial fall in ionized calcium fails to elicit an appropriate parathyroid response when compared to normal newborns. States of maternal hypocalcemia, hypercalcemia, hypomagnesemia, and hypermagnesemia predispose the neonate to calcium abnormalities. Hypoalbuminemia leads to a factitious hypocalcemia and can be corrected by the following formula:

$$\text{Corrected } Ca^{2+} = [Ca^{2+}] + [0.8 \times (\text{normal albumin} - \text{current albumin})]$$

Seriously diminished cardiac function results from decreased ionized calcium levels. Rate, rhythm, contractility, and afterload all are dependent on the maintenance of ionized calcium within a physiologic range. The range at which ionized calcium remains physiologic also is dependent on other variables such as adrenergic activity, preload, and oxygen delivery. Left ventricular contractility increases with calcium administration in the hypocalcemic state; however, when calcium is given to a normocalcemic individual, blood pressure elevations are more likely due to increased peripheral resistance. Calcium chloride boluses can be dangerous, resulting in acute cardiac decompensation in digitalized or hypokalemic individuals. Calcium will only benefit a cardiac arrest associated with hyperkalemia or caused by hypoglycemia-induced arrhythmias. When calcium therapy is required, calcium gluconate should be administered slowly, preferably by continuous infusion into high-flow veins. The calcium repletion dose is 20 mg/kg per dose, with 10% calcium gluconate providing 9 mg of calcium per milliliter and

10% calcium chloride providing 27 mg of calcium per milliliter.

Although hypocalcemia is more common in the neonatal population, many disease states in neonates can result in hypercalcemia. The clinical expression of familial hypercalcemic hypocalciuria is variable and is related to a neonatal state of hyperparathyroidism, which requires initial aggressive resuscitation and may potentially necessitate parathyroidectomy. Patients receiving hyperalimentation or vitamin supplements can develop hypercalcemia secondary to hypervitaminosis A. Those receiving hyperalimentation also are susceptible to hypercalcemia resulting from hypophosphatemia. Primary and tertiary hyperparathyroidism can cause hypercalcemia. Hyperthyroid individuals, during periods of immobilization, are subject to hypercalcemia, and hypothyroidism can cause hypercalcemia secondary to associated calcitonin insufficiency. Solid tumors, which can cause hypercalcemia secondary to paraneoplastic syndromes, are not as common in infants and children as in adults, but tumors with metastases to bone and multiple myeloma may cause hypercalcemia in children. Hypercalcemia can predispose patients to pancreatitis as a result of increased pancreatic duct permeability.

Chloride is the major anion of the ECF, and its intake and output parallel that of sodium. It follows electrochemical gradients created largely by movement of sodium via passive diffusion. Active transport occurs in the ascending limb of the loop of Henle. Though chloride is not directly involved in the regulation of acid-base homeostasis, as adjustments are made in the levels of bicarbonate, chloride often shifts in a reciprocal fashion. Chloride must be given in addition to potassium in order to correct hypokalemia, and chloride administration is necessary to correct most forms of metabolic alkalosis. Prompt administration of potassium and sodium chloride results in excretion of bicarbonate into the urine and correction of the alkalosis. Renal correction of metabolic alkalosis results in reabsorption of chloride in excess of sodium and potassium. The measurement of chloride is necessary for calculation of the anion gap. The concentration of sodium is greater than the sum of the concentrations of chloride and potassium, thus resulting in an anion gap of 8 to 16 mEq/L under normal conditions. This is due to the presence of unmeasured anions, which exceed the concentration of unmeasured cations.

Magnesium plays a major role in intracellular enzymatic activity and is the fourth most abundant cation in the body. It is a crucial cofactor in glycolysis and also in the stimulation of ATPases. Sixty percent of the body's total magnesium is bound in bone, with only one third of this freely exchangeable. The remaining magnesium is intracellular, the majority in muscle and liver, and is bound to proteins, RNA, and ATP. Extracellular magnesium is maintained at a low level within a narrow physiologic range and is freely interchangeable with the bone pool. Absorption of magnesium occurs in the upper gastrointestinal tract by a mechanism that is enhanced by vitamin D, parathyroid hormone, and increased sodium absorption. It remains incomplete, however, with only one third being absorbed. Repletion of magnesium can be given enterally or parenterally at doses of 0.5 mEq/kg 2 to 3 times a day.

Pediatric Metabolism

Much of the improved survival noted in the field of pediatric surgery can be attributed directly to our increased understanding of the acute metabolic response to injury in children. We now understand that surgery presents a small injury insult to the child and that it is the underlying condition that determines the magnitude of the response. This response is catabolic by nature; is in direct competition with somatic, anabolic growth; and varies among children depending on age, organ maturity, and severity of the insult. The following discussion attempts to present what is known about the acute metabolic stress response as it relates to infants and children.

The brain and erythrocytes are primarily dependent on glucose for energy metabolism. During periods of starvation, cerebral metabolism allows for the use of ketone bodies as a source of fuel. Neonates have a higher glucose requirement when compared to adults secondary to the larger neonatal brain mass relative to body weight. Adequate use of glucose depends on the functional maturity of a variety of digestive and metabolic enzyme systems. The balance between insulin, which stimulates glycogen synthesis, and the counter-regulatory hormones, which stimulate glycogenolysis, regulates the immediate production and metabolism of glucose. An alternative source of glucose is hepatic gluconeogenesis from lactate, glycerol, pyruvate, and amino acids such as alanine and glutamine. Although many tissues are capable of gluconeogenesis, only the liver has the capacity to release glucose into the blood stream. The rate at which glucose is released from hepatic glycogen stores is roughly equivalent to the level of glucose use by the brain, and leaves little reserve for other energy requirements of the neonate. The counter-regulatory response to hypoglycemia results in decreased insulin levels relative to increased glucagon, catecholamines, and cortisol. This generates lactate, glycerol, and alanine as primary precursors for the liver to generate more glucose.

Early features of the acute metabolic response to injury include the release of cytokines such as tumor necrosis factor, interleukin-1 and -6, and increased counter-regulatory hormones associated with selective insulin and growth hormone (GH) resistance. As a result, the catabolism of protein, carbohydrate, and fat occurs to provide essential intermediates to fuel the ongoing response. Contrary to starvation metabolism, increasing the level of nutritional repletion cannot reverse this catabolic response. As long as the acute metabolic stressor is not appropriately addressed, the cytokine and counter-regulatory hormone response will continue to drive the system. Furthermore, the liver undergoes a reprioritization of metabolite flow that results in increased generation of acute-phase reactants such as C-reactive protein (CRP) and glucose from catabolized amino acids, while decreasing production of the constitutive proteins albumin and prealbumin (PA). Key enzyme systems may be deficient or functionally immature in neonates. In a recent study in adult and neonatal rabbits, neonates could not restore endotoxin-reduced hepatic ATP levels by 24 hours, whereas adult animals could. Adult animals were able to increase pyruvate generation, a response that also was lacking in the neonates.

Insulin increases glycogen synthesis, lipogenesis, and protein synthesis, and, in combination with insulin-like growth factor-1 (IGF-1), is essential for somatic growth in children. Acute metabolic stress is accompanied by cytokine-induced increases in cortisol, glucagon, and catecholamines, known as counter-regulatory hormones because they oppose the anabolic effects of insulin. Glucagon stimulates glycolysis, glycogenolysis, and gluconeogenesis. Increased glycolysis results in increased lactate and pyruvate as precursors for hepatic gluconeogenesis. Cortisol stimulates gluconeogenesis and proteolysis, which provides alanine and glutamine as further precursors for hepatic gluconeogenesis. The catecholamines stimulate glycogenolysis, lipolysis, and hypermetabolism as well as inhibiting glucose secretion from the pancreas. This entire response system results in a hyperglycemic, catabolic organism that cannot be converted to anabolic metabolism by simply increasing the amount of nutrition. Both term and premature infants can mount a counter-regulatory response to surgically induced injury. The response is short lived and can be blunted with fentanyl anesthesia. However, the response in premature infants appears to be delayed in onset and lasts longer when compared to that in term infants.

A predominant feature of serious illness in neonates is decreased feeding tolerance that results in decreased energy substrate with which to mount a response. The infant then must rely on mobilization of endogenous stores, a process that is particularly precarious for the premature infant with less muscle and adipose mass. Normal anabolic metabolism is counterproductive in the stressed stated, and, as the demands for substrate mobilization increase, anabolic hormone effects are markedly attenuated. Counter-regulatory hormones lead to a relative suppression of the anabolic effects on insulin, GH, and IGF-1. The stressed infant is in a state of insulin

resistance defined by increased glucose production, lipolysis, fatty acid oxidation, and proteolysis, as well as decreased glucose uptake and storage despite elevated glucose, amino acid, and insulin levels.

Septic and acute injury states in adults are characterized by a decreased ability to utilize glucose despite increased serum concentrations. Just giving increased levels of insulin cannot easily reverse this hyperglycemia. During sepsis, providing insulin fails to decrease hepatic gluconeogenesis despite adequate glucose concentrations. Insulin promotes protein anabolism both by encouraging protein synthesis and by decreasing proteolysis. Despite the presence of proteolysis during the acute metabolic stress response, the anabolic effect of insulin is still intact, because large doses of insulin in burned adults have been shown to increase protein synthesis relative to controls.

Normally, GH decreases protein catabolism, increases protein synthesis and fatty acid mobilization by stimulating the conversion of free fatty acids to acetyl-coenzyme A, decreases glucose oxidation, and stimulates glycogen deposition. The anabolic effects of GH are related to IGF-1. During periods of acute metabolic stress, IGF-1 levels markedly decrease while levels of inhibitory IGF-1–binding proteins increase. Substrate mobilization effects of GH—increased lipolysis and fatty acid oxidation—then predominate while protein anabolic effects are inhibited. Exogenous GH can reverse the catabolic effects in moderately stressed adults and burned children. In a recent study in neonates with gastroschisis or necrotizing enterocolitis, exogenous GH given for 7 days did not elicit an anabolic response. It did, however, improve the use of lipid substrate in both term and premature infants. Because somatic growth is an anabolic phenomenon and under normal conditions accounts for up to 30% to 40% of energy expenditure in term and premature infants, a unique situation exists relative to stressed adult patients. Stressed infants and children need fewer calories than their normal maintenance requirements during the acute metabolic stress response period. This is contrary to the adult situation, and only recently has the concept changed in infants. Measured energy expenditure (MEE) in a septic or stressed infant is markedly decreased when compared to controls, to a level near the basal metabolic rate. This situation is contrary to that in stressed adult patients, in whom MEE is markedly increased. As the stress response abates, MEE slowly increases, primarily as a result of increased energy requirement for somatic growth.

Normally the liver secretes many constitutive visceral proteins, including albumin, transferrin, PA, and retinol-binding protein. These proteins account for the early nitrogen losses during the acute metabolic stress response. Studies in infants have demonstrated a precipitous drop in visceral protein concentrations in response to the acute metabolic stress response. Return of these proteins to their

beneficial for a few days to weeks to supplement enteral nutrition but rarely can be used as the sole source of nutrition in infants and children. Solution osmolality should not exceed 600 mOsm/L, and dextrose concentrations should not exceed 12.5%. The addition of lipid can decrease the irritative effects of hypertonic carbohydrate infusion.

The use of peripheral hyperalimentation prevents the complication of central vein thrombosis as well as the technical complications associated with the placement of a central venous catheter. The short-term use of percutaneously placed femoral catheters has been established as a safe alternative for TPN delivery, with a low catheter infection rate of 2%. Percutaneously placed central venous catheters may have a lower infection rate when compared to catheters placed surgically via cutdown.

Cycling of TPN in infants on long-term hyperalimentation is safe and effective, and the cyclic administration of carbohydrates to some extent mimics the intermittent nature of oral feeding. When the TPN is cycled off, serum glucose and insulin concentrations fall, lipid oxidation increases, and lipid storage decreases. All of these factors have possible benefit in reducing liver dysfunction, a complication frequently observed in infants receiving long-term TPN.

A substantial number of randomized, prospective trials have compared TPN with enteral nutritional delivery in acutely stressed high-risk patients, including children. Meta-analysis of eight of these trials showed significant reduction in septic complications (18% vs. 35%) in the enterally fed versus parenterally nourished patients. A study of burn patients demonstrated significantly increased mortality (63% vs. 26%) in the group randomized to receive TPN supplementation versus enteral feeds alone. Studies in adult trauma patients have shown that the infection rate of enterally fed patients is significantly lower than that of parenterally fed patients, as determined by fewer cases of pneumonia and fewer intra-abdominal abscesses. These data would support the preferential use of enteral nutrition to the degree that it is clinically feasible: If the gut works, use it. Parenteral nutrition remains an important clinical option until the gut can tolerate nutritional delivery to meet the needs of the patient. Some enteral feeds should be initiated even in small amounts as soon as possible to maintain the integrity of intestinal barrier function.

Indications for Supplemental Nutrition

Criteria for identifying children who are malnourished differ somewhat in various published reports. In general, the following surveillance criteria can be used to identify children who are malnourished or likely to require supplemental nutritional support:

1. Interval or total weight loss of greater than 5% during the past 3 to 6 months in older children

2. Weight-to-height ratio less than or equal to 90% or weight-to-height percentile less than or equal to 10th percentile

3. Serum albumin concentration less than or equal to 3.2 g/dL

4. A decrease in current percentile for weight of at least two percentile rank during the last 3 to 6 months in older children (weight of 75th or 95th percentile drops to 25th or 50th percentile)

5. Voluntary food intake of less than 70% of estimated requirements for 5 days for well-nourished patients

6. Anticipated gut dysfunction for more than 5 days for well-nourished patients

Overfeeding

Overfeeding occurs when the administration of calories or specific substrate exceeds the requirements to maintain metabolic homeostasis. These requirements, which vary according to the patient's age, state of health, and underlying nutritional status, are substantially altered during periods of injury-induced acute metabolic stress. Excess nutritional delivery during this period can further increase the metabolic demands of an acute injury and place an added burden on the lungs and liver. The result is not only exacerbation of pulmonary and hepatic pathophysiologic processes but also increase in the risk of mortality. It is important, therefore, to ensure that caloric intake does not exceed demand during the period of acute metabolic stress response in critically ill infants and children.

Child Abuse

Any physician dealing with children should be aware of how children who have been abused can present. In most cases, the children are from lower socioeconomic status backgrounds and the parents are often very young. Children who are physically abused tend to be less than 3 years of age, whereas those who are sexually abused average 10 to 12 years of age. Abuse can take many forms, and often an innocent-appearing injury, on further questioning, is just one of a large series of injuries. Clues to the diagnosis of child abuse would include a marked delay in seeking help for a very significant injury, extremely poor hygiene in the child, and severe lack of emotion from the child. Most commonly, fractures, burns, and head trauma comprise most of the injuries. Radiographs showing fractures of various age, bruises of various age noted on physical exam, or burns with sharply demarcated edges are red flags. Injuries with mechanisms that would require maturity on the part of the infant beyond his or her years are suspicious. A stocking-glove distribution of a burn is suspicious for a dip injury. In addition, a history that changes from witness to witness or over time in the same witness, parental response that is out of proportion to the injury, or a mother who is either far removed from the child psychologically or too attached for the circumstances are worth noting. Any perineal trauma or injury should be suspected as potential abuse.

Once a physician suspects child abuse, he or she is legally and ethically obligated to report the situation and ensure the safety of the child. Typically, in most children's hospitals, there is a team well versed in researching the circumstances. If no such team exists, contacting the local social services department and filing a report immediately is mandatory. If the situation is so serious that the child is in immediate jeopardy, admission to the hospital and observation until the circumstances can be investigated may be necessary. The goal is to identify the problem, and not necessarily to punish the family as much as to provide positive intervention, while protecting the child.

Conclusion

Care of the pediatric surgical patient has improved significantly over the past few decades. A thorough knowledge of physiologic differences between children and adults, as well as improvements in fluid and electrolyte resuscitation and advances in nutrition, have been particularly useful in improving outcomes in the infant who has had surgery. The goal of this chapter has been to briefly review many of these issues to provide the physician who intermittently deals with pediatric surgical patients a background from which to operate. Those whose practice is composed primarily of children should actively seek more information from more detailed pediatric surgical subspecialty textbooks.

Bibliography

Anand KJ, Brown MJ, Bloom SR, Aynsley-Green A: Studies on the hormonal regulation of fuel metabolism in the human newborn infant undergoing anaesthesia and surgery. Horm Res 1985;22:115.

Anand KJ, Hansen DD, Hickey PR: Hormonal-metabolic stress responses in neonates undergoing cardiac surgery. Anesthesiology 1990;73:661.

Anand KJ, Hickey PR: Halothane-morphine compared with high-dose sufentanil for anesthesia and postoperative analgesia in neonatal cardiac surgery. N Engl J Med 1992;326:1.

Brooks DC, Bessey PQ, Black PR, et al: Insulin stimulates branched chain amino acid uptake and diminishes nitrogen flux from skeletal muscle of injured patients. J Surg Res 1986;40:395.

Chellis MJ, Sanders SV, Webster H, et al: Early enteral feeding in the pediatric intensive care unit. JPEN J Parenter Enteral Nutr 1996;20:71.

Chen KB: Clinical experience of percutaneous femoral venous catheterization in critically ill preterm infants less than 1,000 grams. Anesthesiology 2001;95:637.

Chwals WJ: Metabolism and nutritional frontiers in pediatric surgical patients. Surg Clin North Am 1992;72:1237.

Chwals WJ, Bistrian BR: Role of exogenous growth hormone and insulin-like growth factor I in malnutrition and acute metabolic stress: a hypothesis. Crit Care Med 1991;19:1317.

Chwals WJ, Fernandez ME, Charles BJ, et al: Serum visceral protein levels reflect protein-calorie repletion in neonates recovering from major surgery. J Pediatr Surg 1992;27:317.

Chwals WJ, Fernandez ME, Jamie AC, Charles BJ: Relationship of metabolic indexes to postoperative mortality in surgical infants. J Pediatr Surg 1993;28:819.

Chwals WJ, Fernandez ME, Jamie AC, et al: Detection of postoperative sepsis in infants with the use of metabolic stress monitoring. Arch Surg 1994;129:437.

Chwals WJ, Sobol WT, Charles BJ, Hinson WH: A comparison of total body water measurements using whole-body magnetic resonance imaging versus tritium dilution in primates. J Surg Res 1992;52:378.

Evain-Brion D: Hormonal regulation of fetal growth. Horm Res 1994;42:207.

Fomon SJ: Requirements and recommended dietary intakes of protein during infancy. Pediatr Res 1991;30:391.

Fong Y, Moldawer LL, Shires GT, Lowry SF: The biologic characteristics of cytokines and their implication in surgical injury. Surg Gynecol Obstet 1990;170:363.

Friedman B, Kanter G, Titus D: Femoral venous catheters: a safe alternative for delivering parenteral alimentation. Nutr Clin Pract 1994;9:69.

Herndon DN, Barrow RE, Kunkel KR, et al: Effects of recombinant human growth hormone on donor-site healing in severely burned children. Ann Surg 1990;212:424.

Herndon DN, Barrow RE, Stein M, et al: Increased mortality with intravenous supplemental feeding in severely burned patients. J Burn Care Rehabil 1989;10:309.

Kasoff SS, Lansen TA, Holder D, Filippo JS: Aggressive physiologic monitoring of pediatric head trauma patients with elevated intracranial pressure. Pediatr Neurosci 1988;14:241.

Kemp L, Burge J, Choban P, et al: The effect of catheter type and site on infection rates in total parenteral nutrition patients. JPEN J Parenter Enteral Nutr 1994;18:71.

Kudsk KA, Croce MA, Fabian TC, et al: Enteral versus parenteral feeding: effects on septic morbidity after blunt and penetrating abdominal trauma. Ann Surg 1992; 215:503.

Letton RW, Chwals WJ, Charles B, et al: Endotoxin-induced hepatocyte energy status and metabolic compensation in adult verses neonatal rabbits. Surg Forum 1996;42:683.

Letton RW, Chwals WJ, Jamie A, Charles B: Early postoperative alterations in infant energy use increase the risk of overfeeding. J Pediatr Surg 1995;30:988.

Letton RW, Chwals WJ, Jamie A, Charles B: Neonatal lipid utilization increases with injury severity: recombinant human growth hormone versus placebo. J Pediatr Surg 1996;31:1068.

Lucas A, Bloom SR, Aynsley-Green A: Gut hormones and 'minimal enteral feeding.' Acta Paediatr Scand 1986;75:719.

Moore FA, Feliciano DV, Andrassy RJ, et al: Early enteral feeding, compared with parenteral, reduces postoperative septic complications: the results of a meta-analysis. Ann Surg 1992;216:172.

Reichman BL, Chessex P, Putet G, et al: Partition of energy metabolism and energy cost of growth in the very low-birth-weight infant. Pediatrics 1982;69:446.

Sakurai Y, Aarsland A, Herndon DN, et al: Stimulation of muscle protein synthesis by long-term insulin infusion in severely burned patients. Ann Surg 1995;222:283.

Shulman RJ, Pokorny WJ, Martin CG, et al: Comparison of percutaneous and surgical placement of central venous catheters in neonates. J Pediatr Surg 1986;21:348.

Talbot FB: Basal metabolism standards for children. Am J Dis Child 1938;55:455.

Taylor AF, Lally KP, Chwals WJ, et al: Hormonal response of the premature primate to operative stress. J Pediatr Surg 1993;28:844.

Thompson AE: Pulmonary artery catheterization in children. New Horiz 1997;5:244.

Tueting JL, Byerley LO, Chwals WJ: Anabolic recovery relative to degree of prematurity after acute injury in neonates. J Pediatr Surg 1999;34:13.

CHAPTER 29

The Morbidly Obese Surgical Patient

Walter J. Pories, M.D., F.A.C.S. and Jayme E. Locke, M.D.

As of 1998, over 39 million Americans were considered obese, and greater than 5 million of those were considered *morbidly obese*, which is defined as exceeding ideal body weight by at least 100 lb. Americans devote $99.2 billion of health care expenditures to the treatment of obesity. Not only is obesity expensive, it is also associated with an increase in morbidity and mortality, especially in the morbidly obese. Morbidly obese patients suffer increased risks for developing coronary heart disease, cerebrovascular disease, congestive heart failure, hypertension, diabetes mellitus, cancers, pulmonary insufficiency, pseudotumor cerebri, stress incontinence, gastroesophageal reflux, and infertility, just to name a few conditions. The morbidly obese also suffer socially because often they are viewed as inferior and lacking self-restraint. They are less likely to be hired, find a mate, or be given educational opportunities. As a result of the health risks and social stigmas from which the morbidly obese suffer, many have tried dieting, exercise, behavioral therapies, and even medications to overcome their obesity. While these techniques have proved effective in some moderately obese patients, they almost always fail in the morbidly obese.

Pathophysiology of Morbid Obesity

Morbid obesity is a complex and serious problem. It is a disease that highlights how little the scientific community knows about obesity. We do not understand the pathophysiology of the disease or its causes. We do not understand how morbid obesity causes comorbidities such as hypertension, pulmonary failure, pseudotumor cerebri, and infertility, nor do we understand why the morbidly obese are immunosuppressed and more prone to have infections, or why their clinical signs are unreliable. Using a simplistic model, morbid obesity can be defined as a disorder of energy balance that occurs when food-derived energy chronically exceeds energy expenditure. This results in excess calories being stored as triglycerides in adipose tissue. There are exceptions to this definition, however, because some individuals chronically exceed their energy requirements yet remain remarkably thin, pointing to a role for the efficiency of metabolism in the disease of morbid obesity. Why these aberrations occur continues to perplex the scientific community. Somewhere within this volume of missing information lies the cure for the disease of morbid obesity.

Over the years, many theories about the pathophysiology of morbid obesity have surfaced. Many have been proven in animal models but have not been convincing in humans. Physiologically, it has been shown that the human body is able to maintain the fine balance between energy expenditure and energy storage by relying on an internal set point or "lipostat." This lipostat, located in the hypothalamus, senses the amount of energy stores and then is able to regulate both food intake and energy expenditure. The lipostat senses the body's energy stores by communicating with adipocytes through an antiobesity factor known as leptin. Leptin binds receptors in the hypothalamus near the "lipostat." It has been shown in animals that binding of these receptors results in an inhibition of appetite, an increase in energy expenditure, an increase in physical activity, and an increase in heat production. Work in humans on the role of leptin has not been as convincing. Even at this early stage, however, the basic physiology of energy balance points to possible hypotheses about morbid obesity. Perhaps the disease is the result of an aberrant lipostat or lack of leptin.

More recently, the peptide hormone ghrelin, which serves as an endogenous ligand for the growth hormone, was discovered to be primarily produced in the stomach. Receptors for ghrelin have been located in the pituitary, hypothalamus, and brainstem, suggesting that ghrelin may prove to be the link between the stomach and the hypothalamic-pituitary axis. Animal studies have shown that daily administration of ghrelin to mice and rats causes a dose-dependent increase in food intake and weight gain. Ghrelin is effective at reducing fat utilization, and therefore may be one of the signals to the hypothalamus when an increase in metabolic efficiency is required.

Comorbidities

These hypotheses regarding pathophysiology do not account for the comorbidities seen with morbid obesity. It has been proposed that increases in intra-abdominal pressure in the morbidly obese account for the comorbidities, including hypertension, venous stasis, thromboembolism, and even diabetes mellitus. The theory points to basic pathophysiology, suggesting that the increase in intra-abdominal pressure decreases venous return to the heart. Decreased venous return results in stasis, which leads to thromboembolic disease. Furthermore, decreased venous return also results in less blood volume or stretch sensed by the atrial receptors of the heart. This results in renal compensation, leading to increased volume and hypertension. Finally, decreased venous return eventually causes an increase in afterload on the heart that with time can cause the heart to fail and pulmonary insufficiency to ensue.

While researchers have more evidence to support the mechanisms for the comorbidities of hypertension, venous stasis, thromboembolism, and pulmonary insufficiency, they have not acquired sufficient evidence to support a relationship between increased intra-abdominal pressure and diabetes mellitus. It is hypothesized, however, that

decreased venous return with subsequent decrease in cardiac output results in decreased blood flow to the islet cells of the pancreas. Lacking proper blood flow and thus oxygen and nutrients, the islet cells cannot perform their routine function of producing insulin adequately. Ultimately, this manifests itself as diabetes mellitus in the morbidly obese patient. Despite the logic behind the hypothesized etiology of the comorbidities in the morbidly obese, the relationship between obesity and diabetes still is a puzzle that has yet to be completely solved. Why, for example, are there both thin diabetics and obese diabetics, and why are there obese patients who are euglycemic?

Multifactorial Etiology of Morbid Obesity

It has long been known that aberrant physiologic processes are not the only triggers for morbid obesity. The etiology of the disease is multifactorial; genetic factors have been identified in twin studies that demonstrate remarkable concordance in the degree of obesity between identical twins reared apart. Also, it is known that environment plays an enormous role in the pathogenesis of obesity, because it has been shown that many Asians who immigrate to the United States have a higher incidence of obesity than those who remain in their native land. Furthermore, normal-weight individuals have been shown to develop morbid obesity after suffering a hormonal imbalance resulting from diseases such as Cushing's syndrome and hypothyroidism, medications such as steroids and antidepressants, cessation of smoking, pregnancy, trauma, and stress.

The Body Mass Index

An individual is considered to be morbidly obese when his or her body mass index (BMI [kg/m^2]) exceeds 35. This is the equivalent of 45.4 kg or 100 lb in excess of ideal body weight. The BMI cutoff of 35 is significant because it is at this point that risk for morbidity and mortality sharply increases. It is important to note that the BMI merely represents the relationship between height and weight. It is unable to differentiate between muscle and fat, and it does not incorporate or take into account the importance of body fat distribution, which is considered a more important risk factor for morbidity and mortality than the BMI alone. For example, an extremely muscular individual, such as a college football player, who weighs 308 lb (140 kg) at a height of 5 feet 8 inches (1.72 m), has a BMI of 47 kg/m^2 based on weight and height, despite having only 7% body fat as measured with hydroimmersion. While this individual would qualify for bariatric surgery based on BMI alone, he would not be a good candidate.

Accordingly, other ways to measure body fat continue to be sought. Two such ways are impedance and hydroimmersion. There is a question about the accuracy of the impedance technique, and hydroimmersion is not clinically useful or practical. The limitations of these methods highlight the importance of using sound clinical judgment along with objective measurements.

Bariatric Surgery

Bariatric surgery, arguably one of the great surgical advances of the last century, has benefited a previously forgotten group of afflicted individuals, but also has demonstrated how little we know about the operations and how they work. Furthermore, we do not understand how changing the intestinal "plumbing" corrects diabetes or hypertension, and we do not understand why some of these patients develop severe vitamin and mineral deficiencies several years after surgery and others do not. Despite these gaps and others in our medical knowledge, bariatric surgery remains the only effective therapy for long-term control of morbid obesity and, probably more importantly, its comorbidities. According to a National Institutes of Health Consensus Conference on the surgical treatment of obesity, patients with a BMI greater than 40 without comorbidities or a BMI greater than 35 with comorbidities are candidates for bariatric surgery. These patients must be highly motivated to comply with postoperative follow-up, must understand the procedure and the risks involved, and must maintain realistic expectations about the operative results. Contraindications to bariatric surgery include high operative risk that cannot be properly managed, ongoing substance abuse, significant uncontrolled psychiatric diseases such as depression and suicide attempts, and failure to understand the procedure. Lack of family support is a relative contraindication.

Bariatric procedures can be divided into those procedures that restrict the stomach's capacity for food, those that cause malabsorption by interfering with digestion, and a combination of both. By far the most commonly performed bariatric operation in the United States is the gastric bypass. The gastric bypass operation, along with other less common procedures, is outlined below and depicted in Figure 29–1.

Gastric Restrictive Procedures

Vertical banded gastroplasty

Vertical banded gastroplasty (Fig. 29–1A) limits intake by reducing the total stomach volume to 30 mL and delays emptying by decreasing the diameter of the outlet. The small outlet is buttressed by a strip of nonexpandable synthetic material. The greatest weight loss from vertical banded gastroplasty is seen during the first year

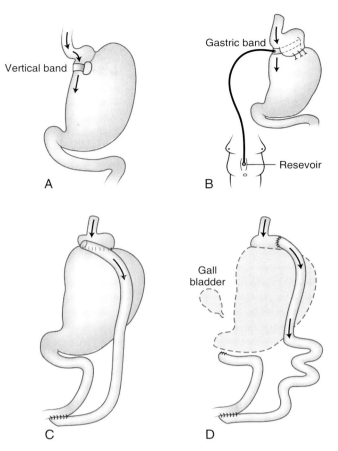

FIGURE 29–1 **A,** Vertical banded gastroplasty. **B,** Gastric banding. **C,** Roux-en-Y gastric bypass. **D,** Biliopancreatic diversion.

following surgery. Weight loss after the procedure gradually stabilizes, and then several years out there is a tendency toward weight gain. The patients most likely to fail with this procedure and continue to experience weight gain are the sweet eaters. These patients consume high-caloric liquid or meltable foods that quickly traverse the stoma. Vertical banded gastroplasty procedure is associated with a high rate of late complications, including obstruction as well as staple line disruption and occlusion of the gastric outlet as a result of erosion or tipping of the synthetic band, causing most surgeons to abandon the procedure. Other complications include ulcer formation in the gastric pouch, subphrenic abscess formation, and stomal obstruction secondary to stricture formation and band migration or erosion. Although this procedure is purely restrictive and does not exclude the stomach or duodenum, it is still important to supplement these patients with multivitamins, especially B complex vitamins.

Gastric banding

Gastric banding (Fig. 29–1B), currently being evaluated for Food and Drug Administration approval, limits intake by creating a small proximal gastric reservoir with a limited outlet. The reservoir is made by applying a small belt just below the esophagus. This belt contains a small bladder that can be inflated or deflated through a small subcutaneous reservoir, allowing the outlet diameter to be adjusted. This procedure offers several advantages to the patient because it avoids vitamin and mineral deficiencies, is performed laparoscopically through minimal incisions, and can be adjusted in the outpatient setting to suit the patient. Weight losses following this surgery have been reported to be as high as 55% to 65% at 3 years out. Again failures are most commonly seen in those patients considered to be sweet eaters. Complications include solid food intolerance, slipping of the band, stomach perforation during the operative dissection, intra-abdominal infection, and pulmonary embolism. In some series, as many as one third of the patients have required reoperation.

Gastric Malabsorptive Procedure: Jejunoileal Bypass

From 1954 until well into the 1970s, jejunoileal bypass was the standard surgical treatment for obesity because it produced significant weight loss in patients. However, the jejunoileal bypass no longer is employed as a surgical treatment for morbid obesity because the severe malabsorption resulted in serious and occasionally fatal nutritional complications, including diarrhea, metabolic imbalances, liver failure, kidney stones, immune complex reactions, and hypoproteinemia.

Combined Gastric Restriction and Malabsorption

Roux-en-Y gastric bypass

The Roux-en-Y gastric bypass (Fig. 29–1C) limits intake by generating a 10- to 30-mL proximal stomach pouch and delays emptying with an 8- to 10-mm gastroenterostomy.

It interferes with absorption by excluding the antrum, the duodenum, and 40 to 100 cm of proximal jejunum from contact with food. This procedure has been shown to be successful even in those patients classified as sweet eaters, primarily because it produces a dumping syndrome upon consumption of a high-sugar meal. Our version, the Greenville Gastric Bypass, has produced significant and maintainable weight loss up to 14 years in duration (Table 29–1).

The perioperative mortality is about 1%, but may rise to 10% in high-risk patients. The serious perioperative complication rate is 10%, and includes wound infections, anastomotic leaks, stenosis of the gastrojejunostomy, subphrenic abscess, and pulmonary emboli. Late side effects are primarily nutritional, including deficiencies of vitamins B_6 and B_{12}, calcium, and iron. Despite these risks, gastric bypass surgery is considered the gold standard for bariatric surgery. It has low mortality and excellent outcomes, including full remission of type 2 diabetes mellitus in 83%, control of hypertension in 50%, and reversal of cardiopulmonary failure and pseudotumor cerebri. In addition, fertility is often restored, physical fitness improved, and socioeconomic status raised.

Biliopancreatic diversion

Biliopancreatic diversion (Fig. 29–1D), also known as the Scopinaro operation, was designed to produce greater weight loss than gastric bypass alone by combining features of gastric and intestinal bypass with a cholecystectomy, and a gastric resection with a partial gastrectomy and an extensive exclusion of the small bowel. Loss of 70% of excess weight is achievable and maintainable up to 15 years with this procedure. Complications include gastric perforation, anastomosis leak, wound dehiscence and infection, stomal ulcers, protein malnutrition, and anemia resulting from iron, folate, and vitamin B_{12} deficiencies. The role for this procedure, still questioned by many, is not clear; the benefits do not appear to justify the risks.

Table 29–1
Weight loss in 608 morbidly obese patients after the Greenville Gastric Bypass*

	Mean Weight (lb)	% Excess Weight Loss	BMI (kg/m²)
Preoperation	304.4 (198–615)	0.0	49.7 (33.9–101.6)
1 yr	192.2 (104–466)	68.9 (10.3–124)	31.5 (19.1–69.3)
5 yr	205.4 (107–512)	57.7 (−14.6–115.9)	33.7 (19.6–7.16)
10 yr	206.2 (130–388)	54.7 (−0.9–103.1)	34.7 (22.5–64.7)
14 yr	204.7 (158–270)	49.2 (7.2–80.9)	34.9 (25.9–54.6)

BMI, body mass index.
*Data collected over 14 years with 97% follow-up. Ranges in parentheses.

Duodenal switch

The duodenal switch, a new procedure still under evaluation, includes the resection of the gastric greater curvature, division of the duodenum at the pylorus, and a roux-en-Y reconstruction. The operation appears to have the same outcomes as the gastric bypass.

Perioperative Care

Controlling Risk

Wound risk

Morbidly obese surgical patients have a diminished resistance to infection. Immunosuppression, comorbidities such as diabetes mellitus, and poor hygiene all contribute to their increased susceptibility for wound infections. Further complicating the picture, it is of note that morbidly obese patients tend to not manifest the classic signs of inflammation. It is documented that, by postoperative day 30, 8.7% of patients have suffered minor infections, 3% have suffered severe infection, and 2.5% have suffered from intra-abdominal abscess. The morbidly obese patient may not manifest the usual postoperative danger signs. The astute surgeon thus must be suspicious of persistent tachycardia greater than 120 beats/min, fever greater than 39°C, or worsening illness despite normal vital signs, all of which warrant a limited upper gastrointestinal study to rule out infection even if the patient looks well. In particular, the first 24 hours postoperatively are important because of the increased risk for a leak or intra-abdominal infection. In order to reduce the number of infections, most surgeons now give prophylactic antibiotics.

In addition to wound infections, these patients also are more prone to wound dehiscence and hernias. These phenomena are believed to occur secondary to increased intra-abdominal pressure, and the belief that the tissues of the morbidly obese do not have the same tensile strength as their thinner counterparts. These complications can be minimized by securely closing the abdomen with strong, broad bites of fascia.

The occurrence of wound problems and hernias has been reduced sharply, from 25% to 2%, with the advent of laparoscopic procedures.

Respiratory risks

The respiratory effects of obesity are complex and influenced by the degree of obesity and type of body fat distribution, either central or peripheral. The expiratory reserve volume in the morbidly obese is significantly decreased secondary to small airway closure. In addition, the mechanical effects of fat distribution on lung volume result in a 30% reduction of vital capacity and total lung capacity in the morbidly obese. The work required of morbidly obese patients to breathe increases dramatically compared to their nonobese counterparts, secondary to abnormal chest elasticity, an increase in chest wall and airway resistance, abnormal diaphragmatic position, upper airway resistance, and a need to eliminate a higher daily production of CO_2. The physiology is well illustrated in the obesity-hypoventilation, or pickwickian, syndrome with its hypersomnolence, sleep apnea, right-sided heart failure, and polycythemia.

In general the morbidly obese patient is hypoxemic. These patients suffer from a wide alveolar-arterial gradient as a result of ventilation-perfusion mismatching. There is alveolar collapse and airway closure at the bases, causing functional residual capacity to fall substantially when the patient is supine or under anesthesia. The morbidly obese also suffer from obstructive sleep apnea secondary to local accumulation of fat in the tracheopharyngeal area. These airway obstruction episodes interrupt sleep and are associated with hypoxia and hypercapnia. Over time, this can lead to pulmonary hypertension and ultimately right-sided heart failure or cor pulmonale. Continuous positive airway pressure at night, which produces significant diuresis, and losing weight can help reduce or eliminate this condition. Furthermore, polycythemia can develop in the morbidly obese secondary to prolonged hypoxia as a compensatory mechanism. This fact, along with diminished levels of antithrombin III and circulating fibrinolytic activity, places the morbidly obese at high risk for developing thromboembolic disease.

Postoperatively, poor respiratory outcome is twice as likely in morbidly obese compared to nonobese patients. Thoracic and upper abdominal incisions further complicate the respiratory effects on these patients. In addition, vertical band gastroplasty and gastric band patients are at increased risk for aspiration pneumonia postoperatively. This increased risk can be attributed to a higher volume of gastric fluid, lower than normal fasting gastric pH, increased intra-abdominal pressure, and higher incidence of gastro-esophageal reflux disease in obese patients. The airway of the morbidly obese surgical patient is difficult to control. Thus patients whose weight exceeds 400 lb often have a tracheostomy placed, and pain control strategies in these patients must avoid or minimize use of agents that cause respiratory depression. Pulse oximetry to monitor the patient and early physical mobilization will reduce the respiratory risks of the postoperative morbidly obese patient and expedite his or her recovery.

Cardiac risks

The adverse cardiovascular risks of morbid obesity are numerous. Morbid obesity results in an increase in total blood volume and resting cardiac output, both of which increase directly with the amount of weight beyond ideal body weight. The increase in cardiac output is due to an increase in stroke volume, because the heart rate tends to remain unchanged. The cardiac output increases to serve the metabolic requirements, specifically an increase in mean oxygen consumption, of excessive fat. The morbidly obese normotensive patient also experiences a decrease in systemic vascular resistance.

It has been reported that the morbidly obese have a decrease in the number of β-adrenergic receptors on their myocardium. This phenomenon results in impaired left ventricular contractility and a decrease in the ejection fraction both at rest and during physical activity. Because these patients have increased preloads from excess volume and reduced ventricular distensibility from left ventricular hypertrophy secondary to hypertension, their left ventricular filling pressure is elevated. Consequently, fluid loading in these patients may be poorly tolerated.

In general, signs of cardiac failure in the morbidly obese are unreliable and physical exams are difficult to perform. Thus these patients may need to be monitored in an intermediate intensive care unit by nurses comfortable with caring for bariatric surgery patients.

Anesthetic risks

The morbidly obese surgical patient is at greater risk while under general anesthesia compared to nonobese patients. In addition to difficulty with venous access and patient positioning, the obese surgical patient has a challenging airway to maintain. The obese patient's anatomy may make intubation difficult because of a large tongue and excessive pharyngeal tissue. As stated previously, patients who weigh in excess of 400 lb may require tracheostomies to facilitate airway management prior to the bariatric procedure. Anesthesia consults can be helpful. Induction of anesthesia results in a 50% reduction in functional residual capacity. This increases the patient's risks for small airway closure, ventilation-perfusion abnormalities, and hypoxemia.

Useful studies in the evaluation of the morbidly obese surgical patient include baseline blood pressure, complete blood cell count, electrolytes, metabolic panel, glucose, clotting indices, electrocardiogram (ECG), chest radiograph, and an arterial blood gas determination. Benzodiazepines along with a histamine$_2$ antagonist or proton pump inhibitor often are used preoperatively. The antacid may prevent aspiration pneumonitis. Sedatives deserve caution in the morbidly obese patient suffering from obesity-hypoventilation syndrome, secondary to the excessive somnolence and airway obstruction associated with this syndrome.

During the operation, the morbidly obese surgical patient should be monitored with an arterial line for blood pressure, ECG, pulse oximetry, capnography, and neuromuscular blockade, at the least. If intubation is difficult, then "awake

fiberoptic intubation" can be performed. The obese surgical patient, however, is at risk for hypoxia while under anesthesia, and it is for this reason that 50% inspired oxygen concentration may be useful initially. Opioids must be used with caution unless the patient is going to be ventilated postoperatively. Short-acting opioids are better choices than long.

Finally, the postoperative management of the morbidly obese surgical patient can be complicated by the anesthetic risk of hypoxia and hypercarbia. These risks can be assessed by evaluating the arterial blood gas values. The risk of hypoxia can be reduced by aiding gas exchange via having the patient in a semirecumbent position or sitting up. Also, encouraging early mobility and ambulation in addition to low-dose heparin therapy may provide excellent prophylaxis against deep venous thrombosis and pulmonary embolism.

Abdominal catastrophe

Intra-abdominal complications following bariatric surgery can be catastrophic for the patient. Immediate postoperative complications usually result from intraoperative incidents. Although rare (once in a career), these events may include stapling the nasogastric tube into the anastomosis, incorrect anastomotic connections, or injury to the esophagus or stomach.

The most feared complications that occur early postoperatively include anastomotic leaks and infections in the left upper quadrant. Clinical manifestations of either of these complications warrant immediate exploratory laparotomy. In addition to these early complications, the morbidly obese also suffer from complications seen in other general abdominal surgery, such as wound infection, dehiscence, ileus, cardiopulmonary failure, pulmonary embolus, pneumonia, and myocardial infarction.

Long-term complications include high rates of cholelithiasis following rapid postoperative weight loss and incisional hernias. Specifically, gastric banding bariatric surgery is associated with stoma complications, band erosion, partial gastric outlet obstruction, and gastric perforation. Gastroplasty patients are at risk for ruptured staple lines, band erosions, and outlet stenoses postoperatively. Finally, gastric bypass patients may suffer from staple line failures, internal hernias, and gastric distention.

Nutritional Support

Despite having excess body fat stores and large lean body stores, morbidly obese patients are at risk for developing protein-energy malnutrition in response to the metabolic stress of the postoperative period. The stressed obese patient will mobilize more protein and less fat versus a nonobese counterpart. Lipolysis and fat oxidation will be inhibited, causing a shift in the preferential use of carbohydrates.

This results in excessive protein breakdown to fuel gluconeogenesis and provide the necessary carbohydrate energy source. Because morbidly obese patients are using increasing amounts of carbohydrates for fuel, their respiratory quotients will increase substantially.

The nutritional requirements for the postoperative bariatric surgery patient are much different from the general requirements listed above for the postoperative morbidly obese patient. In general, because bariatric operations interfere with absorption of food, these patients can suffer from vitamin deficiencies in addition to those deficiencies discussed above. In order to avoid peripheral neuropathy, Wernicke-Korsakoff syndrome, and malnutrition, these patients should be supplemented postoperatively with vitamin B_{12} and thiamine. Female patients, in general, should have their diets supplemented with calcium to prevent bone demineralization, and menstruating women should receive iron supplements to avoid anemia.

Summary

Morbid obesity is a serious and grave disease that handicaps those individuals afflicted with it. The disease is associated with major health problems, such as hypertension, diabetes mellitus, heart disease, and pulmonary insufficiency. While we still do not fully understand this disease and its progression, we have continued to attempt to treat it. Conservative treatments have failed, and thus bariatric surgery has become the treatment of choice for morbid obesity. These operations have resulted in a wide range of outcomes, from desired weight loss to curing diabetes mellitus type 2, again pointing out how little we know about morbid obesity. The care of these patients and their comorbidities is difficult, yet, as we explore this new frontier, we must become more efficient and knowledgeable about the care of the morbidly obese surgical patient.

Bibliography

Albrecht RJ, Pories WJ: Surgical intervention for the severely obese. Best Practice Res 1999;10:149.

Baltasar M, Bou R, Cipagauta LA, et al: "Hybrid" bariatric surgery: bilio-pancreatic diversion and duodenal switch—preliminary experience. Obes Surg 1995;5:419.

Cotran RS, Kumar V, Collins T: Environmental and nutritional pathology. *In* Cotran RS, Kumar V, Collins T, Robbins SL (eds): Robbins Pathologic Basis of Disease (6th ed). Philadelphia: WB Saunders, 1999:452.

Gastrointestinal surgery for severe obesity. NIH Consensus Development Conference. NIH Consens Statement 1991;9(1).

Hunter JD, Reid C, Noble D: Anesthetic management of the morbidly obese patient. Hosp Med 1998;59:481.

Marik P, Varon J: The obese patient in the ICU. Crit Care 1998;113:492.

Merlino G, Scaglione R, Carrao S, et al: Association between reduced lymphocyte beta-adrenergic receptors and left ventricular dysfunction in young obese subjects. Int J Obes Metab Disord 1994;18:699.

Mokdad AH, Serdula MK, Dietz WH, et al: The spread of the obesity epidemic in the United States, 1991–1998. JAMA 1999;282:1519.

Pories WJ, Beshay JE: Surgery for obesity: procedures and weight loss. *In* Fairburn CG, Brownell KD (eds): Eating Disorders and Obesity: A Comprehensive Handbook (2nd ed). New York: Guilford Press, 2002.

Ramon RA, Pories WJ: Surgical treatment of morbid obesity. Endocr Pract 1995;1:265.

Rose DK, Cohen MM, Wigglesworth DE: Critical respiratory events in the postanesthesia care unit: patient, surgical, and anesthetic factors. Anesthesiology 1994;81:410.

Sugerman HJ, Starkey JV, Birkenhauer R: A randomized prospective trial of gastric bypass vs. vertical banded gastroplasty for morbid obesity and their effects on sweets v. non-sweet eaters. Ann Surg 1987;205:613.

Tschop M, Smiley D, Helman ML: Ghrelin induces adiposity in rodents. Nature 2000;407:908.

Wolf AM, Colditz GA: Current estimates of the economic cost of obesity in the United States. Obes Res 1998;6:97.

CHAPTER 30

The Diabetic Surgical Patient

Christopher P. Johnson, M.D. and Irene O'Shaughnessy, M.D.

Diabetes is currently classified according to pathogenesis. Type 1, or immune-mediated, diabetes previously was referred to as insulin-dependent diabetes mellitus. Type 1 diabetes is characterized by absence of insulin production and predilection for ketoacidosis. Type 2, or non–immune-mediated, diabetes (previously referred to as non–insulin-dependent diabetes mellitus) is characterized mainly by defective action of insulin. Some patients display features of both types. Type 2 diabetes accounts for 90% of all cases. Many type 2 diabetics can be managed by a combination of diet and/or oral agents. However, under conditions of stress, insulin often is required.

Diabetics undergoing surgery are at increased risk for postoperative complications for two major reasons: (1) the existence of secondary complications that are related to the long-term effects of diabetes and (2) adverse effects of short-term hyperglycemia. The latter has been shown to increase postoperative infection two- to fivefold. These observations are now supported by experimental evidence showing that impaired phagocytosis and wound healing occur at plasma glucose levels greater than 240 mg/dL.

The goals of diabetic management in the perioperative period should be twofold: (1) recognition and management of secondary diabetic complications along with assessment of cardiovascular risk, and (2) attainment of physiologic glucose regulation (100 to 200 mg/dL) in a manner that is safe and yet practical.

Metabolic Effects of Surgery and Anesthesia

The physiologic stress associated with surgical procedures leads to a catabolic response. Increased secretion of counter-regulatory hormones such as epinephrine, cortisol, and glucagon promotes hyperglycemia and worsens diabetic control. Interestingly, general anesthesia further exacerbates these changes, whereas spinal or epidural anesthesia has minimal effects on glucose regulation. Therefore, it is helpful to have an understanding of the different anesthetic techniques that could be applied for a given surgical procedure.

The most common complication in diabetics undergoing surgery is dehydration secondary to hyperglycemia and osmotic diuresis. This may be associated with poor tissue perfusion and ischemia to vital organs. The most dangerous complication is hypoglycemia, which may go unrecognized. Unfortunately, in order to avoid hypoglycemia, there tends to be a permissive attitude toward hyperglycemia, which may be associated with additional adverse effects including nosocomial infection and increased length of hospitalization.

Preoperative Evaluation

The preoperative evaluation should include a review of the diabetes history. Classification into type 1 or 2 diabetes along with history of insulin usage and adverse reactions is helpful. The average daily dose of insulin represents a good starting point for estimating insulin needs in the perioperative period.

Recent glycemic control should be reviewed. Fasting blood sugars greater than 200 mg/dL and glycosylated hemoglobin values in excess of 10% indicate poor control. Ideally, good diabetic control with glycosylated hemoglobin values less than 8% should be achieved prior to elective procedures, but this is not always possible. Referrals for outpatient evaluation and preoperative testing are generally recommended. In any case, rapid preoperative control of diabetes usually can be attained within a few hours using a glucose-insulin infusion if necessary.

It is important to recognize patients who are managed with long-acting agents such as chlorpropamide or Ultralente insulin. Such individuals can be switched to shorter acting agents for safer perioperative management, although this is not essential with careful perioperative monitoring and glucose administration.

Finally, preoperative evaluations should include an assessment of diabetic complications such as retinopathy, nephropathy, neuropathy, and macrovascular (including coronary) disease. Table 30–1 indicates common perioperative complications associated with these conditions.

Perioperative Management

Major Procedures

Blood glucose concentrations normally are maintained within a narrow physiologic range because of a balance between hepatic glucose production and peripheral utilization. The average glucose production rate is 5 to 10 g/hr (2.0 mg/kg/min) for adults. This is achieved through dietary intake or hepatic gluconeogenesis. Therefore, an intravenous infusion of 5% dextrose at 100 mL/hr (5 g/hr) delivers a necessary amount of glucose to minimize catabolism.

All diabetics managed with insulin should receive insulin during major surgical procedures. Any procedure that requires a general anesthetic, lasts 2 or more hours, or invades a major body cavity can be considered major for purposes of this discussion. Type 2 diabetics not currently managed with insulin but with fasting blood sugar levels higher than 180 mg/dL or glycosylated hemoglobin values of 10% or greater also should receive insulin during surgery.

The safest and most rational way to manage diabetics undergoing major surgery is with the use of continuous intravenous insulin. Numerous factors, including hypothermia, make the absorption of subcutaneous insulin (including that delivered continuously) erratic and unreliable. Bolus injections of intravenous insulin as a means of routine control are also inappropriate because of the short biologic half-life of regular insulin (5 to 6 minutes).

There are two accepted methods for delivering intravenous insulin. The glucose-insulin-potassium method is simple and safe. It is probably the preferred method for most patients undergoing relatively uncomplicated procedures (Box 30–1). Most patients can be maintained in a physiologic blood glucose range by infusion of 1.0 to 2.0 units of regular insulin per hour. The initial rate can be determined by considering the patient's average daily dose of insulin and adjusting for current glycemic control. For individuals receiving less than 50 units of insulin per day, a starting rate of 1.0 U/hr is reasonable, whereas those receiving more than 50 U/day should be started at 1.5 U/hr. Additional modifications are made as indicated in Box 30–1.

Table 30–1

Perioperative complications in diabetic patients undergoing surgery

Diabetic Complication	Possible Outcome
Retinopathy	Intraocular bleeding related to anticoagulants
Nephropathy	Prolonged insulin effect (hypoglycemia)
	Contrast- or antibiotic-related toxicity
Neuropathy	Cardiac arrhythmias (bradycardia)
	Hypotension
	Urinary retention
	Increased susceptibility to pressure sores
	Gastroparesis
Macrovascular disease	Myocardial infarction
	Congestive heart failure
	Stroke

Box 30–1

Perioperative Management Using Combined Glucose-Insulin-Potassium Infusions

General guidelines
- Use 5% dextrose with electrolytes as needed.
- Add regular insulin to this solution as indicated below.
- Infuse at 100 mL/hr.

Initial insulin estimation
- For patients treated with diet, oral agents, or insulin <50 U/day, add 10 U/L.
- For patients treated with >50 U/day, add 15 U/L.

Modifications based on current glycemic control (most recent blood sugar)
- Blood glucose >180 mg/dL: increase insulin by 5 units.
- Blood sugar <120 mg/dL: decrease insulin by 5 units.
- Supplemental subcutaneous doses of regular insulin may be given.

For patients undergoing complex procedures such as coronary bypass grafting or renal transplantation, separate glucose and insulin infusions provide greater flexibility and improved control (Table 30–2). For safety reasons, it is important to "piggyback" the insulin infusion line into the glucose-containing solution. An assessment of coexisting conditions or factors such as obesity, infection, steroid therapy, and renal failure should be made to estimate initial insulin needs. The latter is associated with an increased half-life (prolonged action) for insulin.

The safety and success of combined or separate glucose-insulin infusions is dependent on repeated, accurate measurements of blood glucose levels along with awareness of factors that modulate insulin sensitivity. During the surgical procedure and in the immediate postoperative period, these measurements should be done hourly. A bedside monitoring system (glucose meter) is essential, as is proper education of the nursing staff.

Minor Procedures

An increasing percentage of operations are being performed on outpatients. These include relatively extensive procedures such as laparoscopic cholecystectomy and various types of plastic and reconstructive surgery. Although it is never wrong or incorrect to manage these patients with glucose-insulin infusions, simpler methods often will suffice. Patients who are managed with oral hypoglycemic agents usually can be managed by checking pre- and postprocedure blood glucose levels. Occasionally one or two doses of insulin as indicated in Table 30–3 may be necessary. For insulin-treated patients taking less than 50 U/day, it is best to hold the morning dose of insulin and treat as indicated in Table 30–3. Most type 1 diabetics and all type 2 diabetics receiving greater than 50 U/day should receive one half of their total morning dose as intermediate-acting insulin. Short-acting insulin generally should be avoided.

Table 30–2
Guidelines for separate glucose and insulin infusions

General guidelines
- Administer 5% dextrose (with electrolytes as needed) at 100 mL/hr (5 g/hr).
- Mix 25 U regular insulin in 250 mL saline (0.1 U/mL).
- Piggyback the insulin infusion to the maintenance fluids containing glucose.

Initial insulin estimation
- For patients treated with diet, oral agents, or insulin dose < 50 U/day, starting rate is 1 U/hr.
- For patients receiving >50 U/day, starting rate is 1.5 U/hr.

Modifications based on current glycemic control (most recent blood sugar)

Blood Glucose (mg/dL)	Insulin Rate (U/hr)
<80	0
80–100	0.5
100–140	1.0
140–180	1.5
180–220	2.0
220–260	2.5
260–300	3.0
300–340	4.0
>340	5.0

Anticipate further adjustments based on the following parameters:
- Obesity, liver disease, trauma, burns (1.5 × selected dose)
- Severe infection, steroid therapy (2.0 × selected dose)
- Renal transplantation (2.0 × selected dose)
- Coronary bypass (3.5 × selected dose)

Adapted from Gavin LA: Perioperative management of the diabetic patient. Endocrinol Metab Clin North Am 1992;21:457.

Table 30–3
Guidelines for diabetes management during minor procedure and for outpatients

For patients receiving oral agents
- Hold AM dose
- Check blood glucose before and after procedure
- Give evening dose of oral agent if diet anticipated
- Supplement with regular insulin as indicated below

For type 1 diabetics and type 2 >50 U insulin/day
- Consider glucose-insulin infusions
- Administer ½ total morning dose as intermediate-acting insulin
- Monitor every 1–2 hr
- Supplement with insulin as indicated below

For type 2 diabetics <50 U insulin/day
- Hold all AM insulin
- Supplement with insulin as indicated below

Supplemental regular insulin

Blood Glucose (mg/dL)	SC Insulin Dose
<120	0
120–160	4
161–200	6
201–240	8
>240	10

- Administer 5% dextrose at 100 mL/hr whenever insulin is given.

Postoperative Management

In the postoperative period, patients will transition from a catabolic phase, requiring intravenous glucose and fluid and electrolyte support, to an anabolic or recovery phase. However, the transition period is variable in length because it is dependent on many factors, such as the preoperative condition, type of surgical procedure, and occurrence of postoperative complications. However, it should be emphasized again that the latter could be the result of poor diabetes control.

Many diabetic patients suffer from gastroparesis, which further hinders good diabetes control. Thus continuous insulin infusions often are preferred in the postoperative period. Simply by increasing or decreasing the rate of infusion, one can quickly make adjustments for the numerous postoperative variables that can impact blood glucose control. Separate glucose and insulin infusions provide greater flexibility than combined infusions.

Both are superior to traditional subcutaneous insulin regimens, which are associated with more dramatic swings in blood glucose levels.

During reintroduction of oral intake, it is preferable to continue a glucose-insulin infusion supplemented with small doses of subcutaneous regular insulin. The insulin can be given immediately before or after the meal and dosed according to ingested carbohydrates. A good rule of thumb for surgical patients is 1 unit of regular insulin per 10 g of carbohydrates. Once food tolerance is established, patients generally can be returned to their preoperative regimen, unless a major change has occurred such as initiation of steroid therapy. Some patients previously managed with oral agents may require a prolonged period of supplemental insulin (Table 30–4).

Lispro insulin (Humalog) is a newer rapid-acting insulin analog that may have potential advantages in the treatment of hyperglycemia. However, its use has been limited on an inpatient basis. Lispro insulin generally should be administered within 15 minutes before a meal because its peak action occurs at 60 to 90 minutes after subcutaneous injection.

Enteral and Parenteral Nutrition

Diabetic patients may require tube feedings or total parenteral nutrition (TPN) during prolonged postoperative recoveries. The insulin requirements for these situations can be estimated based on the previous insulin regimen, degree of stress, and carbohydrate intake. Most tube feeding formulations consist of 12% to 16% carbohydrates. Therefore, full-strength tube feedings when given at 100 mL/hr provide 12 to 16 g/hr of carbohydrates, requiring 1.2 to 1.5 units of insulin per hour. This should be added to a basal rate of approximately 1.0 to 1.5 U/hr (Box 30–2) to obtain a final rate of 2 to 3 U/hr.

Patients who are initiated at less than full-strength feedings at 100 mL/hr should have their insulin adjusted for the percentage difference. Insulin can be given as a continuous infusion or in divided doses of NPH (two thirds)/regular (one third) and adjusted as indicated in Box 30–2 and Table 30–2.

The carbohydrate content of TPN, at 25%, is almost double that of tube feedings. Therefore, 100 mL/hr of 25% dextrose delivers 25 g/hr. This may require substantially more insulin, as indicated in Box 30–2. An insulin infusion either separate or mixed with TPN should always be used when TPN is administered. Although a separate insulin infusion provides better control, it is safer to infuse 25% dextrose and insulin together in the same bag.

Table 30-4

Guidelines for postoperative management

Maintain insulin infusion (or sliding scale for minor procedures)

For patients previously treated with diet and oral agents

- Oral agents alone if glucose <180 mg/dL
- Oral agents plus sliding scale (see Table 30-3) if blood glucose >180 mg/dL

For insulin-treated patients

- Resume 75%–80% of usual regimen—if normal food intake is anticipated.
- Alternatively, select new dose based on 75%–80% of previous 24-hr insulin dosage (adjust according to anticipated intake)
- Needs may be higher during persistent stress, infection, steroid therapy
- The new dose can be given at breakfast (25%), lunch (25%), and dinner (25%) as regular insulin and 25% at bedtime as intermediate insulin.
- Either regimen (preoperative insulin dose or new dose) can be adjusted by blood glucose values obtained before a meal.

Blood Glucose (mg/dL)	Adjustment of Regular Insulin
<80	4 U less
81–120	3 U less
121–180	no adjustment
181–240	2 U more
240–300	3 U more
>300	4 U more

A relatively stable regimen should be established prior to discharge.

Adapted from Gavin LA: Perioperative management of the diabetic patient. Endocrinol Metabol Clin North Am 1992;21:457.

Emergency Operations, Ketoacidosis, and Hyperosmolar Coma

Diabetics may present for emergency operations. Common scenarios include acute abdominal conditions such as perforated appendicitis, diverticulitis, and cholecystitis, along with manifestations of peripheral vascular disease such as wet gangrene. Acute surgical conditions may be associated with ketoacidosis in type 1 diabetics and hyperosmolar nonketotic coma in type 2 diabetics.

Ketoacidosis occurs in a setting of relative or absolute insulin deficiency and is associated with hepatic oxidation of free fatty acids. Symptoms include anorexia, nausea, vomiting, and abdominal pain (which can mimic a surgical illness). Treatment of ketoacidosis consists of an initial insulin bolus of 10 to 15 units, followed by an infusion of 0.1 U/kg/hr. Adjustments are made according to hourly blood glucose levels. Once the levels fall to less than 250 mg/dL, a glucose-containing fluid (e.g., 5% dextrose) should be included in the rehydration fluids. One should usually delay surgery until metabolic control is achieved. Significant fluid, electrolyte, and acid-base abnormalities occur in ketoacidosis. The average fluid deficits are 3 to 5 L. Potassium supplementation may not be needed initially, but generous amounts typically are required as blood glucose levels fall. Unless the initial pH is less than 6.9, bicarbonate supplementation is not recommended because this can compromise oxygen delivery by shifting the oxygen-hemoglobin dissociation curve. Children are

Box 30-2

Guidelines for TPN in Diabetic Patients

Standard TPN (25% dextrose) at 100 mL/hr delivering 25 g/hr carbohydrate

Insulin requirements

- Estimated basal rate (1.0–1.5 U/hr)
- For 25 g/hr, increase by 3 U/hr (total 4.0–4.5 U/hr)
- Modify according to previous regimen, stress, etc.
- May distribute insulin in TPN bags by dividing total amount of insulin/day by volume of TPN (L/day)

especially prone to cerebral edema during treatment of ketoacidosis.

Adults with type 2 diabetes are prone to hyperosmolar coma. Residual insulin secretion in these patients is usually enough to prevent full activation of the ketogenic machinery in the liver. Typically, blood glucose levels in the several hundreds to 1000 mg/dL range are seen in association with severe volume depletion and increased serum osmolarity. Fluid deficits are typically 10 to 12 L. Patients are at risk for hyperviscosity syndromes with thrombotic complications. Treatment for hyperosmolar coma should address the profound fluid and electrolyte deficits, in addition to hyperglycemia.

Bibliography

Brandt MR, Kehlet H, Binder C, et al: Effects of epidural analgesia on the glucoregulatory endocrine response to surgery. Clin Endocrinol 1976;5:107.

Gavin LA: Perioperative management of the diabetic patient. Endocrinol Metab Clin North Am 1992;21:457.

Hirsch IB, McGill JB, Cryer PE, et al: Perioperative management of surgical patients with diabetes mellitus. Anesthesiology 1991;74:346.

Pomposelli JJ, Baxter JK, Babineau TJ, et al: Early postoperative glucose control predicts nosocomial infection rate in diabetic patients. JPEN J Parenter Enteral Nutr 1998;22:77.

CHAPTER 31

The Immunologically Compromised and Transplant Surgery Patient

Darrell A. Campbell, Jr., M.D. and Juan D. Arenas, M.D.

Operative procedures performed on immunocompromised patients are not new to surgery. Decades ago, the immunocompromised state was usually the sequela of malnutrition or related to the disease process, and postoperative wound and infectious complications were common. The malnourished surgical patient is less a problem in the modern era, but, as medicine has changed dramatically, new complexities have arisen. Organ transplantation is more and more a feature of current surgical practice, and the acquired immunodeficiency syndrome epidemic has produced legions of immunocompromised patients as well. What is clear is that the immunocompromised state changes the surgical playing field, and optimal results in these patient populations are achieved only through a complete understanding of the biology and the drugs commonly involved. This chapter focuses on the immunocompromised organ transplant recipient.

Transplantation

The purpose of this review is to focus on the immunocompromised patient, rather than the technical transplant procedure itself. Nonetheless, a few general comments are appropriate. First, it should be emphasized that the pace of antirejection drug development is extremely rapid, and results are constantly improving. Although there are some differences, a good rule of thumb is that 1-year graft survival rates for kidney (cadaveric donor), heart, pancreas, lung, and liver all approximate 80%, while 1-year graft survival rates for living donor kidney transplant are well over 90%. The survival curves generally flatten out after 1 year, and the "half-life" (the point at which 50% of recipients have lost the graft beyond 1 year) for kidneys, for example, is quite long, being 7.2 years for cadaveric donors and 13.5 years for living-related donors. The point is that the immunocompromised state is compatible with long life and, as many studies have shown, good quality of life as well.

Another important point to make is that the general strategy of drug development over the past few years has been to use more drugs at lower doses. This is in contrast to the early days of transplantation, when azathioprine and huge doses of steroids (the only drugs available) were given, although they were not particularly effective by today's standards; also, the steroids were attended by all the usual complications of steroid administration, most commonly infection, hypertension, pancreatitis, aseptic necrosis of the hip, cataracts, and poor or absent wound healing.

Modern immunosuppression uses far lower doses of steroids, and from two to four other agents that act at different points in the cycle of immune responsiveness. In some cases, it is possible to withdraw steroid immunosuppression completely. This strategy has produced more effective immunosuppression and less infection than was previously the case.

A final general point is that, in the case of the organ transplant recipient, the immunosuppressive burden is not just a function of the immunosuppressive drugs used, but is also a function of the underlying disease process (e.g., uremia) and the toll it has taken on the recipient, as well as the propensity of the immunosuppressive drugs to activate latent viruses, prominently cytomegalovirus (CMV) but also Epstein-Barr virus (EBV). These viruses themselves produce immunosuppression, thus resulting in a synergistic assault on the immune system. Rescue from over-immunosuppression frequently involves drug dose reduction and also therapy targeted toward the offending activated virus.

Immune Responsiveness to Antigen

Before discussing the important immunosuppressive agents, it is helpful to review briefly the cycle of immunologic events that occur after implantation of an allograft. This is perhaps best done by focusing on the antigen-presenting cell, of donor origin, and a subset of T lymphocytes, the T4 or helper/inducer subset, from the recipient. This interaction involves recognition of foreign class II antigen determinant on the donor cell by T4 cells, and also many important receptor-ligand interactions. As the result of "activation" of T4 cells, soluble mediator molecules are released, most notably interleukin-2 (IL-2), that in turn drive proliferation of the T8 or suppressor/cytotoxic subset of T lymphocytes. Importantly, only a very small fraction of T8 cells, those that have recognized donor foreign class I antigen and consequently have expressed an IL-2 receptor, respond to IL-2. The result is donor-specific clonal expansion of specifically cytotoxic T8 cells, which then initiate graft injury. IL-2 and its receptor thus play a dominant role in the clonal expansion process.

There are two intracellular enzymes and two cell surface structures that are important in the consideration of immune responsiveness and immunosuppression. Calcineurin is an intracellular enzyme that, when activated, causes the T-cell production and release of IL-2. TOR, or "target of rapamycin," is another cytosolic enzyme that, when activated (e.g., by IL-2), triggers cell cycle progression from G to S phase, and results in mitosis and clonal expansion. Both enzymes can be pharmacologically inhibited, as is discussed below.

An important cell surface structure is the IL-2–binding receptor, which appears on the cell surface of class I activated T8 cells, and which can be blocked by monoclonal antibody. Finally, the T3 lymphocyte is a pan–T cell antigen (present on all T cells) in close association with the T-cell antigen-receptor complex. Antibodies are available that recognize T3, and these are important in the treatment of acute rejection.

Maintenance Immunosuppression

Maintenance immunosuppression protocols are designed to act at different points in the cycle of immune responsiveness, with the exception of steroids, which can be considered more "general" immunosuppressants. The typical immunosuppressive regimen used at the University of Michigan for kidney transplant recipients is shown in Table 31–1 and includes three drugs: prednisone, a calcineurin inhibitor, and mycophenolate. Beginning with a rather large dose (500 mg) of intravenous methylprednisolone (Solu-Medrol) intraoperatively, the steroid doses are tapered rapidly. A general goal is to reduce the dose to 10 mg of prednisone orally by 3 months postoperatively.

Calcineurin Inhibitors

Calcineurin inhibition is the mainstay of most immunosuppressive protocols. Calcineurin inhibitors (cyclosporine, tacrolimus) produce significant side effects (Table 31–2), the most important of which are nephrotoxicity, hyperglycemia, and neurotoxicity. Blood levels should be monitored regularly in order to decrease the incidence of these complications. At our center we use a whole-blood high-performance liquid chromatography assay. The desired ranges for drug levels at our institution are shown in Table 31–3.

Cyclosporine

Cyclosporine (Sandimmune), a fungal product, was the first calcineurin inhibitor introduced into clinical practice, and is largely responsible for the tremendous improvement in transplant results over the past two decades. A microemulsion formulation (Neoral) has significantly increased the absorption of the drug. This formulation is not dependent on bile flow, as is Sandimmune, an important factor in liver transplantation.

Tacrolimus

Tacrolimus (FK-506, Prograf) is a calcineurin inhibitor that also acts to block IL-2 production and release, but that is far more potent than cyclosporine. Tacrolimus and cyclosporine cannot be used in combination because their

Table 31–1
Adult renal transplant immunosuppression regimen at the University of Michigan

Day Post-transplant	Oral Prednisone Dose	Cyclosporine	Mycophenylate
1	50 mg bid	3mg/kg PO bid*	1.0 gm PO bid
2	40 mg bid		
3	30 mg bid		
4–6	20 mg bid		
7–14	30 mg qd		
15–21	25 mg qd		
22–28	20 mg qd		
29+	Reduce 2.5 mg/wk until 10 mg qd		

In cases of delayed graft function, cyclosporine is held and only initiated when the serum creatinine has decreased 25% in a 24-hour period. During this interval, the patient is treated prophylactically with goat anti–T cell antibody (Thymoglobulin).

effects are additive. Tacrolimus also produces nephrotoxicity, hyperglycemia, and neurotoxicity.

Mycophenolate Mofetil

Mycophenolate mofetil (MMF, CellCept) commonly is used as a maintenance therapy in combination with prednisone and a calcineurin inhibitor. MMF interferes with DNA and RNA synthesis, and thus inhibits the rapid cell proliferation needed for clonal expression. Importantly, the effects of MMF are selective for lymphocytes, allowing other cells (e.g., polymorphonuclear leukocytes) to proliferate normally.

MMF produces some degree of marrow suppression, unlike calcineurin inhibitors, but does not produce nephrotoxicity, hyperglycemia, or neurotoxicity. Gastrointestinal side effects are common but usually respond to dose reduction.

Interleukin-2 Receptor Blockade

Some transplant programs routinely add IL-2 receptor blockade to their maintenance protocol. Basiliximab (Simulect) is a humanized monoclonal antibody that recognizes the high-affinity (55-kD) form of the IL-2 receptor, which is expressed in response to antigen stimulation. Simulect is administered intravenously on days 1 and 4 following transplantation and is associated with remarkably few side effects. Using this regimen, receptor blockade lasts for 30 to 45 days.

TOR Inhibition

Rapamycin (sirolimus) is a fungal product that inhibits the action of TOR. A synthetic analog (SDZ-RAD) also has

Table 31–2
Side effects of immunosuppressive medication

			Side Effects			
Drug	Nephrotoxicity	Hyperglycemia	Neurotoxicity	Lipid	BM Depression	GI
Prednisone	–	+ +	–	–	–	–
Cyclosporine	+ +	+	+ +	+	–	–
Tacrolimus	+ +	+	+ +	+	–	–
Mycophenolate	–	–	–	–	+ +	+ +
Sirolimus	–	–	–	+ +	+	–
Simulect	–	–	–	–	–	–

BM, bone marrow; GI, gastrointestinal.

Table 31–3
Adult renal transplant target cyclosporine (Neoral) levels at the University of Michigan

Post-Transplant Month	Cyclosporine (Neoral) Level*
First	225–275 ng/mL
Second	175–225 ng/mL
Third and subsequent	125–175 ng/mL

As measured by whole-blood high-performance liquid chromatography.

been developed. Sirolimus is an effective agent by itself, but, importantly, it appears to act in a synergistic way with calcineurin inhibitors, producing potent immunosuppression. In contrast to the calcineurin inhibitors, sirolimus produces neither nephrotoxicity, hyperglycemia, nor neurotoxicity. It does, however, produce significant elevations of plasma cholesterol and triglycerides and may exacerbate the nephrotoxicity of cyclosporine.

Relevant to the subject of the surgical patient on sirolimus, it is important to note that TOR inhibitors have an inhibitory effect on mesenchymal cell proliferation, whereas calcineurin inhibitors do not, and in fact are known to induce upregulation of fibrogenic cytokines. Inhibition of mesenchymal cell proliferation has a salutary effect on fibrosis and scarring of allograft blood vessels, a feature of chronic rejection. Interestingly, the antiproliferative effect also may be advantageous in the nontransplant setting; coronary stents impregnated with sirolimus have been used recently in an attempt to delay or prevent stenosis of such conduits. In our clinical experience, wound healing also has been delayed by administration of this drug.

Acute Rejection

In approximately 25% of cases, an acute rejection episode, or "breakthrough" rejection, occurs in patients on the described maintenance protocols. Most patients, regardless of organ transplant type, do not display clinical signs of rejection; rather, it is a biochemical or biopsy diagnosis. In the case of kidney transplantation, a serum creatinine rise of 0.3 mg/dL or more in a 24-hour period, in the absence of cyclosporine toxicity, is suggestive of rejection and should prompt a biopsy.

The treatment of an acute rejection episode begins with high-dose steroid administration, typically Solu-Medrol 250 mg IV each day for 3 days. Approximately 50% of patients treated in this way respond. For those patients in whom steroids are not sufficient, more aggressive antirejection therapy is indicated. Either a mouse

monoclonal or goat polyclonal antibody is administered daily for 10 to 14 days. The mouse monoclonal antibody, OKT3, recognizes the T3 determinant on all T cells, effectively removing them from the circulation and resulting in profound immunosuppression while the antibody is being administered. This treatment is successful in reversing rejection in 95% of cases. The goat polyclonal antibody is similarly successful, but recognizes a wide variety of T-cell determinants.

Infection

When a surgical specialist is faced with operating on a patient with a functioning organ transplant, the immediate question involves the patient's susceptibility to infection. This question is particularly germane when the procedure to be done is an elective one, and the balance is between the risk of infection and the possible gain from the procedure.

The transplant recipient with a stable course is not particularly at higher risk for surgical site infection, provided that the procedure is not overly long, that prophylactic antibiotics are administered, and that no chronic unresolved infection exists at the time of surgery. This conclusion is somewhat counterintuitive but has been borne out by considerable clinical experience. The wound infection rate in renal transplant patients with an otherwise uncomplicated course was 1.6%, for example, and all were superficial infections; the rate was 0.7% if diabetic patients were excluded. The overall infection rate for clean general surgical cases in nonimmunosuppressed patients was 1.8% by contrast. Many other groups have reported similar findings. These data indicate that the relatively low levels of immunosuppression that are induced in an uncomplicated transplant case are not sufficient to result in an increase in bacterial wound infection. This is in marked contrast to an earlier era, when transplant patients commonly received 30 to 40 mg of prednisone per day as maintenance therapy.

Apart from bacterial wound infections, there is no denying that immunosuppressed patients are at higher risk for various viral or fungal pathogens. The propensity to develop such infections depends upon what has been referred to as the "net state of immunosuppression." This is a function of drug dose, timing, and duration; whether or not various mucocutaneous surfaces have been violated (drainage catheters, endotracheal tubes); the state of protein-calorie malnutrition; and whether or not the patient is infected with an immunomodulating virus, such as CMV, EBV, hepatitis B, hepatitis C, or human immunodeficiency virus. When elective surgery is proposed, prudence would dictate that the surgery be postponed until the active state of infection has resolved. The majority of opportunistic fungal infections in transplant patients occur in the setting of concomitant viral infection.

Infectious patterns have been observed that relate to the time of the transplant procedure. In the first post-transplant month, for example, blood stream infections from contaminated lines or bacterial pneumonia in the intubated patient are most common. In the 1- to 6-month period after transplant, infections from various immunomodulating viruses are prominent, as are opportunistic infections with *Pneumocystis carinii* and fungi. Postoperative infections are less common after 6 months, unless the net immunosuppressive burden is increased because of recurrent rejection and its attendant drug therapy, or because chronic infection with an immunomodulating virus has developed. In these cases, opportunistic infection with *Cryptococcus neoformans*, *P. carinii*, *Listeria monocytogenes*, or *Nocardia asteroides* may occur.

Issues in Clinical Management

Drug Interactions

The surgical specialist operating on the transplant patient may need to add drugs to the therapeutic regimen. Certain drugs may markedly affect the levels of immunosuppressants, and thus must be used cautiously. Cyclosporine and tacrolimus are metabolized by the hepatic cytochrome P-450 3A isozyme system. Drugs that increase the activity of this system, such as rifampin, isoniazid, and nafcillin, result in faster degradation and lower levels of both cyclosporine and tacrolimus for this reason. Other drugs slow the activity of cytochrome P-450, which results in higher levels of the calcineurin inhibitors. Such drugs as erythromycin, clarithromycin, azithromycin, ketoconazole, itraconazole, and fluconazole have this effect. Levels of cyclosporine and tacrolimus should be closely monitored when these drugs are administered.

Another important interaction involves nephrotoxicity. Trimethoprim-sulfamethoxazole (TMP-SMZ) and fluoroquinolones exacerbate cyclosporine- or tacrolimus-induced nephrotoxicity at higher doses, although they are well tolerated and almost universally used at lower doses. Aminoglycoside antibiotics likewise have a synergistic effect with cyclosporine or tacrolimus in producing nephrotoxicity.

Prophylactic Antibiotics, Antivirals, and Antifungals

Transplant patients commonly receive one single-strength tablet of TMP-SMZ daily for several months following transplantation. This regimen drastically reduces the incidence of most urinary tract infections, *P. carinii* and certain unusual respiratory pathogens (*L. monocytogenes*,

N. asteroides, and *Toxoplasma gondii*). Transplant patients also receive prophylactic antiviral drugs, either ganciclovir or acyclovir, for months following transplant to prevent CMV infection or other herpetic infections. The development of symptomatic CMV infection at any time after transplant dictates intravenous ganciclovir for 2 to 4 weeks. Oral nystatin is administered routinely to prevent candidal infection, reserving intravenous fluconazole for particularly high-risk situations.

Antibiotic prophylaxis prior to elective surgery is usually accomplished with cefazolin or cefotaxime in transplant recipients.

Life-threatening Infection

If a transplant patient develops a life-threatening infection of any kind, it is important to reduce levels of immunosuppressive medication. In the case of kidney or pancreatic transplantation, where loss of the organ is not incompatible with life, our practice is to discontinue all medications except for 10 mg of prednisone daily until the infection has been controlled, at which point they may be gradually reinstated. In the case of heart, lung, or liver transplantation, this is a more difficult decision, and some kind of compromise between a low-dose immunosuppressive regimen, close monitoring, and aggressive antibiotic support must be developed.

Adjusting the Perioperative Dose of Steroids

We do not adjust the dose of prednisone upward in preparation for elective surgery. This would increase the chance of infection and is not needed from a hemodynamic standpoint as long as the patient is receiving at least 10 mg of prednisone daily. The patient should, however, take the usual dose of oral prednisone prior to surgery with a sip of water.

The Abdominal Examination in Immunosuppressed Transplant Patients

Inflammation or frank peritonitis in the otherwise healthy individual is manifested by fever, tachycardia, diminished bowel sounds, guarding, and rebound tenderness. Because immunosuppressive agents, predominantly steroids, interfere with the inflammatory response, these findings may be less obvious or absent altogether in transplant patients. In such cases, clinical management has as its base a heightened index of suspicion and relies heavily on ancillary diagnostic aids. An abdominal computed tomography scan is a sensitive screen for the presence of free air and intraperitoneal fluid. If the latter is detected and otherwise unexplained, an aggressive approach with needle aspiration is advisable. Diagnostic laparoscopy is increasingly popular to help make difficult clinical decisions in this patient population.

Bibliography

Abraham RT: Mammalian target of rapamycin: immunosuppressive drugs uncover a novel pathway of cytokine receptor signaling. Curr Opin Immunol 1998;10:330.

Abraham RT, Wiederrecht G: Immunopharmacology of rapamycin. Annu Rev Immunol 1996;14:483.

Brunn JN: Postoperative wound infection: predisposing factors and the effect of a reduction in the dissemination of staphylococci. Acta Med Scand 1970;514(Suppl):3.

Cecka JM: The UNOS Scientific Renal Transplant Registry—2000. In Cecka JM, Terasaki PL (eds): Clinical Transplants 2000. Los Angeles: UCLA Immunogenetics Center, 2001.

First MR: Case 1: persistent acute rejection after kidney transplantation. Transplantation 2001;71:1697.

Fishman J, Rubin R: Infection in organ transplant recipients. N Engl J Med 1998;338:1741.

Kamath S, Dean D, Peddi VR, et al: Efficacy of OKT3 as primary therapy for histologically confirmed acute renal allograft rejection. Transplantation 1997;64:1428.

Knight RJ, Burrows L, Bodiany C: The influence of acute rejection on long-term renal allograft survival: a comparison of living and cadaveric donor transplantation. Transplantation 2001;72:69.

Kovarik JM, Moore R, Wolf P, et al: Screening for basiliximab exposure-response relationships in renal allotransplantation. Clin Transplant 1999;13(1 Pt 1):32.

Kremer B, Henne-Bruns D, Broelsch-Houssin CE: Atlas of Liver, Pancreas, and Kidney. New York: Theime Medical Publishers, 1994.

Kyriakides GK, Simmons RL, Najarian JS: Wound infections in renal transplant wounds: pathogenetic and prognostic factors. Ann Surg 1975;186:770.

Morris RE, Cao W, Huang X: Rapamycin inhibits vascular smooth muscle DNA synthesis in vitro and suppresses narrowing in arterial allografts and in balloon injured carotid arteries: evidence that rapamycin antagonizes growth factor action on immune and non-immune cells. Transplant Proc 1995;27:430.

Rubin RH: Infection in the organ transplant recipient. In Rubin RH, Young LS (eds): Clinical Approach to Infection in the Compromised Host. New York: Plenum Medical Book Company, 1994:629.

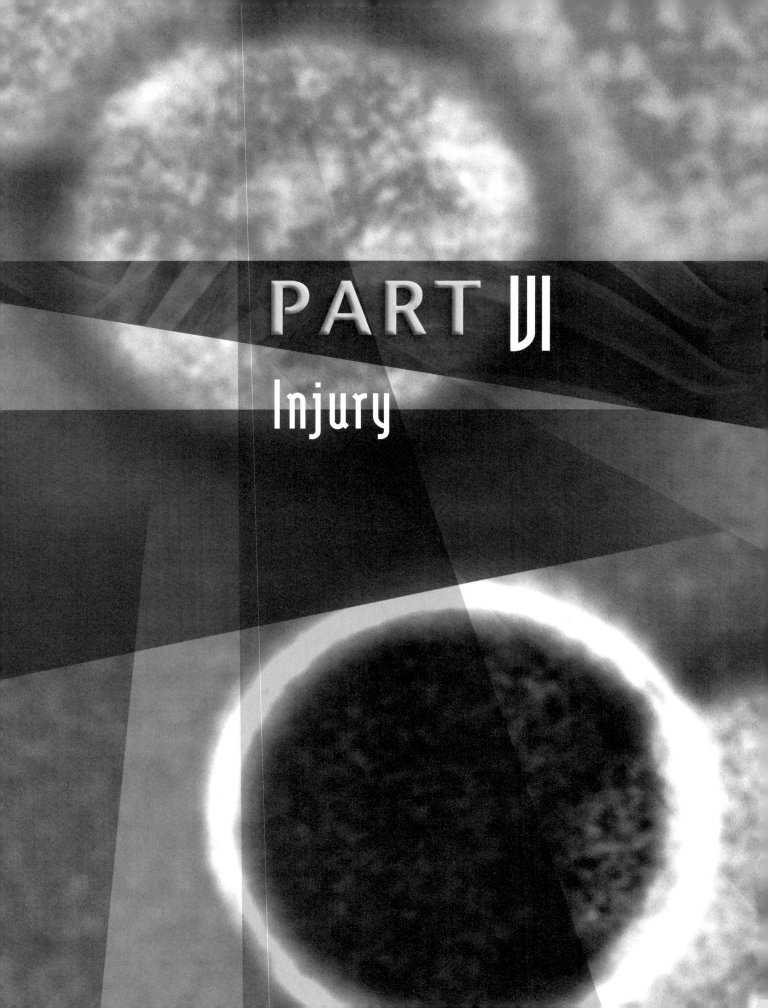

PART VI

Injury

CHAPTER 32

Metabolic Response to Trauma

Marcus Spies, M.D. and David N. Herndon, M.D.

Pathophysiology of Metabolism in Trauma and Burns

Hypermetabolism

The hypermetabolic response after major trauma and burns is characterized by a hyperdynamic circulatory response with increased body temperature, oxygen and glucose consumption, CO_2 production, glycogenolysis, proteolysis, and lipolysis and futile substrate cycling, leading to erosion of lean body mass, muscle weakness, immunodepression, and poor wound healing. This systemic reaction to severe trauma includes a severe increase in resting energy expenditure (REE) to more than 150% of normal levels predicted from standards for size, age, sex, and weight. A study in 25 severely burned children indicated that this hypermetabolic stress response may persist beyond the initial recovery and wound healing time up to 1 year after injury. Hypermetabolism leads to depletion of protein and fat stores, resulting in degradation of body protein, which can be clinically measured as loss of lean body mass and muscle wasting. Beside these effects, which jeopardize recovery and rehabilitation, hypercatabolic patients experience immune suppression with decreased resistance to infection and poor wound healing. The exact genesis of this phenomenon remains unclear, but increased heat loss from the burn wound, increased β-adrenergic activity, and the post-traumatic systemic inflammatory response are important contributing factors.

Energy Requirements

Predictive equations have been developed to estimate REE. In burned children, body surface area, body weight and the predicted basal energy expenditure (PBEE) obtained from the Harris-Benedict equation correlate with measured REE. Energy expenditure becomes maximal at burn sizes over 40% of total body surface area (TBSA) and remains elevated for months after injury despite closure of the burn wound. In smaller injuries, such as a 10% TBSA third-degree burn, minimal effect on metabolic regulation or food intake has been observed. Equations depending on burn size overestimate caloric requirements in patients with large burns, which may put them at risk by exposing them to caloric excess. On average, REE equals $1.29 \times$ PBEE in fed burn patients, which leaves PBEE as the single most powerful predictor of REE in burn patients (Fig. 32–1). However, because there may be considerable variations in this relation, the most accurate determination of REE is obtained by indirect calorimetry, which can be easily obtained using a commercially available calorimeter.

Extensive studies at the U.S. Army Institute of Surgical Research demonstrated that REE might be 200% to 300% greater than predicted basal values in severely burned adults. However, because these patients underwent conventional treatment without early excision or occlusive dressings, measured REE values were much higher than in later studies in patients receiving early excision and occlusive dressings. Despite restricted data, observations

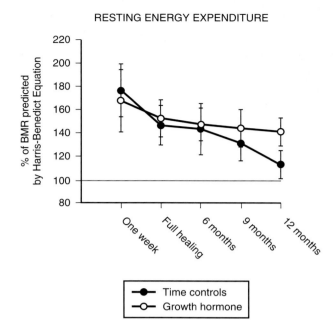

RESTING ENERGY EXPENDITURE

FIGURE 32–1 Hypermetabolism persists over a prolonged period of time. Resting energy expenditure measured as a percentage of the predicted basal metabolic rate (BMR) remained elevated in burned children for up to 12 months. (Adapted from Hart DW, Wolf SE, Mlcak R, et al: Persistence of muscle catabolism after severe burn. Surgery 2000;128:312.)

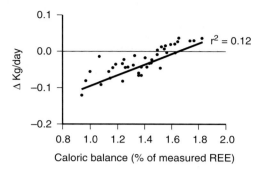

FIGURE 32–2 Linear correlation between total body weight and caloric delivery indexed to measured resting energy expenditure (REE). Caloric delivery at approximately 1.5 × REE was able to achieve maintenance of total body weight. (Adapted from Hart SW, Wolf SE, Herndon DN, et al: Energy expenditure and caloric balance after burn: increased feeding leads to fat rather than lean mass accretion. Ann Surg 2002;235:152.)

made in adults and in children treated with early excision and occlusive dressing are similar: PBEE is the most important predictor of REE, and burn size over 40% TBSA is not related to REE. The average REE (in the fed state) is about 1.3 to 2 × PBEE.

To assess the total caloric requirements, knowledge of the relationship between total energy expenditure (TEE) and REE is essential. In 15 burned children in whom TEE was determined over the whole hospital course by the double-labeled water technique with concomitant REE determination by indirect calorimetry, TEE was $1.33 \pm 0.27 \times$ PBEE, and $1.18 \pm 0.17 \times$ REE in the fed state. TEE was significantly correlated with measured REE ($r^2 = 0.92$). After incorporation of the average activity factor, calculated as the difference between TEE and REE, into a predictive equation based on the measured value of REE, the average energy requirement to maintain energy balance was 1.55 × PBEE. In another study at our institution, a linear correlation could be established between the change in total body weight and actual caloric intake. At a caloric delivery, maintenance of body weight could be achieved (Fig. 32–2). Caloric intake above 1.5 × REE, however, led to increased accretion of fat mass in burn patients. This nutritional goal of 1.5 × REE is significantly lower than that of the commonly used formulas for severely burned patients. Common formulas with

caloric intakes of approximately 2 × PBEE provide excess caloric intake, which in some patients exceeds their actual requirements by more than 70%. Therefore, it seems clinically reasonable to aim for an average caloric intake of 1.5 × PBEE. Although generated in children, the above data are similar to the values for predicted TEE in adults. Close and strict monitoring of individual tolerance to caloric intake is necessary, and adjustments have to be made according to the monitoring of blood glucose and triglyceride concentrations, as well as body weight changes over time.

Changes in Substrate Metabolism

Despite appropriate nutritional support, alterations in the metabolism of specific substrates occur after major burn. This includes changes in intracellular substrate oxidation and the availability of energy substrates.

Carbohydrate metabolism

GLUCOSE. Glycogenolysis and gluconeogenesis in the liver are supply processes for glucose as an energy substrate. Glycogenolysis, or the breakdown of stored glycogen, involves essentially no "net" loss of lean body mass, but represents "delayed" oxidation of ingested glucose. In contrast, gluconeogenesis, or the production of new glucose, is a complex reaction sequence of many intermediate steps, which basically has to reverse glycolysis and thereby has to overcome the energy barriers of this chemical reaction. Although a variety of substrates can serve as gluconeogenic precursors, lactate is the most important one.

Because most lactate is derived from glycolysis of glucose, the resynthesis of glucose from lactate is a cyclic reaction, known as the Cori cycle. Under anaerobic conditions, the Cori cycle is able to maintain a glucose supply sufficient to provide a certain amount of energy by glycolysis, although "net" glucose formation is not increased. However, by using fat oxidation in the liver to supply the needed energy, the Cori cycle serves as a mediator for energy transfer from adipose tissue to muscle, in situations in which the muscle is unable to fully rely on fat oxidation. The Cori cycle in normal subjects accounts for approximately 10% to 15% of the total glucose production in fasting; excess levels of lactate resulting from altered peripheral metabolism of glucose increase the quantitative importance of this metabolic pathway in stress states.

Another gluconeogenic substrate is glycerol. In a normal, lean subject, glycerol contributes about 3% of the total glucose produced during a short fasting period. However, during stimulation of fat mobilization, such as during long fasting periods or severe burn, glycerol may contribute as much as 20% of the total glucose production.

Alanine and glutamine account for 50% to 60% of the total amino acids released from muscle. In nonacidotic conditions, glutamine uptake by the kidney is minimal; rather, glutamine is taken up by the mucosal cells of the small intestine and converted to alanine. Alanine is the major amino acid precursor for gluconeogenesis. Alanine is released from muscle in far greater quantities than it is present in muscle protein. It has been suggested that pyruvate, resulting from the glycolytic catabolism of glucose, is transaminated and the resulting alanine is released into the blood stream, to be reincorporated into glucose by the liver. This metabolic cycle is analogous to the Cori cycle in that alanine results in no new "net" glucose production. The nitrogen required for the transamination of pyruvate is derived from amino acids, which are oxidized by muscle, including the branched-chain amino acids valine, leucine, and isoleucine, as well as aspartate and glutamate. This process transfers ammonia from muscle to liver in the nontoxic form of alanine.

CHANGES OF GLUCOSE PRODUCTION IN CRITICAL ILLNESS. Glucose production is increased in almost all critically ill patients, including those with severe burn, in whom glucose flow is elevated three- to sixfold. The regulation of glucose production is similar in most critical ill patients. Gluconeogenesis is elevated, particularly from alanine; glycogenolysis is also stimulated subsequent to carbohydrate intake. Increased gluconeogenesis from amino acids leads to diminished availability of these amino acids for maintenance of body protein synthesis and homeostasis. The resulting nitrogen loss, primarily by excretion as urea, results in progressive depletion of body protein stores.

CONNECTION BETWEEN GLUCONEOGENESIS AND MUSCLE AMINO ACID RELEASE. A distinct feature of critical illness metabolism is increased protein breakdown compared to that in normal individuals who are fed comparable levels of protein and calories. The resulting increased release of amino acids, including gluconeogenic amino acids, from the muscle is a systemic response to injury. Alanine release from the muscle was found to be elevated in burned as well as unburned legs of severely burned patients. Consequently, it has been suggested that elevated plasma alanine levels may induce glucose formation by the liver at an increased rate. However, plasma amino acid concentrations, including gluconeogenic amino acids, are generally below normal in burn patients. A study in normal volunteers showed that increased alanine delivery to the liver did not stimulate glucose production. Glucose infusion increased alanine release from muscle, indicating that pyruvate availability may be rate limiting for the peripheral formation of alanine. Thus the increase in total glucose production in critical illness appears not to be due to an increased rate of alanine delivery to the liver. Rather, the high rate of glucose production and thus glucose uptake into the muscle drives the rate of peripheral release of alanine. How low concentrations of amino acids could stimulate gluconeogenesis in the liver remains unclear. However, it can be concluded that direct stimulating factors in the liver are more important than peripheral metabolic changes to determine the rate of glucose production.

REGULATION OF GLUCOSE PRODUCTION. Plasma insulin levels are usually normal or slightly elevated in burn patients. The fact that the basal rate of gluconeogenesis is elevated despite normal or elevated plasma insulin levels has been defined as hepatic insulin resistance. Increased plasma glucose concentrations, as are frequently found in burned patients, would normally directly inhibit glucose production. When glucose is infused into burn patients, gluconeogenesis is suppressed to some extent, but the residual endogenous glucose production is higher than in normal volunteers because of hepatic "insulin" and "glucose" resistance. In studies trying to determine the role of hormonal factors for these findings, increased gluconeogenesis could not be explained by increased catecholamine levels, because adrenergic blockade in burned guinea pigs further increased glucose production. This unexpected increase in glucose production could be explained on the basis of the effect of catecholamine blockade on fatty acid metabolism.

In contrast to adrenergic blockade, blocking glucagon secretion shows a pronounced effect on glucose production in burn patients, demonstrating the preeminent role of glucagon as a stimulator of glucose production in burned patients. When infusing somatostatin, an inhibitor of glucagon and insulin secretion, with insulin supplementation to maintain preexistent basal levels, burn-induced elevated glucagon levels are lowered to normal levels and glucose production decreases and remains depressed throughout the infusion. The role of corticosteroids as simulators of glucose production in burn has not yet been thoroughly evaluated; however, the results of hormone infusion experiments indicate that cortisol may play an important role by enhancing and prolonging the effectiveness of glucagon.

REGULATION OF LIPOLYSIS. In normal healthy humans, fat is the major reserve fuel storage. These fat stores can be depleted if needed without any great harm to existing body structures. This contrasts clearly with protein reserves, which consist mostly of structural proteins or functional protein, and whose degradation renders the body especially susceptible to post-traumatic stress. Thus lipids represent the physiologically most desirable endogenous energy source, which can easily be metabolized by most tissue as fatty acids, so limited carbohydrate reserves are preserved for the central nervous system and red blood cells. Additionally, the brain can partially adapt to use ketone bodies (β-hydroxybutyrate and acetoacetate) as an energy substrate. The mobilization and use of fat might be part of an optimal "stress" response. The general stress response includes the release of hormones promoting mobilization of fat depots. However, elevated lactate levels resulting from muscle glycolysis (another catecholamine effect) stimulate re-esterification within the adipose tissue, thus balancing stimulated lipolysis. Other stress response–related factors, such as a decrease in pH and hyperglycemia, both inhibit lipolysis and stimulate re-esterification of fatty acids. Stress-related hypoperfusion of adipose tissue might further prevent effective mobilization of fat reserves. Despite these common regulatory factors, the stimulation of lipolysis is a fundamental part of the metabolic stress response. This event is mediated by increased adrenergic activity, and β-adrenergic blockade in patients acutely reduces the rate of release of free fatty acids (FFAs). However, tachyphylaxis of β-blocking agents may preclude a long-term effect on FFA levels.

Excess peripheral release of FFAs in severe trauma leads to the awkward situation in which over 70% of FFAs are not used as an energy source, but rather are re-esterified into triglyceride. The increased supply of FFAs leads to an increased rate of triglyceride synthesis, predominantly in the liver. In normal metabolic conditions, a proportionate rate of triglyceride synthesis and very-low-density lipoprotein (VLDL) triglyceride secretion leads to a refueling of peripheral storage depots in fat cells. However, in post-traumatic stress this export of VLDL triglycerides by the liver is impaired, leading to deposition of fat in the liver, even with absence of significant hepatic fatty acid synthesis. Delivery of FFAs to the liver is diminished by insulin and glucose administration, resulting in a decreased hepatic triglyceride production. This fits the clinical observation that fat deposition in the liver of critically ill patients is related to the severity of the illness and not to the content or quantity of the nutritional support.

GLUCOSE UTILIZATION. Blood glucose levels are tightly regulated, but rates of glucose uptake and consumption vary greatly. Glucose supply determines the extent of its use as a major fuel; glucose is the major energy source after a carbohydrate-rich meal, and glucose oxidation accounts only for 25% of total carbon dioxide production after several hours of fasting. The brain and erythrocytes, depending entirely on glucose as an energy source and having a relatively constant glucose uptake under normal conditions, may use more than 50% of the total glucose uptake during fasting. However, the absolute amount utilized does not explain the observed changes in the rate of glucose oxidation in different physiologic and pathologic conditions. Although the liver might play a role in the disposition of a glucose load, the overall rate of glucose uptake by the individual is determined by muscle tissue, which constitutes about 40% of the body mass. In the resting postabsorptive state, glucose uptake in muscle is minimal, but with hyperglycemia or exercise, the rate of glucose uptake by the muscle will increase. This implies an important role of changes in muscle glucose metabolism in overall energy metabolism, and the mechanism of its regulation.

In post-traumatic stress, the normal ability of insulin to regulate peripheral glucose uptake is diminished. This insulin resistance, which is evident at submaximal doses in all circumstances, can be overcome by pharmacologic doses of insulin. However, in septic patients insulin effectiveness is diminished. Peripheral insulin resistance has been attributed to an impaired ability to oxidize glucose. Stable isotope studies, however, indicate that pyruvate oxidation is unimpaired and the total rate of glucose oxidation is significantly increased, both in the basal state and during glucose infusion. High lactate concentrations in these patients result from a mass-action effect secondary to a high rate of glycolysis, and are not due to impaired pyruvate oxidation. In addition, the stimulation of glucose oxidation in septic patients by dichloroacetate, a specific pyruvate dehydrogenase stimulator, showed no effect on leucine oxidation, indicating that the alterations in amino acid oxidation and protein kinetics in patients are not directly related to the rate of glucose oxidation.

IMPLICATIONS FOR NUTRITIONAL SUPPORT. The relative availability of endogenous substrates (glucose and fatty acids) determines their share in energy production in critical illness. Because fatty acids make up for the balance between energy requirement and availability of glucose, an excess release of fatty acids in critically ill patients leads to re-esterification of up to 70% of FFAs in the liver, contributing to fat infiltration of the liver. Thus the availability of glucose determines the extent of re-esterification of fatty acids; abundant glucose levels decrease FFA oxidation and stimulate re-esterification.

With regard to exogenously administered nutritional support, this means that carbohydrate intake controls the rate of glucose oxidation and fat oxidation. Thus, at rates below caloric requirements, exogenous glucose is an optimal energy substrate. However, fat oxidation in stress is usually minimized, and glucose is the main energy source in stress situations. A carbohydrate-rich diet leads to an improved net balance of amino acids in muscle when compared to a diet based on fat as the caloric source (Fig. 32–3). This effect may be due to stimulated endogenous insulin production.

The addition of fat to nutritional formulas of severely traumatized patients may be dangerous. Fat transported as VLDL triglycerides after burn is a consequence of peripheral lipolysis and not due to increased de novo synthesis of fatty acids following an increased carbohydrate challenge. Thus it can be surmised that de novo synthesis of fatty acids is of minor importance for fat deposition in the liver compared to peripheral lipolysis. However, additional delivery of dietary fat would likely lead to decompensation of a system running on overload. It therefore seems advisable to deliver non-protein calories mainly as carbohydrates, supplemented only by essential fatty acids to avoid deficiencies.

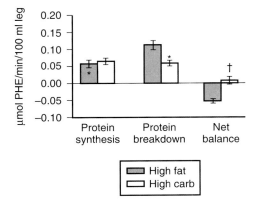

FIGURE 32–3 Muscle protein synthesis and breakdown with high-fat or high-carbohydrate dietary intervention. Calculations of protein synthesis, protein breakdown, and net balance for 13 subjects in each arm of the dietary crossover. *p <0.05; *p <0.01. Carb, carbohydrate; PHE, d_5-phenylalanine. (Adapted from Hart DW, Wolf SE, Zhang XJ, et al: Efficacy of a carbohydrate diet in catabolic illness. Crit Care Med 2001;29:1318.)

Protein requirements

Major trauma, burns, and sepsis lead to early and rapid catabolism of structural body protein. Whereas muscle protein breakdown is increased, "acute-phase" proteins are produced in the liver. Amino acids are required for synthesis of proteins during the wound-healing process and for increased immunologic activity. The net catabolism of muscle may be so prominent that lean body mass in the critically ill patient cannot be preserved. To minimize protein catabolism, administration of dietary protein and/or amino acids is fundamental. To achieve this goal, a higher than normal intake of protein seems beneficial because even the stress of simple bed rest may increase the protein requirement to maintain nitrogen balance. However, this effect is limited, because a protein intake of more than 1.5 g/kg/day does not demonstrate any additional benefit. Therefore, dietary protein provision of 1.2 to 1.5 g/kg/day seems reasonable in adults. Because of their higher normal protein requirement, a higher protein intake of 2 g/kg/day can be recommended in children; an additional increase of protein intake to up to 3 g/kg/day has failed to show any additional advantage. The administration of proteins should contain a well-balanced mixture of amino acids for both adults and children.

Recently more interest has focused on the importance of different amino acids in stress situations. Glutamine has been considered as conditionally essential in trauma. Muscle free glutamine levels decrease during injury, and most likely serve as reservoir to fulfill the requirement of immunocompetent cells after trauma. Although the intracellular glutamine concentration has been proposed as a key regulator of protein synthesis, exogenous administration of glutamine does not show a beneficial effect, and the body seems to depend on de novo synthesis of glutamine. Other amino acids, such as arginine and histidine, have also been promoted as showing specific, unique "pharmacologic" effects; however, convincing experimental evidence in humans is not yet available.

The Hormonal Response to Trauma

The nervous system plays a major role in the activation of the stress response to trauma. Several mechanisms are involved. The limbic system is activated by fear, by emotion, and via thalamic relay of peripheral nociceptive stimuli. Hypoxemia, hypercapnia, and hypotension alter cardiovascular and respiratory reflexes regulated by the brainstem. Bacterial endotoxins and other inflammatory mediators, such as interleukin-1 (IL-1) and tumor necrosis factor (TNF)-α, directly stimulate the hypothalamus, cause a reset of the thermoregulation set point, and alter endocrine function.

Catecholamines are the main mediators of the stress response to trauma or burn. They are released from sympathetic nerve endings (norepinephrine) and the adrenal medulla (epinephrine). Catecholamine production following thermal injury is under hypothalamic control. Norepinephrine levels increase 2- to 10-fold in proportion to burn size. The increase in plasma catecholamines and the metabolic rate are closely correlated. Catecholamine levels remain elevated until wound healing is complete. Catecholamine action is facilitated by cortisol secretion.

Catecholamines act via α-, β_1, and β_2 adrenoreceptors. Epinephrine accelerates hepatic gluconeogenesis, hepatic glycogenolysis, adipocyte lipolysis (via β_1 adrenoreceptors), and muscle proteolysis in order to increase substrate availability for gluconeogenesis and to maintain blood glucose levels.

As mentioned above, insulin levels usually are normal or slightly elevated after burn. However, stress hormone induced insulin resistance counteracts most anabolic effects, such as hypoglycemia, lipogenesis, glycogenesis, increased protein synthesis and decreased gluconeogenesis.

Paradoxically, glucagon levels are elevated following burn despite a decreased glucagon secretion as a result of insulin and hyperglycemia. Glucagon secretion is stimulated by elevated catecholamines, glucocorticoids, and hypoglycemia. Despite the existing hyperglycemia and hyperinsulinemia, glucagon release is stimulated and maintained by an increased sympathetic nervous activity and elevated catecholamine levels. In animal studies, infusion of TNF stimulated increased glucagon release without changing insulin or catecholamine levels.

Glucocorticosteroid substitution is crucial for the survival of adrenal- or pituitary-deficient patients in critical illness. In severely burned patients, cortisol secretion rises up to 10-fold normal levels. The circadian rhythm of plasma cortisol levels is disrupted after burn. Although adrenocorticotropic hormone (ACTH) secretion increases proportionally to burn size, its pulsatile production and short half-life make it difficult to interpret the ACTH-cortisol relationship correctly during trauma. The hypothalamic corticotrophin-releasing hormone triggers ACTH release, but antidiuretic hormone and IL-1 also may stimulate ACTH secretion. ACTH plasma levels are elevated initially after burn, and then return to normal, but lose their circadian rhythm. ACTH plasma levels after major burns often no longer correlate with cortisol levels.

Cortisol, glucagon, and the catecholamines are characterized as counter-regulatory, anti-insulin, or stress hormones, which all are elevated after injury and have synergistic effects. Cortisol stimulates gluconeogenesis, increases proteolysis and alanine synthesis, sensitizes adipocytes to the action of lipolytic hormones (catecholamines), and has an anti-inflammatory action. It causes insulin resistance. Cortisol facilitates the action

of catecholamines and helps stabilize the cardiovascular system during stress. In synergism with catecholamines and glucagon, cortisol diverts glucose utilization from skeletal muscle to central organs such as the brain. As a group, the stress hormones generally cause hyperglycemia. Glucagon increases hepatocyte cyclic AMP and promotes gluconeogenesis, glycogenolysis, lipolysis, and ketogenesis in the liver. Catecholamines cause increased glycogenolysis, hepatic gluconeogenesis, and gluconeogenic precursor mobilization; promote lipolysis and peripheral insulin resistance; and inhibit insulin release. Glucagon and catecholamines synergize to promote gluconeogenesis. After their combined infusion in normal volunteers, gluconeogenesis is more prolonged than if each is infused alone, and combined infusion simulates the metabolic response to injury.

The mechanisms of synergy of cortisol, glucagon, and the catecholamines are varied. Cortisol may induce inhibition of catechol O-methyltransferase and block reuptake of catecholamines by the sympathetic nerve endings. Cortisol increases the total number of β receptors by inducing increased transcription of β-adrenergic receptor messenger RNA, thus increasing the efficacy of catecholamines as adrenoreceptor agonists. In conjunction with glucagon-induced increased intracellular cyclic AMP levels by a non–β receptor mechanism, this leads to increased systemic glucose availability.

Not only stress hormones affect the hypermetabolic response after trauma. Follicle-stimulating hormone (FSH) and luteinizing hormone (LH), regulated by hypothalamic luteinizing hormone-releasing hormone, are altered with injury. FSH levels are decreased in males and females after burn and sensitively indicate the degree of burn trauma. LH levels remain below normal following burn. Amenorrhea is common in female burn patients, although estrogen levels may be as high as during ovulation. In premenopausal women, progesterone levels are decreased after burn and lack the rise usually seen in the secretory phase of the menstrual cycle. Males show high to very high estradiol levels postburn. These changes most likely are due to synthesis in the adrenal gland in both sexes. Levels of adrenal androgens such as dehydroepiandrosterone sulfate and dehydroepiandrosterone are low postburn, which may influence the innate immune response. Decreased testosterone production in males after burn is burn size dependent and is associated with histologic changes in the male gonads such as interstitial atrophy, absence of spermatogenic and Leydig cells, and hyalinization of the basement membranes of the seminiferous tubules. Hypospermia is common, but spontaneous recovery can be expected.

Prolactin levels increase after burn in both men and women, but to a greater extent and for a longer time in women. Hyperprolactinemia causes impotence in men and prevents pregnancy during lactation in women. Postburn impotence is common and can be long lasting.

Influence of Environmental Changes and Wound Closure

The metabolic rate is increased by at least 50% with burn size greater than 20% to 30% TBSA and even more in larger burns (over 40% TBSA) or with presence of burn wound sepsis. Increasing the ambient temperature up to 33°C can attenuate the hypermetabolism significantly. Lower ambient temperatures increase metabolic rate and catecholamine production and are related to increased mortality. At a temperature range of 30° to 33°C, the metabolic expenditure required to maintain core temperatures at 38° to 39°C is minimized. With closed treatment techniques, slightly lower ambient temperatures, about 28°C, are tolerated. Shivering and the evaporative water loss add to the increased energy expenditure. Although increasing ambient temperature will attenuate hypermetabolism and increase patient comfort, the underlying altered metabolic state, with thermogenic futile substrate cycling, will continue and requires additional nutrition support.

The hypermetabolism associated with severe burns may also be modulated by the chosen treatment strategy. In our patient population, the incidence of sepsis was associated with an increase in protein catabolism. In this context, early burn wound excision, within 48 hours of injury, as a preventive measure for infection and sepsis may well have a mitigating effect on protein catabolism. However, in the absence of sepsis, early excision and grafting has not been shown to be effective in the prevention of burn-related hypermetabolism.

Nutritional Modulation

Even in patients with moderate-size burns, up to 30% weight loss has been observed despite maximal oral intake. Wound healing is limited and mortality increases with weight losses exceeding 20% of preburn weights. Tissue breakdown may liberate as much as 30 g of nitrogen per day. This can be limited by adequate dietary carbohydrate. A patient's appetite rarely exceeds preburn levels, and voluntary eating almost meets protein or caloric requirements only in those with small burns. This observation led to parenteral supplementation of nutrition, but this did not improve mortality or indices of immunity. This may be the result of a negative effect of parenteral nutrition on the immune system. Early and immediate enteral nutrition can be administered safely, limits postburn hypermetabolism, and preserves intestinal mucosal integrity, thereby limiting bacterial translocation. Enteral feeding, applied as soon as possible and consisting of about 20% protein and 50% carbohydrate, with the

remainder as low linoleic fats, will help prevent weight loss. Polymeric diets are preferable to the more expensive elemental diets. Quantities required can be estimated by the feeding formulas described elsewhere. If expense or availability precludes the use of more sophisticated feeding preparations, cow's milk has been used extensively with good effect.

Hormonal Modulation

After major trauma, the control of body metabolism is taken over by the sympathetic adrenal axis. The levels of thyroid-stimulating hormone and thyroid hormone, the main regulating hormone of normal-state metabolism, decrease, with a negatively correlated increase of norepinephrine and epinephrine. Neither triiodothyronine (T_3) treatment in burn patients nor thyroxine (T_4) treatment in trauma patients improves survival, and T_3 treatment may well be disadvantageous by inhibiting T_4 secretion. This syndrome of hypermetabolism and low thyroid hormone levels in trauma or critical illness is also known as sick euthyroid syndrome.

Growth Factors and Cytokines

Growth factors and cytokines are considered together because both have a combination of mitogenic, angiogenic, activating, or chemotactic effects on the cell of origin and/or on other cells. Cytokines, particularly IL-1, interleukin-6 (IL-6), and TNF, are the principle messengers that are responsible for many of the events occurring both at the burn wound site and systemically. In addition, many growth factors are released from damaged tissues at the wound site, where they exert local and systemic effects.

Disruption of the vascular endothelium by wounding exposes blood cells to collagen, which precipitates a cascade of events ultimately leading to blood clotting, inflammation, and repair. Platelet degranulation, endothelial damage, and leukocytes contribute to a pool of growth factors and cytokines at the wound site, which subsequently regulate enzymatic degradation, phagocytosis, chemotaxis, angiogenesis, and re-epithelialization. Growth factors and cytokines produced locally at the wound site may spill over into the circulation, where they are carried to distal organs or tissues and stimulate the production of other mediators, growth factors, and cytokines distally. By disseminating these distal tissue mediators into the circulation, more target tissues become involved by a cascading mechanism (Fig. 32–4). It is by this mechanism that cytokines contribute to the activation of catabolism and the hepatic acute-phase response. Predominantly, IL-1 and TNF-α induce type I acute-phase reactant production, whereas IL-6 activates synthesis of type II acute-phase proteins. This shift of protein synthesis in the liver results in a

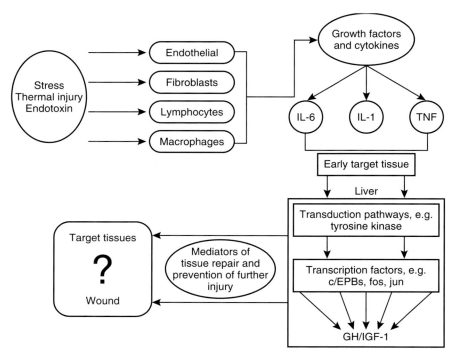

FIGURE 32–4 Stress induces the release of inflammatory mediators from injured tissue. These mediators are disseminated systemically via the circulation and trigger the activation of stress response genes in distal tissues, such as the liver. The protein products of these genes (e.g., recombinant human growth hormone [rhGH] and insulin-like growth factor-1 [IGF-1]) regulate wound repair and prevent further injury in target tissues, such as the wound and other organs. (Adapted from Spies M, Muller MJ, Herndon DN: Modulation of the hypermetabolic response after burn. *In* Herndon DN [ed]: Total Burn Care [2nd ed]. Philadelphia: WB Saunders, 2002:368.)

reduction in production of constitutive proteins, such as albumin, prealbumin, transferrin, and retinol-binding protein, thus diminishing the pool of available functional transport proteins.

The growth hormone/insulin-like growth factor system

Growth hormone (GH) and insulin-like growth factor-1 (IGF-1) levels are decreased following burn injury. Net protein catabolism during the flow phase postburn is caused by an accelerated rate of protein breakdown with a simultaneous failure to increase synthesis sufficiently to compensate. It is well established that GH is a potent anabolic agent and can induce stimulation of net protein synthesis directly or indirectly through the action of IGF-1, and IGF-1 has been shown to increase transmembrane amino acid transport in vitro. The effects of GH include increased appetite, decreased nitrogen losses, increased retention of nitrogen and potassium, weight gain, more rapid wound healing, increased oxygen utilization, and decreased respiratory quotient. These effects are in addition to its well-known linear growth-promoting effect.

GH promotes protein synthesis by increasing the cellular uptake of amino acids and accelerating nucleic acid translation and transcription, thereby enhancing cell proliferation. Fatty acids are released from the hydrolysis of fat for conversion to acetyl coenzyme A, an essential energy-producing molecule for the tricarboxylic acid cycle. Through the preferential use of adipose tissue for energy production, there is a decrease in body fat with the result that protein is spared from catabolism. GH treatment of obese dieters allows lean body mass conservation at the expense of adipose stores. GH also decreases cellular uptake of glucose, thereby exacerbating or precipitating hyperglycemia, which then triggers insulin release. There is decreased sensitivity to insulin at the cellular level; and this causes increased insulin resistance and hyperglycemia.

Growth hormone when given to GH-deficient children promotes active growth and rapidly improves nitrogen balance and increases muscle mass. GH seems to have a more marked anabolic action in those whose protein balance is catabolic. No improvement in muscle mass or strength was detected in young adults undergoing exercise training; while non-trained subjects showed improved net protein balance through an increased rate of whole-body protein synthesis with no change in protein degradation. Further, the protein catabolic effect of prednisone, a glucocorticoid, was prevented by the concomitant administration of GH.

GH anabolic action appears to be primarily mediated by an increase of protein synthesis. Brachial artery infusion of GH in both normal and postoperative patients revealed a direct effect of GH on skeletal muscle, and also acts to stimulate insulin-like growth factor synthesis. GH administration increases IGF-1 blood concentration via increased IGF-1 production by the liver. GH also increases IGF-1 production in other tissues, such as skeletal muscle and cartilage, where IGF-1 may exert an autocrine/paracrine action. The efficacy of growth hormone in treating critically ill patients has been questioned from two prospective, double-blind, randomized placebo-controlled multicenter trials, in which the mortality rate of critically ill adults receiving 0.1 mg/kg/day rhGH was 39% and 44%, respectively, compared to 20% and 18% with placebo. In the survivors, the length of intensive care, hospital stay, and mechanical ventilation were prolonged. Most deaths were related to multi-organ dysfunction, septic shock, or uncontrolled infection, suggesting a possible immune modulating effect. Growth hormone may exert anti- as well as proinflammatory effects, suggesting an effect on immune function in hypermetabolic patients depending on the underlying clinical situation. These findings could not be reproduced in pediatric burn patients. In a controlled study in 263 pediatric burn patients, no increase in septic complications or organ dysfunction could be observed. The mortality rate was 2% in both GH-treatment group (0.2 mg/kg/day) and placebo. In a randomized, prospective, double-blinded study on 28 severely burned children receiving either 0.2 mg/kg/day rhGH or placebo, no increase in mortality (8% vs. 7%) or sepsis (20% vs. 26%) could be shown. Serum IGF-1 and IGFBP-3 levels increased with rhGH treatment, while serum TNF-α and IL-1β levels, as well as acute phase proteins (CRP and serum amyloid-A) were decreased. In 54 adult burn patients, Knox et al. showed a decrease in mortality from 37% for placebo controls to 11% for patients receiving 0.1 mg/kg/day rhGH from 37% in placebo controls. In another study of adult burn patients receiving standard conservative treatment there was an 8% mortality rate with rhGH (0.167 mg/kg/day) compared to 44.5% for those receiving placebo.

Growth hormone effects in burns

While the beneficial metabolic effects of growth hormone in burns have been known for some time, the wound healing potential of GH has only recently been investigated. An extensive prospective randomized, double-blinded clinical trial has examined the basic mechanisms of protein anabolism, hyperglycemia and wound healing in massively burned children and adolescents.

GH (0.2 mg/kg/day) increased protein turnover with increases in both protein synthesis and breakdown, but with synthesis exceeding breakdown in a group of severely burned ($\approx$70% TBSA) hypermetabolic adolescents. This resulted in a net reduction in protein loss of 50% compared to controls. Whole body and isolated limb assessments were performed using N15 lysine stable isotope technique. GH treatment raised leg blood flow significantly. This increase in peripheral blood flow did not cause an increase in cardiac index, which was raised equally in both groups to twice the normal range. Urinary nitrogen excretion was also decreased.

GH causes hyperglycemia by induction of insulin resistance and inhibition of glucose uptake relative to the availability of insulin as shown in a placebo controlled study

in severely burned adolescents receiving GH (0.2 mg/kg/day). As counter-regulation, plasma levels of insulin then increase to maintain euglycemia. Clinically, about one-third of patients treated with GH require therapeutic insulin for two to three days, after which time borderline hyperglycemia persists but not at a level requiring insulin.

GH significantly elevated plasma levels of catecholamines, glucagon and insulin above the already elevated levels found in severely burned patients. Catecholamines and glucagon are typically considered to be catabolic hormones and mediators of the postburn catabolic response. An increase in these mediators might have been expected to increase the hypermetabolic response and its associated protein catabolism, however, as has already been shown, protein anabolism, not catabolism, is induced by GH in burn injury. As insulin infusion has been shown to significantly increase plasma catecholamine levels, it was felt that GH induced insulin resistance led to hyperinsulinemia and then to subsequent elevation of catecholamine levels. In turn, catecholamines or growth hormone or both can stimulate glucagon release, even though they are not the primary stimulus for glucagon release. The reversal of the insulin:glucagon ratio, typically seen in burned patients, was maintained in the GH-treated group. The increase in free fatty acid levels was not surprising, as both catecholamines and GH serve to stimulate lipolysis and release free fatty acids into the circulation. It is significant that metabolic rate/resting energy expenditure was not increased by these hormonal changes as would be expected if the increases in the stress hormone levels were clinically significant.

Improvements in systemic energy and substrate metabolism improve the burn patient's ability to react to additional stressors during acute hospital course. Enhanced host-nonspecific resistance against bacterial infection has been demonstrated. Takagi et al. showed that treating burned mice with 4 mg/kg rhGH before exposure to lethal amounts of herpes simplex virus type 1 mortality could significantly reduce mortality by restoring the burn suppressed IFN-γ response, reducing burn induced suppressor macrophages, and increasing the production of cytostatic macrophages.

Another serious postburn complication in children is growth retardation with severe delays in both height and weight growth development. This growth delay persists for as long as three years post-injury without any "catch-up" growth afterwards. With major illnesses a profound change in growth patterns may result. Growth changes can be transient, disappearing after resolution of the illness, or permanent, such as with intrinsic defects of endocrine function or with pathologic states, like chronic renal failure. In other serious medical conditions, after reconvalescence, the patient experiences a period of explosive growth and growth returns to comparable peer-group patterns. This "catch-up" growth spurt has been observed in other severe trauma conditions. However, this does not occur in pediatric burn patients. Nail and hair growth are attenuated during the catabolic phase of burn response and evidence is mounting that a bony lesion exists which is of an aplastic nature. The exact mechanism of this growth retardation is unknown. Adequate nutrition is required for normal growth. It may be that these patients continue to expend energy stores on the damaged integument, thus leaving few resources for growth. A recent study on severely burned children receiving rhGH during their acute hospitalization, showed a marked improvement in their rate of linear growth between 6 months and 2 years post-injury compared to placebo-treated controls. Similar effects could be demonstrated in a group of growth-retarded children with chronic steroid therapy for juvenile chronic arthritis. In severe burns, bone formation has been found to be markedly reduced. Pediatric burn patients treated with 0.2 mg/kg/day rhGH showed an increase of IGF-1 and IGFBP-3 of 229% and 187%, respectively, compared to placebo. Serum osteocalcin remained below normal levels, while type I procollagen propeptide levels rose to low normal levels. The inhibitory IGF binding protein 4, however, was markedly elevated, suggesting a mechanism by which improved bone formation may be prevented despite increased IGF-1 and IGFBP-3 levels. Besides marked improvement of muscle catabolism long-term administration of growth hormone demonstrated a significant attenuation of the osteopenic changes seen after burn (Fig. 32–5).

GH has many uses in patients who are catabolic, malnourished, or have received severe trauma such as burn. Its more widespread availability and application will benefit many, and ultimately reduce costs. GH acts both directly and indirectly via IGF-1 production in the liver and elsewhere. IGF-1 serum levels are decreased in burn patients. This is consistent with the observation that hepatic IGF-1 secretion is directly impaired despite normal pituitary GH secretion in many disease states, and that simultaneous use of GH and IGF-1 gives enhanced anabolic effects in normal humans.

GH given to septic patients has failed to increase IGF-1 levels. Also, the IGF-1 response to GH treatment is attenuated with increasing severity of trauma or burn. These facts have led to speculation that IGF-1, alone or in combination with GH, may achieve better results in malnourished, septic burn patients. Early animal work has been most encouraging, though at present conclusive human data are lacking.

β-Adrenergic Receptor Agents

The hyperdynamic circulatory response to burn injury, stimulated by up to 10-fold increased catecholamine levels, is involved in the increase of energy expenditure.

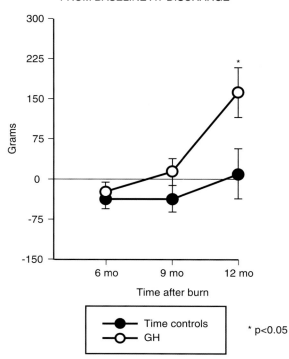

CHANGES IN BONE MINERAL CONTENT
FROM BASELINE AT DISCHARGE

FIGURE 32–5 Reversal of burn-induced osteoporosis with recombinant human growth hormone (rhGH). Changes of bone mineral content measured by serial dual-energy x-ray absorptiometry (DEXA) scans. (Adapted from Hart DW, Herndon DN, Klein G, et al: Attenuation of post traumatic muscle catabolism and osteopenia by long-term growth hormone therapy. Ann Surg 2001;233:827.)

Tachycardia of 120 to 150 beats/min continues for many weeks in massively burned patients. Cardiac dysfunction commonly contributes to mortality, with myocarditis, cardiomyopathy, and focal myocardial ischemia often found at autopsy.

A number of more recent and extensive studies have shown that limited β blockade can be safely used in severely burned patients. Propranolol, 2 mg/kg/day, was given intravenously to 18 patients with burns of 70% ± 30% of TBSA for 5 days. Heart rate was decreased by 20%, left ventricular work index by 22%, and rate-pressure product by 36%. Plasma glucose, FFA, triglyceride, and insulin levels remained unchanged. Catecholamine levels were not affected by nonselective β blockade. Continuous hemodynamic monitoring showed a significant decrease of the pressure-work index and rate-pressure product by β-adrenergic blockade in septic burn patients, leading to improvement of cardiac index, oxygen delivery index, and oxygen consumption.

Selective β_1 blockade is a metabolically inert, cardiovascularly safe way to limit the postburn hyperdynamic cardiovascular response. Therefore, metoprolol would appear to be the drug of choice for the often-encountered problem of burn-induced hypertension. Increased excitability and marked tachycardia are found in almost all patients with large burns, and β blockade is indicated for these patients.

Selective β₂-adrenergic receptor agonists have known protein anabolic effects. Clenbuterol, a totally selective β₂-agonist, has structural similarities to epinephrine and is well known to promote protein anabolism in normal animals via β₂-adrenergic receptor activation. Postsurgical rats and burned rats showed increased muscle mass and body weight with clenbuterol, with evidence that hypermetabolism was also increased.

Anabolic Steroids

Another class of anabolic agents, the steroid hormones, have not been as extensively investigated in burned patients. Substances in this group include oxandrolone, testosterone, and dehydroepiandrosterone sulfate. Particularly attractive is their combination with anabolic proteins because of their different binding characteristics and potential synergistic effects.

Steroid hormones rely on translocation into the nucleus, where they can modulate transcription events. Healthy adult males given 200 mg testosterone intramuscularly showed a twofold increase in muscle protein synthesis. This effect was caused not by changes in the inward transport of amino acids, but by increases in the protein synthesis rate through more efficient reutilization of the intracellular amino acids. At present, the systemic side effects of testosterone restrict its clinical use in burn care.

Oxandrolone, a synthetic testosterone analog with potent anabolic effects, shows only minimal androgenic side effects. Oxandrolone is administered orally, which is more attractive to clinicians and patients compared to frequent GH or testosterone injections. This anabolic steroid has been used as adjunctive therapy to promote weight gain in chronically ill and debilitated patients. Oxandrolone has been shown to improve weight gain in patients with acquired immunodeficiency syndrome wasting myopathy and has been used in the treatment of children with growth disorders. When given to healthy adult males, short-term oral oxandrolone (5 days at 15 mg/day) increased muscle protein synthesis, whereas protein breakdown remained unchanged. The uptake of amino acids did not change, whereas outward transport of amino acids decreased, indicating an improved cellular reutilization of amino acids. Simultaneously, androgen receptor messenger RNA levels in the skeletal muscle were significantly increased, thus suggesting a potential mechanism of action. In burn patients with 30% to 50% TBSA burns, oxandrolone improved weight gain. In a

randomized, double-blind, placebo-controlled trial, adult patients with 40% to 70% TBSA burns received oxandrolone at 20 mg/day. Treated patients showed a significantly improved weight gain during a 3-week period without major liver dysfunction or other complications. Additionally, a standardized donor site healed in 9 ± 2 days, versus 13 ± 3 days for placebo. In malnourished burned children, oxandrolone reversed the decrease in muscle protein net balance compared to controls. This is thought to be due to improved protein metabolism and an increased protein synthesis efficiency (Fig. 32–6). Thus the therapeutic application of oxandrolone seems very promising.

Hormone Antagonists

Alternative approaches to modulate the post-traumatic hypermetabolic response are being investigated. These involve agents that antagonize known mediators of

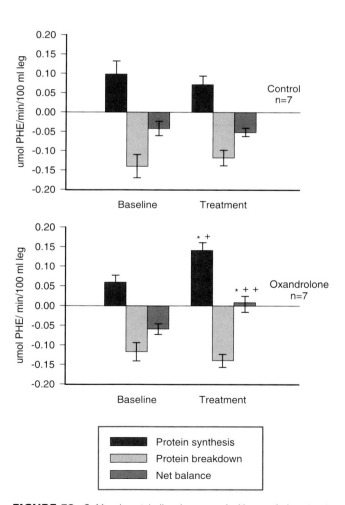

FIGURE 32–6 Muscle catabolism is reversed with oxandrolone treatment. Calculations shown for muscle protein synthesis, protein breakdown, and net protein balance. (Adapted from Hart DW, Wolf SE, Ramzy PI, et al: Anabolic effects of oxandrolone following severe burn. Ann Surg 2001; 233:556.)

hypermetabolism and protein catabolism, such as glucocorticoids and cytokine-blocking agents. Glucocorticoid synthesis inhibitors (e.g., ketoconazole) or glucocorticoid receptor blockers (e.g., mifepristone) may be valuable and effective treatment adjuncts not only for anticatabolic effects, but also for beneficial effects on immune function.

Summary

The hypermetabolic response to trauma and burns can be influenced by environmental warming, infection control, and the use of topical or systemic agents affecting local and systemic inflammation. The catabolism persisting beyond complete wound closure can be limited only by immediate and adequate enteral nutrition supplemented with protein, ω-3 fatty acids, arginine, and glutamine. Hormonal intervention or pharmacologic intervention with β-adrenoreceptor agents and other anabolic agents improves wound closure and reverses the protein catabolism associated with hypermetabolism. By combining these therapeutic modalities with early surgical treatment of the burn wound, mortality and morbidity of burn victims has been significantly improved over the last decades.

Bibliography

Aarsland A, Chinkes D, Wolfe RR, et al: Beta blockade lowers peripheral lipolysis in burn patients receiving growth hormone: rate of hepatic very low density lipoprotein triglyceride synthesis secretion remains unchanged. Ann Surg 1996;223:777.

Abribat T, Brazeau P, Davignon I, Garrel DR: Insulin-like growth factor-1 blood levels in severely burned patients: effects of time post injury, age of patient and severity of burn. Clin Endocrinol 1993;39:583.

Alexander JW, MacMillan BG, Stinnett JD, et al: Beneficial effects of aggressive protein feeding in severely burned children. Ann Surg 1980;192:505.

Andres R, Cader G, Zierler KL: The quantitatively minor role of carbohydrate in oxidative metabolism of skeletal muscle in intact man in the basal state: measurements of oxygen and glucose uptake and carbon dioxide and lactate production in the forearm. J Clin Invest 1956;35:671.

Asch MD, Feldman RJ, Walker HL, et al: Systemic and pulmonary hemodynamic changes accompanying thermal injury. Ann Surg 1973;178:218.

Auichbau SV, Malyafuna EL, Pashalenka AN, et al: Reflexes from carotid bodies upon the adrenals. Arch Int Pharmacol Ther 1969;129:156.

Aulick LH, Hander EH, Wilmore DW, et al: The relative significance of thermal and metabolic demands on burn hypermetabolism. J Trauma 1979;19:559.

Aulick LH, Wilmore DW: Increased peripheral amino acid release following burn. Surgery 1979;85:560.

Aun F, Medeiros-Neto GA, Younes RN, et al: The effect of major trauma on the pathways of thyroid hormone metabolism. J Trauma 1983;23:1048–1050.

Baron PW, Barrow RE, Pierre EJ, Herndon DN: Prolonged use of propranolol safely decreases cardiac work in burned children. J Burn Care Rehabil 1997;18:223.

Barr PO, Birke G, Liljedahl SO, et al: Oxygen consumption and water loss during treatment of burns with warm dry air. Lancet 1968;1:164.

Barrow RE, Wang CZ, Evans MJ, Herndon DN: Growth factors accelerate epithelial repair in sheep trachea. Lung 1993;171:335.

Becker RA, Vaughn GM, Goodwin CW Jr, et al: Plasma norepinephrine, epinephrine and thyroid hormone interactions in severely burned patients. Arch Surg 1980;115:439.

Becker RA, Vaughn GM, Goodwin CW, et al: Interactions of thyroid hormones and catecholamines in severely burned patients. Rev Infect Dis 1983;5:S908.

Becker RA, Vaughn GM, Ziegler MG, et al: Hypermetabolic low tricoelathyranine syndrome of burn injury. Crit Care Med 1982;10:870.

Berger JR, Pall L, Hall CD, et al: Oxandrolone in AIDS-wasting myopathy. AIDS 1996;10:1657.

Bessey PQ, Jiang ZM, Johnson DJ, et al: Posttraumatic skeletal muscle proteolysis: the role of the hormonal environment. World J Surg 1989;13:465.

Bessey PQ, Watters JM, Aoki TT, Wilmore DW: Combined hormonal infusion simulates the metabolic response to injury. Ann Surg 1984;200:260.

Beutler B, Cerami A: Cachectin: more than a tumor necrosis factor. N Engl J Med 1987;316:379.

Black PR, Brooks DC, Bessey PQ, et al: Mechanisms of insulin resistance following injury. Ann Surg 1982;196:420.

Blackburn GL, Maini BS, Pierce EC: Nutrition in the critically ill patient. Anesthesiology 1977;47:181.

Bondy CA, Underwood LE, Clemmons DR, et al: Clinical uses of insulin-like growth factor-1. Ann Intern Med 1994;120:593.

Bortz WM, Paul P, Haff AG, et al: Glycerol turnover and oxidation in man. J Clin Invest 1972;51:1537.

Boulivare SD, Tamborlane WV, Matthews LS, Sherwin RS: Diverse effects of insulin-like growth factor 1 on glucose, lipid and amino acid metabolism. Am J Physiol 1992;262(Endocrinol Metab 25):E130.

Brent GA, Hershman JM: Thyroxine therapy in patients with severe non thyroidal illnesses and low serum thyroxine concentration. J Clin Endocrinol Metab 1986;63:1.

Brizio-Molteni L, Molteni A, Warpeha RL, et al: Prolactin, corticotropin, and gonadotropin concentrations following thermal injury in adults. J Trauma 1984;24:1.

Bruno LP, Stern PJ, Wyrick JD: Skeletal changes after burn injuries in an animal model. J Burn Care Rehabil 1988;9:148.

Byrne TA, Morrissey TB, Gatzen C, et al: Anabolic therapy with growth hormone accelerates protein gain in surgical patients requiring nutritional rehabilitation. Ann Surg 1993;218:400.

Carter WJ, Dang ASQ, Faas FG, et al: Effects of clenbuterol on skeletal mass, body composition and recovery from surgical stress in senescent rats. Metabolism 1991;40:855.

Chance WT, Von Allmen D, Benson D, et al: Clenbuterol decreases catabolism and increases hypermetabolism in burned rats. J Trauma 1991;31:365.

Choo JJ, Horna MA, Little RA, et al: Anabolic effects of clenbuterol on skeletal muscle are mediated by beta-2 adrenoreceptor activation. Am J Physiol 1992;263(Endocrinol Metab 26):E50.

Chwans WJ, Bistrian BR: Role of endogenous growth hormone and insulin-like growth factor 1 in malnutrition and acute metabolic stress: a hypothesis. Crit Care Med 1991;19:1317.

Cioffi WG, Gore DC, Rue LW, et al: Insulin-like growth factor-1 lowers protein oxidation in patients with thermal injury. Ann Surg 1994;220:309.

Clark MA, Plank LD, Hill GL: Wound healing associated with severe surgical illness. World J Surg 2000;24:648.

Clemmons DR: Insulin-like growth factor binding proteins and their role in controlling IGF actions. Cytokine Growth Factor Rev 1997;8:45.

Clemmons DR, Synder DK, Williams R, Underwood LE: Growth hormone administration conserves lean body mass during dietary restriction in obese subjects. J Clin Endocrinol Metab 1987;64:878.

Cori CFU: Mammalian carbohydrate metabolism. Physiol Rev 1931;11:143.

Cuppage FE, Brizio-Molteni L, Molteni A, et al: Aspects of systemic pathologic changes after thermal trauma. In Dolecek R, Brizio-Molteni L, Molteni A, et al (eds): Endocrinology of Thermal Trauma. Philadelphia, Lea & Febiger, 1990:383.

Curreri PW, Richmond D, Marvin J, et al: Dietary requirements of patients with major burns. J Am Diet Assoc 1974;65:415.

Dahn MS, Lange MP, Jacobs LA: Insulin-like growth factor-1 production is inhibited in human sepsis. Arch Surg 1988;123:1409.

Daly JM, Lieberman MD, Goudfine J, et al: Enteral nutrition with supplemental arginine, RNA, and omega-3 fatty acids in patients after operation: immunologic, metabolic, and clinical outcome. Surgery 1992;112:56.

Daughaday WH, Hall K, Salmon WD, et al: On the nomenclature of the somatomedins and insulin-like growth factors [letter to the editor]. J Clin Endocrinol Metab 1987;65:1075.

DebRoy MA, Wolf SE, Zhang XJ, et al: Anabolic effects of insulin-like growth factor in combination with insulin-like growth factor binding protein-3 in severely burned adults. J Trauma 1999;47:904.

Deibert DC, DeFronzo RA: Epinephrine-induced insulin resistance in man. J Clin Invest 1980;65:717.

Demling RH, DeSanti L: Oxandrolone, an anabolic steroid, significantly increases the rate of weight gain in the recovery phase after major burns. J Trauma 1997;43:47.

Demling RH, Orgill DP: The anticatabolic and wound healing effects of the testosterone analog oxandrolone after severe burn injury. J Crit Care 2000;15:12.

Diem E, Schmid R, Schneider WHF, Spona J: The influence of burn trauma on the hypothalamus pituitary axis in normal female subjects. Scand J Plast Reconstr Surg 1979;13:17.

Dinarello CA, Cannon JG, Wolff SM, et al: Tumor necrosis factor (cachectin) is an endogenous pyrogen and induces production of interleukin 1. J Exp Med 1986;163:1433.

Dinarello CA, Conno JG, Wolff SM: New concepts on pathogenesis of fever. Rev Infect Dis 1988;10:168.

Dolecek R, Adamkova M, Sotornikova T, et al: Endocrine response after burn. Scand J Plast Reconstr Surg 1979;13:9.

Dolecek R, Zavada M, Adamkova M, et al: Endocrine response in burned subjects: insulin, somatotropin, renin, angiotensin-11, ACTH and LH. Burns 1974;1:43.

Dong Y-L, Hung KF, Xia ZF, Chung DH, et al: Impact of exogenous insulin-like growth factor-1 on hepatic energy metabolism in burn injury. Arch Surg 1993;128:703.

Durkot NJ, Wolfe RR: Effects of adrenergic blockade on glucose kinetics in septic and burned guinea pigs. Am J Physiol 1984;241:R222.

Edwards CK, Ghiasuddin SM, Yunger LM, et al: In vivo administration of recombinant growth hormone or gamma interferon activates macrophages: enhanced resistance to experimental Salmonella typhimurium infections is correlated with generation of reactive oxygen intermediates. Infect Immunol 1992;60:2514.

Edwards CK, Lorence RM, Dunham DM, et al: Hypophysectomy inhibits the synthesis of tumor necrosis factor (alpha) by rat macrophages: partial restoration by exogenous growth hormone of interferon (gamma). Endocrinology 1991; 128:989.

Egdahl RH: The differential response of the adrenal cortex and medulla to bacterial endotoxin. J Clin Invest 1959;38:1120.

Elsasser TH, Fayer R, Rumsey TS, Hartnell GF: Recombinant bovine somatotropin blunts plasma tumor necrosis factor-(alpha), cortisol, and thromboxane-B2 responses to endotoxin in vivo. Endocrinology 1994;134:1082.

Exton JH: Gluconeogenesis. Metabolism 1975;21:945.

Felig P: The glucose-alanine cycle. Metabolism 1973;22:179.

Felig F, Wahren J: Influence of endogenous insulin secretion on splanchnic glucose and amino acid metabolism in man. J Clin Invest 1971;59:1702.

Ferrando AA, Chinkes DL, Wolfe SE, et al: Acute dichloroacetate administration increases skeletal muscle free glutamine concentrations after burn. Ann Surg 1998;2:249.

Ferrando AA, Chinkes DL, Wolf SE, et al: A submaximal dose of insulin promotes net skeletal protein synthesis in patients with severe burns. Ann Surg 1999;1:11.

Ferrando AA, Tipton KD, Doyle D, et al: Testosterone injection stimulates net protein synthesis but not tissue amino acid transport. Am J Physiol 1998;275:E864.

Finkelstein JW, Roffward HP, Boyer RM, et al: Age-related change in the twenty-four hour spontaneous secretion of growth hormone. J Clin Endocrinol Metab 1972;35:665.

Fleming RYD, Rutan RI, Jahoor F, et al: Effect of recombinant human growth hormone on catabolic hormones and free fatty acids following thermal injury. J Trauma 1992;32:698.

Fraser CM, Potter PC, Chung FZ, et al: Glucocorticoid regulation of human lung beta-adrenergic receptor density occurs at the level of gene transcription. Fed Proc 1987;46:1463.

Fredholm BB: The effect of lactate in canine subcutaneous adipose tissue in situ. Acta Physiol Scand 1971;81:110.

Fryburg DA, Gelfand RA, Barrett EJ: Growth hormone acutely stimulates forearm muscle protein synthesis in normal humans. Am J Physiol 1991;260(Endocrinol Metab 23):E499.

Gamrin L, Essen P, Forsberg AM, et al: A descriptive study of skeletal muscle metabolism in critically ill patients: free amino acids, energy rich phosphates, protein, nucleic acids, fat, water, and electrolytes. Crit Care Med 1996;24:575.

Gann DS, Egdahl RH: Responses of adrenal corticosteroid secretion to hypotension and hypovolemia. J Clin Invest 1965;44:1.

Ganong WF: The stress response: a dynamic overview. Hosp Pract (Off Ed) 1988;23:155, 161, 167.

Garber AJ, Karl IE, Kipnis DM: Alanine and glutamine synthesis and release from skeletal muscle. IV. B-adrenergic inhibition of amino acid release. J Biol Chem 1976;251:851.

Gelfand RA, Glichman MG, Castellino P, et al: Measurement of L-^{14}C-leucine kinetics in splanchnic and leg tissues in humans. Diabetes 1988;37:1365.

Gelfand RA, Hutchinson-Williams KA, Bonde AA, et al: Catabolic effects of thyroid hormone excess: the contribution of adrenergic activity to hypermetabolism and protein breakdown. Metabolism 1987;36:562.

Goran MI, Broemeling L, Herndon DN, et al: Estimating energy requirements in burned children: a new approach derived from measurements of resting energy expenditure. Am J Clin Nutr 1991;54:35.

Goran MI, Peters EJ, Herndon DN, et al: Total energy expenditure in burned children using the doubly labeled water technique. Am J Physiol 1990;259:E576.

Gore DC, Ferrando A, Barnett J, et al: Influence of glucose kinetics on plasma lactate concentration and energy expenditure in severely burned patients. J Trauma 2000;49:673.

Gore DC, Honeycutt D, Jahoor F, et al: Effect of exogenous growth hormone on glucose utilization in burn patients. J Surg Res 1991;51:518.

Gore DC, Honeycutt D, Jahoor F, et al: Effect of exogenous growth hormone on whole-body and isolated limb protein kinetics in burned patients. Arch Surg 1991;126:38.

Gottschlich MM, Jenkins M, Warden GD, et al: Differential effects of three enteral dietary regimens on selected outcome variables in burn patients. JPEN J Parenter Enteral Nutr 1990;14:225.

Hart DW, Herndon DN, Klein G, et al: Attenuation of post traumatic muscle catabolism and osteopenia by long-term growth hormone therapy. Ann Surg 2001;233:827.

Hart DW, Wolf SE, Chinkes DL, et al: Determinants of skeletal muscle catabolism after severe burn. Ann Surg 2000;232:455.

Hart DW, Wolf SE, Herndon DN, et al: Energy expenditure and caloric balance after burn: increased feeding leads to fat rather than lean mass accretion. Ann Surg 2002;235:152.

Hart DW, Wolf SE, Mlcak R, et al: Persistence of muscle catabolism after severe burn. Surgery 2000;128:312.

Hart DW, Wolf SE, Ramzy PI, et al: Anabolic effects of oxandrolone following severe burn. Ann Surg 2001;233:556.

Hart DW, Wolf SE, Zhang XJ, et al: Efficacy of a carbohydrate diet in catabolic illness. Crit Care Med 2001;29:1318.

Herndon DN: Mediators of metabolism. J Trauma 1981;21:701.

Herndon DN, Barrow RE, Rutan TC, et al: Effect of propranolol administration on hemodynamic and metabolic responses of burned pediatric patients. Ann Surg 1988;208:484.

Herndon DN, Barrow RE, Stein M, et al: Increased mortality with intravenous supplemental feeding in severely burned patients. J Burn Care Rehabil 1989;10:309.

Herndon DN, Hart DW, Wolf SE, et al: Reversal of catabolism by beta-blockade after severe burns. N Engl J Med 2001;345:1223.

Herndon DN, Nguyen TT, Gilpin DA: Growth factors: local and systemic. Arch Surg 1993;128:1227.

Herndon DN, Nguyen TT, Wolfe RR, et al: Lipolysis in burned patients with severe burns after beta-blockade. J Burn Care Rehabil 1992;13:1301.

Herndon DN, Ramzy PI, DebRoy MA, et al: Muscle protein catabolism after severe burn: effects of IGF-1/IGFBP-3 treatment. Ann Surg 1999;229:713.

Herndon DN, Stein MD, Rutan TC, et al: Failure of TPN supplementation to improve liver function, immunity, and mortality in thermally injured patients. J Trauma 1987; 27:195.

Herndon DN, Ziegler ST: Bacterial translocation after thermal injury. Crit Care Med 1993;21:S50.

Hiyama DT, Von Allmen D, Rosenblum L, et al: Synthesis of albumin and acute phase proteins in perfused liver after burn injury in rats. J Burn Care Rehabil 1991;12:1.

Hollyoak MA, Muller MJ, Meyer NA, et al: Beneficial wound healing and metabolic effects of clenbuterol in burned and non-burned rats. J Burn Care Rehabil 1995;16:233.

Honeycutt D, Barrow R, Herndon DN: Cold stress response in patients with severe burns after beta-blockade. J Burn Care Rehabil 1992;13:181.

Horber FF, Haymond MW: Human growth hormone prevents the protein catabolic side effects of prednisone in humans. J Clin Invest 1990;86:265.

Huang KF, Chung DH, Herndon DN: Insulin-like growth factor-1 (IGF-1) reduces gut atrophy and bacterial translocation after severe burn injury. Arch Surg 1993;128:47.

Hume DM, Egdahl RH: The importance of the brain in the endocrine response to injury. Ann Surg 1959;150:697.

Inoue T, Saito H, Fukushima R, et al: Growth hormone and insulin-like growth factor-1 enhanced host defense in a murine sepsis model. Arch Surg 1995;130:1115.

Jahoor F, Desai M, Herndon DN, Wolfe RR: Dynamics of the protein metabolic response to a burn injury. Metabolism 1988;37:330.

Jahoor F, Hernond DN, Wolfe RR: Role of insulin and glucagons in the response of glucose and alanine kinetics in burn-injured patients. J Clin Invest 1986;78:807.

Jahoor F, Shangraw RE, Miyoshi H, et al: Role of insulin and glucose oxidation in mediating the protein catabolism of burns and sepsis. Am J Physiol 1989;27:E323.

Jeffries MK, Vance ML: Growth hormone and cortisol secretion in patients with burn injury. J Burn Care Rehabil 1992;13:391.

Jeschke MG, Barrow RE, Herndon DN: Recombinant human growth hormone treatment in pediatric burn patients and its role during the hepatic acute phase response. Crit Care Med 2000;28:1578.

Joshi VV: Effects of burns on the heart. JAMA 1970;211:2130.

Kalsner S: Mechanism of hydrocortisone potentiation of responses to epinephrine and norepinephrine in rabbit aorta. Circ Res 1969;24:383.

Kappel M, Hansen MB, Diamant M, Pedersen BK: In vitro effects of human growth hormone on the proliferative responses and cytokine production of blood mononuclear cells. Horm Metab Res 1994;26:612.

Kavach AGC, Rossell S, Sandor P: Blood flow, oxygen consumption and free fatty acid release in subcutaneous adipose tissue during hemorrhagic shock in control and phenoxybenzamine-treated dogs. Circ Res 1970;26:733.

Keller U, Kraenzlin W, Stauffacher W, Arnaud M: B-adrenergic stimulation results in diminished protein breakdown, decreased amino acid oxidation and increased protein synthesis in man [abstract]. JPEN J Parenter Enteral Nutr 1987;11(suppl):7S.

Kimbrough TD, Shernan S, Ziegler TR, et al: Insulin-growth factor-1 response is comparable following intravenous and subcutaneous administration of growth hormone. J Surg Res 1991;51:472.

Klein GI, Herndon DN, Langman CB, et al: Long-term reduction in bone mass following severe burn injury in children. J Pediatr 1995;126:252.

Klein GL, Herndon DN, Rutan TC, et al: Bone disease in burn patients. J Bone Miner Res 1993;8:337.

Klein GL, Wolf SE, Langman CB, et al: Effect of therapy with recombinant human growth hormone on insulin-like growth factor system components and serum levels of biochemical markers of bone formation in children after burn injury. J Clin Endocrinol Metab 1998;83:21.

Knox J, Demling R, Wilmore D, et al: Increased survival after major thermal injury: the effect of growth hormone therapy in adults. J Trauma 1995;39:526.

Kupfer SR, Underwood LE, Baxter RC, Clemmons DR: Enhancement of the anabolic effects of growth hormone and insulin-like growth factor 1 by use of both agents simultaneously. J Clin Invest 1993;91:391.

Kupper TS, Deitch EA, Baker CC, Wong WC: The human burn wound as a primary source of interleukin-1 activity. Surgery 1986;100:409.

Lephart ED, Baxter CR, Parker CR Jr: Effect of burn trauma on adrenal and testicular steroid hormone production. J Clin Endocrinol Metab 1987;64:842.

Liao W, Rudling M, Angelin B: Growth hormone potentiates the in vivo biological activities of endotoxin in the rat. Eur J Clin Invest 1996;26:254.

Lieberman SA, Butterfield GE, Harrison D, Hoffman AR: Anabolic effects of recombinant human insulin-like growth factor-1 in cachectic patients with acquired immunodeficiency syndrome. J Clin Endocrin Metab 1994;78:404.

Liljedahl SO, Gemzell CA, Plantin LO, Birke G: Effect of human growth hormone in patients with severe burns. Acta Chir Scand 1961;122:1.

Linares HA: Autopsy findings in burned children. In Carvajal HF, Parks DH (eds): Pediatric Burn Management: Burns in Children. Chicago: Year Book Medical Publishers, 1988:298.

Lipman RL, Raskin P, Love T: Glucose intolerance during decreased physical activity in man. Diabetes 1972;21:101.

Little S: Effect of thyroid hormone supplementation on survival after bacterial infection. Endocrinology 1985;117:1431.

Low JF, Herndon DN, Barrow RE: Growth hormone ameliorates growth delay in burned children: a 3 year follow-up study. Lancet 1999;354:1789.

MacGorman LR, Rizza R, Gerich JE: Physiological concentrations of growth hormone exert insulin like and insulin antagonistic effect on both hepatic and extra hepatic tissues in man. J Clin Endocrinol Metab 1981;53:556.

Martin PM, Wooley JH, McCluskey J: Growth factors and cutaneous wound repair. Prog Growth Factor Res 1992;4:25.

McDonald WS, Sharp CW, Deitch EA: Immediate enteral feeding in burn patients is safe and effective. Ann Surg 1991;213:177.

McManson JM, Smith RJ, Wilmore DW: Growth hormone stimulates protein synthesis during hypocaloric parenteral nutrition. Ann Surg 1988;208:136.

Michie HR, Wilmore DW: Sepsis, signals, and surgical sequelae: a hypothesis. Arch Surg 1990;125:531.

Miles JM, Nissen SL, Genrich JE, Haymond MW: Effects of epinephrine infusion on leucine and alanine kinetics in humans. Am J Physiol 1984;247:E166.

Minifee PK, Barrow RE, Abston S, et al: Improved myocardial oxygen utilization following propranolol infusion in adolescents with postburn hypermetabolism. J Pediatr Surg 1989;24:806.

Mjaawand M, Unneberg K, Larsson J, et al: Growth hormone after abdominal surgery attenuated forearm glutamine, alanine, 3-methyhistidine and total amino acid effluse in patients receiving total parenteral nutrition. Ann Surg 1993;217:413.

Mochizuki H, Trocki O, Dominioni L, et al: Mechanism of prevention of postburn hypermetabolism and catabolism by early enteral feeding. Ann Surg 1984;200:297.

Mochizuki H, Trocki O, Dominioni L, et al: Reduction of postburn hypermetabolism by early enteral feedings. Curr Surg 1985;42:121.

Moller S, Jensen M, Stevensson P, Skakkebaek H: Insulin-like growth factor-1 (IGF-1) in burn patients. Burns 1991; 17:279.

Molteni A, Warpeha RL, Brizio-Molteni L, et al: Circadian rhythms of serum aldosterone, cortisol and plasma renin activity in burn injuries. Ann Clin Lab Sci 1979;9:518.

Moore FA, Feliciano DV, Andrassy RJ, et al: Early enteral feeding, compared with parenteral, reduces post operative septic complications: the results of a meta-analysis. Ann Surg 1992;216:172.

Morimoto A, Murakami N, Nakamori T, Watanabe T: Multiple control of fever production in the central nervous system of rabbits. J Physiol 1988;397:269.

Moshage H: Cytokines and the hepatic acute phase response. J Pathol 1997;181:257.

Muller MJ, Gilpin DA, Biolo G, Herndon DN: Biosynthetic human growth hormone: current and potential applications in amino acids in cancer and critical illness. In Latifi R (ed): Amino Acids in Critical Care and Cancer. Austin: RG Landes Co, 1994.

Neely AW, Petra AB, Holloman GH, et al: Researches on the cause of burn hypermetabolism. Ann Surg 1974;179:290.

Newsholme EA, Crabtree B: Substrate cycles in metabolic regulation and in heat generation. Biochem Soc Symp 1976;41:61.

Newsome T, Mason AD, Pruitt BA: Weight loss following thermal injury. Ann Surg 1973;178:215.

Nordenboos J, Hansbrough JF, Gutmacher H, et al: Enteral nutritional support and wound excision and closure do not prevent postburn hypermetabolism as measured by continuous metabolic monitoring. J Trauma 2000;49:667.

Ogle CK, Ogle JD, Mao JM, et al: Effect of glutamine on phagocytosis and bacterial killing by normal and pediatric burn patient neutrophils. JPEN J Parenter Enteral Nutr 1994;18:128.

Patterson BW, Nguyen T, Pierre E, et al: Urea and protein metabolism in burned children: effect of dietary protein intake. Metabolism 1997;46:573.

Pierre EJ, Barrow RE, Hawkins HL, et al: Effects of insulin on wound healing. J Trauma 1998;44:342.

Popp MB, Silverstein EB, Srivastaver LS, et al: A pathophysiologic study of the hypertension associated with burn injury in children. Ann Surg 1981;193:817.

Prader A: Catch-up growth. Postgrad Med J 1978;54 (Suppl):133.

Ramirez RJ, Wolf SE, Barrow RE, Herndon DN: Growth hormone treatment in pediatric burns: a safe therapeutic approach. Ann Surg 1998;228:439.

Reiss W, Pearson E, Artz CP: The metabolic response to burns. J Clin Invest 1956;35:62.

Roe CF, Kinky J: The influence of human growth hormone on energy sources in convalescence. Surg Forum 1962; 13:369.

Rosenfeld RG, Attie KM, Frane J, et al: Growth hormone therapy of Turner's syndrome: beneficial effect on adult height. J Pediatr 1998;132:319.

Rowe JW, Young JB, Minaker KL, et al: Effect of insulin and glucose infusions on sympathetic nervous system activity in normal man. Diabetes 1981;30:219.

Rutan RI, Herndon DN: Growth delay in postburn pediatric patients. Arch Surg 1990;125:392.

Rutan R, Herndon DN: Justification for the use of growth hormone in a pediatric burn center. In Proc 26th Meeting American Burn Association, Orlando, FL, 1994.

Rutan T, Herndon DN, Van Osten T, Abston S: Metabolic rate alterations in early excision and grafting versus conservative treatment. J Trauma 1986;26:140.

Saito H, Tracki O, Alexander JW, et al: The effect of route of nutrient administration on the nutritional state, catabolic hormone secretion, and gut mucosal integrity after burn injury. JPEN J Parenter Enteral Nutr 1987;11:1.

Sakurai Y, Zhang X-J, Wolfe RR: Short-term effects of tumor necrosis factor on energy and substrate metabolism in dogs. J Clin Invest 1993;91:2437.

Sanka J: Dehydroepiandrosterone: metabolic effects. Acta Univ Carol Med Monogr 1976;71:146.

Schmidt KH, Bruchelt G, Koslowski L: Granulocyte function: current knowledge and methods of assessment. J Burn Care Rehabil 1985;6:261.

Schulman GI, Williams PE, Liljenquist JE, et al: Effect of hyperglycemia independent of changes in insulin or glucagons on lipolysis in the conscious dog. Metabolism 1980;29:317.

Shamoon H, Hendler R, Sherwin RS: Synergistic interactions among anti-insulin hormones in the pathogenesis of stress hyperglycemia in humans. J Clin Endocrinol Metab 1981;52:1235.

Sheffield-Moore M, Urban RJ, Wolf SE, et al: Short-term oxandrolone administration stimulates net muscle protein synthesis in young men. J Clin Endocrinol Metab 1999;84:2705.

Shorwell MA, Kilbeg MS, Oxender DL: The regulation of neutral amino acid transport in mammalian cells. Biochim Biophys Acta 1983;737:267.

Singh KP, Prassad R, Chari PS, Dash RJ: Effect of growth hormone therapy in burn patients on conservative treatments. Burn 1998;24:733.

Sonhoff HS, Pearson E, Artz CP: An estimation of nitrogen requirements for equilibrium in burn patients. Surg Gynecol Obstet 1961;112:159.

Soroff HS, Pearson E, Green NL, Artz CP: The effect of growth hormone on nitrogen balance at various levels of intake in burned patients. Surg Gynecol Obstet 1960;111:259.

Soroff HS, Rozin RR, Mooty J, et al: Role of human growth hormone in the response to trauma: metabolic effects following burns. Ann Surg 1967;166:739.

Spies M, Wolf SE, Barrow RE, et al: Modulation of type I and II acute phase reactants with insulin-like growth factor-1/binding protein-3 complex in severely burned children. Crit Care Med 2002;30:83.

Strock LL, Singh H, Abdullah A, et al: The effect of insulin-like growth factor-1 on postburn hypermetabolism. Surgery 1990;108:161.

Stuart CA, Shangraw RE, Prince MJ, et al: Bed-rest induced insulin resistance occurs primarily in muscle. Metabolism 1988;37:802.

Takagi K, Suzuki F, Barrow RE, et al: Growth hormone improves immune function and survival in burned mice infected with herpes simplex virus type 1. J Surg Res 1997;69:166.

Takagi K, Suzuki F, Barrow RE, et al: Growth hormone improves the resistance of thermally injured mice infected with herpes simplex virus type 1. J Trauma 1998;44:517.

Takala J, Ruokonen E, Webster NR, et al: Increased mortality associated with growth hormone treatment in critically ill adults. N Engl J Med 1999;341:785.

Tanner JM, Hughes CPR, Whitehouse RH: Comparative rapidity of response of height, limb muscle and limb fat to treatment with human growth hormone in patients with and without growth hormone deficiency. Acta Endocrinol 1977;84:681.

Tessari P, Inchiostro S, Biolo G, et al: Differential effects of hyperinsulinemia and hyperaminoacidemia on leucine-carbon metabolism in vivo. J Clin Invest 1987;79:1062.

Thompson JC, Marx M: Gastrointestinal hormones. Curr Probl Surg 1984;7:80.

Touati G, Prieur AM, Ruiz JC, et al: Beneficial effects of one-year growth hormone administration to children with juvenile chronic arthritis on chronic steroid therapy. I. Effects on growth velocity and body composition. J Clin Endocrinol Metab 1998;83:403.

Trocki O, Mochizuki H, Dominioni L, Alexander JW: Intact protein versus free amino acids in the nutritional support of thermally injured animals. JPEN J Parenter Enteral Nutr 1986;10:139.

Turner WW, Ireton CS, Hunt JL, Baxter CR: Predicting energy expenditures in burned patients. J Trauma 1985;259:11.

Unger RH, Orci L: Glucagon and the A cell: physiology and pathophysiology. N Engl J Med 1981;304:1518.

VanVliet G, Bosson D, Craen M, et al: Comparative study of the lipolytic potencies of pituitary-derived and biosynthetic human growth hormone in hypopituitary children. J Clin Endocrinol Metab 1987;65:876.

Vaughn GM, Becker RA, Allen JP, et al: Cortisol and corticotrophin in burned patients. J Trauma 1982;22:263.

Voerman HJ, Strack RVS, Groeneveld ABJ, et al: Effects of recombinant human growth hormone in patients with severe sepsis. Ann Surg 1992;216:648.

Vogel AV, Peake GT, Rada RT: Pituitary-testicular axis dysfunction in burned men. J Clin Endocrinol Metab 1985;60:658.

Warden GD, Heimbach DM: Burns. *In* Schwartz SL (ed): Principles of Surgery. New York: McGraw-Hill, 1999:232.

Warwick-David J, Lowrie DB, Cole PJ: Growth hormone is a human macrophage activating factor: priming of human monocytes for enhanced release of H_2O_2. J Immunol 1995;154:1909.

Weissman C: The metabolic response to stress: an overview and update. Anesthesiology 1990;73:308.

Wildmueller HG, Spaeth AE: Intestinal metabolism of glutamine and glutamate from the lumen as compared to glutamine from the blood. Arch Biochem Biophys 1975;171:662.

Wilmore DW, Lindsey CA, Moylan JA, et al: Hyperglucagonaemia after burns. Lancet 1974;1:73.

Wilmore DW, Long JM, Mason AD, et al: Catecholamines: mediators of hypermetabolic response to thermal injury. Ann Surg 1974;180:653.

Wilmore DW, Long JM, Skreen RW, et al: Studies of the Effect of Variations of Temperature and Humidity on Energy Demands of the Burned Soldier in a Controlled Metabolic Room. (Annual Report 1973, Report Control Symbol MEDDH-288 [R]). Ft. Sam Houston, TX: U.S. Army Institute of Surgical Research, 1973.

Wilmore DW, Mason AD, Johnson DW, Pruitt BA: Effects of ambient temperature on heat production and heal loss in burn patients. J Appl Physiol 1975;38:593.

Wilmore DW, Moyland JA Jr, Bristow BF, et al: Anabolic effects of growth hormone and high caloric feedings following thermal injury. Surg Gynecol Obstet 1974;138:875.

Wilmore DW, Orcutt TW, Mason AD Jr, Pruitt BA: Alterations in hypothalamic function following thermal injury. J Trauma 1975;15:697.

Wilson DM, McCauley E, Brown DR, Dudley R: Oxandrolone therapy in constitutionally delayed growth and puberty. Bio-Technology General Corporation Cooperative Study Group. Pediatrics 1995;96:1095.

Wise JK, Hendler R, Felig P: Influence of glucocorticoids on glucagons secretion and plasma amino acid concentrations in man. J Clin Invesst 1973;52:2774–2782.

Wolf SE, Barrow RE, Herndon DN: Growth hormone and IGF-1 therapy in the hypercatabolic patient. Clin Endo Metab 1996;132:158–161.

Wolfe BM, Walker BK, Shaul DB, et al: Effect of total parenteral nutrition on hepatic histology. Arch Surg 1988;123:1084.

Wolfe RR: Caloric requirements of the burned patient. J Trauma 1981;21:712.

Wolfe RR, Allsop JR, Burke JF: Glucose metabolism in man: responses to intravenous glucose infusion. Metabolism 1979;28:221.

Wolfe RR, Durkot MJ: Evaluation of the role of the sympathetic nervous system in the response of substrate kinetics and oxidation to burn injury. Circ Shock 1982;9:395.

Wolfe RR, Durkot MJ, Allsop JR, et al: Glucose metabolism in severely burned patients. Metabolism 1979;28:1031.

Wolfe RR, Goodenough RD, Burke JF, et al: Response of protein and urea kinetics in burn patients to different levels of protein intake. Ann Surg 1983;197:163.

Wolfe RR, Herndon DN, Jahoor F, et al: Effect of severe burn on substrate cycling by glucose and fatty acids. N Engl J Med 1987;317:403.

Wolfe RR, Herndon DN, Peters EJ, et al: Regulation of lipolysis in severely burned children. Ann Surg 1987;206:214.

Wolfe RR, Jahoor F, Hart WH: Protein and amino acid metabolism after injury. Diabetes Metab Rev 1989;5:149.

Wolfe RR, Jahoor F, Herndon DN, et al: The glucose alanine cycle: origin of control [abstract]. JPEN J Parenter Enteral Nutr 1985;9:107.

Wolfe RR, Jahoor F, Herndon DN, et al: Isotopic evaluation of the metabolism of pyruvate and related substrates in normal adult volunteers and severely burned children: effect of dichloroacetate and glucose infusion. Surgery 1991;110:54.

Wolfe RR, Shaw JH: Inhibitory effect of plasma free fatty acids on glucose production in the conscious dog. Am J Physiol 1984;246:E181.

Wolfe RR, Shaw JH, Durkot MJ: Effect of sepsis on VLDL kinetics: responses in basal state and during glucose infusion. Am J Physiol 1985;248:E732.

Wolfe RR, Shaw JH, Jahoor F, et al: Response to glucose infusion in humans: role of the changes in insulin concentration. Am J Physiol 1986;250:E306.

Yarasheski KE, Campbell JA, Rennie MK, et al: Effect of strength training and growth hormone administration on whole-body and skeletal muscle leucine metabolism. Med Sci Sports Exerc 1990;22:505A.

Young FG: Insulin and insulin antagonists. Endocrinology 1963;73:654.

Yu Y-M, Wagner DA, Walesreswski JC, et al: A kinetic study of leucine metabolism in severely burned patients: comparison between a conventional and branched chain amino acid-enriched nutritional therapy. Ann Surg 1988; 207:421.

Yurt RW, McManus AT, Mason AD, Pruitt BA: Increased susceptibility to infection related to extent of burn. Arch Surg 1984;119:183.

Zawacki BE, Spitzer KW, Mason AD Jr: Does increased evaporative water loss cause hypermetabolism in burn patients. Ann Surg 1970;171:236.

CHAPTER 33

Thermal Injury

Leopoldo C. Cancio, M.D., Pamela A. Howard, M.D., Albert T. McManus, Ph.D., Cleon W. Goodwin, M.D., and Basil A. Pruitt, Jr., M.D.

Trauma, thermal or mechanical, elicits a biphasic response on the part of every organ system, the magnitude of which is proportional to the severity of the injury. The burn patient has been termed the "universal trauma model" because the magnitude and duration of these systemic responses and their predictable, sigmoidal relationship to the extent of the burn (Fig. 33–1) readily lend themselves to study. This chapter reviews the scientific basis for the care of patients with severe thermal injury in the following areas: burn shock; inhalation injury; metabolism and nutrition; immunology; and infection. Since World War II, integrated basic and clinical research in these areas, performed at multidisciplinary burn centers, has succeeded in greatly reducing mortality following thermal injury. Many of the studies conducted in burn patients and burn models have had direct application to the understanding and treatment of patients with other forms of injury.

Burn Wounds

The burn wound is the central problem in the care of the burn patient. Its successful management, from resuscitation through definitive surgery and rehabilitation, is the key to a satisfactory outcome. The depth of injury is a function of the temperature applied and the duration of application. Keratinocyte death following thermal injury may occur via heat fixation, apoptosis, and/or accidental cell death. Three zones in the burn wound have been described: a necrotic zone of coagulation; an ischemic zone of stasis; and an inflamed zone of hyperemia. This concept

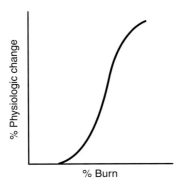

FIGURE 33–1 Idealized sigmoidal dose-response curve describes the effect of burn size on the magnitude and duration of postburn physiologic changes, morbidity, and mortality. (From Pruitt BA Jr: The universal trauma model. Bull Am Coll Surg 1985;70:2–13, with permission.)

emphasizes the fact that meticulous patient care is needed to prevent the zone of stasis from progressing to frank necrosis owing to edema, malperfusion, desiccation, or infection. Furthermore, rescue of apoptotic cells, reversal of tissue ischemia, or prevention of secondary, mediator-induced injury may in the future represent valid strategies for salvaging this "zone of stasis."

Clinically, burn wounds are classified according to their depth as partial-thickness (first and second degree) burns or full-thickness (third degree) burns; no technology has emerged to replace the trained observer for assessing burn depth (Table 33–1). Accurate determination of the burn size is more important than the burn depth during resuscitation. An initial estimate of burn size can be made with the

"rule of nines" and then refined using the Lund-Browder chart. (Burn size, for purpose of resuscitation formulas [see below], etc. includes second and third degree burns only.)

Burn Shock

Pathophysiology

Shock occurs following cutaneous thermal injury to 10% to 20% (or more) of the total body surface area (TBSA) and mandates prompt, adequate fluid resuscitation. Immediately following injury there is a decrease in the cardiac output of about 50% accompanied by a near-doubling of the systemic vascular resistance (SVR) and an even greater increase in pulmonary vascular resistance (PVR) (Fig. 33–2). In patients resuscitated using the Brooke formula (see below), the SVR then decreases to below the normal range by 6 to 8 hours after the burn, reaching 50% of normal by 36 hours. An elevated PVR generally persists until 48 hours after the burn. Concomitantly, the cardiac output is restored to 80% of normal by 6 to 8 hours after the burn and becomes supranormal by 36 hours. The plasma and blood volumes (Fig. 33–3) gradually decrease despite physiologically appropriate resuscitation, reaching a nadir of approximately 80% of predicted normal by 18 to 24 hours. The plasma volume is restored later than the cardiac output (i.e., by 54 hours). Blood volume, on the other hand, is not fully restored, indicating that thermal destruction of red blood cells (RBCs) has occurred.

Table 33–1
Classification of burn depth

Parameter	First Degree	Second Degree	Third Degree
Typical cause	Sunlight; brief exposure to hot liquids; brief flash burns	Limited exposure to hot liquid, flash, flame, or chemical agent	Prolonged contact with flame, hot liquid, hot object, or chemical agent; high-voltage electricity
Color	Red	Pink or mottled red	Dark brown, charred, translucent with visible thrombosed veins, or pearly white
Surface	Dry	Blisters or moist weeping surface	Dry and inelastic
Sensation	Painful	Very painful	Insensate surface
Depth	Epidermis	Epidermis and portions of the dermis	Epidermis, dermis, and possibly deep structures
Time to healing*	A few days	One week or more	Heals by contraction and scar formation

*In the absence of excision and grafting.
Modified from Sabiston DC Jr (ed): Textbook of Surgery (15th ed). Philadelphia: WB Saunders, 1997:222, with permission.

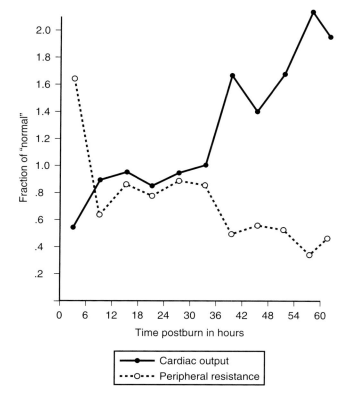

FIGURE 33–2 Changes in cardiac output and in peripheral vascular resistance during resuscitation. (From Pruitt BA Jr, Mason AD Jr, Moncrief JA: Hemodynamic changes in the early postburn patient: the influence of fluid administration and of a vasodilator [hydralazine]. J Trauma 1971;11:36–46, with permission.)

Based on these parameters it can be seen that burn shock is the result of both elevated vascular resistance (increased afterload) and hypovolemia (decreased preload). The postburn decrease in cardiac output and increase in vascular resistance are not uniformly distributed among the various organs, which results in differential changes in regional blood flow. The small intestine may be particularly vulnerable to such decreases; furthermore, aggressive fluid resuscitation and restoration of cardiac output may fail to restore blood flow fully in the mesenteric circulation.

A myocardial depressant factor of burn shock, affecting intrinsic myocardial contractility, has been postulated as an additional mechanism of impaired cardiac output after a burn. Demonstration of impaired contractility ex vivo has depended on the preparation used. Adams and colleagues have reported such contractility changes by means of a modification of the isolated, coronary-perfused heart (Langendorff preparation). Cioffi et al., by contrast, found that fluid resuscitation prevented postburn decrements in isolated papillary muscle function. More relevantly, such decrements have not been demonstrated in vivo; for example, Goodwin et al. documented hypercontractile left ventricular function during burn shock in patients by means of echocardiography.

The hypovolemia that occurs after thermal injury is caused primarily by a loss of plasma volume into the interstitium in both burned and unburned tissues, resulting in edema formation. Transcapillary fluid flux (J_v) is determined by three forces: microvascular permeability, hydrostatic pressure, and colloid osmotic pressure. Each of these forces is affected by thermal injury and contributes to plasma loss and edema formation. More precisely, this

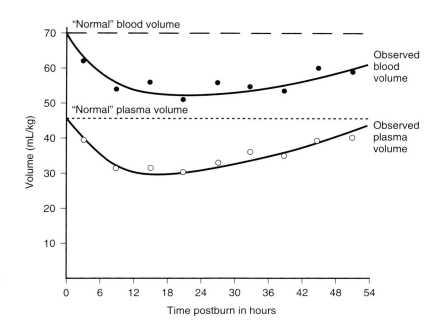

FIGURE 33–3 Blood and plasma volume changes during resuscitation. (From Pruitt BA Jr, Mason AD Jr, Moncrief JA: Hemodynamic changes in the early postburn patient: the influence of fluid administration and of a vasodilator [hydralazine]. J Trauma 1971;11:36–46, with permission.)

process can be described by the following equation (the Starling equilibrium).

$$J_v = L_p S \left[(P_c - P_i) - \sigma(COP_p - COP_i) \right]$$

where P and COP are hydrostatic and colloid osmotic pressures, respectively; subscripts c, p, and i denote capillary, plasma, and interstitial, respectively; σ is the capillary reflection coefficient for protein; L_p is the hydraulic conductivity (permeability) of the capillary membrane; and S is the surface area available for fluid exchange. The product $L_p S$ is called the capillary filtration coefficient.

Changes in these Starling forces occur rapidly after a burn. Water, albumin, sodium, and RBCs accumulate within minutes in burned skin, and the process of edema formation continues throughout the first 24 to 48 hours. Arturson showed that the rate of edema formation, the capillary filtration coefficient, and dilation of resistance vessels all increase most rapidly during the first 5 to 10 minutes after a burn. The ratio of the concentration of a particle in lymph to its concentration in plasma (C_L/C_P) is related to the capillary reflection coefficient (i.e., the permeability) for that particle. By measuring the C_L/C_P for dextrans of various molecular weights, Arturson found that the greatest increase in permeability occurred in large molecules; that this change was maximal 1 to 3 hours after the burn; that it worsened with increased burn depth; and that it gradually resolved as the wound healed. Morphologically, these permeability changes are associated with the opening of intercellular junctions between endothelial cells, with the formation of large numbers of vacuoles (which may transport macromolecules), and with no change in the number of vesicles.

These changes do not entirely explain the increased permeability; hence impaired regulation of endothelial permeability by the connective tissue of the interstitium may also play a role. Pitt et al. determined the relative contribution to edema formation of pressure and permeability changes during the first 3 hours after a burn. Thermal injury caused a near-doubling of capillary pressure, from 24 mmHg to 47 mmHg, by 30 minutes after a burn secondary to a decrease in precapillary resistance with no change in postcapillary resistance. The C_L/C_P and lymph flow increased throughout the 3-hour study. Until about 2 hours after the burn, most of the increase in fluid flux was explained by pressure increases; thereafter permeability increases were of greater importance.

The estimated effective "driving pressure" for edema formation during the initial postburn period is enormous, about 250 to 300 mmHg, and cannot be entirely accounted for by the above-mentioned changes in permeability and hydrostatic pressure. Lund et al. therefore measured the interstitial hydrostatic pressure, P_i, and found it to be reduced by thermal injury: from −1 mmHg to about −25 mmHg. Fluid resuscitation rapidly restored this value to normal; conversely, isolating the skin from the circulation

(e.g., with a plastic barrier) facilitated a further decrease in P_i to −135 mmHg. They also compared changes in the P_i to changes in the interstitial colloid osmotic pressure, COP_i. P_i changes predominated after 10 seconds of exposure, whereas COP_i changes predominated, reaching −133 mmHg, after 60 seconds of exposure. Combined, these changes in P_i and COP_i create a "dermal imbibition pressure" or "suction," which is likely the result of burn-induced ultrastructural changes in interstitial collagen and hyaluronan.

Aside from direct thermal injury to the endothelium and interstitium, several mediators have been implicated in the process of edema formation. Histamine is increased in proportion to the burn size within 1 minute of thermal injury and causes vasodilation of the resistance vessels. Histamine, as well as serotonin and bradykinin, cause endothelial cell contraction and the appearance of intercellular junctions. The endothelial changes seen following histamine exposure are morphologically similar to those seen following thermal injury.

Other mediators of local and systemic injury after a burn include prostaglandins, complement, neutrophils, nitric oxide (NO), and the proinflammatory cytokines. Systemic release of these mediators and generalized hypoproteinemia induce edema formation in unburned tissue following burns in excess of about 25% TBSA. Using lung and prefemoral (flank) lymph fistulas in sheep, Demling et al. defined the effect of a 30% TBSA burn on microvascular permeability in unburned tissues. There was an increase in lung lymph flow (Q_L) but no increase in the C_L/C_P, suggesting no increase in pulmonary microvascular permeability. In contrast, there was an increase in both Q_L and C_L/C_P in the flank areas, the latter resolving by 12 hours after the burn. The burn tissue Q_L was persistently elevated for the duration of the 60-hour study, and the C_L/C_P remained elevated for 48 hours. Thus, it appears that unburned soft tissue microvascular permeability resolves before that of burned soft tissue.

Resuscitation

Three factors laid the foundation for the development of fluid resuscitation formulas for burn shock: (1) recognition that burn shock involves a gradual loss of large volumes of plasma into the interstitium, with resulting hemoconcentration and hypovolemic shock; (2) recognition that these losses were proportional to the burn size; and (3) the widespread availability of plasma transfusions during World War II. The Coconut Grove fire of 1942 allowed Oliver Cope, Francis D. Moore, and colleagues to document experience with a formula based on burn size that provided equal volumes of physiologic saline and plasma. Evans then incorporated the patient's weight into an equation that provided 1 ml colloid (plasma, plasma substitute, or whole blood)/kg/% burn, 1 ml normal saline/kg/%TBSA, and 2000 ml of 5% glucose in water during the first 24 hours after the burn. The original Brooke formula was a modification of this one and employed 1.5 ml lactated Ringer's solution/kg/% burn, 0.5 ml colloid/kg/% burn, and 2000 ml of 5% glucose in water. Half of this volume was given during the first 8 hours after the burn and half during the second 16 hours, in consonance with the observation that plasma volume changes were most rapid during the earlier period.

In subsequent studies, the amount of colloid given during the first 24 hours after a burn, which varied between 0% and 50% of the total volume infused, had no greater effect on augmenting the plasma volume than did an equal volume of crystalloid. Furthermore, the use of colloid immediately after a burn was associated with the accumulation of extravascular lung water as edema fluid was reabsorbed, beginning on postburn day 3. These findings gave rise to the modified Brooke formula, which we currently use. A dose of 2 ml lactated Ringer's solution/kg/% TBSA is administered during the first 24 hours after the burn. During the second 24 hours the administration of colloid becomes effective; a 5% albumin solution is given at a dose of 0.3 to 0.5 ml/kg/% burn to reduce the total volume infused (0.3 ml/kg/% burn for patients with 30% to 50% burns, 0.4 ml/kg/% burn for patients with 51% to 70% burns, and 0.5 ml/kg/% burn for patients with more than 70% burns). In children weighing less than 30 kg, the surface-area/weight ratio is higher, and the volume requirements per %burn are therefore greater. Thus, for children the modified Brooke formula predicts a need for 3 ml lactated Ringer's solution/kg/%TBSA for the first 24 hours after a burn as well as 5% glucose and 0.5 N saline in water at a maintenance rate. The Parkland formula, which estimates fluid requirements as lactated Ringer's solution (4 ml/kg/% burn for the first 24 hours after a burn) was based on the observation that the functional extracellular fluid volume, transmembrane potential, and other indices could be restored more rapidly with a higher rate of fluid administration.

The various formulas provide only an initial estimate of fluid requirements, which must be continually revised based primarily on the hourly urine output. A urine output of 30 to 50 ml/hr in adults or 1 ml/kg/hr in children (weighing less than 30 kg) should be achieved by changes of about 20% in the lactated Ringer's infusion rate every 1 to 2 hours. It is as important to decrease the fluid administration rate as it is to increase it, as needed, to avoid complications associated with excessive edema formation. Typically, the actual volume is greater than that predicted by the formulas. In one review, 2.88 ml/kg/% burn was the final dose administered under the modified Brooke formula. In a recent multicenter review of experience with 50 patients, 5.2 ml/kg/% burn was the final dose given under the Parkland formula. These data suggest that the Parkland formula overestimates the requirements of most patients,

and that its use may lead to excessive edema. However, no randomized controlled trial comparing resuscitation formulas has been reported to date.

The desire to limit fluid intake and recognition of the importance of sodium repletion have led to studies of various hypertonic saline solutions for burn shock resuscitation. Several authors have argued that hypertonic saline solutions containing approximately 250 mEq of sodium per liter reduce water requirements without increasing sodium requirements during burn resuscitation. In contrast, Huang et al. reported no sustained fluid-sparing effect, a twofold increase in mortality, and a fourfold increase in acute renal failure for patients receiving a 290 mEq/L solution versus historical controls receiving lactated Ringer's solution. A recent Cochrane Collaboration review of such regimens found four randomized controlled trials in critically ill patients. The pooled relative risk of death in burn patients was 1.49 [95% confidence interval (CI) 0.56 to 3.95], so these trials must be considered inconclusive. Various beneficial effects have been reported in animal models for 7.5% hypertonic saline/6% dextran 70 solution (HSD) as a pharmacologic adjunct to standard resuscitation regimens, including improved cardiac function and regional blood flow as well as reduced lipid peroxidation. However, HSD has provided early (8 to 12 hours), but not sustained, fluid-sparing effects in large animal models. Consequently, its role in resuscitation after a burn remains to be defined.

Some have proposed a revision of resuscitation goals to include endpoints such as oxygen delivery and consumption or the intrathoracic blood volume. These approaches have led to fluid resuscitation volumes that in one report were 1.5 times those predicted by the Parkland formula and to urine outputs that in another report exceeded 150 ml/hr, three times the maximum recommended by the Brooke formula. There are no data to support these measures; furthermore, the devastating effects of large resuscitation volumes—such as the abdominal and extremity compartment syndromes and respiratory failure secondary to airway edema—are strong arguments against them. To be sure, a small number of patients fail to respond in the customary manner to standard resuscitation regimens and therefore manifest progressively severe acidosis, fluid requirements in excess of 6 ml/kg/% burn, and/or oliguria despite escalating fluid doses. In these patients, pulmonary artery catheterization and measuring the indices of cardiac function may permit more rapid, precise determination of the appropriate fluid infusion rate and identification of patients who, following adequate volume loading, would benefit from an inotrope or afterload reduction.

A pharmacologic approach to reducing the fluid resuscitation requirements of the thermally injured patient would be desirable. High-dose ascorbic acid (66 mg/kg/hr) has been shown by Tanaka and colleagues to reduce lipid peroxidation, vascular permeability, edema in both burned and unburned tissue, and fluid resuscitation requirements in animal models; similar results were recently reported in a trial that included 37 patients. In animal models, intravenous ibuprofen improved intestinal blood flow during burn shock and improved blood flow while reducing edema formation in the burn wound.

Burn shock is associated with important end-organ effects. Edema underneath constricting full-thickness eschar may impair arterial inflow and cause neuromuscular damage in a burned extremity. The progressive diminution of arterial flow, assessed hourly by Doppler flowmetry in the extremities, is an indication for urgent escharotomy. As a consequence of early alterations in gastroduodenal mucosal blood flow, and in the absence of antacid therapy, gastroduodenal stress ulceration (Curling's ulcer) was clinically recognized in 12% of burn patients. Endoscopically, gastric ulceration was visualized in 86% of patients studied with burns of more than 35% of the TBSA; mucosal damage was seen within hours of the burn in some. This complication is effectively prevented with antacids or histamine (H_2)-receptor antagonists. Recent experience suggests that proton-pump inhibitors are also effective. Thermal injury also causes an increase in intestinal permeability, which is increased on day 2 in patients who later develop infection. In animal models, this increased permeability is associated with the translocation of microorganisms and their products, which may lead to systemic inflammation, multiple system organ failure, and/or infection. Nonocclusive mesenteric ischemia and infarction, causing necrosis of a variable extent of small or large bowel, is a rare but potentially devastating complication of thermal injury. Diagnostic peritoneal lavage may be helpful for identifying ischemic bowel.

Inhalation Injury

Approximately one third of patients admitted to burn centers have sustained smoke inhalation injury. Using multiple logistic regression analysis, Shirani et al. established that inhalation injury independently increases the risk of death in burn patients over that predicted by age and burn size alone by a maximum of 20%. Inhalation injury also increases the risk of pneumonia; in turn, pneumonia acts independently to increase the risk of death by a maximum of 40%. These additive contributions to mortality risk are greatest at the midrange of age and burn size. Rue et al. documented significant recent improvements in the survival of patients with inhalation injury, comparing cohorts from 1980–1984 and 1985–1990. As is discussed below, the use of high-frequency percussive ventilation was one of the factors associated with improved survival in the later cohort. Despite these advances, smoke inhalation remains a major cause of morbidity and mortality in thermally injured patients.

Inhalation injury can be classified anatomically as producing (1) injury to the upper airways, including the glottis; (2) injury to the lower airways and pulmonary parenchyma; and/or (3) systemic toxicity by inhaling toxic gases such as carbon monoxide and cyanide. Inhalation of toxic gases is the leading cause of immediate fire-induced death and is discussed separately, although the three classes of inhalation injury frequently coincide.

Upper airway injury may cause life-threatening airway obstruction soon after injury. If this process is properly managed, upper airway edema usually resolves without sequelae in a few days. Subglottic injury, on the other hand, may cause more significant changes in lung function and may be more difficult to manage. Subglottic injury is a chemical injury caused by inhaling the toxic products of incomplete combustion. Smoke has a low heat-carrying capacity; as a result, direct thermal injury to the subglottic airways and pulmonary parenchyma is rare; it usually requires exposure to superheated steam.

Smoke

A large number of toxic compounds are present in smoke, the composition of which is highly variable; it depends on the composition of the burning material and the temperature of the fire. Smoke composition also changes during the course of the fire. Toxic gases, heat, and oxygen deficiency interact to produce severe injury or death at the scene of major structural fires. Davies reviewed a simulation of a 1981 nightclub fire in which temperatures of 1160°C and lethal ambient levels of oxygen (<6%), carbon dioxide, carbon monoxide, and cyanide were rapidly reached in the structure. The ability of victims to escape the fire would have been further impeded by dense smoke—which greatly reduced visibility—and by high levels of severely irritating hydrogen chloride gas.

Several autopsy studies indicate that the toxic gas of greatest importance in fire deaths is carbon monoxide, with lethal levels of carboxyhemoglobin (COHb) (>50%) having been found in most of the nonsurvivors. In contrast, the true incidence of severe cyanide poisoning in fire victims is a matter of debate. Cyanide has a short half-life in vivo and can be either generated or consumed postmortem. For example, Barillo et al. retrospectively reviewed fire fatality data from the state of New Jersey. Altogether 195 of 433 casualties (45%) had lethal (≥50%) COHb levels; and 31 of 364 (8.5%) had lethal (>3 mg/L) cyanide levels. Only 8 of 364 (2.2%) had lethal cyanide levels but a sublethal COHb level. Contrary findings were reported by Baud et al. There are some clinical and laboratory data to support the concept that sublethal doses of CO combined with sublethal doses of cyanide can act synergistically to produce increased toxicity.

Other common toxic smoke constituents include aldehydes (including formaldehyde and acrolein), ammonia, hydrogen sulfide, sulfur dioxide, hydrogen chloride and fluoride, phosgene, nitrogen dioxide, and organic nitriles. Particulate material is an essential component of smoke as well. Removal of solid-phase material from smoke using filters with 0.3 μm diameter pores essentially eliminates the pathophysiology of smoke inhalation injury in some models. Persistent free radicals are also present in smoke. The origin and composition of smoke greatly influence the pathophysiology of the injury and the outcome of studies in this field.

Diagnosis of Inhalation Injury

Early diagnosis of inhalation injury is important to identify patients who merit close intensive care unit (ICU) observation and possibly prophylactic intubation, and who may require special resources such as high-frequency percussive ventilation. Clinical findings in one series included facial burns (96% of patients), wheezing (47%), carbonaceous sputum (39%), rales (35%), dyspnea (27%), hoarseness (26%), tachypnea (26%), and cough and hypersecretion (26%). However, no one physical or historical finding is sufficiently sensitive or specific for a definitive diagnosis. Chest radiographs are routinely obtained but only to provide a baseline, as they are normal on admission in 92% of patients with inhalation injury. Shirani et al. reported an accurate multiple logistic predictor of inhalation injury based on the presence or absence of closed-space injury, the presence or absence of facial burns, the percent of the TBSA burned, and age. In practice, though, an invasive procedure is necessary for the definitive diagnosis of inhalation injury. Patients should also be evaluated for the specific findings of toxic inhalation, as discussed below.

Most often, flexible fiberoptic bronchoscopy is used to diagnose subglottic inhalation injury. When performed by qualified personnel, fiberoptic evaluation of the larynx may permit conservative management of mildly symptomatic patients in an ICU who otherwise might have undergone intubation. Fiberoptic bronchoscopy also permits emergency intubation using the endoscope in patients with difficult airways who are at risk of imminent airway loss. Less commonly, xenon-133 lung scanning is used in questionable cases. Patients with bronchoscopy-negative but xenon-133-positive inhalation injury appear to have a milder injury than those who are bronchoscopy-positive in that the risk of pneumonia, though still increased over that of patients without inhalation injury, is lower in the former group.

Pathophysiology of Inhalation Injury

The morphologic changes seen at several time points following subglottic exposure of sheep to various doses of smoke have been described. Inhalation injury caused necrosis and sloughing of respiratory tract epithelium beginning 15 minutes after exposure. Less severe injury featured loss of cilia. With severe injury (high smoke doses), full-thickness ulceration of the epithelial surface was seen occasionally. Mucus production was increased by 12 hours. Beginning 2 hours after injury and peaking at 24 hours, there was an acute inflammatory reaction featuring neutrophilic infiltration into the airways, with extensive formation of pseudomembranes. Ultimately, these pseudomembranes nearly occluded the major airways of many of the sheep. Atelectasis developed distal to terminal airways obstructed by debris and edema, associated with subsequent bacterial colonization at 72 hours and followed by pneumonia. Parenchymal changes were less prominent than airway changes. Alveolar edema was a delayed phenomenon, seen after 24 hours. Vascular endothelial changes were not found in this model. Electron microscopy revealed changes in type I and type II (surfactant-producing) pneumocytes.

Ventilation-perfusion (V_A/Q) mismatch is a principal cause of hypoxia in a variety of conditions, including inhalation injury. Nieman et al. used a unilateral (one-lung) inhalation injury model to address this question during the immediate postinjury period. Pulmonary vascular resistance increased in the uninjured lung but not in the injured lung. There was a gradual increase in blood flow to the injured lung, which reached significance 2 hours after the injury. These findings suggest that mediators released by smoke inhalation cause vasoconstriction in uninjured segments, whereas other processes cause impairment of local vasoconstriction in injured lung segments.

The effect of inhalation injury on V_A/Q matching was rigorously defined by Shimazu et al. in ovine studies using the multiple inert gas elimination technique (MIGET). Smoke caused time- and severity-related decreases in the partial pressure of oxygen (PaO_2). This hypoxia was associated with an increase in blood flow distribution to low V_A/Q compartments ($0 < V_A/Q < 0.1$) at the expense of blood flow to normal V_A/Q compartments ($0.1 < V_A/Q < 10$). The likely explanation for these changes is the airway obstruction observed histologically.

Clinically significant pulmonary edema is infrequently seen acutely in patients with inhalation injury. One possible reason is concomitant cutaneous thermal injury, which causes elevations in pulmonary vascular resistance that persist for 48 hours after a burn and prevent increases in pulmonary hydrostatic pressure at the capillary level. When present before 48 hours after a burn, such pulmonary edema may indicate a more severe injury. Potential causes of pulmonary edema after inhalation injury include increased endothelial and/or alveolar permeability as well as increased hydrostatic pressure.

Herndon et al. described increases in lung lymph flow (Q_L), the lymph/plasma protein concentration ratio (C_L/C_P), and lung transvascular protein flux at 12 hours after injury in sheep, consistent with an increase in lung endothelial permeability to protein. These findings were refined by studies in which the endothelial surface area was held constant by maximizing the pulmonary venous pressure. In one such study the contribution of hydrostatic pressure was determined as well. Endothelial permeability increases were more prominent than pressure increases at 24 hours, whereas the reverse was true at 48 hours. Increased alveolar permeability to aerosolized radioactive tracers has also been documented.

Using in vivo microscopy, Nieman et al. observed focal atelectasis within minutes of wood smoke inhalation—even before the appearance of significant cellular infiltration or broncheolar obstruction. Most likely this represented a smoke-induced increase in alveolar surface tension, reflecting rapid decreases in the quantity and quality of surfactant. These authors also found that wood smoke but not cotton smoke caused these changes in surface tension, and that in vitro surfactant replacement restored surface tension following injury.

Secondary Lung Injury

A hematogenous route for secondary lung injury following smoke inhalation is probable. Unilateral smoke exposure causes increases in contralateral lung microvascular permeability. Ablation of the bronchial circulation attenuates smoke-induced changes in pulmonary vascular resistance, lung lymph flow, endothelial permeability, the wet/dry weight ratio, and oxygenation.

Neutrophils contribute to secondary lung injury following inhalation injury. Preinjury leukocyte depletion with nitrogen mustard has been reported to attenuate smoke-induced changes in pulmonary artery pressure, pulmonary vascular resistance, pulmonary lymph flow, the PaO_2/FiO_2 ratio, plasma conjugated dienes, and the consumption of antiprotease in lung lymph. A synthetic antiprotease (gabexate mesilate) given after injury had similar protective effects. Tasaki et al. evaluated the effect of sulfo Lewis C, a putative ligand of E-selectins. Free-radical production by granulocytes was increased after smoke exposure in both treated and untreated groups, but the treatment improved oxygenation and reduced the V_A/Q mismatch.

A monoclonal antibody against L-selectin, LAM1-3, attenuated late but not early increases in lung lymph flow. In another study, this drug also preserved the PaO_2/FiO_2 ratio and the lung wet/dry weight ratio. Antibodies to interleukin-8, a neutrophil chemotactic factor, decreased the permeability of the alveolar capillary membrane to protein.

Pentoxifylline, an anticytokine that inhibits multiple steps in neutrophil-mediated inflammation, was evaluated

by Ogura et al. in an ovine model. Beneficial effects included improved oxygenation and V_A/Q matching (by MIGET), lower lung wet/dry weight ratios, and reduced levels of polymorphonuclear neutrophils (PMNs), protein, and conjugated dienes in bronchoalveolar lavage fluid and levels of conjugated dienes in plasma.

Oxygen-derived free radicals are found in smoke and, more importantly, are produced by neutrophils, macrophages, and other cells following injury. They have been extensively implicated in the pathophysiology of inhalation injury. For example, Demling et al. found in a rat model that the degree of lung lipid peroxidation (malondialdehyde levels) correlated with mortality, as did the degree of decrease in lung catalase levels. These authors also noted increased lung lipid peroxidation following smoke inhalation by sheep, along with decreased plasma catalase and glutathione levels.

Thus, pulmonary injury decreases systemic levels of circulating antioxidants. After smoke inhalation, free iron release, leading to increased hydroxyl radical production, may be a mechanism of oxidative injury. Platelet-activating factor (PAF) acts via multiple pathways to activate neutrophils and platelets and to cause increased production of eicosanoids and free radicals. An antagonist of PAF, given before or after inhalation injury, prevented smoke-induced increases in blood, lung, and bronchoalveolar lavage fluid levels of malondialdehyde.

Nitric oxide (NO) may also play a role in secondary injury following smoke inhalation. In addition to its role as a vasodilator, NO serves as a chemotactic factor for neutrophils and combines with oxygen-derived species to form peroxynitrite. Treatment with N^G-nitro-L-arginine methyl ester (L-NAME) or induction of neutropenia reduced indices of oxidative injury and lung permeability to ^{125}I-albumin in a rat model of inhalation injury and systemic inflammation (peritonitis). Similarly, mercaptoethylguanidine (MEG), an inhibitor of inducible NO synthetase and a free-radical scavenger, reduced indices of oxidative injury and the intrapulmonary shunt fraction in smoke-injured sheep. With combined smoke and cutaneous thermal injury, MEG reduced the microvascular permeability of lung but not of burned tissue.

Eicosanoids may contribute to the pathogenesis of a V_A/Q mismatch and edema following inhalation injury. Levels of thromboxane B_2 (metabolite of thromboxane A_2, a potent vaso- and bronchoconstrictor) were increased in tracheobronchial exudates and, to a lesser extent, in lung lymph. Levels of 6-keto-prostaglandin $F_{1\alpha}$ (metabolite of prostacyclin, a vasodilator) were elevated in plasma and lymph. In smoke models featuring high levels of acrolein, lipoxygenase inhibition decreased smoke-induced increases in lung lymph flow, lymph protein flux, and the wet/dry weight ratios. This implicates leukotrienes in the pathogenesis of pulmonary edema following inhalation of acrolein. Smoke also increased the activity in the lung of phospholipase A_2 (PLA_2), the enzyme responsible for production of the eicosanoid precursor arachidonic acid.

Because inhalation injury is commonly followed by pneumonia, its effect on immune function has been investigated. Alveolar macrophages obtained by bronchoalveolar lavage (BAL) from smoke-injured sheep demonstrated reduced phagocytosis and killing of *Pseudomonas aeruginosa* following ingestion. Such macrophages also demonstrated reduced phagocytosis of apoptotic PMNs. PMNs incubated in media conditioned by smoke-exposed alveolar macrophages showed increased apoptosis rates. Similarly, alveolar macrophages obtained by BAL from smoke-injured rabbits showed decreased adherence and phagocytosis of opsonized bacteria. On the other hand, they showed increased basal production of superoxide and lipopolysaccharide (LPS)-stimulated release of tumor necrosis factor. Hence smoke injury decreased the essential functions of leukocytes while increasing potentially deleterious functions.

Systemic Effects of Inhalation Injury

Inhalation injury also affects other organs; for example, regional blood flow to the splanchnic organs is selectively decreased independent of changes in cardiac output or systemic oxygen delivery. Because severe inhalation injury and extensive cutaneous burns frequently coincide, the interrelationship of the two injuries is clinically relevant. Patients with inhalation injury often require more resuscitation fluid than those without; for example, one group of patients resuscitated with the modified Brooke formula (which estimates 2 ml/kg/% burn) actually required more than 5 ml/kg/% burn/24 hr. The addition of smoke injury to a 15% to 18% TBSA burn caused oxygen consumption to become delivery-dependent without causing changes in oxygenation. This combined injury model also featured an increase in fluid balance and lymph flow in burned tissue, unburned tissue, and lung.

Conversely, cutaneous burns may increase the extent of pulmonary dysfunction following smoke inhalation. For example, Clark et al. noted that 12% of patients with inhalation injury alone required endotracheal intubation versus 62% of those with both inhalation injury and burns. Tasaki et al. evaluated the effect a severe inhalation injury (carboxyhemoglobin level 90%), with or without a 40% full-thickness scald injury, had on the pulmonary function of sheep. The smoke-plus-burn group demonstrated more extensive hemodynamic changes and higher lung malondialdehyde levels than the smoke-only group, but there was no difference during the 48-hour study in the PaO_2, lung wet/dry weight ratio, or V_A/Q mismatching by MIGET. A longer observation period or a more severe cutaneous injury relative to the inhalation injury may have revealed greater differences.

Treatment

Approximately 19% of patients admitted to a burn center require intubation for longer than 24 hours. In burn patients who require prolonged translaryngeal intubation, the common practice is conversion to a tracheostomy after approximately 14 days, although earlier tracheostomy may be required for adequate pulmonary toilet. The timely identification and removal of obstructing tracheobronchial casts and clots is critically important to the survival of smoke-injured patients. Predischarge pulmonary function testing may be used to screen patients for upper airway sequelae of inhalation injury and prolonged intubation, with definitive diagnosis by fiberoptic bronchoscopy.

The most important recent developments in the care of patients with inhalation injury include improved methods of lung-protective mechanical ventilation. In 1991 Cioffi et al. described the use of high-frequency percussive ventilation with the volumetric diffusive respiration ventilator (VDR-4; Percussionaire, Sandpoint, ID, USA) as prophylactic therapy for patients with severe inhalation injury. In a comparison with recent historical controls, 54 smoke-injured patients treated with the VDR within 24 hours of intubation experienced a halving of mortality and a near-halving of the pneumonia rate. In a baboon model of inhalation injury, Cioffi et al. compared VDR, high-frequency oscillatory ventilation, and conventional volume-controlled ventilation. The VDR group demonstrated a lower barotrauma index (versus the conventional group) and decreased parenchymal damage (versus both groups). Subsequent clinical reports have confirmed the VDR ventilator's ability to improve oxygenation and ventilation with less barotrauma. Bearing in mind that a primary pathophysiologic feature of inhalation injury is small airway obstruction with a resultant V_A/Q mismatch, atelectasis, and pneumonia, VDR ventilation likely recruits and maintains the patency of these small airways. In addition, high-frequency molecular motion may enhance gas exchange, and the percussive effect may enhance clearance of secretions and debris (F.M. Bird, personal communication).

Two porcine studies employing perfluorocarbon for partial liquid ventilation (PLV) following inhalation injury have yielded differing results. In a 24-hour study in which the perfluorocarbon was instilled immediately after injury, PLV was associated with improved compliance, oxygenation, and survival compared to that seen with conventional ventilation. On the other hand, in a more realistic 72-hour study in which the drug was instilled 2 or 6 hours after injury, opposite results were obtained. Thus, a clinical role for PLV following inhalation injury remains to be defined.

Inhaled β_2-agonists are used as needed in patients with inhalation injury who develop bronchospasm. Inhaled heparin, by reducing the formation of obstructing hemorrhagic casts of the small and large airways, may improve survival following smoke inhalation. In a clinical study in children with inhalation injury, the combination of nebulized heparin alternating with nebulized N-acetyl-cysteine reduced mortality and reintubation rates compared with those of historical controls. We currently use inhaled heparin in intubated patients with acute inhalation injury.

By means of the MIGET technique, Ogura et al. showed that inhaled NO following smoke inhalation in an ovine model improved perfusion of well ventilated lung compartments while reducing blood flow to true shunt and low V_A/Q compartments. This led to a statistically significant but clinically modest improvement in oxygenation.

Carbon Monoxide

Carbon monoxide is produced by the incomplete combustion of many fuels, especially cellulosics such as wood, paper, and cotton. The predominant toxic effect of CO is its binding to hemoglobin to form carboxyhemoglobin (COHb), thereby making hemoglobin unavailable for the transport of oxygen. In addition, COHb shifts the oxygen-hemoglobin dissociation curve to the left and makes its shape less sigmoidal and more hyperbolic (Haldane effect). Thus, oxygen bound to hemoglobin does not dissociate as readily at the capillary level. Finally, CO binds to hemoglobin 200 to 250 times more avidly than does oxygen. These changes cause "CO hypoxia," that is, reduced delivery of oxygen to the tissues. The most vulnerable tissues are those of the central nervous system and the heart. Evidence in support of this concept was provided by a study in which total body asanguineous hypothermic perfusion, by removing all of the COHb, resuscitated comatose dogs within 20 minutes.

In addition, CO binding to intracellular cytochromes and other metalloproteins (e.g., myoglobin) appears to contribute to CO toxicity. Such extravascular binding accounts for 10% to 15% of total body CO stores and may explain the two-compartment pharmacokinetics that have been observed for COHb elimination. In a study that supports this concept, animals were bled and then transfused with COHb-poisoned RBCs to a mean COHb level of 64%, with no ill effect. Spectrophotometrically, the binding of CO to mitochondrial cytochrome c oxidase (cytochrome a,a_3, the terminal cytochrome on the electron transport chain) and its reversal by oxygen at 3 atm has been demonstrated. Despite the elimination of COHb from the blood by oxygen therapy, there was a delay in recovery of phosphocreatine levels, intracellular pH, and cytochrome c oxidase oxidation levels. Cytochrome c oxidase (complex IV) activity in lymphocytes of patients was inhibited by CO poisoning both acutely and several days after eliminating COHb from the blood. Electron transport chain dysfunction, induced by CO binding, may also cause "leakage" of electrons, the generation of superoxide, and mitochondrial oxidative stress; restoration of tissue oxygenation may, in addition, cause a reoxygenation injury. CO also binds to myocardial and skeletal muscle myoglobin, which may impede transport of oxygen in muscle cells.

Patients with CO exposure present with findings referable to the central nervous and cardiovascular systems. The changes range in severity from mild constitutional symptoms, to compensatory tachycardia and tachypnea, to coma, seizures, dysrhythmias, myocardial ischemia, and hypotension. The classic findings of cherry-red lips, cyanosis, and retinal hemorrhages are, in fact, rarely seen. Patients with preexisting cardiac or pulmonary disease may be particularly vulnerable to CO poisoning. The fetus is also vulnerable because the affinity of fetal hemoglobin for CO is greater than that of adult hemoglobin. A delayed neuropsychiatric syndrome, with onset 3 to 240 days after exposure, has been observed. It consists of cognitive and personality changes, parkinsonism, incontinence, dementia, and/or psychosis; spontaneous resolution occurs in many.

Pulse oximeters fail to distinguish between oxyhemoglobin and COHb and give falsely high oxygen saturation (SpO_2) readings in patients with CO poisoning. Arterial blood gas analyzers, which estimate the arterial oxygen saturation (SaO_2) based on measurement of the dissolved PaO_2, also fail to detect elevated levels of COHb. Therefore, the diagnosis of CO poisoning requires direct determination of COHb levels in arterial (or venous) blood by co-oximetry. Magnetic resonance imaging of the brain and other modalities have been used to evaluate symptomatic patients; common findings include lesions of the globus pallidus and other basal ganglia, deep white matter, and the cerebral cortex.

For male adults the half-life of COHb when breathing room air is 240 minutes, when breathing 100% oxygen at 1 atm 47 minutes, and when breathing 100% oxygen at 2.5 atm 22 minutes. The half-life for female subjects is about 30% lower at each pressure. Accordingly, the mainstay of treatment of CO poisoning is 100% oxygen until levels are lower than 10% to 15% and, if clinically indicated, mechanical ventilation. The additional decrement in the half-life gained by the use of hyperbaric oxygen has been the primary rationale for its use. The ability of hyperbaric oxygen to accelerate the dissociation of CO from cytochrome a,a_3 and to increase tissue PO_2 despite impaired hemoglobin function are also cited. However, there have been no well designed, randomized trials of this therapy. Moreover, hemodynamically unstable burn patients are at increased risk of significant complications during hyperbaric oxygenation (e.g., progressive hypovolemia, seizures, aspiration).

Cyanide

Cyanide is produced during the combustion of synthetics such as plastics, foam, varnishes, and paints and of some natural fibers such as wool and silk. Cyanide binds to cytochrome *c* oxidase at a site distinct from that which binds CO, producing dose-dependent inhibition of mitochondrial electron transport. Clinical findings include dyspnea, tachypnea, vomiting, bradycardia, hypotension, coma, and seizures. Diagnosing cyanide poisoning is difficult because no rapid assay is widely available, although several have been described. According to Baud et al., in patients with smoke inhalation but without burns, an elevated lactate level (10 μmol/L) demonstrated a sensitivity of 87% and a specificity of 94% for toxic cyanide levels (40 μmol/L). Also, an elevated mixed venous saturation, indicative of a failure of mitochondrial oxygen utilization, is indicative of cyanide toxicity but is not universally seen.

Cyanide is metabolized by rhodanese (rhodanase), which catalyzes the donation of sulfur from the sulfane pool to cyanide to form nontoxic thiocyanate. The half-life of cyanide in humans varies from 1 to 3 hours. There are three approaches to treating cyanide poisoning. Amyl and sodium nitrite oxidize hemoglobin to methemoglobin, which chelates cyanide to form cyanomethemoglobin (cyanmethemoglobin) but also reduces the oxygen-carrying capacity. The drugs are also vasodilators and can cause hypotension, so they should be used with caution in patients with concomitant CO poisoning or burn shock. Sodium thiosulfate provides sulfur for the detoxification of cyanide by rhodanese and is free of significant side effects. Finally, hydroxocobalamin (hydroxycobalamin) is a cyanide chelator without significant side effects; unfortunately, it is not currently available in the United States in the doses required to treat cyanide toxicity. Our current practice is to consider the use of sodium thiosulfate for patients with smoke inhalation who have persistent, unexplained metabolic acidosis despite adequate fluid resuscitation and cardiopulmonary support.

Metabolism and Nutrition

One of the striking changes seen in patients during the weeks following extensive thermal injury is profound weight loss and erosion of the lean body mass. This phenomenon occurs despite the provision of adequate calories to meet greatly increased metabolic demands and adequate protein to maintain a positive nitrogen balance. This section reviews the pathophysiology and management of the hypermetabolic response to injury.

Prior to the introduction of high-calorie nutrition for thermally injured patients during the 1970s, dramatic postburn weight loss was common. Extensively burned (> 40% TBSA) patients had the largest weight loss and the latest occurring weight nadir. The maximum weight loss in this group was 22% of the preburn weight, which occurred 8 weeks after the burn; subsequent initiation of weight gain was associated with wound closure. Wilmore et al. then demonstrated the feasibility of high-calorie feeding (up to 8000 kcal of combined enteral and parenteral nutrition in some cases). An increase in caloric intake did not cause an increase in oxygen consumption (Vo_2), but the respiratory quotient (RQ) increased from 0.80 to 1.01 with the provision of 6000 kcal—indicating a transition from the use of body fat stores to that of exogenous carbohydrates and fat deposition.

Metabolic Rate and Caloric Requirements

Metabolic requirements were defined, and the effects of environmental and body temperature on the metabolic rate were evaluated. Using an environmental chamber, Wilmore et al. determined that the metabolic rate increased in a curvilinear fashion as the extent of burn increased, up to a maximum of about 75 kcal/m²/hr. Increasing the ambient temperature from 25°C to 33°C was associated with a modest (approximately 10%) decrease in the metabolic rate of patients with extensive burns (60% TBSA or more). In essence, postburn hypermetabolism appeared to be temperature-sensitive but not temperature-dependent. Control subjects with intact skin were able to decrease their skin temperature (through vasoconstriction) in response to moderate environmental cooling and thus to maintain their core temperature without an increase in the metabolic rate. In contrast, patients with large burns could not compensate in this manner; their core-to-skin heat conductance was abnormally high, and environmental cooling resulted in a slight increase in the metabolic rate above already high levels.

Carlson et al. revisited the effect of burn size on metabolic rate during the late 1980s. They measured the metabolic rate (resting energy expenditure, REE) in 62 patients on postburn days 5 to 19 during 1987–1989 and compared these data to the REE for 43 patients during 1972–1973. The age- and sex-specific preburn basal metabolic rate (BMR) was estimated using the Fleisch equation.Whereas Wilmore et al. had found a curvilinear relationship between the percent TBSA burned and the metabolic rate, in this study the relationship was linear. Furthermore, the metabolic rate was lower than in the previous study at the midrange of burn sizes. This improvement may reflect better control of the bacterial and wound factors driving hypermetabolism: better isolation techniques; more effective use of topical antimicrobials; and earlier, more frequent burn wound excision. The following formula summarizes these findings

Predicted REE (kcal/m²/24 hr) = BMR * (0.89142 + 0.01335 * %burn)

where the BMR can be obtained from the Fleisch equation. This predicted REE can then be multiplied by an activity factor (usually 1.25) to estimate energy requirements (i.e., caloric needs) in burn patients.

The effect of environmental temperature on the metabolic rate was updated by Kelemen et al. during the 1990s. The REE was measured in burn patients and controls at ambient temperatures of 22°, 28°, 32°, and 35°C. The REE was 1.5 times the BMR and was independent of burn size at ambient temperatures of 32° and 35°C. A further increase in the metabolic rate, which was correlated with burn size, was seen at 28° and 22°C. This study demonstrated a centrally mediated component of postburn hypermetabolism (which is maximal in patients with burns as small as 20%) and a temperature-sensitive component that increases as the burn size increases. These studies also indicate the importance of keeping burn patients warm by any means necessary: Not only are they at great risk for hypothermia, but "normal" environmental temperatures further increase an already elevated metabolism.

As the burn wound heals, the REE decreases. Milner et al. measured the REE in 20 patients weekly until the wounds were closed or the patient was discharged and compared these results to the REE predicted by the above (Carlson) equation. During the first 30 days after the burn, the predicted and measured REEs were similar. After 30 days the postburn day influenced the measured REE, as follows.

$$\text{Measured REE} = \text{BMR} * (0.274 + 0.0079 * \%\,\text{burn} - 0.004 * \text{PBD}) + \text{BMR}$$

However, the coefficient of variation (r^2) for this equation was only 0.42, which makes it too inaccurate for clinical use. Thus, the best estimate for REE after day 30 is made by indirect calorimetry. At the time of discharge, the measured REE was still 25% above the normal BMR, even though the wounds were closed.

These findings were recently extended by Hart et al., who measured the REE, the lean body mass by dual-energy x-ray absorptiometry, and isolated leg protein kinetics 6, 9, and 12 months after burn in children. The REE remained elevated above the Harris-Benedict prediction and gradually fell throughout the 12-month period. The net protein balance in the leg remained abnormally low, and the lean body mass continued to fall until 9 months after the burn. The protein balance returned to normal and the lean body mass began to rise at 12 months. Thus hypermetabolism and catabolism persisted long after discharge in these patients.

Nitrogen Requirements

The clinician must also meet the burn patient's nitrogen requirements. In burn patients, the rates of whole-body protein synthesis and breakdown are increased above those of uninjured subjects and correlate with the percent of TBSA burned. In a 35% TBSA canine model, Wolfe et al. determined the contributions of various substrates to the total V_{O_2}. Following injury, oxidation of total carbohydrates, plasma glucose, total fat, plasma free fatty acids, and amino acids increased. Fat oxidation was the major source of energy production both before and after injury (70% of V_{O_2}). Amino acid oxidation contributed 16.5% before injury and 18.5% after injury. In other words, oxidation of the various substrates rose proportionately following injury.

There is some evidence that provision of high levels of protein intake in burn patients may have beneficial effects on immune function or on net protein synthesis. Although protein requirements are commonly estimated such that a nonprotein kilocalorie/nitrogen ratio of 150:1 is provided, actual nitrogen requirements are highly variable. The nitrogen intake required to maintain a positive balance declines over time, as the burn wound heals. Matsuda et al. found that a kilocalorie/nitrogen ratio of 100:1, compared with a ratio of 150:1, was necessary to maintain a positive nitrogen balance in patients with large burns. Because of this variability and because urinary nitrogen losses comprise the major route of nitrogen excretion, it is important to measure 24-hour urinary nitrogen losses once a week in patients with large burns. The nitrogen balance is then calculated; small deficits can be made up by an increase in the enteral feeding rate, and large deficits are made up by boluses of a protein formula. Milner et al. found that the urinary urea nitrogen (UUN), which is easily measured, closely predicts ($r = 0.936$) the total urinary nitrogen (TUN), which is not easily measured.

$$\text{TUN}_{\text{predicted}} = \text{UUN} * 1.25$$

Waxman et al. measured protein losses across open burn wounds and found them to be significant. During the first week after the burn, the 24-hour protein loss in grams is

$$\text{Wound losses}_{\text{predicted}} = 0.3 * \text{BSA} * \%\,\text{burn} * 0.8$$

where BSA is body surface area in square meters and %burn is the percentage of the total body surface area burned. After the first postburn week, protein is lost at approximately one third this rate.

$$\text{Wound losses}_{\text{predicted}} = 0.1 * \text{BSA} * \%\,\text{burn} * 0.8$$

The 0.8 factor in both formulas is a correction factor for the use of topical antimicrobials. Waxman et al. found that silver sulfadiazine cream decreased protein losses.

These formulas are commonly used to estimate protein losses across the burn wound. Finally, an estimate of 2 g/day is commonly used for losses via the fecal route. These three major routes of nitrogen excretion (urine, wound, fecal) allow us to write the following equations.

$$\boxed{\text{Nitrogen balance = nitrogen intake – nitrogen output}}$$

$$\boxed{\text{Nitrogen output} = \text{TUN}_{predicted} + \text{wound losses}_{predicted} + \text{fecal losses}_{predicted}}$$

Water Requirements

In extensively burned patients, the fluid infused during resuscitation typically produces a 15% to 20% increase in body weight and a corresponding increase in total body sodium. The infusion of large volumes of lactated Ringer's solution with a sodium concentration of 130 mEq/L for resuscitation commonly reduces the serum sodium to levels that approach 130 mEq/L at the end of resuscitation, even though total body sodium is greatly increased. Following resuscitation, fluid therapy should be adjusted to permit excretion of the excess sodium and a return to preburn weight by the eighth to tenth postburn day. Furthermore, thermal destruction of the cutaneous barrier to evaporation results in an increase of insensible water loss, the volume of which is a function of burn size. After resuscitation is completed, hypernatremia due to inadequate replacement of those losses is the most common electrolyte abnormality in burn patients. Insensible water loss can be estimated by the following formula

$$\boxed{\text{Insensible water loss (ml/hr)} = (25 + \%\text{burn})\text{BSA}}$$

where BSA equals body surface area in m^2. In addition, resetting the hormonal control mechanisms for plasma tonicity may result in a syndrome of inappropriate secretion of antidiuretic hormone (SIADH). Thus, the serum sodium concentration must be carefully monitored, and water intake must be adjusted accordingly to avoid dangerous hyper- or hyponatremia.

Route, Method, and Timing of Nutrition

Augmentation of oral intake with enteral or parenteral nutrition is commonly required in adult patients with burns in excess of 30% TBSA, as they are unable to consume enough orally to meet their needs. Despite early studies in which parenteral nutrition was used to augment caloric and nitrogen intake maximally, the immunosuppressive effects of parenteral nutrition and the benefits of enteral feeding have led most surgeons to employ the enteral route whenever possible. Some burn centers provide enteral nutrition via gastric tubes, reporting a low incidence of complications therefrom. However, discontinuation of gastric feedings because of gastric ileus or to avoid perioperative aspiration may reduce the caloric supply. For these reasons and to minimize the risk of gastric aspiration, we prefer to place a nasoenteral tube past the pylorus and into the jejunum if possible. Bedside fluoroscopy (C-arm) or endoscopy is employed to facilitate nasoenteral tube placement, as needed. Also, initiation of enteral feeding immediately after the burn is recommended by some; however, net absorption of tube feeds may be sufficiently low that predicted caloric needs are not met for several days. Therefore we initiate enteral feeding at the close of the first 48 hours after the burn, once return of bowel function and resolution of ileus have occurred.

Mechanisms of Postburn Hypermetabolism

The mechanisms responsible for postburn hypermetabolism have been explored. Because patients with extensive burns and those with thyrotoxicosis share an elevated metabolic rate, Cope et al. studied thyroid function in hypermetabolic burn patients. Measurements of protein-bound iodine and ^{131}I uptake were normal. These results were confirmed by later authors, who agreed that hyperthyroidism is not the cause of postburn hypermetabolism.

In the presence of normal thyroid function, Cope et al. suggested that catecholamines might be responsible for postburn hypermetabolism. Indeed, Wilmore et al. found that urinary catecholamine excretion correlated well with the metabolic rate in burn patients. This relationship was curvilinear, such that the metabolic rate did not exceed 2.5 times normal despite further increases in catecholamines. In some patients an increase in metabolic rate due to environmental cooling led to an increase in catecholamine excretion. Other patients (all of whom later died) became hypothermic and exhibited decreased catecholamine production following environmental cooling. β-Blockade with propranolol decreased the metabolic rate in burn patients, whereas α-blockade did not; epinephrine infusion increased it in normal subjects. Thus, catecholamines are important mediators of postinjury hypermetabolism.

Infusion of the three counterregulatory ("stress") hormones—cortisol, glucagon, epinephrine—in normal subjects during a 4-day period reproduced many of the metabolic responses seen following injury, and these hormones appeared to act synergistically. The metabolic changes included increases in minute ventilation, V_{O_2}, V_{CO_2}, metabolic rate, urinary nitrogen excretion, glucose and insulin levels, and endogenous glucose production. Skeletal muscle intracellular glutamine concentrations were lower during stress hormone infusion, whereas free amino acid levels in arterial blood and forearm amino acid efflux were unchanged; thus hormonal changes alone do not reproduce all features of postinjury skeletal muscle proteolysis.

Later work evaluated the role of the pro-inflammatory cytokines in postinjury metabolism. For example, infusion of tumor necrosis factor (TNF) into animals produced changes such as hypotension, decreased skeletal muscle transmembrane potential, increased lactate efflux from the extremities, and increased stress hormone levels in a dose-responsive manner. The proinflammatory cytokines appear to influence the hypothalamic-pituitary-adrenocortical (HPA) axis. Intravenous TNFα stimulated ACTH and corticosterone secretion in a dose-dependent fashion, an effect that was inhibited by a corticotropin-releasing hormone (CRH) antiserum. Antibodies to interleukin-6 (IL-6), TNF, and IL-1 receptor each blocked the production of ACTH following lipopolysaccharide infusion, although at different time points. Several mechanisms have been proposed to explain how the inflammatory cytokines cross, or produce changes on the other side of, the blood-brain barrier. In addition, peripheral inflammation may activate the HPA axis via nociceptive, visceral, or somatosensory afferent neurons.

Following resuscitation, the elevated metabolic rate is associated with a striking elevation in the cardiac output as well, up to a maximum of about 20 L/m. To explain this phenomenon, leg blood flow and leg oxygen consumption were determined in patients with and without extensive leg burns but with equal total burn sizes. Leg oxygen consumption was similarly elevated in both groups, but leg blood flow, glucose uptake, and lactate production were markedly increased in the burned legs. Thus, a systemic signal that controls total body oxygen consumption regulates the metabolic rate of the leg, whereas the local burn wound controls leg blood flow as well as glucose and lactate metabolism. On the other hand, blood flow to the muscles of the limb is relatively unchanged, regardless of the presence or absence of leg burns or the total burn size; thus, the increased leg blood flow following leg burns is primarily directed to the wound itself. Release of the gluconeogenic precursor alanine from the leg—an index of skeletal muscle proteolysis—was increased in burn patients and correlated with total burn size and V_{O_2} but not with leg burn size or leg blood flow. Increased blood flow to the burn wound is associated with abnormal responses to external elevation of the core temperature. Normal subjects and burn patients with unburned legs responded to core temperature elevation by increasing their leg blood flow. Those with burned legs, however, could not augment leg blood flow. This points to abnormal vasomotor control of the burn wound vasculature due to maximal vasodilation or to denervation.

Mechanisms of Postburn Muscle Cachexia

Recently, Hart et al. found that net protein breakdown across the isolated leg correlated with increasing age, weight, time to definitive surgery, and REE. Catabolism also increased with burn size until it plateaued at 40% TBSA. This TBSA plateau is analogous to, but higher than, that observed for REE by Kelemen et al. At the molecular level, the breakdown of myofibrillar proteins (actin and myosin) proceeds as follows: (1) they are released from the myofibrils; (2) they are tagged with a marker protein, ubiquitin; and (3) they enter and are degraded by a barrel-shaped proteolytic particle, the 26S proteasome. Several mediators are known to be elevated in burn patients, especially cortisol, although TNFα and IL-1 have also been implicated in this process. In the case of the cytokines, this effect probably involves the upregulation of ubiquitin genes. Thermal injury also results in the upregulation of ubiquitin-conjugating enzyme ($E2_{14k}$), which may be a rate-limiting enzyme in the process, and in an increased rate of ubiquination of proteins. Thermal injury activates skeletal muscle apoptosis as well.

Anabolic Strategies

Despite careful support of calorie and nitrogen requirements, patients with extensive burns are catabolic throughout the wound-healing phase and beyond and sustain continued erosion of the lean body mass. This phenomenon may have several undesirable consequences, such as impaired wound healing, respiratory muscle weakness, difficulty performing physical and occupational therapy, prolonged hospitalization, and delayed return to work. Several approaches have been taken to prevent such catabolism, including provision of human growth hormone (GH), insulin-like growth factor-I (IGF-I), insulin, and oxandrolone.

Recombinant GH has been reported to decrease donor site healing times and hospital length of stay in burned children. These improvements require a GH dose that is associated with increased levels of IGF-I. GH stimulates hepatocyte production of IGF-I and in this way likely exerts its anabolic effect. IGF-I administration promotes glucose uptake and decreases whole-body protein breakdown in thermally injured patients. Insulin plus 50% glucose reduces donor-site healing time in adults. Initially, large doses of insulin and glucose were used, but more recently lower insulin doses have been given such that exogenous glucose was needed in only half of the patients.

The anabolic steroid oxandrolone combined with a high-protein diet increased the weight-gain rate and decreased the rehabilitation hospital length of stay of patients undergoing postburn rehabilitation. In acutely burned patients, its use was associated with more rapid healing of donor sites, decreased net weight loss, a more positive nitrogen balance, and no change in metabolic rate compared to what was found with a placebo.

Immunonutrition

Following the demonstration of enhanced immune function in burned children receiving high amounts of protein intake by Alexander et al., there has been much interest in developing "immune-enhancing diets" (IEDs). The primary components of commercially available IED formulas are glutamine, arginine, and omega-3 fatty acids. Glutamine is a major precursor for hepatic gluconeogenesis and for the production of glutathione (GSH) and nucleic acids. It fuels rapidly dividing cells in the intestinal mucosa and the immune system. It also fuels fibroblasts and stimulates production of collagen by fibroblasts. Following thermal injury in adults, the net production of glutamine in isolated leg skeletal muscle is decreased, and alanine production is increased. Under these conditions, alanine becomes the major vehicle for interorgan nitrogen transfer, and glutamine becomes a "conditionally essential" amino acid. This relative glutamine scarcity, as well as increased requirements, may impair lymphocyte, macrophage, and neutrophil function as well as gut barrier function and energy charge.

Arginine is another frequent IED component. There is evidence that arginine supplementation improves wound healing by increasing the production of NO by inducible NO synthetase. NO, in turn, may improve wound healing by increasing GH release and by activating fibroblasts. In addition, arginine supplementation may downregulate postburn production of the proinflammatory cytokines as a consequence of NO-induced reduction of mRNA expression. After burn injury in guinea pigs, dietary arginine (given in a dose of 2% of total calories) improved T-cell immune function and the mortality rate. Several other reports have confirmed a beneficial effect on T-cell proliferation, particularly CD3+ and cytotoxic (CD8+) T cells.

Omega-3 fatty acids, particularly α-linolenic acid, are frequent IED components. Unlike omega-6 fatty acids, these fatty acids are not converted by cyclooxygenase into prostaglandins. Because of their location on the cell membrane, fatty acids are in a position to influence a variety of signaling processes, such as those involving protein kinase C. The net effect of the omega-3 fatty acids on immune function includes downregulation of proinflammatory cytokine production, decreased PMN chemotaxis, decreased L-selectin and adhesion molecule expression, and decreased production of NO and superoxide.

Clinical trials of IEDs in critically ill patients and burn patients have yielded mixed results. Thus, despite enticing preclinical studies, the precise role of IEDs in burn patient care remains to be defined.

Immune Function

Thermal injury causes many changes in immune function that may predispose the patient to infection. Because infection is the leading cause of death in patients with thermal injury who are admitted to burn centers, elucidation of a complete picture of these immunologic changes is critical.

Neutrophils

Neutrophils play a central role in the innate immune response (e.g., to bacteria and fungi). Moore et al. described in vivo complement-mediated, systemic activation (i.e., "priming") of neutrophils following burns. They documented increased neutrophil expression of receptors for the complement opsonins C3b and iC3b, which is indicative of neutrophil activation. This increase in expression was monophasic, as seen in a systemic rather than a localized etiology for activation. C5a is a potent activator of such expression, and neutrophils exposed to C5a (zymosan), but not to a synthetic peptide, showed decreased chemotaxis—a selective response typical for neutrophils activated by C5a. Also, plasma levels of C3a were increased, consistent with activation of the complement system. The same group showed that low-dose endotoxin, elevations of which have been described in burn patients soon after injury, is capable of causing such activation as well. (Furthermore, in contrast to some reports, neutrophil function was preserved in these patients, including both phagocytosis and killing of staphylococci.) In addition to C5a and endotoxin, other agents that may prime neutrophils include TNFα, granulocyte/macrophage colony stimulating factor (GM-CSF), PAF, and IL-8. Systemic neutrophil activation is potentially harmful, not only because it may impair chemotaxis but because it may lead to endothelial and end-organ damage.

One feature of postburn neutrophil function is a supranormal oxidative burst. Cioffi et al. documented an increase in cytosolic oxidase activity in both unstimulated and stimulated neutrophils from thermally injured patients. Similarly, Dobke et al. described greater uptake of oxygen by unstimulated neutrophils of burn patients than by the neutrophils of control subjects. On the other hand, stimulation caused an increase of lesser magnitude in burn patient neutrophils than in control neutrophils. This difference may reflect the fact that the latter group used a stimulus that was dependent on cell-surface receptors.

Another feature of postburn neutrophil function is abnormal locomotion. Maderazo et al. correlated increased hydrogen peroxide levels in burn patient neutrophils with evidence of abnormal microtubule assembly (capping with concanavalin A) and attributed the observed defect in neutrophil locomotion to autooxidative damage to microtubules. Hasslen et al. described increased levels of stably polymerized actin in postburn neutrophils, whereas normal motility requires cyclic polymerization and depolymerization of actin. An alternate explanation was provided by Krause et al., who ascribed decreased chemotaxis (in blunt trauma patients) to postinjury release of immature neutrophils into the circulation.

T Lymphocytes

T lymphocytes play a central role in adaptive immunity because of their ability to recognize and respond to antigens presented by monocytes, macrophages, and dendritic and other cells. Examples of burn-induced failure of adaptive immunity include prolonged skin allograft survival, an inhibited delayed-type hypersensitivity reaction, and reduced peripheral blood lymphocyte proliferation in the mixed lymphocyte reaction. Such immunosuppression may be explained by decreases in T-cell number or by alterations in function.

With respect to numeric changes, it is well known that thermal injury is associated with leukocytosis, lymphopenia, and monocytosis, including a decrease in the total number of T cells. Several investigators have found a decrease in the helper/suppressor ($CD4^+/CD8^+$) T-cell ratio after a burn; the decrease in $CD4^+$ is variably seen with or without a lesser decrease in the $CD8^+$ count. This change, when seen later in the patient's course, has been associated with an increased frequency of sepsis and mortality. The finding of a decreased helper/suppressor ratio was later questioned by several groups on the grounds that burn injury produces morphologically abnormal granulocytes and monocytes, which may have been indistinguishable from lymphocytes when assessed by earlier flow cytometric techniques. When such abnormal nonlymphocytes were excluded, Burleson et al. found that the helper/suppressor ratio was preserved following burn in a rat model, decreasing only after induction of a burn wound infection.

The process that leads to decreased T-cell numbers following injury may involve T-cell apoptosis. Increased expression of Fas (CD95) and Fas ligand on peripheral blood mononuclear cells, specifically on macrophages, has been described in a group of critically ill patients with multisystem organ failure. These changes were associated with T-cell lymphopenia and increased mortality. It is proposed that macrophage-derived Fas ligand induces T-cell apoptosis, leading to lymphopenia and anergy. Also, glucocorticoids may cause T-cell apoptosis in burn models. Indeed, infusion of hydrocortisone in normal humans reproduced the T-helper cell/suppressor ratio changes seen in burn patients. Recently, postburn glucocorticoid- and Fas ligand-induced apoptosis of $CD4^-/CD8^+$ T cells and B cells in gut-associated lymphoid tissues was described. In contrast, glucocorticoids, but not Fas ligand, were responsible for postburn apoptosis of lymphocytes in the thymus and spleen.

Functional derangements may also explain T-cell failure after burns. Xu et al. evaluated the ability of purified burn patient T cells to take up tritiated thymidine (a functional assay) in response to three conditions: spontaneously; following mitogen (phytohemagglutinin, or PHA) stimulation; following antigen stimulation. In each case

and analogous to Burleson's findings, the removal of nonlymphocytic cells corrected these measures of T-cell function to normal levels. Zapata-Sirvent and Hansbrough examined the time sequence of antigen expression on the surface of T cells from burn patients. Certain antigens—HLA-DR, IL-2 receptor (CD25), transferrin receptor (CD71)—are associated with T-cell activation. These authors found a decrease in the activation antigens as early as day 1 after the burn, which may be indicative of impaired cell-mediated immunity. Others, however, have described increases in the activation markers CD25, CD69, and CD71. In an effort to arrive at a unifying hypothesis, Deitch et al. proposed that burn injury may cause early, nonspecific activation of the cellular immune system, which in turn may impair later specific T-cell responses to a challenge.

Another cause of T-cell functional failure following burn is decreased production of IL-2. IL-2 is principally a product of T lymphocytes and specifically of $CD4^+$ T-helper cells; activation of T lymphocytes via the T-cell receptor (TCR) causes IL-2 production. IL-2, in turn, stimulates T-cell clonal expansion (blastogenesis) in response to a mitogen and enhances nonspecific (natural killer cell) and specific T-cell cytotoxicity. Wood et al. and others found that IL-2 production by burn patient lymphocytes in response to a mitogen was decreased, with further decreases during sepsis. As expected, blastogenesis was concomitantly decreased and correlated with the IL-2 levels. IL-1 stimulates IL-2 release from T cells, but these decreases in IL-2 production were associated with increased IL-1 levels. In burned mice, maximal impairment of IL-2 production preceded maximal impairment of the T-cell response to a mitogen and maximal mortality after cecal ligation and puncture; mortality rates were correlated with rates of suppression of IL-2 production and the mitogen response. Replacement with recombinant IL-2 (rIL-2) restored the T-cell response to mitogens and improved survival in this model.

Changes in IL-2 receptor (IL-2R, CD25) production also occur after burns. IL-2R is a product of a gene activated by IL-2. Teodorczyk-Injeyan et al. found that mitogen-induced expression of IL-2R on peripheral blood mononuclear cells (PBMCs) of burn patients was decreased. Recombinant IL-2 served to upregulate IL-2R expression, but these receptors appeared to be low-affinity, nonfunctional receptors.

An important mediator of T-cell immunosuppression after a burn is prostaglandin E_2 (PGE_2). PGE_2 inhibits T-cell function in vitro, including IL-2 production and consequently T-cell activation. Postburn inhibition of PGE_2 production by indomethacin improves IL-2 production by splenocytes and improves the mitogen responsiveness of peripheral blood mononuclear cells.

Two functionally distinct types of $CD4^+$ T-helper cells, Th1 and Th2, have been described in terms not of their cell-surface markers but of the cytokines they produce. Th1 cells produce cytokines such as IL-2, TNFβ, and interferon-γ (IFNγ). Th2 cells produce cytokines such as IL-4, IL-5, IL-6, and IL-10. Broadly speaking, selective activation of Th1 cells enhances cell-mediated immunity, whereas selective activation of Th2 cells enhances humoral immunity. A shift in the helper-cell phenotype from Th1 to Th2 has been observed following injury. One effect of this shift is a decrease in total T-cell numbers because of decreased IL-2 production.

Several mediators have been implicated in this shift in phenotype from Th1 to Th2. For example, PGE_2 and IL-4 induce the Th2 phenotype. Burn injury decreases production of IL-12 by macrophages, whereas IL-12 induces the Th1 phenotype. Th2-derived IL-10 decreases Th1 cytokine production, as do burn-associated mediators such as norepinephrine and glucocorticoids. IL-12 production in burned mice was inhibited by Th2-derived cytokines (in particular, IL-4). It has been proposed that the shift from Th1 to Th2 phenotype may reflect a "compensatory anti-inflammatory response syndrome" (CARS), which occurs following the initial systemic inflammatory process unleashed by the burn.

The clinical relevance of the Th1/Th2 paradigm has been explored. IL-10 is a product of Th2 cells and inhibits Th1 function. Stimulated T cells from burn and trauma patients produced more IL-10 than did the T cells from normal subjects, indicating a shift in these patients to the Th2 phenotype. The same shift was seen in burned mice. In patients, increased IL-10 production was associated with infection. In burned mice, anti-IL-10 antibody improved survival after cecal ligation and puncture.

In contrast, IL-12 induces the Th1 phenotype; production of IL-12 by PBMCs is reduced following injury. IL-12 replacement in the mouse burn model increased survival following cecal ligation and puncture.

Monocytes and Macrophages

Monocytes and dendritic cells, considered part of the innate immune system, also play a critical role in adaptive immunity by presenting foreign antigens to T lymphocytes in the context of expressed major histocompatability complex (MHC) class II (HLA-DR) antigens. Burns have been associated with various abnormalities in monocyte/macrophage function, including reduced phagocytic capacity, decreased presentation of antigens to T lymphocytes, and increased cytokine production. Thus, impaired monocyte/macrophage function may result in impaired T-cell function. Several groups have now described decreased expression of HLA-DR antigens on the blood monocytes of burn patients, particularly in association with infection or mortality.

B Lymphocytes

Plasma levels of immunoglobulin (Ig), particularly IgG, have been noted to decrease following thermal injury in humans. Decreased in vivo levels may arise from decreased production, increased losses across the burn wound or into the interstitium, increased consumption, and/or burn excision with associated blood loss and transfusion. Thus, subsequent studies have focused on the function of the antibody-producing B lymphocytes. The results of these in vitro studies have been quite variable with respect to IgG and IgM production, regardless of whether it is spontaneous or in response to stimulation. The question is further complicated by the fact that B cells are dependent on T-cell help; thus, changes in cellular immunity influence humoral immunity as well.

Schlüter et al. documented impairment of B-cell activation, proliferation, and differentiation in burn patients. B-cell numbers were unchanged. In contrast, B-cell proliferation in response to *Staphylococcus aureus* strain Cowan I (SAC) was suppressed during weeks 2 to 4 after the burn. The same was true of IgM synthesis in response to pokeweed mitogen or SAC. Diminished IgG production was seen throughout the postburn course. IL-4-induced B-cell activation, measured by CD23 levels, was decreased during weeks 2 to 5. sCD23, a B-cell growth and differentiation marker, was also reduced. This is in contrast to the findings of Schlüter et al. with respect to T cells, mentioned above, which showed increased activation (CD25 levels) but decreased responsiveness to mitogens.

Meyer et al. studied B-cell function in mice following thermal injury. In their model, there was no change in the number of IgG- and IgA-producing B cells at day 5 after a burn and an increase in the number of IgM-producing cells. On the other hand, LPS-induced IgG and IgA production by 10^5 lymphocytes was increased, and IgM production was decreased. In subsequent studies, specific IgM production against the bacterial cell-wall antigen peptidoglycan polysaccharide was increased on postburn day 1 but had decreased by postburn day 8. PGE_2 suppressed, and indomethacin restored, most of these B-cell functions. An exception was IgG synthesis, which was increased by PGE_2 and reduced by indomethacin. Likewise, PGE_2 promoted IL-4-induced IgE and IgG_1 synthesis by B lymphocytes in another study.

Transforming growth factor-β (TGFβ), a cytokine whose levels increase following thermal injury, decreases T- and B-cell proliferation. In one study, addition of TGFβ to splenocytes harvested 8 days after a burn led to decreased IgG and IgM production, decreased B-cell number, and decreased IgM-secreting cells. In contrast, the total amount of IgM produced per IgM-specific cell was increased; hence, this cytokine appears to act by limiting proliferation, not individual cell function.

Infection

Improvements in the care of burn patients—including fluid resuscitation, stress ulcer prophylaxis, and nutritional support—have only highlighted the role of infection as the leading cause of death in burn patients. At the same time, advances in burn wound care have largely overcome the problem of invasive gram-negative burn wound infection, such that the location and microbiology of lethal postburn complications have shifted.

Invasive Bacterial Burn Wound Infection

The conquest of invasive gram-negative burn wound infection is an example of successful integration of clinical and laboratory research. Prior to the introduction of topical mafenide acetate (Sulfamylon) cream in 1964, invasive bacterial infection was the leading cause of death in burn patients. The burn wound, a rich pabulum of devascularized tissue extensively exposed to the environment, provides an ideal medium for the growth of pathogens. Multiple characteristics, including a motile flagellum and the production of toxins, hemolysins, and proteolytic enzymes, made *Pseudomonas* the most common invasive pathogen.

To address this problem, referred to as "burn wound sepsis," a model of invasive *Pseudomonas* burn wound infection was developed. Anesthetized rats underwent a 20% TBSA full-thickness scald injury. This injury is uniformly survivable in the absence of microbial inoculation, but inoculation with 10^8 colony-forming units (CFU) of certain strains of *Pseudomonas* made the injury highly lethal and reproduced the typical trajectory of clinical burn wound infection. Several hours after inoculation, microorganisms proliferated within the devascularized eschar and penetrated the surface, tracking along hair follicles. Bacterial counts built up at the viable–nonviable tissue interface and then invaded viable tissue, causing secondary necrosis of granulation tissue and underlying uninjured tissue. Such invasion was accompanied by bacteremia and visceral (spleen, liver, kidney, lung) infection as well. In contrast, it was possible to seed the burn wound hematogenously with intravenously injected *Pseudomonas* at appropriate bacteremic doses in only a small number of cases. Thus, the proliferation of gram-negative microorganisms in the burn wound was established as the inciting event of invasive burn wound sepsis.

This concept supported the testing of topical antibacterial agents. Mafenide, a drug used previously to prevent gas gangrene in war wounds, was shown to convert a uniformly lethal burn wound infection into a uniformly survivable one if it was applied to the experimental wound within 24 hours of seeding. Topical mafenide was soon thereafter introduced to the clinic, with an immediate and remarkable impact on mortality. Comparing conventional exposure therapy (1962–1963) with mafenide topical therapy (1964–1966), Pruitt et al. reported a decrease in all-cause mortality from 38% to 20%, a decrease in the incidence of burn wound sepsis from 22% of patients to 2%, and a decrease in burn wound sepsis-induced death as a percentage of total deaths from 59% to 10%. The decrement in all-cause mortality was, as one might expect, greatest in the midrange burn size (30% to 60% TBSA burned).

Mafenide is structurally related to the sulfonamide class of antibiotics, but its mechanism of action is distinct. Mafenide has an unequaled record of efficacy against *Pseudomonas*. None of the 8500 strains analyzed over a 25-year period (1967–1992) at the U.S. Army Burn Center were resistant to mafenide at concentrations employed topically (A.T. McManus, unpublished data). Similarly, in a 10-year review of *Staphylococcus aureus* and *Pseudomonas* sensitivity to various topical agents, no other agent—including povidone-iodine, silver sulfadiazine, gentamicin, nitrofurazine, silver nitrate, and hydrogen peroxide—demonstrated superior efficacy against these organisms.

Mafenide concentrations in the burn wound decline to subinhibitory concentrations within about 10 hours, mandating application at least twice daily. Following systemic absorption, mafenide, which has a 10- to 15-minute half-life, is rapidly converted to a nonbacteriostatic metabolite. Both compounds are carbonic anhydrase inhibitors, so the twice-daily use of mafenide may be associated with metabolic acidosis, particularly in patients with extensive partial-thickness burns, decreased glomerular filtration rate (it is cleared renally), and impaired ventilation. The ability of mafenide to penetrate avascular tissue makes it useful not only for treatment of full-thickness burn wounds and infected burn wounds but also for preventing suppurative chondritis of burned ears.

The other major approach to preventing invasive burn wound infection is the use of various formulations of silver, an element with a long history as an antimicrobial. The "oligodynamic" action of silver includes bacterial cell wall disruption, disruption of key bacterial enzymes such as cytochromes, and interaction with nucleic acids.

Moyer et al. introduced silver nitrate ($AgNO_3$) into burn care in 1965. A 0.5% solution of $AgNO_3$ (29.4 mEq/L) was shown to be an effective topical antimicrobial, without epidermal toxicity. By contrast, a 1.0% solution was tissue-toxic, and a 0.1% solution lacked antibacterial activity. This fact underscores the importance of the dressing technique when $AgNO_3$ is used. Moyer et al. described thick dressings that employ six to eight layers of four-ply gauze. The dressings are kept "continuously wet" with $AgNO_3$ solution by reapplication every 3 to 4 hours and are changed at least once (preferably twice) daily. Evaporative water loss causes an increase in $AgNO_3$ concentration in the dressing, so the concentration may reach tissue-toxic levels. Another complication of $AgNO_3$ therapy is loss of sodium, chloride, potassium, and other ions, which follow the concentration gradient from the body into the hypotonic soak solution. Frequent electrolyte determinations are therefore necessary. Finally, and in contrast to mafenide, the precipitation of silver salts that occurs upon contact with burn wound chloride ions and proteins limits the efficacy of $AgNO_3$ to surface contamination only; it has no efficacy against established infection.

Silver sulfadiazine is a water-insoluble compound that forms when $AgNO_3$ reacts with sulfadiazine, a topical antibiotic that suffers from a significant resistance pattern. Silver sulfadiazine is devoid of the side effects seen with $AgNO_3$. Studies employing radioactive silver salts and radioactive sulfa compounds demonstrated that Ag^+, but not sulfadiazine, enters the bacterial cell wall and combines with bacterial DNA. Furthermore, silver sulfadiazine dissociates at a moderate rate, in essence serving as a slow-release formulation of Ag^+. A possible consequence of silver sulfadiazine use is selection of bacteria capable of transferring plasmids that confer resistance, not only to sulfonamides but also to clinically important antibiotics such as aminoglycosides. Unlike mafenide, penetration by silver sulfadiazine cream into eschar is limited, which may explain the observed discrepancies between in vitro and in vivo efficacy. Moreover, silver sulfadiazine use is occasionally associated with a decrease in the white blood cell and granulocyte counts, a phenomenon attributed to toxicity to bone marrow granulocyte/macrophage progenitor cells. This effect rarely requires cessation of silver sulfadiazine therapy; the problem usually resolves despite continued use.

A recent addition to the burn wound armamentarium is a dressing coated with elemental silver. Silver nylon cloth (Swift Textile Metalizing Corp., Hartford, CT, USA; Argentum Medical, Lakemont, GA, USA) effectively prevented invasive burn wound infection in a rat model. Its therapeutic efficacy was enhanced by applying weak direct current to the silver cloth, with the cloth acting as an anode; this serves to liberate Ag^+ from the cloth. Acticoat (Westaim Biomedical, Fort Saskatchewan, Alberta, Canada) is another silver-impregnated dressing. A binary alloy of silver (97%) and oxygen is sputtered onto a polyethylene mesh. Water is applied approximately every 6 hours, and the dressing is changed once every 48 to 72 hours. This dressing provides continuous release of Ag^+ and may also release complexes of non-ionic Ag as well (R. Burrell, personal communication). In a clinical study, Acticoat compared with $AgNO_3$ resulted in a decreased incidence of infection (defined as $> 10^5$ organisms per gram of tissue from burn wound biopsy specimens).

Fungal Burn Wound Infection

With the control of invasive gram-negative burn wound infection, invasive fungal infection has attained greater prominence. Comparing the eras before (1960–1963) and after (1964–1969) the introduction of mafenide, there was an increase in fungal burn wound infection on postmortem examination of burn wounds at our institution, from about 8% to about 30%. This suggested that elimination of bacterial burn wound infection may have enabled the emergence of opportunistic fungal infection. Creation of an isolation ward in 1983 (see Infection Control, below) was associated with a further decrease in bacterial, but not fungal, burn wound infections. Of 141 patients with fungal burn wound infections, 21 died of disseminated disease; the most commonly involved organs were lungs, heart, kidneys, and brain. Improved survival among patients with invasive infection by true fungi (but not by *Candida*) was noted following institution of a more aggressive approach to surgical excision of infected wounds in 1978. The incidence of invasive fungal burn wound infection has decreased from 44 cases for the 7-year period 1982–1989 to 24 cases for the 7-year period 1989–1995.

Candida sp. comprise the most common colonizers of the burn wound, but they rarely cause invasive infection; in fact, such invasion may indicate the collapse of host defenses and is often a preterminal event. By contrast, the filamentous or true fungi are more aggressive invaders of the subcutaneous tissues. These organisms can be broadly classified by their morphologic appearance on wound biopsy specimens. *Aspergillus* and *Fusarium* are currently the most common fungal organisms causing invasive wound infection at our institution; they feature long, filamentous hyphae that branch at 45-degree angles. In contrast, the Phycomycetes (primarily *Mucor*, *Absidia*, and *Rhizopus*) feature broad, nonseptate hyphae that branch widely. The Phycomycetes invade rapidly and frequently spread along and cross fascial planes. Thus, it is not surprising that amputation was required in 26 of 63 patients who required surgery for burn wound infections caused by these organisms.

Diagnosis and Treatment of Burn Wound Infection

Regardless of the causative organism, burn wound infection is best diagnosed by histopathologic examination of biopsy specimens. Quantitative cultures of wound biopsies are sensitive but not specific for infection: A low quantitative culture count is a reliable indicator that infection is not present, but a high count correlates poorly with infection. In other words, cultures cannot distinguish between true infection and heavy colonization, whereas the natural history and treatment of these entities are divergent. In addition, culture results are obtained slowly, but a rapid section technique for biopsy histopathology can be performed in as little as 4 hours.

Patients with known or suspected burn wound infection require aggressive care in an ICU. Gram-negative infections are treated with twice-daily application of mafenide acetate cream, institution of two broad-spectrum antipseudomonal intravenous antibiotics, and subeschar injection (clysis) of one half the daily dose of an antipseudomonal broad-spectrum penicillin (e.g., piperacillin) diluted in a volume appropriate for the size of the involved wound. Clysis is repeated 8 to 12 hours later, and the wound is then primarily excised to fascia. Eradication of gram-negative infection in 10 of 19 patients treated by clysis and excision was described.

In the rat burn wound infection model, subeschar clysis with antipseudomonal penicillins improved survival, even at doses that were ineffective if given systemically. Other antibiotics tested were not therapeutic.

Fungal burn wound infections are treated with intravenous amphotericin B (preferably the liposomal form) and wide excision without use of subeschar clysis. The utility of the newer triazole antifungal agents such as itraconazole and voriconazole is not yet known.

Other Infections

The declining incidence of burn wound infection has heightened the importance of other infections, especially pneumonia and bacteremia, in burn patients. Shirani et al. determined for the period 1980–1984 that pneumonia and inhalation injury each independently increased mortality over that predicted by age and burn size alone; this effect was maximal at the midrange of age and burn size. Postinhalation injury pneumonia typically develops beginning 5 to 6 days after the burn, whereas pneumonia in patients without inhalation injury presents somewhat later in the hospital course. Kaplan-Meier analysis of the risk of pneumonia in intubated burn patients showed that this risk was negligible during the first week of intubation; the incremental risk thereafter was constant; and there was no difference in risk between those with or without inhalation injury. Bacteremia in burn patients may be particularly common during burn wound manipulation, including dressing changes and excisions.

In 1979 there was a 21% incidence of bacteremia during burn wound manipulation. The incidence was 40% during tangential excision; but these episodes were not associated, per se, with evidence of direct harm to the patients. In a later study there was a decrease in bacteremia, which may reflect advances in wound care, patient isolation, and other factors. Bacteremia was seen only in patients with burns of more than 40% TBSA, and it was less common during the first 10 postburn days than thereafter.

The diagnosis of suppurative thrombophlebitis should be considered in burn patients with sepsis of unclear etiology, particularly in those with evidence of hematogenous pneumonia. Local signs of infection are frequently absent, so all previously cannulated veins should be carefully examined. The presence of pus in the vein and a positive culture from the pus or vein lumen confirms the diagnosis. At the U.S. Army Burn Center the incidence of suppurative thrombophlebitis has greatly decreased in association with a strict policy of changing the sites of all intravenous cannulas every 3 days.

Infection Control

In addition to effective topical antimicrobial therapy, other factors have contributed to the reduction in infection-related mortality in burn patients. Redesign of the U.S. Army Burn Center in 1983 to permit isolation of patients with extensive wounds and an increased emphasis on hygiene was associated with reduced mortality and a lower incidence of bacteremia; moreover, endemic strains of multidrug-resistant *Providencia* and *Pseudomonas* were eliminated. Furthermore, the increased mortality previously associated with bacteremia in the open ward was not observed following conversion to an isolation ward. This environmental change was also associated with a striking reduction in the incidence of bacterial burn wound infection, whereas the incidence of fungal burn wound infection remained constant. As noted above, the incidence of fungal burn wound infection subsequently decreased during the 1990s.

Our current approach to infection control and surveillance is as follows. Mafenide acetate cream is applied to the burn wound in the morning and silver sulfadiazine cream in the evening; the advantages of each agent are thereby realized and the side effects minimized. Thrice-weekly cultures of wounds, sputum, urine, and stool are obtained. These surveillance cultures are used in part as a quality-control tool in the ICU to ensure that patient isolation is maintained and to identify cross-contamination with resistant organisms promptly if it is not. Furthermore, when infection is diagnosed, antibiotics are selected based on existing surveillance data.

The antibiotic choice is refined based on the results of cultures of material obtained at the time the infection is diagnosed. Most frequently, vancomycin is used for *Staphylococcus aureus* infections, whereas gram-negative infections are treated with a broad-spectrum antipseudomonal penicillin or amikacin. Pseudomonal or mixed gram-negative infections are usually treated with a combination of these gram-negative agents. Quinolones are occasionally used for uncomplicated urinary tract infections. Cephalosporins are not commonly used, as they may select for β-lactamase-positive gram-negative organisms (as well as for methicillin-resistant *Staphylococcus aureus* and vancomycin-resistant *Enterococcus*). Rather, cephalosporins and carbepenems are held in reserve in case multidrug-resistant organisms require treatment. Prophylactic antibiotics are not used, except perioperatively. Perioperative antibiotics include vancomycin and amikacin: one dose of each immediately before the procedure.

The surgical treatment of the wound may also affect the incidence of infection and the survival of burn patients. The traditional method, in which wounds were grafted once eschar separation occurred and granulation tissue formed, gave way during the early 1980s to tangential excision of deep partial-thickness burns and excision to fascia of extensive full-thickness burns. In some patient groups, the mortality rate has improved for those who undergo burn wound excision within the first 72 hours after injury.

In the absence of sufficient donor sites from which to obtain autologous skin grafts, biologic dressings such as cadaver allograft may be used to close the excised wound temporarily. Such dressings reestablish skin barrier function; in particular, they prevent desiccation-induced necrosis of the wound surface and prevent contamination of underlying tissue with exogenous bacteria. In areas of allograft adherence, wound bacteria counts decrease. Effective closure of a portion of the wound has also been reported to be associated with improved immune function. However, if allograft is placed over nonviable tissue, subgraft suppuration occurs and the grafts do not adhere. Every biologic dressing must be inspected on a daily basis. If suppuration occurs underneath the grafts, they should be removed and replaced as frequently as necessary until suppuration ceases and the biologic dressing becomes adherent. Synthetic skin substitutes, which are more likely to develop submembrane suppuration than are naturally occurring biologic dressings, can be safely applied at the time of burn wound excision but should not be applied to wounds with retained nonviable tissue.

Conclusions

Programs of integrated clinical and laboratory research conducted at burn centers have expanded our understanding of the pathophysiology of burn injury and have provided the rationale for unprecedented improvements in burn care. Resuscitation regimens designed to address the blood volume, cardiac, and microvascular responses to injury have essentially eliminated burn shock and early postburn organ failure. Similarly, the development of reliable diagnostic modalities and the use of new ventilator technology have tamed inhalation injury. On the basis of studies that have described the neurohormonal responses to burn injury, metabolic and nutritional support regimens have been developed that preserve lean body mass and accelerate convalescence. Additionally, knowledge of the immunologic changes that occur after burn injury has been applied to improve the diagnosis and treatment of life- and limb-threatening infections in burn patients. In the aggregate, these improvements in care have reduced burn patient morbidity and have increased their survival,

such that the extent of burn (43%) associated with 50% mortality in a 21-year-old at the midpoint of the twentieth century has almost doubled to 82% today. The scientific approach to burn research at centers with closely integrated laboratory and clinical programs ensure the success of future studies that will produce even greater improvements in burn patient outcomes.

Bibliography

Adams HR, Baxter CR, Izenberg SD: Decreased contractility and compliance of the left ventricle as complications of thermal trauma. Am Heart J 1984;108:1477–1487.

Agostini JC, Ramirez RG, Albert SN, et al: Successful reversal of lethal carbon monoxide intoxication by total body asanguineous hypothermic perfusion. Surgery 1974;75:213–219.

Alexander JW: Immunonutrition: the role of omega-3 fatty acids. Nutrition 1998;14:627–633.

Alexander JW, MacMillan BG, Stinnett JD, et al: Beneficial effects of aggressive protein feeding in severely burned children. Ann Surg 1980;192:505–517.

Arturson G: Microvascular permeability to macromolecules in thermal injury. Acta Physiol Scand Suppl 1979;463:111–122.

Aukland K, Reed RK: Interstitial-lymphatic mechanisms in the control of extracellular fluid volume. Physiol Rev 1993;73:1–78.

Aulick LH, Wilmore DW: Increased peripheral amino acid release following burn injury. Surgery 1979;85:560–565.

Aulick LH, Wilmore DW, Mason AD Jr, Pruitt BA Jr: Depressed reflex vasomotor control of the burn wound. Cardiovasc Res 1982;16:113–119.

Aulick LH, Wilmore DW, Mason AD Jr, Pruitt BA Jr: Influence of the burn wound on peripheral circulation in thermally injured patients. Am J Physiol 1977;233:H520–H526.

Aulick LH, Wilmore DW, Mason AD Jr, Pruitt BA Jr: Muscle blood flow following thermal injury. Ann Surg 1978;188:778–782.

Badley AD, McElhinny JA, Leibson PJ, et al: Upregulation of Fas ligand expression by human immunodeficiency virus in human macrophages mediates apoptosis of uninfected T lymphocytes. J Virol 1996;70:199–206.

Barillo DJ, Goode R, Esch V: Cyanide poisoning in victims of fire: analysis of 364 cases and review of the literature. J Burn Care Rehabil 1994;15:46–57.

Basadre JO, Sugi K, Traber DL, et al: The effect of leukocyte depletion on smoke inhalation injury in sheep. Surgery 1988;104:208–215.

Barrow RE, Ramirez RJ, Zhang XJ: Ibuprofen modulates tissue perfusion in partial-thickness burns. Burns 2000;26:341–346.

Baud FJ, Barriot P, Toffis V, et al: Elevated blood cyanide concentrations in victims of smoke inhalation. N Engl J Med 1991;325:1761–1766.

Baxter CR: Fluid volume and electrolyte changes of the early postburn period. Clin Plast Surg 1974;1:693–709.

Becker WK, Cioffi WG Jr, McManus AT, et al: Fungal burn wound infection: a 10-year experience. Arch Surg 1991;126:44–48.

Bernardini R, Kamilaris TC, Calogero AE, et al: Interactions between tumor necrosis factor-alpha, hypothalamic corticotropin-releasing hormone, and adrenocorticotropin secretion in the rat. Endocrinology 1990;126:2876–2881.

Bessey PQ, Watters JM, Aoki TT, Wilmore DW: Combined hormonal infusion simulates the metabolic response to injury. Ann Surg 1984;200:264–281.

Bidani A, Wang CZ, Heming TA: Early effects of smoke inhalation on alveolar macrophage functions. Burns 1996;22:101–106.

Biolo G, Fleming RY, Maggi SP, et al: Inhibition of muscle glutamine formation in hypercatabolic patients. Clin Sci 2000;99:189–194.

Brown SD, Piantadosi CA: In vivo binding of carbon monoxide to cytochrome c oxidase in rat brain. J Appl Physiol 1990;68:604–610.

Brown SD, Piantadosi CA: Recovery of energy metabolism in rat brain after carbon monoxide hypoxia. J Clin Invest 1992;89:666–672.

Bunn F, Roberts II, Tasker R, Akpa E: Hypertonic versus isotonic crystalloid for fluid resuscitation in critically ill patients (Cochrane review). *In* Cochrane Database of Systematic Reviews [computer file] 2000;4.

Burleson DG, Vaughn GK, Mason AD Jr, Pruitt BA Jr: Flow cytometric measurement of rat lymphocyte subpopulations after burn injury and burn injury with infection. Arch Surg 1987;122:216–220.

Calvano SE, Albert JD, Legaspi A, et al: Comparison of numerical and phenotypic leukocyte changes during constant hydrocortisone infusion in normal humans with those in thermally injured patients. Surg Gynecol Obstet 1987;164:509–520.

Calvano SE, Barber AE, Hawes AS, et al: Effect of combined cortisol-endotoxin administration on peripheral blood leukocyte counts and phenotype in normal humans. Arch Surg 1992;127:181–186.

Carlson DE, Cioffi WG Jr, Mason AD Jr, et al: Resting energy expenditure in patients with thermal injuries. Surg Gynecol Obstet 1992;174:270–276.

Casley-Smith JR, Window J: Quantitative morphological correlations of alterations in capillary permeability, following histamine and moderate burning, in the mouse diaphragm; and the effects of benzopyrones. Microvasc Res 1976;11:279–305.

Chouaib S, Fradelizi D: The mechanism of inhibition of human IL-2 production. J Immunol 1982;129:2463–2468.

Chrousos GP: The hypothalamic-pituitary-adrenal axis and immune-mediated inflammation. N Engl J Med 1995;332:1351–1362.

Chu CS, McManus AT, Pruitt BA Jr, Mason AD Jr: Therapeutic effects of silver nylon dressings with weak direct current on Pseudomonas aeruginosa-infected burn wounds. J Trauma 1988;28:1488–1492.

Cioffi WG, deLemos RA, Coalson JJ, et al: Decreased pulmonary damage in primates with inhalation injury treated with high-frequency ventilation. Ann Surg 1993;218:328–337.

Cioffi WG, DeMeules JE, Gamelli RL: The effects of burn injury and fluid resuscitation on cardiac function in vitro. J Trauma 1986;26:638–642.

Cioffi WG, Gore DC, Rue LW III, et al: Insulin-like growth factor-1 lowers protein oxidation in patients with thermal injury. Ann Surg 1994;220:310–319.

Cioffi WG Jr, Burleson DG, Jordan BS, et al: Granulocyte oxidative activity after thermal injury. Surgery 1992;112:860–865.

Cioffi WG Jr, Rue LW III, Graves TA, et al: Prophylactic use of high-frequency percussive ventilation in patients with inhalation injury. Ann Surg 1991;213:575–582.

Clark WR, Bonaventura M, Myers W: Smoke inhalation and airway management at a regional burn unit: 1974–1983. Part I. Diagnosis and consequences of smoke inhalation. J Burn Care Rehabil 1989;10:52–62.

Clark WR, Bonaventura M, Myers W, Kellman R: Smoke inhalation and airway management at a regional burn unit: 1974 to 1983. II. Airway management. J Burn Care Rehabil 1990;11:121–134.

Coburn RF: The carbon monoxide body stores. Ann NY Acad Sci 1970;174:11–22.

Coburn RF, Mayers LB: Myoglobin O_2 tension determined from measurement of carboxymyoglobin in skeletal muscle. Am J Physiol 1971;220:66–74.

Coburn RF, Ploegmakers F, Gondrie P, Abboud R: Myocardial myoglobin oxygen tension. Am J Physiol 1973;224:870–876.

Cope O, Nardi GL, Quijano M, et al: Metabolic rate and thyroid function following acute thermal trauma in man. Ann Surg 1953;137:165–174.

Cui XL, Iwasa M, Iwasa Y, Ogoshi S: Arginine-supplemented diet decreases expression of inflammatory cytokines and improves survival in burned rats. JPEN J Parenter Enteral Nutr 2000;24:89–96.

Czaja AJ, McAlhany JC, Pruitt BA Jr: Acute gastroduodenal disease after thermal injury: an endoscopic evaluation of incidence and natural history. N Engl J Med 1974;291:925–929.

Davies JW: Toxic chemicals versus lung tissue—an aspect of inhalation injury revisited: the Everett Idris Evans memorial lecture—1986. J Burn Care Rehabil 1986;7:213–222.

Davis CF, Moore FD, Rodrick ML, et al: Neutrophil activation after burn injury: contributions of the classic complement pathway and of endotoxin. Surgery 1987;102:477–484.

Deitch EA, Landry KN, McDonald JC: Postburn impaired cell-mediated immunity may not be due to lazy lymphocytes but to overwork. Ann Surg 1985;201:793–802.

Demling R, Ikegami K, LaLonde C: Increased lipid peroxidation and decreased antioxidant activity correspond with death after smoke exposure in the rat. J Burn Care Rehabil 1995;16:104–110.

Demling R, LaLonde C, Ikegami K: Fluid resuscitation with deferoxamine hetastarch complex attenuates the lung and systemic response to smoke inhalation. Surgery 1996;119:340–348.

Demling RH: Enteral glutamine administration prevents the decrease in cell energy charge potential produced in ileum after a skin burn in the rat. J Burn Care Rehabil 2000;21:275–279.

Demling RH, Orgill DP: The anticatabolic and wound healing effects of the testosterone analog oxandrolone after severe burn injury. J Crit Care 2000;15:12–17.

Demling RH, DeSanti L: Oxandrolone, an anabolic steroid, significantly increases the rate of weight gain in the recovery phase after major burns. J Trauma 1997;43:47–51.

Demling RH, Knox J, Youn YK, LaLonde C: Oxygen consumption early postburn becomes oxygen delivery dependent with the addition of smoke inhalation injury. J Trauma 1992;32:593–599.

Demling RH, Kramer G, Harms B: Role of thermal injury-induced hypoproteinemia on fluid flux and protein permeability in burned and nonburned tissue. Surgery 1984;95:136–144.

Desai MH, Mlcak R, Richardson J, et al: Reduction in mortality in pediatric patients with inhalation injury with aerosolized heparin/N-acetylcystine therapy. J Burn Care Rehabil 1998;19:210–212.

DiVincenti FC, Pruitt BA Jr, Reckler JM: Inhalation injuries. J Trauma 1971;11:109–117.

Dobke MK, Deitch EA, Harnar TJ, Baxter CR: Oxidative activity of polymorphonuclear leukocytes after thermal injury. Arch Surg 1989;124:856–859.

Eagon RG, McManus AT: The effect of mafenide on dihydropteroate synthase. J Antimicrob Chemother 1990;25:25–29.

Eaves-Pyles T, Alexander JW: Comparison of translocation of different types of microorganisms from the intestinal tract of burned mice. Shock 2001;16:148–152.

Elgjo GI, Mathew BP, Poli de Figueriedo LF, et al: Resuscitation with hypertonic saline dextran improves cardiac function in vivo and ex vivo after burn injury in sheep. Shock 1998;9:375–383.

Elgjo GI, Poli de Figueiredo LF, Schenarts PJ, et al: Hypertonic saline dextran produces early (8–12 hrs) fluid sparing in burn resuscitation: a 24-hr prospective, double-blind study in sheep. Crit Care Med 2000;28:163–171.

Elgjo GI, Traber DL, Hawkins HK, Kramer GC: Burn resuscitation with two doses of 4 mL/kg hypertonic saline dextran provides sustained fluid sparing: a 48-hour prospective study in conscious sheep. J Trauma 2000;49:251–265.

Engrav LH, Colescott PL, Kemalyan N, et al: A biopsy of the use of the Baxter formula to resuscitate burns or do we do it like Charlie did it? J Burn Care Rehabil 2000;21:91–95.

Ernst A, Zibrak JD: Carbon monoxide poisoning. N Engl J Med 1998;339:1603–1608.

Evans IE, Purnell OJ, Robinett PW, et al: Fluid and electrolyte requirements in severe burns. Ann Surg 1952;135:804–817.

Faist E, Kupper TS, Baker CC, et al: Depression of cellular immunity after major injury: its association with posttraumatic complications and its reversal with immunomodulation. Arch Surg 1986;121:1000–1005.

Faist E, Mewes A, Baker CC, et al: Prostaglandin E_2 (PGE_2)-dependent suppression of interleukin alpha (IL-2) production in patients with major trauma. J Trauma 1987;27:837–848.

Fang CH, Sun X, Li BG, et al: Burn injuries in rats upregulate the gene expression of the ubiquitin-conjugating enzyme $E2_{14k}$ in skeletal muscle. J Burn Care Rehabil 2000;21:528–534.

Ferrando AA, Chinkes DL, Wolf SE, et al: A submaximal dose of insulin promotes net skeletal muscle protein synthesis in patients with severe burns. Ann Surg 1999;229:11–18.

Fitzpatrick JC, Jordan BS, Salman N, et al: The use of perfluorocarbon-associated gas exchange to improve ventilation and decrease mortality after inhalation injury in a neonatal swine model. J Pediatr Surg 1997;32:192–196.

Fukuda T, Kim DK, Chin MR, et al: Increased group IV cytosolic phospholipase A2 activity in lungs of sheep after smoke inhalation injury. Am J Physiol 1999;277:L533–L542.

Fukuzuka K, Edwards CK III, Clare-Salzer M, et al: Glucocorticoid and Fas ligand induced mucosal lymphocyte apoptosis after burn injury. J Trauma 2000;49:710–716.

Fukuzuka K, Edwards CK III, Clare-Salzler M, et al: Glucocorticoid-induced, caspase-dependent organ apoptosis early after burn injury. Am J Physiol 2000;278:R1005–R1018.

Gamelli RL, Paxton TP, O'Reilly M: Bone marrow toxicity by silver sulfadiazine. Surg Gynecol Obstet 1993;177:115–120.

Gilpin DA, Barrow RE, Rutan RL, et al: Recombinant human growth hormone accelerates wound healing in children with large cutaneous burns. Ann Surg 1994;220:19–24.

Goebel A, Kavanagh E, Lyons A, et al: Injury induces deficient interleukin-12 production, but interleukin-12 therapy after injury restores resistance to infection. Ann Surg 2000;231:253–261.

Goodwin CW, Dorethy J, Lam V, Pruitt BA Jr: Randomized trial of efficacy of crystalloid and colloid resuscitation on hemodynamic response and lung water following thermal injury. Ann Surg 1983;197:520–531.

Gough DB, Moss NM, Jordan A, et al: Recombinant interleukin-2 (rIL-2) improves immune response and host resistance to septic challenge in thermally injured mice. Surgery 1988;104:292–300.

Graves TA, Cioffi WG, McManus WF, et al: Fluid resuscitation of infants and children with massive thermal injury. J Trauma 1988;28:1656–1659.

Grube BJ, Marvin JA, Heimbach DM: Therapeutic hyperbaric oxygen: help or hindrance in burn patients with carbon monoxide poisoning? J Burn Care Rehabil 1988; 9:249–252.

Hales CA, Musto S, Hutchison WG, Mahoney E: BW-755C diminishes smoke-induced pulmonary edema. J Appl Physiol 1995;78:64–69.

Harms BA, Bodai BI, Kramer GC, Demling RH: Microvascular fluid and protein flux in pulmonary and systemic circulations after thermal injury. Microvasc Res 1982;23:77–86.

Harrington DT, Jordan BS, Dubick MA, et al: Delayed partial liquid ventilation shows no efficacy in the treatment of smoke inhalation injury in swine. J Appl Physiol 2001;90:2351–2360.

Hart DW, Wolf SE, Chinkes DL, et al: Determinants of skeletal muscle catabolism after severe burn. Ann Surg 2000;232: 455–465.

Hart DW, Wolf SE, Mlcak R, et al: Persistence of muscle catabolism after severe burn. Surgery 2000;128:312–319.

Hasselgren PO, Fischer JE: Muscle cachexia: current concepts of intracellular mechanisms and molecular regulation. Ann Surg 2001;233:9–17.

Hasslen SR, Ahrenholz DH, Solem LD, Nelson RD: Actin polymerization contributes to neutrophil chemotactic dysfunction following thermal injury. J Leukoc Biol 1992;52:495–500.

Herlihy JP, Vermeulen MW, Joseph PM, Hales CA: Impaired alveolar macrophage function in smoke inhalation injury. J Cell Physiol 1995;163:1–8.

Herndon DN, Barrow RE, Kunkel KR, et al: Effects of recombinant human growth hormone on donor-site healing in severely burned children. Ann Surg 1990;212:424–431.

Herndon DN, Barrow RE, Rutan RL, et al: A comparison of conservative versus early excision: therapies in severely burned patients. Ann Surg 1989;209:547–553.

Herndon DN, Traber LD, Linares H, et al: Etiology of the pulmonary pathophysiology associated with inhalation injury. Resuscitation 1986;14:43–59.

Herndon DN, Traber DL, Niehaus GD, et al: The pathophysiology of smoke inhalation injury in a sheep model. J Trauma 1984;24:1044–1051.

Holm C, Melcer B, Horbrand F, et al: Intrathoracic blood volume as an end point in resuscitation of the severely burned: an observational study of 24 patients. J Trauma 2000;48:728–734.

Huang PP, Stucky FS, Dimick AR, et al: Hypertonic sodium resuscitation is associated with renal failure and death. Ann Surg 1995;221:543–557.

Hubbard GB, Langlinais PC, Shimazu T, et al: The morphology of smoke inhalation injury in sheep. J Trauma 1991;31: 1477–1486.

Huston DP: The biology of the immune system. JAMA 1997;278: 1804–1814.

Ikeuchi H, Sakano T, Sanchez J, et al: The effects of platelet-activating factor (PAF) and a PAF antagonist (CV-3988) on smoke inhalation injury in an ovine model. J Trauma 1992;32:344–350.

Isago T, Noshima S, Traber L, et al: Analysis of pulmonary microvascular permeability after smoke inhalation. J Appl Physiol 1991;71:1403–1408.

Ischiropoulos H, Mendiguren I, Fisher D, et al: Role of neutrophils and nitric oxide in lung alveolar injury from smoke inhalation. Am J Respir Crit Care Med 1994;150:337–341.

Kelemen JJ III, Cioffi WG Jr, Mason AD Jr, et al: Effect of ambient temperature on metabolic rate after thermal injury. Ann Surg 1996;223:406–412.

Kelly JL, Lyons A, Soberg CC, et al: Anti-interleukin-10 antibody restores burn-induced defects in T-cell function. Surgery 1997;122:146–152.

Kikuchi Y, Traber LD, Herndon DN, Traber DL: Unilateral smoke inhalation in sheep: effect on left lung lymph flow with right lung injury. Am J Physiol 1996;271: R1620–R1624.

Kim SH, Hubbard GB, Worley BL, et al: A rapid section technique for burn wound biopsy. J Burn Care Rehabil 1985;6:433–435.

Kimura R, Traber L, Herndon D, et al: Ibuprofen reduces the lung lymph flow changes associated with inhalation injury. Circ Shock 1988;24:183–191.

Krause PJ, Woronick CL, Burke G, et al: Depressed neutrophil chemotaxis in children suffering blunt trauma. Pediatrics 1994;93:807–809.

Lachocki TM, Church DF, Pryor WA: Persistent free radicals in woodsmoke: an ESR spin trapping study. Free Radic Biol Med 1989;7:17–21.

Laffon M, Pittet JF, Modelska K, et al: Interleukin-8 mediates injury from smoke inhalation to both the lung endothelial and the alveolar epithelial barriers in rabbits. Am J Respir Crit Care Med 1999;160:1443–1449.

LaLonde C, Knox J, Youn YK, Demling R: Burn edema is accentuated by a moderate smoke inhalation injury in sheep. Surgery 1992;112:908–917.

LaLonde C, Nayak U, Hennigan J, Demling R: Plasma catalase and glutathione levels are decreased in response to inhalation injury. J Burn Care Rehabil 1997;18:515–519.

LaLonde C, Picard L, Youn YK, Demling RH: Increased early postburn fluid requirements and oxygen demands are predicative of the degree of airways injury by smoke inhalation. J Trauma 1995;38:175–184.

Lederer JA, Rodrick ML, Mannick JA: The effects of injury on the adaptive immune response. Shock 1999;11:153–159.

LeVoyer T, Cioffi WG Jr, Pratt L, et al: Alterations in intestinal permeability after thermal injury. Arch Surg 1992;127:26–30.

Llovera M, Carbo N, Lopez-Soriano J, et al: Different cytokines modulate ubiquitin gene expression in rat skeletal muscle. Cancer Lett 1998;133:83–87.

Lund T, Goodwin CW, McManus WF, et al: Upper airway sequelae in burn patients requiring endotracheal intubation or tracheostomy. Ann Surg 1985;201:374–382.

Lund T, Onarheim H, Wiig H, Reed RK: Mechanisms behind increased dermal imbibition pressure in acute burn edema. Am J Physiol 1989;256:H940–H948.

Lyons M, Clemens LH: Energy deficits associated with nasogastric feeding in patients with burns. J Burn Care Rehabil 2000;21:371–374.

Lyons A, Goebel A, Mannick JA, Lederer JA: Protective effects of early interleukin 10 antagonism on injury-induced immune dysfunction. Arch Surg 1999;134: 1317–1324.

Lyons A, Kelly JL, Rodrick ML, et al: Major injury induces increased production of interleukin-10 by cells of the immune system with a negative impact on resistance to infection. Ann Surg 1997;226:450–460.

Maderazo EG, Woronick CL, Albano SD, et al: Inappropriate activation, deactivation, and probable autooxidative damage as a mechanism of neutrophil locomotory defect in trauma. J Infect Dis 1986;154:471–477.

Maldonado MD, Venturoli A, Franco A, Nunez-Roldan A: Specific changes in peripheral blood lymphocyte phenotype from burn patients: probable origin of the thermal injury-related lymphocytopenia. Burns 1991;17: 188–192.

Manetti R, Parronchi P, Giudizi MG, et al: Natural killer cell stimulatory factor (interleukin 12 [IL-12]) induces T helper type 1 (Th1)-specific immune responses and inhibits the development of IL-4-producing Th cells. J Exp Med 1993;177:1199–1204.

Matsuda T, Kagan RJ, Hanumadass M, Jonasson O: The importance of burn wound size in determining the optimal calorie:nitrogen ratio. Surgery 1983;94:562–568.

Matylevitch NP, Schuschereba ST, Mata JR, et al: Apoptosis and accidental cell death in cultured human keratinocytes after thermal injury. Am J Pathol 1998;153:567–577.

McDonald WS, Sharp CW Jr, Deitch EA: Immediate enteral feeding in burn patients is safe and effective. Ann Surg 1991;213:177–183.

McIrvine AJ, O'Mahony JB, Saparoschetz I, Mannick JA: Depressed immune response in burn patients: use of monoclonal antibodies and functional assays to define the role of suppressor cells. Ann Surg 1982;196:297–304.

McManus AT, Denton CL, Mason AD Jr: Mechanisms of in vitro sensitivity to sulfadiazine silver. Arch Surg 1983;118:161–166.

McManus AT, Mason AD Jr, McManus WF, Pruitt BA Jr: A decade of reduced gram-negative infections and mortality associated with improved isolation of burned patients. Arch Surg 1994;129:1306–1309.

McManus WF, Goodwin CW Jr, Pruitt BA Jr: Subeschar treatment of burn-wound infection. Arch Surg 1983;118:291–294.

McManus WF, Mason AD Jr, Pruitt BA Jr: Subeschar antibiotic infusion in the treatment of burn wound infection. J Trauma 1980;20:1021–1023.

Milner EA, Cioffi WG, Mason AD, et al: A longitudinal study of resting energy expenditure in thermally injured patients. J Trauma 1994;37:167–170.

Milner EA, Cioffi WG, Mason AD Jr, et al: Accuracy of urinary urea nitrogen for predicting total urinary nitrogen in thermally injured patients. JPEN J Parenter Enteral Nutr 1993;17:414–416.

Miro O, Casademont J, Barrientos A, et al: Mitochondrial cytochrome c oxidase inhibition during acute carbon monoxide poisoning. Pharmacol Toxicol 1998;82:199–202.

Molloy RG, Nestor M, Collins KH, et al: The humoral immune response after thermal injury: an experimental model. Surgery 1994;115:341–348.

Moore FD Jr, Davis C, Rodrick M, et al: Neutrophil activation in thermal injury as assessed by increased expression of complement receptors. N Engl J Med 1986;314:948–953.

Moss NM, Gough DB, Jordan AL, et al: Temporal correlation of impaired immune response after thermal injury with susceptibility to infection in a murine model. Surgery 1988;104:882–887.

Moyer CA, Brentano L, Gravens DL, et al: Treatment of large burns with 0.5% silver nitrate solution. Arch Surg 1965;90:812–867.

Mozingo DW, McManus AT, Kim SH, Pruitt BA Jr: Incidence of bacteremia after burn wound manipulation in the early postburn period. J Trauma 1997;42:1006–1011.

Nakanishi T, Nishi Y, Sato EF, et al: Thermal injury induces thymocyte apoptosis in the rat. J Trauma 1998;44:143–148.

Newsome TW, Mason AD Jr, Pruitt BA Jr: Weight loss following thermal injury. Ann Surg 1973;178:215–217.

Niehaus GD, Kimura R, Traber LD, et al: Administration of a synthetic antiprotease reduces smoke-induced lung injury. J Appl Physiol 1990;69:694–699.

Nieman GF, Clark WR Jr: Effects of wood and cotton smoke on the surface properties of pulmonary surfactant. Respir Physiol 1994;97:1–12.

Nieman GF, Clark WR Jr, Goyette D, et al: Wood smoke inhalation increases pulmonary microvascular permeability. Surgery 1989;105:481–487.

Nieman GF, Clark WR Jr, Paskanik AM, et al: Unilateral smoke inhalation increases pulmonary blood flow to the injured lung. J Trauma 1994;36:617–623.

Nieman GF, Clark WR Jr, Wax SD, Webb SR: The effect of smoke inhalation on pulmonary surfactant. Ann Surg 1980;191:171–181.

Nishimura T, Yamamoto H, deSerres S, Meyer AA: Transforming growth factor-beta impairs postburn immunoglobulin production by limiting B-cell proliferation, but not cellular synthesis. J Trauma 1999;46:881–885.

Ochoa JB, Strange J, Kearney P, et al: Effects of L-arginine on the proliferation of T lymphocyte subpopulations. JPEN J Parenter Enteral Nutr 2001;25:23–29.

Ogle CK, Ogle JD, Mao JX, et al: Effect of glutamine on phagocytosis and bacterial killing by normal and pediatric burn patient neutrophils. JPEN J Parenter Enteral Nutr 1994;18:128–133.

Ogura H, Cioffi WG, Okerberg CV, et al: The effects of pentoxifylline on pulmonary function following smoke inhalation. J Surg Res 1994;56:242–250.

Ogura H, Saitoh D, Johnson AA, et al: The effect of inhaled nitric oxide on pulmonary ventilation-perfusion matching following smoke inhalation injury. J Trauma 1994;37:893–898.

Orellano T, Dergal E, Alijani M, et al: Studies on the mechanism of carbon monoxide toxicity. J Surg Res 1976;20:485–487.

Papathanassoglou DE, Moynihan JA, McDermott MP, Ackerman MH: Expression of Fas (CD95) and Fas ligand on peripheral blood mononuclear cells in critical illness and association with multiorgan dysfunction severity and survival. Crit Care Med 2001;29:709–718.

Pellegrini JD, De AK, Kodys K, et al: Relationships between T lymphocyte apoptosis and anergy following trauma. J Surg Res 2000;88:200–206.

Perlstein RS, Whitnall MH, Abrams JS, et al: Synergistic roles of interleukin-6, interleukin-1, and tumor necrosis factor in the adrenocorticotropin response to bacterial lipopolysaccharide in vivo. Endocrinology 1993;132:946–952.

Piantadosi CA, Sylvia AL, Jobsis-Vandervliet FF: Differences in brain cytochrome responses to carbon monoxide and cyanide in vivo. J Appl Physiol 1987;62:1277–1284.

Pierre EJ, Barrow RE, Hawkins HK, et al: Effects of insulin on wound healing. J Trauma 1998;44:342–345.

Pitt RM, Parker JC, Jurkovich GJ, et al: Analysis of altered capillary pressure and permeability after thermal injury. J Surg Res 1987;42:693–702.

Pruitt BA: Advances in fluid therapy and the early care of the burn patient. World J Surg 1978;2:139–150.

Pruitt BA Jr: Phycomycotic infections. Probl Gen Surg 1984;1: 664–678.

Pruitt BA Jr, Goodwin CW Jr, Pruitt SK: Burns: including cold, chemical, and electric injuries. In Sabiston DC Jr (ed): Textbook of Surgery: The Biological Basis of Modern Surgical Practice. Philadelphia: WB Saunders, 1997:221–252.

Pruitt BA Jr, Mason AD Jr, Moncrief JA: Hemodynamic changes in the early postburn patient: the influence of fluid administration and of a vasodilator (hydralazine). J Trauma 1971;11:36–46.

Pruitt BA Jr, McManus AT, Kim SH, Goodwin CW: Burn wound infections: current status. World J Surg 1998;22: 135–145.

Pruitt BA Jr, O'Neill JA Jr, Moncrief JA, Lindberg RB: Successful control of burn-wound sepsis. JAMA 1968;203: 1054–1056.

Roper RL, Conrad DH, Brown DM, et al: Prostaglandin E$_2$ promotes IL-4-induced IgE and IgG1 synthesis. J Immunol 1990;145:2644–2651.

Rue LW, Cioffi WG, Mason AD Jr, et al: The risk of pneumonia in thermally injured patients requiring ventilatory support. J Burn Care Rehabil 1995;16:262–268.

Rue LW III, Cioffi WG, Mason AD, et al: Improved survival of burned patients with inhalation injury. Arch Surg 1993;128:772–780.

Sachse C, Prigge M, Cramer G, et al: Association between reduced human leukocyte antigen (HLA)-DR expression on blood monocytes and increased plasma level of interleukin-10 in patients with severe burns. Clin Chem Lab Med 1999;37:193–198.

Saito H, Trocki O, Wang SL, et al: Metabolic and immune effects of dietary arginine supplementation after burn. Arch Surg 1987;122:784–789.

Sakurai H, Johnigan R, Kikuchi Y, et al: Effect of reduced bronchial circulation on lung fluid flux after smoke inhalation in sheep. J Appl Physiol 1998;84:980–986.

Sakurai H, Schmalstieg FC, Traber LD, et al: Role of L-selectin in physiological manifestations after burn and smoke inhalation injury in sheep. J Appl Physiol 1999;86: 1151–1159.

Sakurai H, Traber LD, Traber DL: Altered systemic organ blood flow after combined injury with burn and smoke inhalation. Shock 1998;9:369–374.

Sayeed MM: Alterations in cell signaling and related effector functions in T lymphocytes in burn/trauma/septic injuries [editorial]. Shock 1996;5:157–166.

Sayeed MM: Signaling mechanisms of altered cellular responses in trauma, burn, and sepsis: role of Ca^{2+}. Arch Surg 2000;135:1432–1442.

Schaffer M, Barbul A: Lymphocyte function in wound healing and following injury. Br J Surg 1998;85:444–460.

Schenarts PJ, Bone HG, Traber LD, Traber DL: Effect of severe smoke inhalation injury on systemic microvascular blood flow in sheep. Shock 1996;6:201–205.

Schenarts PJ, Schmalstieg FC, Hawkins H, et al: Effects of an L-selectin antibody on the pulmonary and systemic manifestations of severe smoke inhalation injuries in sheep. J Burn Care Rehabil 2000;21:229–240.

Schiller WR, Bay RC: Hemodynamic and oxygen transport monitoring in management of burns. New Horiz 1996;4: 475–482.

Schlüter B, Konig W, Koller M, et al: Differential regulation of T- and B-lymphocyte activation in severely burned patients. J Trauma 1991;31:239–246.

Schlüter B, Konig W, Koller M, et al: Studies on B-lymphocyte dysfunctions in severely burned patients. J Trauma 1990;30: 1380–1389.

Shi HP, Efron DT, Most D, et al: Supplemental dietary arginine enhances wound healing in normal but not inducible nitric oxide synthase knockout mice. Surgery 2000;128:374–378.

Shimazu T, Ikeuchi H, Sugimoto H, et al: Half-life of blood carboxyhemoglobin after short-term and long-term exposure to carbon monoxide. J Trauma 2000;49:126–131.

Shimazu T, Yukioka T, Ikeuchi H, et al: Ventilation-perfusion alterations after smoke inhalation injury in an ovine model. J Appl Physiol 1996;81:2250–2259.

Shirani KZ, McManus AT, Vaughan GM, et al: Effects of environment on infection in burn patients. Arch Surg 1986;121:31–36.

Shirani KZ, Pruitt BA Jr, Mason AD Jr: The influence of inhalation injury and pneumonia on burn mortality. Ann Surg 1987;205:82–87.

Soejima K, McGuire R, Snyder NT, et al: The effect of inducible nitric oxide synthase (iNOS) inhibition on smoke inhalation injury in sheep. Shock 2000;13:261–266.

Soejima K, Traber LD, Schmalstieg FC, et al: Role of nitric oxide in vascular permeability after combined burns and smoke inhalation injury. Am J Respir Crit Care Med 2001;163:745–752.

Solomon V, Madihally S, Yarmush M, Toner M: Insulin suppresses the increased activities of lysosomal cathepsins and ubiquitin conjugation system in burn-injured rats. J Surg Res 2000;93:120–126.

Tabata T, Meyer AA: Effects of burn injury on class-specific B-cell population and immunoglobulin synthesis in mice. J Trauma 1993;35:750–755.

Tanaka H, Matsuda T, Miyagantani Y, et al: Reduction of resuscitation fluid volumes in severely burned patients using ascorbic acid administration: a randomized, prospective study. Arch Surg 2000;135:326–331.

Tasaki O, Goodwin CW, Saitoh D, et al: Effects of burns on inhalation injury. J Trauma 1997;43:603–607.

Tasaki O, Mozingo DW, Ishihara S, et al: Effect of sulfo Lewis C on smoke inhalation injury in an ovine model. Crit Care Med 1998;26:1238–1243.

Teodorczyk-Injeyan JA, Sparkes BG, Mills GB, et al: Impaired expression of interleukin-2 receptor (IL2R) in the immunosuppressed burned patient: reversal by exogenous IL2. J Trauma 1987;27:180–187.

Teodorczyk-Injeyan JA, Sparkes BG, Mills GB, Peters WJ: Immunosuppression follows systemic T lymphocyte activation in the burn patient. Clin Exp Immunol 1991;85: 515–518.

Tokyay R, Zeigler ST, Kramer GC, et al: Effects of hypertonic saline dextran resuscitation on oxygen delivery, oxygen consumption, and lipid peroxidation after burn injury. J Trauma 1992;32:704–713.

Tracey KJ, Lowry SF, Fahey TJ III, et al: Cachectin/tumor necrosis factor induces lethal shock and stress hormone responses in the dog. Surg Gynecol Obstet 1987;164:415–422.

Tredget EE, Shankowsky HA, Groeneveld A, Burrell R: A matched-pair, randomized study evaluating the efficacy and safety of Acticoat silver-coated dressing for the treatment of burn wounds. J Burn Care Rehabil 1998;19:531–537.

Utsunomiya T, Kobayashi M, Herndon DN, et al: A mechanism of interleukin-12 unresponsiveness associated with thermal injury. J Surg Res 2001;96:211–217.

Waxman K, Rebello T, Pinderski L, et al: Protein loss across burn wounds. J Trauma 1987;27:136–140.

Wilmore DW: Metabolic response to severe surgical illness: overview. World J Surg 2000;24:705–711.

Wilmore DW, Aulick LH, Mason AD, Pruitt BA Jr: Influence of the burn wound on local and systemic responses to injury. Ann Surg 1977;186:444–458.

Wilmore DW, Curreri PW, Spitzer KW, et al: Supranormal dietary intake in thermally injured hypermetabolic patients. Surg Gynecol Obstet 1971;132:881–886.

Wilmore DW, Long JM, Mason AD Jr, et al: Catecholamines: mediator of the hypermetabolic response to thermal injury. Ann Surg 1974;180:653–669.

Wilmore DW, Mason AD Jr, Johnson DW, Pruitt BA Jr: Effect of ambient temperature on heat production and heat loss in burn patients. J Appl Physiol 1975;38:593–597.

Wolfe RR, Durkot MJ, Wolfe MH: Effect of thermal injury on energy metabolism, substrate kinetics, and hormonal concentrations. Circ Shock 1982;9:383–394.

Wood JJ, Grbic JT, Rodrick ML, et al: Suppression of interleukin 2 production in an animal model of thermal injury is related to prostaglandin synthesis. Arch Surg 1987;122: 179–184.

Wood JJ, Rodrick ML, O'Mahony JB, et al: Inadequate interleukin 2 production: a fundamental immunological deficiency in patients with major burns. Ann Surg 1984;200:311–320.

Xu DZ, Deitch EA, Sittig K, et al: In vitro cell-mediated immunity after thermal injury is not impaired: density gradient purification of mononuclear cells is associated with spurious (artifactual) immunosuppression. Ann Surg 1988;208:768–775.

Yamamoto H, Hayes YO, deSerres S, et al: Burn injury induces a biphasic immunoglobulin M response to bacterial antigen. J Trauma 1995;39:279–284.

Yamamoto H, Siltharm S, deSerres S, et al: Effect of cyclooxygenase inhibition on in vitro B-cell function after burn injury. J Trauma 1996;41:612–621.

Yasuhara S, Kanakubo E, Perez ME, et al: The 1999 Moyer award: burn injury induces skeletal muscle apoptosis and the activation of caspase pathways in rats. J Burn Care Rehabil 1999;20:462–470.

Zapata-Sirvent RL, Hansbrough JF: Temporal analysis of human leucocyte surface antigen expression and neutrophil respiratory burst activity after thermal injury. Burns 1993;19: 5–11.

Zedler S, Bone RC, Baue AE, et al: T-cell reactivity and its predictive role in immunosuppression after burns. Crit Care Med 1999;27:66–72.

Zedler S, Faist E, Ostermeier B, et al: Postburn constitutional changes in T-cell reactivity occur in CD8+ rather than in CD4+ cells. J Trauma 1997;42:872–881.

Zhang J, Piantadosi CA: Mitochondrial oxidative stress after carbon monoxide hypoxia in the rat brain. J Clin Invest 1992;90:1193–1199.

Zwadlo-Klarwasser G, Kauhl W, Schmitz C, Hettich R: Influence of severe burn injury on the expression of RM 3/1 and HLA-DR antigens in human blood monocytes. J Burn Care Rehabil 1996;17:287–293.

CHAPTER 34

Physicochemical Injuries

Mark A. Grevious, M.D. and Raphael C. Lee, M.D., Sc.D., Ph.D.

Terminology used to discuss electrical injury is often confusing, which seriously impedes advancement in treatment concepts. The use of misleading terms such as "entrance wound," "exit wound," "flash burn," and "electrical contact burn" are a few examples that reflect the degree of confusion. The prime objective of the trend toward molecular medicine is to devise ways to reverse or correct molecular pathophysiology caused by injury or disease processes. To apply this strategy to electrical injuries, it is necessary to know the precise biophysical mechanisms of the injury process. Traditionally, refinement in the understanding of the pathology of disease has resulted from more precise use of descriptive terminology.

The term *physicochemical* is used here to reference chemical damage driven by physical forces acting at the molecular level. This would include heat-induced molecular changes, such as macromolecule denaturation; electrical force effects, such as electroconformational coupling and membrane electroporation; frostbite-related ice crystallization leading to membrane disruption; and biomolecular ionization effects such as that caused by toxic doses of ionizing irradiation. In this chapter, an attempt is made to describe the molecular basis and biologic consequences of several types of electrical injuries.

Electrical Injuries

Patients presenting with electrical injury manifest a wide range of clinical signs and symptoms. The effects of electricity on the body are so dependent on dose, anatomic path, duration of exposure, and frequency that each case is a diagnostic challenge. A basic understanding of electricity is essential for properly evaluating and managing these patients.

Passage of electrical current through tissue can produce damaging effects by two fundamentally different mechanisms. One generally appreciated mechanism is thermal burn caused by the Joule heating consequences of current passage. The other mechanism is the direct action of electrical forces on the electrically charged or electrically polarized components of tissue. Both mechanisms ultimately lead to alteration in molecular conformation and/or disruption of macromolecular structures such as proteins or the lipid bilayer of membranes. A fundamental distinction between heat- and electrical force–mediated molecular effects is the mechanism of energy transmission to the molecule(s). In contrast to thermal forces, which are random in direction and over time average to zero, electrical forces produce effects on macromolecules by direct vectorial electrical coupling.

Another important distinction between electrical force effects and heating effects is that tissue structures with dimensions of a macromolecule or larger are influential in electrical effects. For example, the vulnerability of a cell to electrical damage is related to its physical dimensions (Fig. 34–1), whereas vulnerability to supraphysiologic temperatures is not. In addition, because of the nature of the coupling between electrical energy and certain material properties, electrical effects are frequency dependent. For human contacts, strong frequency dependence of damage mechanisms does not occur until the frequency is at or above the order of 10,000 cycles/sec (i.e., 10 kHz), as summarized in Table 34–1. Therefore, when the vast majority of electrical injury involves commercial electrical power that has operating frequencies between 0 and 60 Hz, the effects of frequency can be neglected.

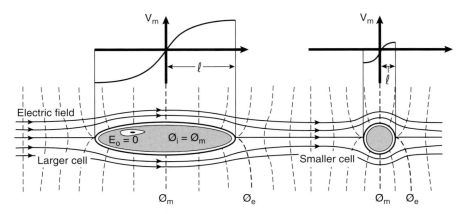

FIGURE 34–1 Distribution of current flow and electrical force lines (solid) around cells exposed to the same applied uniform electrical field. The current (and field lines) are solid. Lines of constant voltage (dashed) run perpendicular to the field lines. In effect, the cell membrane blocks flow of current into the cytoplasm; thus there are no solid or dashed lines in the cytoplasm, which is isopotential throughout. The voltage difference across the membrane depends on the position of the membrane and the physical size of the cell (i.e., $\Delta V_m \sim E_o \frac{1}{2}$). Large cells experience larger maximum induced transmembrane potentials because the voltage drop across the length of the cell scales with the length of the cell in the direction of the field lines.

Characteristically, the cell damage sustained following exposure to strong electrical forces is quite different from that of a cell injured by pure supraphysiologic temperatures. The pathophysiologic significance of these differences is substantial. First, the distribution of injury through the cell is different. This is a consequence of the structure of cells, as illustrated in Figure 34–1. Because the cytoplasm and extracellular fluids have similar ionic strength, they are both good electrical conductors relative to pure water or oils. The electrical resistivity of the cell membrane, however, is characteristically 10^6- to 10^8-fold greater than the surrounding media. Thus the cell can be described as an insulating shell with a highly conductive interior and exterior. Consequently, electrical current established in the extracellular space is to a large degree shielded from the cytoplasm by the electrically insulating cell membrane. This shielding limits the voltage drop within the cytoplasm. If the membrane were a perfect insulator, the voltage in the cytoplasm would be uniform throughout. With current flowing around the cell, a voltage gradient is established along the external surface of the cell, which sets up an "induced" transmembrane potential that varies according to location along the membrane. This induced transmembrane potential will range from zero at the axis of symmetry to a maximum at the extreme projections of the cell in the direction of the current passage. There are several reviews of this subject. Conceptually; the maximum induced transmembrane potential will scale with the total voltage drop along the outer surface of the cell. However, the magnitude of the induced transmembrane potential depends on the size, geometry, and orientation of the cell with respect to the field.

Because cellular membranes are very thin in comparison to the overall dimensions of the cell, the electrical

Table 34–1
Important frequency ranges of electrical injury

Frequency Regimen	General Applications	Biologic Effect
Low frequency (DC, 10 kHz)	Commercial electrical power	Joule heating; destructive cell membrane potentials
Radiofrequency 10 kHz to 10 MHz	Electrothermy, electrocautery	Joule heating; dielectric heating of proteins
Microwave 10 MHz to 10 GHz	Microwave heating	Dielectric heating of water
Light 10^{13} Hz	Vision; laser applications	Molecular heating
10^{14} hertz and higher	Ionizing radiation (ultraviolet, x-ray, cosmic, alpha, electronic, gamma radiation)	Generation of reactive oxygen intermediates

DC, direct current.

field strength established in the membrane is manyfold greater than the field strength along the outer surface of the cell. For example, a 1-cm-long cell in an electrical field of 150 V/cm will briefly experience a peak (because real membranes will not tolerate such potentials) induced transmembrane potential magnitude on the scale of tens of volts. Assuming a membrane thickness of 10 nm, the corresponding peak electrical field magnitude within the plasma membrane is 7.5×10^7 volts/cm, which is of sufficient strength to denature proteins and permeabilize the membrane (electroporation).

Electroporation

Bilayer lipid membranes become structurally altered when the transmembrane potential magnitude becomes too large. Structural defects or "pores" are formed in the membrane that effectively permeabilize the membrane to ions and molecules as large as DNA. This electrically driven pore formation process, termed *electroporation*, typically occurs with sub-millisecond kinetics. The molecular physics responsible for electroporation is still debated, but in general involves the transport of water into molecular-scale pores in the cell membrane (Fig. 34–2) until the size of the pore exceeds a critical size (beyond which it is energetically favorable for expansion rather than pore closure). Supraphysiologic transmembrane potentials of greater than 400 to 600 mV are required to induce pores in the lipid bilayer. Unlike the rupture of a soap bubble following pinprick, the growth of pores in the bilayer lipid component of mammalian cell membrane is thought to be restricted by membrane proteins, which represent approximately 30% of the total membrane mass. The kinetics of pore formation is transmembrane potential dependent within a characteristic range of 10^{-2} to 10^{-1} msec. Electropores can be transient or stable.

When a 1-cm-long skeletal muscle cell is placed in a saline conducting medium with a 150-V/cm applied electrical field, the membrane is rapidly electroporated, resulting in a large increase in membrane electrical conductivity (Fig. 34–3). As the conductivity of the membrane increases toward that of the cytoplasm, the membrane electrical field decreases and the cytoplasm field strength increases, both approaching that of the externally applied field. The drop in the membrane field strength limits further membrane permeabilization. Although the intracellular field strength reaches that of the extracellular field, the intracellular membranes are not electroporated because of the relative small size of intracellular organelles. Unlike thermal injury, in which all membranes and macromolecules are affected, damage resulting from electrical forces is typically restricted to the plasma membrane.

Electroconformational Protein Denaturation

Membrane protein typically spans the entire thickness of the membrane, which means that the membrane protein will experience the entire transmembrane voltage drop. Membrane proteins are composed of amino acids with acidic and basic side groups that can be acted upon directly by an intense intramembrane electrical field. In addition to this mechanism, charged side groups form electrical dipoles, which can align along the length of the transmembrane protein to create a large dipole moment that can also be acted upon by the field. Typically each amino acid unit contributes an electrical dipole moment of about 3.5 Debye (D) to the entire protein. In the α-helical structure of protein, many small peptide dipoles are aligned almost perfectly to form a larger dipole on the order of 120 D across the cell membrane. In general, a molecule under a strong electrical field will tend to shift to a greater dipole moment in the direction of the field.

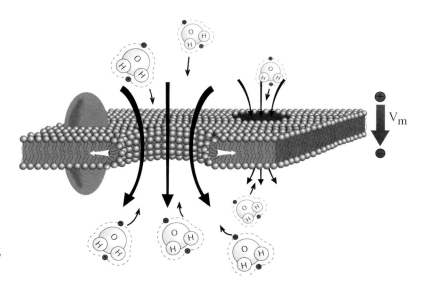

FIGURE 34–2 Schematic illustrating the effect of large electrical fields on cell membrane structure. Although the molecular mechanics are not all known, field-driven hydration of aqueous pores is part of the process. In addition, direct electrical force–mediated damage, such as electroconformational coupling, occurs.

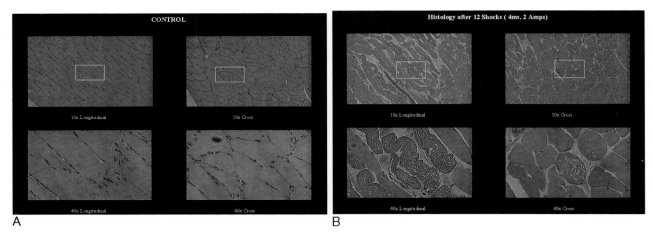

FIGURE 34–3 Histologic appearance of electroporated rat hindlimb skeletal muscle can be appreciated in these photomicrographs (H&E, 400× magnification). **A**, Control skeletal muscle tissue. **B**, Skeletal muscle that has received 12 electrical field pulses of 150 V/cm, 4 msec in duration and separated by 10 seconds to allow thermal relaxation. Maximum temperature rise was 3°C.

This can be realized in several ways: (1) induced dissociation of ionizable side groups; (2) induced separation of electrical charges along the macromolecule; (3) alignment of weak dipoles in a cooperative fashion between subunits or monomers of a protein complex; (4) reorientation of permanent dipoles on the protein within the direction of the field; and (5) induction of electrical dipoles by the applied field, but changing conformational state associated with a higher dipole moment or induction of dipoles as a result of polarizability of the protein. The magnitude of the effect of alteration of the α-helical conformation on the protein's dipole strength can be appreciated by realizing that the random coil or β-helical structures have relatively negligible dipole strength.

When the membrane field strength becomes sufficiently intense, then the dielectrical forces acting on the molecule can actually carry out destructive changes that are not spontaneously reversible. An example of this can be seen in a model wherein the shape of the induced action potential is altered following a 500-mV electrical shock to a frog skeletal muscle cell membrane. The alteration is consistent with loss of function of the potassium channel. In principle, these types of alterations can lead to functional neuromuscular and sensory types of disorders. A therapeutic strategy to correct this problem must return the membrane protein to its native state. If the primary structure of the protein is intact, in theory it might be possible for the molecule to spontaneously return to its native stable state. Increasing the membrane temperature as much as possible without heat damaging the lipid bilayer can influence the rate at which this occurs.

Thermal Injury

Thermal burn is the term most often applied to the damaging supraphysiologic temperature effects caused by heating tissue. It is generally appreciated that the burn injury manifestations are related to damage to proteins and cellular organelle structures. The alteration in protein structure leads to changes in tissue optical properties, which explain the grossly visible changes in tissue. To understand thermal burns, we must first recall that temperature, as defined by Boltzmann, is a measure of the kinetic energy of a moving object. The relationship is defined by

$$T = \frac{kinetic\ energy}{k_B} \qquad \text{[Eqn.1]}$$

where the term T is the absolute temperature (°K) of the object and k_B is Boltzmann's constant. Specifically, the time-averaged speed v of a monoatomic molecule in free solution at temperature T is defined by the relationship

$$k_B T \approx mv^2 \qquad \text{[Eqn.2]}$$

where m is the mass of the molecule with a speed v. As temperature rises, both the molecular momentum transfer between colliding molecules and the frequency of intermolecular collisions increase. When sufficient energy is transmitted, alteration in molecular conformation can take place. As a consequence, at supraphysiologic temperature the probability that proteins and other macromolecules will lose their native structure increases.

There are two conceptually different potential outcomes for the denatured protein that depend on the initial molecular structure and configuration. The first possibility occurs when the native folded state of the protein, held by intramolecular bonds, is different from the most favored configuration if no bonds were needed to maintain the native folded state. When this protein is heated, the intermolecular bonds are broken and it denatures to one of several preferred lower energy states from which it will not spontaneously return to the native conformation.

Conceivably, if the primary structure of the protein is undamaged, it may be plausible to reconfigure the protein using a method similar to the chaperon-assisted mechanisms that established its initial folding after biosynthesis. The second possibility occurs when the native folded state of the protein is the same as the most preferred protein conformation in the absence of intramolecular cross-links. Because the preferred configuration of a non–cross-linked protein is temperature dependent, the protein will heat denature into conformations that are different from the preferred conformations at normal operating temperature.

The speed of the transition from natural to denatured states is governed by the Arrhenius rate equation, which states that, when the kinetic energy of the molecule exceeds a threshold magnitude E, transition to the denatured state will occur. For a large number of molecules at temperature T, the fraction with a kinetic energy above E is governed by the Maxwell-Boltzmann relation:

$$\Gamma = \exp\left(\frac{-E}{k_B T}\right) \qquad \text{[Eqn. 3]}$$

where k_B is Boltzmann's constant. Because the strength of bonds retaining the folded conformation of macromolecules is very dependent on the nature of the chemical bonds, the value of E is dependent on molecular structure. Despite this complexity, the net rate of denaturation of cellular structures containing many different proteins is also often describable in terms of Equations 2 and 3. For example, the accuracy of these equations in describing thermal damage to cell membranes has been reported. Even the thermal injury to intact tissues such as human skin is reasonably described by this simple Equation 3.

It has been known for more than 50 years that the rate at which damage accumulates in heated skin can be estimated by convolving Equation 3 with the temperature history. The resulting expression is called the "damage equation":

$$\frac{d\Omega}{dt} = A * \Gamma \qquad \text{[Eqn. 4]}$$

where Ω is a parameter reflective of the extent of damage, and A is a frequency factor that describes how often a configuration from which reaction is possible occurs, which is also very dependent on molecular structure. The shape of the curve predicted by Equation 4 is indeed the same as the human experimental skin temperature–time scald burn curve measured by Henriques and Moritz. This temperature-time curve shape has also been obtained for heat damage to isolated cells.

Because the bilayer lipid component of the cell membranes is held together only by forces of hydration, the cell membrane is probably the structure most vulnerable to thermal trauma. Even at temperatures of only 6°C above normal (i.e., 43°C), the kinetic energy of the molecules in the cell membrane can exceed the hydration energy barrier, which holds phospholipids in the membrane as a supramolecular assembly (Fig. 34–4). In effect, the warmed membrane goes into solution in the surrounding water, rendering the membrane freely permeable to small ions.

Microwave and Radiofrequency Injuries

Microwave and radiofrequency electrical fields change polarity very fast as defined by their frequency regimen (see Table 34–1). Their biologic effects are frequency dependent, and at high levels of exposure they can cause tissue damage. Individuals experiencing these electrical fields do not feel an electrical "shock" sensation because the field is changing direction in a shorter time than that required to establish enough transmembrane potential across nerve and muscle membranes to cause an action potential. Instead, they complain of a heat sensation and suffer burns. The therapeutic technique of radiofrequency hyperthermia operates according to the same mechanism.

Exposure to an alternating electrical field causes polar molecules to rotate. These rotational oscillations will be constrained by viscous drag interactions between neighboring molecules and by structural bonding with adjacent structures. Radiofrequency fields are absorbed by macromolecules. Smaller molecules such as water, when not bound, are able to follow the field well into the gigahertz frequency range. If the amplitude of the field strength is constant, the heating rate increases with frequency until the viscous drag on the rotating molecules prevents keeping up with the field. Microwave ovens are tuned to couple as efficiently as possible with the water. With frequencies above 1 GHz, the dielectric heating rate decreases with increasing frequency. Because small salt ions in solution also respond to the field, there is Joule heating as well. However, microwave heating is more significant because tissue water content is much higher than dissociated salt content.

Most commonly, microwave fields are transmitted when the person is near to a microwave antenna. At low frequency the epidermis is a highly resistive barrier. In the microwave regimen, the electrical power readily passed the epidermis in the form of capacitive coupling with very little energy dissipation. Consequently, the epidermis is not burned. Because microwave penetration into physiologic solutions has a characteristic depth on the order of 1 cm, microwave electrical injuries produce burns in the dermis and subcutaneous tissue. Fat is usually spared because of its low water content and because lipids are nonpolar. Tissue damage can occur that is essentially due to heating. Electroporation effects are not expected.

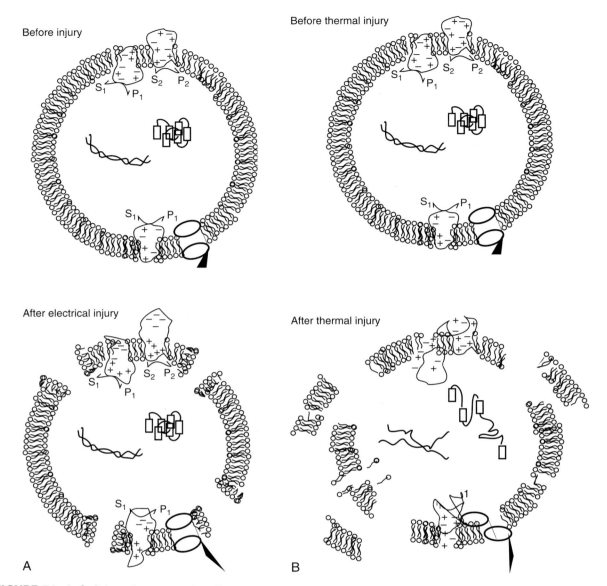

FIGURE 34–4 A, Schematic representation of heat-induced damage to the cell. Membrane lysis and protein denaturation take place to an extent dependent on the thermal history. Membrane integrity is most heat labile, and DNA is one of the most heat-stable components. **B**, Schematic representation of the cell damage caused by brief exposure to large electrical fields typical of those occurring in high-voltage electrical shock. Here "brief" implies insufficient time to cause significant heating. The direct damage in the form of electroporation and electroconformational denaturation of proteins is limited to the membrane. Internal organelles and proteins are spared.

Radiation Injury

Radiation injury occurs following tissue exposure to damaging levels of ionizing particle beam and electromagnetic irradiation, both of which alter atomic structure, which mediates the damaging chemical reactions. Tissue heating has no role in the tissue damage caused by ionizing irradiation. The most common radiation burn is excessive ultraviolet light exposure during sunbathing. Ionizing ultraviolet light can only penetrate the very thinnest layer of the epidermis. Higher frequency electromagnetic fields,

such as x-rays or gamma rays, have sufficient energy to penetrate the entire body. Mechanistically, electromagnetic waves of frequency greater than ultraviolet light can energetically couple at the atomic level, leading to the formation of unpaired electrons in the outer electron orbitals. Such high-energy irradiation acting upon biologic tissues produces protein, polysaccharide, and lipid damage. The reactive species from photoionization of water are primarily hydroxyl ions, which are very reactive against biologic macromolecules. The reaction with biologic macromolecules leads to altered chemical bonding and molecular structure and ultimately blocks function. The hydrogen bonds of DNA and other proteins are particularly vulnerable. This vulnerability permits use of radiation for cancer therapy and for other conditions in which cell proliferation is to be blocked.

Because many free radicals have no net electrical charge, free radicals have free access to the lipid bilayer. Damage to the cell membrane leading to increased permeability results from heavy exposure. The precise molecular mechanics of membrane permeabilization are still under investigation. Some investigators suggest that it is related to desaturation of membrane lipids. The lipids in the membrane bilayer have protons stripped from their carbon backbone, leading to desaturation and bends in the structure. Polyunsaturated fatty acids require greater molecular excluded volume and will self-aggregate by lateral diffusion in the lipid bilayer. Aggregation leads to bilayer instability and poration.

Radiation "burns" also occasionally result as a complication of cancer radiotherapy. Skin wounds develop in heavily irradiated areas as a result of loss of epidermal and dermal cell proliferation potential. In addition, the effects of loss of vascular capillary function with resulting edema and inflammation are manifested in tissue breakdown. Loss of proliferation potential and the loss of expression of other proteins are a manifestation of cellular genetic damage from reactive oxygen intermediate–mediated DNA cleavage. At doses in excess of 80 to 100 gray, even postmitotic cells are lethally injured by bilayer membrane permeabilization. Susceptibility to radiation injury is variable from one patient to the next. The injury mechanism is very different from that of thermal burns. The thermal energy absorbed by even lethal radiation doses is insufficient to raise the surrounding water temperature measurably. Molecular medicine strategies to correct the underlying problems would be very different when considering heat-mediated and ionizing radiation–induced cell injury.

Similarities

Vulnerability to thermal damage depends on molecular structure and strength of bonds, not on cell size or shape. Thus the susceptibility to heat damage is quite similar across different tissues. The damage that occurs is permeabilization of the cellular membranes, protein denaturation, and other secondary consequences. Visual inspection of thermally burned tissue reveals that changes in tissue optical properties result because the optical properties of tissues depend on the macromolecular conformation. Thus the visible changes that occur in heat burn are useful in assessing the viability of injured tissue. This is not the case for damage by electrical force effects.

In contrast to what is found for thermal injury, cell size and tissue structure are very important in determining vulnerability to electrical force damage. The long axes of most skeletal muscle cells and nerve axons are oriented approximately parallel to the direction of the field lines. Human forearm skeletal muscle cells can approach 8 cm in length, and nerves cells are much longer. The transmembrane potentials experienced by these cells and peripheral nerve axons would be significantly larger than those experienced by non–parallel-oriented skeletal muscle cells or experienced by smaller cell types such as fibroblasts or circulating blood cells. From this perspective, it is not surprising that skeletal muscle and nerve cells are the most frequently damaged in electrical injury. Cardiac myocytes and vascular endothelial cells are connected together in a way that in principle creates a large cell effect. The injury is primarily at the site of the cell membrane. Macroscopically the tissues appearance does not resemble thermal injury because denaturation of proteins generally does not occur.

Loss of membrane integrity is common to cells injured by electrical force and by secondary heating effects. Ionic compartmentalization, as permitted by the cell membrane, is essential for the chemical processes of life. The work required to move solvated ions across a pure planar phospholipid bilayer in an aqueous environment approaches $60 \, k_B T$, indicating the strong impediment to passive ion diffusion across the lipid bilayer. However, cell membranes are typically 30% protein. Roughly, these protein effects combine to make the mammalian cell membrane approximately 1 million times more conductive to ions than the pure lipid bilayer. Approximately 60% to 90% of the metabolic energy expended by cells is used to maintain the gradients.

When the lipid bilayer structure is damaged, protein ion pumps cannot keep pace with the increased diffusion of ions across the membrane. Under these circumstances, the metabolic energy of the cell will be quickly exhausted, leading to biochemical arrest and necrosis. The types of burn injury discussed have in common the capacity to disrupt the transport barrier function of the cell membrane through structural alterations. Loss of cell membrane integrity occurs at supraphysiologic temperatures, in frostbite injuries, in free radical–mediated radiation injury, in barometric trauma, and in electrical shock. Ischemia-reperfusion injury, which is mediated by the effects of superoxide free radicals on the plasma membrane, is probably the most common cause and is a substantial factor in many common medical illnesses.

Considering structural stability, it is quite fortunate that cell membranes contain large proteins. In a pure surfactant membrane (i.e., a liposome), a defect sufficiently large to cause a conducting pore will expand until the entire structure ruptures. Surface tension is responsible for causing the defect to expand. This is similar to a pinprick of a soap bubble. Because cell membranes also contain large proteins, some of which are anchored together in the intracellular and extracellular space by other proteins, the defects in the membrane can become stable. Ultrastructural examination of electroporated cell membranes has demonstrated that stable structural defects occur in cell membranes. These studies demonstrated that stable pore diameters might be in the range of 0.1μ, which is large enough to pass any biologic macromolecules.

Molecular Repair

This discussion immediately raises two questions: First, what are the strategies to seal biologic cell membranes? Second, how soon must the sealing occur to prevent cell death? In an aqueous environment, at concentrations above the critical micelle concentration (CMC), surfactant compounds spontaneously self-assemble into supramolecular lamellae called membranes. The most familiar example is the formation of bubbles when water containing detergent is agitated. Biologic lipid membranes are supramolecular assemblies of surfactants, which spontaneously aggregate in an aqueous environment. Structures that orient the surfactant, as with the loop used to create bubbles, can trigger rapid formation of a supramolecular surfactant assembly (the bubble membrane forming across the loop). What is required to form closed membrane structures is a suitably high surfactant concentration in an aqueous environment, the correct range of temperature, and time.

Resealing of permeabilized cell membranes is an important capability of cells. Fusigenic proteins are macromolecules that induce sealing of porated cell membranes following exocytosis. They act to reduce surface tension that prevents flow of phospholipid across the defect to induce membrane fusion. The action of fusigenic proteins indicates that it is possible to seal damaged cell membranes using macromolecular templates. This has also been accomplished using synthetic surfactants, such as poloxamer 188 at a sub-CMC concentration of 0.1 mM (our previous studies indicated that this sub-CMC concentration was quite effective), to seal cells against loss of calcein dye postelectroporation. Other researchers have reported similar observations.

Summary

Advances in burn care have resulted from the development of strategies to interrupt processes that lead to secondary tissue damage and systemic illness. A logical extension of this effort is to focus on initial molecular consequences of physicochemical trauma with the goal of finding strategies that restore intact proteins to their native conformation, excisionally repair damaged nucleic acids, and seal damaged cell membranes. This could, in effect, directly reverse the damage and mitigate the harmful effects of the physicochemical injury.

Acknowledgments

The authors gratefully acknowledge the following support, which has been vital to our research efforts: National Institutes of Health Grant # R01 GM53113 (Dr. Lee), the Electric Power Research Institute.

Bibliography

Blackmore J: Ludwig Boltzmann, His Later Life and Philosophy, 1900–1906. Book One: A Documentary History. Boston: Kluwer Academic Publishers, 1995.

Canaday D, Li P, Weichselbaum R, et al: Membrane permeability changes in gamma-irradiated muscle cells. Ann N Y Acad Sci 1994;720:153.

Chang DC, Reese TS: Changes in membrane structure induced by electroporation as revealed by rapid-freezing electron microscopy. Biophys J 1990;58:1.

Chen W, Lee RC: Altered ion channel conductance and ionic selectivity induced by large imposed membrane potential pulse. Biophys J 1994;67:6.

Cooper MS: Electrical cable theory, transmembrane ion fluxes, and the motile responses of tissue cells to external electrical fields. Presented at the 7th Annual Conference of the IEEE/Engineering in Medicine and Biology Society, "Bioelectric Interactions," Chicago, 1986.

Cravalho EG, Toner M, Gaylor D, Lee RC: Response of cells to supraphysiologic temperatures: experimental measurements and kinetic models. *In* Lee RC, Cravalho EG, Burke JF (eds): Electrical Trauma. New York: Cambridge University Press, 1992:281.

DeFelice LS: Introduction to Membrane Noise. New York: Plenum, 1981.

Gaylor DG, Prakah-Asante A, Lee RC: Significance of cell size and tissue structure in electrical trauma. J Theor Biol 1988;133:223.

Gershfeld NL, Murayama M: Thermal instability of red blood cell membrane bilayers: temperature dependence of hemolysis. J Membr Biol 1968;101:62.

Halliwell B, Gutteridge J (eds): Free Radicals in Biology and Medicine (2nd ed). Oxford, UK: Clarendon Press, 1991.

Henriques FC, Moritz AR: Studies of thermal injury V: the predictability and the significance of thermally induced rate processes leading to irreversible epidermal injury. Arch Pathol 1947;43:489.

Horgan J: In the beginning.... Sci Am 1991;264:117.

Jagger J: Solar-UV Actions on Living Cells. New York: Praeger, 1985.

Karlsson JO, Cravalho EG, Borel Rinkes IH, et al: Nucleation and growth of ice crystals inside cultured hepatocytes during freezing in the presence of dimethyl sulfoxide. Biophys J 1993;65:2524.

Lee RC: Tissue injury from exposure to power frequency electrical fields. *In* JC Lin (ed): Advances in Electromagnetic Fields in Living Systems, Vol 1. New York: Plenum Press, 1994:81.

Lee RC, Gaylor DC, Bhatt D, Israel DA: Role of cell membrane rupture in pathogenesis of electrical trauma. J Surg Res 1988;44:709.

Lee RC, Kolodney MS: Electrical injury mechanisms: electrical breakdown of cell membranes. Plast Reconstr Surg 1988;80:672.

Lee RC, Myerov A, Maloney C: Promising therapy for cell membrane damage. Ann N Y Acad Sci 1994;720:239.

Lee RC, River P, Pan FS, et al: Surfactant-induced sealing of electropermeabilized skeletal muscle membranes in vivo. Proc Natl Acad Sci U S A 1992;89:4524.

Lieber RL, Fazeli BM, Botte MJ: Architecture of selected wrist flexor and extensor muscle. J Hand Surg (Am) 1990;15:244.

Litster JD: Stability of lipid bilayers and red blood cell membranes. Phys Lett 1975;53(A):193.

Moussa NA, McGrath JJ, Cravalho EG, Asimacopoulos PJ: Kinetics of thermal injury in cells. J Biomech Eng 1977;99:155.

Moussa NA, Tell NE, Cravalho EG: Time progression of hemolysis of erythrocyte populations exposed to supraphysiologic temperatures. J Biomech Eng 1979;101:213.

Padanilam JT, Bischof JC, Lee RC, et al: Effectiveness of poloxamer 188 in arresting calcein leakage from thermally damaged isolated skeletal muscle cells. Ann N Y Acad Sci 1994;720:111.

Parsegian A: Energy of an ion crossing a low dielectric membrane: solutions to four relevant problems. Nature 1969;221:844.

Pizzagrello DJ, Witcofski RL: Basic Radiation Biology. Philadelphia: Lea & Febiger, 1967.

Powell KT, Weaver JC: Transient aqueous pore in bilayer membranes: a statistical theory. Bioelectrochem Bioenerg 1986;15:211.

Reilly JP: Scales of reaction to electric shock: thresholds and biophysical mechanisms. Ann N Y Acad Sci 1994;720:21.

Rocchio CM: The kinetics of thermal damage to an isolated skeletal muscle cell. S.B. Thesis, Massachusetts Institute of Technology, Cambridge, 1989.

Schanne OF, Ceretti ERP: Impedance Measurements in Biological Cells. New York: John Wiley & Sons, 1978.

Tanford C: Physical Chemistry of Macromolecules. New York: John Wiley & Sons, 1961:635.

Taylor GI, Michael DH: On making holes in a sheet of fluid. J Fluid Mech 1973;58:625.

Tsong TY: Electroporation of cell membranes. Biophys J 1991;60:297.

Tsong TY, Astumian RD: Electroconformational coupling and membrane protein function. Prog Biophys Mol Biol 1987;50:1.

Tsong TY, Gross CJ: Reversibility of thermally induced denaturation of cellular proteins. Ann N Y Acad Sci 1994;720:65.

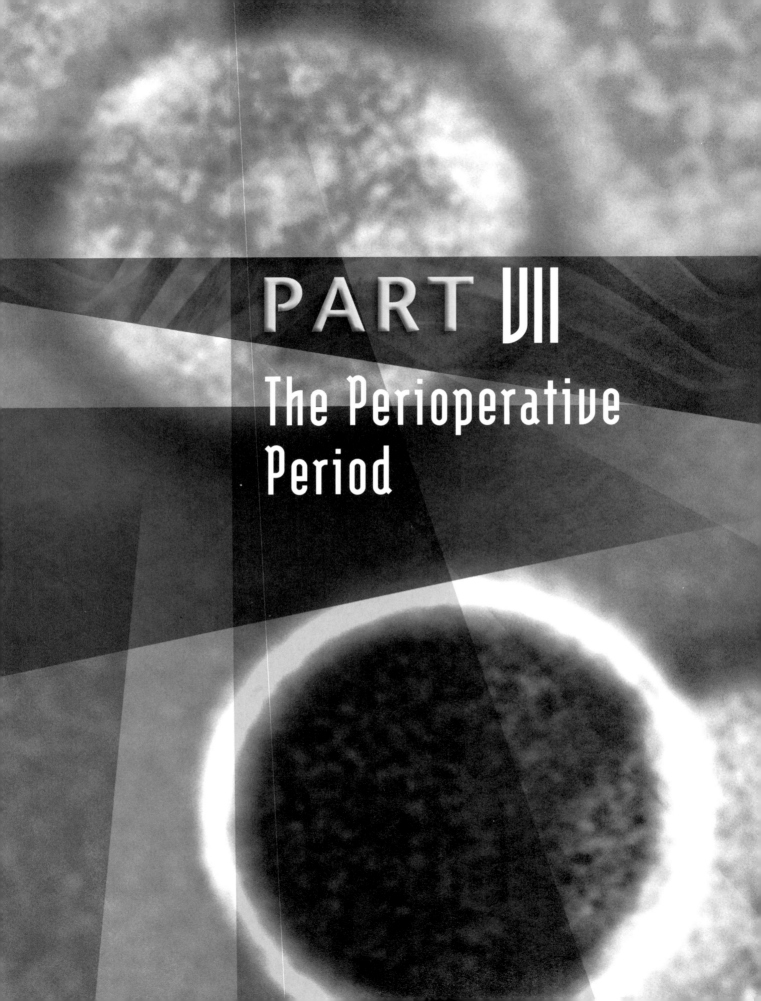

PART VII
The Perioperative Period

CHAPTER 35

Perioperative Fever and Hypothermia

Margaret F. Brock, M.D. and Thomas E. Nelson, Ph.D.

Thermoregulation

Humans, being homeotherms, require maintenance of core temperature within a narrow range for normal metabolic function. This range is maintained by the thermoregulatory system within 0.2°C of normal, which is about 37°C. Even minor deviations may result in cellular and tissue dysfunction. Core temperature is best measured in the pulmonary artery, tympanic membrane, distal esophagus, or nasopharynx. Hypothermia is classified as mild with a core temperature of 32.2° to 35°C, moderate with a temperature of 28° to 32.2°C, or severe with a core temperature below 28°C. Hyperthermia is an increase of core body temperature above normal values. Fever is an elevated core body temperature mediated by an increase in the hypothalamic thermoregulatory set point.

The thermoregulatory system consists of three phases: afferent thermal sensing, central regulation, and efferent responses (Fig. 35–1).

Afferent Thermal Sensing

Anatomically and physiologically distinct cold and warm receptors are located both peripherally and centrally. Receptors in the skin surface, deep abdominal and thoracic tissues, spinal cord, hypothalamus, and other parts of the brain each contribute approximately 20% of input to autonomic temperature control. Cold information travels mostly via A delta fibers, and warm signals through unmyelinated C fibers. Input is transmitted primarily via the spinothalamic tracts in the anterior spinal cord to the hypothalamus, the primary thermoregulatory control center.

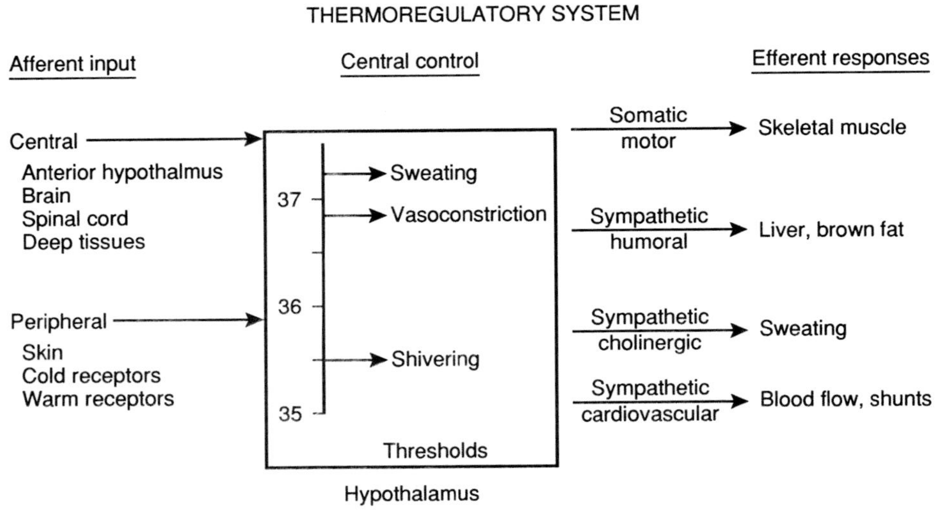

THERMOREGULATORY SYSTEM

FIGURE 35–1 The three main components of the thermoregulatory system: afferent input, the hypothalamic integrating and regulating system, and the efferent responses. (Modified from Flacke WE, Flacke JW: Temperature: homeostasis and unintentional hypothermia. *In* Gravenstein N, Kirby RP [eds]: Complications in Anesthesiology. Philadelphia: Lippincott–Raven, 1996:118.)

Central Regulation

After being preprocessed in the spinal cord and other parts of the central nervous system, integrated thermal inputs from the skin surface, neuraxis, and deep tissues are compared in the hypothalamus with set threshold temperatures for each thermoregulatory response (see Fig. 35–1). Heat- and cold-sensitive neurons in the preoptic area of the anterior hypothalamus integrate the afferent thermal information. The information is relayed to the posterior hypothalamus, which controls the effector response. Each response is characterized by a threshold, gain, and maximal response intensity (Fig. 35–2). The threshold is the core temperature that triggers a certain thermoregulatory response at a particular mean skin temperature. The gain is the slope of the response versus the deviation of core temperature from the threshold. The maximum intensity is the intensity at which the response does not increase with further deviation in core temperature. The interthreshold range of 0.2°C is bounded by the sweating threshold on the upper end and vasoconstriction at the lower end. This range or set point is a thermoneutral zone in which no thermoregulatory autonomic response is elicited.

The means of determination of threshold temperatures is uncertain, but appears to be mediated by norepinephrine, dopamine, 5-hydroxytryptamine, acetylcholine, prostaglandin E_1, and neuropeptides. Human studies have demonstrated diurnal variation of the set point in both sexes, as well as monthly variation in women. Women's sweating and vasoconstriction thresholds are 0.3° to 0.5°C higher than in men. Central regulation is intact in infants, and is even somewhat intact in premature infants. It is frequently impaired in the elderly or extremely ill persons.

Efferent Responses

Behavioral responses depend primarily on input from the skin surface. In contrast, autonomic responses are roughly 80% determined by input from core structures. In the conscious human, behavioral modification (such as increased motor activity, dressing warmly, or adjusting ambient temperature) is the most important effector mechanism.

Cold responses

Energy-efficient mechanisms such as vasoconstriction are maximized before less efficient responses such as shivering are activated. The major autonomic defense against cold is vasoconstriction of arteriovenous shunts located primarily in the toes and fingers. These shunts, 100 μm in diameter, are functionally and anatomically distinct from the skin's nutrient capillaries, which are 10 μm in diameter. The gain of this response is steep, in that control of flow through the shunts is on or off. Local α-adrenergic sympathetic nerves mediate this response, while circulating catecholamines have a minimal impact. Thermoregulatory vasoconstriction does not usually cause a systemic hemodynamic change, because only about 10% of cardiac output travels via these shunts.

Shivering is relatively ineffective because it increases metabolic heat production only 50% to 100% in adults. Shivering does not occur in infants, who depend on nonshivering thermogenesis, which can double heat production in the neonate. Nonshivering thermogenesis is mediated by

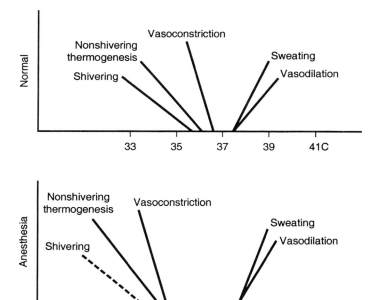

FIGURE 35-2 Activation of thermoregulatory effector responses is triggered at specific threshold temperatures. Under general anesthesia, the threshold temperatures for activation of cold-effector responses are decreased and those for activation of warm-effector responses are increased. (Modified from Sessler DI: Temperature monitoring. *In* Miller RD [ed]: Anesthesia [4th ed]. New York: Churchill Livingstone, 1994:1367.)

β_3-adrenergic receptors on nerves that terminate in brown adipose tissue. This specialized adipose tissue contains large numbers of mitochondria, equipped with a unique uncoupling protein, thermogenin. Metabolic heat production is increased without producing mechanical work because oxidative metabolism is uncoupled to phosphorylation. Heat is produced instead of ATP. In the adult, brown fat is present only in small amounts, so nonshivering thermogenesis increases heat production by less than 10% to 15%. Nonshivering thermogenesis also occurs in the skeletal muscle in the adult. Norepinephrine is the primary control for nonshivering thermogenesis in both brown fat and skeletal muscle.

There is evidence (primarily in animal studies) that hormonal thermogenesis, or non-norepinephrine and non–brown fat thermogenesis, is important in adults and large mammals. This thermogenesis may be induced by substrates such as epinephrine, glucagon, thyroid hormones, peptidergic hormones, and steroid hormones.

On the molecular level, heat production in skeletal muscle is of metabolic origin, resulting from hydrolysis of ATP. Calcium ion recycling is thought to be the major mechanism for skeletal muscle heat production. During contraction, Ca^{2+} is released from storage in the sarcoplasmic reticulum (SR) into the myoplasm. It is returned to the SR by the sarcoendoplasmic reticulum calcium pump (SERCA 1), which translocates two calcium ions for each ATP converted to ADP + P_i + heat. In resting muscle there exists a 10,000-fold calcium concentration gradient from SR to myoplasm, resulting in constant leak from the SR storage site. The released calcium is immediately pumped back inside the SR, generating heat. If the rate of leak from the SR exceeds the return to the lumen, metabolic rate is increased directly by elevated myoplasmic $[Ca^{2+}]$ via activation of enzymes and indirectly by calcium recycling as described above. Thermogenesis by calcium recycling is demonstrated in the heater organ of certain endothermic fish. These cells contain a hypertrophied SR and large numbers of mitochondria. The hypertrophied SR provides an increased surface area to the Ca^{2+}-ATPase, which is the key protein in the heat generation pathway of thermogenic cells.

Warm responses

Sweating is the major mechanism for dissipation of heat when the core temperature exceeds its threshold. It is an active process mediated by postganglionic, cholinergic nerves. Active vasodilation is mediated by an unidentified factor released from sweat glands. The threshold for vasodilation is similar to the sweating threshold, but the gain is less. Maximum sweating intensity occurs at a temperature well below that causing maximum cutaneous vasodilation.

Heat Balance

The total amount of heat maintained in the body is the heat balance. This is decreased by evaporation of sweat and increased by metabolic heat production. Depending on the ambient temperature, body heat content may be increased or reduced by radiation, convection, and conduction. Heat gain may be obligatory, including basal metabolic rate or energy cost of maintaining the body's normal homeostasis; or facultative, depending on thermoregulatory mechanisms to restore heat balance.

Seventy-five percent of heat loss at rest depends on convection, radiation, and conduction (Fig. 35–3). Convection occurs when the insulating layer of air next to the skin is disturbed. Loss resulting from radiation is proportional to the fourth power of the temperature difference between the body and other environmental surfaces. Conduction heat loss is proportional to the amount of heat transferred between two adjacent surfaces. The remaining 25% of heat loss is via evaporation of insensible water, primarily from the respiratory tract or from evaporation of sweat.

Thermal Compartments

The human body consists of a well-perfused core compartment, in which temperature remains relatively uniform, and a peripheral compartment, in which temperature is nonhomogeneous and variable over time. The core compartment comprises 50% of the body mass and consists of the head and trunk, while the arms and legs make up the peripheral compartment. In a moderate climate, a temperature gradient of 2° to 4°C is maintained between the core and periphery by tonic thermoregulatory vasoconstriction.

Heat flows relatively slowly to the periphery and is mediated by blood-borne convection of heat and conduction of heat from adjacent tissues. Accumulation of heat in the periphery is enhanced by local tissue metabolism and reduced by regional cutaneous heat loss to the atmosphere. To maintain a thermal steady state, all metabolic heat must be dissipated to the environment.

Thermoregulation During General Anesthesia

Behavioral thermoregulation is lost during general anesthesia. In normal individuals, general anesthetics do not induce hypothermia or hyperthermia; they just depress the thermoregulatory system (Fig. 35–4). Direction of core temperature change depends on the ambient temperature. Autonomic thermoregulatory control is inhibited in a dose-dependent manner by all intravenous and inhaled anesthetics tested so far. The normal interthreshold range is increased from approximately 0.2° to 4.0°C as a result of a slight increase in warm-response thresholds and a marked decrease in cold-response thresholds (see Fig. 35–2). The volatile agents, characterized by desflurane, increase the sweating threshold approximately 1°C and decrease the vasoconstriction and shivering thresholds 2° to 4°C. The approximately 1° vasoconstriction-to-shivering range remains unchanged; therefore, patients rarely shiver during general anesthesia. Nitrous oxide decreases the shivering threshold and decreases the vasoconstriction threshold to a lesser extent than equipotent doses of volatile anesthetic. Vasoconstriction thresholds are similarly reduced by anesthetics in infants, but are reduced about 1°C further in people ages 60 to 80 years. Nonshivering thermogenesis is inhibited in both adults and infants.

The intravenous agents propofol, alfentanil, and dexmedetomidine produce a marked decrease in the vasoconstriction and shivering thresholds as well as a slight increase in the sweating threshold. Meperidine is efficacious in treatment of shivering because it decreases the shivering threshold to a greater extent. Midazolam has little effect on thermoregulation.

Neuromuscular blocking agents have a quaternary ammonium structure, which prevents penetration of the blood-brain barrier. They have no central effect, but block muscle heat generation. The anticholinergic drug atropine has the peripheral effect of inhibiting sweating. In warm, ambient temperatures this effect may decrease the body's capacity to dissipate heat.

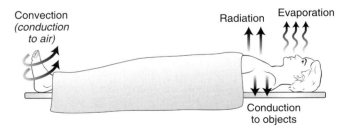

FIGURE 35–3 Mechanisms of heat loss from the body.

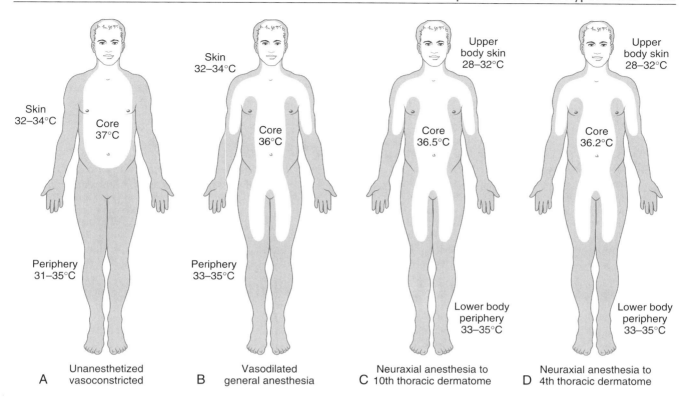

| A | Unanesthetized vasoconstricted | B | Vasodilated general anesthesia | C | Neuraxial anesthesia to 10th thoracic dermatome | D | Neuraxial anesthesia to 4th thoracic dermatome |

FIGURE 35–4 Unanesthetized, vasoconstricted patient (**A**). Cartoon depicting redistribution hypothermia after induction of general anesthesia (**B**). Also shown is redistribution hypothermia after induction of neuraxial anesthesia to the 10th thoracic dermatome (**C**) and the 4th thoracic dermatome (**D**).

Thermoregulation During Regional Anesthesia

Above the level of the block, both epidural and spinal anesthesia decrease the trigger thresholds for vasoconstriction and shivering about 0.6°C. This decrease is unlikely to be due to recirculation of drug to the brain, because the reduction is similar with all local anesthetics regardless of their half-lives and with either spinal or epidural anesthesia.

At leg temperatures in typical operation room environments, most ascending thermal signals originate in cold receptors, so tonic cold signals dominate. Regional anesthesia blocks all thermal information, primarily cold signals, from the lower body. This may be interpreted by the brain as relative leg warming, resulting in reduction of the vasoconstriction and shivering thresholds. In support of this theory, a leg skin temperature of 38°C reduces the threshold the same amount. Therefore, major regional anesthesia appears to reduce the thresholds by producing elevation of apparent rather than actual leg temperature.

Regional anesthetic-induced reduction in the shivering threshold is proportional to the number of segments blocked (see Fig. 35–4). Both the maximum intensity and gain of the shivering response are reduced. Therefore, even when triggered, thermoregulatory defenses are less effective during regional anesthesia.

Supplemental systemic analgesic and sedative medications further impair thermoregulatory control. The effect is worse in the elderly and those with preexisting illness.

Because thermal perception and behavioral response is determined primarily by temperature, core hypothermia may not trigger a perception of cold during regional anesthesia. The patient may experience a perception of warmth even as thermoregulatory responses, including shivering, are activated.

Perioperative Mild Hypothermia

Hypothermia develops during anesthesia as a result of exposure to a cold operating room accompanied by anesthetic impairment of thermoregulation. As discussed above, heat is transferred to the environment in four ways: radiation, conduction, convection, and evaporation (see Fig. 35–3). Radiation and convection contribute the most to perioperative heat loss.

Phases of Development

Intraoperative hypothermia develops in three phases: an initial rapid decrease in core temperature as body heat is redistributed to the periphery, followed by a slow, linear reduction in core temperature, and finally a core temperature plateau (Fig. 35–5). Each phase is due to a different mechanism.

Redistribution phase

The initial rapid decrease in core temperature is due primarily to redistribution of body heat from the core to the periphery (see Fig. 35–4). This occurs during the first 1 to-1.5 hours of anesthesia. Net loss of heat to the environment contributes very little to the decrease. This redistribution occurs during both regional and general anesthesia. During general anesthesia, vasodilation occurs as a result of reduction in the vasoconstriction threshold and direct peripheral vasodilation. During neuraxial anesthesia, there is also central impairment of thermoregulation as well as a block of peripheral sympathetic and motor nerves. Core heat flows down the temperature gradient, normally maintained by tonic thermoregulatory vasoconstriction of arteriovenous shunts, from the core to the periphery. Core temperature is decreased about 0.8°C during regional anesthesia because redistribution is limited to the legs. This is in contrast to the 1° to 1.5°C loss occurring with induction of

general anesthesia. In both regional and general anesthesia, the magnitude of loss depends on the patient's initial body heat content, magnitude of the core-to-periphery gradient, and body morphology. Obese patients redistribute less heat than thin individuals because they are normally more vasodilated to dissipate metabolic heat, and consequently have a higher than normal peripheral temperature.

Linear phase

During this phase, heat loss exceeds metabolic heat production. This net loss occurs with both regional and general anesthesia. The exact cause of the 15% to 40% reduction of metabolic rate during general anesthesia is not established; however, decreased brain metabolism and the use of mechanical ventilation, which spares the diaphragm and chest wall muscles, contribute.

Cutaneous heat loss is mediated by the four mechanisms listed above: radiation, conduction, convection, and evaporation (see Fig. 35–3). The magnitude of heat loss during this phase is greater in infants and children because of their larger body surface area. Larger surgical incisions increase the risk of hypothermia, and warm operating rooms decrease the risk of hypothermia.

RADIATION. Radiation usually contributes the most to the linear phase. Radiation is the transfer of heat between surfaces by photons and does not depend on the temperature of the intervening air. The extent of heat loss depends on both the difference to the fourth power of the object's temperatures in degrees Kelvin and the object's emissivity. Emissivity describes an object's ability to absorb and emit heat. Black bodies emit and absorb heat perfectly and have an emissivity of 1. All colors of human skin have an emissivity of 0.95 for infrared light. Loss of heat from large surgical incisions as a result of radiation is more pronounced than that from small incisions.

CONDUCTION AND CONVECTION. Conduction is the direct transfer of heat between adjacent surfaces, so heat transfer is directly proportional to (1) the difference in temperature between the surface and the skin, and (2) the strength of the insulation between them. Cool intravenous fluids cause loss of heat via conduction as they are warmed to body temperature by the blood and surrounding tissue. As described above, convection occurs when air movement disturbs the insulating layer of air adjacent to the skin surface. Flow of heat is increased in proportion to the square root of the air velocity. In the typical operating room the velocity is nearly 20 cm/sec, so convection is the most important source of heat loss during anesthesia.

EVAPORATION. Normally nonsweating evaporative skin losses and respiratory evaporative losses are small, accounting for approximately 5% and 10% of heat loss,

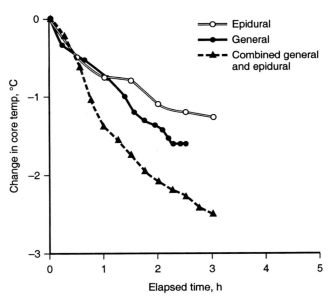

EFFECT OF DIFFERENT MODES OF ANESTHESIA ON LOSS IN CORE TEMPERATURE*

Epidural
General
Combined general and epidural

FIGURE 35–5 Typical patterns of hypothermia during general anesthesia, epidural anesthesia, and combined general and epidural anesthesia. (Adapted from Sessler DI: Perioperative heat balance. Anesthesiology 2000;92:580.)

respectively. Evaporative loss can be substantial from surgical incisions, and core hypothermia is greater with larger incisions. Evaporation of skin preparation solutions also contributes to heat loss. The largest loss occurs with warm or cold alcohol-based solutions, and the smallest loss with radiant warming and water-based solutions.

Core temperature plateau phase

The core temperature plateau usually occurs after 2 to 4 hours of general anesthesia. This plateau can be passive or actively maintained.

PASSIVE PLATEAU. A passive plateau occurs when heat loss equals heat production and thermoregulatory defenses are not activated. This rarely develops in anesthetized patients, but may occur in patients covered over a large surface with effective insulation during operations with small surgical incisions.

ACTIVE PLATEAU. During an actively maintained plateau, thermoregulatory vasoconstriction decreases heat loss and alters the distribution of heat within the body. This thermoregulatory response is activated when the core temperature reaches between 34° and 35°C. Most of the effect of shunt vasoconstriction is to prevent further flow of heat from the core to the periphery. Core temperature is maintained at the expense of the periphery. Cutaneous heat loss is only slightly decreased, so peripheral tissues gradually cool. A thermal steady state is not achieved, and body heat content and mean body temperature decrease.

During neuraxial anesthesia there is no active core temperature plateau, because there is impairment of the central vasoconstriction threshold as well as continued peripheral nerve block in the lower body. This directly prevents vasoconstriction and shivering below the level of the block. Vasoconstriction and shivering in the unblocked upper body triggered by core hypothermia is often insufficient to prevent further hypothermia. Serious hypothermia can occur during prolonged surgeries with large incisions. In addition to inhibition of autonomic response, behavioral response is also affected. Patients may not feel cold and so may not complain.

Use of limb tourniquets in adult patients can induce a core temperature plateau. However, the distal tissues become extremely cold, so a considerable drop in core temperature can occur upon release of the tourniquet.

Combined Regional and General Anesthesia

Combined regional and general anesthesia can result in profound hypothermia. During the redistribution phase, patients become rapidly hypothermic as heat is redistributed to all four extremities, and during the linear phase, patients cool at the higher rate seen with general anesthesia. Both neuraxial and general anesthesia reduce the vasoconstriction threshold; therefore, vasoconstriction occurs later and at a lower core temperature. Heat production by shivering is inhibited by general anesthesia. When the patient is sufficiently hypothermic to reach the vasoconstriction threshold, peripheral nerve block directly prevents vasoconstriction in the legs. Therefore, core temperature continues to decrease throughout surgery because an effective plateau cannot be achieved.

Consequences of Mild Perioperative Hypothermia (Box 35-1)

Benefits

In many animal species, 1° to 3°C of hypothermia provide protection against cerebral ischemia and hypoxemia. Mild hypothermia is far more efficacious in providing protection than barbiturate coma and high-dose isoflurane, which produce comparable reductions in cerebral metabolic rate. The increased protective action of hypothermia may be explained by events other than reduced metabolic rate, such as decreased release of excitatory amino acids. Because of this protective effect, mild hypothermia may be indicated in surgery apt to cause cerebral ischemia, including carotid artery surgery and neurosurgery. In a pilot trial of mild intraoperative hypothermia during cerebral aneurysm surgery, patients with subarachnoid hemorrhage were noted to have a non–statistically significant decrease in neurologic deterioration at 24 and 72 hours postoperatively and a greater incidence of good long-term outcomes. Currently, a multicenter trial is underway to determine the statistical benefit of mild intraoperative hypothermia in patients with acute aneurysmal subarachnoid hemorrhage. Core temperatures near 32°C improved the outcome in patients with traumatic brain injury. Mild hypothermia impedes the triggering of malignant hyperthermia (MH) and, once triggered, lessens its severity. Recovery is facilitated and mortality is decreased by mild hypothermia in patients with adult respiratory distress syndrome.

Complications

Wound infections are a major cause of morbidity and are among the serious complications of surgery and anesthesia. Perioperative hypothermia increases the risk of wound infection by directly impairing immune function and triggering thermoregulatory vasoconstriction with subsequent decline in wound oxygen delivery. In a prospective, randomized clinical trial in patients undergoing colorectal surgery, mild intraoperative hypothermia tripled the incidence of wound infection, significantly delayed wound healing, and prolonged hospitalization by 20%. Protein wasting and decreased synthesis of collagen are associated

Box 35–1

Consequences of Hypothermia on Organ System Function

Cardiovascular

Mild: Increased cardiac output, tachycardia, increased SVR, catecholamine release central redistribution of blood–CHF

Moderate: Decreased cardiac output, bradycardia, hypotension

Severe: Ventricular dysrhythmias

ECG: Sinus bradycardia, prolonged P-R interval, QRS complex, and Q-T interval; T-wave inversion; below 30°C, ventricular ectopy; below 31°C, J or Osborn wave; below 28°C, ventricular fibrillation

Pulmonary

Mild: Increased respiratory rate

Moderate: Decreased respiratory rate and tidal volume, increased PVR, decreased hypoxic pulmonary vasoconstriction, increased anatomic dead space, decreased ventilatory response to hypercarbia and hypoxemia, decreased mucociliary function

Renal

Mild: Increased RVR, decreased RBF and GFR, "cold diuresis" resulting from increased central blood volume

Moderate: Diuresis resulting from decreased renal tubular sodium reabsorption

Severe: Oliguria and azotemia

Hematologic

Mild: Hemoconcentration, increased blood viscosity, left shift of oxyhemoglobin dissociation curve (decreased oxygen availability)

Moderate: Thrombocytopenia, disseminated intravascular coagulation (increased bleeding risk)

Metabolic

Mild: Hyponatremia, hyperkalemia; hyperglycemia resulting from decreased glucose utilization with inhibition of release and cellular uptake of insulin; decreased metabolic rate (increased shivering)

Moderate: Metabolic acidosis (decreased tissue perfusion)

Drug disposition

Mild: Decreased hepatic blood flow and metabolism, decreased renal blood flow excretion, increased solubility of anesthetics, increased duration of muscle relaxants

Neurologic

Mild: Increased CVR, decreased CBF and CMRO; cerebral blood flow decreases 6%–7% per 1°C decrease in temperature; decreased MAC

34°C: amnesia; 30°C: obtundation; 26°C: loss of papillary and deep tendon reflexes; 18°C: isoelectric EEG

Gastrointestinal

Mild: Decreased intestinal motility with increased risk of full stomach

Moderate: Ulcers of stomach, ileum, and colon; hemorrhagic pancreatitis

Immune

Mild: Impaired chemotaxis and phagocytosis of granulocytes, decreased motility of macrophages, decreased antibody production, decreased oxidative killing by neutrophils (increased risk wound infection); decreased collagen deposition (poor wound healing)

CBF, cerebral blood flow; CHF, congestive heart failure; CMRO, cerebral metabolic rate of oxygen; CVR, cerebrovascular resistance; ECG, electrocardiogram; EEG, electroencephalogram; GFR, glomerular filtration rate; MAC, minimum alveolar concentration; PVR, pulmonary vascular resistance; RBF, renal blood flow; RVR, renal vascular resistance; SVR, systemic vascular resistance.

Modified from Young CC, Sladen RN: Treatment of the hypothermic patient. In Atlee JL (ed): Complications in Anesthesia. Philadelphia, WB Saunders, 1999:450.

with hypothermia; both delay wound healing even in patients without infection. Because the thermoregulatory thresholds are 1°C lower in the elderly, it is extremely important to prevent hypothermia to impede increased protein breakdown or decreased protein synthesis.

Both platelet activity and the enzymes of the coagulation cascade are impaired by mild hypothermia. A prospective, randomized clinical trial showed that hypothermia significantly increased the blood loss and need for allogeneic blood transfusion in patients undergoing elective hip arthroplasty. Morbid cardiac outcomes have been attributed to mild hypothermia. This consequence of hypothermia is serious, because myocardial ischemia is a leading cause of perioperative death. A prospective, randomized, controlled trial of over 300 patients undergoing major noncardiac surgery found that maintenance of normothermia reduced the incidence of angina, myocardial infarction, ventricular tachycardia, and cardiac arrest. The metabolism of many drugs is decreased by mild hypothermia. The duration of action of the muscle relaxants vecuronium and atracurium, as well as propofol, is significantly prolonged. The pharmacodynamics of the volatile anesthetics is also affected by hypothermia. The minimum alveolar concentration is reduced about 5%/°C. At core temperatures lower than 20°C, no anesthesia is required to prevent movement in response to skin incision. As expected with decreased metabolism, the postoperative recovery period is significantly prolonged by mild intraoperative hypothermia. Emergence from anesthesia may be delayed as a result of impairment of the central nervous system, slowed hepatic or renal clearance of anesthetics or muscle relaxants, and impaired ventilatory response to hypoxemia and hypercarbia.

In the postoperative period, the sensation of cold and the presence of shivering are both physiologically and psychologically stressful to the patient. Some patients report the thermal discomfort as being worse than surgical pain. Shivering is associated with substantial activation of the sympathetic nervous system, including increases in plasma catecholamines, systemic blood pressure, and heart rate. However, in two prospective, randomized, controlled studies, shivering has been shown not to correlate with adverse cardiac outcomes. In the elderly postoperative patient, shivering occurs with low intensity and frequency, increasing the metabolic rate by an average of only 40% versus 400% in younger patients.

Skin surface warming, clonidine (75 µg IV), physostigmine (0.04 mg/kg), magnesium sulfate (30 mg/kg), or meperidine (12.5 mg IV) can be used to treat postoperative shivering.

Treatment and Prevention

During surgery, most patients do not reach a level of hypothermia adequate to trigger thermoregulatory vasoconstriction. Because the skin is the chief source of heat loss perioperatively, techniques to limit this loss are most important. Ambient temperature is the most important factor in determining the rate of loss by radiation and convection from the skin as well as evaporation from surgical incisions. The optimal temperature to maintain normothermia needs to be greater than 23°C, which is uncomfortable to operating room personnel.

Forced-air warming systems are the best method to maintain normothermia intraoperatively. These are most effective when used intraoperatively in the vasodilated patient, because the applied heat is more effectively distributed to the core. Postoperatively, thermoregulatory vasoconstriction is no longer opposed by the vasodilatory effects of general anesthesia. Therefore, the transfer of cutaneously applied heat to the core is reduced. Patients receiving major neuraxial blockade may still be vasodilated postoperatively and therefore rewarm more quickly with forced-air warming. If time allows, active prewarming for 30 minutes can diminish the initial redistribution of core heat to the periphery by increasing body heat content.

A single layer of passive insulation in the form of cotton blankets or surgical drapes reduces heat loss about 30%. Its effectiveness is primarily determined by the amount of surface area covered. This is most effective for shorter and less extensive operations. Applying more than one layer or prewarming the cotton blankets adds little benefit.

Heating and humidifying inspired gases is relatively ineffective, because only 10% of body heat is lost via the respiratory system. Heat loss via conduction becomes significant when large amounts of refrigerated blood or room-temperature crystalloid are administered. These losses can be minimized by fluid warmers. When large amounts of fluids need to be administered rapidly, high-volume systems, with strong heaters and low resistance, are useful.

Severe Hypothermia

Deliberate Severe Intraoperative Hypothermia

During cardiac and certain neurosurgical procedures, severe hypothermia is induced to provide protection against cardiac and cerebral ischemia. Whole-body metabolic rate decreases by approximately 8%/°C. At 28°C the metabolic rate is close to half the normal rate. This confers protection against tissue ischemia by allowing aerobic metabolism to continue during periods of decreased oxygen supply. Hypothermia also provides protection via membrane stabilization and decreased release of toxic metabolites.

All organ function is affected by severe hypothermia (see Box 35–1). Blood gas interpretation becomes difficult in the hypothermic patient, because the pH of blood increases 0.015 units with each 1°C decrease in temperature.

This occurs because carbon dioxide is more soluble in blood and plasma bicarbonate concentration increases as more carbonic acid is ionized. Blood gases may be interpreted using the pH-stat method, which mimics compensatory methods of hibernating homeotherms. This method aims to keep constant arterial pH at 7.40 and arterial carbon dioxide tension at 40 mm Hg at any given temperature.

The alpha-stat strategy allows pH to vary with body temperature, which mimics poikilotherms. This method aims to keep a constant ratio of [OH⁻]:[H⁺] at 16:1. Blood pH is regulated to keep the stage of dissociation of the imidazole moiety of histidine constant. Histidine is present in many enzyme systems, whose function is optimal when the ratio of [OH⁻]:[H⁺] is 16:1. This ratio occurs during different pH values at different temperatures. Alpha-stat is used most often during adult cardiopulmonary bypass, because cerebral blood flow autoregulation appears to remain intact. pH-stat is associated with improved neurologic outcome in children during deep hypothermic circulatory arrest, because cerebral blood flow becomes pressure dependent.

Accidental Severe Hypothermia

Severe hypothermia occurs commonly in the elderly, neonates, or unconscious and immobile people exposed to cold. Associated conditions include alcoholism, drug addiction, mental illness, endocrine deficiency states, malnutrition, uremia, severe infection, stroke, myocardial infarction, cirrhosis, and pancreatitis. If not treated, the patient experiences fatal multisystem organ failure, including intractable ventricular dysrhythmias, congestive heart failure, pneumonia, stroke, and pancreatitis (see Box 35–1).

Patients with severe hypothermia must be actively rewarmed. This is best done by active core rewarming. In the severely hypothermic patient, heating and humidifying air, warming intravenous fluids with heat exchanged, and peritoneal lavage with heated dialysate achieve core rewarming. Cardiopulmonary bypass is the best method to rewarm patients with hemodynamic instability or circulatory arrest. Most rhythm disturbances are difficult to treat at temperatures below 28°C. At 27°C, defibrillation is ineffective in treatment of ventricular fibrillation. Temperature must be raised to 28° to 30°C before defibrillation is effective.

Perioperative Fever

Definition of Fever

Fever is a regulated increase in body temperature resulting from the elevation of the set point temperature. Exogenous pyrogens (e.g., endotoxin) and the consequently produced endogenous pyrogens, including interleukin-1, tumor necrosis factor, interferon-α, and macrophage inflammatory protein-1, activate it. Several theories exist on how pyrogens activate the hypothalamus. These include carrier-mediated transport of cytokines into the brain, and passage of pyrogenic messages from the blood to the brain by crossing the capillaries at the organum vasculosum of the laminae terminalis, which lack a blood-brain barrier. These blood-borne pyrogens cause the release of prostaglandins in the preoptic area that may mediate passage of pyrogenic messages from the blood to the brain. Vagally mediated signals to brainstem noradrenergic cell groups, which transmit signals to the preoptic area, also trigger release of prostaglandins. Thermoregulatory response thresholds are increased because pyrogens decrease the firing rate in preoptic warm-sensitive neurons. The cold defenses, vasoconstriction and shivering, are activated until the core temperature reaches the new set point. Defervescence is initiated when the presence of pyrogens decreases and the reduced set point results in recovery of the heat loss defenses, vasodilatation and sweating.

Differential Diagnosis of Perioperative Fever

The differential diagnosis of perioperative fever includes allergic reactions, transfusion reactions, infection, noninfectious inflammation, deep venous thrombosis, pulmonary embolism, blood in the fourth cerebral ventricle, major trauma, tumor resection, autoimmune disease, metabolic diseases such as pheochromocytoma and thyrotoxicosis, drug-induced causes such as MH, anticholinergic effect, cocaine or tricyclic antidepressants, and iatrogenic causes such as increased room temperature and excess warming blankets.

Fever is uncommon intraoperatively because of anesthetic-induced inhibition of the warm responses. Paralysis during general and regional anesthesia prevents shivering, which is probably a chief block to the development of fever. Postoperative fever, mostly stemming from wound infections, remains a major problem.

The increased metabolic rate associated with fever results in increased oxygen consumption leading to increased heart rate, stroke volume, and cardiac output. Acidosis and myocardial ischemia can occur if metabolic demand exceeds oxygen delivery. Compensatory thermoregulatory responses of sweating and vasodilatation can result in decreased intravascular volume and preload, causing further decrease in oxygen delivery. Electrolyte abnormalities occur with excessive perspiration. There is a rightward shift in the oxygen-hemoglobin dissociation curve; therefore, hemoglobin has a lower affinity for oxygen. Neurologic injury after ischemia or status epilepticus may be worse because of the increase in cerebral metabolic rate and increased cerebral blood flow.

Treatment

Fever is best managed by treating the underlying cause. Antibiotics and nonsteroidal anti-inflammatory drugs are useful for infectious and noninfectious fevers, respectively. Excessively high core temperatures (over 39°C) may need to be actively cooled. Methods include skin surface cooling, which may trigger thermoregulatory responses such as shivering or vasoconstriction, resulting in cardiac stress. Other means include cooled intravenous solutions; ice-water lavage into the surgical wound, bladder, stomach, or rectum; and cardiopulmonary bypass.

Malignant Hyperthermia

Definition

MH is a pharmacogenetic disease that predisposes to an anesthetic agent-induced life-threatening, hypermetabolic state. MH is inherited as an autosomal dominant trait with variable penetrance. Patients presenting with a family history of MH must be considered susceptible to the disease. Most individuals with MH have no clinical signs of the disease until they are exposed to certain anesthetic agents. The underlying cause of MH is a defect in regulation of calcium in skeletal muscle, and at present this is linked to mutation in either the voltage-gated calcium channel (*DHPR*) or the ryanodine receptor (*RYR1*) calcium channel genes. Two malignant hyperthermia–susceptible (MHS) families have been reported with linkage to mutations in the *DHPR* gene, while 50% to 80% of families have linkage to mutations in the *RYR1* gene. Currently, over 30 different mutations in the *RYR1* gene have linked to MH in a large number of unrelated families. These mutations predispose to an increase in myoplasmic calcium when exposed to the "trigger" anesthetic agents, and, depending on the amount of rise in myoplasmic calcium level, the response may be a large (up to fivefold) increase in oxygen consumption and skeletal muscle contracture. Unabated, this calcium-induced hypermetabolic state will fulminantly lead to acidosis and electrolyte disturbances incompatible with life.

Clinical Presentation

The trigger drugs for MH include all potent volatile anesthetics and succinylcholine. Safe and adequate anesthesia can be provided for MHS individuals. Safe agents include barbiturates, narcotics, propofol, nitrous oxide, and local anesthetics. The identification of MH in a family is almost always by a clinical episode in the proband. The clinical features of MH can vary from individual to individual and may be influenced by the genotype and the environment, especially the mode of anesthesia. The most potent MH trigger would be simultaneous administration of a volatile agent and succinylcholine, which could produce an immediate global skeletal muscle rigidity and cardiac arrest secondary to hyperkalemia. The same drugs in another MHS patient may produce masseter muscle rigidity, tachycardia, and increased metabolism. While in these cases an immediate onset of MH is apparent, in other patients the onset may be insidious over several minutes or may occur in the postanesthesia care unit. Intraoperatively, the most common early signs of MH include increases in carbon dioxide production, which in the spontaneously breathing patient is associated with hyperpnea, and tachycardia. Skeletal muscle rigidity occurs in some patients, and a rapid rise in body temperature is often one of the late signs. Reduced mortality and morbidity from MH are associated with an early diagnosis and rapid treatment onset.

Treatment

Treatment includes stopping trigger agents; administration of 100% oxygen; administration of dantrolene, 2 mg/kg initially, followed by 1 mg/kg until definite signs of therapeutic response are noted; and, following determination of arterial blood gas values, appropriate correction of respiratory and metabolic acidosis. If temperature is rising or elevated, then aggressive cooling measures should be undertaken. The MH clinical syndrome may produce profound rhabdomyolysis, and appropriate fluid management is critical to prevent renal failure. Recrudescence as high as 25% has been reported, and, consequently, the patient should be closely monitored over 48 hours.

Counseling

The discovery of MHS in a family should be followed by counseling regarding the seriousness of the disease, its inheritance, and the need to wear Medic Alert identification for MH. Family members should be informed about diagnostic testing, which is done only at specialized centers that perform in vitro contracture testing of fresh, surgically removed skeletal muscle. Muscle fascicles are mounted in a contracture chamber and exposed to halothane and caffeine, and the contracture response to these two drugs is used to identify MHS in an individual. The MH muscle contracture test is 98% specific and 76% sensitive. Details about MH and the current diagnostic centers can be found on the web site of the Malignant Hyperthermia Association of the United States (*www.mhaus.org*).

Bibliography

Antognini JF: Hypothermia eliminates isoflurane requirements at 20°C. Anesthesiology 1993;78:1152.

Block BA: Thermogenesis in muscle. Annu Rev Physiol 1994; 56:535.

Boulant JA, Bignall KE: Hypothalamic neuronal responses to peripheral and deep-body temperatures. Am J Physiol 1973;225:1371.

Boulant JA, Demieville HN: Responses of thermosensitive preoptic and septal neurons to hippocampal and brain stem stimulation. J Neurophysiol 1977;40:1356.

Boulant JA, Hardy JD: The effect of spinal and skin temperatures on the firing rate and thermosensitivity of preoptic neurones. J Physiol 1974;240:639.

Buggy DJ, Crossley AW: Thermoregulation, mild perioperative hypothermia and postanesthetic shivering. Br J Anaesth 2000;84:615.

Burton AC: Human calorimetry: the average temperature of the tissues of the body. J Nutr 1935;9:261.

Cheng C, Matsukawa T, Sessler DI, et al: Increasing mean skin temperature linearly reduces the core-temperature thresholds for vasoconstriction and shivering in humans. Anesthesiology 1995;82:1160.

Chinet A, Decrouy A, Even PC: Ca++-dependent heat production under basal and near-basal conditions in the mouse soleus muscle. J Physiol (Lond) 1992;455:663.

Cork RC, Vaughan RW, Humphrey LS: Precision and accuracy of intraoperative temperature monitoring. Anesth Analg 1983;62:211.

Davatelis G, Wolpe SD, Sherry B, et al: Macrophage inflammatory protein-1: a prostaglandin-independent endogenous pyrogen. Science 1989;243:1066.

Dawkins MJ, Scopes JW: Non-shivering thermogenesis and brown adipose tissue in the human new-born infant. Nature 1965;206:201.

Eger EL II, Johnson BH: MAC of I-653 in rats, including a test of the effect of body temperature and anesthetic duration. Anesth Analg 1987;66:974.

Emerick TH, Ozaki M, Sessler DI, et al: Epidural anesthesia increases apparent leg temperature and decreases the shivering threshold. Anesthesiology 1994;81:289.

Faries G, Johnston C, Pruitt KM, et al: Temperature relationship to distance and flow rate of warmed IV fluids. Ann Emerg Med 1991;20:1198.

Frank SM, Fleisher LA, Breslow MJ, et al: Perioperative maintenance of normothermia reduces the incidence of morbid cardiac events: a randomized clinical trial. JAMA 1997;277:1127.

Frank SM, Higgins MS, Breslow MJ, et al: The catecholamine, cortisol, and hemodynamic responses to mild perioperative hypothermia: a randomized clinical trial. Anesthesiology 1995;82:83.

Glosten B, Sessler DI, Faure EAM, et al: Central temperature changes are poorly perceived during epidural anesthesia. Anesthesiology 1992;77:10.

Hales JRS: Skin arteriovenous anastomoses: their control and role in thermoregulation. In Johansen K, Burggrem W (eds): Cardiovascular Shunts: Phylogenetic, Ontogenetic and Clinical Aspects. Copenhagen: Munksgaard, 1985:433.

Hardy JD, Milhorat AT, DuBois EF: Basal metabolism and heat loss of young women at temperatures from 22 degrees C to 35 degrees C. J Nutr 1941;21:383.

Heier T, Caldwell JE, Sessler DI, et al: Mild intraoperative hypothermia increases duration of action and spontaneous recovery of vecuronium blockade during nitrous oxide-isoflurane anesthesia in humans. Anesthesiology 1991;74:815.

Hemingway A, Price WM: The autonomic nervous system and regulation of body temperature. Anesthesiology 1968;29:693.

Hervey GR: Thermoregulation. In Emslie-Smith D, Paterson C, Scratcherd T, Read N (eds): Textbook of Physiology (11th ed). Edinburgh: Churchill Livingstone, 1988:510.

Hindman BJ, Todd MM, Gelb AW, et al: Mild hypothermia as a protective therapy during intercranial aneurysm surgery: a randomized prospective pilot trial. Neurosurgery 1999;44:23.

Hynson JM, Sessler DI: Intraoperative warming therapies: a comparison of three devices. J Clin Anesth 1992;4:194.

Hynson JM, Sessler DI, Moayeri A, et al: Absence of nonshivering thermogenesis in anesthetized adult humans. Anesthesiology 1993;79:695.

Jansky L: Humoral thermogenesis and its role in maintaining energy balance. Physiol Rev 1995;75:237.

Jessen C, Feistkorn G: Some characteristics of core temperature signals in the conscious goat. Am J Physiol 1984;247:R456.

Joris J, Ozaki M, Sessler DI, et al: Epidural anesthesia impairs both central and peripheral thermoregulatory control during general anesthesia. Anesthesiology 1994;80:268.

Kim J-S, Ikeda T, Sessler DI, et al: Epidural anesthesia reduces the gain and maximum intensity of shivering. Anesthesiology 1996;84:1327.

Kor T: Hyperthermia. In Atlee JL (ed): Complications in Anesthesia. Philadelphia: WB Saunders, 1999:452.

Kurz A, Kurz M, Poeschl G, et al: Forced-air warming maintains intraoperative normothermia better than circulating-water mattresses. Anesth Analg 1993;77:89.

Kurz A, Plattner O, Sessler DI, et al: The threshold for thermoregulatory vasoconstriction during nitrous oxide/isoflurane anesthesia is lower in elderly than in young patients. Anesthesiology 1993;79:465.

Kurz A, Sessler DI, Annadata R, et al: Meperidine slightly increases the sweating threshold, but markedly decreases the vasoconstriction and shivering thresholds [abstract]. Anesthesiology 1995;83(3A):A169.

Kurz A, Sessler DI, Lenhardt R: Perioperative normothermia to reduce the incidence of surgical-wound infection and shorten hospitalization. N Engl J Med 1996; 334:1209.

Lazar HL: The treatment of hypothermia. N Engl J Med 1997; 337:1545.

Lenhardt R, Marker E, Goll V, et al: Mild intraoperative hypothermia prolongs postanesthetic recovery. Anesthesiology 1997;87:1318.

Lenhardt R, Negishi C, Sessler DI: Perioperative fever. Acta Anaesth Scand Suppl 1997;111:325.

Leslie K, Sessler DI: Reduction in the shivering threshold is proportional to spinal block height. Anesthesiology 1996; 84:1327.

Leslie K, Sessler DI, Bjorksten AR, et al: Mild hypothermia alters propofol pharmacokinetics and increases the duration of action of atracurium. Anesth Analg 1995;80:1007.

Lopez M, Sessler DI, Walter K, et al: Rate and gender dependence of the sweating, vasoconstriction, and shivering thresholds in humans. Anesthesiology 1994;80:780.

Marion DW, Penrod LE, Kelsey SF, et al: Treatment of traumatic brain injury with moderate hypothermia. N Engl J Med 1997;336:540.

Matsukawa T, Sessler DI, Sessler AM, et al: Heat flow and distribution during induction of general anesthesia. Anesthesiology 1995;82:662.

Michelson AD, MacGregor H, Barnard MR, et al: Reversible inhibition of human platelet activation by hypothermia in vivo and in vitro. Thromb Haemost 1994;71:633.

Nelson TE: Porcine malignant hyperthermia: critical temperatures for in vivo and in vitro responses. Anesthesiology 1990;73:449.

Nelson TE: Heat production during anesthetic-induced malignant hyperthermia. Biosci Rep 2001;21:169.

Orkin FK: Physiologic disturbances associated with induced hypothermia. In Gravenstein N, Kirby RR (eds): Complications in Anesthesiology (2nd ed). Philadelphia: Lippincott–Raven, 1996:131.

Ozaki M, Kurz A, Sessler DI, et al: Thermoregulatory thresholds during epidural and spinal anesthesia. Anesthesiology 1994;81:282.

Ozaki M, Sessler DI, Suzuki H, et al: Nitrous oxide decreases the threshold for vasoconstriction less than sevoflurane or isoflurane. Anesth Analg 1995;80:1212.

Passias TC, Mekjavic IB, Eiken O: The effect of 30% nitrous oxide on thermoregulatory responses in humans during hypothermia. Anesthesiology 1992;76:550.

Pierau F-K, Wurster RD: Primary afferent input from cutaneous thermoreceptors. Fed Proc 1981;40:2819.

Plattner O, Semsroth M, Sessler DI, et al: Lack of nonshivering thermogenesis in infants anesthetized with fentanyl and propofol. Anesthesiology 1997;86:772.

Poulos DA: Central processing of cutaneous temperature information. Fed Proc 1981;40:2825.

Schmied H, Kurz A, Sessler DI, et al: Mild hypothermia increases blood loss and transfusion requirements during total hip arthroplasty. Lancet 1996;347:289.

Sessler DI: Central thermoregulatory inhibition by general anaesthesia. Anesthesiology 1991;75:5573.

Sessler DI: Temperature monitoring. In Miller RD (ed): Anesthesia. New York: Churchill Livingstone, 1994:1363.

Sessler DI: Perioperative thermoregulation and heat balance. Ann N Y Acad Sci 1997;813:757.

Sessler DI: Perioperative heat balance. Anesthesiology 2000;92:578.

Sessler DI: Temperature monitoring. In Miller RD (ed): Anesthesia. New York: Churchill Livingstone, 2000:1367.

Sessler DI, McGuire J, Sessler AM: Perioperative thermal insulation. Anesthesiology 1991;74:875.

Sheffield CW, Sessler DI, Hopf HW, et al: Centrally and locally mediated thermoregulatory responses alter subcutaneous oxygen tension. Wound Rep Reg 1997;4:339.

Simon E: Temperature regulation: the spinal cord as a site of extrahypothalamic thermoregulatory functions. Rev Physiol Biochem Pharmacol 1974;71:1.

Staab DB, Sorenson VJ, Fath JJ, et al: Coagulation defects resulting from ambient temperature-induced hypothermia. J Trauma 1994;36:634.

Todd NM, Warner DS: A comfortable hypothesis reevaluated: cerebral metabolic depression and brain protection during ischemia. Anesthesiology 1992;76:161.

van Oss CJ, Absolom DR, Moore LL, et al: Effect of temperature on the chemotaxis, phagocytic engulfment, digestion and O_2 consumption of human polymorphonuclear leukocytes. J Reticuloendothel Soc 1980;27:561.

Villar J, Slutsky AS: Effects of induced hypothermia in patients with septic adult respiratory distress syndrome. Resuscitation 1993;26:183.

Vitez TS, White PF, Eger EI II: Effects of hypothermia on halothane MAC and isoflurane MAC in the rat. Anesthesiology 1974;41:80.

Walpoth BH, Walpoth-Aslan BN, Mattle HP, et al: Outcome of survivors of accidental deep hypothermia and circulatory arrest treated with extracorporeal blood warming. N Engl J Med 1997;337:1500.

Washington DE, Sessler DI, Moayeri A, et al: Thermoregulatory responses to hyperthermia during isoflurane anesthesia in humans. J Appl Physiol 1993;74:82.

Wass CT, Lanier WL, Hofer RE, et al: Temperature changes of $\geq 1°C$ alter functional neurologic outcome and histopathology in a canine model of complete cerebral ischemia. Anesthesiology 1995;83:325.

Wyss CR, Brengelmann GL, Johnson JM, et al: Altered control of skin blood flow at high skin and core temperatures. J Appl Physiol 1975;38:839.

CHAPTER 36

Nutrition

Joshua M.V. Mammen, M.D. and Josef E. Fischer, M.D.

The previous century witnessed dramatic improvements in numerous areas of medicine, including antibiotics, blood transfusions, critical care, anesthesiology, transplantation, and cardiopulmonary bypass. To this extensive list must be added nutritional support, which has played a substantial role in improving our care of the surgical patient. While the history of nutritional supplementation extends back to the ancient Egyptian nutrient enemas, the most important contributions occurred more recently, particularly during the latter half of the 20th century. Dudrick and colleagues performed seminal work in Rhoads' laboratory at the University of Pennsylvania by maintaining puppies on total parenteral nutrition (TPN). An equally important advance was Aubiniac's subclavian venipuncture, which enabled the administration of hypertonic dextrose to support a calorie:nitrogen ratio that would support nitrogen equilibrium. The initial overwhelming acceptance of parenteral nutrition has been tempered recently by more critical evaluation of its effect on patient outcome. Additionally, new interest has developed in the field of nutritional pharmacology, in which specific nutrients are utilized to address specific disease states. Recent studies that have demonstrated a clear benefit for the enteral route of nutritional support, which has replaced parenteral nutrition in patients whose gastrointestinal tract is functional.

Protein

Protein is the most important nutrient because it is required for all organic functions. The synthesis and degradation of protein are energy-requiring processes, with degradation providing only one fourth of the energy required for synthesis. Because of this, the utilization of protein as a source of energy is physiologically wasteful.

Amino Acids

Amino acids are utilized in three major ways by the body: (1) protein synthesis, (2) catabolic reactions leading to either urea or carbon dioxide, and (3) synthesis of nonessential amino acids and other small molecules (i.e., purines and pyrimidines).

Basic structure

The central components of amino acids are an amino group and a carboxyl group attached to a carbon atom from which a side chain extends. The side chain is composed of one or more carbon atoms, except for glycine, in which the side chain is a hydrogen atom. The amino acids are further classified as optically active isomers that rotate polarized light to the left (levorotatory or L-form) or to the right (dextrorotatory or D-form). Amino acids are also classified based on electrical charge and side chain.

Essential and conditionally indispensable amino acids

Essential amino acids have a carbon skeleton that cannot be synthesized by the body, but requires an external source. The classic examples are valine, leucine, isoleucine, lysine, methionine, phenylalanine, threonine, and tryptophan. Cysteine and tyrosine are synthesized from methionine and tryptophan, respectively, and hence are conditionally indispensable. For those individuals with low synthetic rates, particularly infants, or increased demands, histidine, proline, hydroxyproline, glutamine, and arginine are also conditionally indispensable. Thus, in critical illness, the majority of amino acids are either essential or conditionally indispensable.

Transport

Several transport systems have been suggested to allow for transport of amino acids into cells, although only a few cell lines have been examined to date:

1. A system: an energy- and sodium-dependent system with an affinity for neutral amino acids; stimulated by insulin

2. L system: a sodium-independent system transporting branched-chain and aromatic amino acids as well as methionine and histidine; exchanges for intracellular amino acids and is competitive

3. Two transport systems for basic amino acids

4. Transport system for dicarboxylic amino acids

Different metabolic conditions likely modify amino acid transport, thereby producing physiologic changes.

Turnover: synthesis and degradation

The synthesis of protein is an energy-requiring process, which leads from DNA to messenger RNA to charge transfer RNA to polysomes to amino acids. In protein degradation, amino acids are catabolized to ammonia, urea, carbon dioxide, glucose, and energy. All of the indispensable amino acids except those with branched chains (valine, leucine, and isoleucine) are degraded in the liver. Skeletal muscle has a major role in branched-chain amino acid catabolism. Of the 20 amino acids, 12 are transaminated to an α-ketoacid, which is then converted to glucose or oxidized to carbon and high-energy phosphate by the tricarboxylic acid cycle. The branched-chain amino acids are transaminated with pyruvate to alanine and with glutamate to glutamine. Oxidative deamination is a less important pathway. A final protein degradation pathway involves urea synthesis, in which the liver and the kidney are involved (arginosuccinic acid cycle) (Fig. 36–1).

Regulation of amino acid levels within organs, including muscle

Skeletal muscle contains the majority of the amino acids in the body. Glutamine comprises 50% to 60% of white, fast-twitch and mixed muscles. Within 20 hours of an operative procedure or trauma, a large portion of the glutamine store has been depleted, and it is only replaced up to 8 weeks later. The importance of this phenomenon of rapid depletion followed by slow refilling of glutamine stores is unclear at this time. Some success has been achieved in preventing glutamine depletion by using glutamine supplementation in parenteral nutrition, but no clinical significance has been demonstrated.

The regulation of muscle protein synthesis and degradation differs in white, fast-twitch muscle and red, slow-twitch muscle. Protein synthesis is modulated by insulin, amino acid supplementation, branched-chain amino acid concentration, and likely human growth hormone, somatomedin, and insulin-like growth factor-1. Normally, 60% to 100% of daily nitrogen retention is due to the postprandial branched-chain amino acid uptake into skeletal muscle. In sepsis, protein synthesis rate is decreased partially as a result of a concomitant decrease in branched-chain amino acids. Insulin-mediated protein synthesis is depressed in muscle. Muscle proteolysis is mainly in white, fast-twitch muscle, with 3-methylhistidine (3-MH) being a major marker. Stimuli for catabolism include glucagon, steroids, epinephrine, interleukin-1 (IL-1), tumor necrosis factor (TNF), and interleukin-6 (IL-6).

Muscle proteolysis includes lysosomal and nonlysosomal, calcium-dependent and calcium-independent, and energy-requiring and non–energy-requiring pathways.

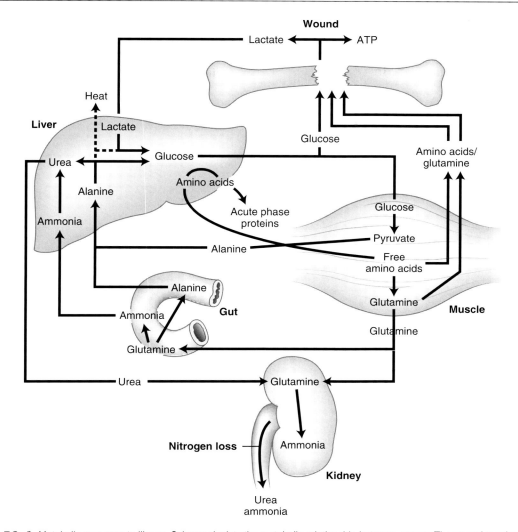

FIGURE 36–1 Metabolic response to illness. Scheme depicts the metabolic relationship between organs. The wound requires glucose, arginine, and likely glutamine. The movement of amino acids from muscle to the liver results in acute-phase protein production to fight infection. (Adapted from Bessey PQ: Metabolic response to critical illness. *In* Wilmore DW, Cheung LY, Harken AH, et al (eds): Scientific American Surgery, Section II, Subsection 11. New York: Scientific American, 1996. Copyright Scientific American, Inc. All rights reserved.)

The ubiquitin pathway is one of the most important of the energy-requiring pathways. Proteolysis in white, fast-twitch muscles is a result of the disruption of Z bands by calcium release of myofilaments, with the subsequent degradation of the released myofilaments by the ubiquitin-proteasome system.

Roles of the Kidney

In protein metabolism, the kidney produces urea from ammonia via the argininosuccinate cycle, produces ammonia from glutamine for urinary acid-base balance, and metabolizes other amino acids. The kidney also acts as a minor source of glucose.

Total Integration of Body Protein

A 70-kg man contains 10 to 11 kg of protein, with 250 to 300 g, or 3%, of turnover every day. The largest portion of turnover is from the intestines, resulting from sloughed enterocytes and the secreted digestive enzymes. All but 1 g of nitrogen is absorbed after the digestion of amino acids. Most of the daily amino acids available to the body are provided by proteolysis (50 to 70 g), with only 25 g provided by absorption. Most of the amino acids are then resynthesized into proteins if an adequate amount of calories are available; 50 g is used daily for muscle, 20 g for plasma proteins, 8 g for hemoglobin, 20 g for white blood cells, and a few grams for skin. The amount of protein turnover

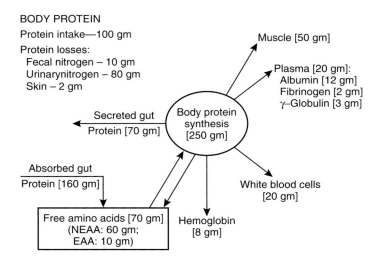

BODY PROTEIN

Protein intake—100 gm

Protein losses:
Fecal nitrogen – 10 gm
Urinarynitrogen – 80 gm
Skin – 2 gm

Muscle [50 gm]

Plasma [20 gm]:
Albumin [12 gm]
Fibrinogen [2 gm]
γ–Globulin [3 gm]

Secreted gut Protein [70 gm]

Body protein synthesis [250 gm]

Absorbed gut Protein [160 gm]

White blood cells [20 gm]

Free amino acids [70 gm] (NEAA: 60 gm; EAA: 10 gm)

Hemoglobin [8 gm]

FIGURE 36–2 Daily two of amino acids in a 70 kg man. Total body protein synthesis in 250 g per 24 hours of which 50 g is muscle. Proteolysis contributes approximately the same. Nitrogen equilibrium is the result with adequate energy. (Adapted from Munro HN: Parenteral nutrition: metabolic consequences of bypassing the gut and liver. *In* Clinical Nutrition Update: Amino Acids. Chicago: American Medical Association, 1977:141.)

decreases with age. The neonate has 25 g/kg/day of protein turnover, while the adult rate is 3 g/kg/day. The turnover rate does not change appreciably with the amount of lean body mass. Caloric source plays a role in determining protein synthesis. Carbohydrates increase muscle protein synthesis mediated by insulin, while albumin synthesis is not increased as much. Lipids increase hepatic and visceral protein synthesis, but do not increase muscle protein synthesis to the same degree as carbohydrates (Fig. 36–2).

Protein Requirements

The normal recommended daily protein allowance is 0.8 g/kg or between 56 and 60 g of protein per day. This amount of intake is often doubled in industrialized countries. Sepsis or other stress increases the requirements to between 1.5 and 2 g/kg/day as a result of an increased amount of proteolysis. In healthy adults, only one fifth of the protein intake needs to be essential amino acids, because most amino acids are recycled. The percentage increases with various stresses. Infants require 40% to 50% of intake to be composed of essential amino acids.

Calories

Energy Sources

The major sources of energy are proteins, carbohydrates, and fats. Amino acids normally provide 15% of energy, with branched-chain amino acids contributing 6% to 7% by being oxidized directly to a high-energy phosphate,

bypassing glucose. The remaining amino acid component is provided via gluconeogenesis. Of the remaining percentage of energy, 70% to 75% is provided by the direct oxidation or metabolism of fat into ketone bodies in the liver. Abnormal body states may preferentially use different energy sources.

The respiratory quotient (RQ) aids in estimating the utilization of caloric sources. The RQ is the ratio of carbon dioxide produced to oxygen consumed. With carbohydrate utilization, the RQ is 1, while an RQ of 0.7 indicates fat utilization. An RQ of less than 0.7 indicates ketogenesis (Table 36–1).

Calorie:Nitrogen Ratio

In a normal individual, a calorie:nitrogen ratio of 100:1 to 150:1 is necessary for protein synthesis. In sepsis, the ratio required decreases to 100:1, while in uremia, a ratio between 300:1 and 400:1 is needed.

Carbohydrates

Carbohydrate stores are virtually depleted after a greater than 24-hour fast, with liver glycogen depleted and only small amounts of muscle glycogen remaining. In the Krebs tricarboxylic acid cycle, glucose is completely oxidized to produce a larger amount of high-energy phosphate than in the incomplete oxidation of anaerobic glycolysis that produces lactate. Glucose is the "gold standard" for protein sparing, with at least 400 calories required in 24 hours. Glucose can reduce the degree of proteolysis up to 50%. Numerous cell types, including neural tissue, red blood

Table 36–1

Differences in metabolic responses in starvation and stress*

	Starvation	Stress Hypermetabolism
Resting energy expenditure	↓	↑↑
Respiratory quotient	Low (0.65)	High (0.85)
Mediator activation	–	+++
Regulatory responsiveness	++++	+
Primary fuels	Fat	Mixed
Proteolysis	+	+++
Branched-chain oxidation	+	+++
Hepatic protein synthesis	+	+++
Ureagenesis	+	+++
Urinary nitrogen loss	+	+++
Gluconeogenesis	+	+++
Ketone body production	++++	+

*Patients fall in continuum between extremes of starvation and stress.

cells, and white blood cells, prefer to utilize glucose as an energy source. Excessive glucose levels can lead to hepatic steatosis, poor neutrophil function, and increased infectious complications. The maximal rate of glucose oxidation is 4 to 5 mg/kg/min; thus total glucose intake should not exceed that amount.

Carbohydrate sources other than glucose have not been widely used. Fructose is suspected to cause lactic acidosis, and its utilization requires the expenditure of high-energy phosphate in the pentose phosphate shunt to convert it to glucose. Xylitol is hepatotoxic. Glycerol in high doses may result in renal failure, but it shows promise in lower doses because it can be sterilized in solution and has a low osmolality.

Fats

In starvation, the majority of calories are provided by fat, which is converted to ketone bodies produced in the liver. Steroids, catechols, glucagons, and some cytokines promote lipolysis, while insulin is an inhibitor. Fat as 25% of non-protein calories in normal or moderate stress conditions seems to be optimal for hepatic protein synthesis. The "fat overload syndrome" of fever, back pain, chills, pulmonary insufficiency, and impairment of the reticuloendothelial system (particularly as a result of ω-6-polyunsaturated long-chain fatty acids) should be avoided by limiting fat intake to no more than 2 g/kg/day. Infants can tolerate up to 4 g/kg/day.

Alternative or Nonconventional Fuels

Glutamine shows promise as a supplement because it provides energy for enterocytes. Numerous studies have shown only a minimal change in nitrogen balance with administration of glutamine, although in cases of severe stress it has been shown to decrease hospital stay, decrease infections, and improve nitrogen balance. The advantages have been attributed to maintenance of the gut barrier function, although gut and hepatic protein synthesis may also be involved. The ketone bodies (acetoacetate, propionate, and butyrate) are another area of investigation because of their potential benefits as substitutes for enterocyte energy sources in place of glutamine.

Energy requirements

The amount of resting energy expended is determined by measuring the patient's expired gas using indirect calorimetry. Errors tend to increase with high ventilatory settings. The Harris-Benedict equation, with a correction for activity, may be used to measure basal energy expenditure (BEE):

Men: BEE = 66.5 + [13.7 × wt (kg)] + [5.0 × ht (cm)] – [6.7 × age (yr)]

Women: BEE = 655.1 + [9.56 × wt (kg)] + [1.85 × ht (cm)] – [4.68 × age (yr)]

This equation tends to overestimate calorie requirements.

Catabolism

Hormones

Insulin inhibits lipolysis, increases nitrogen in muscles, and increases protein synthesis and fat storage in the liver. Growth hormone also has an anabolic role, likely through insulin-like growth factor-1. Glucagon, catecholamines, and steroids promote proteolysis and gluconeogenesis while increasing hepatic protein synthesis.

Cytokines

Cytokines, materials produced by macrophages and T lymphocytes, were extensively investigated during the last decade, with most of the attention focused on IL-1, IL-2, IL-6, TNF, and interferon-γ. Steroids appear to be a major mediator in proteolysis, with TNF perhaps serving as a permissive factor or a cofactor. TNF may act to trigger other cytokines in a cytokine cascade. IL-1 and IL-6 are certainly also promoters of catabolism. Enterocytes are not only the targets of cytokines, but may also be the source of IL-1, IL-6, and TNF (Table 36–2).

Nitric Oxide

The synthesis of nitric oxide in mammalian cells was first described in 1993; since that time myriad physiologic roles have been described for the compound. Nearly every human cell type is capable of producing nitric oxide. Nitric oxide is an unstable compound and has a half-life of only a few seconds or less. L-Arginine is the sole substrate for nitric oxide synthesis, with reduced nicotinamide adenine dinucleotide phosphate acting as a nitric oxide donor and citrulline formed as a coproduct. Nitric oxide synthetase has three isoforms, with inducible nitric oxide synthetase as the most physiologically important. In addition to serving a role in vasodilatation and neurotransmission, nitric oxide likely has a major function in infection and inflammation by promoting hepatic protein synthesis, killing pathogens, and regulating cell death and apoptosis.

Malnutrition

Causes of Inadequate Nutrition

Lack of food remains a cause of malnutrition in poor areas, particularly in alcoholics. However, the etiology of inadequate nutrition usually is anorexia secondary to cancer, sepsis, or liver disease, or poor intake resulting from obstruction of the gastrointestinal tract secondary to cancer or stricture. Poor absorption may occur secondary to scleroderma, motility disorders, pseudo-obstruction, major gastric resection, short-bowel syndrome, gastrointestinal fistulas, inflammatory bowel disease, or protein-losing enteropathies.

Methods of Assessment

Measurement of lean body mass

The ultimate objective of nutritional support is to promote the accumulation of lean body mass. Measurement of lean body mass, however, is a significant challenge.

DISPLACEMENT. The most sensitive method is displacement of water volume by various parts of the body. However, this method is not practical in most institutions and for many patients.

EXCHANGE OF LABELED IONS. This method determines the amount of lean body mass by measuring the exchangeable potassium and the content of extracellular water by calculating total exchangeable sodium. A ratio of exchangeable sodium to exchangeable potassium of greater than 1.22:1 indicates the presence of increased extracellular water and decreased body mass that occurs in malnutrition.

NEUTRON ACTIVATION ANALYSIS. The body is bombarded by activated neutrons, and nitrogen is measured.

TOTAL-BODY COUNTERS. These measure the spontaneous decay of naturally occurring isotopes that indicate lean body mass. They require patients to remain immobile in counting machines for prolonged periods of time.

MAGNETIC RESONANCE IMAGING. This may serve as an accurate measure of lean body mass.

History and physical examination

Malnutrition should be suspected in patients with significant weight loss, anorexia, weakness, difficulty with normal activities, or illness that prevent adequate nutrition intake. A weight loss of 5% to 10% in 1 month or a 10% to 20% loss in 6 months significantly increase complications of surgery. On physical examination, the patient should be inspected for thenar atrophy, loose skin, edema, weakness, loss of body fat, and pallor. Anthropometric measurements are often limited by interobserver variability resulting from changes in hydration and age. However, a physician's subjective evaluation has prognostic value.

Useful clinical tests

NITROGEN BALANCE. This is determined by measuring urinary and gastrointestinal losses with respect to nitrogen intake. In patients not receiving enteral nutrition,

Table 36–2
Sources and targets of cytokines and other peptide regulatory factors

Regulatory Factor*	Sources	Target Tissues/Cells
Interleukins (ILs)		
IL-1α, IL-1β (endogenous pyrogen, lymphocyte-activating factor, leukocyte endogenous mediator, hemopoietin-1)	Monocytes/macrophages; many endothelial, epithelial, and hematopoietic cells	Thymocytes, T and B cells, hematopoietic cells, fibroblasts, chondrocytes, receptors in brain and liver, hepatocytes
IL-2 (T-cell growth factor)	T cells	T and B cells, thymocytes, natural killer cells
IL-3 (multipotential colony-stimulating factor, hematopoietic growth factor)	T cells, myelomonocytic cells	Hematopoietic cells, pre–B cells
IL-4 (B-cell stimulating factor 1, B-cell growth factor I)	T cells, mast cells	T and B cells, mast cells, other hematopoietic cells
IL-5 (T-cell replacing factor, eosinophil differentiation factor, B-cell growth factor II, eosinophil colony-stimulating factor, IgA-enhancing factor)	T cells	B cells, eosinophils, thymocytes
IL-6 (B-cell stimulating factor 2, interferon-β$_2$, hepatocyte-stimulating factor, hybridoma growth factor, B-cell differentiation factor, 26-kd protein)	Monocytes/macrophages, T cells, fibroblasts, epithelial cell types	T and B cells, fibroblasts, hepatocytes, hematopoietic stem cells
IL-7 (lymphoprotein-1, pre–B-cell growth factor)	Stomal cells, thymus	Pre–B cells, thymocytes
IL-8	Macrophages, neurotrophils, endothelial cells, hepatocytes, fibroblasts	Neutrophils, fibroblasts
IL-9	T cells	Lymphoid cells, myeloid cells
IL-10	Monocytes/macrophages, B cells, T-helper cells	Macrophages, cytokines, antigens, IL-1 receptors
IL-11	Lung stromal cells, bone marrow stromal cells	Progenitor cells, B cells
IL-12	Monocytes/macrophages, B cells, skin Langerhans' cells	T-cell growth factor, cytokines
IL-13	T-helper cells	Monocytes, endothelial cells, B cells
IL-14	B cells	B cells (B-cell growth factor)
IL-15	Mononuclear cells, muscle	T cells, B cells
Tumor Necrosis Factors (TNFs)		
TNF (TNF-α, cachectin)	Monocytes/macrophages, lymphocytes, natural killer cells, glial cells, Kupffer cells	Endothelial cells, monocytes/ macrophages, neutrophils, fibroblasts, receptors in liver, muscle, lung, gut, kidney
Lymphotoxin (TNF-β)	Monocytes/macrophages	? Same receptors as TNF
Interferons		
Interferon-α (leukocyte interferon)	Monocytes/macrophages	Multiple immune cells
Interferon-β (fibroblast interferon)	Fibroblasts, epithelial cells	Multiple immune cells
Interferon-β$_2$ [see IL-6]		
Interferon-γ (immune interferon, macrophage-activating factor)	Multiple cell types (antigen-antibody reaction)	T and B cells, phagocytic cells

Table continued on following page

Table 36-2
Sources and targets of cytokines and other peptide regulatory factors—*Continued*

Regulatory Factor*	Sources	Target Tissues/Cells
Insulin-like Growth Factors (IGFs)		
IGF-1 (somatomedin C)	Fibroblasts, astrocytes, other neuronal and nonneuronal cells	Most cell types (necessary for cell survival), muscle and cartilage, precursor cells
IGF-2 (somatomedin A)	Astrocytes	Most cell types

*The terms in parentheses are alternative terms that have been, and in some cases still are, used for the same substance or group of substances.
Note: This is only a partial and likely outdated list, because new cytokines are being discovered constantly.
Adapted from Bessey PQ: Metabolic response to critical illness. In Wilmore DW, Cheung LY, Harken AH, et al (eds): Scientific American Surgery, Section II, Subsection 11 New York: Scientific American, 1996.

stool nitrogen is assumed to be 1 g/day. Total nitrogen output can be calculated by adding 2 to 3 g of nitrogen for insensible losses to the measured urinary urea nitrogen. Alternatively, one can add less than 1 g to total urea nitrogen measured by chemiluminescence.

NITROGEN BREAKDOWN. The urinary excretion of 3-MH, is used to estimate nitrogen turnover. 3-MH is a product of actin and myosin and reflects lean body mass turnover. It also may reflect intestinal protein turnover.

INDIRECT CALORIMETRY. Metabolic charts are used to estimate caloric demands with the patient in the resting state. An additional 15% must be added for activity.

DELAYED CUTANEOUS HYPERSENSITIVITY OR ANERGY. Anergy by itself cannot be used to determine malnutrition, because other disease states also lead to immunologic defects. However, malnutrition can lead to a state of anergy. An increase in surgical complications in patients who are anergic is well documented.

FUNCTIONAL STUDIES OF MUSCLE. Other means are useful to identify functional malnutrition. Tests used include handgrip dynamometry and rate of recovery from fatigue after electrical stimulation of the ulnar nerve. Correlation with outcome has not been shown, but a correlation with postoperative complications has been demonstrated.

Considerations for Initiating Nutritional Support

The following factors, while not exclusive, should be considered when beginning perioperative nutritional support: (1) premorbid state, (2) nutritional status, (3) age, (4) duration of starvation, (5) degree of expected surgical insult, (6) duration until normal intake is resumed, (7) unplanned weight loss of 15% or more, and (8) serum albumin of less than 3 g/100 mL. Elderly patients in particular must be treated with caution. Patients up to 60 years of age can generally tolerate a fast of 10 to 14 days; this should not be interpreted as advocating absence of nutrition for 14 days. However, patients 70 years or older should not fast for greater than 7 days, and those over 80 years old should not fast for more than 5 or 6 days.

Routes of Administration

The routes of nutritional administration are enteral, into the stomach or, preferably, small intestine; or parenteral, into the circulatory system. Recent studies have demonstrated that, in several disease states, enteral nutrition provides improved results over parenteral nutrition. A seminal study demonstrating a survival advantage in burned children involved increasing the percentage of feedings delivered to the intestine. Numerous studies have demonstrated improved outcome in patients with blunt or penetrating trauma when using early enteral nutrition. In several conditions such as liver transplantation, bowel resection in well-nourished patients, and pancreatitis, enteral nutrition has not been demonstrated to have a benefit.

Factors justifying the use of enteral therapy over parenteral therapy for nutritional support include (1) enteral nutrition is less costly; (2) enteral nutrition appears to improve and protect hepatic function; (3) enteral nutrition mimics the normal route of nutrition, so that the liver can process, store, and release nutrients in a physiologic fashion; (4) "gut mucosal integrity" is maintained; and (5) enteral nutrition has indirect beneficial effects on noncontiguous mucosa. Recent studies have suggested that the full benefits of enteral feeding may be achieved by a relatively small percentage of total calories (20% to 30%) given enterally.

Enteral Nutrition

Translocation Hypothesis

The role of the gut in ameliorating the deleterious effects following injury was first suggested by the inhibition of hypercatabolism in guinea pigs with enteral feeding immediately following burn. A delay of feeding of only 24 hours resulted in catabolism and weight loss. Teleologically, translocation may exist as a method to prime the immune system with small amounts of endotoxin, or a means of immune surveillance of potential pathogens. However, greatly increased translocation may occur in burns or other significant injury, possibly leading to the overwhelming of normal protective mechanisms. The bacteria are no longer arrested and "cleared" by mesenteric lymph nodes, but rather enter the portal circulation and contribute to hepatic failure. Although this theory is popular, it is still not clear that restoration of gut mucosal integrity is responsible for the benefits ascribed to enteral feeding. Other theories demonstrate the importance of the enteral route in maintaining gut-associated lymphoid tissue, and in this manner contributing to a proposed body-wide mucosal immunity.

Enterocyte-Specific Nutritional Substrates

Glutamine

Glutamine was first described as a significant energy source of the small intestine in 1974. Glutamine uptake is predominantly by enterocytes from both the basolateral membrane and lumen, although lymphocytes and macrophages may also play a role. The gut absorbs the substance from plasma across the basolateral membrane and by using system B, a brush-border mucosal transporter, for transport from the lumen. The gut increases glutamine synthetase to synthesize glutamine from ammonia. Glutamine may play a role in maintenance of small intestinal mucosa when taken orally, but results are conflicting with respect to parenteral administration, and the potential of glutamine as an energy source for tumors is of deep concern.

Short-chain fatty acids

Acetoacetate, propionate, and butyrate are produced by the fermentation of pectin by colonic bacteria. Ten percent of acetoacetate is used locally, with 90% exported; 50% of propionate is used locally, with 50% exported; and 80% of butyrate is used locally, with only 20% exported. The major fuel for colonocytes is butyrate, followed by acetoacetate, L-glutamine, and D-glucose. Short-chain fatty acids provide approximately 70% of the energy for colonocytes. A deficiency of these fatty acids may result in disruption of the colonic barrier.

General Principles of Enteral Feeding

The stomach prevents the entry of an excessive osmotic load to the small intestine by inhibiting gastric motility upon receiving a bolus. Gastric contents then pass through the pylorus as they become isosmotic after gastric secretion of dilutional material. The small bowel is the principal area of nutrient absorption; protein is usually absorbed within 120 cm and carbohydrates are typically absorbed prior to the mid-jejunum. Simple sugars and dipeptides are preferred if the bowel is short or function is poor. Fat absorption is more difficult because of the additional mixing and processing required by bile and pancreatic enzymes. Calcium, iron, and other metals are absorbed principally in the duodenum.

Practicalities of Enteral Feeding

In the past, enteral nutrition was avoided because of fear that the gastrointestinal tract was nonfunctional during severe injury. However, recent observations indicate that ileus is usually limited to the stomach and colon. In fact, nutrition provided beyond the ligament of Treitz is well tolerated in patients with head trauma and laparotomy, who are prone to gastroparesis. In burn patients, early enteral feeding aids in preventing gastroparesis. Even if total nutritional requirements cannot be provided enterally, benefit can be obtained by providing at least 20% of calories and protein through the gut. Most patients can tolerate nasogastric feeding via a no. 10 French Silastic catheter, and aspiration may be reduced by placing the tip of the tube distal to the ligament of Treitz. A small-bore tube is used to decrease the risk of esophageal stricture, reflux, or necrosis of the nasal ala. The position of the tube should be confirmed by measuring pH (if in the stomach), by fluoroscopy, or by plain film. Air insufflation is inadequate because the sound may be transmitted to the left lung or esophagus. The patient should always be kept at a 30-degree angle to decrease the risks of aspiration and reflux.

Administration

For gastric feedings, first osmolality and then volume is increased. In small intestinal feeding, volume is increased and then osmolality. The small bowel does not generally tolerate feeds with concentrations greater than 500 mOsm. For safety, osmolality should be kept below 375 mOsm.

Available Enteral Diets

Many forms of enteral diets are available, including formulas that are similar to blenderized food and formulas that contain simpler nutritional elements. Specialty formulas have been created that contain substrates required during physiologic stress, and may include arginine, ω-3 fatty acids, nucleotides, glutamine, and branched-chain amino acids.

Complications

In addition to aspiration, another major complication in enteral feeding is diarrhea caused by hyperosmolar solutions. The resulting diarrhea can lead to dehydration, electrolyte imbalance, and hyperglycemia. Additionally, continuation of feeds may lead to pneumatosis intestinalis, bowel necrosis, and perforation. To reduce the incidence of these complications, resuscitation should be completed prior to feeding and the osmolality of feeds to the small bowel should be relatively iso-osmolar.

Parenteral Nutrition

In the following discussion of parenteral administration of nutrients, three major assumptions are made regarding the content:

1. The protein is a mixture of synthetic single amino acids made from bacterial cultures.

2. The caloric source is hypertonic dextrose.

3. The fat is made of 10% or 20% soy or safflower oil emulsions.

Peripheral Administration

The peripheral route is used primarily in hospitals without established nutritional support programs. It is useful in cases in which parenteral nutrition will be limited or is perhaps not required. The patient's veins are usually quickly depleted, and the risk of phlebitis is high. Caloric requirements are satisfied with a 10% or 20% fat emulsion given with amino acids and 5% dextrose.

Central Administration

With the central route of hyperalimentation, the catheter is usually in the superior vena cava (though sometimes in the inferior vena cava), allowing for administration of hyperosmolar solutions using greater than 10% dextrose. A team approach of nurses, physicians, and pharmacists operating under a strict protocol is required for a safe and effective program.

Requirements for Nutrition

Generally, patients receive 35 kcal/kg/day of protein, with a safe requirement being 1.7 g of protein equivalent/kg/day. Hepatic protein synthesis is likely optimized with fat composing 20% to 25% of nonprotein calories. Adequate vitamins and trace minerals should be administered, although actual required amounts are still not clearly defined (Table 36–3).

Indications for Parenteral Nutrition

Indications for parenteral nutrition are summarized in Box 36–1.

Table 36–3
Suggested dosage of vitamins and trace metals during severe illness

Vitamin	Suggested Dosage (mg/day)
Water soluble	
Thiamine	25
Riboflavin	25
Niacin	200
Pantothenic acid	50
Pyridoxine	50
Folic acid*	2.5
B_{12}†	5
Fat soluble	
A†	5000 μg
D†	400 μg
E†	100 μg
K*	10
Trace Metal	
Zinc	10–20
Copper	0.5–2.0
Chromium	20 μg
Selenium	70–150 μg
Manganese	2–2.5
Iron	25

*Inactivated (oxidized) by addition to hypertonic glucose–amino acid solutions.
†Sufficient stores of these vitamins exist so that deficiency states are unlikely during short-term (2 to 4 weeks) parenteral nutrition. In practice, however, it is wise to provide them.

Box 36-1

Indications for Parenteral Nutrition

Primary therapy

Efficacy shown*

- Gastrointestinal cutaneous fistulas
- Renal failure (acute tubular necrosis)
- Short bowel syndrome
- Acute burns
- Hepatic failure (acute decompensation superimposed on cirrhosis)

Efficacy not shown

- Crohn's disease
- Anorexia nervosa

Supportive therapy

Efficacy shown*

- Acute radiation enteritis
- Acute chemotherapy toxicity
- Prolonged ileus
- Weight loss preliminary to major surgery

Efficacy not shown

- Before cardiac surgery
- Prolonged respiratory support
- Large wound losses

Areas under intensive study

Patients with cancer

Patients with sepsis

This indicates that randomized prospective trials or similar investigations have suggested that such nutritional intervention results in changed (improved) outcome.

Primary therapy: efficacy shown

GASTROINTESTINAL-CUTANEOUS FISTULAS. Patients with gastrointestinal-cutaneous fistulas present a classic rationale for the use of parenteral nutrition because, as enteral intake increases, fistula output correspondingly increases. TPN has increased the rates of spontaneous fistula closure, although in major centers the mortality rate in fistula treatment has not been reduced. However, patients are in better nutritional condition if surgical correction is required. Enteral nutrition can also aid in fistula closure. If output increases with increased oral intake, 20% to 30% of calories are provided enterally, with the remainder provided parenterally.

RENAL FAILURE. TPN decreases mortality in patients with acute renal failure, particularly when using essential amino acids. If dialysis is not clearly indicated, a formula of essential amino acids and hypertonic saline is utilized so dialysis may be avoided. Essential amino acids are used to decrease the accumulation of potassium and blood urea nitrogen. Once dialysis is well established, a mixture of essential and nonessential amino acids may be used, because these are being lost.

SHORT-BOWEL SYNDROME. Major causes of this syndrome are multiple small bowel resections for Crohn's disease or major enterectomy for mesenteric thrombosis or volvulus. TPN allows survival of these patients for approximately 10 years. Small-bowel hypertrophy may allow a patient to decrease or discontinue TPN. Hypertrophy in 1 or 2 years will usually allow a patient with 2.5 feet of small bowel to end reliance on TPN.

BURNS. The decline in burn mortality since the late 1960s is likely due to the initiation of aggressive nutritional support. High-protein diets not only improve survival, but also improve the patient's immunologic condition. Nutritional support is now initiated within the first 3 hours of the burn patient's arrival and maintained throughout multiple surgical procedures. Parenteral nutrition is used when enteral nutrition is inadequate to meet caloric requirements. Nutritional pharmacology continues to play a major role, particularly with the use of ω-3 fats in fish oil to produce the E_3 family of prostaglandins and thromboxanes, which are less catabolic than the prostaglandin E_2 family. A product known as Impact will, under certain circumstances, decrease the sepsis rate, lower the number of days of bacteremia, decrease mortality, and shorten hospital stay.

HEPATIC FAILURE. Improved survival in hepatic failure is shown with proper aggressive parenteral nutrition. Patients with liver disease are often more susceptible to stress as a result of malnourishment from alcoholism and decreased food intake. Protein is an important nutrient in these individuals, but may lead to hepatic encephalopathy. According to the unified hypothesis, portal shunting (functional or anatomic) resulting from decreased hepatic function leads to an imbalance of amino acid precursors of central monoamine neurotransmitters, which leads to derangement of central nervous system neurotransmitters. The imbalance can be addressed by TPN solutions with increased branched-chain amino acids and decreased amounts of aromatic amino acids, which compete for entry across the blood-brain barrier. Such solutions have been shown to be at least as effective as lactulose and neomycin in treating hepatic encephalopathy, with some studies demonstrating improved survival.

Primary therapy: efficacy not shown

INFLAMMATORY BOWEL DISEASE. In inflammatory bowel disease, intake of oral nutrition may result in diarrhea, protein-losing enteropathy, bleeding, and abdominal pain. Bowel rest and parenteral nutrition may be useful in inducing remission, especially if disease is limited to the small bowel, in which case the remission rate is 75%. In a long-term study, however, only 26% of patients avoided surgery after 15 months. Patients in whom almost total removal of affected bowel is required can be maintained on long-term home TPN. Long-term TPN is not recommended for ulcerative colitis because definitive surgical correction is available. Instead, up to 2 weeks of parenteral nutrition will decrease inflammation, making surgery technically easier.

Supportive therapy: efficacy shown

ACUTE RADIATION ENTERITIS OR CHEMOTHERAPY TOXICITY. Radiation enteritis or chemotherapy toxicity may prevent adequate oral intake. Parenteral nutrition may allow for survival until the gastrointestinal tract recovers. Home parenteral nutrition may be indicated in patients with significant postradiation intestinal stricture.

PROLONGED ILEUS. TPN may be required for a prolonged ileus until it resolves.

Supportive therapy: efficacy probably present

WEIGHT LOSS PRELIMINARY TO MAJOR SURGERY. A significant review of the literature has not demonstrated a case for TPN prior to major surgery. However, a subset of patients who have lost greater than 15% of their body weight and have associated immunologic compromise are at increased risk of surgical complications. As a group, the patients at risk can be identified, but individual patient identification is more challenging. A history of 10% to 15% weight loss coupled with an albumin level of less than 3 g/100 mL places these individuals in a high-risk group. The number of septic complications, in particular, is dramatically decreased, particularly in the most malnourished patients, by even a short duration (7 to 10 days) of parenteral nutrition. An ideal period of time for preoperative TPN is 5 to 7 days. An early study indicated a trend toward improved outcome after only 3 days.

MALIGNANT DISEASE. TPN, particularly with overfeeding, can lead to tumor growth. Therefore, preoperative parenteral nutrition should not exceed 5 days.

CARDIAC SURGERY. Cardiac cachexia, which increases the complications and mortality of cardiac surgery, may respond to nutritional support. However, animal studies suggest that the period required for improvement may be prolonged, perhaps as long as 6 weeks. This limits its use.

RESPIRATORY FAILURE AND REQUIREMENTS FOR PROLONGED RESPIRATORY SUPPORT. Nutritional support is necessary to ensure adequate energy substrate for the muscles of respiration. Overproduction of carbon dioxide, making weaning more difficult or requiring intubation, may occur when depleted septic patients are given large loads of glucose suddenly. Despite its notoriety, this remains a rare occurrence.

LARGE WOUNDS. Nutritional support may aid in healing of large wounds, especially when large amounts of protein are lost.

Areas under intense study

PATIENTS WITH CANCER. Cancer patients typically have significant weight loss as a result of an altered central nervous system satiety center. Mechanical obstruction may also play a role. A major difficulty in performing clinical trials in this area is finding patients who are uniform in nutritional status, type of cancer, and stage. Current research in this area is attempting to identify inhibitors of cell growth to utilize in conjunction with TPN. Preoperative nutritional therapy decreases morbidity and mortality in patients with esophageal cancer and gastric cancer. Postoperative nutritional support also appears to decrease septic complication and length of stay of cancer patients.

SEPSIS. Sepsis is a major cause of surgical mortality. It involves a state of proteolysis, with the flow of amino acids to the liver resulting in increased protein synthesis. In addition, insulin resistance and gluconeogenesis are present. Branched-chain amino acids have been utilized as an energy source, thereby avoiding glucose, to stimulate protein synthesis and decrease muscle proteolysis. No improvement in outcome has been demonstrated, but an improvement in amino acid flux and lowered requirement for insulin are present.

Complications of Parenteral Nutrition

Technical complications

TECHNICAL COMPLICATIONS OF CATHETER PLACEMENT

1. Pneumothorax, which is more common in elderly and cachectic patients; internal jugular lines should be considered in high-risk patients

2. Arterial lacerations; keep needle no steeper than 10 degrees to horizontal

3. Hemothorax caused by leakage from subclavian vein or superior vena cava

4. Mediastinal hematoma

5. Nerve injury to brachial plexus

6. Hydrothorax caused by administration of fluid from malpositioned catheter into thoracic cavity

7. Sympathetic effusions

8. Thoracic duct injury in left-sided cannulation

9. Air embolism caused by poor technique and improperly positioned, poorly hydrated patient

10. Catheter embolism, usually involving shearing of the catheter by the needle

LATE TECHNICAL COMPLICATIONS

1. Erosion of catheter into bronchus, right atrium, or other structures

2. Subclavian thrombosis; requires thrombolytic therapy followed by anticoagulation

3. Septic thrombosis; if antibiotics and anticoagulation fail, axillary and/or subclavian vein can be excised (rare) or, more likely, Fogarty catheter embolectomy performed

Metabolic complications

The metabolic complications of TPN are due to deficiencies, disorders of glucose metabolism, and electrolyte abnormalities.

PLASMA ELECTROLYTE ABNORMALITIES.
Electrolyte abnormalities are not uncommon. At least 50 mEq sodium, 40 mEq potassium, 90 to 100 mEq phosphorus, and 28 to 32 mEq of calcium and magnesium should be provided daily to patients on TPN. Acetate should be added in patients with acidosis, and potassium chloride in patients with large gastric output.

If potassium chloride fails to correct hypokalemia (paradoxical aciduria), arginine hydrochloride or dilute hydrochloric acid may be required.

TRACE METAL DEFICIENCIES
Zinc deficiency. This may occur in individuals who are very catabolic or suffer from severe diarrhea. 3 to 6 mg of elemental zinc is needed per day in patients with normal bowel movements, and up to six times that amount in patients with diarrhea. A deficiency of zinc is characterized by a perioral pustular rash, darkened skin creases, and neuritis.

Copper deficiency. This may present as a microcytic anemia.

Chromium deficiency. This occurs only in patients on long-term TPN with minimal to no oral intake. Chromium is necessary for proper glucose utilization. The daily minimum is 15 to 20 µg of chromium. Deficiency presents as brittle diabetes, peripheral neuropathy, and encephalopathy. To treat this deficiency, 150 µg of chromium per day for several days is required.

Selenium deficiency. Deficiency is manifested by abnormalities of basement and plasma membranes. Selenium is ubiquitous, making deficiency very rare.

Biotin deficiency. This occurs only with no oral intake.

ESSENTIAL FATTY ACID DEFICIENCY.
The deficiency can be prevented by administration of soybean or safflower fat emulsion. Deficiency is characterized by dry, flaky skin with small, reddish papules and alopecia.

DISORDERS OF GLUCOSE METABOLISM
Hypoglycemia. This may occur when a rapid glucose infusion is suddenly decreased.

Hyperglycemia. This often is caused by a too-rapid increase of the TPN infusion. The most common cause of sudden hyperglycemia is sepsis. Hyperglycemia may antedate sepsis by 24 hours and is an early warning sign.

Diabetes mellitus. Adult-onset diabetes is not difficult to control with insulin and amino acids. Hyperosmolar nonketotic coma is a complication in which blood glucose concentrations are greater than 700 mg/dL, resulting in dehydration, fever, obtundation, and coma. Treatment is large volumes of saline followed by insulin. Potassium is also required.

Liver function derangements. Any type of TPN may result in elevated liver enzymes, although hyperbilirubinemia is rare and usually associated with sepsis. Hepatic steatosis has been attributed to all components of parenteral nutrition, but the etiology is likely derangements in the portal insulin-to-glucagon molar ratio. This is more serious and often irreversible in pediatric patients, leading to cirrhosis and hepatic failure, which is rare in adults.

Septic complications: catheter infection

The bacterial catheter sepsis rate is related to catheter care and can be reduced to less than 1%. Catheter sepsis correlates with the lack of catheter protocol, degree of colonization of the pericatheter skin, gram-positive organisms obtained at other sites, and candidemia. A catheter with surrounding skin colonization of greater than 10^3 organisms/cm^2 should be removed. In patients who develop a new fever, the current TPN bag should be removed with the tubing and be sent for culture. Blood cultures and a full work-up should then be performed to evaluate the source of fever. If the fever remains for 8 hours, the catheter should be removed and the tip sent for culture. If a septic catheter is removed, more than 24 hours of antibiotics is unnecessary unless the fever persists. Changing a catheter over a guidewire is acceptable only if the infection is at another site.

Prevention of catheter complications

The catheter should be placed with adequate assistance in a well-hydrated patient who is lightly sedated. A subclavian approach is preferred because of improved dressing maintenance. The patient is positioned with a roll placed vertically between the shoulder blades, arms at the sides, head relaxed, and the bed in 15 degrees of Trendelenburg position. The incidence of septic complications is significantly lower if diligent sterile technique is followed. After the patient is prepped and draped, the vein is located with a no. 22 needle through which lidocaine has been infiltrated along the expected tract and periosteum. The insertion site is 1 cm medial and 1 cm caudad to the midpoint of the clavicle. The needle should be no more than 10 to 15 degrees to the horizontal as one aims 1 cm above the sternal notch. After the vein is located, the larger needle is inserted into the vein and blood should be flowing freely. The patient is asked to perform a Valsalva maneuver, at which point the guidewire is inserted. If the wire cannot be inserted smoothly, both the wire and needle should be removed simultaneously. If the wire is inserted without difficulty, the tract is then dilated over the wire and the catheter is inserted over the wire. The wire is then removed. The catheter is sutured in place with 3-0 or 4-0 monofilament suture. Blood backflow and easy infusion should be ensured. A confirmatory chest radiograph is mandatory.

Other Considerations

Pediatric patients

The nutritional requirements for children are quite different from those for adults because of their immature enzyme systems and the large percentage of viscera compared to lean body mass. Children have a much higher protein requirement than adults, and caloric needs are proportionally larger as well. Fats can be administered at 4 g/kg in infants, which is double the maximum for adults. Vitamins and trace metals are also necessary, but potential toxicity must be monitored. Aggressive nutritional therapy has increased survival in meconium ileus, gastroschisis, and neonatal enterocolitis.

Home hyperalimentation

Patients have been treated at home with mostly parenteral nutrition for decades, with a mean catheter life of 7 years in a well-run program. TPN is normally cycled overnight, and numerous alarms assist the vigilance of the patient. Most home TPN patients have lost a large portion of their small bowel from Crohn's disease or as a result of a midgut volvulus or mesenteric thrombosis. Other indications include sprue, pseudo-obstruction, chronic radiation enteritis, and scleroderma. The catheters are placed either through a percutaneous or open method, often into a small branch of the axillary vein. Complications from home TPN include sepsis, nutritional deficiencies, and infection of the catheter exit site.

Summary

The field of nutritional support has increased dramatically over the last few decades. As the understanding of various disease states improves, nutrition will become tailored to address specific concerns. In the coming years, nutritional therapy may become as specialized and as focused for the specific illness as pharmaceuticals.

Bibliography

Alexander JW, MacMillan BG, Stinnett JD, et al: Beneficial effects of aggressive protein feeding in severely burned children. Ann Surg 1980;192:505.

Aubiniac R: Une nouvelle voie d'injection oude ponction veineuse: la voie sousclaviculaire. Semin Hop Paris 1952;28:3445.

Barbul A: Arginine. In Fischer JE (ed): Surgical Nutrition (2nd ed). Boston: Little, Brown, 1996:411–422.

Billiar TR, Simmons RI: Nitric oxide. In Fischer JE (ed): Surgical Nutrition (2nd ed). Boston: Little, Brown, 1996:443–458.

Blackburn GL, Bistrian BR, Maini BS, et al: Nutritional and metabolic assessment of the hospitalized patient. JPEN J Parenter Enteral Nutr 1977;1:11.

Bodoky G, Haranyi L, Pap A, et al: Effect of enteral nutrition in exocrine pancreatic function. Am J Surg 1991;161:144.

Bower RH, Cerra FB, Bershadsky B, et al: Early enteral administration of a formula (Impact) supplemented with arginine, nucleotides, and fish oil in intensive care unit patients: results of a randomized prospective clinical trial. Crit Care Med 1995;23:436.

Buzby GP, for the Veterans Affairs Total Parenteral Nutrition Cooperative Study Group: Perioperative total parenteral nutrition in surgical patients. N Engl J Med 1991;325:525.

Campbell SK, Kudsk KA: "High tech" metabolic measurements: useful in daily clinical practice? JPEN J Parenter Enteral Nutr 1988;12:610.

Cerra FB: Metabolic and nutritional support. *In* Mattox KL, Feliciano DV, Moore EE (eds): Trauma (3rd ed). Stamford: Appleton & Lange, 1996:1155.

Chance WT, Balasubramanian A, Fischer JE: Neuropeptide Y and the development of cancer anorexia. Ann Surg 1995;221:579.

Christensen HN: Role of amino acid transport and counter transport in nutrition and metabolism. Physiol Rev 1990; 70:43.

Daly JM, Reynolds J, Thom A, et al: Immune and metabolic effects of arginine in the surgical patient. Ann Surg 1988;208:512.

Detsky AS, Baker JP, O'Rourke K, Goel V: Perioperative parenteral nutrition: a meta-analysis. Ann Intern Med 1987;107:195.

Detsky AS, McLauglin JR, Baker JP, et al: What is subjective global assessment of nutritional status? JPEN J Parenter Enteral Nutr 1987;11:8.

Dudrick SJ, Wilmore DW, Vars HM, et al: Long-term total parenteral nutrition with growth, development, and positive nitrogen balance. Surgery 1968;64:134.

Enia G, Sicuso C, Alati G, Zoccali C: Subjective global assessment of nutrition in dialysis patients. Nephrol Dial Transplant 1993;8:1094.

Fan ST, Lo CM, Lai ECS, et al: Perioperative nutritional support in patients undergoing hepatectomy for hepatocellular carcinoma. N Engl J Med 1994;331:547.

Fang CH, Tiao G, James JH, et al: Burn injury stimulates multiple proteolytic pathways in skeletal muscle, including the ubiquitin-energy-dependent pathway. J Am Coll Surg 1995;180:161.

Fong Y, Lowry SF: Cytokines and the cellular response to injury and infection. *In* Wilmore DW, Cheung LY, Harken AH, et al (eds): Scientific American Surgery, Volume 2, Section II. New York: Healtheon/ WebMD, 2000:1–21.

Food and Nutrition Board, National Research Council: Recommended Dietary Allowances (10th ed). Washington, DC: National Academy of Sciences, 1989.

Galandiuk S, O'Neill M, McDonald P, et al: A century of home parenteral nutrition for Crohn's disease. Am J Surg 1990;159:540.

Gamble JL: Physiological information gained from studies on the life rate ration. Harvey Lect 1947;42:247.

Garrel DR, John N, deJonge LHM: Should we use the Harris and Benedict equations? Nutr Clin Pract 1996;11:99.

Hall JC, O'Quigley J, Giles GR, et al: Upper limb anthropometry: the value of measure variance studies. Am J Clin Nutr 1980;33:1846.

Hasse JM, Blue LS, Liepa GU, et al: Early enteral nutrition support in patients undergoing liver transplantation. JPEN J Parenter Enteral Nutr 1995;19:437.

Hasselgran PO: Glucocorticoids and muscle catabolism. Curr Opin Clin Nutr Metab Care 1999;2:201.

Hershko A, Ciechanover A: The ubiquitin system for protein degradation. Annu Rev Biochem 1992;61:761.

Heslin MJ, Latkany L, Leung D, et al: A prospective, randomized trial of enteral feeding after resection of upper gastrointestinal malignancy. Ann Surg 1997;226:567.

Holter A, Fischer JE: The effects of perioperative hyperalimentation on complications in patients with carcinoma and weight loss. J Surg Res 1977;23:31.

Hunter DC, Jaksik T, Lewis D, et al: Resting energy expenditure in the critically ill: estimates versus measurements. Br J Surg 1988;75:875.

Hwang T-L, Hwang S-L, Chen M-F: The use of indirect calorimetry in critically ill patients—the relationship of measured energy expenditure to Injury Severity Score, Septic Severity Score, and APACHE II Score. J Trauma 1993;34:247.

Jenkins M, Gottschlich M, Alexander JW, Warden GD: Effect of immediate feeding on the hypermetabolic response following severe burn injury. JPEN J Parenter Enteral Nutr 1989; 13(Suppl 1):12s.

Jones TN, Moore FA, Moore EE, et al: Gastrointestinal symptoms attributed to jejunostomy feeding after major abdominal trauma—a critical analysis. Crit Care Med 1989; 17:146.

Kinsella JE, Lokesh B, Broughton S: Dietary polyunsaturated fatty acids and eicosanoids: potential effect on the modulation of inflammatory and immune cells: an overview. Nutrition 1990;6:24.

Kudsk KA, Croce MA, Fabian TC, et al: Enteral versus parenteral feeding: effects on septic morbidity after blunt and penetrating abdominal trauma. Ann Surg 1992; 215:503.

Kudsk KA, Minard G, Croce MA, et al: A randomized trial of isonitrogenous enteral diets after severe trauma: an immune-enhancing diet reduces septic complications. Ann Surg 1996;224:531.

Kudsk KA, Teasley-Strausburg KM: Enteral and parenteral nutrition. *In* Irwin RS, Gera FB, Ripple JM (eds): Intensive Care Medicine (4th ed). New York: Lippincott-Raven, 1998:2243–2261.

Li J, Kudsk KA, Gocinski B, et al: Effects of parenteral nutrition on gut-associated lymphoid tissue. J Trauma 1995;39:44.

Li S, Nussbaum MS, McFadden DW, et al: Addition of L-glutamine to total parenteral nutrition (TPN) and its effects on portal insulin, glucagons and the development of hepatic steatosis in rats. J Surg Res 1991;48:421.

Long CL, Lowry SR: Hormone regulation of protein metabolism. JPEN J Parenter Enteral Nutr 1990;14:555.

Mayer RJ, Arnold J, Laszlo L, et al: Ubiquitin in health and disease. Biochim Biophys Acta 1991;1089:141.

McCamish MA, Bouunous G, Geraghty ME: History of enteral feeding: past and present perspective. *In* Rombeau JL, Rolandelli RH (eds): Clinical Nutrition: Enteral and Tube Feeding (3rd ed). Philadelphia: WB Saunders, 1997:1.

McDonald WS, Sharp CW Jr, Deitch EA: Immediate enteral feeding in burn patients is safe and effective. Ann Surg 1991;213:177.

Mester M, Tompkins RG, Gelfand JA, et al: Intestinal production of interleukin 1α during endotoxemia in the mouse. J Surg Rec 1993;54:584.

Meyer TA, Noguchi Y, Ogle CK, et al: Endotoxin stimulates IL-6 production in intestinal epithelial cells: a synergistic effect with PGE$_2$. Arch Surg 1994;129:1290.

Meyer TA, Tiao GM, James JH, et al: Nitric oxide inhibits LPS-induced IL-6 production in enterocytes. J Surg Res 1993;58:570.

Miller JJ, Venus B, Mathru M: Comparison of the sterility of long-term central venous catheterization using single lumen, triple lumen, and pulmonary artery catheters. Crit Care Med 1984;12:634.

Moore EE, Jones TN: Benefits of immediate jejunostomy feeding after major abdominal trauma—a prospective, randomized study. J Trauma 1986;26:874.

Moore FA, Moore EE, Jones TN, et al: TEN versus TPN following major abdominal trauma—reduced septic morbidity. J Trauma 1989;29:916.

Morris SM Jr, Billiar TR: New insights into the regulation of inducible nitric oxide synthesis. Am J Physiol 1994;82:7738.

Munro HN: Parenteral nutrition: metabolic consequences of bypassing the gut and liver. *In* Clinical Nutrition Update: Amino Acids. Chicago: American Medical Association, 1977:141.

Nathans AB, Ding JW, Marshall JC, et al: The gut as a cytokine generating organ: small bowel TNF-α production during systemic endotoxemia [abstract]. Presented at the 14th Annual Meeting of the Surgical Infection Society, Toronto, April 1994.

Naylor CD, O'Rourke K, Detsky AS, Baker JP: Parenteral nutrition with branched-chain amino acids in hepatic encephalopathy: a meta-analysis. Gastroenterology 1989;97:1033.

Nelson KM, Long CL: Physiological basis for nutrition in sepsis. Nutr Clin Pract 1989;4:6.

Pelham LD: Rational use of intravenous fat emulsions. Am J Hosp Pharm 1981;38:198.

Pemberton LB, Lyman B, Lander V, et al: Sepsis from triple vs. single-lumen catheters during total parenteral nutrition in surgical or critically ill patients. Arch Surg 1986;121:591.

Pikul J, Sharp MD, Lowndes R, et al: Degree of postoperative malnutrition is predictive of postoperative morbidity and mortality in liver transplant patients. Transplantation 1994;57:469.

Pomposelli JJ, Baxter JK, Babineau TJ, et al: Early postoperative glucose control predicts nosocomial infection rate in diabetic patients. JPEN J Parenter Enteral Nutr 1998;22:77.

Raff T, Hartmann B, Germann G: Early intragastric feeding of seriously burned and long-term ventilated patients: a review of 55 patients. Burns 1997;23:19.

Rombeau JL, Lew JL: Intestinal fuels: implications for improvement of intestinal growth and function. *In* Fischer JE (ed): Surgical Nutrition (2nd ed). Boston: Little, Brown, 1996:385–410.

Rose WC, Haines WJ, Warner DJ: The amino acid requirements of man: the role of lysine, arginine, and tryptophan. J Biol Chem 1954;206:421.

Russell D, Leiter LA, Witwell J, et al: Skeletal muscle function during hypocaloric diets and fasting: a comparison with standard nutritional assessment parameters. Am J Clin Nutr 1933;37:133.

Shiloni E, Corondao E, Freund HR: The role of total parenteral nutrition in the treatment of Crohn's disease. Am J Surg 1989;157:180.

Shizgal HM: Body composition. *In* Fischer JE (ed): Surgical Nutrition. Boston: Little, Brown, 1993:3–18.

Stabile BE, Borzatta M, Stubbs RS: Pancreatic secretory responses to intravenous hyperalimentation and intraduodenal elemental and full liquid diets. JPEN J Parenter Enteral Nutr 1984;8:377.

Studley HO: Percentage of weight loss: a basic indicator of surgical risk in patients with chronic peptic ulcer. JAMA 1936;106:458.

Stuehr DJ, Marletta MA: Mammalian nitrate biosynthesis: mouse macrophages produce nitrite and nitrate in response to *Escherichia coli* lipopolysaccharide. Proc Natl Acad Sci U S A 1985;82:7738.

Tiao G, Fagan J, Roegner V, et al: Energy-ubiquitin-dependent muscle proteolysis during sepsis in rats is regulated by glucocorticoids. J Clin Invest 1996;97:339.

Tiao GM, Fagan JM, Samuels N, et al: Sepsis stimulates non-lysosomal, energy-dependent proteolysis and increases ubiquitin mRNA levels in rat skeletal muscle. J Clin Invest 1994;94:2255.

Weir JB de V: New methods for calculating metabolic rate with special reference to protein metabolism. J Physiol 1949;109:1.

Wicks C, Somasundaram S, Bjarnason I, et al: Comparisons of enteral feeding and total parenteral nutrition after liver transplantation. Lancet 1994;344:837.

Williams AB, deCourten-Myers GM, Fischer JE, et al: Sepsis stimulates release of myofilaments in skeletal muscle by a calcium-dependent mechanism. FASEB J 1999;13:1435.

Windmueller HG, Spaeth AE: Uptake and metabolism of plasma glutamine by the small intestine. J Biol Chem 1974;249:5070.

Windsor JW, Hill GL: Weight loss with physiologic impairment: a basic indicator of surgical risk. Ann Surg 1988;207:290.

Wolfe R, Allsop J, Burke J: Glucose metabolism in man: responses to intravenous glucose infusion. Metabolism 1979;28:210.

Wolfe RR, Shaw JHF: Glucose and FFA in kinetics in sepsis: role of glucagons and sympathetic nervous system activity. Am J Physiol 1985;248:E236.

Zeiderman MR, McMahon MJ: The role of objective measurement of skeletal muscle function in preoperative patients. Clin Nutr 1989;8:161.

Ziegler TR, Young LS, Benfall K, et al: Clinical and metabolic efficacy of glutamine-supplemented parenteral nutrition after bone marrow transplantation: a randomized, double-blind, controlled study. Ann Intern Med 1992; 116:821.

CHAPTER 37

Hematology and Hemostasis

*Christopher P. Michetti, M.D., F.A.C.S., Kirsten Huber, M.D., Ph.D.,
and Samir M. Fakhry, M.D., F.A.C.S.*

Portions of this chapter have been reprinted from Fakhry SM, Rutherford
EJ, Sheldon GF: Hematologic principles in surgery. *In* Townsend CM,
Beauchamp RD, Evers BM, Mattox KL (eds): Sabiston's Textbook of
Surgery: The Biological Basis of Modern Surgical Practice (16th ed).
Philadelphia: WB Saunders, 2001:68.

G iven the surgeon's almost daily encounters with
blood, a thorough understanding of hematology
and mechanisms of hemostasis is critical for the
practicing surgeon. In this chapter, we review the basic
principles of hematology, the cellular elements of the
blood, and the principles of primary and secondary
hemostasis. Additionally, a discussion of red blood cell
development and hemoglobin metabolism provides the
basic science necessary for understanding the clinical
concepts of anemia and oxygen delivery. The emerging
relationship between coagulation and sepsis is explored,
and a review is provided of the most common disorders
of hemostasis seen in the surgical patient. A basic and
practical discussion on the evaluation of bleeding in the
pre-, intra-, and postoperative periods follows. The chapter
concludes with a discussion of the various hemoactive
drugs commonly in use at the present time.

Hematopoiesis: Blood Composition and Formation

The blood is composed of two components: the plasma
and the cellular elements. The plasma represents the soluble
fraction and accounts for 55% of the total blood volume;
plasma volume can be estimated as roughly 7% to 8% of
the total body weight. The plasma bathes the tissues in
nutrients and soluble ions, and carries proteins (such as
albumin, complement, immunoglobulins, and enzymes)
to their places of action. The cellular fraction represents
45% of the blood volume and is divided into three major
cell types: erythrocytes, leukocytes, and megakaryocytes.
Each cell line, however, can be traced back to a single
pluripotent stem cell. Erythrocytes (red blood cells)

function primarily to carry oxygen to tissues. Leukocytes (white blood cells) are a broad class with a variety of more specialized cells, whose primary function involves host defense and immunity. The last major cell type is the megakaryocyte. Platelets and endothelial cells are derived from this committed lineage and are critical to the mechanisms of hemostasis.

Under normal conditions, the production, release from the bone marrow, and survival of the cellular elements in the peripheral blood are highly regulated. At any given time, a set of morphologically and functionally normal cells is available to maintain homeostasis. During stress, injury, and disease states, regulatory mechanisms shift, leading to both quantitative and qualitative changes in the differential count of circulating blood cell types.

The complex process of blood formation is called hematopoiesis (*hemat* = blood and *poiesis* = formation). Hematopoiesis is an ongoing, lifelong process in the bone marrow in the adult. The generation of blood elements begins in the yolk sac of the embryo by gestational day 19 and continues throughout the first trimester of development. Extramedullary hematopoiesis (outside the bone marrow) begins during the third gestational month in the fetal liver. The spleen, kidneys, thymus, and lymph nodes are responsible for a minor role in hematopoiesis during fetal development. After birth, the lymph nodes assume a primary function in the proliferation and differentiation of leukocytes and lymphocytes, while the bone marrow takes over as the major source of blood cell production. Similarly, the liver and spleen assume a critical role in the reticuloendothelial system for the destruction and turnover (apoptosis) of aged and dysfunctional cellular elements.

Pluripotent stem cells residing in the bone marrow are the source of all blood cell types. They give rise to two multipotential stem cells, the lymphoid and myeloid cells. These in turn differentiate into specific cell types called committed unilineage progenitors, which develop into the blood cells in their final form.

Erythropoiesis: Life of the Red Blood Cell

The normal red blood cell is a biconcave disk approximately 7 to 7.5 μ in diameter, containing a fluid volume of 80 to 100 fL. It is the major component of the cellular compartment of the blood, with a circulating life of about 100 to 120 days. Its primary role is to deliver oxygen to the tissues for cellular metabolism and carry dissolved carbon dioxide to the lungs for elimination. The red cell is dependent upon the hemoglobin molecule to perform its role in human biology. Because the red blood cell contains no nucleus, it is incapable of synthesizing new proteins or lipids while in circulation. Its entire complement of hemoglobin

is made during the process of differentiation. This is discussed in more detail in the section on Hemoglobin below.

The erythrocyte begins life as a pluripotent stem cell in the bone marrow. The committed progenitor forms two distinct colonies of cells in response to the hormone erythropoietin: burst-forming units–erythroid and colony-forming units–erythroid (CFU-e). In response to erythropoietin, interleukin-3, interleukin-4, and granulocyte-macrophage colony-stimulating factor, the CFU-e are spurred into cycle, giving rise to the first erythrocyte precursor, the pronormoblast. The pronormoblast is a large nucleated cell with a high nuclear-to-cytoplasmic ratio, giving it a bluish tone on hematoxylin-eosin staining. During the normoblast maturation, 65% of the red cell's hemoglobin is synthesized. Finally, the reticulocytes are formed, no longer containing a nucleus but with residual RNA and mitochondria, synthesizing 35% of the red cell's hemoglobin. They continue to mature for around 2 days in the marrow before making their way to the sinuses and peripheral circulation, where they spend another day in final maturation. Reticulocytes represent about 1% of the entire red blood cell mass, but will be seen in higher concentrations following substantial blood loss. Each pronormoblast yields the formation of 8 to 32 mature erythrocytes.

The concentration of circulating erythrocytes in the blood ranges from 3.8 to 5.9 million cells per microliter of blood, with a hemoglobin concentration ranging from 12 to 17 g/dL and a hematocrit of 35% to 52%. The normal range is broad, varying between men and women, between young and old, and with respect to altitude. Induced erythropoiesis, leading to the expansion of red cell mass, occurs in response to hypoxia, blood loss, and a variety of hormones and disease states.

The most important mediator of erythropoiesis is erythropoietin. Erythropoietin is a hormone produced by the kidney in response to hypoxia. This hormone stimulates the pluripotent stem cells in the bone marrow to mature. Although CFU-e progenitors are only minimally responsive to erythropoietin, the CFU-e cells have many erythropoietin receptors, which are not present on the more differentiated reticulocytes and erythrocytes. The bone marrow is capable of increasing the production of red cells by 5 to 10 times normal under the influence of erythropoietin. However, because of the rate-limiting factor of iron availability, the upregulation is usually only two to three times normal. Additionally, in patients with chronic renal failure, or following a nephrectomy, the ability to generate a vigorous erythropoietin response is impaired.

Unique Metabolic Pathways of the Red Blood Cell

The red blood cell does not possess the structures required for DNA synthesis or replication, nor for transcription and translation of proteins. Cellular viability hinges on the cell's ability to generate ATP through the utilization of glucose. Without the pathways described below, the cell would not be able to maintain its membrane integrity and deformability, proper ionic gradients, or the ability to maintain hemoglobin in its reduced form for the transport and delivery of oxygen.

The most critical pathway to survival is the Embden-Meyerhof pathway for glycolysis. However, three other pathways are important to the survival of the red cell: the hexose monophosphate shunt (also called the pentose shunt), the Rapoport-Luebering shunt, and the methemoglobin reductase pathway. Glucose is the primary fuel of the erythrocyte. It enters the cell through facilitated diffusion from the plasma, and through glycolysis ultimately is converted to lactate and pyruvate. This process uses 2 moles of ATP and produces 4 moles of ATP, for a net gain of 2 ATP molecules. The rate-limiting step is controlled by the activity of phosphofructokinase, which converts fructose 6-phosphate to fructose 1,6-phosphate. This enzyme is inhibited by high concentrations of ATP, which signal the "fed" state. Conversely, high concentrations of AMP signal an "energy-starved" state, favoring continued glycolysis. The energy generated by glycolysis is utilized by the Na^+-K^+ ATPase pump to regulate cell membrane potentials.

Maintenance of the appropriate redox potential is essential for the red blood cell to complete its function of oxygen delivery. This requires the integration of the three aforementioned pathways. The hexose monophosphate shunt must generate reducing equivalents to protect the hemoglobin molecule from oxidation injury. The methemoglobin reductase pathway is required to maintain heme iron in the reduced ferrous (Fe^{2+}) state, which is the form able to combine with oxygen. Finally, the Rapoport-Luebering shunt maintains the correct concentration of 2,3-diphosphoglycerate (2,3-DPG) needed to combine with deoxyhemoglobin and provide for the release of oxygen to the tissues. Because the level of 2,3-DPG in stored red cells falls rapidly, affinity for oxygen is enhanced, such that transfused blood may release oxygen less efficiently to the tissues. Clinically this is usually not of concern because levels of 2,3-DPG rebound quickly in circulation. It may, however, be important in cases of massive transfusion. The red cell ultimately dies as its enzyme systems burn out. The inability to continue glycolysis sufficient to maintain membrane gradients leads to changes in membrane permeability and the cell's ultimate destruction. More than 90% of red cells with altered membrane characteristics are destroyed by the macrophages of the reticuloendothelial system (spleen, liver, and marrow). As the cells are destroyed, the hemoglobin molecule is further degraded. The iron is largely conserved, redistributed to the marrow, and incorporated into new hemoglobin.

Hemoglobin: Characteristics, Synthesis, Degradation, and Function

The hemoglobin molecule binds oxygen and transports it to tissues. It is composed of four polypeptide globin chains, each bound by iron to a single heme moiety. Although four types of globin chains are synthesized (α, β, δ, and γ), the major form of hemoglobin in the adult, HbA_1, is composed of two α-globin chains, two β-globin chains, and one heme prosthetic group. Greater than 97% of hemoglobin in the adult is the HbA_1 type. Each hemoglobin molecule binds 4 molecules of oxygen in a positively cooperative manner, meaning that binding of each oxygen molecule progressively increases hemoglobin's affinity for each successive oxygen molecule. Conversely, as each molecule of oxygen is released to the tissues, dissociation of the next is easier. Each gram of hemoglobin can carry 1.34 mL of oxygen.

The majority of red cell destruction occurs by macrophages of the reticuloendothelial system in the spleen, liver, and bone marrow. The hemoglobin molecule is reduced to its globin, iron, and heme components. Carbon monoxide is generated upon cleavage of the porphyrin ring of the heme moiety to yield biliverdin. The CO_2 is transported to the lungs as carboxyhemoglobin and eliminated. The biliverdin is then reduced to bilirubin (unconjugated), which binds to albumin and is carried to the liver for conjugation with bile acids. After conversion to urobilinogen by intestinal flora, it is excreted in the feces or recycled in small quantities by the enterohepatic circulation. Some of the reabsorbed urobilinogen may spill out into the urine.

Normally, intravascular breakdown of red blood cells accounts for a small portion of hemoglobin turnover. This increases when there is a condition of active hemolysis. In this case, free hemoglobin is released into the circulation. The hemoglobin dissociates into two dimers, which immediately bind haptoglobin in the plasma in a 1:1 ratio. The haptoglobin-hemoglobin complexes are carried to the liver, where extravascular breakdown continues. The complex prevents free hemoglobin from being filtered by the kidneys and reabsorbed by the proximal tubules. Clearance of complexes from the circulation to the liver occurs in as few as 10 minutes. However, in cases of severe active hemolysis, haptoglobin stores may become depleted. In this case, the free hemoglobin is filtered by the kidney, reabsorbed by the tubules, and broken down into biliverdin and iron. Some iron-containing tubule cells eventually may spill into the urine. Haptoglobin is an acute-phase reactant, meaning it is upregulated during periods of stress, inflammation, or tissue injury. Thus even during periods of active hemolysis, the haptoglobin levels may be within normal limits.

The characteristics of the hemoglobin-oxygen dissociation curve are critically important to the understanding of oxygen transport. This curve demonstrates how various environmental conditions influence oxygen uptake and delivery. It has been graphically presented as a sigmoid curve with the percentage of oxygen-saturated hemoglobin plotted versus the partial pressure of oxygen (PO_2). The P_{50} (point where 50% of hemoglobin is saturated with oxygen) in humans is 26 mm Hg. The steepest part of the curve provides for dramatic changes in oxygen saturation in relation to very small changes in PO_2. This is evident when one considers that the PO_2 in the arteries is roughly 100 mm Hg, whereas in the veins it is 40 mm Hg. These correspond to oxygen saturations of 100% in the arteries and 75% in the veins, suggesting that 25% of oxygen was taken up by the tissues. By shifting the curve to the right, hemoglobin's affinity for oxygen is decreased. Therefore, more oxygen is released to the hypoxic tissues. If the curve shifts to the left, the oxygen is more tightly bound to hemoglobin, and less likely to be released to the tissues. During conditions of stress, tissue oxygen demand is high. There is an increase in tissue metabolism, body temperature rises, PO_2 is low, partial pressure of carbon dioxide (PCO_2) is high, lactate levels rise, and pH drops. The curve shifts to the right, facilitating oxygen release from hemoglobin to the oxygen-starved tissues. Conditions resulting in a rightward shift of the curve are increased hydrogen ion concentration (lower pH), PCO_2, temperature, and 2,3-DPG. A decrease in these factors results in a leftward shift. Conditions of acidosis are more favorable to oxygen uptake by tissues than is alkalosis. This may be especially important when deciding whether or not one should "treat" acidosis by the administration of exogenous bicarbonate.

Primary Hemostasis: Platelets and Endothelium

Function

Hemostasis is a complex process of interdependent physiologic events whose purpose is the control of bleeding. It can be divided into two broad stages: primary and secondary hemostasis. Primary hemostasis involves the initial clot formation by adherence of platelets to the damaged vessel wall. Secondary hemostasis includes initiation of the coagulation cascade, thrombin generation, and fibrin deposition.

Components

The main components of primary hemostasis are platelets and endothelial cells. Platelets are 1.5- to 3.5-μm discoid blood cells without nuclei or DNA that are formed from bone marrow megakaryocytes. Their key elements are their secretory granules, contractile cytoskeleton, and outer proteoglycan coat, which contains membrane receptors.

The intracellular granules are of two types, alpha granules and dense granules (or dense bodies). Alpha granules contain platelet thrombospondin, fibrinogen, fibronectin, platelet factor 4, von Willebrand's factor (vWf), platelet-derived growth factor (PDGF), factors V, X, and VIII, and many other proteins. Dense granules contain ATP, ADP, GTP, GDP, other phosphates, calcium, and serotonin. After platelet activation, these contents are released, and so the presence of platelet-specific proteins in the serum is an indication of platelet activation.

The endothelium is now recognized as a metabolically active tissue that plays a substantial role in coagulation and inflammation. The endothelium functions to maintain a nonthrombogenic surface in normal blood vessels, and keep a steady state between the continuous processes of coagulation and fibrinolysis. Although the normal endothelium is nonthrombogenic, it secretes a subendothelial matrix that, when exposed to the plasma, is highly thrombogenic. Another function of the endothelium (and megakaryocytes) is production of vWf. Stores of vWf are released into the subendothelium when the endothelium is damaged. This initiates platelet adhesion, leading to degranulation and further adhesion. Primary hemostasis is further enhanced by the initial vasoconstriction of the damaged vessels.

Mechanism

The first step in primary hemostasis is adhesion of circulating platelets to subendothelial collagen in the damaged vessel wall. Adhesion initially depends on the binding of subendothelial vWf to the platelet glycoprotein (gp) Ib-α receptor, part of the Ib-IX-V complex, which is its principal receptor. The initial binding of vWf to the glycoprotein complex does not irreversibly tether the platelets to the endothelium. Definitive adhesion is dependent on subsequent binding of integrin receptors. The bleeding disorders resulting from deficiency of gp Ib-IX-V (Bernard-Soulier syndrome) and vWf (von Willebrand's disease [vWD]) demonstrate the critical role of these substances in platelet adhesion and hemostasis.

Next, the adherent platelets are activated by exposure to collagen and other components of the damaged vessel wall. Mediators of activation include thrombin, ADP, epinephrine, and thromboxane A_2 (TXA_2). Thrombin is the most potent physiologic platelet agonist. It causes degranulation and activates phospholipase A_2, which acts on cell membrane phospholipids to produce arachidonic acid (AA). Cyclooxygenase (COX) converts AA to prostaglandins G_2 and H_2, and then to TXA_2, which all are released from platelets and cause vasoconstriction and platelet aggregation. Activated platelets also undergo a shape change, mediated by the protein actin.

Activation also causes degranulation, during which platelets release the contents of their alpha and dense granules into the extracellular environment. ADP is released and induces further platelet deformation and aggregation. Growth factors such as PDGF and transforming growth factor-β are released to induce tissue growth and repair. Clotting factors are emitted to aid in secondary hemostasis. In fact, about 20% of all factor V is within platelets, and this portion may be more important to the clotting mechanism that serum factor V levels. In addition to granule contents, products of AA metabolism are released. The most important of these is TXA_2, which stimulates vasoconstriction and aggregation to enhance primary hemostasis.

As platelets are reversibly bound and activated, cohesion and aggregation occur, with formation of the platelet plug and stronger linking to the vessel wall. This process involves binding of various agonists to platelet surface membrane receptors. ADP is an important agonist and was the first one recognized. Its key role in hemostasis is evident by the development of new ADP antagonist drugs, which are used to prevent thrombosis. These agonists continue to activate the platelets, and allow binding of the gp IIb/IIIa integrin in the platelet wall to ligands such as vWf and fibrinogen. This step is required for thrombus formation because it immobilizes the clot on the vessel wall. Fibrinogen is the major ligand for gp IIb/IIIa, which it binds on activated platelets only. By binding fibrinogen or vWf, platelets are joined to form a thrombus. These aggregated platelets then provide a surface for the enzymatic reactions of the coagulation system, and the formation of fibrin.

Fibrin, formed by cleavage of fibrinogen by thrombin, cross-links with the aid of activated factor XIII (factor XIIIa), resulting in a more stable clot. The clot retracts and becomes smaller within minutes of formation.

Secondary Hemostasis: Coagulation Cascade

Following the initiation of the hemostatic process by the interaction of platelets and the vessel wall, the so-called coagulation cascade is activated and ultimately leads to formation of a stable fibrin clot. Inactive precursors are sequentially converted to their active forms and lead to a cascade effect with progressively larger amounts of coagulation factors produced. Fibrin monomers are

generated as the final product of the cascade and are cross-linked to form the final stable clot. Normal coagulation involves the interaction of many elements and under normal conditions is limited to the locale of the vessel wall injury through a complex series of inhibitory and regulatory substances, through feedback loops, and by the diluting effect of the blood flowing through the affected area.

Until recently, coagulation was understood to involve two "pathways": intrinsic and extrinsic (Fig. 37–1). The intrinsic pathway did not require interaction with the injured vessel wall and posited the activation of factor XII as the initiating event for coagulation. Activated factor XII then activated factor XI, which in turn activated factor IX. A complex of activated factor VIII (factor VIIIa) and activated factor IX (factor IXa) with calcium and phospholipid then activated factor X. Activated factor X (factor Xa) then converted prothrombin to thrombin, which in turn converted fibrinogen to fibrin. Factor XIIIa converted the fibrin monomers into a cross-linked fibrin clot in the presence of calcium. In the extrinsic pathway, coagulation is initiated when circulating factor VII interacts with subendothelial tissue factor (TF) in the presence of calcium. Subendothelial TF is exposed to the circulation as a result of endothelial injury. The activated factor VII (factor VIIa)–TF complex activates factor X. Factor Xa then converts prothrombin to thrombin, and the reaction proceeds as described previously to generate a stable fibrin clot.

It is not clear that the intrinsic pathway plays a major role in vivo. Inadequate levels of some of its key components, while rendering standard coagulation tests abnormal,

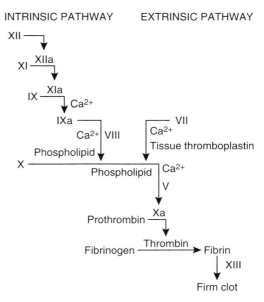

FIGURE 37–1 Classical depiction of the blood coagulation cascade. (From Flacke WE, Flacke JW: Temperature homeostasis and unintentional hypothermia. In Gravenstein N, Kirby KP [eds]: Complications in Anesthesia. Philadelphia: Lippincott-Raven, 1996:118.)

do not routinely result in a clinically significant bleeding disorder. This inconsistency is exemplified by deficiency of factor XII, which is not associated with a bleeding tendency in humans, whereas deficiencies of factor VIII or factor IX exhibit the pronounced bleeding disorders known as hemophilia A and B, respectively. However, the importance of the TF pathway as the predominant mechanism for in vivo coagulation is supported by recent research. The distribution of TF in the subendothelial layer, the epidermis, and myoepithelial cells constitutes a "hemostatic envelope." Injury puts TF into contact with factor VII, thus initiating coagulation. The TF–factor VIIa complex catalyzes the activation of factor IX to factor IXa. As mentioned above, the TF–factor VIIa complex also can directly convert factor X to factor Xa, converting prothrombin to thrombin. The relatively small amounts of thrombin formed by the direct activation of factor X to factor Xa cannot account for observed hemostatic effects. Although rapid inactivation of the TF–factor VIIa–factor Xa complex by TF pathway inhibitor occurs locally, there is sufficient activity of the complex to activate factors VIII and IX, thereby perpetuating the cascade. Factor IXa creates a complex with factor VIIIa, calcium, and phospholipid. This complex activates factor X to factor Xa and produces large amounts of thrombin, which in turn catalyzes the production of significant fibrin from fibrinogen. The activation of factor X to factor Xa by the factor VIIIa–factor IXa–phospholipid complex appears to be the predominant

mechanism for generation of thrombin in vivo (Fig. 37–2). Thrombin then cleaves fibrinogen to fibrin while activating factor XIII. The factor XIIIa cross-links fibrin, resulting in a stable clot. Thrombin also contributes to the initiation of fibrinolysis, as is discussed later. This concept of a single coagulation pathway (TF pathway) is most consistent with current data and observed clinical syndromes and should replace the older concept of two pathways.

Fibrinolysis and Regulation of Thrombosis

The fibrinolytic system acts to break down fibrin and dissolve thrombus, allowing wound healing. It provides a balance to the thrombotic mechanism, and maintains a level of homeostasis within the hemostatic system. The main mechanism of fibrinolysis is the breakdown of fibrin into soluble fragments by the proteolytic enzyme plasmin. Plasmin binds fibrin, and degrades it by cleaving it at multiple sites, resulting in fibrin split products (FSPs). Plasminogen is the precursor to plasmin. It is converted to plasmin by tissue plasminogen activator (tPA), which is released from endothelial cells near the site of injury. Although this reaction is inefficient in the general circulation, in the presence of a fibrin clot it is rapid. Thus fibrin is both the substrate and regulator of its own destruction. Urokinase, eponymously named because of

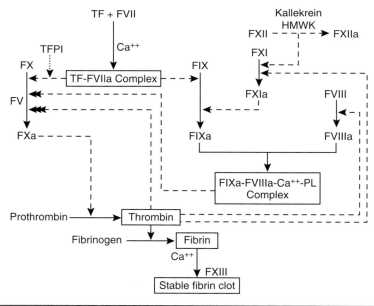

TF: Tissue factor
PL: Phospholipid
HMWK: High-molecular weight
       kininogen Williams-Fitzgerald
       Flaujeac factor

TFPI: Tissue factor pathway inhibitor
·······▶: Negative effect
‑ ‑ ▶: Positive effect

FIGURE 37–2 Contemporary depiction of the blood coagulation cascade.

its high concentration in the urine, is a plasminogen activator that is not fibrin specific. That is, it converts plasminogen to plasmin in the circulation and not just on the clot. It is also the main activator of fibrinolysis in the extravascular space. Urokinase is formed from the single-chain urokinase plasminogen activator precursor.

α_2-Antiplasmin (α_2-AP) is the main inhibitor of plasmin, but also can bind plasminogen. Plasmin is inhibited by α_2-AP when in the circulation, but its degradation is prevented when bound to the fibrin clot. This ensures localized, and not systemic, fibrinolysis. Fibrinolysis is kept in check by several inhibitors of plasminogen activation. These include plasminogen activator inhibitor type 1 (PAI-1) and thrombin-activatable fibrinolysis inhibitor (TAFI).

Laboratory Evaluation

No single test confirms fibrinolysis, but the process can be inferred by laboratory evaluation of several factors along with the clinical scenario. One can measure levels of fibrinogen, FSPs, plasminogen, plasminogen activators, and plasmin inhibitors. Thromboelastography (TEG) also can be useful. The thrombin time (TT) is prolonged in fibrinolysis, and is useful in monitoring the fibrinolytic state during fibrinolytic therapy. Bleeding complications from such therapy are more common when the fibrinogen level is less than 100 mg/dL, and when FSPs are greater than 100 U/dL. Fresh frozen plasma (FFP) can be used to replenish fibrinogen levels and reduce coagulopathy in such situations.

Coagulation and Sepsis

Sepsis is the coexistence of the systemic inflammatory response syndrome with a known or presumed infectious source. Severe sepsis is defined as sepsis with failure of one or more organ systems.

Role of Coagulation in Sepsis

There is increasing evidence of the interrelationship of the coagulation system with the inflammatory response. Acute inflammation causes expression of TF, which activates the coagulation cascade, increases fibrin formation, and increases expression of adhesion molecules that promote inflammation directly.

Thrombin binds to thrombomodulin, and this complex activates protein C. Activated protein C (APC) then causes feedback inhibition of thrombin formation by inhibiting activated factor V (factor Va) and factor VIIIa. In addition, APC inhibits TF and thus downregulates the coagulation cascade. APC also enhances fibrinolysis by inactivating PAI-1, and preventing activation of TAFI.

APC is found in the highest concentrations in the microcirculation, where it functions to quickly clear the capillary bed of thromboses. APC activity is decreased in up to 85% of patients with severe sepsis. As a result, microvascular thrombosis occurs, leading to end-organ congestion and eventually failure.

APC also has more direct anti-inflammatory effects, such as inhibition of nuclear factor κB, tumor necrosis factor, and leukocyte adhesion molecules.

Modulation of Coagulation as Therapy for Sepsis

Given the role of APC in modulation of the coagulation and inflammation involved in sepsis, it is now evident that a subclinical coagulopathy plays a more important role in sepsis than previously thought. Indeed, administration of recombinant human APC has been shown to reduce mortality in severely septic patients.

Disorders of Bleeding and Coagulation

Acquired Disorders

Vitamin K deficiency

Vitamin K is a necessary cofactor in the γ-carboxylation of glutamate residues of factors II, VII, IX, and X as well as protein C and protein S. Therefore, these factors are referred to as the vitamin K–dependent factors. Without vitamin K, these coagulants cannot bind calcium properly and thus are not active. The causes of vitamin K deficiency are many. Dietary intake may be poor, or the intake may be adequate but malabsorbed. Vitamin K is a fat-soluble vitamin, so any factor that causes decreased fat emulsification by bile salts can lead to malabsorption (e.g., biliary obstruction, decreased bile salt formation, cholestasis, biliary fistula). Antibiotic causes include oral antibiotics that can kill vitamin K–producing bacteria in the gut, or cephalosporin antibiotics containing the N-methylthiotetrazole side chain (e.g., cefoperazone, cefotaxime, cefamandole, moxalactam). Other etiologies include parenteral alimentation without vitamin K supplementation, renal insufficiency, and hepatic dysfunction.

Vitamin K may be given orally or parenterally to correct coagulopathy from deficiency or to reverse the effects of warfarin.

Anticoagulant drugs

Drugs that affect hemostasis are abundant and their numbers increase each year (see Table 37–1). More detailed

Table 37–1
Hemoactive drugs

Coagulation Cascade	Platelets	Fibrinolytics/Thrombolytics
Heparin	Aspirin	Urokinase (Abbokinase)
Warfarin (Coumadin)	Ibuprofen	Streptokinase (Kabikinase, Streptase)
Enoxaparin (Lovenox)	Tirofiban (Aggrastat)	tPA, Alteplase (Activase)
Dalteparin (Fragmin)	Anagrelide (Agrylin)	Bivalirudin (Angiomax)
Danaparoid (Orgaran)	Dipyridamole (Persantine)	Anistreplase (Eminase)
Lepirudin (Refludan)	Eptifibatide (Integrilin)	Reteplase (Retavase)
Antithrombin III (Atnativ, Thrombate III)	Clopidogrel (Plavix)	Tenecteplase (TNKase)
	Cilostazol (Pletal)	
	Abciximab (Reopro)	
	Ticlopidine (Ticlid)	

information on hemoactive drugs can be found later in this chapter.

Thrombocytopenia

Thrombocytopenia is generally defined as a platelet count less than $100,000/mm^3$. Bleeding is more common after surgery or injury, with counts from 50,000 to $100,000/mm^3$. However, spontaneous bleeding usually does not occur until the count drops below 20,000, and is common with counts below 10,000.

The etiology of thrombocytopenia may be (1) decreased production of platelets; (2) increased use, consumption, or sequestration of platelets; or (3) dilution. Decreased production may occur with various oncologic disorders or after chemotherapy. Consumption of platelets may occur in sepsis, disseminated intravascular coagulation (DIC), or thrombotic thrombocytopenic purpura, and sequestration can occur in the spleen. Dilutional thrombocytopenia is possible after massive transfusion. In addition, many drugs can cause thrombocytopenia through an immune mechanism, whereby antibodies are formed to platelet glycoproteins. Examples of such drugs are quinidine, sulfa drugs, histamine$_2$-antagonists, oral hypoglycemics, gold salts, rifampin, and heparin. The most common of these is heparin. Chronic alcohol consumption may lead to alcohol-induced thrombocytopenia.

Clinical manifestations of thrombocytopenia include cutaneous petechiae or purpura, mucosal bleeding, easy bruising, and excessive bleeding after surgery or injury. Management involves correcting or reversing the underlying cause if one is found. Transfusion of platelet concentrates is indicated for active bleeding associated with thrombocytopenia, and to keep platelet counts above 10,000 to $20,000/mm^3$. If an invasive procedure or surgery is necessary in a thrombocytopenic patient, transfusion is most beneficial in providing hemostasis when given just before or during the procedure. Multiple platelet transfusions often lead to formation of alloantibodies, thus decreasing the efficacy of repeated administration. Platelet transfusion is not indicated for empiric or prophylactic treatment during massive transfusion or resuscitation, unless there is clinical evidence of microvascular bleeding, or a prolonged bleeding time.

Hypothermia

Hypothermia is a common but often overlooked cause of coagulopathy in surgical patients. It is often related to shock and massive transfusion. As body temperature decreases, the rate of all biologic enzymatic reactions slows. Because the coagulation cascade consists of a series of proteolytic enzymes, hypothermia slows the process of coagulation. As a result, clotting is significantly slowed. Coagulation enzyme activity and platelet function are significantly altered in trauma patients with a core temperature less than 34°C compared to those with core temperatures above 34°C. This defect is not detected by the prothrombin time (PT)/partial thromboplastin time (PTT), because blood samples are warmed to 37°C prior to testing. Hypothermia also causes decreased thromboxane production, resulting in platelet dysfunction, microvascular bleeding, and a prolonged bleeding time.

Typically, coagulopathy from hypothermia occurs in the perioperative setting, when patients receive large volumes of fluid during prolonged procedures, or in patients with hemorrhagic shock receiving massive resuscitation. The result is diffuse nonmechanical or "nonsurgical" bleeding, for which the only treatment is rapid rewarming of the patient. Transfusion of FFP and platelets in an attempt to stop bleeding usually worsens the hypothermia and exacerbates the coagulopathy. Management usually requires quick completion or abbreviation of the procedure without definitive treatment, packing of bleeding areas, and transport to the intensive care unit for rewarming. This "damage control" technique commonly is used in exsanguinating trauma patients, in whom core temperatures less than 32°C are usually associated with death. Patients are returned to the operating room for definitive care later after rewarming and resuscitation are complete.

Consumptive coagulopathy

In certain conditions, bleeding is caused by a decrease in platelets and/or coagulation factors resulting from their consumption in the microvasculature, a condition known as consumptive coagulopathy. Accelerated fibrin deposition occurs, decreasing the fibrinogen level, and platelets become trapped, causing thrombocytopenia. Hypofibrinogenemia concurrent with thrombocytopenia in a bleeding patient is good evidence for a consumptive coagulopathy. Fibrinolysis is induced, resulting in increased fibrin degradation products in the blood.

There are many etiologies of consumptive coagulopathy, with the principle example being the syndrome of DIC. The distinction between DIC and the other etiologic conditions listed below is ill defined, and one or more of the processes may be overlapping.

SEPSIS OR INFECTION. These conditions are a common cause of postoperative thrombocytopenia. The mechanism is unclear, but may in part be due to endotoxin-induced aggregation and destruction of platelets in the microvasculature, or by direct activation of the coagulation cascade. Also, APC is deficient and so formation of microthrombi is not inhibited.

SHOCK, TRAUMA, BURNS, AND PANCREATITIS. These conditions cause release of thromboplastic substances that increase thrombin formation and consumption of coagulation factors. They also can lead to thrombocytopenia. In addition, inadequate tissue perfusion incites the inflammatory response, which leads to coagulopathy.

TRAUMATIC BRAIN INJURY. Injured brain tissue releases its rich stores of thromboplastin, which leads to hypercoagulability by accelerating fibrin formation and microvascular thrombosis. Coagulation substrates are consumed and further clotting is impaired.

OBSTETRIC EMERGENCIES. Placental abruption, amniotic fluid embolism, dead fetus, eclampsia, septic abortion, and hydatidiform mole all can cause release of thromboplastic substances that increase thrombin formation and consumption of coagulation factors.

DISSEMINATED INTRAVASCULAR COAGULATION. DIC is an acquired coagulation disorder that involves diffuse activation of the coagulation system, with fibrin deposition in the microvasculature, platelet aggregation, and thrombosis. The severity ranges from subclinical or low grade to severe and life threatening. Clinically DIC is manifested by generalized bleeding, and end-organ failure results from the diffuse microvascular thrombosis. The more severe form can lead to multiple organ system failure and death. Mortality is increased in septic or severely injured patients with DIC.

A variety of clinical conditions are associated with DIC. In addition to all of the processes listed above, DIC may be associated with massive transfusion, hemolysis, liver disease, and malignancy (including leukemia). The pathophysiologic process in DIC is initiated through inflammatory mechanisms and cytokines, especially interleukin-6. The systemic formation of fibrin results from three mechanisms. First, TF activates factor VII, and the TF–factor VIIa complex mediates formation of thrombin, with subsequent conversion of fibrinogen to fibrin and activation of platelets. Second, the natural anticoagulant mechanisms operating via antithrombin III (ATIII), protein C, and TF pathway inhibitor all are impaired in DIC. This leads to a shift in the hemostatic balance toward thrombosis. Finally, fibrin clearance is decreased because of a relative excess of PAI-1, which inhibits plasmin formation and fibrinolysis.

Diagnosis of DIC is made by the combination of clinical findings and certain supportive laboratory tests. There is no specific test that confirms or rules out the diagnosis. Clinically one suspects DIC in patients with a generalized coagulopathy, bleeding, and the presence of an inciting factor or disease associated with DIC. The patient usually has a low or decreasing platelet count and prolonged PT/PTT. FSPs may be present in the plasma, and coagulation inhibitors such as ATIII may be deficient. Fibrinogen levels may be low in severe DIC, but, because fibrinogen is an acute-phase reactant, its production is increased as part of the stress response, and levels may be normal. The D-dimer assay is the most sensitive test for DIC, being abnormal in up to 94% of patients with a diagnosis of DIC. In many patients with coagulopathy who are suspected of having DIC, hypothermia needs to be considered as the primary etiology of the bleeding disorder, especially if sepsis is not present.

Treatment of DIC centers around treatment of the underlying disease process. Symptomatic treatment is generally futile if the proinflammatory impetus is not addressed concomitantly. Several strategies have been investigated as specific therapy for DIC.

Anticoagulation has been used as an attempt to halt the underlying hypercoagulation in DIC. Currently there have been no controlled studies showing any benefit of unfractionated or low-molecular-weight heparin (LMWH) in DIC. One randomized, double-blind, placebo-controlled trial in healthy humans showed that unfractionated heparin (UFH) and LMWH improved laboratory measures of coagulation in endotoxin-induced coagulation in humans. This has not been confirmed in patients with DIC. ATIII-independent thrombin inhibitors such as desirudin currently are being studied.

Platelet and FFP transfusion has no benefit when used prophylactically in patients with DIC. However, benefit exists for patients with active bleeding and those undergoing invasive procedures. In the latter case, such transfusions are best given just prior to, or during, the procedure to maximize the chances of hemostasis before the platelets and coagulation factors are consumed.

As mentioned previously, ATIII levels are low in patients with DIC. Administration of high doses of ATIII has shown some efficacy in the subgroup of patients with septic shock, with improved symptoms of DIC, organ function, and mortality. This therapy may hold promise for the future.

Antifibrinolytics such as ε-aminocaproic acid (EACA) have improved bleeding in specific oncologic disorders and fibrinolytic syndromes, but not in DIC. Their use cannot be recommended in DIC.

Hepatic failure

The liver is the site of synthesis for all coagulation factors except factor VIII, so, in hepatic failure, synthesis of these and other proteins is decreased. Cirrhotics produce less fibrinogen, but also make an abnormal form of fibrinogen with impaired clotting ability. Poor oral intake, malabsorption, or biliary obstruction may lead to vitamin K deficiency and impaired synthesis of the vitamin K–dependent factors by the liver. These patients usually have a prolonged PT, a normal to slightly elevated PTT, and low fibrinogen levels (as demonstrated by a prolonged TT). Correction of the coagulopathy may be effected by administration of desmopressin acetate (DDAVP) in cirrhotics, transfusion of FFP, or replacement of vitamin K as the situation dictates.

Liver trauma

Severe liver injury can cause coagulopathy through several mechanisms. In such cases massive transfusion is often required, leading to both dilutional thrombocytopenia and hypothermia. If a large percentage of the liver is damaged, production of coagulation factors may be decreased, and clearance of profibrinolytic substances is reduced, impairing coagulation.

Renal failure

Renal failure causes a qualitative platelet defect, attributable to decreased platelet adhesiveness and aggregation.

The mechanism of this dysfunction is not known, but the effects can be reversed with dialysis (most effective), DDAVP, cryoprecipitate, and conjugated estrogens. DDAVP reduces bleeding complications after a number of procedures in renal failure patients. It can be given intravenously in a dose of 0.3 μg/kg in uremic patients, and can help to decrease the bleeding time, as do cryoprecipitate and conjugated estrogens. Conversely, dialysis patients with chronic renal failure can have a defect in fibrinolysis that correlates with the severity of the renal dysfunction, leading to thrombotic complications.

Congenital Disorders

Hemophilia A

Hemophilia A is an X-linked recessive disorder resulting from factor VIII deficiency, and is the most common congenital bleeding disorder. Its pattern of inheritance makes it almost universally a disease in males, occurring in about 1 in 10,000 male births, and a carrier state in females. Bleeding tendency correlates inversely with factor VIII levels. Spontaneous bleeding may occur with levels less than 5%, and those patients with higher levels (mild disease) tend to bleed abnormally after surgery or injury. Carriers generally have levels greater than 50% and do not have clinical manifestation of the disease. A factor VIII level of at least 30% is needed for surgical hemostasis. Hemophilia A patients will have a prolonged PTT and decreased factor VIII levels. The PT and bleeding time are normal. Normal vWf levels distinguish hemophilia from vWD, because both have low factor VIII levels.

Treatment of bleeding is with factor VIII replacement. Although FFP and cryoprecipitate both contain factor VIII in low levels (5 to 10 times higher in cryoprecipitate vs. FFP), the preferred treatment is transfusion of pooled factor VIII concentrate. Since 1984, factor VIII concentrates have been treated to inactivate human immunodeficiency virus, hepatitis, and other viruses, making viral infection unlikely. DDAVP may temporarily raise factor VIII levels in patients with mild hemophilia A.

About 10% to 20% of hemophiliacs develop inhibitors (immunoglobulin G [IgG] antibodies) to factor VIII, usually in response to factor VIII infusions. Treatment can be complicated, and detection of such inhibitors requires a mixing study.

Hemophilia B

Hemophilia B, or Christmas disease, is an X-linked disorder of factor IX deficiency. Clinical manifestations are similar to those in patients with hemophilia A, and the severity of symptoms correlates inversely with factor IX levels. Laboratory studies reveal an abnormal PTT and low factor IX levels, with a normal PT and bleeding time.

Treatment is with factor IX concentrates, aimed at increasing levels up to 50% of normal, because higher levels may actually cause arterial and venous thromboses. Like hemophilia A, inhibitors may develop, and can be detected with a mixing study.

von Willebrand's disease

vWD is an inherited bleeding disorder caused by deficiency or dysfunction of vWf, which facilitates platelet adhesion to damaged endothelium and also stabilizes factor VIII in the blood. There are three types of vWD. Type 1 is characterized by a partial deficiency in levels of vWf, and type 3 refers to complete absence of vWf. Type 2 vWD has several subtypes, but all refer to a qualitative defect in vWf, which is present in normal quantity. vWD generally is characterized by low levels of factor VIII coagulant activity and a prolonged bleeding time. Symptoms are similar to those caused by platelet dysfunction, and include mucosal bleeding, epistaxis, petechial hemorrhage, menorrhagia, and prolonged bleeding after surgery.

Diagnosis may be difficult because of the lack of any one test with sufficient sensitivity and specificity. The PT/PTT and bleeding time may be prolonged. Types 1 and 3 vWD have reduced levels of factor VIII:c and vWf antigen. Factor VIII:c is reduced because vWf is the major serum carrier for circulating factor VIII. Other tests include the vWf ristocetin cofactor assay, which measures the ability of vWf to aggregate platelets in the presence of the antibiotic ristocetin, or the vWf collagen-binding activity assay.

Treatment of vWD varies according to the specific subtype. DDAVP, a synthetic vasopressin analog, causes release of factor VIII and vWf into the plasma, and can cause correction of abnormal bleeding times and levels of vWf and factor VIII. Because endothelial stores of vWf may take up to 48 hours to reaccumulate, repeated doses of DDAVP are sometimes less effective, though this problem is less frequent in patients with type 1 vWD. DDAVP is ineffective in type 3 vWD because of absence of significant stores of vWf, and is contraindicated in type 2 vWD because it can cause thrombocytopenia and increase bleeding.

Transfusion of cryoprecipitate can be used to treat or prevent bleeding associated with all types of vWD. FFP contains 5 to 10 times less vWf and factor VIII than cryoprecipitate, and therefore is not effective unless given in large volumes. Factor VIII–vWf concentrates also are available for bleeding patients with vWD unresponsive to DDAVP. These, unlike cryoprecipitate, are virus inactivated, and risk of infection transmission is less of a concern. Factor VIII–vWf concentrates are believed by some to be the treatment of choice for types 2 and 3 vWD. Adjunctive therapy also can be given with the antifibrinolytic agents EACA (50 to 60 mg/kg every 4 to 6 hours) and tranexamic acid (20 to 25 mg/kg every 8 to 12 hours).

Other congenital deficiencies

Several other rare congenital deficiencies exist, including deficiencies of factors V, VII, X, XI, XII, and XIII; prekallikrein; high-molecular-weight kininogen (HMWK); and proteins C and S. Most are autosomal recessive and heterogeneous in their phenotypic expression. Protein C and S deficiencies, and APC resistance (associated with the factor V Leiden mutation), predispose to venous thrombosis.

Evaluation of Bleeding and Coagulation

Preoperative Period

All patients who are to have surgery should have a thorough screening for bleeding abnormalities as part of their history and physical examination. Diagnosis of most disorders is made predominately by clinical evaluation, with laboratory studies used only in certain circumstances.

The patient should be questioned about his or her bleeding history. One should ask about known bleeding disorders, bruising tendency, excessive bleeding during medical or dental procedures, prolonged menorrhea, gastrointestinal (GI) bleeding, or repeated or severe epistaxis. Primary hemostatic defects (platelets) manifest as excessive bleeding from cuts or mucosal surfaces, or easy bruising. Secondary defects (factor deficiencies) usually have hemarthroses or intramuscular hematomas.

A medication history should be obtained to determine the use of oral anticoagulants such as warfarin, aspirin, and nonsteroidal anti-inflammatory drugs (NSAIDs), among others. One should specifically ask if the patient is taking these drugs or any over-the-counter products, because many patients may not consider agents such as aspirin a medication, and may fail to mention them. Finally, one should ask about medical conditions that may affect hemostasis, such as alcohol abuse, liver or kidney dysfunction, or a family history of hemophilia or other disorder.

Physical examination may reveal bruising, joint abnormalities, petechiae, purpura, ecchymosis, telangiectasia, hepatosplenomegaly, or malnutrition. These findings would increase suspicion of an underlying coagulation disorder.

Laboratory testing should not be done routinely on patients with a normal hematologic history and physical exam. Current data do not support routine screening laboratory evaluation preoperatively in patients without a history of abnormal bleeding or clinical indications of a bleeding disorder. In addition, the PT, PTT, and bleeding time have a low yield in revealing occult bleeding disorders or in predicting clinically significant perioperative bleeding, and may have false-positive results. Indications for specific tests should be based on the history and physical exam and the existence of other processes that may alter hemostasis, such as the systemic inflammatory response syndrome, sepsis, malnutrition, or organ failure.

The following is a list and description of the laboratory tests most commonly used in the investigation of bleeding abnormalities:

Prothrombin time—This test is done by adding a thromboplastin, containing TF, phospholipid, and calcium, to citrated plasma and measuring the time in seconds until a fibrin clot is formed compared to a control. The PT measures the activity of the extrinsic pathway (factor VII) and the common pathway (fibrinogen and factors II, IX, and X). It is used to monitor warfarin therapy, and affected by depletion of the vitamin K–dependent factors (factors II, VII, IX, and X and proteins C and S).

International normalized ratio (INR)—The INR is used to adjust for individual lab variation in the PT, using the formula INR = (log patient PT/log control PT) to the power of *c*, where *c* is the international sensitivity index. The thromboplastin used in individual laboratories is thus calibrated against a reference thromboplastin.

Partial thromboplastin time—The PTT is done by adding a partial thromboplastin (mixture of phospholipids), an activating substance, and calcium chloride to citrated plasma. It measures the activity of the intrinsic pathway (HMWK, prekallikrein, and factors VIII, IX, XI, and XII) and the common pathway (fibrinogen and factors II, IX, and X). Only factor VII is not measured by the PTT. It is used to monitor heparin therapy because heparin affects the intrinsic pathway but not factor VII of the extrinsic pathway.

Platelet count—This is a quantitative measure of circulating platelets. Counts less than $50,000/mm^3$ increase bleeding from cut surfaces, and counts less than $20,000/mm^3$ may be associated with spontaneous bleeding.

Bleeding time—The bleeding time is the only test that measures platelet function and primary hemostasis. However, because of variation in the performance of the test and the methods used, it is relatively insensitive and nonspecific in identifying platelet function abnormalities. In addition, the test may not predict surgical bleeding.

Thrombin time—The TT is determined by adding thrombin to citrated plasma with or without calcium. The TT measures the time for conversion of fibrinogen to fibrin, which is induced by thrombin. It is prolonged when fibrinogen is deficient (<100 mg/dL) or abnormal; in the presence of circulating anticoagulants, including FSPs and heparin; and during excessive fibrinolysis. Its high sensitivity to exogenous anticoagulants such as heparin limits its usefulness in hospitalized patients, but it can be used to detect low levels of circulating heparin, which do not cause changes in the PTT.

Fibrinogen—Fibrinogen is a large protein that is cleaved by thrombin to produce fibrin monomers. These then cross-link to form a fibrin clot in the presence of factor XIII. Thus, as clotting increases (i.e., fibrin is formed), the fibrinogen level decreases. Low levels may be seen with consumptive conditions such as DIC, sepsis, severe traumatic brain injury, and obstetric emergencies, or with overanticoagulation by thrombolytic agents. However, fibrinogen is an acute-phase reactant that may be elevated in response to physiologic stress, producing normal levels even while its consumption is accelerated.

Thromboelastography—TEG analyzes various characteristics of clot formation in a sample of whole blood, and converts these data to graphic form by computer analysis. A unique thromboelastogram tracing is depicted based on the rate of clot formation, fibrin cross-linking, and platelet-fibrin interaction. By measuring various parameters of the tracing, TEG provides an assessment of platelet function, coagulation enzyme activity, and the overall degree of coagulability. It can also identify primary fibrinolysis, consumptive coagulopathy, anticoagulant therapy, and even the effect of hypothermia on clotting. TEG is used frequently during cardiopulmonary bypass and liver transplantation and in intensive care settings, as a result of its rapid availability and ability to assess the components of coagulation in an integrated fashion.

Fibrin split products—FSPs are fragments of the fibrin molecule that result from breakdown of fibrin by plasmin during fibrinolysis. The presence of FSPs is not diagnostic in and of itself, but, when added to the clinical scenario, can provide evidence of a consumptive process such as DIC. The D-dimer is a specific form of FSP that is most closely associated with DIC.

Factor assays—Specific coagulation factor levels can be used to diagnose specific diseases or deficiencies. The PT/PTT is not altered until factor levels are significantly depleted. The more common assays are factor VIII for hemophilia A and factor IX for hemophilia B. Other assays may detect deficiencies in factors V, VII, X, XI, XII (Hageman factor), prekallikrein, and HMWK. All are very rare disorders.

Intraoperative Period: Surgical Versus Nonsurgical Bleeding

During surgery, bleeding may arise from direct dissection of tissues and transection of vessels. This is known as "surgical bleeding" because the cause and remedy are surgical in nature. Surgical bleeding is best handled by prevention, with careful attention to dissection and tissue planes. However, when encountered, such bleeding can be stopped by coagulation with electrocautery or suture ligation. Nonsurgical bleeding, also referred to as microvascular bleeding, arises from a disturbance in the clotting mechanism, and is diagnosed clinically by the observation of diffuse oozing of blood from all damaged tissues, including areas that may not have been directly cut or dissected. Treatment is directed at the cause of the coagulopathy, and usually involves termination of the operative procedure.

The most common nonsurgical causes of intraoperative bleeding are hypothermia and thrombocytopenia. The latter usually arises from dilution resulting from massive transfusion, or from DIC.

Postoperative Period

Postoperative hemorrhage must be evaluated in a systematic fashion designed to detect the cause, and thereby direct the treatment, of the bleeding. Evaluation, as always, begins with a detailed history. One should review the operative notes for the exact procedure performed, and any details pertinent to the current situation (e.g., oozing of the liver bed after cholecystectomy). Pre- and postoperative medications should be reviewed for drugs that may affect coagulation, as well as any medical conditions that may influence hemostasis (see Acquired Disorders above). Physical exam should be directed toward localizing the source of the bleeding if possible (e.g., a wound hematoma, fresh blood from a drain), but also toward other signs that may indicate the cause. For example, bleeding from all cut surfaces, intravenous line sites, and needle puncture sites may indicate a coagulation disorder, as opposed to a purely technical problem such as a slipped ligature. Petechiae indicate platelet deficiency or dysfunction. Fever, tachycardia, and tachypnea may point

toward infection or sepsis as the cause of consumptive coagulopathy.

Laboratory tests may help diagnose the cause of the coagulopathy. Platelet count, bleeding time, PT, and PTT help to differentiate primary versus secondary hemostatic problems, and low fibrinogen levels may indicate a consumptive coagulopathy. Note that a hematocrit level does not help to determine the presence of acute bleeding. The intravascular space must first be diluted with fluid either shifted from the interstitial space or added from intravenous administration before the hematocrit will fall. This often takes several hours, by which time the presence of bleeding should be obvious by clinical data, as described below.

The etiology of postoperative bleeding may fall into one of the following broad categories: loss of surgical hemostasis or coagulation disorders. Loss of surgical hemostasis refers to bleeding from the operative site. This may be due to a technical failure such as a slipped ligature or disruption of a vascular anastomosis, or inadequate hemostasis during the procedure. Often the problem stems from vessels on cut surfaces that did not bleed intraoperatively because of vasoconstriction, but that postoperatively, when the patient is warmer and rehydrated, vasodilate and bleed. Loss of surgical hemostasis, when discovered acutely, usually requires a return to the operating room for definitive control. The diagnosis often is made by observing signs and symptoms of hypovolemia, such as tachycardia, restlessness, anxiety, pallor, oliguria, and hypotension. Anxiety and tachycardia are early signs of hemorrhage. An anxious, agitated surgical patient should never be sedated without a thorough evaluation for the causes of this deceptive clinical presentation. Many an inexperienced surgeon has learned this important lesson the hard way. It is also important to remember that a normal blood pressure does not exclude hemorrhage, because up to 30% of the normal blood volume may be lost before hypotension occurs.

Coagulation disorders may arise from a congenital or acquired defect in primary or secondary hemostasis. Primary hemostatic failure denotes a problem with formation of the initial platelet plug. This may be due to a qualitative or quantitative platelet defect. Qualitative defects in platelet dysfunction can be caused by drugs, hypothermia, acute renal failure, or congenital diseases such as vWD. Quantitative abnormalities (thrombocytopenia) can be caused by dilution after massive transfusion, sepsis or major infection, consumptive coagulopathy, chemotherapy, radiation, hemolytic uremic syndrome, thrombotic thrombocytopenic purpura, idiopathic or immune thrombocytopenic purpura, post-transfusion purpura, or drug-induced immune thrombocytopenia (e.g., quinine).

Secondary hemostatic failure refers to a problem with the factors of the coagulation cascade, which also may arise from a qualitative or quantitative abnormality. Decreased production of factors may result from liver failure, or there may be a decreased availability of activated factors as a result of vitamin K deficiency. Existing factors may function abnormally, as with hypothermia, or be inhibited by drugs, as with warfarin and heparin use. The effects of heparin can be reversed with protamine, as described later in this chapter. Note that, although administration of FFP will correct prolongation of the PT, it will not correct bleeding caused by UFH, which prolongs the PTT, or by LMWH. Increased destruction of factors can result from consumptive coagulopathy. Dilution of coagulation proteins by massive fluid or plasma infusion occurs rarely, if at all. Therefore, there is no need to replace factors based solely on the volume of fluids or blood infused.

Hemoactive Drugs

Anticoagulants

Unfractionated heparin

UFH is a glycosaminoglycan that exerts its anticoagulant effect through binding and potentiation of ATIII. ATIII inactivates activated factors II (factor IIa), IXa, and Xa, and inhibits the prothrombinase complex, which consists of factors Xa and Va assembling in the presence of calcium on a phospholipid membrane. Therapy with UFH is gauged by the PTT, which is prolonged by inhibition of the above-noted factors. UFH is not absorbed orally, so it must be given intravenously or subcutaneously. The half-life is about 1 hour. UFH can be reversed by protamine sulfate (see below), which binds and neutralizes the heparin molecule.

Major adverse reactions with UFH include bleeding, thrombocytopenia, and osteoporosis. Heparin may cause a thrombocytopenia, which reverses spontaneously, even with continued use of heparin. Heparin-induced thrombocytopenia (HIT), however, is an IgG-mediated immune disorder that can have severe sequelae in a small percentage of patients. In addition to the low platelet count, HIT can lead to paradoxical arterial or venous thrombosis with their resultant problems. Diagnosis is made with the appropriate clinical scenario plus the presence of heparin antibodies in the serum. Discontinuation of the heparin is mandatory in such cases. If continued anticoagulation is required and warfarin use is not feasible, danaparoid sodium may be used. Lepirudin, a hirudin derivative, is the only drug approved by the Food and Drug Administration (FDA) to treat HIT-related thromboses.

Low-molecular-weight heparin

LMWH is produced by fragmentation of heparin molecules to produce smaller molecules (4000 to 5000 kD vs. 5000 to 30,000 kD). LMWH has reduced binding ability, a longer half-life, and more efficient bioavailability than UFH, accounting for its different physiologic effects. Less binding to plasma proteins leads to a predictable anticoagulant response, which allows therapy without monitoring coagulation tests. Decreased binding to platelets may result in a lower incidence of HIT. The mechanism of action, like UFH, is activation of ATIII. However, whereas UFH affects factors IIa and Xa equally, LMWH's inhibition of factor Xa is two to five times greater than that of factor IIa.

Complications include bleeding, although HIT and osteoporosis are reduced with LMWH. It may be used for prophylaxis (40 mg SQ daily for perioperative elective general surgery; 30 mg SQ bid for major trauma and orthopedic procedures) or treatment. The treatment dose is based on patient weight (1 mg/kg SQ bid).

Warfarin

Warfarin is the most common oral anticoagulant in North America. Its mechanism of action is inhibition of thrombin formation by interfering with the activation and conformational change of the vitamin K–dependent coagulation factors (II, VII, IX, and X). Vitamin K is oxidized and reduced in cyclic fashion while acting as a cofactor for the γ-carboxylation of glutamate residues on the vitamin K–dependent proteins. Warfarin inhibits the enzymes vitamin K epoxide reductase and vitamin K reductase, which are necessary for these reactions, thus decreasing the activation of the vitamin K–dependent factors.

Warfarin also inhibits the natural anticoagulants protein C and protein S through the same mechanism. Because these proteins have shorter half-lives than do factors II, VII, IX, and X, warfarin theoretically causes an initial hypercoagulable state. Although clinical manifestations of this hypercoagulable state are rare in patients without factor deficiencies, this is the rationale for initiating therapeutic levels of anticoagulation with heparin prior to starting warfarin.

Therapy is gauged by the PT and INR. Factor VII has the shortest half-life of the vitamin K–dependent factors (about 6 hours), so prolongation of the PT in the first 2 to 3 days after initiation of warfarin may reflect factor VII inhibition and not full anticoagulation.

Many drugs affect warfarin therapy by reducing its absorption, altering its metabolism in the liver, or changing its clearance. Adverse reactions include bleeding and skin necrosis. The latter has an unknown mechanism and may be more common with concomitant protein C or S deficiency.

Hirudin

Hirudin is a direct thrombin inhibitor originally isolated from the leech *Hirudo medicinalis*, but now genetically engineered. It binds and inactivates thrombin independently of ATIII. Lepirudin is the only hirudin currently approved in the United States. It is indicated for use mainly in patients with HIT. Like heparin, it causes prolongation of the PTT.

Antiplatelet Agents

Aspirin

Aspirin is the classical platelet antagonist. It permanently and irreversibly acetylates the enzyme COX, preventing its binding to AA and subsequent metabolism of AA to TXA_2, thus inhibiting platelet aggregation and plug formation. Because platelets are anucleic and cannot resynthesize COX, new platelets are required before normal platelet function returns. Thus aspirin must be discontinued (e.g., before surgery) for the 8- to 12-day life span of the platelet for its effects to vanish.

ADP inhibitors

Ticlopidine and clopidogrel are inhibitors of ADP-mediated platelet activation and aggregation. They are used primarily in prevention of thrombosis in patients with vascular disease, such as stroke or myocardial infarction. Clopidogrel may be preferred because of its decreased incidence of side effects compared to ticlopidine.

Glycoprotein IIb/IIIa antagonists

Abciximab is the Fab fragment of a monoclonal antibody that binds to the gp IIb/IIIa receptor on activated platelets, thereby inhibiting platelet aggregation and plug formation. It is used in the acute setting to prevent thrombosis associated with percutaneous coronary procedures and refractory unstable angina. Its main adverse effect is thrombocytopenia. Eptifibatide and tirofiban are two newer drugs that reversibly inhibit platelet aggregation. Their effects are reversed within a few hours of discontinuation of the infusion. They are indicated for treatment of unstable angina or non–Q wave myocardial infarction, with an additional indication for eptifibatide for patients undergoing percutaneous coronary procedures.

Phosphodiesterase inhibitors

Inhibition of phosphodiesterase (PDE) results in higher concentrations of cyclic AMP (cAMP) within platelets. This in turn inhibits phospholipase and COX, thus inhibiting thromboxane production and platelet aggregation. Dipyridamole is one such agent with efficacy in prevention of stroke, especially when combined with aspirin. It also has coronary vasodilatory effects, which is the basis for its use in nuclear imaging of the heart.

Pentoxifylline was the first agent approved for treatment of claudication. Its exact mechanism of action remains unclear, but it is reported to increase red blood cell deformability and decrease blood viscosity. Cilostazol is only the second agent that is FDA approved for treatment of claudication. It inhibits prostaglandin E_3, which is the predominant form of PDE within platelets, and selectively inhibits cAMP-PDE.

Nonsteroidal Anti-inflammatory Drugs

Ibuprofen

Ibuprofen blocks prostaglandin metabolism temporarily, by reversibly binding to COX. Its inhibition lasts about 3 to 4 days.

COX-2 inhibitors

Recently it has been recognized that there are two forms of the COX enzyme, COX-1 and COX-2. COX-1, which is constitutively expressed in most tissues, is the catalyst for TXA_2 synthesis, and for prostaglandins in the GI tract. Inhibition of COX-1 is thought to be responsible for the GI side effects of aspirin and NSAIDs. Aspirin inhibits COX-1 more than COX-2.

COX-2 is not detectable in most tissues, but is rapidly upregulated in response to inflammatory and other stimuli. COX-2 is involved mainly in synthesis of prostacyclin. Selective COX-2 inhibitors, such as celecoxib and rofecoxib, retain anti-inflammatory and analgesic properties while sparing most of the GI and bleeding side effects of the COX-1 enzyme.

Shortly after their introduction in 1999, these agents became some of the most widely prescribed medications in the United States. However, the COX-2 inhibitors can have undesirable renal and cardiovascular side effects similar to those of traditional NSAIDs, and should be used with caution in certain patient populations. Also, because COX-2 inhibitors prevent prostacyclin synthesis while preserving TXA_2, there is a theoretical risk of increased thrombosis. However, this has not yet been proven clinically.

Thrombolytics

Streptokinase

Streptokinase is not an enzyme per se, but a glycoprotein produced by β-hemolytic streptococcal bacteria. It binds to plasminogen both on the fibrin clot and systemically; then this streptokinase-plasminogen complex activates other plasminogen molecules to form plasmin. Because of its bacterial derivation, it is highly immunogenic, and so cannot be used repeatedly in the same patient.

Urokinase

Urokinase is a plasminogen activator found in urine that converts plasminogen to plasmin. Like streptokinase, urokinase acts systemically and therefore poses a higher risk of bleeding complications.

Tissue plasminogen activator

tPA binds to fibrin, and there it cleaves fibrin-bound plasminogen to plasmin. It has little effect on plasminogen in the systemic circulation, but still has significant systemic bleeding risks. The original human tPA has been produced in a recombinant form that is not antigenic, and does not produce allergic reactions like the nonsynthetic form. Other thrombolytic agents include the second-generation agent anistreplase (anisoylated plasminogen streptokinase activator complex), and the third-generation drug reteplase. Bioengineering techniques have improved many features of the newer thrombolytics, but a major goal continues to be development of a drug that has high clot specificity with few systemic effects and little bleeding risk.

Procoagulants

DDAVP (desmopressin)

DDAVP is a synthetic vasopressin analog that causes release of factor VIII and vWf from the endothelium into the plasma, and can cause correction of abnormal bleeding times and levels of vWf and factor VIII. It is used to treat bleeding complications associated with type I vWD and platelet dysfunction resulting from renal failure.

ε-Aminocaproic acid

EACA is an antifibrinolytic agent that inhibits lysis of clots. It binds plasminogen, preventing its adherence to fibrin and conversion to plasmin. It is used in surgical patients mainly to reverse the effects of thrombolytic drugs and in cardiac surgery to reduce bleeding after cardiopulmonary bypass.

Aprotinin

Aprotinin is a serine protease inhibitor that improves platelet function and promotes antifibrinolysis, and also may have complex anti-inflammatory effects. Like EACA, it is used for hemostasis during and after cardiopulmonary bypass.

Protamine sulfate

Protamine is a protein that binds to heparin and neutralizes its anticoagulant effects. The dose is 1 mg of protamine for each 100 units of heparin given. The half-life of heparin must be taken into account when calculating the protamine dose, such that the dose of heparin must be halved for each hour since its injection. So, for example, a 5000-unit bolus of heparin given 3 hours ago would require 6.25 mg of protamine (sequentially halve 5000 three times to get 625, then divide 625 by 100 to get 6.25). Adverse reactions include hypotension, which may be avoided by slow injection over 10 minutes, and a 1% risk of anaphylaxis in patients who have had previous exposure to protamine of NPH insulin. Protamine also has been reported rarely to cause a hypercoagulable state.

Estrogen

Estrogen is used frequently for hormone replacement therapy in postmenopausal women. It has been reported to have cardioprotective effects, but also prothrombotic effects in the venous system. The exact mechanism of the increased risk of venous thrombosis is not clear, but proposed mechanisms are inhibition of fibrinolysis, decreases in natural anticoagulants such as ATIII and protein S, or increases in coagulation factors.

Conclusion

Surgeons rely on the normal functioning of blood to ensure the successful outcomes of their operations and the welfare of their patients. The field of hematology and coagulation is a large and ever-expanding specialty, and most surgeons cannot be expected to master it. We have attempted to provide a practical review of the subject for the practicing surgeon. Consultation with a specialist in the field will help in the more complex situations.

Bibliography

Andrews RK, Shen Y, Gardiner EE, et al: The glycoprotein Ib-IX-V complex in platelet adhesion and signalling. Thromb Haemost 1999;82:357.

Bennett JS: Structural biology of glycoprotein IIb-IIa. Trends Cardiovasc Med 1996;16:31.

Bennett JS: Novel platelet inhibitors. Annu Rev Med 2001;52:161.

Bernard GR, Vincent JL, Laterre PF, et al: Efficacy and safety of recombinant human activated protein C for severe sepsis. N Engl J Med 2001;344:699.

Bick RL, Baker WF: Diagnostic efficacy of the D-dimer assay in disseminated intravascular coagulation (DIC). Thromb Res 1992;65:785.

Broze GJ: The role of tissue factor pathway inhibitor in a revised coagulation cascade. Semin Hematol 1992;29:159.

Dessypris EN: Erythropoiesis. *In* Lee GR, Foerster J, Lukens J, et al (eds): Wintrobe's Clinical Hematology (10th ed), Vol I. Baltimore: Williams & Wilkins, 1999:169.

Eisele B, Lamy M, Thijs LG, et al: Antithrombin III in patients with severe sepsis: a randomized, placebo-controlled, double-blind multicenter trial plus a meta-analysis on all randomized, placebo-controlled, double-blind trials with antithrombin III in severe sepsis. Intensive Care Med 1998;24:663.

Eisenberg JM, Clarke JR, Sussman SA: Prothrombin and partial thromboplastin times as preoperative screening tests. Arch Surg 1982;117:48.

Esmon CT: The roles of protein C and thrombomodulin in the regulation of blood coagulation. J Biol Chem 1989;264:4743.

Fakhry SM, Rutherford EJ, Sheldon GF: Hematologic principles in surgery. In Townsend CM, Beauchamp RD, Evers BM, Mattox KL (eds): Textbook of Surgery: The Biological Basis of Modern Surgical Practice (16th ed). Philadelphia: WB Saunders, 2001:68.

Fourrier F, Chopin C, Huart JJ, et al: Double-blind, placebo-controlled trial of antithrombin III concentrates in septic shock with disseminated intravascular coagulation. Chest 1993;104:882.

Francis JL, Armstrong DJ: Acquired dysfibrinogenaemia in liver disease. J Clin Pathol 1982;35:667.

Frangos SG, Chen AH, Sumpio B: Vascular drugs in the new millennium. J Am Coll Surg 2000;191:76.

Gachet C: Platelet activation by ADP: the role of ADP antagonists. Ann Med 2000;3232:15.

Gewirtz AS, Kottke-Marchant K, Miller ML: The preoperative bleeding time test: assessing its clinical usefulness. Cleve Clin J Med 1995;62:379.

Gewirtz AS, Miller ML, Keys TF: The clinical usefulness of the preoperative bleeding time. Arch Pathol Lab Med 1996;120:353.

Gottsater A, Berg A, Centergard J, et al: Clinically suspected pulmonary embolism: is it safe to withhold anticoagulation after a negative spiral CT? J Intern Med 2001;249:237.

Greinacher A, Eichler P, Lubenow N, et al: Drug-induced and drug-dependent immune thrombocytopenias. Rev Clin Exp Hematol 2001;5:166.

Grinnell BW, Hermann RB, Yan SB: Human protein C inhibits selectin-mediated cell adhesion: role of unique fucosylated oligosaccharide. Glycobiology 1994;4:221.

Grinnell BW, Joyce D: Recombinant human activated protein C: a system modulator of vascular function for treatment of severe sepsis. Crit Care Med 2001;29(Suppl):S53.

Guyton AC, Hall JE: Red blood cells, anemia, and poly-cythemia. In Guyton AC, Hall JE (eds): Textbook of Medical Physiology (10th ed). Philadelphia: WB Saunders, 2000:382.

Hirsh J, Dalen JE, Anderson DR, et al: Oral anticoagulants: mechanism of action, clinical effectiveness, and optimal therapeutic range. Chest 1998;114:445S.

Hirsh J, Warkentin E, Raschke R, et al: Heparin and low-molecular-weight heparin: mechanisms of action, pharmacokinetics, dosing considerations, monitoring, efficacy, and safety. Chest 1998;114:489S.

Ikeda Y: Antiplatelet therapy using cilostazol, a specific PDE3 inhibitor. Thromb Haemost 1999;82:435.

Jurkovich G, Greiser W, Luterman A, et al: Hypothermia in trauma victims: an ominous predictor of survival. J Trauma 1987;27:1019.

Kasper CK: Treatment of factor VIII inhibitors. Prog Hemost Thromb 1989;9:57.

Klopfenstein CE: Preoperative clinical assessment of hemostatic function in patients scheduled for a cardiac operation. Ann Thorac Surg 1996;62:1918.

Komers R, Anderson S, Epstein M: Renal and cardiovascular effects of selective cyclooxygenase-2 inhibitors. Am J Kidney Dis 2001;38:1145.

Landis RC, Asimakopoulos G, Poullis M, et al: The antithrombotic and antiinflammatory mechanisms of action of aprotinin. Ann Thorac Surg 2001;72:2169.

Lethagen S: Desmopressin (DDAVP) and hemostasis. Ann Hematol 1994;69:173.

Leung LLK: Hemostasis and its regulation. In Wilmore DW, Cheung LY, Harken AH, et al (eds): ACS Surgery: Principles & Practice. New York, WebMD Corp, 1999:Chap XII. Available at www.acssurgery.com

Levi M: Pathogenesis and treatment of disseminated intravascular coagulation in the septic patient. J Crit Care 2001;16:167.

Levi M, ten Cate H: Disseminated intravascular coagulation. N Engl J Med 1999;341:586.

Levi M, van der Poll T, ten Cate H, et al: The cytokine-mediated imbalance between coagulant and anticoagulant mechanisms in sepsis and endotoxaemia. Eur J Clin Invest 1997;27:3.

Levy JH, Schwieger IM, Zaidan JR, et al: Evaluation of patients at risk for protamine reactions. J Thorac Cardiovasc Surg 1989;98:200.

Lind SE: The bleeding time does not predict surgical bleeding. Blood 1991;77:2547.

Lorant DE, Topham MK, Whatley RE, et al: Inflammatory roles of P-selectin. J Clin Invest 1993;92:559.

Majerus PW, Tollefsen DM: Anticoagulant, thrombolytic, and antiplatelet drugs. In Hardman JG, Limbird LE, Gilman AG (eds): Goodman & Gilman's The Pharmacological Basis of Therapeutics (10th ed). New York: McGraw-Hill, 2001:1025.

Mannucci PM: How I treat patients with von Willebrand disease. Blood 2001;97:1915.

Mannucci PM, Bettega D, Cattaneo M: Patterns of development of tachyphylaxis in patients with haemophilia and von Willebrand disease after repeated doses of desmopressin (DDAVP). Br J Haematol 1992;82:87.

Mannucci PM, Canciani MT, Rota L, et al: Response of factor VIII/von Willebrand factor to DDAVP in healthy subjects and patients with haemophilia A and von Willebrand disease. Br J Haematol 1981;47:283.

Matthay MA: Severe sepsis—a new treatment with both anticoagulant and antiinflammatory properties. N Engl J Med 2001;344:759.

McAdam BF, Catella-Lawson F, Mardini I, et al: Systemic biosynthesis of prostacyclin by cyclooxygenase (COX)-2: the human pharmacology of a selective inhibitor of COX-2. Proc Natl Acad Sci U S A 1999;96:272.

McVey JH: Tissue factor pathway. Baillieres Clin Haematol 1994;7:469.

Mukherjee D, Nissen SE, Topol EJ: Risk of cardiovascular events associated with selective COX-2 inhibitors. JAMA 2001;286:954.

Murakami K, Okajima K, Uchiba M, et al: Activated protein C prevents LPS-induced pulmonary vascular injury by inhibiting cytokine production. Am J Physiol 1997;272:L197.

Ofosu FA, Nyarko KA: Human platelet thrombin receptors: roles in platelet activation. Hematol Oncol Clin North Am 2000;14:1185.

Opatrny K Jr: Hemostasis disorders in chronic renal failure. Kidney Int Suppl 1997;62:S87.

Pernerstorfer T, Hollenstein U, Hansen J-B, et al: Heparin blunts endotoxin-induced coagulation activation. Circulation 1999;100:2485.

Rodgers RPC, Levin J: A critical reappraisal of the bleeding time. Semin Thromb Haemost 1990;16:1.

Rose EH, Aledort LM: Nasal spray desmopressin (DDAVP) for mild hemophilia and von Willebrand disease. Ann Intern Med 1991;114:563.

Ruggeri ZM: Role of von Willebrand factor in platelet thrombus formation. Ann Med 2000;32(Suppl 1):2.

Scott-Conner CEH, Rigdon EE, Rock WA Jr, et al: Hematology. In O'Leary JP, Capote LR (eds): The Physiologic Basis of Surgery (2nd ed). Baltimore: Williams & Wilkins, 1996:479.

Shapiro MB, Jenkins DH, Schwab CW, et al: Damage control: collective review. J Trauma 2000;45:969.

Taylor FB, Chang A, Esmon CT, et al: Protein C prevents the coagulopathic and lethal effects of Escherichia coli infusion in the baboon. J Clin Invest 1987;79:918.

Valeri CR, Feingold H, Cassidy G, et al: Hypothermia-induced reversible platelet dysfunction. Ann Surg 1987;205:175.

Warkentin TE, Levine MN, Hirsh J, et al: Heparin-induced thrombocytopenia in patients treated with low-molecular-weight heparin or unfractionated heparin. N Engl J Med 1995;332:1330.

Watts DD, Trask A, Soeken K, et al: Hypothermic coagulopathy in trauma: effect of varying levels of hypothermia on enzyme speed, platelet function, and fibrinolytic activity. J Trauma 1998;44:846.

Young E, Wells P, Holloway S, et al: Ex-vivo and in-vitro evidence that low molecular weight heparins exhibit less binding to plasma proteins than unfractionated heparin. Thromb Haemost 1994;71:300.

CHAPTER 38

Transfusion and Replacement Therapy

Todd J. Lucas, M.D. and A. Gerson Greenburg, M.D., Ph.D.

- ▶ What is Anemia?
- ▶ Transfusion of Coagulation Factors
- ▶ The Risks of Transfusion
- ▶ The Transfusion Decision
- ▶ Transfusion Options
    - Allogeneic
    - Autologous
- ▶ Future Options: Red Cell Substitutes
- ▶ Bibliography

"States of the body really requiring the infusion of blood into the veins are probably rare; yet we sometimes meet with cases in which the patient might die unless such operation can be performed; and still more frequently with cases which seem to require a supply of blood, in order to prevent the ill health which usually arises from large losses of the vital fluid, even when they do not prove fatal." This quote from James Blundell's article "Observations on Transfusion of Blood," published in 1828, illustrates the fundamental question of transfusion medicine today: Does this patient need a transfusion? That is, in which patients might a transfusion help prevent death or "ill health"? Once the question of whether the patient needs a transfusion is answered in the affirmative, a related question comes to mind: Should I transfuse this patient? The answer to this incorporates a full knowledge of the risks and benefits of a transfusion and the risks of *not* transfusing. Finally, if the decision to transfuse has been made, the question of what to transfuse must be answered. This chapter attempts to provide a framework for decision making in an area where few absolutes are applicable.

The decision of when to transfuse incorporates two separate but related issues. These are: Would this patient benefit from a transfusion? and Should I transfuse this

patient? The first question relates to the physiologic changes that one could make for the betterment of the patient with the administration of blood or blood products, while the second question balances these benefits with the risks of that action. Although it would be much simpler to adhere to the "10/30" rule that some physicians still promote, doing so ignores the wealth of information that is available about oxygen delivery physiology, tissue oxygen demands, and the significant risks that can accompany transfusions, including infections, transfusion reactions, and immunosuppression. It is clear that, if the physiologic basis for the transfusion "trigger" is understood, we will be able to better serve not only patients as individuals but also the population as a whole through a more judicious use of this limited resource. Unfortunately, for the moment, definition of oxygen kinetics requires some element of invasive monitoring and for the most part is not practical outside of the operating room or intensive care units.

What is Anemia?

The first concept one must understand is that of anemia. Historically defined, it is an absolute number for hemoglobin (Hb) and hematocrit (Hct) that is out of the range of normal, and below which a patient can be officially referred to as anemic (<13 g/dL/39% for men, and <12 g/dL/36% for women, respectively). This definition works well to identify those patients with a low red blood cell (RBC) count, alerting the physician to the presence of an underlying medical condition in need of further investigation and/or treatment. These numbers also allow for an objective indicator of what *may* be occurring physiologically; however, this again must be individualized for each situation. For example, a Hb concentration of 6 g/dL in a healthy 17-year-old male will lead to a much different physiologic state than in an 85-year-old male with severe coronary artery disease and an ejection fraction of 15%. The recommendations for transfusions below a certain value are ways to simplify the decision making for clinicians by making generalizations about what physiologic states usually accompany these values. Although these guidelines are useful to remind a clinician to think about the risks and benefits of transfusion when he or she sees a certain value, a more complete understanding of anemia as a deficiency of oxygen delivery (DO_2) will provide for more timely and better patient care.

A more useful definition of anemia would be *an alteration in the oxygen delivery–oxygen use physiology*. This approach allows patient individualization, deciding if a given patient has impaired tissue perfusion before considering blood or blood product transfusion. Knowing the components that affect global DO_2 thus avoids creation of an oxygen debt (use >> delivery), and knowing a patient's Hb concentration affords the ability to make an appropriate decision regarding transfusion. Global DO_2 is defined in the following equation:

$$DO_2 = \text{cardiac output} \times (1.34 \times \text{Hb} \times \text{Sao}_2) \times 10$$

where SaO_2 is the arterial oxygen saturation. DO_2 is determined by a number of variables, one of which is Hb, an expression of RBC mass. Given the risks assumed to be associated with transfusion, optimizing flow and saturation first is a reasonable paradigm prior to considering transfusion. The details of both cardiac and pulmonary physiology and dysfunction are discussed elsewhere in this book. Simply put, increasing SaO_2 (e.g., with supplemental inspired oxygen) and increasing cardiac output by altering the cardiac output variables of preload, contractility, and afterload will lead to improved DO_2 independent of transfusion. This stated, there are often limits to maximizing cardiac output because of underlying disease processes or the presence of pharmacologic agents (e.g., β-blockers). There are also risks involved with optimizing SaO_2, particularly when a patient is on a ventilator, requiring parameters beyond the range of normal (e.g., high positive end-expiratory pressure in a setting of adult respiratory distress syndrome). It should also be noted from the above equation that Hb plays a major role in determining DO_2 and that transfusion to increase this has a predictable and significant positive affect on DO_2.

The other side of the oxygen kinetics equation is global oxygen consumption (VO_2) at the tissue level. This is illustrated by the following equation:

$$VO_2 = \text{cardiac output} \times 13.4 \times \text{Hb} \times (\text{Sao}_2 - \text{Svo}_2)$$

where SvO_2 is the venous oxygen saturation. Normal values for VO_2 are a rate of 125 to 175 mL/min/m^2, which is about 25% of the global DO_2. Components of the equation can be manipulated to better the patient's situation. Cardiac output (preload, contractility, and afterload),

SaO_2, and arterial oxygen content can all be optimized, sequentially or in parallel, to varying extents to achieve the goal. The amount of oxygen used by the tissue globally may be reflected in the mixed SvO_2. This broad indicator of oxygen consumption, obtained by invasive monitoring, may be useful in some situations. Although mixed SvO_2 is used as an indicator of global VO_2, the reality is that clinicians have no direct control over this element of tissue metabolism. The global oxygen extraction ratio (OER) helps determine the degree of tissue hypoxia. When used in combination with base excess and/or serum lactate or lactic acid measures, a reasonable assessment of the magnitude of tissue hypoxia is possible. The global OER is illustrated by the following equation:

$$OER = VO_2 / DO_2$$

This ratio is normally 0.25 to 0.35. If it exceeds this range by 20% to 30%, it usually indicates tissue hypoxia with a switch to anaerobic metabolism.

Although these numbers can be measured and calculated from data obtained with invasive monitoring, such as a Swan-Ganz catheter, there are many clinical indicators of tissue hypoxia. These include the obvious alterations in vital signs—hypotension and tachycardia—that accompany hemorrhagic hypovolemia but may not be as prominent if the patient is euvolemic. Tachypnea is an effort to compensate for the metabolic acidosis resulting from the anaerobic metabolism of tissues. Many humoral and endocrine mediators are released in response to decreased tissue perfusion. Increased catecholamines and glucagon and decreased insulin secretion preserve a supply of glucose for the heart and brain. Corticotropin (ACTH), aldosterone, growth hormone, antidiuretic hormone, renin, angiotensin, multiple cytokines, and many other substances interact in ways not entirely understood, many of which can be assumed to affect tissue perfusion and metabolism. It is far beyond the scope of this chapter to attempt a discussion of these homeostatic mechanisms and their role in any mismatch between oxygen delivery and use. The acidotic environment resulting from tissue hypoxia induces a number of changes at the cellular level. The sum of these interactions is cellular membrane instability, which leads to cellular edema with eventual loss of structural integrity and finally cell death. This destructive process can be arrested and reversed in the intact cell by providing adequate oxygen delivery and tissue perfusion.

Transfusion of Coagulation Factors

Apart from correcting the anemic state, blood products are also used to correct coagulation deficiencies. Here, too, consideration of the benefits and risks enters the decision-making process. Some physicians would transfuse blood products such as fresh frozen plasma (FFP), platelets, cryoprecipitate, or coagulation factors at predetermined values for a given laboratory test (such as platelets <50,000/μL). However, patients are best served by an individualized approach, again weighing the risk of ongoing bleeding with the benefits of transfusing. This measured approach can be used regardless of the chronicity or etiology of the coagulopathy.

Platelet function can be impaired for two main reasons: there are an insufficient number available to provide the initial step of hemostasis or there are enough platelets available but they have a functional deficiency. The decision to transfuse platelets depends not only on the number of platelets and their function, a rarely evaluated process, but also on the clinical situation: Is the patient going to surgery immediately or bleeding? With an intact vascular system, platelets should be transfused if the count is less than 5000/μL. The risk of spontaneous bleeding increases at this level, with bleeding occurring in the gastrointestinal tract, mucous membranes, urinary tract, or central nervous system. Significant bleeding usually does not occur between 10,000 and 50,000 platelets/μL unless there is associated platelet dysfunction. Patients with platelet counts higher than 50,000/μL usually do not have significant bleeding even with associated platelet dysfunction. In patients with damaged vascular integrity, bleeding times increase at platelet counts less than 100,000/μL. Bleeding in this situation, when the count is greater than 100,000/μL, is associated with platelet dysfunction. The reader should keep in mind that all the above situations assume that all other coagulation parameters are within normal limits and that any bleeding would be attributable to the thrombocytopenia or platelet dysfunction. The benefits of platelet transfusion can be measured by direct observation intraoperatively, stabilized serial Hcts, or improved bleeding times, another rarely measured variable. Aside from the recommendations for platelet transfusion at extremely low levels (<5000/μL), platelet transfusion therapy should be directed by a combination of platelet count and demonstration of need and not by platelet count alone.

The role of specific coagulation factors is not discussed here. However, it is obvious that an insufficient concentration of these, as is the case in many genetic diseases, is associated with an increased risk of bleeding. As with any transfusion decision, the risk of bleeding must be weighed against the risks associated with the transfusion. There are indications for the use of FFP. One use is the correction of clotting in an actively bleeding anticoagulated patient who may require surgery. The international normalized ratio (INR) should be greater than 1.5 or the partial thromboplastin time greater than twice normal before considering this therapy. If the INR is less than 1.5, anticoagulation is unlikely to be contributing to the bleeding. FFP is also

used to treat a variety of isolated factor deficiencies when specific factor concentrates are unavailable. FFP may be used, but not necessarily, for massive transfusion, liver disease, and cardiac surgery. In each of these cases, coagulation factors are usually decreased for specific, almost unique reasons. The need to correct the INR to 1.5 or less with FFP is based on active bleeding or need for surgery and is not an automatic prophylactic replacement per unit of packed RBCs (PRBCs) transfused.

The Risks of Transfusion

To appropriately answer the question of whether to transfuse a patient, the risks of transfusion must also be known. These risks can be divided into three main categories: transfusion reactions, infectious complications, and immunosuppression.

Transfusion reactions can be further divided into hemolytic and nonhemolytic. Nonhemolytic reactions in the most minor form manifest as a low-grade fever, pruritus, and urticaria, and, in the most severe form, as anaphylactic shock and death. These reactions are due to the reaction of antibodies in the recipient's circulation with antigens on donor leukocytes and platelets. The incidence of these reactions is summarized in Table 38–1. The treatment of these reactions is based on their severity. Anaphylactic shock is treated by immediately stopping the transfusion, assessing the patient's airway, and then proceeding per advanced cardiac life support protocol if necessary. The patient should be transferred to an intensive care unit (ICU) and monitored closely for coagulopathies, disseminated intravascular coagulation, and adequacy of resuscitation. Febrile and minor allergic reactions do not necessarily require cessation of the transfusion. Closer monitoring with frequent vital signs, antipyretics, and antihistamines may be used. The severity of a bronchospastic reaction will again guide the therapy. Minor reactions may be treated with inhaled β-agonists; major respiratory compromise requires stopping the transfusion and the use of inhaled epinephrine or intubation. An increased use of leukodepleted PRBCs serves to minimize the frequency of these events.

Hemolytic reactions occur when the recipient's complement cascade is initiated as a result of RBC antigen-antibody interaction. Fatal hemolytic reactions are usually secondary to ABO incompatibilities that are typically the result of clerical errors. The reaction is manifested by tachypnea, hypotension, and an appropriate sense of impending doom by the recipient. Treatment requires stopping the transfusion immediately and providing supportive care. Fatal hemolytic transfusion reactions, although rare, can occur with less than 150 mL of RBCs transfused. There are also delayed hemolytic reactions, again caused by RBC antigen-antibody interactions.

Table 38–1
Risks of blood transfusion

Risk Factor	Estimated Frequency		No. of Deaths per Million Units
	Per Million Units	Per Actual Unit	
Infection			
Viral*			
Hepatitis A	1	1/1,000,000	0
Hepatitis B	7–32	1/30,000–1/250,000	0–0.14
Hepatitis C	4–36	1/30,000–1/150,000	0.5–17
HIV	0.4–5	1/200,000–1/2,000,000	0.5–5
HTLV types I and II	0.5–4	1/250,000–1/2,000,000	0
Parvovirus B19	100	1/10,000	0
Bacterial contamination			
Red cells	2	1/500,000	0.1–0.25
Platelets	83	1/12,000	21
Acute hemolytic reactions	1–4	1/250,000–1/1,000,000	0.67
Delayed hemolytic reactions	1000	1/1000	0.4
Transfusion-related acute lung injury	200	1/5000	0.2

HIV, human immunodeficiency virus; HTLV, human T-cell lymphotrophic virus.
From Goodnough LT, Brecher ME, Kanter MH, AuBuchon JP: Medical progress: transfusion medicine. N Engl J Med 1999;340:440. Copyright 1999 Massachusetts Medical Society. All rights reserved.

These reactions can occur up to several weeks after the transfusion, and their diagnosis can be confirmed by serologic testing.

The infectious complications of transfusion are perhaps the most feared. The incidence of these is also summarized in Table 38–1. These complications are what the public focuses on and are probably the main source of questions that patients ask when discussing transfusions. Although the numbers show that the risk of viral disease transmission per unit transfused is very low, patient and surgeon concern stems from the fact that, if a viral disease (primarily hepatitis or human immunodeficiency virus [HIV]) is contracted, the disease state is often chronic if not ultimately fatal. For example, although initially mild in presentation, post-transfusion hepatitis can progress to chronic liver disease in a third of cases, with a fifth of overall cases developing cirrhosis. The risk of hepatocellular carcinoma is also increased with both hepatitis B and C. The long-term prognosis of HIV transmission, although improved over the past 20 years, is still fatal.

Immunomodulatory effects of blood transfusions became a significant focus of research in the early 1970s when it was noted that preoperative blood transfusions improved the survival of cadaveric renal transplants. Since then, multiple studies have attempted to elucidate an exact relation between transfusions and subsequent aberrations in the human immune response. The observed effects may be associated with the transfused leukocytes. These cells can circulate in the recipient for more than a year. Although the exact mechanisms of these immunomodulatory effects remains unclear, leukocyte-depleted blood may be effective in modulating these events. While many reports cite transfusions as contributory to an increased incidence of wound infections and cancer recurrences, there are many that cast doubt on the clinical significance of transfusion-associated alterations in immune chemistry and the relationship to clinical events. Based on current knowledge, blood transfusion most likely contributes to some degree of immune suppression but the full clinical implications remain unclear. Potential immune suppression should be added to the list of possible adverse events necessitating careful consideration of the transfusion decision.

There are also complications associated with massive transfusions (>10 units PRBCs in a single setting). These include hemostatic abnormalities, hyperkalemia, citrate toxicity, hypothermia, and acidosis. The coagulopathy of massive transfusion results from both coagulation factor deficiency and thrombocytopenia. The coagulation factor deficiency is largely a dilutional effect, arising from the transfusion of PRBC units containing small volumes of plasma. The thrombocytopenia, however, can only be partially accounted for by dilution. The treatment of these deficiencies is replacement with platelets and/or FFP. In massive transfusion situations, it is also important to check the fibrinogen level. If it is below 100 mg/dL, cryoprecipitate transfusion is warranted.

During storage of PRBCs, there are shifts of potassium from within the RBCs to the liquid component of the transfusion, resulting in a potassium concentration of about 80 mEq/L after 3 to 4 weeks of storage. Rapid infusion of PRBC transfusions can lead to a transient, usually clinically insignificant hyperkalemia unless the patient has an underlying reason for decreased potassium excretion, as in renal failure. This can usually be avoided by using fresh blood or washed RBCs. Another complication related to the storage of blood is citrate toxicity. Citrate is the most common anticoagulant used for blood storage. Its mode of action is to bind calcium, making it unavailable to the coagulation cascade. During rapid-infusion, high-volume massive transfusion, high levels of citrate can produce hypocalcemia with side effects including hypotension and depressed cardiac function. If infused rapidly and at cold temperature, cardiac irritability is often manifest.

Patients can generally tolerate 1 unit of PRBCs every 5 minutes without evidence of citrate toxicity. The normally functioning liver will metabolize the excess citrate in that period of time. A more rapid infusion rate requires monitored calcium replacement. The exceptions to this rule are neonates, because of small volumes, and obviously patients with significant liver disease. After 5 weeks of storage, the pH of a unit of PRBC is about 6.6 secondary to the accumulation of lactic and citric acids. When infused, there is a transient metabolic acidosis that is rapidly corrected. Significant persistent acidosis is more likely to be related to under-resuscitation and tissue hypoxia than infused red cells.

Because blood products are stored at 4°C, infusing large quantities rapidly can obviously lead to hypothermia. This in turn leads to coagulopathy and depressed myocardial activity. This side effect of transfusion can be eliminated by warming the blood to 37°C prior to infusion.

The Transfusion Decision

When to transfuse? The benefits of transfusion of blood or blood products include better DO_2, improved tissue perfusion, and improved clotting. The risks associated with transfusion are multiple and significant, although relatively rare. In addition to assessment of the risks of transfusing, one must also consider the risks of *not* transfusing. That is, what are the morbidity and mortality associated with leaving a patient in a physiologic state that could be improved with transfusion? The decision to not transfuse needs to be as active as the decision to transfuse. The clinically defined transfusion trigger is that point where the benefits of transfusion outweigh the risks of transfusion after considering the risks of not transfusing. This point is of necessity different for each individual and depends on his or her overall cardiovascular, pulmonary, and metabolic state.

In an attempt to provide an objective guide that illustrates the decision-making process, Figure 38–1 illustrates an important relationship between DO_2 and VO_2. Note that VO_2 appears to be both independent of and

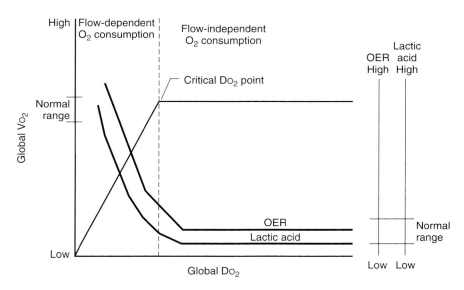

FIGURE 38–1 Schematic representation of the relationship of oxygen delivery (DO_2), oxygen consumption (VO_2), and tissue perfusion reflected by oxygen extraction ratio (OER) and lactic acid levels. Metabolism appears appropriately aerobic and adequate when global VO_2 is independent of DO_2. (Reprinted from Greenburg AG: A physiologic basis for red blood cell transfusion decisions. Am J Surg 1995; 170 [6A Suppl]:44S. Copyright 1995, with permission from the Excerpta Medica Inc.)

dependent on blood flow. That is, the $\dot{V}O_2$ reaches a plateau beyond which increasing the DO_2 does not affect it. If the DO_2 at this point can be assumed to represent adequate tissue perfusion and this point is identified specifically, this information is very useful in arriving at a transfusion decision. This point, defined as the critical DO_2, relates to many aspects of global oxygen kinetics. Two parameters that reflect tissue perfusion begin to change at or near the critical DO_2 point: lactate levels and the slope of the OER. A physiologically defined end point appears to be OER greater than 0.30, increased serum lactate, and a global DO_2 of less than 10 to 12 mL/kg/min. Figure 38–2 illustrates the significant increase in cardiac output required to effect normal-range global DO_2 in the presence of anemia, here defined as decreased global DO_2. If the other variables in the previously noted formula for DO_2 cannot be optimized, then increasing oxygen-carrying capacity with a blood transfusion is indicated.

While a state of tissue hypoxia is more objectively identified in an ICU patient using invasive monitoring and the ability to check mixed venous gases, the clinical reality of blood transfusion applies mostly to patients without that level of access to physiologic parameters. The transfusion trigger for the majority of patients is clinical and empirical, based on the available clinical data and the surgeon's experience. The first piece of information needed is the patient's Hb level. There is little evidence to support the idea that increasing the Hb beyond 10 g/dL improves outcome in any situation. As the Hb concentration decreases, there are more situations when a transfusion, based on clinical information, may be justified.

Some of the factors entering into the decision include the patient's past medical history, comorbid diseases (especially cardiac disease), symptoms, and expected clinical course. The chronicity of the decreased Hb concentration should also be considered. Is the patient's baseline Hb 7 g/dL, or did it drop from 14 to 7 g/dL over the past 8 hours?

Clearly, there are no absolute rules for the decision to transfuse. If rules and guidelines did exist and were generally accepted, they would be used. Indeed, there are at least four different transfusion guidelines available to consider, each well documented and all reflecting "expert opinion" because truly evidence-based data are unavailable. The transfusion decision is all about assessing the odds of improving a patient's outcome by transfusion. Retrospective studies have shown the perioperative mortality to be increased in patients with low preoperative Hb levels, and furthermore this increase is more pronounced in patients with cardiovascular disease. An absolute Hb value for use as a transfusion trigger has not been identified. The general recommendation is to individualize for each patient. Another retrospective study of elderly patients undergoing hip repair looked at postoperative mortality among those receiving and not receiving a transfusion. With equal past medical histories between the groups, no outcome benefit was found to transfusing patients with a Hb less than 8.0 g/dL. This could not be studied for values less than 8 because over 90% of patients falling below that level received a transfusion. Table 38–2 provides some guidelines for establishing clinical transfusion triggers.

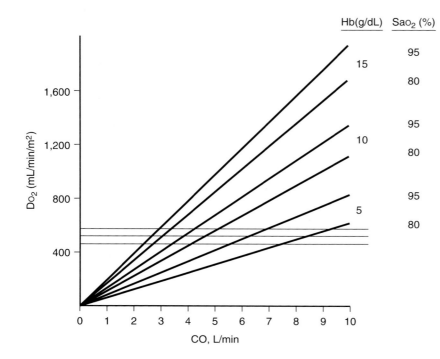

FIGURE 38–2 Changes in oxygen delivery (DO_2) with changes in hemoglobin (Hb) concentration and arterial oxygen saturation (SaO_2). Note the effect of decreased SaO_2 on the need to increase cardiac output (CO) to maintain normal global DO_2. Correction of SaO_2 will measurably decrease CO. (Reprinted from Greenburg AG: A physiologic basis for red blood cell transfusion decisions. Am J Surg 1995; 170 [6A Suppl]:44S. Copyright 1995, with permission from the Excerpta Medica Inc.)

Table 38–2
Clinical transfusion triggers

Hb (g/dL)	Transfusion
>10	None
8–10	Rarely indicated
	• ICU patients with cardiopulmonary status optimized and continued poor oxygen delivery
	• severe cardiac disease with anticipated further blood loss
6–8	Transfusion based on associated risk factors, including:
	• coronary artery disease
	• cerebrovascular disease
	• ongoing blood loss
	• acute vs. chronic decrease in Hb
	• symptoms
<6	Transfusion usually indicated, may be selective in healthy young patients without further bleeding

Hb, hemoglobin; ICU, intensive care unit.

Transfusion Options

Once the decision has been made to transfuse a patient, the questions becomes what and how much to transfuse. There are many different forms of allogeneic and autologous blood products available for use. The specific use is often dictated by the clinical situation; not all products are available for each condition. Table 38–3 summarizes the options.

Allogeneic

Although there are reports of blood transfusions dating back to the 14th century, the overall outcome of pre-20th century transfusions was grim at best. By the early 1900s, once the ABO blood groups were identified, biologically sound transfusion was possible. The science of cross-matching has changed significantly since that time, but the overall goal remains the same: to prevent hemolytic transfusion reactions. ABO typing is the most important test for determining transfusion safety. As mentioned before, most fatal hemolytic reactions are due to ABO incompatibility. The reaction to this incompatibility is quick and dramatic because patients have preexisting antibodies to ABO antigens not present on their own RBCs; they do not require previous exposure to the foreign antigens. The second most common typing test is that for the D antigen in the Rh blood group system; the patient either has it (Rh$^+$) or does not (Rh$^-$). Beyond these two groups, there are multiple other antibody groups (Kell, Kidd, Duffy, Ss, etc.) for which the patient's serum is screened. This is the screening that takes place when a "type and screen" is ordered. If no clinically important RBC antibodies are detected, then the patient may be transfused with any unit of the appropriate ABO/Rh type—a type-specific transfusion.

Occasionally, acute hemorrhage will require the transfusion of blood products in a more timely fashion than can be accomplished with formal type and crossmatching.

Table 38–3
Available blood products

Component	Composition	Approx. Volume (mL)	Shelf Life	Storage Temp. (°C)
Whole blood	RBC, plasma, non-functional WBC, and platelets	525	35 days	1–6
Packed RBCs	RBC, some plasma, non-functional WBC, and platelets	350	42 days	1–6
Platelets (single donor)	Platelets, few RBC, and non-functional WBC equivalent to 6–8 units of random donor platelets	180–350	5 days	20–24
Platelets (random donor)		50	5 days	20–24
Fresh frozen plasma	Plasma, all coagulation factors	220	1 year	−18
Cryoprecipitate	Fibrinogen, factors VIII and XIII, von Willebrand's factor, fibronectin	5–15	1 year	−18

RBC, red blood cells; WBC, white blood cells.

Crossmatched blood can usually be available in 45 minutes unless RBC antibodies are found, in which case it may take several hours. In the most urgent and emergency situations, O-negative blood is immediately available from most blood banks. The risk of significant hemolysis is rare. It is estimated that 0.2% to 0.6% of the population will have RBC antibodies that may cause a delayed hemolytic reaction. Some hospitals have a policy of transfusing O-positive blood in males and O-negative blood in females in acute life-threatening situations. This approach will generally prevent Rh alloimmunization in females of childbearing age, a situation that can lead to hemolytic disease of the fetus. It is a safe practice in males because, even if it is given to Rh⁻ males, they will have very little risk of a reaction unless they have been transfused Rh⁺ blood previously and developed anti-D antibodies. Type-specific, uncrossmatched blood can be available within 15 minutes of the blood bank's receiving the specimen. If possible, this is advantageous because of the relatively short supply of type O blood. Because it is not crossmatched, it is no safer to a patient than type O. Although type O is considered a universal donor, a type O patient is not a universal recipient.

Once the decision has been made to transfuse a patient to improve tissue perfusion, the amount to transfuse becomes the issue. Because the risks of transfusion are per unit, it is obvious that giving 2 units entails twice the exposure and risk of 1 unit. The best approach is to transfuse 1 unit and reassess the need for further transfusion. Sometimes, however, one knows before the transfusion begins that more than 1 unit will be required, as in an elderly trauma patient in hemorrhagic shock. A single unit is expected to increase the Hb by 1 g/dL and the Hct by 3%, assuming there is no ongoing hemorrhage. Knowing this allows one to consider what raising the Hct by 3% will do in terms of vascular volume and Do_2.

A special note is made of the elderly patient with coronary artery disease. Impaired coronary flow limits cardiac function, decreasing the ability to compensate for increased demand by increasing cardiac output. A natural senescence of cardiac function further contributes to this attenuated response. For the patient with coronary artery disease and a decreased Hb concentration, myocardial perfusion becomes very limited, further modulating compensatory responses. Add to this the effects of various cardiac and cardiovascular drugs that also affect the ability to respond to increased demand, and one is left with the sense that the transfusion decision for these patients should be at a slightly lower threshold. Invoking the principle of individualizing the transfusion decision, this is logical.

Other factors to consider when making this decision include expected ongoing blood loss, comorbid diseases, current cardiopulmonary state, and nutritional status. All the components of the patient's situation that drove the decision to transfuse should be reassessed after each unit is transfused to determine the need for subsequent transfusions.

Autologous

The transfusions discussed so far are allogeneic. The transfusion of autologous blood has received much attention lately, especially with the public's knowledge and awareness of a risk for infectious complications. The use of autologous blood has many advantages, including an obviously decreased incidence of infectious complications, no hemolytic reactions, no allergic or anaphylactic reactions, and no graft-versus-host disease. The use of autologous blood products also decreases the use of allogeneic units from the blood bank. The drawbacks of autologous transfusions mainly affect the hospital involved. When patients donate blood for themselves (usually for an impending surgery), there are more procedures required for the collection along with the increased blood tracking needed to make sure these units are given to the correct patient. The risks to the patient of autologous blood donation center primarily around the delays in surgery that are necessary for donation. Most patients who are candidates for elective surgery are candidates for preoperative autologous donation. This preoperative donation should be offered only for patients scheduled for cases that require transfusion greater than or equal to 10% of the time. Autologous transfusion risks, although decreased, are not negligible. The risk of administrative errors remains, as does bacterial contamination. The safest approach is to set one's indications for transfusion at the same point regardless of the blood source.

Cell salvage and intraoperative autologous donation (IAD) are additional forms of autologous red cell transfusion. The former is effective in large blood loss surgery where there is no expected contamination, whereas the latter can be exercised in almost any operation in any time frame. IAD involves removing 1 or 2 units of fresh whole blood, perhaps more, in the immediate preoperative period, often in the operating room. As the blood is removed, the vascular space is filled with a crystalloid, colloid, or combination physiologic solution to maintain vascular volume for the early part of the operation, including the induction of anesthesia. During the early part of the operation, the blood lost is diluted, so there is conservation of the patient's red cells. Red cell mass loss is minimized. When the majority of bleeding has ceased and is under control, the units of autologous whole blood, units that have not left the operating room, can be infused. This is a most effective and safe transfusion concept that deserves wider application in all types of surgery. Where else can the patient get fresh whole blood with minimal risk of clerical error?

In the same vein as the preoperative autologous blood transfusion is the use of a Cell Saver. This is a portable machine capable of collecting a patient's shed blood intraoperatively and allowing it to be transfused. It has all the advantages of autologous donation without the risk of clerical error. The drawback is the cost of using this machine, which is about $600 per case. On a cost basis alone, that would make the Cell Saver effective only if 2 or more units are collected and transfused. Studies have shown that the removal of contaminants from the RBCs, such as fat particles, heparin, C3a, and D dimer, is very effective using the available equipment. The use of the Cell Saver appears to be a safe and effective way to conserve allogeneic blood for transfusion and decreases its risks to the patient. It should be considered preoperatively in all cases where blood loss is significant and subsequent transfusion is usually needed.

Future Options: Red Cell Substitutes

Three classes of "hemoglobin substitutes"—the preferred terminology—have been actively pursued for nearly a century. The most critical efforts have taken place in the last decade of the 20th century when acceptable pure preparations of Hb became available. A great deal of laboratory and clinical testing has been done with a variety of Hb solutions, perfluorocarbons, and Hb encapsulated in liposomes. The latter are nearing early phases of clinical trials.

Perfluorocarbons are interesting chemical compounds capable of carrying a great deal of oxygen dissolved in solution. These diverse molecules are difficult to deal with as "neat liquids" and require composition of a solution with the addition of emulsifiers, electrolytes, and other agents to make them biologically compatible. The emulsions can, if exposed to 100% oxygen, dissolve and deliver sufficient oxygen to hypoxic areas of underperfused tissue, and can also be used in hemodilution techniques. Problems with these emulsions are an incidence of apparent allergic reaction, complement activation, and a relatively poor intravascular persistence. Reticuloendothelial system (RES) clearance is another issue of concern. Resuscitation therapy that could impair host defense mechanisms could be a liability in some situations. Along similar lines, liposome-encapsulated Hb, with or without the addition of agents that will minimize or modulate reperfusion injury, may also deliver oxygen but is rapidly cleared from the circulation, necessitating repeat dosing to achieve an effect. Here again, the RES clearance coupled with the poor intravascular persistence remains an issue to be resolved before clinical trials can be started. Hemoglobin solutions vary as to source of Hb—extracted

from outdated RBCs, bovine, or recombinant—and generally have undergone some form of modification to minimize the normal renal clearance mechanism, thus improving intravascular persistence. Indeed, these modifications also generally effect a right shift of the oxyhemoglobin dissociation curve, enhancing the ability of the Hb to off-load oxygen. This improved ability to off-load oxygen potentially improves tissue perfusion, one goal of transfusion therapy. A host of Hb modifiers and cross-linking agents have been evaluated over the years. Some modifiers also act as cross-linking agents so that a single compound serves both goals.

Studies with stabilized Hb tetramer have been accomplished with fair or unexpected results in clinical Phase III trials. One product, diaspirin cross-linked Hb, was in the middle of a Phase III clinical trial of trauma resuscitation when the trial was abruptly stopped for safety reasons. Another cross-linked Hb, this one without a 64-kD component, completed a Phase II trial with promising results. Patients could receive multiple doses and survive severe hemorrhage with RBC Hb less than 3.0 g/dL—a remarkable feat that confirmed many laboratory observations. Another modified Hb, an oligomer 64 to 512 kD in size, has completed a Phase III trial as a diluent for IAD in cardiac surgery. The results were very encouraging because there was decreased use of all allogeneic blood products for patients who received the test material. A similar trial with bovine Hb–based solution showed similar results.

The toxicity often associated with early Hb solutions (renal failure and coagulopathy) has not been observed with these cleaner, modified, well-manufactured solutions. Some elements of vasoactivity have been noted but do not appear to compromise efficacy. By most standards these solutions meet general safety requirements.

Hemoglobin solutions, even the first-generation products with oxygen-carrying capacity, oncotic pressure, and balanced electrolytes, will have a place in surgery. Although trauma resuscitation may be the most obvious area of application, it is also one of the most difficult to study. Use of these solutions as diluents for IAD is a most seductive concept. With this application, say in cardiac surgery, overall demand on the blood supply, always an issue, is decreased. An added benefit is the availability of more blood and blood products for use in other clinical situations.

Although these solutions are technically not "virus free," they are sterile. Moreover, each one has been tested and has demonstrated multiple log-order decreases in all classes of viruses resulting from the manufacturing process. There is a presumed decreased risk of transmission of infectious disease with these solutions, an added appeal given the generally expressed concern about the safety of the blood supply.

Enormous strides in attaining a useful and usable Hb-based red cell substitute have been accomplished in the past 10 years. Pivotal trials progressively show both safety and efficacy, the latter usually defined as avoidance of allogeneic transfusion. Solutions currently in clinical testing are far superior to their laboratory-scaled predecessors and will gain a place in the surgical armamentarium. Newer generations of solutions with specific properties for specific therapeutic applications will build on these observations, because development is an evolutionary process. One recent analysis indicated that, given a Hb-based solution that carries oxygen, provides oncotic and osmotic forces, and has a balanced electrolyte composition, 60% or more of allogeneic RBC use in elective and urgent surgery can be replaced with such a solution. The benefits accrued to the blood banking system generally and transfusion medicine specifically would be enormous, decreasing patient risk with a presumed beneficial positive patient outcome.

Bibliography

Goodnough LT, Brecher ME, Kanter MH, AuBuchon JP: Medical progress: transfusion medicine. N Engl J Med 1999;340:438.

Gould SA, Moore EE, Hoyt DB, et al: The first randomized trial of human polymerized hemoglobin as a blood substitute in acute trauma and emergent surgery. J Am Coll Surg 1998;187:113.

Greenburg AG: Indications for transfusion. *In* Scientific American Care of the Surgical Patient. New York: Scientific American, 1989:1–19.

Greenburg AG: A physiologic basis for red blood cell transfusion decisions. Am J Surg 1995;170(6A):44S.

Klein H: Immunomodulatory aspects of transfusion: a once and future risk? Anesthesiology 1999;91:861.

Sloan EP, Koenigsberg M, Gens D, et al: Diaspirin cross-linked hemoglobin (DCLHb) in the treatment of severe traumatic hemorrhagic shock. JAMA 1999;282:1857.

CHAPTER 39

Electrolytes and Electrolyte Dysfunction

Mark A. Malangoni, M.D., F.A.C.S. and Charles J. Yowler, M.D., F.A.C.S.

The basics of fluid and electrolyte balance are an essential component of patient management that must be thoroughly understood by all clinicians. Normally, we regulate the variability in our daily intake of water, other fluids, and ions primarily through a complex interaction of endogenous hormones that control renal function. Electrolyte as well as acid-base balance is critical to normal cellular function, and any alteration in this cellular environment can have profound effects on cellular homeostasis and organ function. Diseases, serious injury, and disorders of renal and endocrine function, as well as physician interventions, can result in life-threatening conditions.

This chapter provides the scientific background essential to understanding the regulation of normal fluid, electrolyte, and acid-base balance. Common disorders that are relevant to patient care are presented along with therapeutic solutions to these problems.

Distribution of Body Fluids

Total body water (TBW) is an estimated fraction of total body weight. TBW is increased in individuals who have a relatively greater muscle mass or solid organ weight. In contrast, adipose tissue and bone have a relatively lower water content.

TBW approximates 60% of body weight in adult men and 51% in adult women (Table 39–1). TBW is greater in infants, and decreases resulting from aging are attributed to a decrease in lean body mass and an increase in fat tissue. In thin patients, TBW is 5% to 10% above normal, whereas in obese patients it is decreased by 10% to 20%. TBW is distributed as two-thirds intracellular water (ICW) and one-third extracellular water (ECW). The largest proportion of ICW is located in skeletal muscle. It follows that many women will have a lower percentage of ICW because of a relatively smaller muscle mass.

Extracellular water is composed of interstitial, intravascular, and transcellular components that together constitute approximately 20% of TBW. Interstitial fluid is mainly contained in the acellular tissue matrix and equilibrates rapidly with the remainder of ECW. The intravascular space contains the plasma volume. Transcellular fluids include glandular secretions and cerebrospinal, synovial, pleural, pericardial, peritoneal, and intraocular fluids. The passage of fluids into the transcellular space from other body compartments is very slow. Table 39–2 outlines the distribution of these fluids within the major body compartments.

Table 39-1
Total body water as a fraction of total body weight

Age Group	Fraction of Total Body Weight (kg)
Infants	0.75–0.80
Children	0.65–0.70
Adult males	0.60
Adult females	0.50
Elderly males	0.50
Elderly females	0.45

Composition of Body Fluids

The electrolyte composition of the intracellular fluid (ICF) and extracellular fluid (ECF) differ considerably; however, water diffuses freely across the semipermeable membrane that separates these compartments to balance osmotic forces. Sodium is the most abundant cation in ECF, while potassium is the predominant positively charged ion in ICF. The concentration gradient between these two fluid spaces is maintained by an ATP-dependent sodium-potassium pump, which resides in the cellular membrane. Chloride is the principal anion of ECF, but it is sparse in ICF, where phosphates and other anions provide electrical balance. Proteins also contribute to the electrical charge and osmolality of all fluid compartments (Table 39–3).

Water is evenly distributed throughout all compartments of the body. Therefore, the addition of a given volume of water has little effect on any single body compartment. In contrast, the administration of sodium-containing fluids leads to their even distribution across the entire ECF space.

Table 39-2
Distribution of fluids within major body compartments as a percentage of body weight

Compartment	Distribution by Body Weight (%)	Distribution in Average 70-kg Man (L)
Total body water	60	42
Intracellular fluid	40	28
Extracellular fluid	20	14
Interstitial fluid	14	10
Intravascular fluid	4.5	3.2
Transcellular fluid	1.5	1

Because of the relative size of the component spaces of ECF, most sodium-containing fluids expand the interstitial fluid approximately three times as much as intravascular volume.

The total concentration of diffusible cations and anions on either side of a semipermeable membrane must be equivalent (Gibbs-Donnan equilibrium equation). Therefore, the slight difference in ionic composition of the plasma and interstitial fluid spaces is due to the higher protein content of plasma, which contributes organic anions to this compartment. The greater number of ions in the intracellular space is due to the fact that ionic concentration is expressed in milliequivalents (mEq), which does not fully account for osmotic activity. In addition, some intracellular cations (e.g., magnesium) exist in an undissociated form.

Osmolality is defined as the number of active particles or ions present per unit of volume. Osmolality is generally expressed as milliosmoles per liter (mOsm/L). This differs from other common expressions of concentration such as electrical charge (mEq) or the weight of electrolytes per unit volume (g or mg/100 mL).

The osmotic pressure of ICF and ECF must be equal. Normal osmolality is tightly regulated between 280 and 290 mOsm/L. The total osmotic pressure of a given fluid equals the sum of the osmotic pressures contributed by each solute, including substances that may not freely pass through the pores of a semipermeable membrane, such as proteins. *Tonicity* is a physiologic concept that designates the relationship between osmolality of ECW and ICW. Remember that water is quickly distributed across the cell membrane in response to any perturbation in tonicity in order to maintain osmotic equilibrium between the extracellular and intracellular compartments.

A few practical examples are helpful. The administration of isotonic solutions (lactated Ringer's or 0.9% normal saline) results in little change in water flux. In contrast, hyperglycemia causes an increase in extracellular osmolality resulting in a redistribution of water to the extracellular space. Alcohol and urea increase osmolality in both ICF and ECF, but do not affect tonicity because these substances rapidly equilibrate between extracellular and intracellular spaces. Mannitol does not cross the cell membrane because of its large particle size. Therefore, mannitol administration increases osmolality in the ECF, with a resultant shift of water from the intracellular to the extracellular space.

Normal osmolality is maintained by a variety of mechanisms. Arginine vasopressin (AVP), the human antidiuretic hormone, is synthesized in the hypothalamus and transported to the posterior pituitary. An increase in serum osmolality results in the stimulation of osmoreceptors in the brainstem and the subsequent release of AVP from the posterior pituitary. AVP then increases the reabsorption of

Table 39–3
Electrolyte distribution in various fluid compartments

Electrolyte	Plasma (mEq/L)	Interstitial (mEq/L)	Intracellular (mEq/L)
Na^+	145	144	12
K^+	4	4	150
Ca^{2+}	8	3	Trace
Mg^{2+}	1.5	2	40
Cl^-	105	114	4
HCO_3^-	24	30	12
$HPO_4^{3-} + SO_4^{2-}$	8	3	140
Protein	16	1	40

water by the renal tubular cells. This, along with an increase in water consumption secondary to thirst, results in an increase in TBW and a decrease in osmolality.

Brainstem osmoreceptors are not the only stimulant to AVP release from the pituitary. Baroreceptors stimulate AVP release in response to reduced intravascular volume or decreased mean arterial pressure. Both pain and emotional stress can result in pituitary secretion of AVP. These nonosmotic mechanisms take precedence over the osmoreceptor regulation, and AVP-regulated renal water resorption will dilute ECW osmolality to less than 280 mOsm/L in the presence of hypovolemia, hypotension, and/or pain. Thus, increased TBW and hyponatremia are common findings in patients following surgery or traumatic injury.

Tonicity is influenced mainly by serum sodium concentration. Serum osmolality can be estimated by the following formula:

$$S_{osm} = [2 \times Na^+ \, (mEq/L)] + [glucose \, (mg/100 \, mL)/18] + [urea \, (mg/100 \, mL)/2.8]$$

Sodium is decreased approximately 2 mEq/L for each increase in glucose of 100 mg/dL. Alcohol intoxication can result in hypertonicity from excretion of dilute urine.

Most common electrolyte disorders occur as a result of fluid losses. The electrolyte disturbance is usually due to the volume and type of fluid lost. For instance, ECF deficits resulting from blood loss, interstitial fluid losses, or sequestration of fluid as a result of infection or injury are isotonic because these fluids have sodium concentrations similar to that of plasma. Thus restoration of these volume deficits should be done using isotonic fluids such as lactated Ringer's solution or 0.9% normal saline (Table 39–4). The loss of hypotonic fluids or significant gastrointestinal tract losses should be replaced based on the expected concentration of cations and anions in these fluids (Table 39–5). There is usually little variability between the estimated and actual electrolyte composition of these fluids, making laboratory measurement superfluous.

Third-space fluid losses refer to a shift in distribution of fluid to a site where it no longer contributes to the maintenance of intravascular volume. These losses primarily occur as a result of a shift of water into the interstitial space as well as to other body sites involved with infection, injury, or major operative dissection. These losses are sequestered from the intravascular space and are necessary because of an imbalance in the membrane permeability that results from a disruption of normal homeostasis under

Table 39–4
Composition of commonly used parenteral fluids (mEq/L)

Parenteral Fluid	Na^+	K^+	Ca^{2+}	Cl^-	HCO_3^-	pH
Lactated Ringer's	130	4	2.7	109	28	6.5
0.2% N saline	30	–	–	30	–	4.5
0.45% N saline	77	–	–	77	–	4.5
0.9% N saline	154	–	–	154	–	4.5
3% N saline	513	–	–	513	–	4.5

Table 39–5

Electrolyte composition of common gastrointestinal secretions (mEq/L)

Fluid	Volume/Day (mL)	Na$^+$	K$^+$	Cl$^-$	HCO$_3^-$
Saliva	1200	10-20	20	10	30
Stomach	1500	60	10	120	–
Small intestine	3000	140	4	100	30
Large intestine	400	60	30	40	–
Bile	1000	140	5	100	35
Pancreatic fluid	500	140	5	75	110

these adverse circumstances. Third-space fluid losses generally persist until the pathophysiologic processes that initiated the change return to normal. These distributional fluid shifts result in contraction of the ECF but no net loss of TBW.

The exchange of fluid and solutes between the plasma and interstitial fluid compartments is essential for the support of cellular metabolism. This exchange results in a net flow of these substances, which include albumin and other plasma proteins, from the intravascular space to the interstitium and back to the circulation through the lymphatics in order to maintain physiologic fluid balance. Hydrostatic pressure within the capillaries is a major determinant of the flux of water through the interstitium.

The interstitium consists of an extracellular matrix of collagen fibers, glycosaminoglycans, and fluid (lymph) that forms a hydrated gel phase. Fluids in skin and skeletal muscle comprise more than 50% of the total interstitial volume. Because water and small molecules such as electrolytes, urea, and glucose easily pass through the capillary membrane, the concentrations of these substances in lymph and plasma are approximately equal. Large molecules such as albumin, fibrinogen, and immunoglobulins do not pass as readily through the transcapillary membrane, and, therefore, the plasma concentrations of these substances exceed their concentration in lymph fluid. The *porosity* of the transcapillary membrane is regulated by specific characteristics in different tissues; for example, the liver is very porous but muscle is not. Hormonal and autocrine factors such as histamine and bradykinin also influence membrane porosity.

Edema is an abnormal accumulation of excess fluid in the interstitium. As edema occurs, there is an increased permeability of the transcapillary membrane to plasma proteins so that the serum concentration of these substances diminishes. This counteracts fluid movement from plasma to the interstitium. Diuresis removes the excess interstitial fluid and eventually restores protein distribution to normal.

The complex movement of fluid across the capillary membrane is described by Starling's hypothesis regarding the balance of forces across microvascular membranes. This formula is

$$Q = K_f [(P_c - P_i) - \sigma (COP_p - COP_i)]$$

where Q = the net rate of transcapillary fluid movement (mL/min/100 g); K_f = capillary filtration coefficient, which represents the permeability of the capillary membrane to small solutes in water and, as described above, varies according to tissue and surface area of the membrane; $P_c - P_i$ = the hydrostatic pressure gradient; σ = the reflection coefficient, which represents the ability of capillary membranes to prevent plasma proteins from crossing the membrane; and $COP_p - COP_i$ represents the colloid oncotic pressure gradient. Atrial natriuretic factor and platelet activating factor can affect K_f. $P_c - P_i$ is regulated predominantly by arteriolar and venous vasomotor tone. Under normal conditions, the hydrostatic pressure gradient is approximately 9 mm Hg and the colloid oncotic pressure gradient is approximately 8 mm Hg. The value of σ can vary from 0 to 1. When high capillary membrane permeability is present, σ measures closer to 0. In normal circumstances, σ in skin and skeletal muscle exceeds 0.9.

This complex interaction governing transcapillary fluid movement cannot be simplified by adjusting a single parameter. Autoregulation of fluid movement suggests that, when there is an increase in hydrostatic pressure that leads to net fluid movement into the interstitium, the plasma protein concentration in the interstitium will decrease. This results in a higher oncotic pressure in the plasma, thereby retarding fluid movement. A decrease in plasma colloid oncotic pressure may lead to increased water flow into the interstitium; however, more fluid in the interstitium dilutes the interstitial oncotic pressure and returns oncotic forces to normal. Albumin is the principal determinant of colloid oncotic pressure.

Disorders of Fluid Composition

Hyponatremia

The sodium content in the average adult is approximately 60 mEq/kg. Hyponatremia is defined as a serum Na^+ concentration less than 130 mEq/L. Hyponatremic patients may be hypovolemic, hypervolemic, or euvolemic. A thorough history and physical examination and measurement of both serum and urine electrolytes are required to determine the overall volume status of an individual patient. Only then can a rational treatment plan be outlined.

Hypervolemic hyponatremia occurs secondary to nonosmotic stimulation of AVP release, resulting in increased reabsorption of free water by renal tubular cells. Patients with congestive heart failure, nephrotic syndrome, or cirrhosis have an excess of both sodium and water in the ECF compartment; however, they have a contracted intravascular volume and thus baroreceptors stimulate AVP release. This vascular contraction also results in renal hypoperfusion and decreased glomerular filtration of water, compounding the fluid retention. A similar situation can occur in a patient in hemorrhagic shock or following major surgery if an intravenous solution with inappropriately low salt content (such as 5% dextrose in water [D_5W]) is utilized. Hypotension, pain, and a contracted intravascular volume result in AVP release and tubular reabsorption of water. This can result in either hypervolemic or hypovolemic hyponatremia, depending on the amount of hypotonic solution administered.

Hypovolemic hyponatremia most commonly occurs when increased pathologic losses of sodium-rich body fluids (nasogastric losses, diarrhea, biliary fistulas, etc.) are replaced by inadequate volumes of sodium-deficient fluids. For example, an elderly patient who has severe diarrhea and whose oral intake has been insufficient may present with both a contracted intravascular volume and hyponatremia. A similar situation can occur in a patient with bowel obstruction and large nasogastric losses that are erroneously replaced with sodium-deficient intravenous fluids.

Patients with hypervolemic hyponatremia (appropriate history, edema, and dilute urine) require fluid restriction, not sodium administration. Depending on the clinical situation, giving a diuretic also may assist in correcting the fluid balance. Conversely, the hyponatremic patient with a decreased intravascular volume (appropriate history, poor skin turgor, and a concentrated urine) requires fluid resuscitation with a sodium-rich solution, such as normal saline. The use of a diuretic in this situation would only worsen the fluid deficit and could contribute to renal injury.

Rarely, patients present with symptomatic hyponatremia. Symptoms consist of headache, nausea, emesis,

and weakness, and the serum sodium concentration is usually less than 120 mEq/L. Seizures may rarely occur. Initial treatment consists of administration of hypertonic (3%) NaCl with monitoring of serum sodium levels every 2 hours. Central pontine myelinolysis can occur when correction of serum sodium exceeds 10 to 15 mEq/L over a 24-hour period. Thus the rate of correction should not exceed 0.5 mEq/L/hr. Hypertonic saline infusion should be stopped when the patient is symptom free or serum sodium exceeds 128 mEq/L. Further treatment should consist of fluid restriction or treatment of the syndrome of inappropriate secretion of antidiuretic hormone (SIADH), if present.

Hyponatremia may occur secondary to the inappropriate secretion of AVP (or AVP-like proteins), which is known as SIADH. Potential etiologies of this syndrome include central nervous system disorders (e.g., head trauma, brain tumors, intracranial infections or hemorrhage), pulmonary disorders (e.g., tumors, viral infections), or ectopic AVP production by malignant neoplasms. The diagnosis of SIADH is established by a high urine sodium concentration (>30 mEq/L) and urine osmolality (>400 mOsm/L) in the face of a low serum sodium concentration and serum osmolality. Treatment consists of fluid restriction and diuretic therapy, if needed. Demeclocycline antagonizes the renal action of AVP and can be used for patients with chronic SIADH.

Hyponatremia in the neurosurgical patient also may occur secondary to cerebral salt-wasting syndrome. The mechanism by which cerebral disease leads to renal salt wasting is not well understood. Nevertheless, depressed renal sodium absorption results in the loss of both sodium and water. The diagnosis of cerebral salt wasting is made in the patient who has the laboratory findings of SIADH, but who on clinical exam is obviously volume depleted, unlike the euvolemic or edematous patient with true SIADH. This distinction is important because patients with cerebral salt wasting require volume loading with normal saline, not fluid restriction. Patients with chronic salt wasting may require dietary sodium supplementation as well as rehydration.

Euvolemic hyponatremia occurs in patients with normal renal function who consume massive amounts of water. This disorder is suggested by finding marked hyponatremia in a patient with no history suggestive of abnormal sodium losses and with no physical findings of edema. The condition is often psychogenic in nature, and treatment consists of restriction of free water ingestion.

Hypernatremia

Hypernatremia (serum Na^+ concentration greater than 145 mEq/L) is usually secondary to TBW depletion. This may occur either when water intake is insufficient or when water losses are excessive. Insufficient intake of water may be secondary to obtundation, nausea, or abnormal thirst mechanisms. Elderly patients often present with elevated serum sodium concentrations as a result of poor appetite and reduced fluid intake. Profound hypernatremia usually results from the combination of increased fluid losses and decreased fluid intake. Fever often is overlooked as a source of increased insensible water loss. Insensible water loss averages about 8 to 12 mL/kg/day and increases 10% for every degree of body temperature above 37.2°C.

Hypernatremia may be due to diabetes insipidus following severe head trauma or neurosurgical procedures. In this condition, the secretion of AVP is decreased and renal tubular reabsorption of water is markedly reduced despite a hyperosmolar state. Hypernatremia secondary to diabetes insipidus is diagnosed by determining urine specific gravity and osmolality along with serum osmolality. The finding of a maximally diluted urine (specific gravity <1.005, urine osmolality <200 mOsm/L) in a hypernatremic patient with an elevated serum osmolality (>290 mOsm/L) confirms the diagnosis. Treatment consists of vasopressin given either subcutaneously or by intravenous drip initially, followed by intranasal desmopressin if chronic replacement therapy is required. Moderate hypernatremia is well tolerated, and symptoms rarely develop unless serum sodium levels exceed 160 mEq/L or serum osmolality exceeds 320 mOsm/L. Symptoms of hypernatremia consist of restlessness, irritability, and seizures and are secondary to hyperosmolality.

Rapid correction of severe hypernatremia can result in cerebral edema and herniation. The cells within the brain adapt to chronic hypernatremia by increasing their intracellular osmotic content, thereby correcting their cellular volume. Sudden decreases in extracellular sodium concentration can result in significant cerebral edema.

The water requirement to replace the free water deficit can be calculated using the following formula:

$$\text{Free water requirement (L)} = (\text{actual [Na}^+]/\text{desired [Na}^+] - 1) \times \text{TBW (L)}$$

One third to one half of the water requirement should be administered over 24 hours. The free water deficit is then recalculated and again partially corrected. The goal is to correct the deficit over 48 to 72 hours. For example, a 70-kg patient with a TBW of 42 L (60% of body weight) has a serum sodium of 170 mEq/L:

$$\begin{aligned}\text{Free water requirement (L)} &= [(170/140) - 1] \times 42\ \text{L} \\ &= (1.21 - 1) \times 42\ \text{L} \\ &= 9\ \text{L}\end{aligned}$$

This free water deficit should be replaced with administration of approximately 4 L the first day and recalculation of the deficit in 24 hours. It should be noted that ongoing free water losses (fever, diarrhea, etc.) need to be replaced in addition to the free water deficit.

Hyperkalemia

Extracellular potassium concentration is regulated primarily by renal excretion. The majority of the potassium filtered by the glomerulus is reabsorbed in the proximal tubule, so the net renal excretion of potassium is determined by the amount secreted in the distal tubule and collecting duct of the nephron. Potassium excretion is stimulated by increased urine flow in the distal nephron segments (diuretics), increased sodium delivery to the distal tubule (diuretics), high plasma potassium concentrations, and alkalosis. Aldosterone, AVP, and β-adrenergic agonists also increase renal excretion of potassium. Conversely, renal failure results in marked decreases in renal potassium excretion.

Hyperkalemia usually results from decreased renal function. Serum potassium levels may increase by 0.3 to 0.5 mEq/L/day in noncatabolic patients with acute renal failure. Potassium levels may increase by more than 0.7 mEq/L/day in catabolic patients. The increase in potassium associated with acute renal failure is exacerbated by the treatment of hyperglycemia with insulin or by the administration of β-antagonists.

Cellular destruction also can result in increased serum potassium levels. Crush syndrome may result in lethal potassium concentrations secondary to the release of potassium from necrotic tissue in association with acute renal failure caused by myoglobinuria. Reperfusion of ischemic limbs, tumor lysis syndrome associated with chemotherapy, and use of depolarizing muscle relaxants (succinylcholine) in patients with paralysis, muscular disorders, or burns all may lead to elevated potassium levels.

The clinical features of hyperkalemia are related primarily to cellular membrane depolarization. An electrocardiogram initially will reveal peaked T waves with progression to flattened P waves, prolongation of the QRS complex, and deep S waves as serum potassium level increases. Ventricular fibrillation will occur eventually if potassium levels are not corrected. Concurrently, hyperkalemia also results in muscle paresthesias and weakness that can progress to flaccid paralysis.

The treatment of mild hyperkalemia consists of limiting oral potassium intake and removing any intravenous potassium-containing solutions. Potassium excretion through the gastrointestinal tract can be increased by administering K^+-Na^+ exchange resins such as sodium polystyrene sulfonate (Kayexalate), either orally or as a retention enema. Each gram removes approximately 0.5 mEq of potassium.

More severe hyperkalemia (electrocardiogram changes present) requires more aggressive treatment. The rapid infusion of 10% calcium gluconate will transiently stabilize cellular membranes. Administration of sodium bicarbonate will result in a more alkalotic environment and shift potassium into the ICF space. Further displacement of potassium into the intracellular compartment can be accomplished by administering 50 to 100 mL of 50% glucose with 10 to 20 units of regular insulin. These measures, along with administration of exchange resins, can provide the time required for definitive treatment of the acute hyperkalemia with hemodialysis.

Hypokalemia

Hypokalemia is the most common electrolyte disorder in hospitalized patients. It can occur as a result of decreased potassium intake, increased gastrointestinal potassium loss, or increased renal potassium loss. Hypokalemia can occur secondary to the administration of potassium-free intravenous solutions for prolonged periods. Increased gastrointestinal potassium loss may occur secondary to diarrhea or the presence of mucus-secreting colon tumors, typically villous adenomas. Excess renal losses can occur as a result of chronic metabolic alkalosis, magnesium deficiency, hyperaldosteronism, and chronic diuretic use.

The clinical features of hypokalemia primarily involve the cardiac and muscular systems. Muscle weakness becomes evident at potassium levels below 2.5 mEq/L, and severe hypokalemia may result in paralysis and respiratory arrest. Smooth muscle dysfunction of the gastrointestinal tract can lead to an ileus. Electrocardiographic abnormalities include ventricular ectopy, flattened T waves, depressed ST segments, prominent U waves, and prolongation of the Q-T interval.

The treatment of hyperkalemia requires recognition that the majority of total body potassium is present in the intracellular compartment. Thus a serum potassium deficiency of 1 mEq/L represents a total body deficiency of greater than 100 mEq. Clearly, the most common error made in potassium replacement is underestimation of the dosage required to correct the hypokalemia. Intravenous replacement is required if the patient is unable to ingest oral potassium supplements or if electrocardiogram changes are present. Intravenous replacement should not exceed 10 mEq/hr unless serious cardiac abnormalities are present. Most patients with mild hypokalemia are best treated by oral potassium supplementation.

Hypercalcemia

A comprehensive analysis of calcium homeostasis is beyond the scope of this review of electrolyte disorders. Normal serum calcium levels rely upon the exchange of calcium between bone and the ECF compartment, renal excretion of calcium, and the intestinal absorption of calcium. Parathyroid hormone is central to the control of this balance. Ionized calcium is the physiologically active form of this cation and makes up approximately 45% of total body calcium. Forty percent of serum calcium is bound to proteins, primarily albumin. Total serum calcium concentrations fluctuate directly with serum albumin, but only deficiencies in the ionized component are clinically significant. A decrease in serum albumin concentration of 1 g/dL will decrease total serum calcium by 0.8 mg/dL but usually does not significantly decrease ionized calcium levels. The normal serum concentration of ionized calcium is about 4.5 mg/dL. Acidosis decreases protein binding and increases ionized calcium levels.

Hypercalcemia is most commonly due to hyperparathyroidism, bony metastases, neoplasms that secrete parathyroid hormone–like substances, sarcoidosis, or renal diseases. The clinical features of hypercalcemia depend on both the severity and the chronicity of the disorder. Neuromuscular effects are most common and include muscle fatigue and weakness. Neurologic symptoms include confusion, delirium, and coma, and gastrointestinal complaints include nausea, vomiting, and abdominal discomfort. The electrocardiogram may reveal prolongation of the Q-T interval. Chronic hypercalcemia may result in nephrolithiasis and nephrocalcinosis, and ultimately can result in renal failure.

Severe acute hypercalcemia (>14 mg/dL) represents a true medical emergency because of the associated neuromuscular and cardiac effects. Initial therapy involves increasing renal excretion of calcium through the administration of normal saline and furosemide. Saline restores intravascular volume and increases the glomerular filtration of calcium. Furosemide inhibits calcium and sodium reabsorption, thereby increasing calcium excretion in the urine. Saline and furosemide should be adjusted to maintain a urine output of 200 to 300 mL/hr. During this time, any offending drugs (e.g., thiazides, vitamins A and D, calcium supplements) must be discontinued.

Attention then is directed at reducing calcium release from bone. Surgery is the preferred treatment of severe primary hyperparathyroidism once the patient is stabilized. Patients with chronic diseases associated with increased bone resorption can be treated with bisphosphonates. These agents inhibit bone resorption, bone formation, and osteoclast activity. Pamidronate may be given as a daily infusion of 15 to 45 mg for up to 10 days or as a single infusion of 30 to 90 mg over 24 hours. Seventy to 100% of hypercalcemic patients will become eucalcemic after a single intravenous infusion of 60 to 90 mg. The duration of action of bisphosphonates can be several weeks.

Calcitonin and mithramycin are rarely used since the introduction of the bisphosphonates. Corticosteroids (e.g., prednisone 40 to 100 mg daily) are effective in treating hypercalcemia secondary to sarcoidosis and hematologic cancers, such as multiple myeloma, lymphoma, and leukemia.

Hypocalcemia

Any patient who has a low total serum calcium concentration should have an ionized calcium level determination to verify whether there is true ionized hypocalcemia. This condition may be secondary to thyroid or parathyroid surgery, pancreatitis, vitamin D deficiency, chronic renal failure, or critical illness. The combination of severe hemorrhagic shock with metabolic acidosis requiring vigorous fluid resuscitation commonly results in ionized hypocalcemia.

Neurologic and muscular symptoms predominate. Muscle cramps and paresthesias may progress to tetany and seizures. Confusion may progress to frank delirium and psychosis. Classical physical signs include hyperactive deep tendon reflexes, Chvostek's sign (tetany of the masseter muscle following a tap over the facial nerve), and Trousseau's sign (tetany of the hand when the upper arm is compressed). Electrocardiogram changes include prolongation of the Q-T or ST intervals.

The treatment of mild hypocalcemia is the administration of oral calcium supplements. The addition of oral vitamin D (calcitriol) will increase the rate of intestinal absorption and decrease oral calcium requirements. Severe hypocalcemia is treated by intravenous infusion of 10% calcium gluconate or calcium chloride. Calcium is irritating to veins, and dilute solutions should be administered through a central vein. Initial intravenous therapy consists of 100 mg of elemental calcium over 5 to 10 minutes followed by an infusion of 0.5 to 1.0 mg/kg/hr. The response to therapy varies depending on renal function and acid-base state, and infusions should be adjusted to maintain serum levels at 1.0 mmol/L.

Hypermagnesemia

Approximately half of the total body content of magnesium is confined to bone, and most of the remaining amount is distributed in the intracellular compartment. Only 1% of total body magnesium is in the extracellular compartment, where normal adult serum levels range from 1.7 to 2.4 mg/dL. Magnesium is excreted by the kidneys, and 40% is reabsorbed in the proximal tubule.

Hypermagnesemia is most commonly due to renal failure. Increased consumption of magnesium-containing antacids or laxatives in the presence of acute or chronic renal failure is a common etiology. Hypermagnesemia also may be secondary to the release of magnesium from injured tissues, as in burns, crush injuries, and rhabdomyolysis.

Elevated magnesium levels depress neuromuscular function. Early signs such as loss of deep tendon reflexes may progress to paralysis and coma. Cardiac arrhythmias and arrest can occur at levels exceeding 18 mg/dL.

Treatment typically involves limiting magnesium-containing medications. Calcium antagonizes the acute neuromuscular effects of hypermagnesemia, and intravascular volume expansion and loop diuretics will increase renal excretion. Hemodialysis may be necessary in rare patients with severe increases in serum magnesium and profound renal failure.

Hypomagnesemia

A decreased level of magnesium usually results from the loss of magnesium via the gastrointestinal or renal systems. Malabsorption syndromes, chronic diarrhea, and biliary or pancreatic fistulas can cause magnesium depletion. Fluid from the lower gastrointestinal tract is much richer in magnesium (10 to 14 mEq/L) than fluid from the upper tract (1 to 2 mEq/L).

Diuretic therapy is the most common cause of increased renal loss of magnesium; however, mannitol, aminoglycoside, amphotericin B, and cisplatin therapy also increase renal magnesium excretion. Because magnesium is reabsorbed by the kidney along with calcium and sodium, any condition associated with hypercalcemia or hypercalciuria may increase the renal excretion of magnesium.

Poor magnesium intake may contribute to hypomagnesemia. Chronic alcoholism and protein-calorie malnutrition are associated with decreased stores of total body magnesium. Thus the postoperative patient with restricted oral intake and excessive losses from gastrointestinal or renal sources is especially susceptible to hypomagnesemia if these losses are not replaced.

Magnesium deficiency is associated with a number of cardiac disorders. Normal function of Na^+-K^+ ATPase is dependent on magnesium, so magnesium deficiency results in decreased intracellular potassium concentrations. The electrocardiographic changes of hypomagnesemia mirror those of hypokalemia (prolonged Q-T interval, ST segment depression, and T wave inversion). In a similar manner, magnesium deficiency also predisposes to digitalis-induced arrhythmias. Ventricular arrhythmias associated with hypomagnesemia are resistant to defibrillation unless the magnesium deficiency is corrected. Neuromuscular signs of hypomagnesemia include hyperreflexia and positive Chvostek's and Trousseau's signs. Severe hypomagnesemia may progress to seizures.

Not only is hypomagnesemia associated with hypocalcemia and hypokalemia, but it may directly contribute to the deficiency of the latter two ions. Hypomagnesemia impairs parathyroid hormone release and enhances calcium deposition in bone. Magnesium depletion also increases renal losses of potassium. Thus associated deficiencies in serum calcium and potassium may be difficult to correct without prior correction of the hypomagnesemia.

Severe or life-threatening hypomagnesemia (e.g., cardiac arrhythmias) should be treated with 1 to 2 g of intravenous magnesium sulfate (8 to 16 mEq) over 5 to 10 minutes followed by an infusion of 0.5 to 1.0 g/hr. Because sulfate anion will bind calcium and potassium, both calcium and potassium levels should be monitored. Magnesium oxide is preferred for oral administration because magnesium-containing antacids are poorly absorbed.

Acid-Base Metabolism

Normal cellular function is critically dependent on maintaining body fluid pH within a narrow range (7.35 to 7.45). Deviation in either direction can have profound effects. Control of the net acid flux resulting from dietary intake, by-products of cellular metabolism, and pathophysiologic events occurs mainly through two physiologic buffering systems.

The bicarbonate buffering system is the most important buffer system and is the major physiologic buffer in the ECF compartment. The buffering capacity of this system is related to its ability to regulate arterial partial pressure of carbon dioxide ($PaCO_2$) through changes in alveolar ventilation. Other important buffers include proteins and phosphates, which play a major role in maintaining intracellular pH. Hemoglobin is the major intracellular buffer for the red blood cells.

Buffer systems consist of a weak acid or base and its associated salt. They quickly reduce the effect of any acid or base added to the system and moderate changes in pH. For example, acids combine with bicarbonate, producing the sodium salt of the acid and carbonic acid:

$$HCl + NaHCO_3 \leftrightarrow NaCl + H_2CO_3 \leftrightarrow H_2O + CO_2$$

The lungs rapidly excrete the carbon dioxide produced.

The kidney contributes to the maintenance of acid-base balance by excreting the anions associated with acid production as well as by regeneration of bicarbonate used to buffer the acid load. The kidneys provide bicarbonate through reabsorption in the proximal tubule, which is accelerated by ECF deficits, increased $PaCO_2$, decreased potassium, and mineralocorticoid activity. Bicarbonate also can be generated in the distal tubule. Aldosterone causes hydrogen ion to be excreted in exchange for reabsorption of sodium ion. The excretion of hydrogen ion into the urine along with ammonia and weak anions allows bicarbonate to be restored to the ECF.

Any change in hydrogen ion concentration in body fluids results in a compensatory response to restore pH to normal. The function of the bicarbonate buffer system is expressed in the Henderson-Hasselbalch equation:

$$pH = pK + \log_{10} BHCO_3/H_2CO_3$$
$$= 6.1 + \log_{10} (27 \text{ mEq/L}/1.35 \text{ mEq/L} = 20/1)$$
$$= 6.1 + 1.3 = 7.4$$

It is important to understand that pH is determined by the *ratio* of CO_2 to bicarbonate rather than by the absolute concentrations of either molecule. When acid is added to the system, the decreasing bicarbonate concentration must be balanced by increased alveolar ventilation in order for the 20:1 ratio to be maintained. The renal system affects compensation more slowly by increasing excretion of acid salts and retention of bicarbonate.

Disorders of Acid-Base Balance

Acidemia is defined as pH less than or equal to 7.35 and alkalemia as pH greater than or equal to 7.45. When a disturbance in acid-base balance is identified (usually by measurement of arterial blood gases), one must determine whether the perturbation is due primarily to a metabolic or to a respiratory component. This is simply decided by comparison of pH and $PaCO_2$. If these values change in the same direction (e.g., decreased pH and decreased $PaCO_2$), the disorder is primarily metabolic. In contrast, if the pH and $PaCO_2$ change in opposite directions, then a respiratory acid-base disorder is contributing to the abnormality.

Metabolic Acidosis

Metabolic acidosis results from either (1) acid production that exceeds the ability of the renal system to excrete acid and regenerate bicarbonate or (2) the loss of bicarbonate from the gastrointestinal tract or the kidneys. When metabolic acidosis is present, calculation of the anion gap is useful to define the underlying disease process. The anion gap represents the difference between measured cations and measured anions in the intravascular space and can be calculated by the following formula:

$$\text{Anion gap} = Na^+ (\text{mEq/L}) - [Cl^- (\text{mEq/L}) + HCO_3^- (\text{mEq/L})]$$

The anion gap represents unmeasured anions such as proteins, phosphates, and sulfates plus lactate and other organic anions. The normal anion gap ranges from 10 to 15 mEq/L. The anion gap is reduced approximately 2.5 mEq/L for every 1-g/dL fall in albumin, because of a diminished contribution of albumin to organic anions.

The common causes of metabolic acidosis are listed in Table 39–6. Lactic acidosis is the most common reason for metabolic acidosis in hospitalized patients and is usually due to inadequate tissue perfusion as a result of shock or hypoxemia. Rarely, lactic acidosis can occur as a result of

Table 39–6
Common causes of metabolic acidosis

Cause	Mechanism	Treatment
Anion gap		
Lactic acidosis	Poor tissue perfusion or hypoxemia	Restoration of perfusion; correction of hypoxemia
Diabetic ketoacidosis	Increased glucagons:insulin ratio with production of ketoacids; dehydration	Administration of insulin; restoration of intravascular volume
Renal failure	Retention of fixed acids	Administration of $NaHCO_3$; low-protein diet; dialysis
Salicylates, methanol, ethylene glycol, paraldehyde, toluene	Addition of fixed acids	Enhance excretion; possible dialysis
Non–Anion Gap		
Saline administration	Renal HCO_3^- loss	Administer alternative fluid
Diarrhea or other loss of gastrointestinal fluid	Gastrointestinal HCO_3^- loss	Replacement of fluid volume and electrolytes
Proximal renal tubular acidosis; acetazolamide	Decreased reabsorption of HCO_3^-	Stop acetazolamide
Distal renal tubular acidosis	Failure of renal HCO_3^- production	Administer alkali

poisoning from carbon monoxide or cyanide. Patients who have anion gap metabolic acidosis should always have measurement of serum lactate, ketones, and glucose levels because these are common causes of this disorder.

Acidosis associated with a normal anion gap is most commonly due to loss of bicarbonate from the gastrointestinal tract or the kidneys. Metabolic acidosis resulting from gastrointestinal tract losses is associated with renal compensation (in the presence of normal renal function), as evidenced by a urine pH of 5 or less. Renal tubular acidosis leads to a decreased capacity to excrete acid and a defect in urinary ammonium excretion. Distal renal tubular acidosis is due to a decreased capacity of the kidneys to generate bicarbonate.

The treatment of metabolic acidosis depends on the underlying cause (see Table 39–6). Bicarbonate should be given cautiously because any resultant increase in pH will result in a shift of the oxyhemoglobin disassociation curve to the left, which interferes with oxygen delivery at the cellular level. Sodium bicarbonate administration is useful when acidosis is severe (pH ≤ 7.15), or resistance develops to exogenous catecholamine administration in the presence of a low pH (usually pH ≤ 7.2). When indicated, sodium bicarbonate should be given as a bolus (2 ampules or approximately 90 mEq intravenously) over several minutes followed by a continuous infusion (3 ampules sodium bicarbonate in 1 L D_5W) to maintain pH greater than 7.2. Blood pH, sodium, and bicarbonate levels should be measured frequently to guide treatment.

Metabolic Alkalosis

Metabolic alkalosis can result from (1) loss of acid from the gastrointestinal tract or urine or (2) gain of bicarbonate either from an exogenous source or because of loss of chloride-rich (or bicarbonate-poor) fluids. The kidney normally compensates for metabolic alkalosis by limiting reabsorption of bicarbonate in the proximal tubule. Respiratory compensation is limited because the hypoxemia that accompanies hypoventilation stimulates breathing.

Causes of metabolic alkalosis can be divided into chloride-responsive and chloride-resistant groups (Table 39–7). The urine chloride concentration is low in chloride-responsive metabolic alkalosis (≤ 15 mEq/L) and represents a deficiency in chloride as the cause. In contrast, urine chloride concentration in chloride-resistant alkalosis exceeds 15 mEq/L. Chloride-resistant alkaloses do not have a chloride deficit as their cause and they do not respond to chloride-containing solutions. The primary defect in these disorders is increased renal excretion of acid and bicarbonate reabsorption. ECF volume is normal or increased in chloride-resistant states. Treatment involves the correction of potassium deficits and therapy directed at the underlying disorder.

Chloride-responsive forms of metabolic alkalosis are associated with ECF deficits. The prototype disorder for chloride-responsive metabolic alkalosis is prolonged vomiting or nasogastric suction as a result of pyloric obstruction. There is volume depletion and loss of hydrogen, potassium,

Table 39-7
Causes of metabolic alkalosis

Type	Mechanism	Treatment
Chloride responsive		
Vomiting; nagogastric suction	Loss of chloride	Restore intravascular volume; give normal saline
Diuretics	Loss of chloride	Restore intravascular volume; give normal saline and KCl
Chloride resistant		
Primary hyperaldosteronism; Cushing's syndrome; exogenous steroids	Stimulation of Na^+/H^+ and Na^+/K^+ exchange in the distal tubule	Replace potassium; treat underlying disorder; spironolactone
Severe potassium depletion	Impaired chloride reabsorption	Replace potassium
Excessive administration of alkali	Renal failure; massive transfusion; milk-alkali syndrome	Stop alkali

and chloride ions. The volume deficit stimulates sodium reabsorption from the proximal tubule. Bicarbonate is reabsorbed with sodium in order to maintain electroneutrality, which aggravates the alkalosis. *Hypokalemia is actually due to renal loss of potassium* rather than loss of potassium from the gastrointestinal tract. This is related to the exchange of potassium for sodium in the distal tubule, which also encourages excretion of hydrogen ion in exchange for sodium and results in a paradoxical aciduria. Chloride-responsive alkaloses are treated by the administration of isotonic (0.9% N) sodium chloride, which repletes the chloride deficit and restores intravascular volume. Once the volume deficit begins to correct, as evidenced by an increased urine output, giving potassium chloride should treat the hypokalemia. Diuretics enhance chloride excretion even in chloride-deficient patients, so urine electrolyte determinations may be spurious unless diuretics are withheld for at least 24 hours prior to measurement.

The clinical manifestations of metabolic alkalosis are uncommon. When symptoms do occur, they are usually due to excessive neuromuscular excitability and include paresthesias, carpopedal spasm, or lightheadedness. Ventricular arrhythmias may occur when pH is 7.55 or greater. The need to administer exogenous acid is uncommon; however, if pH is 7.55 or greater, the administration of a dilute hydrochloric acid (HCl) solution is indicated. Either 0.1% N or 0.2% N HCl is administered at a rate of 25 to 50 mL/hr. Serum pH, $PaCO_2$, and electrolytes should be measured every 6 hours. This will control metabolic alkalosis temporarily; however, treatment of the underlying disorder should be instituted as soon as possible for complete correction.

Respiratory Acid-Base Disorders

Respiratory acid-based disorders are classified as either acute or chronic. This depends on the extent to which renal compensation reverses the pH alterations induced by the primary respiratory disorder. Renal compensatory mechanisms usually require 2 to 3 days for maximal effect.

Respiratory Acidosis

Acute increases in $PaCO_2$ result in dramatic changes in serum pH. This reflects the limited capacity of nonbicarbonate intracellular buffering systems to correct pH abnormalities. Chronic elevation of $PaCO_2$ stimulates renal resorption of bicarbonate and hydrogen excretion, which tends to normalize the pH.

The normal respiratory drive attempts to maintain normal $PaCO_2$. Thus respiratory acidosis is usually due to suppression of the respiratory drive by medications or underlying pulmonary dysfunction. Patients receiving mechanical ventilation develop an elevated $PaCO_2$ as a result of hypoventilation, an increased dead space, or an increase in the rate of CO_2 production as a result of the excess provision of carbohydrates.

Respiratory acidosis is usually manifest by headache, restlessness, blurred vision, and anxiety, which can progress to delirium and coma. Treatment should be directed at reversing the underlying cause and usually involves increasing minute ventilation. The administration of bicarbonate is not indicated.

Box 39–1

Causes of Respiratory Alkalosis

- Pain
- Fever
- Sepsis
- Cirrhosis
- Hypoxia
- Shock
- Severe head injury
- Salicylates

Respiratory Alkalosis

Respiratory alkalosis is manifested by a low $PaCO_2$, while the pH can vary. It is due to increased minute ventilation that can result from a variety of causes (Box 39–1). Persistent hypocapnia reduces acid excretion and bicarbonate reabsorption in the proximal tubule.

Respiratory alkalosis rarely produces symptoms. When alkalosis is acute and severe, the sudden increase in pH leads to a reduction of ionized calcium as a result of increased calcium binding to circulating plasma proteins. This manifests as neuromuscular irritability with circumoral or peripheral paresthesias, cramping, or carpopedal spasm. Confusion also can occur. Cardiac arrhythmias may result if the increase in pH is rapid and profound.

Bibliography

Ayus J, Carmelo C: Sodium and potassium disorders. *In* Grenvik A (ed): Textbook of Critical Care (14th ed). Philadelphia: WB Saunders, 2000:853.

Carlstadt F, Lind L: Hypocalcemic syndromes. Crit Care Clin 2001;17:139.

Dacey M: Hypomagnesemic disorders. Crit Care Clin 2001;17:155.

Gennari JF: Hypokalemia. N Engl J Med 1998;339:451.

Harrigan M: Cerebral salt wasting. Crit Care Clin 2001;17:125.

Mullins RJ: Fluids, electrolytes, and shock. *In* Townsend CM (ed): Textbook of Surgery (16th ed). Philadelphia: WB Saunders, 2001:45.

Nathens AB, Maier RV: Acid-base problems. *In* Cameron JL (ed): Current Surgical Therapy (7th ed). St. Louis: Mosby, 2001:1321.

Shires GT III, Shires GT: Fluid and electrolyte management of the surgical patient. *In* Schwartz S (ed): Principles of Surgery (7th ed). New York: McGraw-Hill, 2001:92.

Zaloga G, Roberts P: Calcium, magnesium, and phosphate disorders. *In* Grenvik A (ed): Textbook of Critical Care (14th ed). Philadelphia: WB Saunders, 2000:862.

CHAPTER 40

Thromboembolic Disease

James O. Menzoian, M.D., F.A.C.S. and Joseph D. Raffetto, M.D., F.A.C.S.

Superficial Venous Thrombosis

Thrombosis of the superficial venous system was always believed to be a benign and self-limiting disease, usually treated with bed rest, local heat, leg elevation, and aspirin or some anti-inflammatory agent. However, recent data suggest that this treatment may be inadequate in some patients.

The superficial system is composed of the greater saphenous vein and the lesser saphenous vein along with their respective tributaries. The characteristics of these veins are somewhat different from those of the veins of the deep system. The superficial venous system veins are not surrounded by skeletal muscle and thus are not compressed and emptied by the action of the calf muscle pump. Instead, these superficial veins have much thicker walls, which contain more smooth muscle cells and therefore have a well-developed intrinsic system for emptying. Valvular incompetence in the walls of the superficial veins results in the development of varicosities, which can be in the trunks of the greater and lesser saphenous veins or in their tributaries. These varicosities can contribute to the development of superficial phlebitis.

Pathogenesis

Varicose veins

Patients with varicose veins are susceptible to the development of superficial venous thrombosis (SVT). It is presumed that this is due to stasis of blood. These patients present with a painful "knot" at the site of a prominent varicosity. There is often local heat and tenderness and sometimes a discoloration to the skin that resembles cellulitis. These patients are very uncomfortable as a result of pain and require analgesics for pain control.

Local trauma

SVT can develop as a result of local trauma caused by an extremity injury from a variety of causes. Often there is bruising of the skin in conjunction with a palpable venous cord. Other forms of local trauma include an intravenous catheter in an upper extremity vein. This is usually a self-limiting problem that improves once the catheter is removed. In some instances, the local thrombosis is severe, and there also can be associated skin trauma, usually caused by local extravasation of the infused material, that can result in a skin slough. Septic phlebitis can occur at the site of an intravenous catheter. The usual treatment is removal of the catheter and intravenous antibiotics; in some rare instances, removal of the septic vein is necessary if the patient does not respond to the usual therapy and if there is evidence of ongoing infection.

Coexistent conditions

If there is no apparent explanation for the presence of SVT, the possibility of other coexistent conditions should be evaluated. Sometimes the first manifestation of a hypercoagulability syndrome is the development of SVT. There is a long list of such conditions that can be diagnosed with a blood test and are easily treated, usually with coumadin. SVT also is associated with vasculitis, such as polyarteritis nodosa and Buerger's disease. Also, some patients with repeated bouts of SVT, often at different sites, have been found to have a malignancy. This association was first suggested by Trousseau in 1865.

Diagnosis and Treatment

In the past, the diagnosis of SVT was based solely on the physical exam. The presence of a painful, tender area directly over a prominent superficial vein was thought to be enough. If the SVT was below the knee, treatment was bed rest, local heat, analgesics, and anti-inflammatory agents such as aspirin. If the SVT was above the knee, with the possible risk of direct extension to the sapheno-femoral junction, patients were treated in the remote past with surgical ligation of the saphenofemoral junction. In more recent times, this surgical procedure was abandoned in favor of treatment with heparin.

Recent studies have clearly demonstrated that SVT, in some patients, is associated with deep venous thrombosis (DVT). Attempts at developing a typical risk profile of which patients are more likely to have associated DVT have been unsuccessful. It was previously believed that the most significant risk for the progression of SVT to DVT was the presence of clot in the greater saphenous vein at or near the saphenofemoral junction or in the lesser saphenous vein at or near the popliteal vein, resulting in direct clot propagation into the deep system. Recent data from many centers now show that, although there can be contiguous clot extending from the superficial to the deep venous system, there is also the frequent development of DVT at noncontiguous sites in the deep venous system. There have been attempts to correlate the site of the SVT and the likelihood of the subsequent development of DVT, but these data remain somewhat controversial.

Because of this association of SVT and DVT, which ranges from 17% to 40% in incidence, a thorough evaluation of patients with SVT becomes critical. The modern standard for this evaluation is duplex ultrasound. We recommend that all patients with SVT undergo a full duplex evaluation, not only to confirm the diagnosis of SVT but also to evaluate the patient for the presence of coexistent DVT. A complete duplex evaluation of the entire leg is important because of the possibility of DVT not only at a site contiguous with the SVT but also at noncontiguous sites remote from the SVT.

An association between SVT and clinically silent pulmonary embolism (PE) was made in a recent study.

This series involved the routine screening of all patients with SVT for the presence of PE by lung scan. Any patients with documented coexistent SVT and DVT were excluded. Although this study does show an association between SVT and PE, it is not suggested that all patients with SVT have a baseline lung scan unless there is a clinical suspicion of PE. These study results lend more credence to the suggestion that SVT is not always a benign condition. Further such studies will be necessary before routine lung scans can be suggested for patients with SVT.

If the evaluation of a patient with SVT reveals the presence of DVT, full anticoagulation is suggested along with outpatient warfarin.

Deep Venous Thrombosis

DVT is a significantly more serious clinical problem because of a higher risk for PE and chronic venous insufficiency and the possibility for chronic postphlebitic syndrome with chronic skin changes, chronic edema, and leg ulceration. The incidence of DVT is difficult to assess accurately because of a number of confounding issues. The population studied is a major factor. The screening of outpatients versus hospitalized patients can give varying results. Whom to screen is also a factor because many patients with DVT are asymptomatic. Autopsy studies are biased because they often include an elderly hospitalized patient population with many comorbid conditions. Some estimates place the incidence of DVT in the United States at 250,000 cases per year.

Pathogenesis

As postulated by Virchow, three factors are important in the development of DVT: stasis, increased blood viscosity, and vascular injury. Some combination of these three factors is essential for the development of DVT, but recent evidence shows that different factors are more important in certain individuals. For example, a relatively slight decrease in blood flow in an individual who has an elevated level of activated coagulation factors as a result of recent surgery or the presence of cancer or of inflammatory cells known to activate tissue procoagulants can make the individual more susceptible to clot formation. Likewise, an individual with a significant vascular injury, either local trauma to the femoral vein at the time of hip surgery or a biochemical endothelial injury from factors released at a remote site as a result of surgery or some inflammatory process, could develop DVT with a slight decrease in venous flow. More is being learned about the relative interaction of a variety of factors that result in some combination of Virchow's triad causing venous thrombosis.

Risk Factors

Primary DVT occurs in the absence of any of the usual recognized risk factors and secondary DVT occurs in the setting of the usually recognized risk factors.

Age

The increased incidence of DVT in the elderly could be the result of confounding variables because, along with increasing age, other risk factors increase. These factors include acquired thrombotic states, immobilization, decrease in the action of the calf muscle pump, and anatomic changes in the veins and venous valves.

Immobilization

Immobilization is a major factor in the development of DVT and is apparent in the increased incidence of DVT in patients at bed rest and individuals in a cast. There is also an increase in the reports of DVT in individuals sitting in cramped positions during prolonged airplane flights. One author has coined the phrase "coach class thrombosis" to describe this condition. Again, many coexistent factors may contribute to the development of DVT in this circumstance.

Surgery

It is well documented that, following surgery, patients are at an increased risk for developing DVT. A wide range of risk factors are important and include type of surgery, age of the patient, length of procedure, coexistent medical factors, and the presence of any underlying hypercoagulability factors. In patients who do not receive prophylaxis, the risk of DVT ranges from 20% to 50%.

History of DVT

Patients who have experienced previous DVT are at increased risk for the subsequent development of DVT. The exact reason for this is unclear, but it could be that an underlying abnormality in coagulation is present. Evaluating patients with recurrent DVT for any of the many hypercoagulability syndromes is crucial because, if such a syndrome is found, lifelong treatment would be necessary.

Malignancy

There appears to be a two-way association between DVT and cancer. Patients with DVT often have an underlying malignancy. One report revealed that, among patients with none of the usual risk factors for DVT, 10% will have a malignancy. Conversely, patients with malignancies are at increased risk for developing DVT. Also, patients who receive a diagnosis of cancer within 1 year of their diagnosis of DVT seem to have an advanced stage of their malignancy and a poor prognosis.

Hypercoagulability syndromes

There are now many well-described hypercoagulability syndromes, such as deficiencies of antithrombin III, protein C, protein S, and plasminogen; activated protein C resistance; factor V Leiden gene mutation; anti-cardiolipin antibody and lupus anticoagulant; prothrombin 20210 gene mutation; dysfibrinogenemia; increased levels of plasminogen activator inhibitor; and hyperhomocystinemia. These often first manifest as DVT, and any of these abnormalities are more likely to cause DVT than acute arterial occlusion.

Other risk factors

There are many more risk factors for DVT, including trauma, pregnancy, use of oral contraceptives and estrogen therapy, blood group A, and inflammatory bowel disease, but data supporting these associations are less strong.

Diagnosis

The clinical history and the physical examination of patients with suspected DVT can be helpful but also can be very misleading. It is well known that many misdiagnoses have occurred as a result of both under- and over-diagnosis. Much depends on the clinical situation and the risk factors. It is true that many patients with DVT are asymptomatic and have a normal physical exam. Some of the factors contributing to this include either a partially occluding thrombus or a total occlusion that is well collateralized, resulting in no or little obstruction to flow and thus no subsequent swelling. Also, these veins are often deep in the extremity and cannot be easily palpated. There is evidence that categorizing patients into low, moderate, and high risk based on the usual risk factors as well as the clinical setting can increase the yield of the history and physical exam as well as the diagnostic tests.

Venous duplex ultrasound

Numerous reports from many institutions have shown that using this method to diagnose DVT is fast, accurate, and noninvasive and compares favorably to traditional invasive phlebography. There can be some difficulty in visualizing certain anatomic areas in obese individuals, such as the calf and the area above the inguinal ligament. Visualization of the subclavian vein proximally is difficult because of the overlying bone.

Phlebography

Long considered the gold standard for the diagnosis of DVT, this technique is now seldom used because of the success of duplex ultrasound imaging.

Magnetic resonance venography

This is a relatively new technique that is gaining in popularity, especially for large central veins such as the subclavian, superior vena cava, inferior vena cava (IVC), and iliac veins, where excellent imaging is possible. The contraindications of metallic implants, claustrophobia, and a noncooperative patient still exist.

D-dimer measurement

Degradation of fibrin by the fibrinolytic pathway results in the release of D-dimers, which now can be assayed rapidly and accurately. There are reports of the use of D-dimer levels as a secondary test to support other diagnostic tests, such as an equivocal duplex ultrasound test. If the D-dimer value is at a normal level, then the likelihood of DVT is less. We do not have experience with this test and await further corroborative studies before we suggest its routine use.

Treatment

The treatment of DVT is anticoagulant therapy, starting with heparin, either conventional unfractionated heparin or low-molecular-weight heparin (LMWH), followed by oral anticoagulant therapy. The most widely used oral anticoagulant in North America is warfarin (a 4-hydroxycoumarin compound). Its popularity is the result of its predictable onset and duration of action and its excellent bioavailability.

Pulmonary Embolism

Of the various complications resulting from DVT, PE is considered the most serious. A PE can lead to significant impairment in pulmonary gas exchange as well as hemodynamic instability, possibly resulting in death. The actual incidence of PE is underestimated in our aging population, and reliable estimates vary among the groups of patients studied. In the United States, it is estimated that up to 5 million patients each year have an episode of venous thrombosis, and that 10% will have a PE. The number of fatalities resulting from PE each year ranges from 50,000 to 200,000. Hospital admissions encompass diverse patient diseases that present a risk for DVT and PE, including cardiovascular, pulmonary, surgical, orthopedic, oncologic, genitourologic, and traumatic conditions. It is important to recognize this risk because the incidence of PE is 3.5 per 1000 hospital admissions in tertiary medical centers, and PE accounts for a mortality of 1 per 1000 hospital admissions. Unfortunately, the diagnosis is unsuspected in two thirds of patients dying of PE, and only 30% of patients with autopsy-proven PE as the cause of death have a clinical diagnosis suspected prior to death.

Clinical Manifestations

The signs and symptoms of PE are not specific, may vary with the magnitude of the PE, and require an astute clinician to maintain a high level of suspicion, particularly in patients who are at risk (e.g., the elderly; patients with congestive heart failure or thrombophilia disorders; those with orthopedic, oncologic, and neurologic conditions). The degree, severity, and duration of symptoms are related to the type of PE: minor, moderate, or severe. Sudden and unexplained episodes of hypotension, chest pain, and respiratory insufficiency suggest the possibility of PE. Minor PE may be asymptomatic and inconsequential, and may present with a transient episode of tachypnea and tachycardia usually resolving spontaneously; however, in patients with significant cardiac and pulmonary disease, even these small PEs may manifest in severe symptoms or cause death. Moderate PE may have a more dramatic clinical presentation, often resulting in hypotension, tachycardia, respiratory distress, and chest pain. The most common symptoms experienced are dyspnea and chest pain, occurring in 79% and 65% of patients, respectively. A major PE obstructing more than 50% of the pulmonary outflow tract may result in a catastrophic presentation with refractory hypotension, cardiac arrest, bradycardia, acute right heart failure, and significantly impaired gas exchange. The symptoms and signs are not unique to PE; therefore, in the differential diagnosis of PE, one should include myocardial infarction, cardiogenic shock, hypovolemic shock, sepsis, aortic dissection, tension pneumothorax, ruptured aortic aneurysm, addisonian crisis, pericardial tamponade, pulmonary pathology, and congestive cardiac failure.

Diagnosis

If a high index of suspicion for a PE is entertained, treatment with anticoagulation should be expeditious and not delayed for confirmatory test results, and must be based on clinical judgment, patient risk assessment, symptomatology, and comorbid factors. Additional diagnostic test should be obtained and utilized to either confirm or refute a PE as well as DVT, and the results of such tests dictate the treatment for an acute PE.

Arterial blood gas measurement

The measurement of arterial blood gases is a simple and rapid test in delineating acid-base status and oxygen–carbon dioxide gas exchange. In the hospitalized patient with acute hypoxia in the absence of any cardiac, pulmonary, or metabolic disorders, the diagnosis of PE stands until proven otherwise. Furthermore, when the arterial partial pressure of oxygen is decreased in the setting of respiratory compromise, chest pain, and tachycardia and in the absence of pulmonary pathology on chest radiography, PE should be strongly considered.

Electrocardiography

In the population at risk for PE, an electrocardiogram (ECG) is essential in any patient with chest pain, shortness of breath, and hypotension. An ECG should be performed to evaluate for cardiac disorders of ischemia and dysrhythmias as a possible cause of the patient's symptoms. The most common finding on ECG in patients with acute PE is sinus tachycardia. With massive or multiple submassive PE, the ECG may demonstrate the classical pattern of $S_1Q_3T_3$, T-wave inversion in the right ventricular leads, and right or left axis deviation in approximately 16% of patients.

Chest radiography

A chest radiograph is useful in evaluating for other cardiac and pulmonary abnormalities, such as congestive heart failure, pneumonia, or pneumothorax, that may explain the clinical picture. A chest radiograph lacks sensitivity and specificity in diagnosing a PE, but is a useful companion in the interpretation of lung scintigraphy. Although nonspecific, the chest radiograph may display significant abnormalities in the presence of a PE, including parenchymal abnormalities, pleural effusion, pleural-based opacity (Hampton's hump), diaphragm elevation, decreased pulmonary vascularity, cardiomegaly, and focal oligemia (Westermark's sign).

D-dimer measurement

D-dimer is a protein fragment produced during the breakdown of fibrin, which results from the fibrinolytic action of the plasmin found in thrombus. D-dimer is not specific for venous thromboembolism, and levels may be elevated in conditions such as malignancy, trauma, infections, sepsis, and pregnancy. Newer techniques utilizing enzyme-linked immunosorbent assay to measure D-dimer have high sensitivity, thereby allowing the measurement of small circulating quantities. The absence of D-dimers implies the absence of fibrin degradation and intravascular thrombus, with a high negative predictive value.

Noninvasive venous studies

ULTRASOUND. Ultrasound has become the mainstay for the diagnosis of lower extremity DVT. Ultrasound is extremely useful in patients suspected of having had a PE and those having evidence of acute DVT because the therapy for uncomplicated thromboembolism is anticoagulation. A nondiagnostic ventilation-perfusion scan in the presence of lower extremity venous thrombosis occurs in as many as 10% of patients, thereby avoiding the need for any further pulmonary imaging. However, in the presence of an equivocal ventilation-perfusion scan, a normal duplex ultrasound scan does not exclude the possibility of a PE, necessitating further diagnostic tests.

VENTILATION-PERFUSION SCANNING. A ventilation-perfusion scan utilizes radiopharmaceuticals to assess for alveolar gas exchange that is matched with pulmonary blood flow for a given segment of lung. When a pulmonary embolus obstructs a segmental pulmonary artery, the blood flow is altered despite ventilation of the corresponding lung alveoli. The presence of a normal perfusion lung scan essentially excludes the possibility of a PE. However, an abnormal perfusion lung scan does not necessarily establish the diagnosis of a PE because reductions in pulmonary blood flow can occur with atelectasis, pneumothorax, chronic obstructive pulmonary disease, and emphysema. Perfusion lung scans for PE are interpreted as normal, low, intermediate (or indeterminate), and high probability. In general, and in the absence of other pulmonary diseases, the importance of a corresponding ventilation lung scan is to determine if these perfusion defects are matched or mismatched with a ventilation scan, indicating a low-probability or a high-probability study for PE, respectively. Clinical suspicion of a PE should guide confirmatory diagnostic tests.

The Prospective Investigation of Pulmonary Embolism Diagnosis (PIOPED) group studied the relationship of ventilation-perfusion scanning to pulmonary arteriography. The study found that, when both the clinical suspicion and radiographic probability were high, the diagnostic accuracy of ventilation-perfusion scanning was 96% compared to angiography. Similarly, when the probability for PE was low based on clinical suspicion and ventilation-perfusion scans, there was only a 2% to 9% incidence of angiographically diagnosed PE. The relationship between clinically suspected PE and perfusion scan results was the basis of the Prospective Investigative Study of Acute Pulmonary Embolism Diagnosis (PISA-PED). The PISA-PED study demonstrated that perfusion scanning for PE had positive and negative predictive values of 87% to 94% and 80% to 87%, respectively. Unfortunately, it is not known if a perfusion scan alone is more accurate than a ventilation-perfusion scan, and in the PIOPED study only 13% of patients had high-probability scans and 14% had normal scans. A fair number of patients in the PIOPED trial had intermediate scans and in clinical practice would require additional diagnostics.

PULMONARY ANGIOGRAPHY. Pulmonary angiography is considered the method of choice in the diagnosis of PE, although it should not be used as the initial test in screening for PE. Angiography should be employed only if the clinical status of the patient mandates an absolute diagnosis; if the additional benefits of angiography, including placement of a vena cava filter, lytic therapy, and suction thromboembolectomy, are considered to outweigh the risks; and if other noninvasive test are nondiagnostic or unavailable. Patients undergoing pulmonary angiography require continuous pulmonary, electrocardiographic, and hemodynamic monitoring. Proper patient oxygenation and hydration should be instituted. Common adverse occurrences include catheter-induced rhythm disturbances, which need to be recognized and treated accordingly and in most instances require careful catheter manipulation to treat the dysrhythmia. The reliability and hence the interpretability of pulmonary angiography decreases in the subsegmental arterial level because of the diminished resolution in the smaller caliber vessels. However, clinically significant PEs are usually macroscopic, and angiography has both a sensitivity and a specificity between 95% and 98%. Despite these limitations and the associated risks of angiography in patients with congestive heart failure, renal insufficiency, and pulmonary hypertension, as well as the potential for adverse contrast-induced reactions, pulmonary angiography remains an important diagnostic tool in selected patients with suspected PE and sets a reference standard to which other test are compared.

COMPUTED TOMOGRAPHY AND MAGNETIC RESONANCE ANGIOGRAPHY. Computed tomography (CT) and magnetic resonance angiography (MRA) are noninvasive radiographic modalities gaining widespread use in the diagnosis of PE. Helical CT is based on the principle of direct identification of an embolus in the pulmonary arteries by visualizing an intraluminal filling defect in the presence of iodinated contrast enhancement. The sensitivity and specificity of CT in detecting PE are between 63% and 100% and 78% and 97%, respectively; however, these values are only estimates, and a significant amount of patient selection variability, prevalence, and technical data acquisition methodology influence these results. The utility and accuracy of helical CT in the diagnosis of PE are further influenced by technical artifacts, contrast timing, beam collimation of the suspected lung fields, patient motion artifacts, altered blood flow, and intrinsic pulmonary disease. Despite these limitations, CT imaging techniques and technology are improving, and, in the presence of other pathology, CT proves useful in identifying other causes for indeterminate ventilation-perfusion scans.

MRA has found a number of uses in the noninvasive imaging of the vascular tree, including its use in imaging the pulmonary vasculature to identify and diagnose PE. The sensitivity and specificity of PE detection by MRA are comparable to those of CT, ranging from 75% to 100% and from 95% to 100%, respectively. Limitations of MRA compared to CT are institutional availability, longer data acquisition times, patients requiring metallic monitoring devices, and breath-hold compliance.

Prevention and Risk Assessment

Because of the significant patient impact and cost of venous thromboembolism, it is advantageous to identify patients at risk and reduce or prevent the possibility of PE by judicious prophylaxis against the formation of thrombus. Factors that increase a patient's risk for developing venous thromboembolism include age, medical comorbidities, and type of surgery. Strategies to reduce thromboembolism take into consideration methods to decrease venous stasis, alter the coagulation cascade, or provide prophylaxis against a PE. Because patients present with different physiologic risks and surgical requirements, there will be variability in both the risk of developing thromboembolism and the preventive measure employed to reduce DVT and PE. A recent report reviewed a large body of data and established useful guidelines based on current knowledge of DVT and PE in patients at risk (Table 40–1). In addition, pentasaccharide, a highly selective indirect inhibitor of activated factor X, recently demonstrated significant benefit in preventing venous thromboembolism in patients undergoing total hip replacement.

Treatment

For uncomplicated venous thromboembolism, the mainstay of treatment is anticoagulation with heparin, warfarin, or LMWH. Patients generally are treated with intravenous heparin with concomitant overlap of 3 to 5 days of warfarin, and then continued on warfarin for 3 to 6 months. LMWH is advantageous for not requiring monitoring and can be administered in an outpatient environment in the treatment of DVT. LMWH has been shown to be as effective and free from bleeding complications as unfractionated heparin in the treatment of both DVT and PE. It is important to note that ambulation is safe and does not increase the risk of PE in patients treated for venous thromboembolism. Recurrent episodes of venous thromboembolism should be treated indefinitely with anticoagulation, although an increased risk of bleeding needs to be taken into consideration. Patients who have an absolute contraindication to anticoagulation generally are treated with a vena cava filter to prevent fatal PE (see Filters: Indications, Types, and Risks below).

For complicated PE and/or in the clinical setting of hemodynamic instability or right ventricular failure secondary to massive PE, thrombolytic therapy given systemically can improve outcome. However, patients with either of these two manifestations have increased bleeding complications and a sixfold increase in mortality. The most commonly used thrombolytics are streptokinase, anistreplase, and recombinant tissue plasminogen activator (rtPA). In the event that thrombolytics are contraindicated, pulmonary

Table 40–1

Risk of thromboembolism and prophylaxis

Risk*	Site of Thromboembolic Event				Prevention
	Calf DVT	Prox. DVT	PE	Fatal PE	
Low	2%	0.4%	0.2%	0.002%	None
Minor surgery					
Uncomplicated					
Age <40 yr					
No clinical risk factors					
Moderate	10%–20%	2%–4%	1%–2%	0.1%–0.4%	Unfractionated heparin q12h
Any surgery					*OR*
Age 40–60 yr					LMW heparin
No clinical risk					*OR*
OR					Intermittent compressed device
Major surgery					
Age <40 yr					
No clinical risk					
High	20%–40%	4%–8%	2%–4%	0.4%–1%	Unfractionated heparin q8h
Major surgery					*OR*
Age >60 yr					LMW heparin
No clinical risk					*AND*
OR					Intermittent compressed device
Major surgery					
Age 40–60 yr					
Clinical risks					
OR					
MI					
Medical morbidity					
Very High	40%–60%	10%–20%	4%–10%	1%–5%	Unfractionated heparin
Major surgery					*OR*
Age >40 yr					LMW heparin
Prior DVT/PE					*AND*
OR					Intermittent compression device
Major surgery					*OR*
Malignancy					Warfarin
Hypercoagulable					*OR*
OR					Intravenous dose-adjusted heparin
Major surgery					
Orthopedic					
Fracture					
OR					
Spinal cord injury					
Multiple trauma					

DVT, deep venous thrombosis; MI, myocardial infarction; PE, pulmonary embolus; Prox, proximal.
*Clinical risks: age, congestive heart failure, malnutrition, oral contraceptives, hormone replacement therapy, postpartum status; immobilization, chemotherapy, and neurotic disease.
Adapted from Clagett GP, Anderson FA, Geerts W, et al: Prevention of venous thromboembolism. Chest 1998;114:531S.

embolectomy either surgically or by endovascular techniques can be employed.

Anticoagulation Therapy—Benefits and Risks

Heparin

There are two forms of heparin, standard unfractionated heparin, with a molecular weight of between 5000 and 30,000, and fractionated heparin, with a molecular weight of approximately 7000. The major advantage of LMWH is ease of administration. Standard heparin therapy is given by continuous intravenous infusion and must be carefully adjusted to keep the activated partial thromboplastin time within a prescribed range. LMWH is administered subcutaneously according to a weight-based dosing schedule, and does not require laboratory monitoring. This is possible because of a more predictable anticoagulant response than with standard heparin, a longer plasma half-life, and better bioavailability when administered subcutaneously. Numerous studies have compared standard heparin and LMWH, and the efficacy and safety are comparable. The added advantage is that LMWH can be administered at home without laboratory monitoring, thus being more advantageous and convenient to the patient and having a reduced cost because there is no required hospitalization and monitoring of laboratory tests.

Side effects

The most frequent side effect of heparin therapy is bleeding. Various studies report the incidence of major bleeding to be around 6%. The frequency of bleeding complications does not appear to differ significantly when comparing route of administration (intravenous vs. subcutaneous). Recent studies have demonstrated that the risk of major bleeding complications is diminished in patients treated with LMWH compared with patients treated with standard heparin. The concomitant use of aspirin may increase the likelihood of bleeding complications. Other possible associated risk factors for bleeding include renal failure and female gender.

Thrombocytopenia is also a well-recognized complication of heparin therapy and appears to be more common in patients receiving heparin from a bovine source than a porcine source (15% vs. 6%). There is also a 0.4% possibility of developing arterial or venous thrombosis with heparin-associated thrombocytopenia. Thrombocytopenia develops between 3 and 15 days after the initiation of heparin therapy, but can occur in hours in patients previously exposed to heparin. Once the heparin is discontinued, the platelet count will return to baseline levels in 4 days.

This heparin-associated thrombocytopenia is caused by an immunoglobulin G–heparin–platelet factor 4 immune complex. LMWHs can have immunologic cross-reactivity with standard heparin.

Other complications of heparin therapy include osteoporosis, heparin-induced skin necrosis, alopecia, hypersensitivity reactions, and hypoaldosteronism.

Heparin and pregnancy

Heparin is the anticoagulant of choice for use in pregnancy because it does not cross the placenta and it does not have any untoward effects on the fetus.

Oral Anticoagulants (Warfarin)

Oral anticoagulants such as warfarin induce their anticoagulant effect by inhibition of vitamin K–dependent clotting factors. They are rapidly absorbed from the gastrointestinal tract. There is a variable response rate in patients for a variety of reasons, which can include warfarin resistance, fluctuating levels of vitamin K, diets rich in green vegetables, nutritional fluid supplements rich in vitamin K, fat malabsorption, fever, hyperthyroidism, liver disease, and a variety of drug interactions.

Testing for the efficacy of warfarin has been problematic; comparisons between the results of various laboratories have been very difficult because of an inability to standardize the thromboplastin reagents from various laboratories. To solve this problem, the international normalized ratio (INR) was established. The INR is the prothrombin time ratio that reflects the result that would be obtained if the World Health Organization reference thromboplastin had been used.

Once the patient has been on heparin, warfarin is then started on the same day. The clinical onset of a therapeutic level is variable for all of the reasons noted above. Once a therapeutic level is achieved as measured by the INR, the warfarin is continued for 3 to 6 months. The appropriate INR value is variable depending on the indication for anticoagulation therapy. An INR of between 2 and 3 is appropriate for patients treated for thromboembolic disorders.

The duration of oral anticoagulant therapy is generally between 3 and 6 months. Attempts at reducing the treatment period to 6 weeks have met with a higher likelihood of the development of recurrent thromboembolism.

Side effects

The major complication from oral anticoagulant therapy is bleeding. The level of anticoagulation, use of aspirin, increasing age, and renal failure influence the risk of bleeding. Skin necrosis is a rare complication and usually occurs between the third and eighth day of therapy. This thrombosis of the venules and capillaries in the subcutaneous fat may be associated with protein C deficiency.

Warfarin and pregnancy

Oral anticoagulant drugs pass across the placenta and have teratogenic effects, and should not be used in pregnancy. If anticoagulation is indicated, then heparin is the drug of choice.

Filters: Indications, Types, and Risks

In patients with venous thromboembolism and an absolute contraindication for anticoagulation or thrombolytic therapy, a metallic filter is placed in the IVC to act as a trap for large pulmonary emboli that may otherwise prove fatal. Patients suitable for IVC filter placement include any patient who demonstrates or is at increased risk for bleeding that could jeopardize life or neurologic function if anticoagulation is initiated, as well as patients who have had recurrent PEs despite adequate anticoagulation. Also, filters are indicated if there are any adverse events from chronic anticoagulation therapy, poor medication compliance, failure of a previously placed filter, or severe trauma with prolonged immobilization involving neurologic, pelvic, and long bone fractures and solid organ injury where DVT prevention with anticoagulation is recommended. In addition, patients who have had a successful pulmonary embolectomy or have confirmed DVT in the presence of a paradoxical embolus require IVC filters, and filters are useful as prophylaxis in high-risk patients with poor cardiopulmonary reserve and confirmed DVT. Relative indications for filter placement include free-floating IVC thrombus, DVT in the presence of a patent right-to-left shunt, protection from large thrombus burden treated with thrombolytics or thromboembolectomy, prophylaxis of PE in high-risk orthopedic procedures, and severe cardiopulmonary disease or hypercoagulability disorders in high-risk patients.

Many Food and Drug Administration–approved filters are available for use. The filters available for IVC interruption are designed with two common features: an anchoring system to attach to the IVC and a trapping device to prevent a large embolus from reaching the cardiopulmonary system. Although the filters have different sizes, shapes, delivery systems, construction, and material designs, they have comparable results with respect to protection from PE and complication rates. Recurrent PE after filter placement ranges between 3% and 4%. Complications from different types of IVC filters are listed in Table 40–2 and vary with respect to the design, mechanics, delivery, and possibly the material composition. The major complications of vena caval filter placement include access site thrombosis (2% to 41%); filter-associated IVC thrombosis (0% to 30%); filter migration, both distal (1% to 18%) and proximal (0% to 3.5%); metal fatigue and mechanical failure requiring another filter placement; filter infection (extremely rare); and filter strut penetration with associated organ injury or vessel penetration. In the gravid patient requiring an IVC filter, it is advisable to place the filter in the suprarenal position to avoid potential harm to the nearby uterus by strut perforation. Placement of filters in the suprarenal position has not been associated with an increased risk of IVC thrombosis, renal vein thrombosis, or renal failure, and the incidence of recurrent PE is 4%, similar to

Table 40–2

Inferior vena cava filters, material, and major complications

Filter	Material			Complications		
		PE Recurrence	Fatal PE	IVC Patency	Access Site Thrombosis	Proximal Migration*
Greenfield	Stainless steel	4%	0.7%	90%–98%	19%–41%	3.5%
Greenfield	Titanium alloy	3%	1.6%	97%–100%	2%–8%	0%
Bird's nest	Stainless steel alloy	3%	2.1%	79%–95%	NA	0%
Simon nitinol	Nickel-titanium alloy	4%	1%	75%–93%	11%	0%
Vena Tech	Stainless steel–cobalt alloy	4%	0.4%	70%–92%	8%	1.3%
TrapEase[†]	Nickel-titanium alloy	0%	0%	97%	0%	0%

DVT, deep venous thrombosis; NA, not available; PE, pulmonary embolism.

Proximal migration indicates migration of the filter to the heart or pulmonary artery, or to a position where the filter is no longer functional against a PE.

[†]*Data for TrapEase are at 6-month follow-up.*

From Rousseau H, Perreault P, Otal P, et al: The 6-F nitinol TrapEase inferior vena cava filter: results of a prospective multicenter trial. J Vasc Interv Radiol 2001;12:299, with permission.

that with infrarenal filter placement. Filters of larger diameter, such as the titanium or stainless steel Greenfield filters, are recommended to reduce the risk of caudal migration.

Newer Thrombolytic Drugs

The lytic agents most commonly utilized in United States clinically and in trials are streptokinase, anistreplase, urokinase, tissue plasminogen activator (tPA), and rtPA. (In 1999, the Food and Drug Administration removed urokinase from clinical use and distribution because of the significant theoretical risk of virus contamination.) Thrombolytic agents work directly or indirectly by forming plasminogen-activating complexes that have an active serine protease that cleaves plasminogen bound to thrombus, forming plasmin, and also a serine protease that initiates fibrin lysis, thereby rapidly restoring venous patency. Treatment of DVT with anticoagulation will result in rapid and complete resolution of the thrombus in only 10% of patients. The advantages of directed thrombolysis are the acute alleviation of obstructive symptoms and the theoretical amelioration of the possible long-term effects of post-thrombotic syndromes (e.g., valvular insufficiency with chronic leg edema, venous ulcer, pulmonary hypertension), which occur in about one third of patients. Catheter-directed thrombolysis has been advocated as the initial treatment of choice in patients with acute iliofemoral DVT, especially those at risk for phlegmasia cerulea dolens and the associated complication of limb loss. Clinical benefits of thrombolysis can be expected in greater than 75% of patients, and the majority of these patients will report improved functional status and quality of life.

Although urokinase is no longer available, many of the studies evaluating both venous and arterial disease thrombosis assessed both the efficacy and safety of using urokinase. The National Multicenter Registry for Lower Extremity Deep Venous Thrombosis evaluated catheter-directed thrombolysis with urokinase in 463 symptomatic patients with iliofemoral and femoral-popliteal DVT. Thrombolytic therapy was determined to be most effective in providing complete lysis for patients with acute DVT (less than 10 days of symptoms), and venous patency was found to be both predictive of and dependent on success of thrombus lysis. Because thrombolytic agents have different plasma kinetics, mechanisms of elimination, and potential side effects, it would be unwise to extrapolate clinical data on the use of urokinase in the treatment of venous thromboembolic disease and apply it to tPA and rtPA, which are employed currently in the treatment of DVT. Few studies have begun to investigate tPA and rtPA in treating iliofemoral DVT. A recent study demonstrated that tPA could successfully restore patency in 79% of iliofemoral DVTs treated. However, the study only

examined 24 patients and bleeding was a significant complication, requiring blood transfusion in 25% of the patients. Additional trials with these newer agents to evaluate their effectiveness in clearing venous thrombus will be required to assess safety, efficacy, and long-term prognosis in venous thromboembolic disorders.

Bibliography

Agnelli G, Goldhaber SZ: Thrombolysis for the treatment of venous thromboembolism. *In* Oudkerk M, van Beek EJR, ten Cate JW (eds): Pulmonary Embolism. Vienna: Blackwell Science, 1999:364.

Ascer E, Lorensen E, Pollina RM, et al: Preliminary results of a nonoperative approach to saphenofemoral junction thrombophlebitis. J Vasc Surg 1995;22:616.

Aswad MA, Sandager GP, Pais SO, et al: Early duplex scan evaluation of four vena caval interruption devices. J Vasc Surg 1996;24:809.

Blumenberg RM, Barton E, Gelfand ML, et al: Occult deep venous thrombosis complicating superficial thrombophlebitis. J Vasc Surg 1998;27:338.

Clagett GP, Anderson FA, Geerts W, et al: Prevention of venous thromboembolism. Chest 1998;114:531S.

Comerota AJ, Aldridge SC, Cohen G, et al: A strategy of aggressive regional therapy for acute iliofemoral venous thrombosis with contemporary venous thrombectomy or catheter-directed thrombolysis. J Vasc Surg 1994;20:244.

Comerota AJ, Katz ML, Greenwald LL, et al: Venous duplex imaging: should it replace hemodynamic tests for deep venous thrombosis? J Vasc Surg 1990;11:53.

Comerota AJ, Throm RC, Mathias SD, et al: Catheter-directed thrombolysis for iliofemoral deep venous thrombosis improves health-related quality of life. J Vasc Surg 2000;32:130.

Dalen JE, Haffajee CL, Alpert JS, et al: Pulmonary embolism, pulmonary hemorrhage and pulmonary infarction. N Engl J Med 1977;296:1431.

Ferretti GR, Bosson JL, Buffaz PD, et al: Acute pulmonary embolism: role of helical CT in 164 patients with intermediate probability at ventilation-perfusion scintigraphy and normal results at duplex US of the legs. Radiology 1997;205:453.

Ginsberg JS: Management of venous thromboembolism. N Engl J Med 1996;335:1816.

Ginsberg JS, Kearon C, Douketis J, et al: The use of D-dimer testing and impedance plethysmographic examination in patients with clinical indications of deep vein thrombosis. Arch Intern Med 1997;157:1077.

Goldhaber SZ, Hennekens CH, Evans DA, et al: Factors associated with an antemortem diagnosis of major pulmonary embolism. Am J Med 1982;73:822.

Gupta A, Frazer CK, Ferguson JM, et al: Acute pulmonary embolism: diagnosis with MR angiography. Radiology 1999;210:353.

Hull RD, Raskob GE, Pineo GF, et al: Subcutaneous low-molecular-weight heparin compared with continuous intravenous heparin in the treatment of proximal-vein thrombosis. N Engl J Med 1992;326:975.

Levine M, Gent M, Hirsh J, et al: A comparison of low-molecular-weight heparin administered primarily at home with unfractionated heparin administered in the hospital for proximal deep-vein thrombosis. N Engl J Med 1996; 334:677.

Manganelli D, Palla A, Donnamaria V, et al: Clinical features of pulmonary embolism: doubts and certainties. Chest 1995;107:25S.

Mewissen MW, Seabrook GR, Meissner MH, et al: Catheter-directed thrombolysis for lower extremity deep venous thrombosis: report of a national multicenter registry. Radiology 1999;211:39.

Miniati M, Pistolesi M, Marini C, et al: Value of perfusion lung scan in the diagnosis of pulmonary embolism: results of the Prospective Investigative Study of Acute Pulmonary Embolism Diagnosis (PISA-PED). Am J Respir Crit Care Med 1996;154:1387.

Moser KM: Venous thromboembolism. Am Rev Respir Dis 1990;141:235.

Oudkerk M, van Beek EJR, Reekers JA: Pulmonary angiography: technique, indication and interpretations. *In* Oudkerk M, van Beek EJR, ten Cate JW (eds): Pulmonary Embolism. Vienna: Blackwell Science, 1999:135.

Partsch H, Kechavarz B, Kohn H, et al: The effect of mobilization of patients during treatment of thromboembolic disorders with low-molecular-weight heparin. Int Angiol 1997;16:189.

Partsch H, Kechavarz B, Mostbeck A, et al: Frequency of pulmonary embolism in patients who have iliofemoral deep vein thrombosis and are treated with once- or twice-daily low-molecular-weight heparin. J Vasc Surg 1996;24:774.

The PIOPED Investigators: Value of the ventilation/perfusion scan in acute pulmonary embolism: results of the Prospective Investigation of Pulmonary Embolism Diagnosis (PIOPED). JAMA 1990;263:2753.

Proctor MC, Greenfield LJ: Pulmonary embolism: diagnosis, incidence and implications. Cardiovasc Surg 1997;5:77.

Robbins KC: The plasminogen-plasmin enzyme system. *In* Comerota AJ (ed): Thrombolytic Therapy for Peripheral Vascular Disease. Philadelphia: JB Lippincott, 1995:41.

Schulman S, Granqvist S, Holmstrom M, et al: The duration of oral anticoagulation therapy after a second episode of venous thromboembolism. N Engl J Med 1997;336:393.

Semba CP, Bakal CW, Calis KA, et al: Alteplase as an alternative to urokinase: advisory panel on catheter-directed thrombolytic therapy. J Vasc Interv Radiol 2000;11:279.

Simonneau G, Sors H, Charbonnier B, et al: A comparison of low-molecular-weight heparin with unfractionated heparin for acute pulmonary embolism. N Engl J Med 1997;337:663.

Sorensen HT, Mellemkjaer L, Olsen JH, et al: Prognosis of cancers associated with venous thromboembolism. N Engl J Med 2000;343:1846.

Turpie AGG, Gallus AS, Hoek JA: A synthetic pentasaccharide for the prevention of deep-vein thrombosis after total hip replacement. N Engl J Med 2001;344:619.

Verlato F, Zucchetta P, Prandoni P, et al: An unexpectedly high rate of pulmonary embolism in patients with superficial thrombophlebitis of the thigh. J Vasc Surg 1999;30:1113.

Warkentin TE, Kelton JG: Temporal aspects of heparin-induced thrombocytopenia. N Engl J Med 2001;344:1286.

PART VIII

Infection

CHAPTER 41

Bacterial Infection

Philip S. Barie, M.D., M.B.A., F.C.C.M., F.A.C.S. and
Soumitra R. Eachempati, M.D., F.A.C.S.

Bacteria are ubiquitous in the environment, but only a minority of species is pathogenic in humans. Ironically, the virulence of bacteria, and hence the clinical manifestations of infection, depend more on the characteristics of the host response than any characteristics of the pathogen. Bacterial colonization of the host is commonplace, and precedes most infections, but infection does not occur unless the host is invaded by the pathogen. Bacteria have evolved mechanisms to facilitate colonization and tissue invasion, just as hosts have evolved defenses against infection. Unfortunately, as health care has become increasingly sophisticated, it also has become increasingly invasive, and patients are also increasingly elderly and sick and therefore immunosuppressed. Any breach (e.g., laceration, incision, cannulation, intubation) of natural epithelial barriers to infection (e.g., skin, respiratory mucosa, gut mucosa), increases the potential that host defenses will be unable to contain a localized invasion, and systemic infection will ensue.

Bacterial Pathogenicity

An infection begins when the balance between bacterial invasion and host resistance is upset. That balance favors the microbe, because the growth rate of bacteria far exceeds that of most eukaryotic cells, bacteria are more versatile than eukaryotic cells in substrate utilization and biosynthesis, and the high mutation rate of bacteria combined with their short generation time results in rapid selection of the best adapted organisms. The expression of bacterial virulence is contingent upon the host response. If a pathogen invades tissue, but does not evoke a host response, there is no means to identify clinically the presence of the bacteria, or to distinguish bacterial colonization from tissue invasion.

Bacteria have a single practical objective: to multiply. Teleologically, it disadvantages the pathogen to kill the host, because the death of the host usually means the death of the pathogen. Few bacterial species cause disease consistently in a given host. The most highly evolved or adapted pathogens are those that can sustain nutritional growth and dissemination with the smallest expenditure of energy and least damage to the host. Some bacteria that are poorly adapted to the host synthesize virulence factors (e.g., botulinum, tetanus, and diphtheria toxins) so potent that they threaten the life of the host.

Virulence factors are produced by a microorganism and evoke a response from the host. Examples of virulence factors include toxins, surface proteins that inhibit phagocytosis, and surface receptors that facilitate binding of the bacterium to host cells. Most overt bacterial pathogens have evolved specific virulence factors that allow them to multiply in their host or vector without being killed or expelled by the host's defenses. Many virulence factors are produced only by specific virulent strains of a microorganism. For example, not all strains of *Escherichia coli* secrete the enterotoxins that cause diarrheal illness.

Expression of Bacterial Virulence

Virulence factors in bacteria may be encoded on chromosomal DNA, viral bacteriophage DNA, plasmids, or transposons in either plasmids or the bacterial chromosome. Packages of transmissible genetic material known as "islands" may provide all of the genetic material necessary to encode for resistance, virulence, or other characteristics. Other virulence factors are acquired by bacteria following infection by a bacteriophage, which integrates its genome into the bacterial chromosome by a process called lysogeny. Bacteriophages often provide the source code for toxin production.

The virulence factors of bacteria can be divided into a number of functional types. These include adherence factors, invasion factors, capsules and other surface proteins, and a myriad of toxins.

Adherence and Colonization Factors

To cause infection, many bacteria must first adhere to a mucosal surface. Integral to host defenses are mucosal properties that act to prevent or counteract adhesion and clear the bacterium to the external environment before invasion and clinical illness. Gut mucosa is cleansed of ingested bacteria by mucus from goblet cells, and by normal peristalsis. Secretory immunoglobulin A (IgA) of gut mucosal origin also plays a major role in host defense. Similarly, ciliated respiratory epithelium sweeps inhaled bacteria upward so that they can be expelled by cough. Rapid turnover of epithelial cells—about 48 hours in the case of gut epithelium—means that bacteria have only a brief period to become adherent and invade to establish infection. Thus bacteria have evolved attachment mechanisms, such as pili (fimbriae), that recognize and attach the bacteria to cells. Some examples of piliated, adherent bacterial pathogens are *Pseudomonas aeruginosa*, *Vibrio cholerae*, *E. coli*, *Salmonella* species, *Neisseria gonorrhoeae*, *Neisseria meningitidis*, and *Streptococcus pyogenes*.

Adherence may also occur to extracellular matrix proteins, or even to medical devices. *Staphylococcus aureus* expresses surface proteins that promote attachment to host proteins such as laminin and fibronectin that form part of the extracellular matrix. The protein fibronectin is present on epithelial and endothelial surfaces, possibly to promote cell-cell adhesion and signaling, as well as being a component of blood clots. In addition, most strains express a fibrinogen/fibrin-binding protein, which promotes attachment to blood clots and traumatized tissue. Most strains of *S. aureus* express fibronectin- and fibrinogen-binding proteins. The receptor that promotes attachment to collagen has been associated with strains that cause osteomyelitis and septic arthritis. Mutant strains that are defective in binding to fibronectin and to fibrinogen demonstrate reduced virulence in animal models of endocarditis, suggesting that bacterial attachment to initially sterile vegetations is promoted by fibronectin and fibrinogen.

Adherence and medical device infections

Infections associated with indwelling medical devices such as venous catheters, prosthetic joints, heart valves, and synthetic vascular grafts are most often caused by *Staphylococcus epidermidis* and *S. aureus*. After implantation of a biomaterial, it becomes coated with a biofilm that is a complex mixture of host proteins and platelets known as a glycocalyx, or "slime." Fibrinogen is the dominant component, explaining why staphylococci so readily become adherent to or even incorporated into the biofilm, where they enjoy a protected environment owing to the inability of antibiotics to penetrate. As time passes and the biomaterial becomes increasingly incorporated, the fibrinogen is degraded and no longer promotes bacterial attachment. Instead, fibronectin, which remains intact, becomes the predominant ligand promoting attachment.

Invasion Factors

Some invasive bacteria (e.g., *Rickettsia*, *Chlamydia*) are obligate intracellular pathogens, but most are facultative. Often, multiple gene products participate in the process that leads to cellular invasion by bacteria, but they are poorly characterized for many species, if at all. Some *Shigella* invasion factors are encoded on a 140-KD plasmid that, when conjugated into *E. coli*, gives these noninvasive bacteria the capacity to invade cells.

Capsules and Other Surface Components

Capsule formation (polymerized complex polysaccharides) has long been recognized as an antiphagocytic protective mechanism for bacteria. Encapsulated strains of many bacteria (e.g., pneumococci) are more virulent and more resistant to phagocytosis and intracellular killing than the nonencapsulated strains. Organisms that cause bacteremia (e.g., *Pseudomonas*) are less sensitive than many other bacteria to killing by fresh human serum containing complement, which may be related in part to the amount and composition of capsular antigens.

In general, bacteria that can enter and survive within eukaryotic cells are shielded from humoral antibodies and can be eliminated only by a cellular immune response. The capacity of bacteria to survive and multiply within host cells has great impact on the pathogenesis of the respective infections. Some bacteria and parasites have the ability to survive and multiply inside phagocytic cells. A classic example is *Mycobacterium tuberculosis*, the survival of which seems to depend on the structure and composition of its cell surface. The parasite *Toxoplasma gondii* has the remarkable ability to block the fusion of lysosomes with the phagocytic vacuole. The lysosomal enzymes are therefore unable to destroy the parasite. Other bacteria (e.g., *Legionella pneumophila*, *Brucella abortus*, and *Listeria monocytogenes*) resist killing after phagocytosis by unknown mechanisms. Still other bacteria survive the intracellular milieu by producing phospholipases to dissolve the phagocytic vesicle surrounding them. This appears to be the case for *Rickettsia rickettsii*, which destroys the phagosomal membrane with which the lysosomes fuse. *Legionella pneumophila*, which prefers the intracellular environment of macrophages for growth, appears to induce its own uptake and blocks lysosomal fusion by undefined mechanisms. Other bacteria have evolved to the point that they prefer the low-pH environment within the lysosomal granules.

Most bacterial pathogens do not invade cells, proliferating instead in the extracellular environment enriched by body fluids. Some bacteria (e.g., *V. cholerae*, *Bordetella pertussis*) do not even invade tissue, but rather adhere to epithelial surfaces and cause disease by secreting potent toxins. Although bacteria such as *E. coli* and *P. aeruginosa* are referred to as noninvasive, they frequently spread rapidly to various tissues once they gain access through an artificial portal such as a wound or therapeutic breach in a natural mucosal barrier.

Cell Wall Antigens and Secretory Products

The cell wall also consists of several structural proteins. Using group A streptococci as an example, the R and T proteins may serve as epidemiologic markers, but the M proteins (surface mucoid protein "slime") are clearly virulence factors associated with resistance to phagocytosis. More than 50 types of *S. pyogenes* M proteins have been identified on the basis of antigenic specificity. Both the M proteins and lipoteichoic acid are supported externally to

the cell wall on fimbriae, and the lipoteichoic acid, in particular, appears to mediate bacterial attachment to host epithelial cells. M protein, peptidoglycan, N-acetylglucosamine, and group-specific carbohydrate portions of the cell wall have antigenic epitopes similar in size and charge to those of mammalian muscle and connective tissue. Recently emerging strains of increased virulence are distinctly mucoid, rich in M protein and highly encapsulated.

The capsule of *S. pyogenes* is composed of hyaluronic acid, which is chemically similar to that of host connective tissue and is therefore nonantigenic. In contrast, the antigenically reactive and chemically distinct capsular polysaccharide of *Streptococcus pneumoniae* allows the single species to be separated into more than 80 serotypes. The antiphagocytic *S. pneumoniae* capsule is the most clearly understood virulence factor of these organisms; type 3 *S. pneumoniae*, which produces copious quantities of capsular material, are the most virulent. Unencapsulated *S. pneumoniae* are avirulent. The polysaccharide capsule in *Streptococcus agalactiae* allows differentiation into types Ia, Ib, Ic, II, and III.

The importance of the interaction of streptococcal products with mammalian blood and tissue components is becoming widely recognized. The soluble extracellular growth products or toxins of the streptococci, especially of *S. pyogenes*, have been studied intensely. Streptolysin S is an oxygen-stable cytolysin, whereas streptolysin O is a reversibly oxygen-labile cytolysin; both are leukotoxic. Hyaluronidase (spreading factor) can digest host connective tissue hyaluronic acid as well as the organism's own capsule. Streptokinases participate in fibrin lysis. Streptodornases A through D possess deoxyribonuclease activity; B and D possess ribonuclease activity as well. Protease activity similar to that in *S. aureus* has been shown in strains causing soft tissue necrosis or toxic shock syndrome. This large repertoire of products may be important in the pathogenesis of *S. pyogenes* by enhancing virulence; however, antibodies to these products appear not to protect the host even though they have diagnostic importance.

Three pyrogenic exotoxins of *S. pyogenes* are recognized: types A, B, and C. These toxins act as superantigens by a mechanism that has also been described for staphylococci, in that they do not require processing by antigen-presenting cells. Rather, they stimulate T cells by direct nonspecific binding of class II major histocompatibility complex (MHC) molecules. With stimulation by superantigens, about 20% of T cells may be activated (vs. 1/10,000 T cells stimulated by conventional antigens). The result is massive cytokine release. Reemergence in the late 1980s of these exotoxin-producing strains has been associated with a toxic shock–like syndrome similar in pathogenesis and manifestation to staphylococcal toxic shock syndrome and other forms of invasive disease associated with severe tissue destruction.

Pseudomonas aeruginosa produces many factors that may contribute to its virulence. Almost all strains of *P. aeruginosa* are hemolytic on blood agar plates, and several different hemolysins have been described. Furthermore, *P. aeruginosa* strains isolated from respiratory tract infections produce more hemolysin than do environmental strains, suggesting that this glycolipid hemolysin may play a role in *P. aeruginosa* pulmonary infections.

Several heat-labile protein hemolysins also have been described. One of these hemolysins may be identical to phospholipase C, which is produced by approximately 70% of all clinical strains of *P. aeruginosa*. Phospholipase C, which hydrolyzes lecithin, is of unknown toxicity, and its role in *P. aeruginosa* infections also remains unknown. Some strains of *P. aeruginosa* produce a thermolabile protein (leukocidin), that lyses polymorphonuclear leukocytes (PMNs) but is nonhemolytic. This leukocidin (also called cytotoxin) damages lymphocytes and various tissue culture cells, but, despite its toxicity, the role of leukocidin also remains unknown.

Approximately 90% of *P. aeruginosa* strains produce extracellular proteases. Three separate proteases have been purified; although all are capable of digesting casein, one of them, protease II, also digests elastin. When injected into the skin of animals, purified *P. aeruginosa* proteases induce formation of hemorrhagic lesions, which become necrotic within 24 hours. Toxin A, the most toxic known extracellular protein of *P. aeruginosa*, is produced by 90% of all strains. The toxicity of toxin A has been attributed to its ability to inhibit protein synthesis in susceptible cells. It achieves this by catalyzing the transfer of the ADP-ribosyl moiety of nicotinamide adenine dinucleotide onto elongation factor-2 (EF-2). The resultant ADP-ribosyl–EF-2 complex is inactive in protein synthesis. Evidence suggesting that toxin A may be a major virulence factor of *P. aeruginosa* includes observations that toxin A–deficient mutants are less virulent in several animal models than their toxin A–producing parental strains, as well as the observation that most patients surviving *P. aeruginosa* sepsis have elevated levels of antitoxin A antibody or are infected with strains that produce little or no detectable toxin A in vitro. A second ADP-ribosyltransferase, exoenzyme S, has been described. Exoenzyme S catalyzes the transfer of ADP-ribose onto a number of GTP-binding proteins; however, it does not modify EF-2. Exoenzyme S is produced by about 90% of clinical isolates of *P. aeruginosa*. Transposon-induced exoenzyme S–deficient mutants are less virulent in several animal models than is their S-producing parental strain; thus exoenzyme S may also be involved in the pathogenesis of some *P. aeruginosa* infections.

Endotoxins

Endotoxin, or lipopolysaccharide (LPS), is composed of toxic components of the outer membrane of gram-negative bacteria. The complex is secured to the outer membrane by ionic and hydrophobic forces, and its strong negative charge is neutralized by Ca^{2+} and Mg^{2+} ions. Endotoxin exerts profound biologic effects on the host, and may be lethal. Endotoxin shares many properties with several of the exotoxins elaborated by gram-positive bacteria, but, importantly, it is distinguished by release following cytolysis of bacteria as opposed to the exotoxins that are secreted by gram-positive bacteria.

Although all LPS molecules are similar in chemical structure and biologic activity, some diversity has evolved. The molecular complex can be divided into three regions: (1) the O-specific chains, which consist of a variety of repeating oligosaccharide residues; (2) the core polysaccharide that forms the backbone of the macromolecule; and (3) lipid A, composed usually of a glucosamine disaccharide with attached long-chain fatty acids and phosphate. The polysaccharide portions are responsible for antigenic diversity, whereas the lipid A moiety confers toxicity. Members of the family Enterobacteriaceae exhibit O-specific chains of various lengths, whereas *N. gonorrhoeae*, *N. meningitidis*, and *B. pertussis* contain only core polysaccharide and lipid A.

Host Resistance

Although easily damaged, the skin represents one of the most important barriers of the body to the microbial world, which contains a diverse array of bacteria in enormous numbers. Fortunately, most bacteria in the environment are relatively benign to individuals with normal immune systems. However, in patients who are immunosuppressed, such as individuals receiving cancer chemotherapy or who have acquired immunodeficiency syndrome, opportunistic microbial pathogens can establish life-threatening infections. Normally, microbes in the environment are prevented from entering the body by the skin and mucous membranes. The outermost surface of the skin consists of squamous epithelium, largely comprising dead cells that are sloughed off as new cells are formed beneath. In addition to the skin barrier, mucous membranes of the respiratory, gastrointestinal, and urogenital systems represent other portals through which bacteria can gain access to the host. As with squamous epithelium of the skin, mucosal epithelial cells divide rapidly, and, as the cells mature, they are pushed toward the intestinal lumen and shed. The entire process requires only 36 to 48 hours for complete replacement of the gut epithelium, which diminishes the number of bacteria associated with the epithelium.

The skin surface is a dry, acidic environment. The pores and crevices of the skin also are colonized by the "normal bacterial flora," which ensure competition for pathogens to which the skin is exposed. Similarly, the mucous layer that covers the epithelia contains substances hostile to microbial colonization. Protective concentrations of lysozyme, lactoferrin, and lactoperoxidase in the mucus either kill bacteria or restrict their growth. In addition, the mucus contains secretory immunoglobulins (predominantly secretory IgA) synthesized by plasma cells resident in the submucosal tissue. During the normal course of life, individuals develop local antibodies specific for a variety of intestinal bacteria that colonize mucosal surfaces.

Another mechanism of restricting growth of bacteria that penetrate the skin and mucous membranes is competition for iron. Typically, the amount of free iron in tissues and blood available to bacteria is very low because plasma transferrin binds virtually all free iron in the blood. Similarly, hemoglobin binds iron. Without free iron, bacterial growth is restricted unless the bacteria synthesize siderophores, or receptors for iron-containing molecules that compete for transferrin-bound iron. Such siderophores strip iron from transferrin and present it to the bacteria, which enables them to grow.

The usual response of the host to injury or infection is to incite an inflammatory response. Even a trivial injury can provoke a response, so sensitive are the triggers for inflammation. The point of the response is to repel bacterial invaders, to stop hemorrhage, and to effect tissue repair. The response must be graded, because it would squander biologic resources to respond maximally to a minor challenge. The response must also be self-contained, in order to assure a graded response.

Three major events characterize the initial inflammatory response: activation of coagulation; increased microvascular endothelial permeability with tissue edema formation; and chemotaxis, margination, and transvascular migration of PMNs. The first step in the process is recognition of a foreign antigen, either by specific (e.g., T cells, preformed antibodies) or nonspecific means (e.g., phagocytic cells, alternative pathway of complement, coagulation). The development of inflammation is then amplified in a complex process regulated by cytokines, plasma enzymes (e.g., complement, coagulation, kinin and fibrinolytic pathways), lipid mediators (e.g., prostaglandins, leukotrienes), and mast cell– and platelet-derived mediators. Fast-acting mediators, such as vasoactive amines and bradykinin, modulate the immediate response. Several hours later, mediators such as leukotrienes are involved in the accumulation and activation of phagocytes. Once PMNs have arrived at a site of inflammation, they release mediators that, in turn, control the later accumulation and activation of monocyte/macrophages.

Minor inflammatory responses may be localized by the activation of coagulation. Endothelial injury results in the deposition of fibrinogen and fibronectin; platelets become adherent and activated within the fibrin clot. As the fibrin clot proliferates, red blood cells are entrapped, and blood flow ceases. However, at some difficult-to-define point,

containment is lost and the response becomes systemic, generating fever and an acute-phase hepatic response by the actions of cytokines on the hypothalamus and liver, respectively.

Cytokines are basic regulators of inflammation, including PMN priming and activation, and of synthesis and secretion of cytokines, including interleukin (IL)-1, IL-6, IL-8, tumor necrosis factor-α (TNF-α), and granulocyte-monocyte colony-stimulating factor (GM-CSF). Interleukin-8, a potent chemoattractant, synergizes with interferon-γ (IFN-γ), TNF-α, GM-CSF, and granulocyte colony-stimulating factor to amplify various neutrophil cytotoxic functions. Cytokines also increase microbicidal activity. Interferon-γ and GM-CSF amplify antibody-dependent PMN cytotoxicity. The anti-inflammatory cytokines IL-4 and IL-10 inhibit the production of IL-8 and the release of TNF-α and IL-1. Moreover, some cytokines prolong PMN survival. The acute inflammatory response may be terminated by the secretion of macrophage inflammatory protein-1α from PMNs, signaling mononuclear cell recruitment and clearance of PMNs from the affected tissue.

Other mediators, including bioactive lipids, neuroendocrine hormones, histamine, and adenosine, also regulate inflammation. Bioactive lipids originate mainly from arachidonic acid (Fig. 41–1), which is abundant in cell membranes, and is the substrate for prostaglandin (PG), leukotriene (LT), and lipoxin (LX) synthesis. Leukotriene B_4 is a potent PMN chemoattractant. The vasoactive leukotrienes LTC_4, LTD_4, and LTE_4 increase microvascular permeability and may contribute to ischemia-reperfusion injury. In contrast to LTs, PGs suppress most PMN functions, possibly through their ability to increase intracellular cyclic AMP (cAMP). The lipoxins LXA_4 and LXB_4 are potent inhibitors of PMN microbicidal activity. In many inflammatory conditions, the concentration of platelet-activating factor (PAF) rises in affected tissues. PAF primes superoxide generation and elastase release, and is a potent vasoconstrictor. Injury can be attenuated by PAF antagonists, which may have therapeutic potential.

"Cross talk" effected by cytokines and neurotransmitters between nervous and immune cells, respectively, provides indirect communication between the neuroendocrine and immune systems. Growth hormone, prolactin, β-endorphin, glucocorticoids, and catecholamines regulate PMNs. Growth hormone primes the oxidative burst of human PMN, as does its effector hormone insulin-like growth factor-1, which is also a potent PMN-priming agent. Prolactin, which shares considerable functional and structural similarities with growth hormone, is comparably potent as a priming agent. Glucocorticoids and opioids are generally considered to be immunosuppressive. Containment of the stress response may be the principal role of glucocorticoids. Glucocorticoids impair globally the phagocytic and cytotoxic activities of PMNs and macrophages.

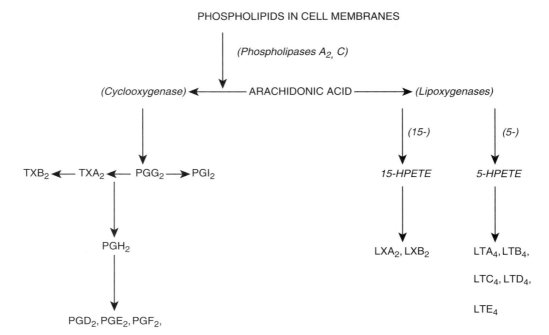

FIGURE 41–1 Prostaglandin synthesis. HPETE, hydroxypentaenoic acid tetradiene; LT, leukotriene; LX, lipoxin, PG, prostaglandin; PGI$_2$, prostacyclin; TX, thromboxane.

Histamine is also a potent inhibitor of PMN microbicidal activity. The interactions between platelets and PMNs are essential for both cell types. Activated platelets can bind to PMNs and stimulate the oxidative burst, whereas platelets themselves synthesize LT. As is the case with PG, many immunosuppressive mediators use cAMP as a second messenger. Increased intracellular cAMP in PMNs is associated with decreased microbicidal activity, whereas cyclic GMP (cGMP) is stimulatory. It is possible that PMN activation/priming may be regulated by the intracellular ratio of cGMP to cAMP.

Neutrophils

Neutrophils are the "initial responders" against infectious agents or "nonself" substances that penetrate the body's physical barriers, including bacteria, fungi, protozoa, and viruses. Although premature forms (e.g., metamyelocytes, nonsegmented [band] neutrophils) can be released from bone marrow in response to maximal stress, it is the segmented PMN that is fully functional. Upon release to the circulation, PMNs are in a nonactivated state and have a half-life of 4 to 10 hours before marginating and entering tissue pools, where they survive for 1 to 2 days. Cells of the circulating and marginated pools exchange freely. Senescent PMNs undergo apoptosis (programmed cell death) prior to removal by macrophages. Viability of PMNs is shorter in individuals suffering from infectious or acute inflammatory diseases when the tissue requirement for newly recruited neutrophils increases considerably,

although inhibition of apoptosis by the anti-inflammatory counter-regulatory response may potentiate inflammation. Subpopulations of neutrophils exist in dormant, activated, and intermediate states. For example, neutrophil priming is a mechanism whereby dormant neutrophils undergo preactivation to enable a more powerful response once a second inflammatory microbial stimulus occurs.

Mature PMNs contain cytoplasmic granules (primary [or azurophil] and secondary [or specific]), which contain numerous antimicrobial or cytotoxic substances (Table 41–1) and a pool of cytoplasmic membrane receptors. Among azurophil granule constituents, myeloperoxidase (MPO) is a critical enzyme in the conversion of hydrogen peroxide to hypochlorous acid. Together with hydrogen peroxide and a halide cofactor, MPO forms the most effective microbicidal and cytotoxic mechanism of PMNs— the myeloperoxidase system. Defensins are small (molecular weight < 4 kD) peptides that are cytotoxic to a broad range of bacteria, fungi, and some viruses; they constitute 30% to 50% of azurophil granule protein. Defensin-mediated toxicity may be due to increased membrane permeability of the target cell, in a manner characteristic of other channel-forming proteins known as perforins. Bacterial permeability-increasing protein is another perforin, which is toxic to gram-negative bacteria but not to gram-positive bacteria or fungi, and can also neutralize LPS by competitive binding with the LPS-LPS-binding protein complex. Lactoferrin sequesters free iron, preventing the growth of surviving ingested organisms. Serine proteases (e.g., elastase, cathepsins) hydrolyze bacterial cell wall

Table 41–1

Contents and biologic effects of neutrophil granules

Functionality	Granule Type		
	Azurophil	Specific	Small Storage
Antimicrobial	Myeloperoxidase Lysozyme Defensins Bactericidal permeability- increasing protein	Lysozyme Lactoferrin	
Neutral proteinases	Elastase Cathepsin G Proteinase 3	Collagenase Complement activator	Gelatinase Plasminogen activator
Acid hydrolases	Cathepsin B Cathepsin D β-D-Glucuronidase α-Mannosidase Phospholipase A_2	Phospholipase A_2	Cathepsin B Cathepsin D β-D-Glucuronidase α-Mannosidase
Cytoplasmic membrane receptors		CR3, CR4 FMLP receptors Laminin receptors	

CR, complement receptor; FMLP, N-formylmethionyl-leucyl-phenylalanine.

proteins, including collagen, proteoglycans, and elastins. Regulation of tissue destruction by proteases is mediated by protease inhibitors such as α1-macroglobulin and α2-antiprotease.

Although azurophil granules function predominantly in the intracellular milieu, to kill and degrade microorganisms, PMN-specific granules can be induced to release their contents extracellularly, thus having an important role in initiating inflammation. Specific granules represent an intracellular reservoir of various plasma membrane components, including cytochrome b_{558} (a component of nicotinamide adenine dinucleotide phosphate [NADPH] oxidase, the enzyme responsible for the production of superoxide anion), receptors for complement fragment iC3b (CR3 and CR4) for laminin, and the formylmethionyl-peptide chemoattractant. In addition, there is also a histaminase capable of the degradation of histamine, a plasminogen activator (responsible for plasmin formation and cleavage of C5a from C5), and others.

The major role of PMNs is phagocytosis of infectious agents. Opsonization is a process in which proteins adsorb to the surface of bacteria or other particles and facilitate adherence to the phagocyte. Specific binding between the bacterium and phagocyte is mediated by immunoadherent receptors, including Fc receptors and complement receptors 1 and 3. Specific binding between particle and phagocyte also may be performed by lectins and lectin receptors (lectinophagocytosis). Phagocytosis comprises several

morphologic and biochemical steps. After adherence to the phagocyte, the process proceeds through ingestion (engulfment), phagosome origination, phagolysosome formation, and killing and degradation of ingested cells or other material. The phagolysosome is formed when cytosolic granules (lysosomes) fuse with the plasma membrane as it invaginates around the microorganism being engulfed. The granules release their contents (degranulate) into the phagolysosome, creating a highly toxic microenvironment. This degranulation normally prevents release of the toxic components into the extracellular milieu. Tissue damage occurs when PMN products are released extracellularly to such an extent that host defenses (antioxidants and antiproteases) in the immediate vicinity are overwhelmed.

Two types of free radicals are produced by PMNs, macrophages, endothelial, and other cells: reactive oxygen intermediates (ROIs) and reactive nitrogen intermediates, including nitric oxide (NO•). During the respiratory burst associated with phagocytosis, oxygen is reduced by the NADPH oxidase electron transport chain to superoxide anion or its protonated form, perhydroxyl radical. Those intermediates are then converted by action of superoxide dismutase to hydrogen peroxide. In addition to causing tissue damage, ROIs also promote the margination of neutrophils by triggering the expression of adhesion molecules on endothelial cells. Hydrogen peroxide (H_2O_2) interacts with the myeloperoxidase contained in PMN azurophil granules to produce hypochlorous acid (HOCl), and thence hypochlorite ion. Hydroxyl radical is formed predominantly by degradation of H_2O_2 catalyzed by Fe^{2+}. Hydroxyl radical and hypochlorite are powerful microbicides and cytotoxins; therefore, neutrophils and other phagocytes protect themselves from autolysis with endogenous reserves of antioxidants such as glutathione and ascorbic acid.

Reactive nitrogen intermediates are formed by oxidation of L-arginine to L-citrulline to yield $NO^\bullet$. This reaction is catalyzed by oxygen-dependent nitric oxide synthase (NOS), of which there are three distinct isoforms. There are two isoforms of constitutive NOS (cNOS): Endothelial cNOS is mostly membrane bound and formed only in endothelial cells, whereas neuronal cNOS is found only in the central nervous system. Activation of soluble guanylate cyclase by $NO^\bullet$ leads to the synthesis of cGMP, which leads to relaxation of vascular smooth muscle, inhibition of platelet adherence and aggregation, inhibition of neutrophil chemotaxis, and signal transduction in the nervous system. Large amounts of $NO^\bullet$, if produced for a prolonged period, cause vasodilatation and hypotension in sepsis. The third isoform of NOS, inducible NOS (iNOS), is not present in resting cells, but instead is induced by cytokines or LPS. Among the cytokines and other mediators upregulating the production of iNOS are IFN-γ, IL-1, IL-6, TNF-α, GM-CSF, and PAF, whereas suppression has been observed with IL-4, IL-8, IL-10, transforming growth factor-β (TGF-β), and others. Once expressed, iNOS generates large amounts of $NO^\bullet$. $NO^\bullet$ may react with superoxide to form the highly toxic peroxynitrite anion ($OONO^-$), which may be transformed in an acid milieu to peroxynitrite acid (a cofactor in microbial killing) and thence to hydroxyl radical.

Regulation of PMN Function

Under normal conditions, PMNs roll along microvascular walls via low-affinity interaction of selectins with specific endothelial carbohydrate ligands. During the inflammatory response, proinflammatory cytokines and other chemotactic factors signal the recruitment of PMNs to sites of infection and/or injury, with subsequent activation of PMN β2-integrins and high-affinity binding to adhesion molecules on the surface of activated endothelial cells. Under the influence of a chemotactic gradient, generated locally and by diffusion of chemoattractants from the infection site, neutrophils penetrate the endothelial layer and migrate through connective tissue to sites of infection (diapedesis), where they congregate and adhere to extracellular matrix components such as laminin and fibronectin.

Adhesion Molecules

The emigration of circulating leukocytes from the blood into inflamed tissues is a "three-step" process. At least four superfamilies of adhesion molecules participate in these events (Table 41–2): the selectins, the integrins, certain members of the immunoglobulin superfamily, and cadherins. Initially, rolling of leukocytes along the vasculature is mediated through transient interactions between selectin proteins and their carbohydrate ligands. Rolling is followed by activation of both neutrophils and endothelial cells, resulting in a high-affinity interaction between integrins and glycoproteins of the immunoglobulin superfamily. Ultimately, extravasation occurs in response to a chemoattractant gradient. In the initial phase of acute inflammation, circulating leukocytes are activated by exposure to inflammatory mediators including complement fragments (C5a), cytokines such as IL-1, IL-8 and TNF-α, LPS, or other chemoattractants, resulting in microvascular sequestration owing to decreased deformability and increased adhesiveness. Endothelial cells are activated similarly, leading to enhanced expression of several adhesion molecules and PAF.

Table 41–2
Characteristics of adhesion molecule interactions

Family	Neutrophil Receptor	Endothelial Receptor	Actions
Selectins	p150sLe^x (CD15), sLe (CD15s), L-selectin	P-selectin (CD62P), E-selectin (CD62E), GlyCAM-1, others	PMN rolling, initial loose attachments
Integrin-immunoglobulin superfamily	LFA-1 (CD11a/CD18), VLA-4 (CD49d/CD29)	ICAM-1 (CD54), ICAM-2, VCAM-1 (CD106)	Firm attachment, homing
Immunoglobulin superfamily	PECAM-1 (CD31), HCAM (CD44)	PECAM-1 (CD31)	Adhesion, migration, binding to connective tissue
Cadherins	Surface-bound proteases (e.g., elastase, cathepsin G)	VE cadherin	Cleavage of VE cadherin opens endothelial tight junctions, facilitating neutrophil migration

GlyCAM, glycosaminoglycan cell adhesion molecule; HCAM, homing cell adhesion molecule; ICAM, intercellular adhesion molecule; LFA, leukocyte function–associated molecule; PECAM, platelet–endothelial cell adhesion molecule; PMN, polymorphonuclear leukocyte; sLe^x, sialylated Lewis antigen X; VCAM, vascular cell adhesion molecule; VE, vascular endothelial; VLA, very late antigen.

The selectin family is composed of three members named according to the cells in which they were discovered. L-selectin (CD62L) is expressed constitutively on leukocytes, and its target cells are activated endothelial cells. E-selectin (CD62E) is produced exclusively by endothelial cells, and its receptors are on PMNs, monocytes, eosinophils, lymphocyte subsets and some tumor cells. P-selectin (CD62P) is preformed and stored for rapid release from platelets and endothelial cells. Its target cells are the same as those for E-selectin.

The integrins, a large family of heterodimeric glycoproteins, are expressed particularly by PMNs. The leukocyte integrins are represented by three heterodimeric molecules: lymphocyte function-associated antigen-1 (LFA-1; CD11a/CD18), CR3 (CD11b/CD18), and CR4 (CD11c/CD18). Each of them contains the same 95-kD CD18 subunit. The intact CD11a/CD18 molecule is LFA-1, and is expressed by lymphocytes, myeloid cells (monocytes, macrophages, and granulocytes), and several other cell types. Complexed CD11b/CD18 is complement receptor type 3 (CR3), whereas CD11c/CD18 is CR4. Two other ligands for LFA-1, intercellular adhesion molecule (ICAM)-1 (CD54) and ICAM-2 (CD102), are members of the immunoglobulin superfamily. CR3 mediates phagocytosis of complement-coated particles. In addition to ICAM-1 and ICAM-2, the platelet–endothelial cell adhesion molecule PECAM-1 (CD31) is another member of the immunoglobulin superfamily. Both ICAM-1 and ICAM-2 are expressed by endothelial cells, whereas PECAM-1 has been identified on PMNs, monocytes, and platelets and is present in large amounts on endothelial cells.

Macrophages and Monocytes

Mononuclear phagocytes—monocytes and macrophages—are also basic to inflammation and immunity. Monocyte differentiation in the bone marrow is rapid (1.5 to 3 days). Peripheral blood monocytes possess migratory, chemotactic, and phagocytic capabilities. Once tissue invasion occurs, peripheral blood monocytes differentiate into tissue macrophages. During migration into tissues, monocytes undergo further differentiation to become multifunctional tissue macrophages. As part of the process of differentiation, cytoplasmic granules are formed with enzyme content similar to those of neutrophils (Table 41–3).

Macrophages are mononuclear phagocytes responsible for numerous homeostatic, immunologic, and inflammatory processes. Macrophages can be divided into inflammatory and fixed-tissue populations. Fixed-tissue macrophages are present in several tissues: skin and connective tissue (histiocytes, Langerhans' cells), liver (Kupffer cells), lung (alveolar macrophages), lymph nodes (free and fixed macrophages), spleen (free and fixed macrophages), bone marrow (fixed macrophages), serous fluids (pleural and peritoneal macrophages), and other tissues. The macrophage

Table 41–3
Selected macrophage products

Microbicidal/Cytotoxic	Reactive oxygen species
	Reactive nitrogen species
	Proteases, acid hydrolases, lysozyme, defensins
Proinflammatory Cytokines	Interleukins-1, -6, and -8
	Tumor necrosis factor-α
	Interferon-gamma
	Macrophage inflammatory proteins
Bioactive Lipids	Prostaglandins
	Thromboxanes
	Leukotrienes
Bioactive Oligopeptides	Glutathione
Complement Factors	C1, C4, C2, C3, C5, factors B, D, H, I, P

population in a particular tissue may be maintained by three mechanisms: influx of monocytes from the circulating blood, local proliferation, and biologic turnover. Under normal steady-state conditions, the renewal of tissue macrophages occurs through local proliferation of progenitor cells and not via monocyte influx.

Fixed-tissue macrophages are relatively quiescent immunologically, having low oxygen consumption, low levels of MHC class II gene expression, and little or no cytokine secretion. However, tissue macrophages retain some proliferative and phagocytic capability. Macrophages, when activated, acquire specific functional activity. There are two stages of macrophage activation, the first being a IFN-γ–primed stage of enhanced MHC II expression, antigen presentation, and oxygen consumption, but reduced proliferative capacity. Other factors, including IFN-α, IFN-β, IL-3, macrophage colony-stimulating factor, GM-CSF, and TNF-α, can also prime macrophages for selected functions. Primed macrophages respond to secondary stimuli to become fully activated, defined by an inability to proliferate, high oxygen consumption (through NADPH oxidase), killing of facultative and intracellular parasites, tumor cell lysis, and maximal secretion of mediators of inflammation, including TNF-α, PGE$_2$, IL-1, IL-6, ROS, and NO$^\bullet$. Agents capable of providing secondary signals are numerous, including LPS, products of gram-positive bacteria, yeast glucans, and GM-CSF.

There is also evidence that activated macrophages can be deactivated. PGE, macrophage deactivating factor, IL-4, calcitonin gene-related peptide, and TGF-β may have this effect. Some effector mechanisms (but not all) are steroid-sensitive.

The Acute-Phase Response

The acute-phase response is a dynamic homeostatic process that involves all of the major systems of the body, in addition to the immune, cardiovascular, and central nervous systems (Box 41–1). Normally, the acute-phase response lasts only a few days. Two physiologic responses are associated closely with acute inflammation. The first involves the alteration of the temperature set point in the hypothalamus and the generation of fever. The second involves alterations in metabolism and gene expression in the liver. Interleukin-1, IL-6, and TNF-α regulate the febrile response through the induction of PGE_2, possibly as a protective mechanism against bacterial infection. At the same time, IL-1 and IL-6 act on the hypophyseal-pituitary-adrenal axis to generate corticotropin (ACTH) and stimulate cortisol production. This provides a negative feedback loop, because corticosteroids inhibit cytokine gene expression.

The second important aspect of the acute-phase response is altered hepatic protein synthesis. Normally, the liver synthesizes numerous plasma proteins at steady-state concentrations. In the acute phase of tissue injury/inflammation, production of several proteins is upregulated, whereas synthesis of others is suppressed. Acute-phase reactants (APRs) thus may be "positive" or "negative." Most positive APRs are induced severalfold over normal concentrations. This group includes fibrinogen, serum amyloid A, and C-reactive protein. Negative APRs

(e.g., albumin) are decreased in plasma concentration during the acute-phase response to allow an increase in the capacity of the liver to synthesize the induced APRs. Although most APRs are synthesized by hepatocytes, a few are produced by other cell types, including monocytes, endothelial cells, fibroblasts, and adipocytes.

APRs contribute to host defense in several ways, including direct neutralization of inflammatory mediators, thereby minimizing tissue damage and facilitating tissue repair. For example, increased synthesis of complement proteins mobilizes PMNs and macrophages. Fibrinogen plays an essential role in hemostasis and the promotion of wound healing. Protease inhibitors neutralize the lysosomal proteases released following the infiltration of activated PMNs and macrophages, thus mitigating the activity of the proinflammatory enzyme cascades. Increased plasma concentrations of metalloproteinases help prevent iron loss during infection and injury, minimizing the amount of heme iron available for bacterial metabolism, and scavenging ROS.

Antibiotic Therapy

Infections remain the leading cause of death in hospitalized patients, and antimicrobial therapy is a mainstay of treatment. However, several trends that impact antimicrobial therapy are apparent. Widespread overuse and misuse of antibiotics have led to an alarming increase in multidrug-resistant pathogens. New, extremely effective agents allow shorter courses of therapy and prophylaxis, which are desirable from the cost perspective and for control of the microbial ecology of the host and the treating institution. However, data indicate that adverse drug reactions remain common events in hospitalized patients, and that antibiotics are second only to analgesic agents in the number of related incidents. Antibiotic agents are potent drugs that have potent adverse effects, and appropriate use requires detailed knowledge of the agents, their properties, and the characteristics (known or presumed) of the infections and microbes being treated.

Principles of Pharmacokinetics

The goal of pharmacologic therapy is an effective response with no toxicity. Accomplishment of the goal requires the prescriber to understand the principles of pharmacokinetics. The relationship between dose and response can be influenced by a variety of factors, including dose, dosing interval, and route of administration. The concentration of drug achieved in tissue is influenced by absorption, distribution, and elimination, which in turn depend on drug metabolism and excretion. The relationship between local drug concentration and effect is defined by several pharmacodynamic principles.

Box 41–1

Selected Acute Phase Proteins

Positive
Serum amyloid A
C-reactive protein
Numerous complement proteins
Ferritin
Fibrinogen
Von Willebrand factor
Protease inhibitors (e.g., α_1-antitrypsin, plasminogen activator inhibitor-1)
Ceruloplasmin
Manganese superoxide dismutase
Lipopolysaccharide-binding protein

Negative
Albumin
Prealbumin
Apolipoproteins A-I, A-II

A few basic concepts of pharmacokinetics are useful to the practitioner. Bioavailability is defined as the percentage of an administered dose of a drug that reaches the systemic circulation. By definition 100% after intravenous administration, bioavailability is an important determinant of drug concentration in blood after oral administration. Oral bioavailability is affected by absorption (affected by product formulation and gastric emptying time), intestinal transit time (affected by diarrhea or ileus), and the degree of hepatic first-pass metabolism. Absorption is also affected by drug interactions and probably by diseases or functional abnormalities of the gastrointestinal mucosa.

Distribution throughout the body may be affected by several factors, including active transport, lipid solubility, ambient pH, and binding to serum proteins (unbound drug can diffuse or be transported more easily to tissues). Antibiotics that are highly protein bound (>90%) include penicillins, cephalosporins, the carbapenem ertapenem, and sulfonamides. The volume of distribution is a proportionality constant that relates to plasma concentration and the amount of drug in the body. It is useful for estimating achievable plasma drug concentrations that result from a given dose. It is a derived parameter that is independent of a drug's clearance or half-life, and it does not have particular physiologic significance, but pathophysiologic conditions can alter significantly the volume of distribution of a drug. Such a reduction in the volume of distribution will result in higher plasma drug levels for a given administered dose. However, the usual physiology of surgical illness—"third space" extravascular volume redistribution and fluid overload, and hypoalbuminemia with consequent decreased drug binding—increases the volume of distribution and will result in lower peak drug concentrations for a given dose. For these reasons, the apparent volume of distribution can vary widely for an individual drug, making dosing a complex matter.

Half-life refers to the amount of time required for the concentration of the drug to reduce by one half, and thus depends on both clearance (affected by organ function, metabolism, and route of excretion) and volume of distribution. If a "loading dose" is not administered intravenously, thereby creating instantly a desired drug concentration, four to five half-lives must elapse before steady-state concentrations are achieved. Interpretation of drug concentration data (e.g., peak and trough antibiotic concentrations) is difficult if the patient is not at a steady state, and even more so in critically ill patients in whom fluctuations in organ function, volume of distribution, and concurrent administration of numerous drugs complicate matters further.

Drug elimination may be by metabolism, excretion, or dialysis. Most drugs are metabolized by the liver to polar compounds that can then be excreted by the kidney. Metabolism, however, does not imply inactivation. For example, metronidazole is degraded to a active bactericidal metabolite with a prolonged half-life. The kidneys are most important for excretion of metabolized drugs, although some drugs are metabolized or conjugated by the kidneys. Renal excretion may occur by filtration or by either active or passive transport. The degree of filtration is determined by molecular size and charge and by the number of functional nephrons. In general, if greater than 40% of administered drug or its active metabolites is eliminated unchanged in the urine, decreased renal function will require a dosage adjustment. The dialyzability of a drug is affected primarily by molecular size.

Principles of Pharmacodynamics

The variation in responses that may be seen when a drug is administered to a heterogeneous patient population can be understood according to the principles of pharmacodynamics, which is the study of the relationships between a drug and its intended effect. The pharmacodynamics of antibiotic therapy are especially complex, because there is not only a drug-patient interaction, but also drug-microbe and microbe-patient interactions to account for. Knowledge of how patient characteristics influence absorption, distribution, and elimination of a drug or how, in the circumstance of antibiotics, the drug interacts with the targeted microbe, can increase the likelihood that the selected drug will be effective and that there will be a salutary clinical response. In turn, antimicrobial effects on bacteria are highly variable. Microbial physiology, inoculum size, microbial growth phase, intrinsic and extrinsic mechanisms of resistance, microenvironmental factors such as the pH at a local site of infection, and the patient's immune response are also important factors.

Specifically, pharmacodynamics relates the concentration of drug in tissue to its effects on biologic systems, but, in the case of antimicrobial therapy, the key drug interaction is not with the host, but with the microbe. Because of microbial ability to develop resistance, mere delivery of drug may not be microbicidal. Factors that may contribute to the development of resistance are the production of drug-inactivating enzymes, alteration of cell surface receptor target molecules, and altered bacterial permeability to antimicrobial penetration. Critical to the microbe-patient interaction is the patient's immune system, both circulating phagocyte function and the function of reticuloendothelial host defenses. Inseparable are drug-patient factors that may influence pharmacokinetics, such as hepatic and renal function, serum albumin concentration, and extracellular volume status.

Antibiotic pharmacodynamics is usually determined by laboratory analysis, so the extrapolation of in vitro results to the patient may also be problematic because the interaction with the host immune system is isolated from the analysis of the drug-microbe interaction. Analyses that may be developed from in vitro study include the minimal inhibitory concentration (MIC), the minimal bactericidal concentration (MBC), and serum bactericidal titer (SBT). The MIC is the minimal drug concentration in serum that is necessary for inhibition of bacterial growth, which may also be expressed as the proportion of the inoculum that is inhibited (MIC_{90} refers to 90% inhibition). Unfortunately, the MIC is not an all-or-none phenomenon. Antibiotics may have an important effect on bacteria at subinhibitory concentrations, and MIC testing may not detect the presence of resistant bacterial subpopulations (a particular problem with gram-positive bacteria). The MBC is used to determine the drug concentration necessary to kill 99.9% of the inoculum, but such information is rarely available clinically. The SBT is the greatest dilution of a patient's serum that kills a standard inoculum of the pathogen. Determination of the SBT is useful in therapy of certain difficult-to-treat infections such as endocarditis or osteomyelitis, and can be used to estimate the synergistic potential of combinations of antibiotics.

Sophisticated analytic strategies draw upon the principles of both pharmacokinetics and pharmacodynamics, for example, by determination of the ratio between the peak serum concentration and the MIC, the duration of time that plasma concentrations remain above the MIC, and the area of the plasma concentration-time curve above the MIC (the "area under the curve", or AUC). With some antimicrobials, antibacterial effects may persist for prolonged periods after plasma drug levels have decreased below the therapeutic range. The persistent inhibition of bacterial growth (but not killing) is known as the postantibiotic effect (PAE). Appreciable PAE can be observed with aminoglycosides and fluoroquinolones for gram-negative bacteria, and with some β-lactam drugs (notably imipenem) against S. aureus, but the clinical relevance of the PAE is uncertain. Through analyses of this type, certain drugs (e.g., aminoglycosides) have been characterized as having concentration-dependent killing, whereby higher peak concentrations increase the efficacy of bacterial killing. Other agents (most β-lactam agents) exhibit bactericidal properties that are independent of concentration; efficacy is determined by the duration of time that plasma concentrations remain above the MIC.

Mechanisms of Bacterial Action Against Bacteria

Cell wall–active agents

The β-lactam antibiotic group consists of penicillins, cephalosporins, monobactams, and carbapenems. Within this group, several agents have been combined with β-lactamase inhibitors to broaden the spectrum and increase the efficacy of the drugs. Activity against cell wall peptidoglycan is crucial to the killing of both gram-positive and gram-negative bacteria by β-lactam antibiotics. Peptidoglycan holds cell walls rigid, and protects against osmotic rupture. A three-stage process characterizes peptidoglycan synthesis: After synthesis of the carbohydrate substrate and transmembrane transport, transglycosylation of disaccharide monomer into peptidoglycan polymer occurs, followed by cross-linking with existing polymer in the cell wall. As part of the cross-linking, a transpeptidation reaction occurs that is sensitive to interdiction by β-lactam agents. Carboxypeptidation and endopeptidation reactions of possible significance for peptidoglycan modification but uncertain importance for antimicrobial susceptibility also occur. Penicillin-binding proteins (PBPs) of four distinct types catalyze those peptidation reactions, and their binding by β-lactam agents (especially the high-molecular-weight PBPs that affect transpeptidation) inhibits the crucial step in cell wall synthesis, probably at the time of cell division. Penicillin-receptor PBPs also transmit a transmembrane signal that induces production of β-lactamases, which are non–membrane-bound PBPs that catalyze hydrolysis of the β-lactam ring.

The highest molecular weight PBP of a given organism is designated PBP1, and so on. If one protein is found subsequently to be more than 1, it is designated by letter suffixes (PBP2a, PBP2b, etc.). They differ in the amounts present in individual species, and in their physiologic roles. They also differ in their binding affinities for different antibiotics, which explains partly why different antibiotics have different antibacterial properties and spectra. No single PBP is the target of β-lactam antibiotics, which usually exert lethality by effects on multiple PBPs simultaneously.

Also active against the cell wall of gram-positive bacteria, vancomycin is a soluble glycopeptide with a complex bactericidal mechanism of action. The drug inhibits synthesis and assembly of the second phase of cell wall peptidoglycan synthesis, and it may also injure protoplasts by altering the permeability of their cytoplasmic membrane. There is some evidence that RNA synthesis may be impaired as well. Vancomycin is rapidly bactericidal, but only on dividing organisms. A PAE persists for about 2 hours. The multiple mechanisms of action, along with a lack of cross-resistance with other antibiotics, may explain why resistance of gram-positive bacteria took several decades to develop. However, resistant staphylococci and enterococci have now emerged because of prolonged or indiscriminate use of vancomycin.

Protein synthesis inhibitors

Several classes of antibiotics, although dissimilar structurally and having widely divergent spectra of activity, exert their effects by binding to bacterial ribosomes to inhibit protein synthesis. Aminoglycosides bind to the bacterial 30S ribosomal subunit. With the exception of slightly better activity against gram-positive cocci possessed by gentamicin, the spectrum of activity for the various agents is identical. Differences among the agents are based upon differences in toxicity, and efficacy based on local resistance patterns. Aminoglycosides kill bacteria most effectively when the peak concentration of antibiotic is high; therefore, a loading dose is necessary and serum drug level monitoring is often performed. Synergistic therapy with a β-lactam agent may be effective because damage to the bacterial cell wall caused by the β-lactam drug enhances intracellular penetration of the aminoglycoside, but not to the extent that a dosage reduction is possible. Serious infections have traditionally required 5 mg/kg/day of gentamicin or tobramycin after a 2-mg/kg loading dose, or 15 mg/kg/day of amikacin after a loading dose of 7.5 mg/kg. Clearance and volume of distribution are variable and unpredictable in critically ill patients, and even higher doses are sometimes necessary. Single-daily-dose protocols (5 to 7 mg/kg day of gentamicin or tobramycin, or 20 to 30 mg/kg/day of amikacin) can obviate these problems in selected patients.

Tetracyclines bind irreversibly to the 30S ribosomal subunit, but, unlike aminoglycosides, they are bacteriostatic agents. Widespread resistance limits their utility in the hospital setting (with the single exception of doxycycline), but they are still prescribed as oral agents. Their antibacterial spectra are essentially identical, and prescribing is a matter of preference. Resistance to one agent implies resistance to all.

Chloramphenicol is a bacteriostatic agent that binds to the 50S ribosomal subunit. This activity leads to bacterial inhibition or death, depending on the organism and the concentration obtained in tissue at the site of infection. A brief resurgence in the use of chloramphenicol was occasioned by the emergence of vancomycin-resistant enterococci. Chloramphenicol also penetrates well into cerebrospinal fluid, and receives occasional usage for meningitis, especially when caused by *Haemophilus influenzae*. The bone marrow toxicity of chloramphenicol is feared, but very rare in actuality. Reversible, dose-related bone marrow toxicity is far more common than aplastic anemia, which occurs in only about 1 in 25,000 courses of therapy. It is one of very few antibiotics that require a dosage reduction in liver disease but not in renal insufficiency.

The macrolide-lincosamide-streptogramin group of antibiotics is structurally diverse but similar in mechanism of action, binding to the 50S ribosomal subunit. Among the macrolides are azithromycin, clarithromycin, and erythromycin. Despite their similarities, substantial differences exist that affect the dosing of macrolides. Clarithromycin has the highest oral bioavailability of the class (55%). Clarithromycin requires dosage reductions for both renal and hepatic insufficiency, whereas azithromycin does not. All macrolides inhibit the function of the cytochrome P450 system; therefore, the possibility of drug interaction is substantial. Clindamycin is a lincosamide

antibiotic that has good antianaerobic activity, and is a preferred choice over vancomycin for prophylaxis of clean surgical cases in penicillin-allergic patients, where the primary concern is the prevention of gram-positive wound infections. The use of clindamycin has been associated with the development of antibiotic-associated colitis caused by overgrowth of *Clostridium difficile*. The streptogramin group of antimicrobials rarely exhibits cross-resistance with other anti-infective agents. Antimicrobial activity depends upon a tertiary complex of two agents with the ribosome. Quinupristin/dalfopristin, the first injectable streptogramin, is a fixed 30:70 ratio admixture. Each component binds to a different site on the 50S ribosomal subunit to form the stable tertiary complex. The drug exhibits rapid bactericidal activity against gram-positive cocci, and a prolonged PAE. Both components are converted rapidly in the liver to active metabolites. Although the elimination half-lives for quinupristin and dalfopristin are approximately 0.9 and approximately 0.75 hours, respectively, the prolonged PAE is approximately 10 hours for S. *aureus* and approximately 9 hours for pneumococci. The clearance for both drugs is similar (0.7 L/kg), as is the volume of distribution (1 L/kg). Less than 20% is excreted by the kidneys. The usual adult dose is 7.5 mg/kg q8h. Dosage reductions for renal dysfunction are not needed, but are necessary in hepatic insufficiency.

Linezolid, an oxazolidinone, is rapidly and extensively absorbed after oral dosing, with absolute bioavailability of approximately 100%. Linezolid distributes readily to well-perfused tissues. The plasma protein binding of linezolid is approximately 31%. Linezolid binds to the bacterial 23S ribosomal RNA of the 50S subunit and prevents the formation of a functional 70S initiation complex, which is an essential component of the bacterial translation process. The mechanism of action is unique; therefore, cross-resistance between linezolid and other classes of antibiotics is unlikely. Linezolid does not induce or inhibit the action of the cytochrome P450 system. No dosage reduction is required for renal or hepatic insufficiency. The drug is broadly active against gram-positive cocci, but is generally reserved for therapy of multidrug-resistant organisms. Linezolid has been associated with thrombocytopenia (incidence of 2% to 3%) when used in doses up to 600 mg every 12 hours, usually for longer than 14 days, but platelet counts recover after cessation of therapy.

Drugs that disrupt nucleic acid biology

The quinolones inhibit bacterial DNA synthesis rapidly by inhibiting DNA gyrase, which serves to fold DNA into a superhelix in preparation for the initiation of replication. Discovery in the 1980s of the fluorine- and piperazinyl-substituted derivatives was followed by explosive use of these drugs. The fluoroquinolones exhibit a broad spectrum of activity, and excellent oral absorption and bioavailability.

These are potent antimicrobial agents, and it is unfortunate that overuse and misuse has led to the widespread development of resistance.

The rifamycins, of which rifampin is widely used clinically, inhibit DNA-dependent RNA polymerase at the β-subunit, which prevents chain initiation. Rifampin is a zwitterion that is soluble in acidic aqueous solution, yet is highly diffusable through lipid membranes and penetrates almost all body tissues well. Rifampin has a unique ability to penetrate living neutrophils and kill phagocytized intracellular bacteria. Oral bioavailability approaches 100% with the usual dose of 600 mg once daily. Rifampin is active against a broad range of microbes, including gram-positive cocci, *Chlamydia* species, and mycobacteria. Unfortunately, the rapid development of resistance relegates this agent to combination therapy in virtually all circumstances. Rifampin is a potent inducer of the hepatic microsomal enzymes, resulting in reduced oral bioavailability and decreased serum half-life for many drugs, including barbiturates, benzodiazepines, calcium channel blockers, chloramphenicol, cyclosporine, digitalis, estrogens, fluconazole, haloperidol, histamine H_2-antagonists, metoprolol, phenytoin, prednisone, propranolol, quinidine, theophylline, and warfarin.

Cytotoxic antibiotics

Metronidazole is highly active against nearly all anaerobic pathogens and against many human protozoal parasites. The most notable exception to the antianaerobic efficacy of metronidazole is a lack of activity in actinomycosis. Potent bactericidal activity is characterized by killing often at the same concentration required for inhibition. Resistance remains extremely rare and of negligible clinical significance. Metronidazole causes DNA damage after intracellular reduction of the nitro group of the drug. Acting as a preferential electron acceptor, it is reduced by low-redox-potential electron transport proteins, decreasing the intracellular concentration of the unchanged drug and maintaining a transmembrane gradient that favors uptake of additional drug. Toxicity is mediated directly by short-lived intermediate compounds or free radicals.

The drug diffuses well into nearly all tissues, including the central nervous system, thus making it an effective agent for deep-seated infections even against bacteria that are not multiplying rapidly. Oral bioavailability is nearly 100%. Adequate serum concentrations are also achieved after rectal administration. Loading doses are no longer recommended. The half-life of the drug is 8 hours owing to the production of an active hydroxy metabolite, permitting q12h dosing. No dosage reduction is required for patients with renal insufficiency, but the drug is dialyzed effectively, and administration should be timed to follow dialysis if twice-daily dosing is used. Pharmacokinetics studies of patients with hepatic impairment performed at higher doses indicate that a dosage reduction of 50% may be necessary, but not if twice-daily dosing is used.

Sulfonamides exert bacteriostatic activity by interfering with bacterial folic acid synthesis, a necessary preliminary step in purine and ultimately DNA synthesis. Resistance is widespread, and the agents are seldom used for infections other than of the urinary tract. The addition of sulfamethoxazole (SMX) to trimethoprim (TMP) in a fixed-dose combination of TMP:SMX of 1:5 prevents the conversion of dihydrofolic acid to tetrahydrofolic acid by the action of dihydrofolate reductase (downstream from the action of sulfonamides), accentuating the inherent bactericidal effects of TMP. The combination is useful in urinary tract infections, acute exacerbations of chronic bronchitis, and *Pneumocystis* infections in immunocompromised patients, and is the treatment of choice for rare infections caused by *Stenotrophomonas maltophilia*. The drug may be used as second-line therapy for many other infections caused by susceptible organisms because tissue penetration is generally excellent. Oral absorption is rapid and bioavailability is nearly 100%. Full doses (15 to 30 mg TMP in three to four divided doses) may be given as long as the creatinine clearance is greater than 30 mL/min, but the drug is not recommended when the creatinine clearance is less than 15 mL/min.

Bacterial Resistance to Antibiotics

Bacteria are adept at developing resistance to antimicrobial agents. In the early antibiotic era, resistance to such drugs as sulfonamides and streptomycin was conferred as the result of single nucleotide mutations of chromosomal origin. The result was single amino acid changes of a bacterial protein, the function of which was crucial but highly specific to the circumstance (e.g., affecting binding of the antibiotic to the bacterium). In the late 1950s, it was first discovered that enteric bacteria had developed resistance to multiple antibiotics concurrently. This resistance was due not to a chromosomal change, but rather to the presence of extrachromosomal DNA that was transmissible by structures called plasmids. Resistance-conferring plasmids are present in virtually all bacteria. Bacteria also contain transposons, which can insert into plasmids and also into the chromosome. Transposon-mediated resistance to most of the major antibiotics has been identified.

Antimicrobial agents exert a strong selective pressure on the development of both chromosomal and plasmid-mediated resistance. Administration of an antibiotic destroys the susceptible bacteria in a population, but may permit resistant clones to emerge and proliferate. From an epidemiologic viewpoint, plasmid-mediated resistance is the most important type because it is transmissible, is stable, and confers resistance to many different classes of antibiotics simultaneously.

In general, bacteria use four different mechanisms to develop resistance to antibiotics. Cell wall permeability to antibiotics is decreased by changes in porin channels (especially important for gram-negative bacteria with complex cell walls, affecting aminoglycosides, β-lactam drugs, chloramphenicol, sulfonamides, tetracyclines, and possibly quinolones). Production of specific antibiotic-inactivating enzymes by either plasmid-mediated or chromosomally mediated mechanisms affects aminoglycosides, β-lactam drugs, chloramphenicol, and macrolides. Alteration of the target for antibiotic binding in the cell wall affects β-lactam drugs and vancomycin, whereas alteration of target enzymes can inhibit β-lactam drugs, sulfonamides, quinolones, and rifampin. Drugs that bind to bacterial ribosomes are also susceptible to alteration of the receptor on the ribosome. Antibiotics may be extruded actively from the cell by "efflux pumps" once entry is achieved in the case of macrolides, lincosamides, streptogramins, quinolones, and tetracyclines.

About 55% of *S. aureus* and 85% of *S. epidermidis* strains are now resistant to methicillin. Methicillin resistance is properly called intrinsic resistance. This form of resistance encompasses all β-lactam drugs, including the cephalosporins. Intrinsic resistance is transmitted chromosomally, causing production of PBP 2a (also referred to as 2′). These bacteria are fully virulent. Affected strains produce penicillinase, and possess a full armamentarium of toxins, including protein A, catalase, coagulase, and DNAse.

The overall prevalence of enterococcal resistance to vancomycin is approximately 30%. Resistance is conferred by three distinct phenotypes, the gene products of which are abnormal peptidoglycans that disrupt vancomycin-binding sites. The *vanA* gene confers resistance to vancomycin and teicoplanin. Organisms with the *vanA* gene represent about 85% of clinical isolates. The *vanB* phenotype confers resistance to vancomycin, but the organisms remain sensitive to teicoplanin; this phenotype represents about 15% of clinical isolates. The *vanC* gene, which is not found in clinical isolates, is expressed constitutively by *Enterococcus gallinarum*.

Two examples highlight the complexity of these effects. Cephalosporin resistance among gram-negative bacilli can be the result of induction of chromosomal β-lactamases after prolonged or repeated exposure to the antibiotic. The extended-spectrum cephalosporins are rendered ineffective when bacteria such as enteric gram-negative bacilli mutate to produce constitutively a β-lactamase that is normally an inducible enzyme. Although resistance to cephalosporins can occur by several mechanisms, the appearance of chromosomally mediated β-lactamases has been identified as a consequence of the

use of third-generation cephalosporins. Resistance rates decline after use is restricted. The induction of an extended-spectrum β-lactamase (ESBL) in *Klebsiella* by ceftazidime was first reported approximately 15 years ago. The mutant bacteria develop resistance rapidly not only to all cephalosporins, but to entire other classes of β-lactam antibiotics as well. It is justifiable, therefore, to restrict the use of ceftazidime, especially in institutions grappling with an ESBL-producing bacterium. The quinolones, carbapenems, aminoglycosides, and possibly cefepime generally retain useful microbicidal activity against ESBL-producing strains.

Resistance Resulting from Altered Receptors

β-*Lactam resistance*

The best-known mechanism of bacterial resistance is the resistance to β-lactams, which is mediated by penicillinase enzymes. Resistance of *E. coli* to penicillin was recognized in 1940, before sufficient penicillin was made to be clinically useful. In the 1940s, resistance of staphylococci was shown to be due to a penicillinase. Because these enzymes also attack other β-lactam compounds such as cephalosporins, carbapenems, and monobactams, they are more appropriately designated β-lactamases. The most important activity of these enzymes is alteration of the β-lactam nucleus. β-Lactamases are widely distributed in nature and are usually classified on the basis of the principal compounds they destroy (e.g., as penicillinases or cephalosporinases). β-Lactamases may be chromosomally or plasmid mediated, and they may be constitutive or inducible.

In gram-positive species, β-lactamases are primarily exoenzymes; that is, they are excreted into the milieu around the bacteria. Virtually all hospital isolates of staphylococci, both *S. aureus* and *S. epidermidis*, have β-lactamases, and 50% to 80% of community-acquired staphylococcal isolates produce β-lactamases. In gram-negative species, both aerobic and anaerobic, β-lactamases are contained in the periplasmic space, thus effectively protecting the PBPs.

In 1974, *H. influenzae* was shown to possess a plasmid-mediated β-lactamase. At present, 10% to 35% of *H. influenzae* strains in the United States produce β-lactamases. The *Haemophilus* β-lactamase is the same structurally as the enzyme found in *E. coli*, *Salmonella* species, *Shigella* species, and *N. gonorrhoeae*. The enzyme has generally been called the TEM enzyme after the initials of the patient from whom an *E. coli* strain containing a plasmid β-lactamase was first isolated. By far the most common plasmid β-lactamase found in nature is TEM-1, which accounts for 75% to 80% of plasmid-mediated β-lactamase resistance worldwide. Recently, new β-lactamases have been found that hydrolyze compounds such as inomethoxy cephalosporin, which are not destroyed by other plasmid-encoded β-lactamases. The new β-lactamases have an altered amino acid composition, which permits binding to the cephalosporin and subsequent hydrolysis. How common these new enzymes will become is unknown, but more than 80 TEM-type enzymes have been described.

Chromosomally mediated β-lactamases are present in many *Enterobacter*, *Citrobacter*, *Proteus*, *Providencia*, and *Pseudomonas* species. All *Klebsiella* species possess a β-lactamase, which acts primarily as a penicillinase and is chromosomally mediated. Constitutively, produced β-lactamases are also present in many anaerobic species. Resistance of *S. pneumoniae* to penicillin has been increasing, and there are now relatively resistant isolates in many parts of the world. Altered PBPs also explain the resistance of some *S. aureus* strains to β-lactamase–stable penicillins (the so-called methicillin-resistant strains). The β-lactams induce synthesis of PBP2a, which does not bind any β-lactam. The β-lactam resistance of coagulase-negative staphylococci is also the result of altered PBPs. Staphylococcal organisms resistant to methicillin are resistant to all penicillins, cephalosporins, and carbapenems.

Vancomycin resistance

Certain transposable genetic elements encode special cell wall–synthesizing enzymes that change the structure of the normal D-Ala-D-Ala side chain in the peptidoglycan assembly pathway. The altered side chain (D-Ala-D-Lac) does not bind vancomycin and allows normal peptidoglycan polymerization to occur in the presence of the drug. Depending upon the nature of the vancomycin resistance gene, high-level resistance can occur to glycopeptides. Thus far, this type of resistance has been found in enterococci but not in multidrug-resistant isolates of *S. aureus*.

Macrolide-lincomycin resistance

Macrolide-lincomycin resistance in clinical isolates of staphylococci and streptococci is due to methylation of two adenine nucleotides in the 23S component of 50S RNA. This resistance is plasmid-mediated, and the resistance is encoded on transposons. Resistance results from induction of an enzyme that is normally repressed. The methylated RNA binds macrolide-lincomycin–type drugs less well than does unmethylated RNA. Induction of resistance varies by species, and in most gram-positive species erythromycin is a more effective inducer of resistance than is clindamycin. The plasmids that mediate macrolide-lincomycin resistance in streptococci and staphylococci have extensive structural similarity, indicating that these plasmids pass readily between these species.

Rifampin resistance

The resistance of bacteria to rifampin is caused by an alternation of one amino acid in DNA-directed RNA polymerase, which results in reduced binding of rifampin. The degree of resistance is related to the degree to which the enzyme is changed, but does not correlate strictly with enzyme inhibition. This form of resistance occurs at a low level in any population of bacteria, so that resistance develops by natural selection during a course of therapy. Naturally-resistant organisms are more common among members of the Enterobacteriaceae.

Quinolone resistance

Quinolone resistance is chromosomally mediated for the most part, primarily by changes in the target sites for the antibiotic (DNA gyrase or topoisomerase IV). Resistance to quinolones can be caused by mutations in DNA gyrase subunits A or B, reduced outer membrane permeability in gram-negative cells, or active efflux "pumps" found in many bacteria. Multiple mechanisms of resistance can occur in a single isolate of bacteria, leading to a higher level of resistance to many fluoroquinolones. The highest level of resistance to the newer fluoroquinolones is most frequently associated with chromosomal mutations, causing amino acid substitutions in a highly conserved region in the A subunit of DNA gyrase.

Quinolone resistance is relatively easy to induce if a sublethal dose is chosen for initial therapy. Resistance to one quinolone may also increase the MIC for the other quinolones against the organism, so a highly active agent given in adequate dosage is essential.

Resistance Resulting from Decreased Entry of a Drug

Tetracycline resistance

Tetracycline resistance is common in both gram-positive and gram-negative bacteria. In most cases it is plasmid-encoded and inducible; however, chromosomal, constitutive resistance is found in some organisms, such as *Proteus* species. Tetracycline resistance in *S. aureus* is due primarily to small multicopy plasmids; chromosomal resistance is rare. Tetracycline resistance is found on nonconjugative plasmids in *Enterococcus faecalis* and on the chromosome of *S. pneumoniae*, *S. agalactiae* (group B streptococci), and oral streptococci. Plasmids mediating tetracycline resistance have moved among *S. aureus*, *S. epidermidis*, *S. pyogenes*, *S. pneumoniae*, and *E. faecalis*. *Clostridium* species such as *C. difficile* harbor chromosomal genes for tetracycline resistance.

Tetracycline resistance is due to a decrease in the concentrations of accumulated drug. Decreased uptake and increased efflux both probably participate. Resistant bacteria bind less tetracycline, and the tetracycline they do accumulate is lost by an energy-dependent process when they are in a drug-free milieu. Plasmid-mediated resistance to tetracyclines can be partially overcome in gram-positive species (but not gram-negative bacteria) by modifying the tetracycline nucleus. Hence, achievable concentrations of minocycline and doxycycline, in particular, will inhibit some tetracycline-resistant streptococci such as S. *pneumoniae*, and some S. *aureus* strains.

Aminoglycoside resistance

In members of the Enterobacteriaceae and in *Pseudomonas* species, the aminoglycosides pass through the cell wall via porin protein-lined channels designed to admit cationic molecules to the periplasmic space. Some members of the Enterobacteriaceae and *P. aeruginosa* appear to be resistant because of altered porin channels, because these bacteria do not take up any drug and do not have aminoglycoside-inactivating enzymes. After uptake, aminoglycosides are then translocated across the cell membrane by an energy-dependent proton-motive force and, in the cytoplasm, bind to ribosomes located just below the membrane. Aminoglycosides bind only to ribosomes actively engaged in protein synthesis. Binding to the ribosomes induces a protein involved in the uptake of the aminoglycosides. In the most important form of aminoglycoside resistance, the drug is modified outside the cell, resulting in poor uptake of the altered compound. Also, all aminoglycosides have free amino and hydroxy groups that are essential for binding to ribosomal proteins. A number of enzymes can acetylate the amino groups and phosphorylate or adenylate the hydroxyl groups and reduce the binding affinity. Many of the genes for aminoglycoside-modifying enzymes are carried on transposons. Alteration of the binding site on the 30S ribosomes is a rare form of resistance. Anaerobic organisms such as *Bacteroides* species are resistant to aminoglycosides because they lack an oxygen-dependent transport system to move the drugs across the cytoplasmic membrane.

Selected Nosocomial Pathogens

Clostridium difficile

Overgrowth of *C. difficile* is the most common identifiable cause of antibiotic-associated colitis (AAC, or "pseudomembranous" colitis). Although ampicillin, cephalosporins, and clindamycin are most commonly associated with AAC, nearly any antibiotic can cause the disorder, including topical or oral therapy and single-dose intravenous prophylaxis. *Clostridium difficile* is clearly a nosocomial pathogen. It is a constituent of normal colonic flora of only 3% of normal adults, but colonization rates of 15% to 36% have been reported in hospitalized patients.

The presentation of AAC ranges from asymptomatic to life-threatening transmural pancolitis with perforation and generalized peritonitis. Most cases of AAC begin with acquisition of exogenous flora by hosts predisposed to superinfection by previous or current antibiotic therapy or mechanical bowel preparation. Acquisition is clearly facilitated by environmental factors and transmission by caregivers. Other fomites include such mundane instruments as bedside commodes and rectal thermometers. Once endemic in the hospital, epidemics are possible.

The diagnosis of AAC is usually made with a latex agglutination test for exotoxin performed on a fresh stool specimen. The false-negative rate for the latex assay is about 10% to 15%, so it may be necessary to repeat the test once in suspicious cases. The positive yield from a third assay after the first two have been negative is only 2%, so such repetitive testing is not generally indicated.

Antibiotic therapy of AAC is not invariably necessary. Some patients with mild disease will improve spontaneously with only withdrawal of the offending antibiotic. If specific therapy is administered, it is desirable to discontinue the offending antibiotic, but not mandatory if it is needed for another serious infection. Resolution of AAC with specific therapy has been reported despite continuation of the putative cause. Oral metronidazole (250 mg q6h) and oral vancomycin (125 mg q6h) have equivalent efficacy (~ 80% cure rate). Higher doses of vancomycin are not necessary. Treatment for 10 to 14 days is sufficient, although the exotoxin assay may remain positive for weeks. Oral metronidazole is the treatment of choice because of cost and the need to decrease vancomycin use and selection pressure for the development of vancomycin resistance. Oral vancomycin may be used for treatment failures or for those patients who are intolerant of oral metronidazole (e.g., gastrointestinal symptoms, metallic taste).

Prevention strategies are essential for avoidance and control of outbreaks, which are unfortunately common. Reduction of the duration of antibiotic therapy is important, both in terms of prolonged therapeutic use of antibiotics and elimination of inappropriate prophylactic use. Hospital staff must be educated regarding the epidemiology of AAC, so they may be cognizant of infection control initiatives and the importance of health care workers as vectors for transmission. Cohorting or isolation of colonized patients is essential, and the use of common equipment such as shared bedside commodes must be curtailed.

Methicillin-Resistant Staphylococcus

First described in 1961, methicillin-resistant *Staphylococcus* (MRS) is now a major worldwide problem. A huge reservoir of staphylococci is resident on normal human hosts. Twenty percent to 40% of adults are carriers of colonizing staphylococci. Health care workers, diabetic patients, dialysis patients, intravenous drug abusers, and patients with chronic skin diseases are potential carriers. Carriers who undergo surgery have higher infection rates. Patient-to-patient transfer occurs via the colonized hands of hospital personnel, or from the inanimate environment.

Diligent, careful, repetitive hand washing by all hospital personnel is essential for avoidance and control of MRS infections, as is adherence to universal precautions and isolation techniques. Isolation or cohorting of patients is mandatory. Timely, accurate identification and reporting of new isolates is essential for effective implementation of infection control measures. Increasing evidence suggests that elimination of the carrier state may be beneficial. Intranasal 2% mupirocin ointment is the most effective agent for eradication of MRS from carriers, but resistance does develop. Oral rifampin may be effective as well. Vancomycin should not be used for attempted eradication of the carrier state, because it should be reserved for first-line therapy of infections.

Vancomycin-Resistant *Enterococcus*

First described in 1988 in Europe, the emergence of vancomycin-resistant *Enterococcus* (VRE) was associated with empirical combination use of vancomycin and ceftazidime for sepsis. Most strains of VRE also exhibit high-level aminoglycoside resistance. Documented risk factors for the acquisition of VRE include prolonged hospitalization, multiple courses of antibiotics (especially third-generation cephalosporins), neutropenia, prior oral or parenteral vancomycin therapy, proximity to another patient with the organism, and increasing severity of either an underlying illness or acute medical comorbidity. Transmission is commonly via fecal-oral spread, either via diarrhea or communal bedpan use. Health care workers are definite disease vectors. Prolonged persistence in the inanimate environment has also been documented.

In addition to the usual infection control practices (education of hospital staff, cohorting or isolation of colonized patients, careful nursing staff assignments, and early detection and prompt reporting of isolates), changes in antibiotic prescribing practices are important measures for reduction of the threat posed by VRE. Prudent vancomycin use is essential. Several studies indicate that vancomycin is often misprescribed. Reduced use of third-generation cephalosporins is equally important, including the elimination of prophylactic use. In contrast to colonization with MRS, attempts to sterilize VRE-colonized patients have invariably failed.

Pseudomonas aeruginosa

Pseudomonas aeruginosa is a motile gram-negative bacillus. Almost all strains are motile by means of a single polar flagellum, and some strains have two or three flagella. The flagella yield heat-labile antigens (H antigens). Clinical isolates usually have pili, which may be antiphagocytic

and probably aid in bacterial attachment, thereby promoting colonization. *Pseudomonas aeruginosa* is a nonfermentative aerobe that derives its energy from oxidation rather than fermentation of carbohydrates. Able to use more than 75 different organic compounds, it can grow on media supplying only acetate for carbon and ammonium sulfate for nitrogen. Furthermore, although an aerobe, it can grow anaerobically, using nitrate as an electron acceptor. In addition to its nutritional versatility, *P. aeruginosa* thrives in moist conditions and resists high concentrations of salt, dyes, weak antiseptics, and many commonly used antibiotics. These properties help explain its ubiquitous nature and contribute to its preeminence as a cause of nosocomial infections. Potential hospital reservoirs include respiratory equipment, endoscopes, cleaning solutions and disinfectants, sinks, mops, food mixers, and flowers in patient rooms. *Pseudomonas* is sometimes present as part of the normal microbial flora of humans (skin, 2%; nasal mucosa, 3%; pharyngeal mucosa, 6%; and feces, 24%). Hospitalization may lead to much higher rates of colonization, especially if natural epithelial barriers have been breached by therapy. Alteration of host antibiotic flora by antibiotic therapy may select for colonization by *Pseudomonas* species. *Pseudomonas aeruginosa* is the fourth most common nosocomial pathogen. The overall incidence of infection is 4 in 1000 hospital discharges, accounting for 10% of all hospital-acquired infections. *Pseudomonas aeruginosa* is the most common pathogen in the intensive care unit, accounting for more than 12% of such infections.

Pseudomonas aeruginosa can cause nearly every conceivable infection, including pneumonia, endocarditis, bacteremia, peritonitis, central nervous system infections, ear and eye infections, bone and joint infections, urinary tract infections, skin and soft tissue infections, and urinary tract infections. *Pseudomonas aeruginosa* has a documented propensity to develop resistance during therapy, particularly during therapy with agents that are potent inducers of ESBL enzymes (i.e., third-generation cephalosporins).

Bibliography

Acar JF, Goldstein FW: Trends in bacterial resistance to fluoroquinolones. Clin Infect Dis 1997;24(Suppl 1):S67.

Behnia M, Robertson KA, Martin WJ: Lung infections: role of apoptosis in host defense and pathogenesis of disease. Chest 2000;117:1771.

Borriello SP: Pathogenesis of *Clostridium difficile* infection. J Antimicrob Chemother 1998;41(Suppl C):13.

Casadevall A, Pirofski LA: Host-pathogen interactions: basic concepts of microbial commensalisms, colonization, infection, and disease. Infect Immun 2000;68:6511.

Craig WA: Pharmacokinetics of antibiotics with special emphasis on cephalosporins. Clin Microbiol Infect 2000;6(Suppl 3):34.

Cunha BA: Antibiotic resistance. Med Clin North Am 2000;84:1407.

De Lancey Pulcini E: Bacterial biofilms: a review of current research. Nephrologie 2001;22:439.

DiPiro JT, Edmiston CE, Bohnen JMA: Pharmacodynamics of antimicrobial therapy in surgery. Am J Surg 1996;171:615.

Dobrindt U, Reidl J: Pathogenicity islands and phage conversion: evolutionary aspects of bacterial pathogenesis. Int J Med Microbiol 2000;290:519.

Ebersole JL, Cappelli D: Acute-phase reactants in infections and inflammatory diseases. Periodontology 2000;23:19.

Falkow S: Perspectives series: host/pathogen interactions. Invasion and intracellular sorting of bacteria: searching for bacterial genes expressed during host/pathogen interactions. J Clin Invest 1997;100:239.

Fleckenstein JM, Kopecko DJ: Breaching the mucosal barrier by stealth: an emerging pathogenic mechanism for enteroadherent bacterial pathogens. J Clin Invest 2001;107:21.

Fontana R, Cornaglia G, Ligozzi M, Mazziariol A: The final goal: penicillin-binding proteins and the target of cephalosporins. Clin Microbiol Infect 2000;6(Suppl 3):34.

Fry DE: The importance of antibiotic pharmacokinetics in critical illness. Am J Surg 1996;172(Suppl):20S.

Gold HS, Moellering RC: Antimicrobial drug resistance. N Engl J Med 1996;335:1445.

Gonzalez LS, Spencer JP: Aminoglycosides: a practical review. Am Fam Physician 1998;58:1811.

Hacker J, Carniel E: Ecological fitness, genomic islands, and bacterial pathogenicity: a Darwinian view of the evolution of microbes. EMBO Rep 2001;2:376.

Hahn HP: The type-4 pilus is the major virulence-associated adhesin of *Pseudomonas aeruginosa*—a review. Gene 1997;192:99.

Hatala R, Dinh T, Cook DJ: Once-daily aminoglycoside therapy in immunocompetent adults: a meta-analysis. Ann Intern Med 1996;124:717.

Heinzelmann M, Scott M, Lam T: Factors predisposing to bacterial invasion and infection. Am J Surg 2002;183:179.

Hellinger WC, Brewer NS: Carbapenems and monobactams: imipenem, meropenem, and aztreonam. Mayo Clin Proc 1999;74:420.

Huebner J, Goldmann DA: Coagulase-negative staphylococci: role as pathogens. Annu Rev Med 1999;50:223.

Kasten MJ: Clindamycin, metronidazole, and chloramphenicol. Mayo Clin Proc 1999;74:825.

Klare I, Werner G, Witte W: Enterococci: habitats, infections, virulence factors, resistances to antibiotics, transfer of resistance determinants. Contrib Microbiol 2001;8:108.

Lamb HM, Figgitt DP, Faulds D: Quinupristin/dalfopristin: a review of its use in the management of serious gram-positive infections. Drugs 1999;58:1061.

Lister PD: Beta-lactamase inhibitor combinations with extended-spectrum penicillins: factors influencing antibacterial activity against Enterobacteriaceae and *Pseudomonas aeruginosa*. Pharmacotherapy 2000;20:213S.

Livermore DM: Beta-lactamase-mediated resistance and opportunities for its control. J Antimicrob Chemother 1998;41(Suppl D):25.

Lyczak JB, Cannon CL, Pier GB: Establishment of *Pseudomonas aeruginosa* infection: lessons from a versatile opportunist. Microbes Infect 2000;2:1051.

Mehrad B, Standiford TJ: Role of cytokines in pulmonary antimicrobial host defense. Immunol Res 1999;20:15.

Michel M, Gutmann L: Methicillin-resistant *Staphylococcus aureus* and vancomycin-resistant enterococci: therapeutic realities and possibilities. Lancet 1997;349:1901.

Moxom ER, Hood DW, Saunders NJ, et al: Functional genomics of pathogenic bacteria. Philos Trans R Soc Lond B Biol Sci 2002;357:109.

Muller A, Rudel T: Modification of host cell apoptosis by viral and bacterial pathogens. Int J Med Microbiol 2001;291:197.

Negri MC, Morosini MI, Blasquez J, Baquero F: Antibiotic resistance in hospital infections: the role of newer cephalosporins. Clin Microbiol Infect 2000;6(Suppl3):95.

Ochman H, Moran NA: Genes lost and genes found: evolution of bacterial pathogenesis. Science 2001;292:1096.

Oliphant CM, Green GM: Quinolones: a comprehensive review. Am Fam Physician 2002;61:455.

Perry CM, Jarvis B: Linezolid: a review of its use in the management of serious gram-positive infections. Drugs 2001;61:525.

Perry CM, Markham A: Piperacillin/tazobactam: an updated review of its use in the treatment of bacterial infections. Drugs 1999;57:805.

Rastogi D, Ratner AT, Prince A: Host-bacterial interactions in the initiation of inflammation. Paediatr Respir Rev 2001;2:245.

Schluger NW, Rom WN: Early responses to infection: chemokines as mediators of inflammation. Curr Opin Immunol 1997;9:504.

Simmons CP, Clare S, Dougan G: Understanding mucosal responsiveness: lessons form enteric bacterial pathogens. Semin Immunol 2001;13:201.

Smith H: What happens to bacterial pathogens in vivo? Trends Microbiol 1998;6:239.

Swain SD, Rohn TT, Quinn MT: Neutrophil priming in host defense: role of oxidants as priming agents. Antioxid Redox Signal 2002;4:69.

van der Poll T: Coagulation and inflammation. J Endotoxin Res 2001;7:301.

Weinstock GM: Genomics and bacterial pathogenesis. Emerg Infect Dis 2000;6:496.

Wilson JW, Schurr MJ, LeBlanc CL, et al: Mechanisms of bacterial pathogenicity. Postgrad Med J 2002;78:216.

Wu YJ, Su WG: Recent developments on ketolides and macrolides. Curr Med Chem 2001;8:1727.

CHAPTER 42

Fungal Infection

Amar Safdar, M.D., M.B.B.S. and Donald Armstrong, M.D.

Human infections are caused by only a fraction of the nearly 250,000 known fungal species. In our ecosystem, fungi are symbiotes and play a critical role in nitrogen fixation. These eukaryotic organisms exhibit low intrinsic virulence, and disease is often accidental. Person-to-person transmission is rare but may occur in skin infections caused by dermatophytes; common examples include "ringworm" (tinea corporis), "athlete's foot" (tinea pedis), and "jock itch" (tinea cruris). Most infections are acquired from the environment, although patients' microflora may serve as an endogenous reservoir. For example, colonization with *Candida* species not only increases the rise of invasive yeast infection in severely immunocompromised patients with cancer or following marrow or solid-organ transplantation, but also poses a serious threat for patients undergoing high-risk surgical procedures. Hematogenous invasion by *Candida* species frequently arises from hosts' orointestinal tract or genitourinary tract. Fungemia caused by *Malassezia furfur* (previously *Pityrosporum* species) complicating patients receiving total parenteral nutrition originates commonly from cutaneous sebaceous gland microflora.

In the past two decades there has been a near-exponential increase in the prevalence of nosocomial blood stream fungal infections in the United States. This is attributed in part to the increasing population of susceptible individuals, such as patients with an underlying neoplasm or transplant recipients. Severe chemotherapy-induced granulocytopenia, prolonged use of broad-spectrum antibiotics, corticosteroids, diabetes mellitus, hemodialysis, presence of an implantable or semi-implantable indwelling intravascular device, and extended stay in a critical care or burn unit are important promoters of systemic mycoses. Patients undergoing complicated surgery are at an additional risk, especially those with prolonged surgical procedures such as abdominopelvic or cardiovascular surgery, and patients with extensive trauma. Changes in hosts' defense against *Candida* during the perioperative period may further increase the risk of systemic yeast invasion. In this chapter, initial discussion is based on the mucocutaneous and invasive mycoses, and then a review of antifungal drugs is presented.

Cutaneous and Mucocutaneous Fungal Infections

Fungal infections involving the skin and related structures are common and seen in all age groups. Tinea capitis is common in children, whereas tinea pedis is the most common fungal infection in adults. Skin infections are especially severe in patients with T-cell–dependent immune dysfunction, such as those with acquired immunodeficiency syndrome (AIDS) or common variable immune deficiency syndrome, and patients with leukemia, lymphoma, and myelodysplastic syndrome. Dermatophytes and *Candida* species are the most common fungi affecting the skin and mucous membranes. *Malassezia* species cause tinea versi-color, a scaling dermatosis with nonpruritic hyperpigmented or hypopigmented macules and plaques found most typically over the trunk and proximal aspects of the extremities. *Malassezia* species have also been implicated in the pathogenesis of seborrheic dermatitis. *Candida* species are common causes of nondermatophyte cutaneous infections in patients with certain risk factors, such as diabetes mellitus, prolonged corticosteroid therapy, severe burns, extended broad-spectrum antibiotic therapy, obesity, poor personal hygiene, and chronic skin maceration. Infrequently, systemic mycosis caused by *Fusarium, Aspergillus, Cryptococcus neoformans, Coccidiodes immitis, Blastomyces dermatitidis, Histoplasma capsulatum,* and other rare opportunistic fungi may present initially as skin lesions. Diagnostic skin biopsy may be considered early in the course of infection because cutaneous manifestations of systemic mold infections are often nonspecific and highly variable in appearance, especially in individuals with compromised immunity.

Dermatophytosis

Dermatophytes are molds that cause disease by invading tissues containing keratin, namely the stratum corneum of the skin, hair, and nails. *Trichophyton, Microsporum,* and *Epidermophyton* are the three genera of medical impor-tance. Species that cause human infections are classified as anthropophilic, geophilic, or zoophilic, depending on whether their major reservoir is humans, the soil, or animals, respectively. The most characteristic lesions of dermatophyte infection are annular, scaling lesions and/or erythematous patches with minimal induration. The mar-gin is typically raised, and the central portion of the lesion shows less inflammation than the periphery.

The anthropophilic dermatophytes are acquired by close human contact, especially in the setting of disadvan-taged socioeconomic situations such as overcrowding, poor personal hygiene, and malnutrition. *Trichophyton capitis, Trichophyton tonsurans,* and *Trichophyton rubrum* are important examples. Anthrophilic dermatophytosis is usually of insidious onset with minimal host inflammatory response. The zoophilic dermatophytes are typically acquired by close household contact with animals, such as puppies and kittens; such exposures lead to infection involving the exposed skin over the face and extremities mostly in children

and young adults. *Microsporon canis* and *Trichophyton mentagrophytes* are common examples. The geophilic dermatophytes such as *Microsporum gypseum, Microsporum fulvum,* and *Microsporum racemosum* tend to cause sporadic or incidental infections. These infections are usually associated with an intense local inflammatory response.

Candidiasis

Candida species are ubiquitous in the environment; they are present in the soil, inanimate objects, and food. *Candida* is part of the human cutaneous, orointestinal, and vaginal microflora. Most systemic *Candida* infections arise from the patient's own microflora. However, person-to-person transmission may lead to nosocomial postsurgical wound infections, endovascular infections, and recalcitrant infec-tion of prosthetic devices. Cutaneous candidiasis can be clinically indistinguishable from dermatophytosis. Yeast skin infections, however, tend to have ill-defined margins and satellite lesions are common, and, unlike in tinea cruris, the scrotum, penis, and vulva are commonly involved. Onychomycosis of the nails (tinea unguium) affects people of any age but is more common in older persons. Usually, there is infection of the skin adjacent to the nail. Non-*Candida* onychomycosis caused by *Acremonium, Aspergillus, Fusarium,* or *Curvularia* species is inseparable in appearance. A single nail involvement and accompany-ing paronychia is highly suggestive of nondermatophyte, *Candida* and non-*Candida* fungal infection.

Among the nearly 150 species of *Candida, C. albicans* is most commonly associated with human infection. In the past decade, the frequency of non-*albicans Candida* oropharyngeal and vaginal yeast infections has increased considerably, especially in high-risk patients with prior exposure to antifungal drugs. The following species may be encountered: *C. glabrata, C. krusei, C. parapsilosis, C. tropicalis, C. lusitaniae, C. guilliermondii,* and the recently identified *C. dubliniensis.* Factors that predispose to superficial candidiasis include poor hygiene, chronic skin maceration, obesity, diabetes mellitus, burns, prolonged exposure to antibiotics and corticosteroids, and cellular immune dysfunction, as in patients with AIDS. Oral candidiasis can present in a number of ways, the most characteristic being "thrush," which is the presence of thick, white, cottage cheese–like or curdlike patches on the tongue and oropharyngeal mucous membrane. Removal of these patches by scraping reveals a raw, bleeding epithe-lial surface. Other forms of oral candidiasis include chronic atrophic candidiasis or "denture sore mouth" in patients with dental plates, presenting with chronic inflammation; acute atrophic candidiasis, presenting as atrophy of the tongue; erosive candidiasis, presenting as shallow ulcera-tions and usually found in persons with human immuno-deficiency virus disease; angular cheilitis, presenting as persistent inflammation and fissures at the corners of the mouth; and *Candida* leukoplakia, presenting as adherent white plaques on the lips, tongue, and buccal mucosa that are difficult to scrape off.

Candida esophagitis usually occurs in patients with advanced AIDS or malignancy and may present as central chest pain, odynophagia, and dysphagia. Herpes simplex, human cytomegalovirus infection, and "aphthous" ulceration of the esophagus are other diagnostic considerations. Untreated *Candida* esophagitis carries severe morbidity and promotes malnutrition, leading to further immunosuppression in patients with AIDS.

Vulvovaginal candidiasis is an extremely common problem. It is most commonly associated with antibiotic therapy, pregnancy, and diabetes mellitus, and it has been estimated that 75% of women develop this infection at some point during their lives. The most characteristic form presents with a thick, white, cottage cheese–like or curdlike discharge, accompanied by intense pruritus. *Candida* balanitis usually begins as vesicles on the penis that evolve into pruritic patches and that often spread to the scrotum, perineum, and buttocks. Intertrigo is a common skin infection caused by *Candida* that typically involves skinfolds, affecting areas under the breast, perineum, and abdominal wall. The warm, moist environment of these areas promotes yeast invasion of the semi-macerated epidermis. The process begins as vesicopustules that rupture, progressing to fissuring of the skin. Satellite lesions are common and observed beyond the advancing border of the rash. *Candida* folliculitis sometimes affects the beard area and must be distinguished from tinea barbae. Widespread *Candida* folliculitis sometimes occurs in severely ill patients who have received multiple antibiotics, and have higher propensity for secondary bacterial infections caused by *Streptococcus* and *Staphylococcus* species.

Chronic mucocutaneous candidiasis is a persistent/refractory yeast infection involving the skin and mucous membranes, including the esophagus. It often leads to scarring and irreversible disfiguration. It most often presents in infancy among children with a congenital immunodeficiency syndrome involving selective defects in T-cell response to *Candida* antigens. This syndrome is rarely encountered in persons over the age of 30 years. Response to prolonged antifungal therapy is limited, and cure is an exception rather than the rule.

Invasive *Candida* Infections

Candidemia

Systemic *Candida* infections are on the rise, and the incidence of nosocomial fungemia has dramatically increased over the past two decades. *Candida* species

account for approximately 90% of all systemic fungal infections and are the fourth leading cause of blood stream invasion reported to the Centers for Disease Control and Prevention's nosocomial infections surveillance programs. Traditionally, *Candida albicans* has been the common species in this setting, but recently the incidence of non-*albicans* candidemia has increased considerably, which includes *C. glabrata* and *C. krusei* (less susceptible species or intrinsically non–fluconazole-susceptible) as well as *C. parapsilosis*, *C. tropicalis*, and *C. lusitaniae* (with variable in vitro resistance to amphotericin B). Nearly all patients with invasive candidiasis have one or more risk factors, as illustrated in Box 42–1. Presence of an indwelling intravascular catheter and prolonged exposure to broad-spectrum antibiotics are the most common promoters of hematogenous candidiasis. During the past two decades, a near-exponential increase in candidemia has been most pronounced in patients being treated in surgical intensive care units.

The orointestinal tract serves as reservoir and portal of blood stream entry in most patients with hematogenous dissemination. Among individuals with chemotherapy-induced neutropenia, accompanying mucosal ulceration has been suggested as an independent risk for fungemia. The indwelling intravascular catheter may be refractory to treatment, and high-grade/sustained fungemia is associated with increased risk of serious metastatic complications, appearing even after the infected device has been removed. Patients undergoing cardiopulmonary bypass surgery may develop early blood stream infection caused by *Candida* species. Another life-threatening complication is endocarditis, which is likely to occur in patients after heart surgery, especially those undergoing prosthetic heart valve placement. Endophthalmitis may result from untreated hematogenous dissemination of *Candida* in as many as 10% to 35% of patients. Funduscopic examination of the retina frequently shows the lesion prior to the onset of the irreversible vision loss. Intracranial fungal aneurysm resulting from *Candida* endocarditis may prove fatal. Patients with implantable pacemaker devices may rarely develop refractory yeast endovascular infections. Purulent *Candida* pericarditis is another uncommon complication that may follow thoracic surgery and requires prompt diagnosis and combined medical (amphotericin B or caspofungin [Cancidas]) and surgical (pericardiectomy) treatment. The overall 4-week attributable mortality in hospitalized candidemic patients approaches 40%, compared to the less than 20% mortality attributed to *Staphylococcus aureus* or *Pseudomonas aeruginosa* hematogenous systemic dissemination.

Systemic Candidiasis

Candida peritonitis is an uncommon but serious complication in patients undergoing chronic peritoneal dialysis.

Box 42–1

Predisposing Factors for Systemic Candidiasis

Extended stay in critical care units
   Surgical >> medical >> neonatal
Indwelling intravascular devices
   Hickman-Broviac, MediPort, and the like
Broad-spectrum antimicrobial therapy
   >2 antibiotics
   >5–7 day
High-risk surgery
   Complicated abdominopelvic surgery
   Cardiothoracic surgery
Hyperalimentation
   Total parental nutrition
Extended duration of hospitalization
   >3 weeks
Trauma
Burns
Severe granulocytopenia
   <100 cells/mm³
   >5-7 day
Candida spp. colonization
   >100,000 colony count
   Multiple body sites
   C. glabrata and C. krusei
Corticosteroids
Antineoplastic radiation and chemotherapy
   Mucosal ulceration
   Neutrophil dysfunction
Extremes of age
Diabetes mellitus
Solid organ transplantation
   Liver
   Heart and lung
Hematopoietic stem cell transplantation
   High-risk, mismatched allogeneic marrow graft
Graft rejection
   Graft-versus-host disease
   Immunosuppressive therapy
Recurrent hematologic malignancy
Refractory leukemia

It may also present as a component of polymicrobial infection in patients with bowel perforation ("complicated surgical peritonitis"), necrotizing pancreatitis, or intra-abdominal abscesses complicating the postoperative course of gastrointestinal tract surgery. Treatment is often difficult and relapsed infections are not infrequent. Patients may present with ruptured infected aneurysm of the abdominal aorta following seeding from hematogenous candidiasis.

Candida osteomyelitis, diskitis, and infection of prosthetic joints may be encountered occasionally. Life-threatening complications such as sternal osteomyelitis and *Candida* mediastinitis following cardiothoracic surgery are on the rise. Treatment of this serious infection with antifungals alone results in an extremely high rate of failure, and the mainstays of effective treatment include emergent sternectomy, extensive infected deep tissue débridement, and delayed wound closure. Occasionally, *Candida* is introduced during the placement of prosthetic joints or other foreign devices results in potentially inextricable infection, such as vertebral osteomyelitis following spine stabilization surgery. This may present as late-onset, insidious postoperative recalcitrant yeast infection, which in the majority of cases requires removal of the infected device along with the administration of appropriate antifungal drugs. Occasionally, in select patients with yeast prosthetic infections who are poor surgical risks, fluconazole has been used safely for extended periods, while leaving the prosthesis in place.

Most cases of invasive *Candida* urinary tract infection follow instrumentation. Commonly, patients belong to either extremes of age; had received broad-spectrum antibiotics, external radiation therapy for cancer, indwelling urethral catheters, or organ transplantation; are diabetics; or were diagnosed with obstructive uropathy. Response to antifungal treatment is often good. *Candida* pneumonia is an exceedingly rare complication observed in profoundly immunocompromised patients with an underlying acute/refractory hematologic malignancy. The present evidence suggests that *Candida* lung infections result from hematogenous seeding rather than direct invasion of the pulmonary parenchyma by aspiration leading to direct lower respiratory tract inoculation. Mortality is near universal. Hepatosplenic or chronic progressive candidiasis is a recently recognized syndrome of disseminated systemic candidiasis that has been described in children and adults after blood or marrow transplantation or following accelerated salvage-chemotherapy for acute hematologic neoplasm. Remitting fever may be the only clinical sign in patients during and/or after the recovery from an extended (2 to 3 weeks') duration of profound granulocytopenia (absolute neutrophil count ≤ 150 cells/mm³) or agranulocytosis. Multiple, microscopic/macroscopic fungal abscesses are present in the liver, spleen, and other organs. Computed tomography scan shows characteristic well-circumscribed hypodense hepatic and splenic lesions that exhibit enhancement following the infusion of intravenous contrast. Treatment requires amphotericin B and/or fluconazole administered for extended periods (3 to 6 months). *Candida* species isolated from surgical wounds are in most instances a component of polymicrobial flora. Patients undergoing surgery involving the oropharynx, gastrointestinal tract, or genitourinary tract, and patients with severe trauma and those being treated in burn units, are at an increased risk for fungal (*Candida*) wound infections.

Antifungal prophylaxis in critically ill surgical patient

Systemic candidiasis has a profound negative impact on the outcome of high-risk surgical patients. The critically ill patients in this setting frequently have one or more promoters leading to hematogenous invasion by *Candida* species, as outlined in Box 42–1. Assisted mechanical ventilation and tracheal intubation among patients in the surgical intensive care unit are considered important risks for systemic candidiasis. The controversy surrounding prophylaxis, or preemptive therapy, with either low-dose amphotericin B or fluconazole is presently unsettled. In most institutions, routine antifungal prophylaxis is not given because of the lack of data suggesting significant clinical efficacy, cost of routine administration of an expensive drug, and above all, concern regarding fluconazole-induced selection pressure, which may lead to increase in the triazole (fluconazole) resistant nosocomial *Candida* isolates.

Endemic Mycosis

Histoplasmosis

Histoplasmosis is a fungal disease caused by *Histoplasma capsulatum*, which is a dimorphic fungus endemic to soil of river valleys throughout the New World, especially the Ohio and Mississippi River valleys, although reports of histoplasmosis are found from all around the world. Bird and bat guano in soil promotes sporulation of *H. capsulatum*. Exploration of caves, archeological sites, or abandoned buildings with poor ventilation promotes inhalation of the infectious spores, and the respiratory tract is the primary site of infection. Immunocompromised patients, especially those with AIDS, those on high-dose corticosteroids therapy, and allogeneic transplant recipients, may develop symptomatic, disseminated infection. In endemic areas, most of the population acquires histoplasmosis without symptoms or with only a vague, flulike illness. Fewer than 10% with acute *H. capsulatum* infection come to medical attention.

Acute pulmonary histoplasmosis typically presents as cough, chest pain, fever, and arthralgias, and frequently occurs after an exposure to a large number of spores. In 5% of cases, mostly women, erythema nodosum or erythema multiforme may be present. Radiographic features are patchy infiltrates with hilar lymphadenopathy. Acute pericarditis occurs in 5% to 10% of patients who develop symptomatic acute histoplasmosis and is commonly manifested by fever and precordial pain. In two thirds, a pericardial friction rub may be heard on examination. Mediastinal lymphadenopathy frequently complicates acute histoplasmosis and occasionally becomes symptomatic. Compression of airways by enlarged lymph nodes predisposes to postobstructive pneumonia and chronic bronchiectasis. Mediastinal lymphadenopathy often evokes suspicion of malignancy, prompting unnecessary surgery. Mediastinal fibrosis (also known as fibrosing mediastinitis) may occur and cause progressive invasion and occlusion of the mediastinal great vessels and airways. Mediastinoscopy with biopsy in this setting can be dangerous because the fibrosis may encase blood vessels and predisposes to massive hemorrhage during surgery. Histoplasmoma, another complication of acute histoplasmosis, presents as a coin lesion with a central core of calcification, which helps to distinguish it from malignancy. Cavitary pulmonary histoplasmosis usually affects persons with underlying chronic obstructive pulmonary disease, especially men. The cavities are nearly always in the upper lobes, and are associated with low-grade fever, dyspnea, productive cough, weight loss, and occasionally night sweats and hemoptysis. Acute pulmonary histoplasmosis heals spontaneously in most cases without treatment. Cavitary pulmonary histoplasmosis is usually a slowly progressive disease. Many of the cavities (10% to 60%) resolve spontaneously; death usually results from the underlying lung disease or from pneumonia. Disseminated histoplasmosis has high mortality (83% to 100%) in untreated individuals.

Progressive disseminated histoplasmosis is classified as acute, subacute, or chronic. Acute progressive disseminated histoplasmosis is seen mainly in immunocompromised patients, especially those with AIDS. Fever, weight loss, lymphadenopathy, organomegaly, skin lesions, anemia, leukopenia, thrombocytopenia, and abnormal liver function tests are common at presentation. Patchy pneumonitis with hilar lymphadenopathy is present on chest radiograph. Multiorgan failure with shock occurs in sever cases. Subacute progressive disseminated histoplasmosis is, by definition, a more subtle illness. Clinical features include oral ulcers that can be easily mistaken for malignancy; other features include gastrointestinal ulcers, chronic meningitis with other central nervous system (CNS) syndromes, and adrenal insufficiency. Laboratory abnormalities are similar to those in the acute form of the disease but tend to be less striking. Chronic progressive disseminated histoplasmosis presents with fever and malaise. A deep, painless mouth ulcer is found in about 50% of cases and is an important clue to diagnosis. Histoplasmosis, like tuberculosis, can affect nearly every organ. Ocular histoplasmosis is relatively common in endemic zones.

Definitive diagnosis depends on isolation and identification of *H. capsulatum* in cultures. Cultures performed on bronchial specimens yield the organism in most (~ 90%) patients with profound immunosuppression. Blood and bone marrow cultures are helpful in patients with disseminated infection but are positive in only about one half of instances. Detection of antibodies to *H. capsulatum* is useful in all forms of histoplasmosis, but nearly 50% of immunosuppressed patients are unable to form detectable antibody response. Complement fixation (CF) serial dilution titers are commonly used, with titers greater than 1:8 suggesting acute infection and titers greater than or equal to 1:32 being consistent with systemic dissemination. Demonstration of *H. capsulatum* polysaccharide antigen in urine and serum is now widely used for diagnosis. The sensitivity is highest (90%) in the presence of a large yeast burden, as occurs in progressive disseminated histoplasmosis. In cases without clinically apparent dissemination, such as acute pulmonary histoplasmosis, the urine antigen test is often negative (80%). Even with cavitary pneumonia, the diagnostic yield is less than 50%. Monitoring the urine antigen level is used as a guide for therapeutic response and for surveillance in immunocompromised patients for future relapse.

Asymptomatic infections do not need treatment. Treatment is reserved for moderately symptomatic acute pulmonary histoplasmosis and for all disseminated infections. Diffuse pulmonary histoplasmosis in the immunocompromised host is treated with amphotericin B. In patients with chronic pulmonary histoplasmosis, itraconazole or amphotericin B can be used. Severe progressive disseminated histoplasmosis is treated with high-dose amphotericin B (induction) followed by 6 to 18 months of maintenance (amphotericin B, or itraconazole) therapy. Treatment of patients with granulomatous mediastinitis is problematic; in patients with severe obstructive symptoms, itraconazole or amphotericin B may be given. Surgery can be useful but is often technically difficult. With appropriate treatment, the mortality rate is decreased to less than 10% for patients with disseminated histoplasmosis.

Coccidioidomycosis

Coccidioidomycosis is a systemic fungal infection caused by *C. immitis*, a dimorphic fungus endemic to the southwestern United States and parts of Central and South America. It is especially important in southern Arizona, central California, southern New Mexico, and west Texas. An estimated 100,000 new cases of coccidioidomycosis occur in the United States each year. Most of these (50% to 70%) are subclinical and most of the clinically apparent infections are mild; a few may present with

disseminated disease. As in histoplasmosis, disseminated coccidioidomycosis is more common in immunosuppressed patients with AIDS or cancer and recipients of hematopoietic stem cell transplant. Among individuals with competent immune systems, disseminated infection is more common in certain races (African-American or Filipino decent) and during pregnancy.

Mild symptoms of cough, malaise, chest pain, headache, and sore throat are common during the acute pulmonary infection, which is often self-limited. A nonpruritic papular rash sometimes occurs early in the illness, and some patients may present with weight loss. In some, especially women, erythema nodosum and erythema multiforme may be present. The triad of fever, arthralgia, and erythema nodosum is known as "desert fever." Elevated sedimentation rate, peripheral blood eosinophilia, and patchy lung infiltrates, hilar lymphadenopathy, and pleural effusions are common. In nearly 8%, thin-walled pulmonary cavities and/or pulmonary nodules (4%) are present on initial examination. Patients with AIDS may present with diffuse, life-threatening pneumonia and systemic inflammatory response syndrome. Individuals with underlying lung disease may rarely present with chronic fibrocavitary *Coccidioides* pneumonia. Acute pulmonary disease resolves spontaneously, and within 2 years nearly 50% of pulmonary cavities may resolve without treatment.

Disseminated infection occurs early after the initial exposure to *C. immitis* and involves the skin, bone, joints, and CNS. A variety of skin lesions are encountered; the knee (arthritis) and vertebrae (osteomyelitis) are common sites of dissemination. The most feared complication is meningitis, which develops within 6 to 24 weeks after acute infection. If untreated, nearly half of patients succumb to disseminated infection. Unaddressed, systemic coccidioidomycosis with meningeal involvement is uniformly fatal.

The diagnosis is usually suspected on the basis of the clinical presentation in a person who resides in or has visited an endemic area. Recent reports highlight the need to consider coccidioidomycosis in returning travelers from the southwestern United States. Definitive diagnosis is made by culture. Presence of the pathognomonic *C. immitis* spherules in bronchoalveolar lavage fluid and/or biopsy specimens is also diagnostic. Serologic diagnosis is based on an immunoglobulin (Ig) M–induced tube precipitin test, which is positive within 2 to 3 weeks after an acute infection. An IgG-based CF test is also commonly used; a high CF titer (≥ 1:32) is consistent with disseminated infection. The CF titer is also used to monitor the response to treatment. The spherule-derived coccidioidin skin test remains positive for life and does not aid in diagnosis; the presence of anergy is associated with poor prognosis. Long-term therapy with amphotericin B or fluconazole is indicated for patients with progressive pulmonary infection, meningeal involvement, or systemic dissemination and those with compromised cellular immune function.

North American Blastomycosis

Blastomycosis is a fungal infection caused by *B. dermatitidis*, which is a thermally dimorphic fungus endemic to the central and southeastern United States and to Canada. Rare cases have been reported from India, Africa, and the Middle East. The infection is asymptomatic in nearly half of patients. If symptoms do occur, they are usually pulmonary in nature. Skin disease, the most common extrapulmonary manifestation, may provide a clue to more extensive disease. The fungus may remain isolated to the lung or it may disseminate into the blood stream. The most common sites of dissemination are the skin, bone, genitourinary tract, and CNS. Direct inoculation rarely occurs. Initial symptoms may include fever, cough, chest discomfort, hemoptysis, and skin lesions. Acute pulmonary blastomycosis can be easily mistaken for influenza or community-acquired pneumonia. As in pulmonary histoplasmosis, the upper lobes are involved, with the exception of hilar lymphadenopathy or pleural effusion. Extrapulmonary complications occur in 20% to 40% of cases. A variety of skin lesions can be present, with the most characteristic, fully developed lesion being a hyperkeratotic plaque that may show central ulceration or scarring, often on the face or extremities. Skin involvement heralds systemic dissemination. Skeletal blastomycosis results in osteolytic lesions, paraspinous abscesses, osteomyelitis, and arthritis. Genitourinary involvement is manifested by urinary obstruction, pyuria, and chronic prostatitis. Meningitis and brain abscesses are relatively common (up to 40%) in patients with compromised immunity as a result of cancer or AIDS.

The most rapid method of diagnosis is visualization of a refractile, broad-based, single budding yeast on KOH mounts of pus, skin scrapings, or sputum. Serologic evaluation for acute and chronic blastomycosis is not recommended. Some patients with blastomycosis recover spontaneously, especially those with local lung infection. However, in most patients therapy is given. Response to itraconazole is excellent (~ 90%) in patients with acute non-CNS blastomycosis. In patients with severe infection, including the CNS, response to amphotericin B ranges from 70% to 90%. Relapses are uncommon.

Cryptococcosis

Systemic infections caused by *C. neoformans* are found throughout the world. *Cryptococcus neoformans* is found in soil and especially in areas where aged bird droppings accumulate, such as common roosting sites in attics and vacant old buildings. Transmission occurs through inhalation of aerosolized yeast. The pulmonary infection is most common, and often self-limited. Meningitis is the most common extrapulmonary complication. The infection is usually contained by intact host defenses. Prior to the AIDS epidemic, about one half of cases of cryptococcal meningitis occurred in elderly patients with apparently normal cellular immunity. Today, systemic cryptococcosis is a frequent opportunistic complication in patients with AIDS. Infection may also involve the kidneys, prostate, bone, pericardium, peritoneum, skin, and other organs. Patients with impaired helper $CD3^+/4^+$ T-lymphocyte function, such as those with AIDS, common variable immunodeficiency syndrome, and idiopathic $CD3^+/4^+$ lymphocytopenia, are at relatively high risk. Other predisposing factors in patients with disseminated cryptococcosis include systemic lupus erythematosus, sarcoidosis, hematologic malignancies (lymphoma and leukemia), hypercortisolism (Cushing's disease and Cushing's syndrome, including patients on high-dose corticosteroid therapy), and suboptimally treated diabetes mellitus.

The most common presentation of disseminated cryptococcosis is meningitis. Onset is usually insidious but can be acute. Headache, fever, stiff neck, malaise, confusion, behavioral changes, and, in advanced cases, stupor or coma may be present. Cranial nerve (CN) involvement is relatively common and is often manifested by impaired hearing (CN VIII) and/or loss of vision (CN II). Increased intracranial pressure and papilledema occurs in up to one third of patients. In 10%, skin lesions similar to cutaneous coccidioidomycosis may present as papular lesions resembling molluscum contagiosum, especially in AIDS. The rapid diagnosis of cryptococcosis is made by an antigen-detection assay using latex agglutination on blood or cerebrospinal fluid (CSF). In addition, direct microscopy with India ink or nigrosin mounts allows observation of the budding encapsulated yeast. Definitive diagnosis is made by culture of appropriate specimens such as CSF, blood, or tracheobronchial secretions. The mortality rate of untreated disseminated cryptococcosis is 70% to 80%.

Pulmonary cryptococcal disease confined to the lungs is often treated with fluconazole for 3 to 12 months. Patients who have undergone thoracic surgery (e.g., lobectomy or wedge resection of a coin lesion) for suspected neoplasm and who are found to have cryptococcosis should be treated with fluconazole because of the theoretical risk of dissemination to the meninges during the manipulation of pulmonary tissue during surgery. Patients with severe or progressive pulmonary disease are treated with amphotericin B alone. In those with CNS infection, a combination of amphotericin B and flucytosine is recommended. Fluconazole may be substituted for amphotericin B in mild cases of meningeal cryptococcosis. With appropriate treatment, the mortality in patients with fungal meningitis is 10% to 15%. In patients with AIDS, mortality may reach 60% despite prompt antifungal treatment; relapse is common (50% to 65%) unless secondary prophylaxis is continued through immune restoration.

Sporotrichosis

Sporotrichosis is encountered most commonly as the syndrome of nodular lymphangitis. Occasionally, inhalation of *Sporothrix schenckii* microconidia can cause pulmonary and systemic infection. This is especially likely to occur in patients with compromised immunity as a result of cancer, transplantation, or AIDS. Pulmonary sporotrichosis sometimes occurs in middle-aged men with an underlying chronic obstructive pulmonary disease or alcoholism, and presents as chronic pneumonia or fibronodular cavitary disease. Chronic disabling *Sporothrix* arthritis is rare. Itraconazole has become the drug of choice for lymphocutaneous sporotrichosis and for milder forms of pulmonary disease. Sixty percent to 80% of patients with osteoarticular sporotrichosis respond to therapy. Amphotericin B is the mainstay of therapy for patients with disseminated, life-threatening infection.

Aspergillosis

Aspergillus species are saprophytic molds found throughout the world. They frequently colonize mucosal surfaces. Invasive aspergillosis is a major cause of morbidity and mortality among the severely immunocompromised. Allergic bronchopulmonary aspergillosis and allergic *Aspergillus* sinusitis are common noninvasive or locally invasive diseases in patients with intact immunity. In hospitals, air-conditioning duct systems, potted plants, tap water, and certain foods such as peppers and other spices may lead to nosocomial exposure to the infectious microconidia, and systemic infections, especially in the severely immunocompromised patients, can be devastating. *Aspergillus fumigatus* is the most frequent cause of human infection (~90%), followed by A. *flavus* (~10%), A. *niger* (~2%), and A. *terreus* (~2%). Primary infection is via inhalation of microconidia, and structural abnormalities of the lower respiratory tract, such as cystic fibrosis, severe bronchiectasis, silicosis, and pneumoconiosis, increase the probability of fungal colonization and occasionally invasive disease. Intact polymorphonuclear leukocyte function is pivotal to host defense against invasive *Aspergillus* species infection. Patients with severe and prolonged (>14 days) chemotherapy-induced granulocytopenia are at the highest risk. Infection spreads to the adjoining tissue either by invasion of vessels, leading to thrombosis and tissue necrosis, or by hematogenous dissemination. Recently, we have described a novel mechanism of fungal propagation along the perineuronal route, and this may be significant in head and neck infections.

Aspergilloma, or fungus ball, may develop within a preexisting lung cavity or in a paranasal sinus.

Pulmonary aspergillomas were formerly encountered most commonly in patients with existing cavitary tuberculosis. Aspergillomas eventually develop in 15% to 25% of tuberculous lung cavities. Presently, the most common predisposing conditions in patients from the developed world are lung cavities resulting from sarcoidosis, healed cases of necrotizing bacterial pneumonia, and chronic *Pneumocystis carinii* infections in patients with AIDS. Patients are often asymptomatic, and occasionally chronic cough, wheezing, weight loss, and hemoptysis may be present. Rarely, severe hemoptysis may represent life-threatening pulmonary hemorrhage caused by the invasion and rupture of bronchial artery, and emergent surgical lobectomy can be life saving. Aspergilloma in a paranasal sinus cavity may lead to recurrent bacterial infection and carries the risk of locally invasive disease. Chronic fungal otitis externa caused by A. *niger* can also lead to refractory infection with permanent loss of hearing. Post-traumatic aspergillosis is encountered most commonly in ophthalmology practice as post-traumatic keratitis or vision-threatening fungal endophthalmitis.

Invasive aspergillosis occurs most commonly in the immunocompromised patient, and the lung (80% to 90%) is the most common site. Acute invasive pulmonary aspergillosis is a fulminant, rapidly progressive infection, often seen in severely neutropenic (absolute neutrophil count $\leq 100/mm^3$) patients with cancer and in transplantation recipients. High-resolution computed tomography of the chest may yield findings highly suggestive of invasive mold infection, which include dense peripheral, pleural-based consolidation with a surrounding area of low attenuation (the "halo sign"); later in the course of disease, as a result of cavitation within the necrotized lung, a "crescent sign" may be seen. Chronic invasive pulmonary aspergillosis is encountered less commonly, and pursues a more indolent course, especially in non-neutropenic individuals with AIDS and nongranulocytopenic allogeneic marrow transplant recipients with chronic graft-versus-host disease and in patients with diabetes mellitus, chronic obstructive pulmonary disease treated with high-dose corticosteroids, chronic alcoholism, or chronic granulomatous disease. Invasive aspergillus sinusitis, especially that involving the sphenoid sinus, can progress to life-threatening intraorbital and/or intracranial infection. Aspergillosis of the CNS presents as brain abscesses and/or arteritis; early surgical débridement is critical in procuring a favorable outcome. Rarely, primary renal aspergillosis may be encountered in susceptible patients, and treatment requires surgical débridement coupled with systemic antifungal therapy.

Histologic evidence of fungal tissue invasion is necessary for the definitive diagnosis of invasive aspergillosis. Unfortunately, a tissue diagnosis is often difficult to secure. Open lung biopsy has higher diagnostic yield, compared with transbronchial tissue samples. Diagnosis is also established on histologic examination by surgical removal of a suspicious cavitary or noncavitary pulmonary lesion. Treatment includes high-dose conventional amphotericin B, lipid-based preparations such as Abelcet and AmBisome, and/or itraconazole along with aggressive surgical resection of the infected tissue. For refractory non-CNS disease, caspofungin (Cancidas) has recently become available in the United States. Voriconazole is the latest (2002) antifungal addition for the treatment of refractory systemic aspergillosis. In patients with acute invasive *Aspergillus* species infection, the overall response to amphotericin B and/or itraconazole is approximately 35% to 45%.

Mucormycosis

The term mucormycosis denotes invasive tissue infection caused by one or another of a diverse group of fungi belonging to the order Mucorales. Mucoraceae species such as *Rhizopus*, *Rhizomucor*, *Absidia*, and *Mucor* are commonly involved. These fungi are ubiquitous in nature and grow rapidly on decaying organic material. *Rhizopus* spores, for example, grow rapidly on bread, leading to frequent household exposure. Infection usually results from inhalation of spores, and occasionally direct inoculation of abraded skin can lead to local and/or systemic infection. Patients with poorly controlled diabetes mellitus, extensive trauma, severe burns, high-dose corticosteroid therapy, hematologic malignancies, chemotherapy-induced granulocytopenia, organ or bone marrow transplantation, and graft-versus-host disease are especially at risk. Polymorphonuclear leukocytes are the main line of defense against these fungi. Mucormycosis is an unusual opportunistic infection in the non-neutropenic patients with AIDS. Patients with chronic renal failure and iron overload who are undergoing deferoxamine chelation therapy are also at increased risk for severe systemic Mucorales infection. Like *Aspergillus*, the Mucoraceae species are notorious for invading the walls of blood vessels, causing infarction and tissue necrosis.

Rhinocerebral mucormycosis commonly presents with facial pain and headaches. Altered mental status is common. Most patients have underlying diabetes mellitus, typically with a recent history of ketoacidosis or hyperosmolar state. Agranulocytosis in patients with acute leukemia is another common predisposition. Initial symptoms and signs may suggest sinusitis or facial cellulitis. The paranasal sinuses have been called "way stations to the brain" for Mucoraceae, because these fungi cause a highly invasive form of fungal sinusitis leading to life-threatening cavernous sinus thrombosis, frontal lobe infarction, and death. The presence of chemosis, conjunctival injection, and proptosis indicates intraorbital extension. Involvement of CN II, V, and VII suggests intracranial extension and predicts poor prognosis.

Pulmonary mucormycosis is seen most commonly in patients with acute leukemia, during periods of prolonged chemotherapy-induced agranulocytosis. Cough, dyspnea, and fever are common. Severe hemoptysis indicates fungal erosion of the wall of a major bronchial or mediastinal blood vessel. Consolidation is present in nearly two thirds of pulmonary cases, and nearly half have evidence of cavitary lesions of the lung. Pulmonary mucormycosis in diabetics, unlike rhinocerebral infection, may follow a subacute or chronic course, and may occasionally present as pulmonary nodules. Other forms of mucormycosis are less common and include cutaneous infections in patients with extensive burns or trauma, gastrointestinal mucormycosis in patients with severe malnutrition, and CNS infection in severely debilitated patients.

The diagnosis of mucormycosis depends on the demonstration in tissue biopsy specimens of broad (10 to 20 μm in diameter), ribbon-shaped, nonseptate hyphae that characteristically branch at right angles, as opposed to the acute-angle branching shown by *Aspergillus* species. Isolation of the causative mold from biopsy specimens is desirable but is frequently not achieved even when the organisms appear to be abundant on histologic examination. Methods for securing tissue include endoscopic paranasal sinus biopsy and transbronchial versus open lung biopsy. Useful serologic methods of diagnosis are not available. Blackening of the nasal mucosa or the palate is an important early clue. Computed tomography scans and/or magnetic resonance images of the sinuses, orbits, and brain are critical for evaluating the extent of the disease. Early and aggressive surgical débridement of necrotic tissue, combined with high-dose amphotericin B therapy, holds the key to a successful outcome for rhinocerebral, invasive pulmonary, and progressive cutaneous mucormycosis. The currently available triazoles, such as itraconazole, have a limited role in the treatment of systemic Mucorales infection. Adjuvant therapy with hyperbaric oxygen and, more importantly, recombinant cytokines (granulocyte, granulocyte-macrophage, and macrophage colony-stimulating factors; interleukin-12; or interferon-γ) is unproven, but may be considered in refractory cases. Untreated rhinocerebral mucormycosis is uniformly fatal.

Discussion of phaeohyphomycosis caused by dematiaceous molds, chromoblastomycosis, and infections caused by *Fusarium* species, *Penicillium marneffei*, and *Paracoccidioides brasiliensis* are not included in this chapter and can be referenced in textbooks on infectious diseases.

Antifungal Drug Therapy

Systemic antifungal therapy has undergone great advances in the past decade. Amphotericin B remains the most broadest spectrum antimicrobial in this category. Two new lipid preparations of amphotericin B are currently in use, Abelcet and AmBisome, and both are associated with significantly reduced nephrotoxicity compared with the conventional amphotericin B deoxycholate (Fungisome). AmBisome also provides additional benefit of reduced untoward side effects that are observed during or right after conventional amphotericin B infusion. The triazole-based compounds (fluconazole and itraconazole) are better tolerated antifungal drugs presently available, and enable oral therapy for certain infections that previously required long-term parenteral amphotericin B. Their major problems are lack of fungicidal action and complex drug-drug interactions. Terbinafine and flucytosine represent two additional classes that have more limited applications for systemic fungal infections. In 2001, an echinocandin/pneumocandin (caspofungin [Cancidas]) became available in the United States for human infections, and in 2002 the first fungicidal broad-spectrum triazole (voriconazole [Vfend]) was approved by the U.S. Food and Drug Administration. The applications of systemic antifungal drug therapy differ sharply according to the underlying mycosis, the patient's condition, and concurrent therapy. There are also important cost considerations in selecting the appropriate treatment option.

Polyenes (Amphotericin B and Nystatin)

Amphotericin B remains a useful drug for life-threatening fungal infection. All polyenes act by rapidly binding to ergosterol in fungal and to a lesser degree mammalian cell membranes. This disrupts the steric integrity of the membrane, permitting influx of sodium and loss of intracellular potassium. Ergosterol binding also disrupts activity of fungal cell membrane oxidative enzymes. In vitro the activity is lethal to most but not all fungal cells. Binding to hosts' renal tubule cells causes a reduction in distal tubule osmotic integrity and the potassium wasting in renal tubular acidosis. Binding to erythrocytes can cause hemolysis, and cardiac arrhythmias may occur as a result of disruption of action potentials across the cell membrane in the conduction pathways of the human heart. The polyenes also act to cause glomerular vessel vasospasm and eventually ischemic renal failure. Interaction with phagocytes and lymphocytes and proinflammatory cytokine release have been suggested to supplement antifungal activity, but may also lead to infusion-related fever, chills, rigors, dyspnea, and local thrombophlebitis. Normocytic anemia may ensue after prolonged administration, resulting from stunted synthesis of erythropoietin by the juxtaglomerular apparatus, and, rarely, amphotericin B can cause severe hypertension.

The most common method of delivery of amphotericin B is to dissolve 50 mg in 1 L of 5% glucose and administer it through a central venous catheter (to avoid thrombophlebitis), infusing over 2 to 3 hours. The daily dose varies from 0.5 to 0.7 mg/kg/day for candidiasis, histoplasmosis, and cryptococcosis to 1.0 to 1.5 mg/kg/day for mucormycosis, aspergillosis, and other invasive filamentous mold infections. There are multiple problems with administration of amphotericin B. At doses of 1 mg/kg/day or more, renal failure supervenes within 1 to 2 weeks. The nephrotoxicity of amphotericin B is paradoxical because the kidneys play only a small role (about 10%) in the excretion of the drug and renal failure does not influence pharmacokinetics. The dose for patients on dialysis is the same as for patients with normal renal function; however, infusion time may be increased to 6 hours or longer to reduce sudden potassium efflux, which may precipitate life-threatening arrhythmia. Amphotericin B is not dialyzable and does not clear with peritoneal dialysis. Nevertheless, patients may require dialysis during administration of the drug to control dangerous hyperkalemia.

Recent advances

There are now three lipid vehicles for amphotericin B (Abelcet, AmBisome, and Amphotec) that all have significant reduction of glomerular toxicity, however tubular toxicity manifested by hypokalemia and hypomagnesemia may still be encountered. All three preparations can be given up to and in excess of 5 mg/kg daily, and infusion-related adverse events are markedly diminished in patients receiving AmBisome. These drugs are useful options for the treatment of fungal infection in patients with underlying renal disease, or those with precarious renal reserves. AmBisome can be given safely up to 10 to 15 mg/kg, but it is unclear whether such heroic doses are more effective than conventional doses. Indeed, there is no evidence that the lipid formulations are more effective than amphotericin B desoxycholate in candidemia, and little evidence of increased efficacy in patients with systemic aspergillosis. The major problem is costs, which may exceed $600/day for AmBisome and $300/day for Abelcet. The third preparation, amphotericin B colloidal dispersion (ABCD, or Amphotec) is not used often because of frequent infusion related reactions and least renal preservation among lipid-based amphotericin B preparations.

Flucytosine

Flucytosine, an antimetabolite, is used mainly for combination therapy with amphotericin B in patients with cryptococcal meningitis. The major toxicity is hematologic. Flucytosine is excreted in the urine, and doses must be reduced in renal failure. Traditional doses of 37.5 mg/kg every 6 hours are now appreciated to be too high, and a reduced dose (25 mg/kg every 6 hours) is generally used. Flucytosine is used only orally in the

United States, though in Europe it can be obtained for intravenous use. Because of rapid emergence of resistance, flucytosine should be used only in combination therapy with amphotericin B or fluconazole for cryptococcosis. Monitoring complete blood count and liver function tests is recommended on a weekly or biweekly basis, unless amphotericin B is given, in which case monitoring should be more frequent. Flucytosine is not recommended for other yeast infections, including *Candida* species or those caused by filamentous fungi.

Allylamines (Terbinafine)

Terbinafine is the only currently available member of its class, squalene oxidase inhibitors. The drug concentrates in the skin and nail beds, and its main use is in the treatment of dermatomycosis and onychomycosis; recently it has been used successfully in sporotrichosis. Terbinafine is well tolerated. A common regimen for toe onychomycosis is to give 500 mg/day for 1 week each month for 6 or longer until there is clear evidence of new noninfected toenail growth.

Azoles and Triazoles (Ketoconazole, Fluconazole, and Itraconazole)

Miconazole and ketoconazole were the first azole antifungals. Fluconazole and itraconazole are triazole-based compounds with an improved tolerability profile. These agents have brought relative safety and convenience of administration for patients with systemic mycoses. All azoles act by binding to and inhibiting the activity of lanosterol 14-α-demethylase, progressively blocking synthesis of ergosterol, which leads to substitution of other intermediate sterols in fungal cell membranes and causes slow breakdown of the steric integrity of the membrane and eventually cell death. Several generations of fungal growth may be required for optimal antifungal effect of these agents to become apparent. Their toxicity is mostly due to the interaction with the mammalian cytochrome P450 (CYP) enzyme complex. Systemic miconazole is no longer used because of toxicity, especially cardiac arrhythmias. Ketoconazole causes hepatic toxicity and impairs the synthesis of several key sterol-based hormones. Adverse effects include hypogonadism, impairment of menstrual cycles, hair loss, and adrenal insufficiency. Hypocholesterolemia has also been reported. The newer drugs in this category, fluconazole and itraconazole, have specificity for fungal enzymes and less hepatotoxicity than ketoconazole.

Itraconazole is somewhat similar to ketoconazole in kinetics, except that one metabolite, hydroxyitraconazole, is biologically active. Itraconazole metabolism is via CYP3A4, an enzyme that is highly vulnerable to drug interactions.

All agents that induce enzyme activity induce enhanced clearance of itraconazole. This includes rifampin derivatives (though less with rifabutin than rifampin). It usually requires 1 to 2 weeks after discontinuing such drugs for the perturbations to decrease. Itraconazole has been successfully used for the treatment of invasive aspergillosis. Patients with other causes of hyalohyphomycosis and phaeohyphomycosis and those with chromoblastomycosis may also respond to prolonged therapy with oral itraconazole. We recommend monitoring of serum drug concentration, especially in patients with suboptimum enteric absorption.

A pernicious problem is the coadministration of drugs that are also metabolized by the CYP3A4 enzyme. These provide substrate competition, which may increase the serum and tissue concentrations of either or both drugs. Many classes of drugs are represented, and, if the practitioner is unaware of these interactions, there can be dangerous consequences. For example, triazolam retention can cause profound somnolence. Lovastatin may accumulate as the acid form, causing rhabdomyolysis. Cyclosporine retention may cause renal failure, drug fever, and myelosuppression. Terfenadine, astemizole, or cisapride retention may cause Q-Tc prolongation and may induce potentially lethal torsade de pointes arrhythmia. Digoxin toxicity may occur. It is imperative to be aware of patients' concurrent medications and make dose adjustment when these compounds are administered.

The pharmacokinetics of fluconazole is predictable, and it has wide tissue distribution in the aqueous phase, with good bioavailability following oral administration. Its use is limited to yeast infections, including *Candida* species other than *C. krusei* (which is intrinsic non-susceptible), *C. neoformans* and *C. immitis*, and second-line azole therapy for other endemic mycosis. Fluconazole resistance, especially among *C. glabrata* and *C. albicans*, has increased during the later half of the 1990s. Prior long-standing triazole exposure has been an important predictor of drug resistance in this setting. In *C. tropicalis* and *C. neoformans*, fluconazole resistance is rare and encountered sporadically.

Recent Advances in Antifungals

Broad-Spectrum Triazoles (Voriconazole, Posaconazole, and Ravuconazole)

The next generation of triazoles has broad-spectrum antimycotic activity against *Candida* species, including fluconazole-resistant *C. albicans* and *C. krusei*; *C. neoformans*; and a wide range of filamentous fungi. Voriconazole (Vfend) shows good in vitro activity against *A. fumigatus, A. flavus, A. niger, A. terreus, Fusarium* species,

Pseudallescheria boydii, Scedosporium apiospermum, dematiaceous molds (black fungi), and the dimorphic fungi, including *B. dermatitidis, C. immitis,* and *H. capsulatum.* In contrast, it is less active against agents of zygomycosis, such as *Rhizopus* species, *S. schenckii,* and *Scedosporium prolificans.* The other agents in advanced stages of development are posaconazole (Schering; SCH-56592) and ravuconazole (Bristol Myers-Squibb; BMS-207147). All are excreted by hepatic clearance. Voriconazole has an unexplained, transient visual toxicity manifested as increased brightness of objects, usually present only during the early phase of therapy. No permanent retinal damage has been demonstrated either in animal experiments or clinical trials. CSF penetration of voriconazole is excellent; levels nearly half those of non–protein-bound serum are recovered from CSF. The suboptimal in vitro activity and its role in clinical mucormycosis need further clinical evaluation.

Echinocandins/Pneumocandins (Caspofungin, Micafungin, Anidulafungin)

The drugs in this novel class of antifungals inhibit the synthesis of β-(1,3)-D-glucan, an integral component of the fungal cell wall, which is absent in the eukaryotic cell. Caspofungin (Candidas) became available in the United States in 2001 for the treatment of non-CNS refractory systemic aspergillosis. Other agents in advanced stages of development include micafungin (Fujisawa; FK-463) and anidulafungin (Ely Lily; LY-303366). They have superb in vitro activity against *C. albicans* and non-*albicans Candida,* including *C. krusei;* notable exceptions are *C. parapsilosis* and *C. guilliermondii.* Activity against *Aspergillus, Paecilomyces* species, *P. boydii, S. apiospermum,* and agents of phaeohyphomycosis such as *Alternaria, Bipolasis, Curvularia,* and *Exophiala* is good. Caspofungin, the currently available echinocandin, has poor activity against *Fusarium, Rhizopus,* and *S. prolificans.* Because of a paucity of the target enzyme, caspofungin has minimal activity against *C. neoformans.* It is well tolerated, with no apparent nephrotoxicity and minimal liver dysfunction. Reversible transaminitis was observed in immunocompromised patients receiving concomitant cyclosporin therapy, and currently not recommended for patients receiving cyclosporin. Because of their large molecular structure, penetration in the CNS is modest, and, until further clinical data become available, these agents should be avoided in patients with intracranial infections. At present these drugs are extremely potent in mucosal candidiasis, and studies of candidemia and other mycoses are in progress. This class is anticipated to provide a major alternative and/or adjuvant in the treatment of otherwise difficult-to-treat invasive fungal infections.

Conclusions

Systemic mycoses are on the rise, especially in critically ill hospitalized surgical patients. Surgical débridement has been recognized as pivotal in the successful outcome of some patients with invasive fungal infections. Therefore, it is imperative that the physicians practicing surgical faculties have an understanding of the natural course and pathogenesis of these infections. It is important to recognize fungal components of the polymicrobial surgical wound and/or prosthetic device infections, which may be refractory to antimicrobial/antifungal therapy alone. Antifungal prophylaxis has received widespread attention and is presently sporadically given at institutions with hybrid prophylaxis protocols. Because of concern for the emergence of resistance among nosocomial *Candida* and other fungal isolates, we recommend that routine prophylaxis with the triazole-based drugs be withheld and preemptive and/or empirical therapy reserved for highly susceptible patients in surgical clinical care units.

Bibliography

Abi-Said D, Anaissie E, Uzun O, et al: The epidemiology of hematogenous candidiasis by different *Candida* species. Clin Infect Dis 1997;24:1122.

Anaissie EJ, Darouiche RO, Abi-Said D, et al: Management of invasive *Candida* infections: results of a prospective, randomized, multicenter study of fluconazole versus amphotericin B and review of literature. Clin Infect Dis 1996;23:964.

Andriole VT: Aspergillus infections: problems in diagnosis and treatment. Infect Agents Dis 1996;5:47.

Antunes PE, Bernardo JE, Eugenio L, et al: Mediastinitis after aorto-coronary bypass surgery. Eur J Cardiothorac Surg 1997;12:443.

Arikan S, Lozano-Chiu M, Paetznick V, et al: In vitro synergy of caspofungin and amphotericin B against *Aspergillus* and *Fusarium* spp. Antimicrob Agents Chemother 2002; 46:245.

Arnavielhe S, Blancard A, Mallie M, et al: Multilocus enzyme electrophoresis analysis of *Candida albicans* isolates from three intensive care units: an epidemiological study. Mycoses 1997;40(5-6):159.

Beck-Sague CM, Jarvis WR: Secular trends in the epidemiology of nosocomial fungal infections in the United States, 1980–1990. J Infect Dis 1993;167:1247.

Berrouane Y, Bisiau H, Le Baron F, et al: *Candida albicans* blastoconidia in peripheral blood smears from non-neutropenic surgical patients. J Clin Pathol 1998;51:537.

Berrouane YF, Herwaldt LA, Pfaller MA: Trends in antifungal use and epidemiology of nosocomial yeast infections in a university hospital. J Clin Microbiol 1999; 37:531.

Blumberg HM, Jarvis WR, Soucie JM, et al: Risk factors for *Candida* bloodstream infections in surgical intensive care unit patients: the NEMIS Prospective Multicenter Study. Clin Infect Dis 2001;33:177.

Chapman SW, Bradsher RW, Campbell GD, et al: Practice guidelines for the management of patients with blastomycosis. Clin Infect Dis 2000;30:679.

Chew FS, Kline MJ: Diagnostic yield of CT-guided percutaneous procedures in suspected spontaneous infectious diskitis. Radiology 2001;218:211.

Clancy CJ, Nguyen MH, Morris AJ: *Candida* mediastinitis: an emerging clinical entity. Clin Infect Dis 1997;25:608.

Conway N, Kothari ML, Lockey E, et al: *Candida* endocarditis after heart surgery. Thorax 1968;23:353.

De Foer C, Fossion E, Vaillant JM: Sinus aspergillosis. J Craniomaxillofac Surg 1990;18:33.

Denning DW: *Aspergillus* species. *In* Mandell GL, Bennett JE, Dolin R (eds): Principles and Practice of Infectious Diseases (5th ed). Philadelphia: Churchill Livingstone, 2000:2674.

Denning DW, Ribaud P, Milpied N, et al: Efficacy and safety of voriconazole in the treatment of acute invasive aspergillosis. Clin Infect Dis 2002;34:563.

Diekema DJ, Messer SA, Hollis RJ, et al: An outbreak of Candida parapsilosis prosthetic valve endocarditis. Diagn Microbiol Infect Dis 1997;29:147.

Dismukes WE: Introduction to antifungal drugs. Clin Infect Dis 2000;30:653.

Edwards JE, Bodey GP, Bowden RA, et al: International conference for the development of a consensus on the management and prevention of severe *Candida* infections. Clin Infect Dis 1997;25:43.

Ellis ME, Al-Abdely H, Sandridge A, et al: Fungal endocarditis: evidence in the world literature, 1965–1995. Clin Infect Dis 2001;32:50.

Fearon JA, Yu J, Bartlett SP, et al: Infections in craniofacial surgery: a combined report of 567 procedures from two centers. Plastic Reconstr Surg 1997;100:862.

Flanagan PG, Barnes RA: Fungal infection in the intensive care unit. J Hosp Infect 1998;38:163.

Galgiani JN, Ampel NM, Catanzaro A, et al: Practice guidelines for the treatment of coccidioidomycosis. Clin Infect Dis 2000;30:658.

Georgopapadakou NH: Update on antifungal targeted to the cell wall: focus on beta-1,3-glucan synthase inhibitor. Expert Opin Invest Drugs 2001;10:269.

Giamarellou H, Antoniadou A: Epidemiology, diagnosis, and therapy of fungal infections in surgery. Infect Control Hosp Epidemiol 1996;17:558.

Godec CJ, Mielnick A, Hilfer J: Primary renal aspergillosis. Urology 1989;34:152.

Gossot D, Validire P, Vaillancourt R, et al: Full thoracoscopic approach for surgical management of invasive pulmonary aspergillosis. Ann Thorac Surg 2002;73:240.

Gouello JP, Asfar P, Brenet O, et al: Nosocomial endocarditis in the intensive care unit: an analysis of 22 cases. Crit Care Med 2000;28:377.

Habicht JM, Matt P, Passweg JR, et al: Invasive pulmonary fungal infection in hematologic patients: is resection effective? Hematol J 2001;2:250.

Habicht JM, Reichenberger F, Gratwohl A, et al: Surgical aspects of resection for suspected invasive pulmonary fungal infection in neutropenic patients. Ann Thoracic Surg 1999;68:321.

Hebrecht R, Letscher-Bru V, Bowden RA, et al: Treatment of 21 cases of invasive mucormycosis with amphotericin B colloidal dispersion. Eur J Clin Microbiol Infect Dis 2001;20:460.

Hogevik H, Alestig K: Fungal endocarditis—a report on seven cases and a brief review. Infection 1996;24:17.

Ikeda M, Kambayashi J, Lawasaki T: Contained rupture of infected abdominal aortic aneurysm due to systemic candidiasis. Cardiovasc Surg 1995;3:711.

Kac G, Durain E, Amrein C, et al: Colonization and infection of pulmonary artery catheter in cardiac surgical patients: epidemiology and multivariate analysis of risk factors. Crit Care Med 2001;29:971.

Kauffman CA, Hajjeh R, Chapman SW, et al: Practice guidelines for the management of patients with sporotrichosis. Clin Infect Dis 2000;30:684.

Kirby RM, McMaster P, Clements D, et al: Orthotopic liver transplantation: postoperative complications and their management. Br J Surg 1987;74:3.

Kralovicova K, Spanik S, Oravcova E, et al: Fungemia in cancer patients undergoing chemotherapy versus surgery: risk factors, etiology and outcome. Scand J Infect Dis 1997;29:301.

Kujath P, Lerch K, Kochendorfer P, et al: Comparative study of the efficacy of fluconazole versus amphotericin B/flucytosine in surgical patients with systemic mycoses. Infection 1993;21:376.

Kurup A, Janardhan MN, Seng TY: *Candida tropicalis* pacemaker endocarditis. J Infect 2000;41:275.

Lee FY, Mossad SB, Adal KA: Pulmonary mucormycosis: the last 30 years. Arch Intern Med 1999;159:1301.

Luzzati R, Amalfitano G, Lazzarini L, et al: Nosocomial candidemia in non-neutropenic patients at an Italian tertiary care hospital. Eur J Clin Microbiol Infect Dis 2000;19:602.

McKinnon PS, Goff DA, Kern JW, et al: Temporal assessment of *Candida* risk factors in the surgical intensive care unit. Arch Surg 2001;136:1401.

Merrer J, Dupont B, Nieszkowska A, et al: *Candida albicans* prosthetic arthritis treated with fluconazole alone. J Infect 2001;42:208.

Michalopoulos A, Stavridis G, Geroulanos S: Severe sepsis in cardiac surgical patients. Eur J Surg 1998; 164:217.

Nasser RM, Melgar GR, Longworth DL, et al: Incidence and risk of developing fungal prosthetic valve endocarditis after nosocomial candidemia. Am J Med 1997;103:25.

Nassoura Z, Ivatury RR, Simon RJ, et al: Candiduria as an early marker of disseminated infection in critically ill surgical patients: the role of fluconazole therapy. J Trauma Injury Infect Crit Care 1993;35:290.

Nieto-Rodriguez JA, Kusne S, Manez R, et al: Factors associated with the development of candidemia and candidemia-related death among liver transplant recipients. Ann Surg 1996;223:70.

Nolla-Salas J, Leon C, Torres-Rodriguez JM, et al: Treatment of candidemia in critically ill surgical patients with intravenous fluconazole. Clin Infect Dis 1992;14:952.

Nolla-Salas J, Sitges-Serra A, Leon-Gil C, et al: Candidemia in non-neutropenic critically ill patients: analysis of prognostic factors and assessment of systemic antifungal therapy. Study Group of Fungal Infection in the ICU. Intensive Care Med 1997;23:23.

Nucci M, Anaissie E: Should vascular catheters be removed from all patients with candidemia? An evidence-based review. Clin Infect Dis 2002;34:591.

Parry MF, Grant B, Yukna M, et al: Candida osteomyelitis and diskitis after spinal surgery: an outbreak that implicates artifical nail use. Clin Infect Dis 2001;32:352.

Patterson TF: Role of newer azoles in surgical patients. J Chemother 1999;11:504.

Patterson TF, Kirkpatrick WR, White M, et al: Invasive aspergillosis: disease spectrum, treatment practices, and outcomes. 13 Aspergillus Study Group. Medicine 2000;79:250.

Penk A, Pittrow L: Role of fluconazole in the long-term suppression therapy of fungal infections in patients with artificial implants. Mycoses 1999;42(Suppl 2):91.

Remsey ES, Lytle BW: Repair of fungal aortic prosthetic valve endocarditis associated with periannular abscess. J Heart Valve Dis 1998;7:235.

Rex JH, Okhuysen PC: Sporothrix schenckii. In Mandell GL, Bennett JE, Dolin R (eds): Principles and Practice of Infectious Diseases (5th ed). Philadelphia: Churchill Livingstone, 2000:2695.

Rex JH, Walsh TJ, Sobel JD, et al: Practice guidelines for the treatment of candidiasis. Clin Infect Dis 2000;30:662.

Rocco TR, Reinert SE, Simms HH: Effects of fluconazole administration in critically ill patients: analysis of bacterial and fungal resistance. Arch Surg 2000;135:160.

Rocco TR, Simms HH: Inadequate proof of adverse outcome due to the use of fluconazole in critically ill patients. Arch Surg 2000;135:1114.

Roger PM, Boissy C, Gari-Toussaint M, et al: Medical treatment of a pacemaker endocarditis due to Candida albicans and to Candida glabrata. J Infect 2000;41:176.

Ryan T, McCarthy JF, Rady MY, et al: Early bloodstream infection after cardiopulmonary bypass: frequency rate, risk factors, and implications. Crit Care Med 1997;25:2009.

Saag MS, Graybill RJ, Larsen RA, et al: Practice guidelines for the management of cryptococcal disease. Clin Infect Dis 2000;30:710.

Safdar A: Progressive cutaneous hyalohyphomycosis due to Paecilomyces lilacinus: rapid response to treatment with caspofungin and itraconazole. Clin Infect Dis 2002;34:1415.

Safdar A, Armstrong D: Infections in patients with neoplastic diseases. In Shoemaker WC, Grenvik M, Ayers SM, Holbrook PR (eds): Textbook of Critical Care (4th ed). Philadelphia, WB Saunders, 2000:715.

Safdar A, Armstrong D: Infectious morbidity in critically ill patients with cancer. Crit Care Clin 2001;17:531.

Safdar A, Armstrong D: Prospective evaluation of Candida species colonization in hospitalized cancer patients: impact on short-term survival in recipients of marrow transplantation and patients with hematological malignancies. Bone Marrow Transplant 2002;30:931.

Safdar A, Bryan CS, Graybill JR: Fungal infections and antifungal therapy. In Bryan CS (ed): Infectious Diseases in Primary Care. Philadelphia: WB Saunders, 2002:493.

Safdar A, Chaturvedi V, Cross EW, et al: Prospective study of Candida species in patients at a comprehensive cancer center. Antimicrob Agents Chemother 2001;45:2129.

Safdar A, Dommers MP, Talwani R, et al: Intracranial perineuronal extension of invasive mycosis—a novel mechanism of disease propagation by Aspergillus fumigatus. Clin Infect Dis 2002;35:e50.

Safdar A, van Rhee F, Henslee-Downey JP, et al: Candida glabrata and Candida krusei fungemia after high-risk allogeneic marrow transplantation: no adverse effects of low-dose fluconazole prophylaxis on incidence and outcome. Bone Marrow Transplant 2001;28:873.

Sawyer RG, Raymond DP, Pelletier SJ, et al: Implications of 2,457 consecutive surgical infections entering year 2000. Ann Surg 2001;233:867.

Schiefer HG: Mycoses of the urogenital tract. Mycoses 1997; 40(Suppl 2):33.

Schrank JH, Dooley DP: Purulent pericarditis caused by Candida species: case report and review. Clin Infect Dis 1995;21:182.

Sharma RR, Gurusinghe NT, Lynch PG: Cerebral infarction due to Aspergillus arteritis following glioma surgery. Br J Neurosurg 1992;6:485.

Singh N, Gayowski T, Singh J, et al: Invasive gastrointestinal zygomycosis in a liver transplant recipient: case report and review of zygomycosis in solid-organ transplant recipients. Clin Infect Dis 1995;20:617.

Stevens DA, Kan VL, Judson MA, et al: Practice guidelines for diseases caused by Aspergillus. Clin Infect Dis 2000;30:696.

Takeda S, Wakabayashi K, Yamazaki K, et al: Intracranial fungal aneurysm caused by Candida endocarditis. Clin Neuropathol 1998;17:199.

Tran LT, Auger P, Marchand R, et al: Epidemiological study of Candida spp. colonization in cardiovascular surgical patients. Mycoses 1997;40(5-6):169.

Tran TL, Auger P, Marchand AR, et al: Perioperative variation in phagocytic activity against *Candida albicans* measured by a flow-cytometric assay in cardiovascular-surgery patients. Clin Diagn Lab Immunol 1997;4:447.

Vindenes H, Bjerkens R: Microbial colonization of large wounds. Burns 1995;21:575.

Wade JJ, Rolando N, Hayllar K, et al: Bacterial and fungal infections after liver transplantation: an analysis of 284 patients. Hepatology 1995;21:1328.

Walsh TJ: Recent advances in the treatment of systemic fungal infections. Methods Find Exp Clin Pharmacol 1987;9:769.

Walsh T, Rex JH: All catheter-related candidemia is not the same: assessment of the balance between the risk and benefits of removal of vascular catheters. Clin Infect Dis 2002;34:600.

Weiss CA, Statz CL, Dahms RA, et al: Six years of surgical wound infection surveillance at a tertiary care center: review of the microbiologic and epidemiological aspects of 20,007 wounds. Arch Surg 1999;134:1041.

Wenzel RP: Nosocomial candidemia: risk factors and attributable mortality. Clin Infect Dis 1995;20:1531.

Yazdanparast K, Auger P, Marchand R, et al: Predictive value of *Candida* colonization index in 131 patients undergoing two different cardiovascular surgical procedures. J Cardiovasc Surg 2001;42:339.

CHAPTER 43

Viral Infections

Donald E. Fry, M.D.

Infections in surgical patients traditionally have been viewed as being of bacterial origin. Prior to 1980, hepatitis B was recognized as causing cirrhosis and its related clinical manifestations, and cytomegalovirus was recognized in immunosuppressed transplantation and oncology patients receiving chemotherapy. "Herpetic" blistering occasionally was seen in severe and sustained surgical illness. In general, viral infections were not viewed as having particular relevance for surgeons engaged in the "everyday" practice of surgery.

In 1981, the identification of young male homosexual patients with *Pneumocystis carinii* pulmonary infection led to the description of the acquired immunodeficiency syndrome (AIDS). Vigorous investigation led to the identification of human immunodeficiency virus (HIV) type 1 as the viral pathogen of AIDS. Serologic and antigen detection

methods have now identified that about 1 million people in the United States are infected with HIV-1, and that an international pandemic of the infection exists. In addition, the number of hepatitis viruses has increased. Because of concerns about occupational risks of acquiring viral infections, increased interest about viral infections in their patients has emerged among surgeons. The role of viruses in oncogenesis and perhaps even atherosclerosis also has brought increased attention to the future of antiviral therapy in the management of surgical patients.

This chapter provides a basic introduction to those viral agents currently understood to have a role in surgical illnesses. The list of viral agents has grown considerably over the last 20 years and likely will grow ever larger in upcoming years. Virology, like bacteriology, will be an important area for understanding diseases of the surgical patient.

Basic Virology

Viruses are the most primitive form of infectious agents. They cause infections in all species of animals and in many species of plants, and even infect bacteria (e.g., bacteriophages). Viruses are obligate intracellular parasites. They contain no cellular machinery for the production of cellular energy and are totally dependent upon the host cell for energy sources in order to produce new viral particles. Viral particles measure 10 to 50 nm in diameter.

All viruses have two basic structural elements; also, some particles may have a third structure. First, all viruses have genetic material that could be viewed as analogous to the chromosomes of animal species. The genetic material may be either DNA (e.g., herpesviruses) or RNA (e.g., hepatitis C). DNA viruses are double stranded, whereas RNA viruses may be either single or double stranded. The second structural element common to all viruses is the nucleocapsid. This shell contains the aforementioned genetic material of the virus, and serves the principal function of protecting the genetic material against environmental degradation. The nucleocapsid is a symmetrical structure that may be either helical or icosahedral in shape; DNA viruses are all icosahedrons, whereas RNA viruses may have either configuration. Because the essential components of a functioning viral unit are only the genetic material and the nucleocapsid, the nucleocapsid may have specific protein receptors on its surface that target the surface of host cells.

A third structure that may exist in some viruses is an envelope that is external to the nucleocapsid. This envelope contains the lipid and carbohydrate components of the plasma membrane taken from the infected host cell when the new viral particle was released. Protein spikes of the virus may protrude through this envelope and are important factors in the virulence of the virus, acting as receptors in adherence to targeted host cells.

The pathogenesis of viral infection depends upon the presence or absence of the envelope, and whether the virus has DNA or RNA as its nuclear material. Viruses with envelopes will fuse the envelope with the plasma membrane of the targeted cell, with the subsequent release of the nucleocapsid into the cytoplasm. Viruses without envelopes are internalized by endocytosis after binding to the plasma membrane of the targeted cell. In both cases, the nucleocapsid is degraded and the genetic material of the virus is released. DNA migrates to the nucleus of the host cell and then begins transcription of messenger RNA for protein synthesis. RNA viruses initiate viral protein synthesis by direct translation from the genetic material of the virus. A third pattern that can occur among retroviruses (e.g., HIV) is discussed separately below.

Human Immunodeficiency Virus Type 1

HIV-1 is one of four groups of retroviruses that are associated with human infection. Prior to the recognition of HIV-1 infection, retroviruses were of uncertain significance in human infection.

The infection is acquired by direct transmission via blood or blood products. Sexual transmission from infected to naïve hosts is the most common route. Intravenous drug abuse using shared drug paraphernalia has been a common route of transmission in urban areas of the world. Vertical transmission from infected mothers to their children during the birthing process remains a route of infection when infected mothers do not receive last-trimester antiretroviral therapy. Blood transfusion had formerly been a route of transmission, but this has been quite infrequent with current screening processes. Occupational transmission among health care workers also has been quite infrequent, but remains a major source of concern.

The understanding of the pathogenesis of HIV-1 infection continues to evolve, but certain features are generally accepted:

Exposure: A critical inoculum of viral particles gains access to the host circulation.

Adherence: CD4$^+$ T cells are the principal target of the virus. Macrophages and dendritic cells are also early targets. The virus adheres to the target cell by binding of the viral glycoprotein 120 surface protein to the CD4 receptor of the T cell.

Membrane Fusion: The viral envelope fuses with the plasma membrane of the target cell and allows release of the nucleocapsid of the virus into the cytoplasm. Degradation of the nucleocapsid releases the viral RNA.

Reverse Transcription: The viral RNA becomes the template for reverse transcription whereby a double-stranded, complementary DNA (cDNA) is produced. The viral RNA does not serve a direct role in viral protein synthesis or replication, but serves the unique role of cDNA synthesis.

cDNA Migration/Incorporation: The viral DNA then migrates from the cytoplasm into the nucleus, where it is incorporated into the chromosomal DNA of the host cell.

Viral Protein Transcription: Transcription of the viral RNA message occurs within the nucleus of the infected cell. Protein synthesis and assembly of new nucleocapsids with viral RNA then occurs within the cytoplasm.

Budding: New viral particles are then budded through the plasma membrane of the host and are released to infect other cells. The envelope of the new virion comes from the plasma membrane of the host cell.

Death of the Host Cell: Death of the host cell occurs when the viral load reaches a critical concentration, resulting in either lysis of the cell or activation of apoptotic mechanisms.

Clinical infection with HIV-1 begins with a typical acute-phase syndrome seen with any acute viremia, characterized by fever, fatigue, and myalgias. Lymphadenopathy and rash may be present. Viral counts may approach 10^6 virions per milliliter of blood. The acute viral syndrome may be quite indolent and not recognizable as a clinically relevant infection, which likely relates to the effectiveness of the host immune response in suppressing the effects of the acute viral dissemination.

The acute phase of the infection is then followed by clinical latency. The latency lasts as long as a full decade before clinical AIDS is present. During this latent period, the loss of CD4+ T cells is contained by antiviral defenses and by production of new T cells. When CD4+ cell losses exceed the production of new cells, then clinical immuno-suppression ensues and manifestations of AIDS become evident.

With clinical AIDS, a full array of clinical illnesses are seen that have potential relevance to the surgeon. Many of the infections are caused by other viruses (discussed below) because of the immunosuppressed state of the host. AIDS also is associated with several different neoplasms and degenerative central nervous system illnesses.

The diagnosis of HIV infection is suspected in patients with potential exposure to the virus. The infection is assessed initially by the detection of antibodies using enzyme-linked immunosorbent assay (ELISA). If positive, a second ELISA is performed. The concurrence of two positive ELISA studies is highly specific and sensitive for the diagnosis. A rapid ELISA is available that also has high sensitivity and specificity. This rapid assay is used when early presumptive diagnosis may dictate clinical decisions, such as the initiation of chemoprophylaxis for percutaneous exposure of a health care worker when HIV is suspected. The Western blot is then used to confirm the ELISA results. If the ELISA is positive and the Western blot is indetermi-nate, then additional testing using polymerase chain reaction (PCR) or culture of the virus may be required.

Clinical AIDS is considered to exist when the HIV-positive patient has a CD4+ cell count of less than 200/μL or has an indicator condition. The indicator conditions, identified in Box 43–1, are commonly infections, and several are discussed subsequently.

Prevention of HIV infection has been addressed principally by efforts at modifying personal high-risk behavior. Certainly, the risks of HIV transmission from transfusion have been reduced by effective screening of the blood supply. Vaccine development continues to be vigorously pursued, but no effective vaccine has yet evolved.

Therapy for established HIV infection has improved the outcomes and the duration of survival for these patients. A host of different agents have been introduced, and combination therapy is the standard for treatment. The drugs can be grouped into four categories:

1. Nucleoside analog reverse transcriptase inhibitors (e.g., zidovudine, or AZT)—these agents interfere with the DNA polymerase of the reverse transcrip-tase enzyme.

Box 43–1

Clinical Conditions That Fulfill the Revised Case Definition for Diagnosis of Clinical AIDS

Any one of the following combined with a positive HIV serology:

Infectious
- Candidiasis of the upper aerodigestive tract (e.g., esophagus, lungs)
- Extrapulmonary coccidioidomycosis
- Extrapulmonary cryptococcosis
- Extrapulmonary coccidioidomycosis
- Cryptosporidiosis
- Extralymphatic cytomegalovirus infection (e.g., non–lymph node, non–spleen or liver)
- Herpes simplex pneumonia or esophagitis
- Extrapulmonary histoplasmosis
- Isoporosis infection
- Kaposi's sarcoma
- Disseminated tuberculosis, or atypical *Mycobacterium* infection
- Nocardiosis
- *Pneumocystis carinii* infection
- *Salmonella* septicemia
- Extraintestinal *Strongyloides* infection
- Toxoplasmosis

Noninfectious
- Invasive cervical cancer
- HIV-associated wasting or dementia
- Primary CNS lymphoma
- Any non-Hodgkin's or B-cell or undifferentiated type of lymphoma
- Progressive multifocal leukoencephalopathy

---

2. Non-nucleoside reverse transcriptase inhibitors (e.g., nevirapine)—these agents are noncompetitive inhibitors of reverse transcriptase by allosteric inhibition.

3. Nucleotide analog reverse transcriptase inhibitors (e.g., adefovir)—once these agents are converted to the diphosphate form intracellularly, they compete with the natural substrates of reverse transcriptase.

4. Protease inhibitors (e.g., saquinavir)—these com-pounds block the cleavage of polyproteins that are necessary in the late stages of viral replication.

The number of available agents totals more than 20, with many more under investigation. Agents are used in combination to try to optimize synergistic interactions between different drugs, drug pharmacology, interactive toxicities, and likelihood of patient compliance. The scope of possible combinations is enormous and is reviewed elsewhere.

Although surgeons are involved in the care of HIV/AIDS patients for routine problems as well as those commonly associated with the disease itself, the biggest concern has been about occupational risks for disease transmission to the surgeon during the care of these patients. Traditionally, blood exposure and percutaneous injury in the operating room have been a fairly common event. With the recognition of the HIV epidemic, great concern has surfaced about occupational infection. Current data underscore that the overall risk of HIV transmission among health care workers from a hollow needlestick is 0.3%. To date, no transmissions have been documented among surgeons from solid needle injury in an operating room environment in the United States.

Table 43–1 summarizes data from the Centers for Disease Control and Prevention regarding documented or probable transmissions of HIV to health care workers since the beginning of the epidemic. Only six surgeons are identified among the probable transmissions, and none have been documented cases. Probable transmissions refer to those cases in which infected individuals had health care exposures to infected patients, but seroconversion from a specific episode was not documented. The documented cases included individuals with an index exposure event who had a negative HIV serology at the time of exposure, and who then seroconverted subsequently. The overall number of cases is likely to be understated, but the important point is that occupational transmission has not been a common event. The risk of HIV infection for the surgeon is low, but it is not zero. Adherence to barrier protection strategies and avoidance of operating room practice that places the surgeon at risk are very important.

Another issue of importance is the HIV-infected surgeon and whether surgical practice should continue. Transmission of HIV infection from a Florida dentist to several patients is the only recognized occurrence among health care workers. Restriction of privileges for HIV-positive physicians is not warranted, especially when current treatments may bring viral counts to very low numbers. Patients and health care workers should be tested and know their HIV status when clinical criteria so dictate, as a matter of their own health. Neither should be tested as a mandatory policy for either the receipt of care, or the privilege of delivering care.

Hepatitis

The hepatitis viruses are a heterogeneous group of viruses that share the liver cell as an exclusive target (Table 43–2). Other viruses may cause a hepatitis syndrome (e.g., cytomegalovirus), but they are not exclusive to liver cells as their pathologic target. Each of the six different hepatitis viruses has different levels of surgical significance, but all are presented here for completeness.

Hepatitis A

Hepatitis A is an RNA virus that is transmitted by the fecal-oral route when contaminated water or food is ingested. The virus adheres to the epithelial cells of the upper aerodigestive tract or even via the salivary glands. The virus is transported by the circulation and binds to the hepatocyte. Host cell penetration results in release of the RNA of the virus into the cytoplasm, where protein

Table 43–1

Details of documented and possible occupational HIV infections acquired by health care workers

Occupation	Documented Cases	Possible Cases
Nurses	23	35
Clinical lab technicians	16	17
Health aide/attendants	1	15
Emergency medical technicians	0	12
Housekeeping/maintenance personnel	2	13
Nonsurgical physicians	6	12
Surgical physicians	0	6
Others	8	28
TOTAL	56	138

Table 43–2

Pertinent information about the currently recognized hepatitis viruses

Virus (Genome)	Route of Transmission	Important Information
Hepatitis A (RNA)	Fecal-oral	Transmitted by ingestion of contaminated food or water
		No chronic infection; only an acute infection
		Vaccine available for prevention, particularly for foreign travelers
Hepatitis B (DNA)	Blood borne, Sexual contact	5% of acute infections result in chronic infection
		1.25 million people in U.S. have chronic disease
		Highly effective (95%) vaccine is available
Hepatitis C (RNA)	Blood borne, Sexual contact	80% of acute infections result in chronic disease
		4 million people in U.S. have chronic infection
		No vaccine is available for prevention
		Leading indication for liver transplantation
Hepatitis D (RNA)	Blood borne	Requires pre-existent hepatitis B infection
		Prevalence in the U.S. unknown
		Primarily a disease of intravenous drug abusers
		No vaccine; all disease is chronic
Hepatitis E (RNA)	Fecal-oral	Primarily a disease of Southeast Asia
		No chronic infection; no vaccine
Hepatitis F (—)	—	Existence of this virus remains unconfirmed
Hepatitis G (RNA)	Blood borne, Transfusion	Many factors of this disease are unknown
		Uncommonly causes cirrhosis as solitary virus
		4 million people chronically carry the virus
		Synergistic pathogen with hepatitis B and C

synthesis occurs and new viral particles are synthesized without a transcriptional phase. Hepatocyte necrosis is the result. Lysed cells release new viral particles to infect adjacent cells, and shedding of the virus into the bile allows the virus to be released external to the host to potentially infect others. Specific immune responses subsequently contain and eradicate the infection, with death of the host being an uncommon result. There is no chronic phase to hepatitis A virus (HAV) infection and there is no postnecrotic cirrhosis.

The diagnosis of HAV infection is suspected by fever, leukocytosis, malaise, and nonspecific right upper quadrant pain. Symptoms begin 2 to 8 weeks following exposure. Jaundice may be pronounced, and hepatomegaly is usually present. Cutaneous excoriation from pruritus is common. Dramatic elevation of levels of aspartate transaminase (AST) and alanine transaminase (ALT) is present. Alkaline phosphatase is mildly elevated. Detection of immunoglobulin M antibody confirms acute infection, and reverse transcriptase–polymerase chain

reaction (RT-PCR) can be used to detect viral RNA. Immunoglobulin G antibody detection is used to establish prior infection in the patients.

Prevention of HAV infection is by avoidance of contaminated food and water. Contaminated oysters and clams can transmit HAV infection. An effective HAV vaccine currently is available and is recommended for individuals traveling to areas with high endemic rates of HAV. Patients with chronic hepatitis B virus (HBV) and hepatitis C virus (HCV) infection are recommended to have HAV vaccination because of the unusually severe infection that results from HAV in this setting.

When clinical infection occurs, supportive care is the only management strategy. Antiviral chemotherapy is being explored for use in HAV infection, but infection inevitably resolves for all but a few patients. Hospitalizations for intravenous volume support may be necessary in severe cases.

HAV rarely is transmitted by transfusion or by percutaneous injury. Because HAV infection has no chronic phase, it poses no significant occupational risk to health care workers. HAV vaccination is not recommended for occupational risks.

Hepatitis B

Causing a disease originally called serum hepatitis, HBV is a DNA virus that is transmitted by the blood-borne route. Sexual contact, intravenous drug abuse, transfusion, and vertical transmission to the newborn are recognized routes of transmission. Effective screening strategies have largely eliminated risks of transfusion.

HBV particles are absorbed across mucous membrane surfaces. Absorbed or intravascularly introduced particles are delivered to the hepatic circulation, bind to hepatocytes, and are internalized into the cells. Because they are DNA viruses, the transcription process occurs in the nucleus, with the protein synthesis and assembly of new virus occurring in the cytoplasm. Cellular injury of the liver is thought to relate more to the robust response of the host immune system than to the cytotoxicity of the infection.

Acute infection is indolent, with only 25% of patients having a clinical hepatitis syndrome. The absence of significant symptoms results in the remaining 75% of patients not appreciating that they have had acute HBV infection. Whether the patient has a clinically apparent infection or not, 5% of all patients develop chronic HBV infection for the remainder of life. Many will have the carrier state with only limited if any progression of the disease. Some will progress to cirrhosis, end-stage liver disease, portal hypertension, and/or hepatocellular carcinoma over the course of 20 or more years. All are infectious to others. Current estimates indicate that 1.25 million people in the United States have chronic HBV infection.

For the symptomatic patient, acute HBV infection is suspected by a clinical syndrome similar to that seen with acute HAV infection. Definitive diagnosis is made by either antigen or antibody detection. The diagnosis of chronic HBV infection commonly is suspected when patients have blood chemistries done for the evaluation of unrelated problems, or with blood donation. Abnormalities of AST and ALT are seen but are commonly only two to three times above normal values in the patient with chronic infection. Both surface and core antibody are detectable. Chronic HBV infection is positive for the surface antigen, and selected chronic HBV infections will be positive for the "e"-antigen. The e-antigen, a degradation product of the core antigen of the virus, is the result of rapid replication of the virus in the liver. These patients have advancing liver disease, have high viral concentrations in blood, and are especially infectious to others.

Prevention of HBV infection is now possible for most people. A highly effective vaccine from recombinant technology can be administered in three intramuscular doses, with the second and third given at intervals of 1 and 6 months after the first. Surface antibody response must be documented after vaccination because 5% of recipients do not respond to the initial course. Repeat vaccination is recommended for nonresponders.

Chronic HBV infection has been treated with interferon-alfa, with response rates of about 25%. Relapse rates of those responding are high. Lamivudine therapy with or without interferon-alfa also has been reported. Again, like interferon-alfa, relapse rates among responding patients have been high.

Occupational risks for HBV infection remain a source of concern for surgeons and other health care workers. It is estimated that as many as 250 health care workers die annually from occupationally acquired chronic HBV infection. Because a single hollow needlestick exposure carries a 30% risk of transmission, vaccination of all surgeons and health care workers is recommended. If successful vaccination has been achieved, the surgeon is protected against occupational HBV infection from blood exposure in the management of patients. However, older surgeons have not accepted HBV vaccination as readily as have younger surgeons, with as many as one third of surgeons in practice for greater than 10 years not having vaccination, and remaining at risk for HBV infection. For surgeons who have been vaccinated but have not seroconverted to the immunized state, strict adherence to infection control practices and barrier precautions is essential.

Are surgeons with chronic HBV infection a risk to their patients? Should surgeons with known chronic HBV infection continue in clinical practice? These questions continue to be a source of debate. Surgeons who have chronic HBV infection and are positive for the e-antigen of HBV have been shown to transmit the infection to patients. Only one report has demonstrated HBV transmission to patients when the surgeons were negative for the e-antigen. In this latter case, the four surgeons in question were believed to be infected with an unusually virulent mutant of the virus. The position of the American College of Surgeons is detailed in Box 43–2. It is recommended that surgeons know their status with respect to HBV infection. Surgeons with chronic HBV infection should know their e-antigen status. For the surgeon who is positive for the e-antigen, an expert panel should be convened to provide direction for the scope of practice that would guard against HBV transmission to patients.

Hepatitis C

HCV has now become the most significant hepatitis virus in the United States. It is estimated that as many as 4 million people have chronic HCV infection in the United States. Its mode of transmission is similar to that of HIV

Box 43–2

Current Position of the American College of Surgeons with Respect to the Hepatitis B–Infected Surgeon

1. Surgeons should continue to utilize the highest standards of infection control, involving the most effective known sterile barriers, universal precautions, and scientifically accepted infection control practices. This practice should extend to all sites where surgical care is rendered.

2. Surgeons have the same ethical obligations to render care to HBV-infected patients as they have to care for other patients.

3. Surgeons with natural or acquired antibodies to HBV are protected from acquiring HBV from patients. All surgeons (and other members of the operating room team) without natural immunity should be vaccinated against HBV as early as possible in their careers.

4. Surgeons who perform invasive procedures without evidence of immunity to HBV should know their hepatitis B surface antigen (HBsAg) status and, if that is positive, should also know their HBeAg status.

5. Surgeons who are infected with HBV (and are HBeAg positive) should seek counsel from an unbiased expert review panel structured to maintain practitioner confidentiality.

and HBV in that it is a blood-borne virus. Intravenous drug abuse, multiple sexual partners, and blood transfusion (especially before 1992) are risk factors.

HCV is an RNA virus. After gaining access to the circulation, it binds to the hepatocyte and the viral RNA is released into the host cell cytoplasm. Viral protein synthesis and replication occur directly from the nuclear RNA template of the infecting virus. Injury of the host liver is thought to be the consequence of the vigorous interaction between the host response and the virus, rather than direct cell lysis by the large numbers of replicated virus.

HCV infection shares common features with HBV infection. Only about 30% of patients with acute HCV infections have a clearly demonstrable acute hepatitis syndrome, leaving the majority of infected individuals without personal knowledge that infection has occurred. Infection commonly is recognized only when the infected individual donates blood or has laboratory studies done for unrelated medical issues.

Unlike HBV infection, acute HCV infection results in chronic disease in 60% to 80% of infected individuals. When the individual has chronic HCV infection, a varied course in seen. Some patients proceed to end-stage liver disease, cirrhosis, portal hypertension, or hepatocellular carcinoma. Others have a clinically indolent course and do not show progression of the liver disease. All patients with chronic HCV infection are potentially infectious to others.

HCV infection is established by either antibody, antigen, or viral RNA detection. An advanced ELISA has been valuable for blood screening and as the first diagnostic study to establish infection. The diagnosis usually is confirmed by the recombinant immunoblot assay (RIBA). RT-PCR studies will document the presence of the viral RNA in blood and usually are reserved for inconclusive RIBA studies. Because antibody seroconversion may require 6 months or longer after acute infection, RT-PCR may be desirable when high-risk exposures have occurred

and patients wish to know whether transmission have occurred prior to the time of antibody seroconversion.

There is currently no vaccine for HCV. The HCV immunoglobulin has not been effective in preventing infection after exposure. No evidence supports postexposure prophylaxis with interferon-alfa. When acute HCV infection is recognized, interferon-alfa therapy may reduce the risk of developing chronic HCV infection.

With established chronic HCV infection, interferon-alfa therapy initially was shown to have some value. Subsequent studies have demonstrated better outcomes with interferon-alfa plus ribavirin. Nearly 40% of treated patients have had demonstrated clearance of the virus by 6 months. Failure of interferon-alfa and ribavirin is associated with pre-existent cirrhosis, high viral counts in serum, and the type 1 genotype. Unfortunately, the type 1 genotype represents the majority of infections in the United States.

Because of the large numbers of patients with chronic HCV infection, it can be expected that surgeons will encounter large numbers of patients in future years with surgical diseases caused by HCV. End-stage liver disease, portal hypertension, and hepatocellular carcinoma likely will be seen more often among the population with chronic HCV infection as the indolent course of the disease unfolds in the decade after the patient developed the acute infection.

HCV infection is an occupational risk for the surgeon. With hollow needlestick injury, it is currently estimated that a risk of 2% exists for transmission. Solid needlestick injuries are likely to have lower seroconversion rates. Nevertheless, occupationally transmitted disease appears to give surgeons a higher incidence of chronic HCV infection than the population in general. Because there is no vaccine for the prevention of HCV infection, only strict adherence to barrier precautions and safe surgical practice in the operating room will prevent occupational infection from occurring.

Several reports have now identified transmission of HCV infection to patients from chronically infected surgeons. The small number of reports is far less than those for HBV infection. Although it is currently not recommended that chronic HCV-infected surgeons have any restriction to surgical practice, this subject will continue to be re-evaluated in upcoming years as new data become available.

Hepatitis D

Hepatitis D virus (HDV) is an incomplete RNA virus that does not appear to cause infection without the presence of coexistent HBV infection. HDV is a blood-borne virus that has been identified primarily among intravenous drug abusers and multiunit transfusion recipients. Infection with HDV is thought to intensify the severity and accelerate the chronology of clinical events associated with the coexistent HBV infection. The diagnosis is made by either antibody detection or RT-PCR to directly identify the viral RNA. The overall incidence of the disease is unknown, and data about effectiveness of antiviral chemotherapy are inadequate at this time. HDV infection has not been documented as an occupationally transmitted pathogen in health care workers. Effective HBV vaccination should eliminate the risk of HDV infection for surgeons.

Hepatitis E

Hepatitis E virus (HEV) is an RNA virus that is transmitted by the fecal-oral route like HAV. It is primarily identified in Southeast Asia but, with global travel, can be seen occasionally in other areas. Like HAV, HEV is associated with an acute hepatitis illness, which can be quite severe but seldom causes death. Also, like HAV infection, HEV infection is not associated with a chronic illness. Infection does not persist after the acute phase is over. It presents no occupational issues for surgeons, but could be a part of the differential diagnosis in patients with jaundice of unknown origin.

Hepatitis F

Although initially reported to be a unique fecal-oral–transmitted hepatitis virus, the existence of this virus has not been confirmed.

Hepatitis G

Hepatitis G virus (HGV) is a unique blood-borne RNA virus that shares considerable genetic homology with the HCV virus. It is transmitted similarly to HBV and HCV. Acute infection is generally occult. HGV infection has an incidence similar to that of HCV infection. It appears to have infrequent clinical significance in the absence of

coexistent HBV or HCV infection. In can only be diagnosed by RT-PCR. Little can be said about specific therapy at this point. HGV has little clinical or occupational risk for surgeons at this time.

Herpesviruses

Herpesviruses are double-stranded DNA viruses that are becoming of increasingly greater interest to surgeons. There are now eight separate species that cause infection in humans (Table 43–3), but many more are identified as pathogens in animals. The transmission of herpesvirus is usually through oral secretions. Infection begins with release of the viral DNA into the host cell's cytoplasm. The DNA enters the nucleus and begins synthesis of viral proteins and new particles.

An important feature of herpesvirus infection is latency. The acute infection is of variable clinical significance, but the virus remains present in specific cell populations for the lifetime of the host. With biologic stress or immunosuppression, reactivation of infection can occur and remains a potential issue for the life of the host. Over 90% of the U.S. population carries one or more latent herpesviruses.

Human Herpesvirus-1

Human herpesvirus (HHV)-1 is commonly known as herpes simplex type 1. It is associated most commonly with cold sores and conjunctivitis. HHV-1 infection involves the skin and mucous membranes. More than 90% of the U.S. population carries the latent virus within the sensory nerve ganglia. Relapsing infection is common.

Table 43–3		
Common names and estimated adult prevalence of eight types of herpesviruses		
HHV Type	**Common Name**	**Adult Prevalence**
1	Herpes simplex-1	>90%
2	Herpes simplex-2, genital herpes, herpes labialis	10%–35%
3	Varicella-Zoster virus	>90%
4	Epstein-Barr virus	>90%
5	Cytomegalovirus	>50%
6	Exanthema subitum, roseola	>95%
7	HHV-7	>85%
8	Kaposi's sarcoma virus	10%–25%

The diagnosis is usually made by clinical criteria. Acute infection can be documented with acute and convalescent antibody titers. The virus can be cultured from vesicles. Acute infection is self-limited. No vaccine is clinically proven for prevention.

Antiviral chemotherapy may be employed for severe conjunctivitis and for central nervous system infection. Reactivation infection can be seen in transplantation patients and in oncology patients receiving chemotherapy, and these patients require antiviral therapy. Inhibitors of DNA polymerase are the treatment of choice, and include acyclovir and valacyclovir. Valacyclovir is absorbed more effectively from the gut and is the agent of choice.

Human Herpesvirus-2

HHV-2, also known as herpes simplex type 2 or genital herpes, is associated with cutaneous and mucous membrane infection of the genital area. Acute infection has the characteristic vesicular lesions. Between 10% and 35% of adults have HHV-2 infection, with the latent virus residing within sensory or autonomic ganglia.

Infection occurs from sexual contact, but the virus also is transmitted vertically from infected mothers to children. Transmission can occur whether the infected individual has clinical evidence of vesicles present or not. Reactivation disease is seen in transplantation patients, induction chemotherapy patients, AIDS patients, and severe trauma patients. The diagnosis is a clinical one that can be confirmed by cultures of the virus or by PCR studies.

Acyclovir therapy is used for symptomatic treatment of reactivation disease in the genital area, and for the patient with nongenital manifestations associated with immunosuppression. Antiviral treatment does not eradicate the virus.

Human Herpesvirus-3

HHV-3 is the varicella-zoster virus. The acute infection occurs following inhalation of droplet secretions that result in the macular-to-vesicular-to-crusted lesions of chickenpox. Severe cases may have pneumonia, hepatitis, or central nervous system infection. Chickenpox is associated with secondary group A streptococcal necrotizing fasciitis. Resolution of the acute infection results in lifetime latency of the virus in the sensory ganglia. In the course of a lifetime, it is estimated that 20% of patients with childhood chickenpox will develop herpes zoster (i.e., shingles) as reactivation disease. Reactivation occurs as painful neuritis with a vesicular rash occurring in a dermatome distribution. Herpes zoster is associated with aging, transplantation, cancer, and corticosteroid therapy. The neuritis is quite painful and may persist long after resolution of the dermatomal rash.

The diagnosis is a clinical one, but can be confirmed by cultures, PCR, or immunofluorescent stains. An effective vaccine for the virus is available and is strongly recommended for all children. Acyclovir/valacyclovir therapy is recommended for immunosuppressed patients with acute infection. It is also recommended for herpes zoster to reduce the longevity of the rash and perhaps the longevity and severity of the neuritis.

Human Herpesvirus-4

HHV-4 is more commonly known as Epstein-Barr virus. Acute infection occurs from contaminated saliva with resultant viral proliferation in the B cell of the regional lymph nodes. Infection begins within 2 weeks of transmission and is characterized by the mononucleosis syndrome of fever, pharyngitis, and lymphadenopathy. Occasional severe infection may include hepatitis, aplastic anemia, and meningoencephalitis. Acute infection usually resolves within a month of onset of symptoms, but the latent virus remains for life within B cells and the salivary glands. About 90% of adults have antibodies to HHV-4.

Diagnosis of HHV-4 infection is made by the identification of heterophile antibodies. In difficult cases, the virus can be cultured, specific viral antigen can be detected, or PCR can be used.

Therapy of the acute infection is symptomatic care only for the vast majority of cases. Antiviral chemotherapy (acyclovir) may be used in unusually severe acute infections. Acyclovir does not affect the latency of the infection. No effective vaccine has been developed as yet.

Relapsing infection with HHV-4 is thought to be in the form of malignancies and lymphoproliferative disorders that are associated with the virus. Burkitt's lymphoma, nasopharyngeal cancer, gastric cancer, thymoma, and salivary gland cancers are associated with HHV-4.

Human Herpesvirus-5

HHV-5 is cytomegalovirus. Transmission of the virus occurs from saliva, vertical transmission at birth, breast milk, organ transplantation, and blood transfusion, as well as by sexual contact. More than 50% of adults carry the latent virus in monocytes and neutrophils. Clinically recognized acute infection is not common. The acute infection presents as a mononucleosis-like syndrome. Neonatal infection is severe and causes cytomegalic inclusion disease. Severe acute cases in older patients may include hepatitis, pneumonitis, myocarditis, and chorioretinitis. Relapsing disease is a particular problem in immunosuppressed transplant patients, who will have gastroenteritis with perforation in addition to hepatitis, interstitial pneumonia, chorioretinitis, and the like. AIDS patients will have manifestations of this infection similar to those seen in the transplant population. Of interest, HHV-5 has even been associated with the pathogenesis of atherosclerosis.

The diagnosis is of greatest concern in transplant, AIDS, and neonatal cases. Viral cultures and PCR are commonly used. Identification of the characteristic inclusions bodies in tissue specimens is most dependable.

Prevention of reactivation disease is of greatest value in transplant patients. Using ganciclovir and acyclovir during the initial 4 to 6 months after transplantation has been useful. Hyperimmune globulin has been of value in kidney transplant patients. With established HHV-5 infection in the immunocompromised patient, ganciclovir is used for therapy.

Human Herpesvirus-6

HHV-6 is the causative virus of roseola. This acute infection is characterized by high fever and a maculopapular rash. The disease is transmitted by oral secretions. Antibody evidence shows nearly ubiquitous evidence of prior infection in the population by age 2, even though only 15% of children have a clinical infection. Latent virus after the acute infection resides in macrophages.

Relapsing disease is seen with immunosuppressed patients and is characterized by a mononucleosis-like syndrome, bone marrow suppression, and interstitial pneumonia. Clinical associations include various cancers, chronic fatigue syndrome, and multiple sclerosis.

The diagnosis in children is usually based upon clinical criteria. The diagnosis is established by acute/convalescent serum antibodies, culture of the virus from lymphocytes, or PCR of plasma or cerebrospinal fluid.

No vaccine is presently available. Antiviral therapy is not proven for this infection, although HHV-6 is thought to be sensitive to ganciclovir and foscarnet.

Human Herpesvirus-7

Infection by HHV-7 is common in children, and presents as a clinical syndrome that is similar to HHV-6. It is transmitted in saliva, and the virus resides and is latent after acute infection in the CD4+ lymphocyte. Reactivation is seen with immunosuppression and is associated with chronic fatigue syndrome and pityriasis rosea. Diagnosis is by several antibody detection methods, and the virus can be cultured. Specific antiviral therapy has not been explored.

Human Herpesvirus-8

HHV-8 is the Kaposi's sarcoma virus. Acute infection produces fever and lymphadenopathy in AIDS patients, but no clinical syndrome is identified in immunocompetent hosts. Lymphocytes are the target cells, and epithelial cells are the latent reservoir. It is thought to be present in 10% to 25% of adults. Transmission occurs by sexual contact, organ transplantation, and blood transfusion. HHV-8 may be synergistic with HHV-4 in oncogenesis.

HHV-8 also is associated with lymphoma, sarcoma, pemphigus, Castleman's disease, and multiple myeloma. Cultures of the virus, PCR, and immunohistochemical staining methods are used for diagnosis. Antiviral therapy is being explored.

Summary

Viruses likely will be pathogens of greater interest to surgeons in the years ahead. The role of viruses in surgical disease is probably greater than is understood at the present time. The explosion in gene research will identify genetic sequences that likely will be of viral origin, and will lead to a greater appreciation of viral particles in oncogenesis, central nervous system diseases, perhaps vascular disease, and other diseases.

Bibliography

Alter MJ: Community-acquired viral hepatitis B and C in the United States. Gut 1993;34(Suppl 2):517.

Alter MJ: Epidemiology of hepatitis C. Hepatology 1997;26(Suppl 1):62S.

American College of Surgeons: Statement on the surgeon and hepatitis B infection. Bull Am Coll Surg 1995;80:33.

Anonymous: Hepatitis C virus transmission from health-care worker to patient. CDR Wkly 1995;5:121.

Atrah H, Ahmed M: Hepatitis C virus seroconversion by a third-generation ELISA screening test in blood donors. J Clin Pathol 1996;49:254.

Beutner KR, Friedman DJ, Forszpaniak C, et al: Valaciclovir compared with acyclovir for improved therapy for herpes zoster in immunocompetent adults. Antimicrob Agents Chemother 1995;39:1546.

Bonino F, Smedile A: Delta agent (type D) hepatitis. Semin Liver Dis 1986;6:28.

Centers for Disease Control: Guidelines for prevention of transmission of human immunodeficiency virus and hepatitis B virus to health-care and public safety workers. MMWR Morb Mortal Wkly Rep 1989;38:1.

Centers for Disease Control: 1993 Revised classification system for HIV infection and expanded surveillance case definition for AIDS among adolescents and adults. MMWR Morb Mortal Wkly Rep 1992;41:1.

Centers for Disease Control and Prevention: Recommendations for follow-up of health care workers after occupational exposure to hepatitis C virus. MMWR Morb Mortal Wkly Rep 1997;46:603.

Centers for Disease Control and Prevention: Recommendations for prevention and control of hepatitis C virus (HCV) infection and HCV-related chronic disease. MMWR Morb Mortal Wkly Rep 1998;47:1.

Committee on Infectious Diseases: Recommendations for the use of live attenuated varicella vaccine. Pediatrics 1995;95:791.

Corey L, Holmes KK: Sexual transmission of hepatitis A in homosexual men: incidence and mechanism. N Engl J Med 1980;302:435.

Deka N, Sharma MD, Mukerjee R: Isolation of the novel agent from human stool samples that is associated with sporadic non-A, non-B hepatitis. J Virol 1994;68:7810.

Dienstag JL, Perrillo RP, Schiff ER, et al: A preliminary trial of lamivudine for chronic hepatitis B infection. N Engl J Med 1995;333:1657.

Division of HIV/AIDS Prevention, National Center for HIV, STD and TB Prevention, Centers for Disease Control and Prevention: Table 17: Documented and possible occupationally acquired AIDS/HIV infection, by occupation, reported through June 2000, United States. *In* HIV/AIDS Surveillance Report, Vol 12. Atlanta, Centers for Disease Control and Prevention, 2000. Available at *www.cdc.gov/hiv/stats/hasr1201/table17.htm*

Esteban JI, Gomez J, Martell M, et al: Transmission of hepatitis C virus by a cardiac surgeon. N Engl J Med 1996;334:555.

Fry DE: Human immunodeficiency virus infection. *In* Fry DE (ed): Surgical Infections. Boston: Little, Brown, 1995:669.

Fry DE: Microbiology of Surgical Pathogens. *In* Fry DE (ed): Surgical Infections. Boston: Little, Brown, 1995:11.

Fry DE: Herpesvirus infection: an emerging nosocomial pathogen? Surg Infect 2001;2:121.

Gottlieb MS, Schroff R, Schanker HM, et al: Pneumocystis carinii pneumonia and mucosal candidiasis in previously healthy homosexual men: evidence of a new acquired cellular immunodeficiency. N Engl J Med 1981;305:1431.

Hanna GJ, Hirsch MS: Antiretroviral therapy of human immunodeficiency virus infection. *In* Mandell GL, Bennett JE, Dolin R (eds): Principles and Practice of Infectious Disease. New York: Churchill Livingstone, 2000;1479.

Harpaz R, von Seidlein L, Averhoff FM, et al: Transmission of hepatitis B virus to multiple patients from a surgeon without evidence of inadequate infection control. N Engl J Med 1996;334:549.

Heptonstall J, and the Incident Investigation Team: Transmission of hepatitis B to patients from four infected surgeons without hepatitis B e antigen. N Engl J Med 1997;336:178.

Hidaku Y, Liu Y, Yamamoto M, et al: Frequent isolation of human herpesvirus 7 from saliva samples. J Med Virol 1993;40:343.

Jones CA, Isaacs D: Human herpes virus-6 infections. Arch Dis Child 1996;74:98.

Koretz RL, Brezina M, Polito AJ, et al: Non-A, non-B posttransfusion hepatitis: comparing C and non-C hepatitis. Hepatology 1993;17:361.

Krugman S, Ward R, Giles JP: The natural history of infectious hepatitis. Am J Med 1962;32:717.

Lee WM: Hepatitis B virus infection. N Engl J Med 1997;337:1733.

Linnen J, Wages J Jr, Zhang-Keck Z-Y, et al: Molecular cloning and disease association of hepatitis G virus: a transfusion-transmissible agent. Science 1996;271:505.

Martin M, Manez R, Linden P, et al: A prospective randomized trial comparing sequential ganciclovir-high dose acyclovir to high dose acyclovir for prevention of cytomegalovirus disease in adult liver transplant recipients. Transplantation 1994;58:779.

McHutchison JG, Gordon SC, Schiff ER, et al: Interferon alfa-2b alone or in combination with ribavirin as initial treatment for chronic hepatitis C. N Engl J Med 1998;339:1485.

Nahmias AJ, Lee FK, Bechman-Nahmias S: Sero-epidemiological and sociological patterns of herpes simplex virus infection in the world. Scand J Infect Dis 1990;69:19.

Niederau C, Heintges T, Lange S, et al: Long-term follow-up of HBeAg-positive patients treated with interferon alfa for chronic hepatitis B. N Engl J Med 1996;334:1422.

Nocera A, Corbellino M, Valente U, et al: Posttransplant human herpes virus 8 infection and seroconversion in a Kaposi's sarcoma affected kidney recipient transplanted from a human herpes virus 8 positive living related donor. Transplant Proc 1998;30:2095.

Okano M: Epstein-Barr virus infection and its role in the expanding spectrum of human diseases. Acta Paediatr 1998;87:11.

Pereira MS, Blake JM, Macrae AD: EB virus antibody at different ages. Br Med J 1969;4:526.

Popejoy SL, Fry DE: Blood contact and exposure in the operating room. Surg Gynecol Obstet 1991;172:480.

Poynard T, Leroy V, Cohard M, et al: Meta-analysis of interferon randomized trials in the treatment of viral hepatitis C: effects of dose and duration. Hepatology 1996;24:778.

Quebbeman EJ, Telford GL, Hubbard S, et al: Risk of blood contamination and injury to operating room personnel. Ann Surg 1991;214:614.

Rakela J, Mosley JW, Redeker AG: The role of hepatitis A virus in fulminant hepatitis. Gastroenterology 1975;69:854.

Reyes GR, Purdy MA, Kim JP, et al: Isolation of a cDNA from the virus responsible for enteric transmitted non-A, non-B hepatitis. Science 1990;247:1335.

Seeff LB, Koff RS: Evolving concepts of the clinical and serologic consequences of hepatitis B virus infection. Semin Liver Dis 1986;6:11.

Shapiro CN: Occupational risk of infection with hepatitis B and hepatitis C virus. Surg Clin North Am 1995;75:1047.

Skiest DJ: Cytomegalovirus retinitis in the era of highly active antiretroviral therapy. Am J Med Sci 1999;317:318.

Slusarczyk J, Hess G, Meyer zum Buschenfelde K-H: Association of hepatitis B e antigen(HBeAg) with the core of the hepatitis B virus. Liver 1985;5:48.

Smith MA, Brennessel DJ: Cytomegalovirus. Infect Dis Clin North Am 1994;8:427.

Smith S, Weber S, Wiblin T, Nettleman M: Cost-effectiveness of hepatitis A vaccination in healthcare workers. Infect Control Hosp Epidemiol 1997;18:688.

Spijkerman IJB, van Doorn L-J, Janssen MHW, et al: Transmission of hepatitis B virus from a surgeon to his patients during high-risk and low-risk surgical procedures during 4 years. Infect Control Hosp Epidemiol 2002;23:306.

Streicher HZ, Reitz MS Jr, Gallo RC: Human immunodeficiency viruses. *In* Mandell GL, Bennett JE, Dolin R (eds): Principles and Practice of Infectious Disease. New York: Churchill Livingstone, 2000:1874.

Stokes J, Berk JE, Malamut LL, et al: The carrier state of viral hepatitis. JAMA 1954;1059.

Wang K-S, Choo Q-L, Weiner AJ, et al: Structure, sequence and expression of the hepatitis delta viral genome. Nature 1986;323:508.

Weller S, Blum MR, Doucette M, et al: Pharmacokinetics of the acyclovir pro-drug valacyclovir after escalating single- and multiple-dose administration to normal volunteers. Clin Pharmacol Ther 1993;54:595.

Wharton M: The epidemiology of varicella-zoster virus infections. Infect Dis Clin North Am 1996;10:571.

Whitley RJ, Gnann JW Jr: Acyclovir: a decade later. N Engl J Med 1992;327:782.

Whitley RJ, Kimberlin DW, Roizman B: Herpes simplex viruses. Clin Infect Dis 1998;26:541.

Williams WW, Hickson MA, Kane MA, et al: Immunization policies and vaccine coverage among adults: the risk for missed opportunities. Ann Intern Med 1988;108:616.

Zajac BA, West DJ, McAleer WJ, Scolnick EM: Overview of clinical studies with hepatitis B vaccine made by recombinant DNA. J Infect Dis 1986;13(Suppl A):39.

PART IX

Anesthesia

CHAPTER 44

General Anesthesia

Randy W. Calicott, M.D. and Deborah M. Whelan, M.D.

S urgery's defining moment was not possible until the issues of pain and infection were addressed. We deal with the former of these in this chapter. Until patients could be rendered insensate to pain, the only common procedures possible were draining of abscesses and amputation of limbs. Anesthesia is defined as "loss of feeling or sensation . . . it is applied especially to loss of the sensation of pain, as it is induced to permit the performance of surgery or other painful procedures."

Preoperative Assessment

Preoperative assessment has become an increasingly critical component of anesthetic management. With the advent of "fiscal responsibility," the luxury of a total work-up during a hospital admission is past. The current trend of same-day surgeries or admissions the day of surgery demands that the work-up for surgical patients be quick, efficient, and thorough.

Laboratory Tests

In the past, as new tests became available, they were ordered frequently and without scientific purpose. This practice of ordering large numbers of laboratory tests purely for data collection has passed. Currently, the practice is to order laboratory tests that are procedure and patient specific. Many institutions now require specific labs to be ordered based on age, procedure to be performed, or medical status of the patient. Sample general guidelines are given in Table 44–1.

Guidelines for Type and Screen (T&S) and Type and Crossmatch (T&C)

Category 1 (no T&S or T&C): The following procedures offer minimal risk to the patient, or are minimally invasive procedures with little or no blood loss: breast biopsy, removal of minor skin or subcutaneous lesions, placement of myringotomy tubes, hysteroscopy, cystoscopy, vasectomy, circumcision, and fiberoptic bronchoscopy.

Category 2 (no T&S or T&C): The following procedures are more invasive and/or have the possibility of less than 500 mL of blood loss to the patient, and therefore present a moderate risk to the patient: diagnostic laparoscopy, dilatation and curettage, fallopian tube ligation, arthroscopy, inguinal hernia repair, laparoscopic lysis of adhesions, tonsillectomy/adenoidectomy, umbilical hernia repair, septoplasty/rhinoplasty, percutaneous lung biopsy, laparoscopic cholecystectomy, and extensive superficial procedures.

Category 3 (T&S or T&C and Hematocrit): The following procedures are significantly more invasive

Table 44-1

General guidelines for preoperative assessment labs: simplified strategy for preoperative testing

Preoperative Condition	Preoperative Test*†												
	HH	CBC	LC	PT/PTT	BT	EC	Cr/BUN	BMP‡	BG	Mg	K	U/A	SGOT/AP
Hypertension	X						X						
Malignancy			L	L									
Radiation therapy			X										
Hepatic disease				X									X
Exposure to hepatitis													X
Renal disease	X			X		X	X	±					
Bleeding disorder	±			X	X								
Diabetes							X	±	X				
Family history of diabetes									X				
Use of digoxin							X				X		
Use of steroids						X		±	X				
Use of anticoagulants	±			X									
Suspected urinary tract infection						±						X	
Hypokalemia or diuretics								±		X	X		
Arrhythmia history										X	X		
Cisplatin										X	X		
History of excessive alcohol consumption													X

*H&H, hemoglobin (M) and hematocrit; CBC, complete blood count; LC, leukocyte count; PT/PTT, prothrombin time/partial thromboplastin time; EC, electrolyte count; Cr/BUN, creatinine/blood urea nitrogen; BMP, basic metabolic panel; BG, blood glucose; Mg, magnesium; K, potassium; U/A, urinalysis; SGOT/AP, serum glutamic-oxaloacetic transaminase/alkaline phosphatase.

†X = obtain; L = obtain for leukemias only; ± = perhaps obtain.

‡Consider BMP as a less expensive alternative to multiple individual tests (e.g., electrolytes, BUN, glucose).

and have the possibility of 500 to 1000 mL of blood loss: hysterectomy, myomectomy, cystectomy, cholecystectomy, laminectomy, hip/knee replacement, nephrectomy, major laparoscopic procedures, and resection/reconstructive surgery of the digestive tract.

Category 4 (T&C and Hematocrit): Highly invasive procedures with the possibility of blood loss greater than 1500 mL are major orthopedic surgery, major reconstructive surgery of the gastrointestinal tract, major genitourinary tract surgery, or major vascular repair.

Category 5 (T&C and Hematocrit): These procedures are again highly invasive and have the possibility of greater than 1500 mL of blood loss: cardiothoracic, intracranial, major oropharyngeal, and major vascular surgery.

Obviously, if the patient has an anticoagulation problem, appropriate blood products should be available for most all procedures.

Airway Evaluation

Inability to secure an airway is one of the quickest ways to end a case before it begins. The airway exam is one of the crucial components of the preoperative visit. The anesthetic concern is the ability to mask ventilate and intubate the patient.

The patient's airway examination includes four measurements. The first is the Mallampati classification (with Samsoon and Young modification). There are four Mallampati classes (Fig. 44–1). The Mallampati class is obtained with the patient's mouth wide open and the tongue protruding without phonation. The second measurement is the thyromental distance. This is the distance from the hyoid or thyroid cartilage to the mental protuberance of the mandible. The distance is measured in fingerbreadths; normal is greater than 6.5 cm or 3 fingerbreadths. The third measurement is the mouth opening, again measured in fingerbreadths. Normal is greater than 2.5 fingerbreadths. The fourth measurement is the sternomental distance and is measured from the sternal notch to the mental protuberance of the mandible with the neck fully extended. Normal is 12 cm or greater. If any of these measurements is less than normal, this implies a potentially difficult intubation.

The American Society of Anesthesiologists (ASA) has become the leader in difficult airway management with the development and generalized implementation of a difficult airway algorithm (Fig. 44–2). The algorithm begins with the recognized and unrecognized difficult intubation.

The patient who has a known difficult airway or one that is labeled difficult by exam can have his or her airway secured by an awake intubation or tracheostomy if deemed necessary. It is the unanticipated difficult airway that is of greatest concern. Patients in this category can be separated into two groups also: the patient who can be ventilated, and the more serious airway emergency patient who cannot be ventilated or intubated.

Anesthetic Considerations

Concurrent Disease States

Cardiovascular

The patient's cardiovascular status is one of the major concerns addressed during the examination of the patient. The functional status needs to be documented by history as well as by laboratory examination. There needs to be documentation of the patient's activity of daily living, chest pain, effective treatment of angina, history of congestive heart failure or myocardial infarction, and current therapy. Any old or new electrocardiographs should be available, as well as the results of other invasive or noninvasive cardiac tests that have been performed. The question that needs to be answered is "What is the patient's functional status, and is it maximal?" A general anesthetic can be safely delivered to patients with severe cardiac disease, but the drugs used must be evaluated for their hemodynamic stability. Drugs such as etomidate and vecuronium, which have no cardiac depressant effects or histamine release, can be used. Current data suggest but do not statistically support increased postoperative morbidity with diastolic pressure greater than 110 mm Hg. Poorly controlled hypertensive patients are more likely to develop intraoperative episodes of myocardial ischemia, arrhythmias, and labile blood pressure. Though again there is no statistically supported increase in long-term morbidity, the subsequent work-up for intraoperative cardiac events may increase morbidity secondary to testing, as well as increase the hospital length of stay and the patient's financial responsibility. Poorly controlled hypertension and elevated diastolic pressures in a presenting patient need to be managed prior to surgery; however, if the patient's condition is deemed emergent, then a minimally stressful induction is indicated.

Pulmonary

Again, the functional status of the patient will need to be determined prior to elective surgery. Has the patient recently been treated for an upper respiratory infection? Is the patient febrile? Is there a productive cough, or is there new-onset wheezing? If so, the surgery, unless emergent or urgent, may need to be delayed approximately 6 weeks secondary to an increased incidence of intraoperative and postoperative reactive airway issues. If the patient has significant reactive airway disease, is he or she on maximum therapy? Has the patient recently been on steroids or intubated and ventilated as a result of pulmonary disease? If the scheduled surgery is for excision of an anterior mediastinal mass, is there significant compression of airway structures? Documentation of any old or new pulmonary function test must be available. General anesthesia and positive pressure ventilation may disrupt a tenuous balance for a patient with advanced chronic obstructive pulmonary disease and precipitate prolonged postoperative ventilatory support. For these patients, when undergoing thoracic or abdominal procedures, an epidural or paravertebral block should be offered to assist with extubation and prevent splinting after surgery.

Cerebrovascular

Neurologic procedures are often performed on patients in whom even small alterations in technique may cause severe morbidity. The neurosurgeon has the misfortune to operate on an organ that cannot accommodate an expanding mass; this results in the manipulation of the cerebrospinal fluid pressure, cerebral blood flow, and cerebral perfusion pressure (mean arterial blood pressure minus the central venous pressure or intracerebral pressure, whichever is greater). Brain and spinal cord injuries often have insufficient perfusion and need blood pressure support. Also, operating conditions should be optimized for

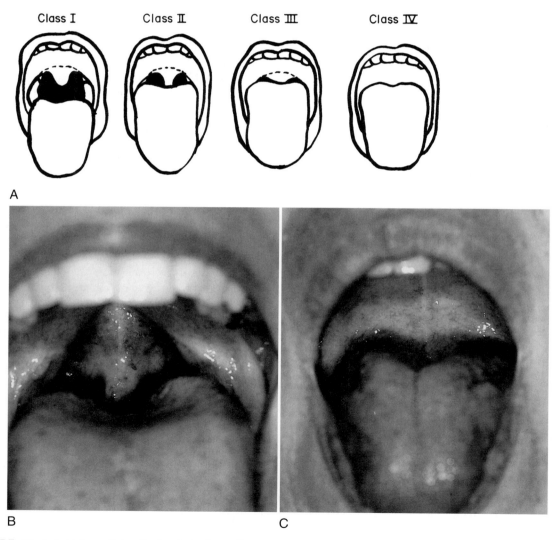

FIGURE 44–1 A, Mallampati classification. A drawing and its corresponding photo below illustrate each class. **B**, Class I is defined as clear visualization of the tonsil pillars and uvula. **C**, Class II is visualization of the arch, uvula, and some of the tonsil pillars.

Figure continued on opposite page

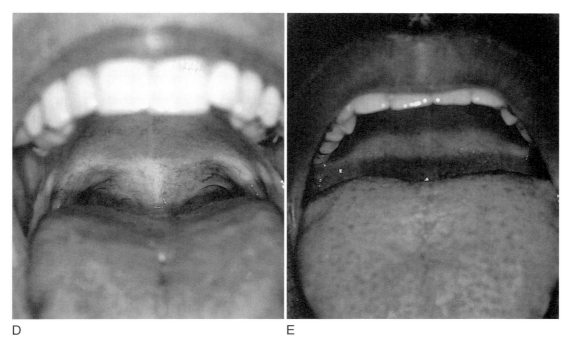

D   E

FIGURE 44–1 *Continued* **D**, Class III is visualization of the soft palate and partial view of the arch. **E**, Class IV is visualization of the hard palate only. (Line drawings from Anaesthesia 1987;42:487. By kind permission of The Association of Anesthetists of Great Britain and Ireland.)

the neurosurgeon, and neuromuscular blockade, hyperventilation, and diuretics are often necessary.

Renal

Patients with end-stage renal disease will be unable to metabolize or eliminate anesthetic drugs by this method. Care should be taken in the selection of agents that will be prolonged in the face of decreased kidney function, such as pancuronium. Even short episodes of hypotension can disrupt flow in an arteriovenous fistula and cause thrombosis; therefore, the fistula site should be monitored throughout the case.

Gastrointestinal

The major concern with any gastrointestinal malady is the presentation of a patient with a "full stomach" and its associated risk of aspiration. Any bleeding in the anterior portion of the alimentary tract predisposes to nausea and vomiting, with subsequent hypovolemia and possibly hypotension upon induction of a general anesthetic. A rapid-sequence induction with cricoid pressure is the safest and preferred technique.

Endocrine

Diabetes is the most common endocrine disorder encountered by anesthesiologists. Patients with diabetes should have blood glucose levels monitored preoperatively, during surgery, and in the postanesthesia care unit.

Oral hypoglycemic agents should be withheld the morning of surgery, and regular insulin doses are usually halved. Longer acting, lente insulin doses may be given or reduced, depending on the anticipated time of surgery. Diabetics often have cardiac, renal, and neurologic abnormalities, along with decreased gastric emptying. A hemodynamically stable rapid-sequence induction is often indicated.

ASA Physical Status

The preoperative assessment culminates in the classification of the patient's ASA physical status. In 1961 the ASA developed a grading system based upon physical status. Initially there were five classifications, but a sixth category was added to address organ procurement patients (Table 44–2). Table 44–3 lists the mortality rates related to the different ASA physical status classifications.

NPO Status

Nil per os (NPO) status is currently undergoing a change in anesthesia. Anesthesiologists, surgeons, and patients are challenging the standard "NPO after midnight" restriction for all patients, regardless of age and scheduled time of procedure. An easy and safe NPO schedule for children of all ages is 2 hours' fast for clear fluids, 4 hours for breast milk, and 6 hours for formula or solids.

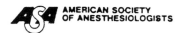

AMERICAN SOCIETY OF ANESTHESIOLOGISTS

DIFFICULT AIRWAY ALGORITHM

1. Assess the likelihood and clinical impact of basic management problems:

    A. Difficult Intubation

    B. Difficult Ventilation

    C. Difficulty with Patient Cooperation or Consent

2. Consider the relative merits and feasibility of basic management choices:

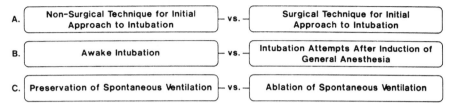

A. Non-Surgical Technique for Initial Approach to Intubation — vs. — Surgical Technique for Initial Approach to Intubation

B. Awake Intubation — vs. — Intubation Attempts After Induction of General Anesthesia

C. Preservation of Spontaneous Ventilation — vs. — Ablation of Spontaneous Ventilation

3. Develop primary and alternative strategies:

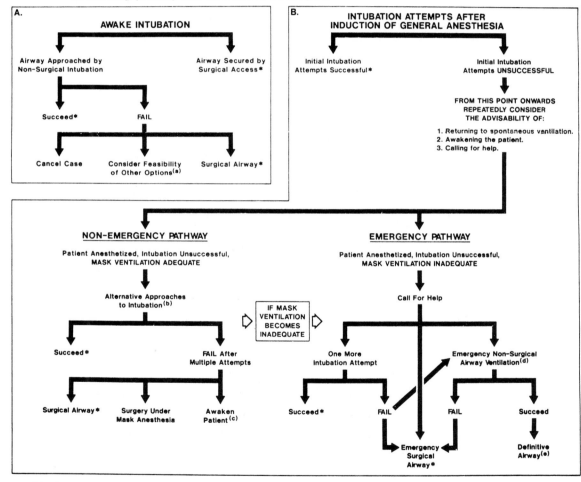

A. AWAKE INTUBATION

Airway Approached by Non-Surgical Intubation — Airway Secured by Surgical Access *

Succeed * — FAIL

Cancel Case — Consider Feasibility of Other Options (a) — Surgical Airway *

B. INTUBATION ATTEMPTS AFTER INDUCTION OF GENERAL ANESTHESIA

Initial Intubation Attempts Successful* — Initial Intubation Attempts UNSUCCESSFUL

FROM THIS POINT ONWARDS REPEATEDLY CONSIDER THE ADVISABILITY OF:
1. Returning to spontaneous ventilation.
2. Awakening the patient.
3. Calling for help.

NON-EMERGENCY PATHWAY

Patient Anesthetized, Intubation Unsuccessful, MASK VENTILATION ADEQUATE

Alternative Approaches to Intubation (b)

Succeed * — FAIL After Multiple Attempts

Surgical Airway * — Surgery Under Mask Anesthesia — Awaken Patient (c)

IF MASK VENTILATION BECOMES INADEQUATE

EMERGENCY PATHWAY

Patient Anesthetized, Intubation Unsuccessful, MASK VENTILATION INADEQUATE

Call For Help

One More Intubation Attempt — Emergency Non-Surgical Airway Ventilation (d)

Succeed * — FAIL — FAIL — Succeed

Emergency Surgical Airway * — Definitive Airway (e)

---

* CONFIRM INTUBATION WITH EXHALED CO_2

(a) Other options include (but are not limited to): surgery under mask anesthesia, surgery under local anesthesia infiltration or regional nerve blockade, or intubation attempts after induction of general anesthesia.

(b) Alternative approaches to difficult intubation include (but are not limited to): use of different laryngoscope blades, awake intubation, blind oral or nasal intubation, fiberoptic intubation, intubating stylet or tube changer, light wand, retrograde intubation, and surgical airway access.

(c) See awake intubation.

(d) Options for emergency non-surgical airway ventilation include (but are not limited to): transtracheal jet ventilation, laryngeal mask ventilation, or esophageal-tracheal combitube ventilation.

(e) Options for establishing a definitive airway include (but are not limited to): returning to awake state with spontaneous ventilation, tracheotomy, or endotracheal intubation.

Table 44-2
ASA physical status classification

ASA Classification	Definition
I	A normal healthy patient
II	A patient with mild systemic disease and no functional limitation
III	A patient with moderate to severe systemic disease that results in some functional limitation
IV	A patient with severe systemic disease that is a constant threat to life and functionally incapacitating
V	A moribund patient who is not expected to survive 24 hours with or without surgery
VI	A brain-dead patient whose organs are being harvested
E	If the procedure is an emergency, the classification is followed by an "E."

Adults may also have clear fluids up to 2 hours prior to surgery, with a 6-hour fast for solids. The concern for a full stomach should be balanced with the concern for a patient becoming significantly dehydrated prior to surgery.

Monitoring

Routine

The ASA set forth the "Standards for Basic Intraoperative Monitoring" on October 21, 1989, with amendments dated October 13, 1993. These standards are as follows:

Standard I: "Qualified anesthesia personnel shall be present in the room throughout the conduct of all general anesthetics, regional anesthetics, and monitored anesthesia care."

Standard II: "During anesthetics the patient's oxygenation, ventilation, circulation, and temperature shall be continually evaluated. The minimal recommendations are electrocardiography (ECG/EKG), pulse oximetry, oxygen analyzer, blood pressure, availability of temperature monitoring, and, if intubated, end tidal capnography."

Invasive

Central venous access can be achieved via the internal jugular, subclavian, or femoral vein depending upon the surgical site. Arterial access is usually via the radial artery, but can be femoral or brachial depending upon surgical site or the patient's peripheral vascular disease or injuries. Transesophageal echocardiography can be used to evaluate cardiac function and therapeutic responses to inotropes.

The indications for invasive monitoring should be based upon therapeutic or diagnostic needs. Pulmonary artery catheterization or transesophageal echocardiography should be considered in patients with significant cardiac history. Large-bore peripheral intravenous access or large-bore central access will be necessary for patients with massive blood loss and subsequent transfusion or fluid shifts requiring large volumes of crystalloids. The requirement of frequent laboratory evaluations may necessitate either central access or arterial line placement. The arterial catheter is also necessary for patients requiring continuous monitoring of blood pressure secondary to significant cardiac disease, hypertension, trauma, or expected large fluid shifts or massive blood loss.

General Anesthesia

Inhalation Agents (Table 44-4)

While most commonly used for maintenance of general anesthesia, inhalation agents may also be employed for induction. This method is usually reserved for pediatric patients and occasionally for patients requiring continued spontaneous ventilation. Each agent has different properties that lend it advantages and disadvantages in various circumstances.

FIGURE 44-2 American Society of Anesthesiologists difficult airway algorithm. (From Practice guidelines for management of the difficult airway: a report by the American Society of Anesthesiologists Task Force on Management of the Difficult Airway. Anesthesiology 1993;78:597, with permission.)

Table 44–3
Mortality rates related to ASA physical status classification

ASA Classification	Mortality Rate (%)
I	0.06–0.08
II	0.27–0.4
III	1.8–4.3
IV	7.8–23
V	9.4–51

Equipotent doses of inhalational agents are measured as minimal anesthetic concentration (MAC). MAC is the percent vapor required to prevent 50% of patients from moving with surgical stimulation.

Intravenous Agents (Table 44–5)

Intravenous agents derive from a variety of pharmaceutical classes, including barbiturates and benzodiazepines. Although these drugs can be used as an infusion for continued unconsciousness, they are typically used for induction. At lower doses these agents can be used for conscious sedation. The use of these agents for sedation or induction requires basic anesthesia monitoring—pulse oximetry, electrocardiogram, and blood pressure. In patients with cardiovascular compromise, induction may result in significant hypotension, respiratory depression, and possibly cardiovascular and pulmonary arrest.

Neuromuscular Blocking Agents (Table 44–6)

The neuromuscular blocking agents are used to facilitate intubation, to allow maximum surgical exposure, or to assist with ventilator support. Any patient who is chemically paralyzed may be conscious but unable to communicate, and therefore may require either general anesthesia or adequate sedation and analgesia.

Narcotics (Table 44–7)

Narcotics provide preoperative, intraoperative, and postoperative analgesia. Because narcotics are not able to provide amnesia, they are not used as sole anesthetics. Again, as with the induction agents, the patient's cardiovascular and pulmonary status may result in cardiovascular and pulmonary arrest if narcotics are used inappropriately.

Airway Control

Central to anesthetic management and safety is control of the patient's airway. Although many surgical procedures can be managed with face mask ventilation alone, often a more secure means of airway support is needed. The two primary methods utilized are endotracheal intubation (Figs. 44–3 through 44–7) and placement of a laryngeal mask airway (Figs. 44–8 and 44–9), with intubation being the more secure method. Once general anesthesia has been induced and the ability to ventilate with a face mask has been verified, a neuromuscular blocking agent is usually given to facilitate intubation. The airway can be secured with a variety of tubes and techniques depending on the surgical needs, the patient's airway, and the need for postoperative ventilation.

Maintenance

After the intubation, the patient generally receives a mixture of volatile agents, narcotics, and nondepolarizing muscle relaxants. The combination of these agents allows the patient to be analgesic, amnestic, and chemically paralyzed, thus allowing maximal surgical exposure and

Table 44–4
Advantages and disadvantages of volatile agents

Agent	Advantages	Disadvantages
Nitrous oxide		Requires that a smaller Fio_2 be used; diffuses into air spaces
Halothane	Excellent for inhalation induction	Sensitizes the heart to catecholamines, with subsequent dysrhythmias
Isoflurane	Inexpensive	Longer acting than desflurane or sevoflurane
Desflurane	Quick induction and emergence	Airway irritant
Sevoflurane	Excellent for inhalation induction	Pleasant odor, thus allowing inhalation induction

Fio_2, fraction of inspired oxygen.

Table 44–5

Intravenous induction agents

Agent	Bolus	Sedation	Metabolism	Elimination	Advantages	Disadvantages
Barbiturates						
Sodium pentothal	3–6 mg/kg	0.5–1.5 mg/kg	Hepatic	Renal	Inexpensive	↓ BP, ↑ HR
Benzodiazepines						
Diazepam	0.3–0.6 mg/kg	0.04–0.2 mg/kg	Hepatic	Renal		Painful injection
Midazolam	0.1–0.4 mg/kg	0.01–0.1 mg/kg	Hepatic	Renal	Less painful injection	
Other Agents						
Ketamine	1–2 mg/kg	5- to 10-mg boluses to effect	Hepatic	Renal	↑ BP, HR, and CO	Nightmares, myocardial depression if catecholamine depleted
Propofol	1–2.5 mg/kg	25–100 µg/kg/min	Hepatic and extrahepatic	Renal		Painful injection
Etomidate	0.2–0.5 mg/kg	2- to 4-mg boluses to effect	Hepatic	Renal	Minimal cardiovascular effects	Painful injection

BP, blood pressure; CO, cardiac output; HR, heart rate.

Table 44–6
Neuromuscular blocking agents

Agent	Dose: Bolus (Infusion)	Time of Onset (Duration)	Metabolism	Elimination	Advantages	Disadvantages
Short Acting						
Mivacurium	0.1–0.2 mg/kg (4–20 μg/kg/min)	2–3 min (20–30 min)	Pseudocholines-terase		Short-acting	Histamine release
Succinylcholine	1–1.5 mg/kg	30–60 sec	Pseudocholines-terase		Short-acting	Hyperkalemia, malignant hyperthermia
Intermediate						
Atracurium	0.5 mg/kg (5–10 μg/kg/min)	Approx. 2 min	Hoffmann degradation Ester hydrolysis 10% renal/biliary	10% unchanged Renal/biliary	Hoffmann degradation Ester hydrolysis	Histamine release Prolonged elimination with ↓ temperature and acidosis
cis-Atracurium	0.15–0.2 mg/kg (1–2 μg/kg/min)	2 min	Hoffmann degradation Ester hydrolysis		Hoffmann degradation Ester hydrolysis No histamine release	↓ Elimination with acidosis and hypothermia
Vecuronium	0.08–0.1 mg/kg (1–2 μg/kg/min)	Approx. 2 min	Small extent by liver	Primarily biliary 25% renal	No cardiovascular changes	Prolonged use (days) causes a polyneuropathy
Rocuronium	0.6–1.2 mg/kg (5–12 μg/kg/min)	90 sec, but with 1 mg/kg, 1 min		Primarily liver Minimal renal excretion	No cardiovascular changes Rapid onset with ↑ dose	
Long Acting						
Pancuronium	0.08–0.12 mg/kg	2–3 min	Liver	Primarily renal 10% bile	Vagal blockade Long acting	Tachycardia and hypertension with large boluses Prolonged action with renal failure

Table 44–7
Narcotics

Narcotics	Preoperative Dose	Intraoperative Dose	Postoperative Dose
Morphine	0.03–0.15 mg/kg	0.1–1 mg/kg	0.03–0.15 mg/kg
Fentanyl	0.5–1.5 μg/kg	2–20 μg/kg	0.5–1.5 μg/kg
Sufentanil		0.25–10 μg/kg	
Remifentanil		0.5–20 μg/kg/min	
Meperidine	0.2–0.5 mg/kg	2.5–5 mg/kg	0.2–0.5 mg/kg

preventing patient movement. Currently there is not a single monitor that can determine the "depth" of anesthesia; therefore, the patient's depth is inferred by vital signs and the response to surgical stimuli. The different stages of anesthesia are illustrated in Figure 44–10. The optimal stage for the majority of surgical procedures is stage 3.

Trauma

The delivery of an anesthetic is usually associated with calm deliberation and planning. Counter to this norm is the often whirlwind pace and excitement involved in a general anesthetic induction for a severe trauma. These patients may present to the operating room with little

more than a few moments' notice. Patients are often unable to give a history, and a physical exam may be reduced to a cursory look, depending on the extremis of the patient. The general anesthetic must be delivered regardless of NPO status or ASA classification.

Airway considerations for the trauma patient may include an uncleared airway and possibly unstable cervical spine, the presence of a hard collar, and distortion of the face and airway as a result of tissue disruption and bleeding. A full stomach is always assumed; therefore, a rapid-sequence induction is necessary in most cases, often utilizing the most experienced laryngoscopist available to secure the airway while another person holds the head in a neutral alignment. Occasionally, with a very tenuous

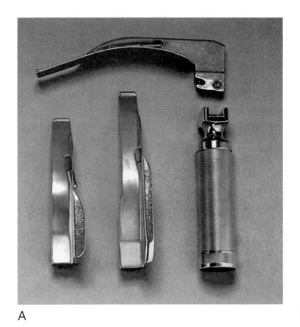

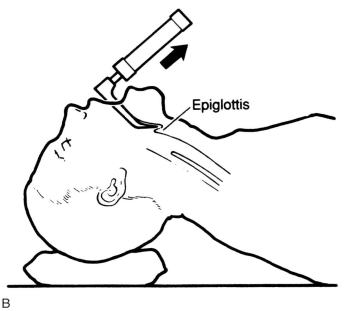

A   B

FIGURE 44–3 **A**, No. 3 and no. 4 Macintosh blades. **B**, The Macintosh blade is inserted with the tip in the vallecula (base of the tongue and epiglottis), and then an upward and forward motion is used to visualize the glottic opening. (**B** from Stone DJ, Gal TJ: Airway management. *In* Miller RD [ed]: Anesthesia [5th ed]. New York: Churchill-Livingstone, 2000:1414, with permission.)

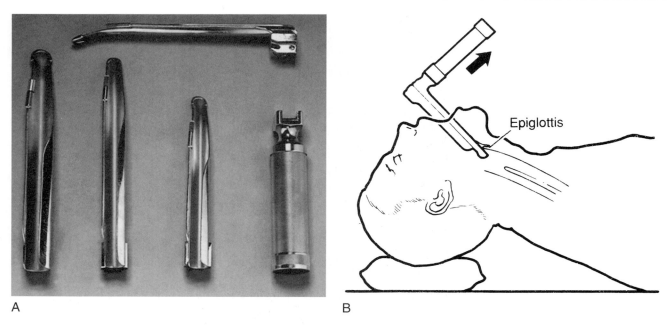

A   B

FIGURE 44–4 A, No. 2, no. 3, and no. 4 Miller blades. **B**, The Miller blade can be inserted in the vallecula or can be used to lift the epiglottis using the same motion as with the Macintosh blades. (**B** from Stone DJ, Gal TJ: Airway management. *In* Miller RD [ed]: Anesthesia [5th ed]. New York: Churchill-Livingstone, 2000:1414, with permission.)

cervical spine and adequate hemodynamics, an awake fiberoptic intubation can be performed.

Anesthetic agents used for induction must meet the demands for speed and hemodynamic stability. Ketamine, which causes a release of catecholamines, is an excellent choice for the hypovolemic patient, usually preventing the fall in blood pressure associated with a general induction.

Muscle relaxation can be achieved rapidly with succinylcholine or high-dose rocuronium (1.0 to 1.2 mg/kg). Intubating conditions will be achieved within 60 seconds for succinylcholine and 90 seconds for high-dose rocuronium. Once the airway is secured, additional intravenous access and any appropriate invasive monitoring are obtained.

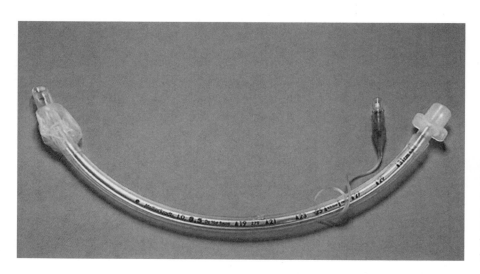

FIGURE 44–5 Endotracheal tube. The standard is a low-volume, high-pressure cuffed endotracheal tube. A variety of endotracheal tubes are available, the choice being dependent upon the surgical needs of the patient. Double-lumen tubes are available for cases requiring lung isolation.

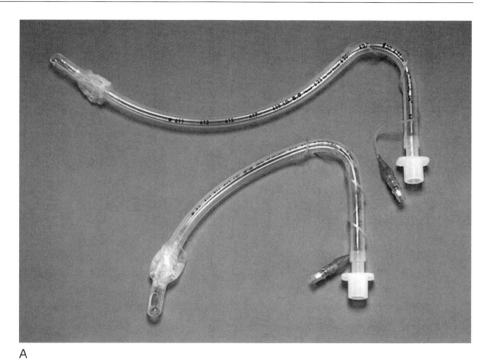

A

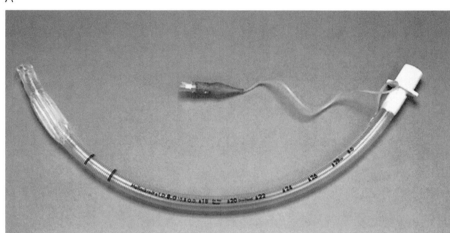

B

FIGURE 44–6 Some specially designed tubes. **A**, The nasal RAE (top) and the oral RAE (bottom). **B**, The reinforced endotracheal tube, which is indicated when the surgical field is the airway or near the airway, and there will be possible manipulations of the endotracheal tube or a high probability of tube kinking.

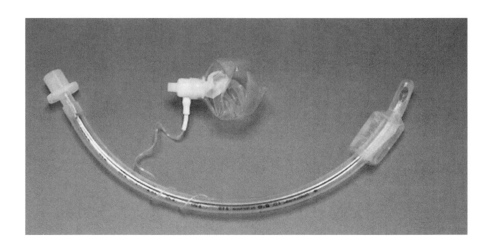

FIGURE 44–7 The high-volume, low-pressure endotracheal tube, used when prolonged ventilation is anticipated.

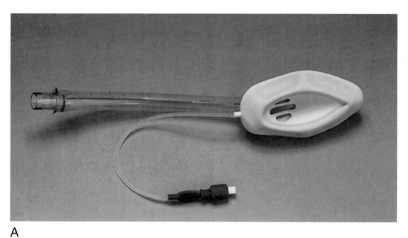

A

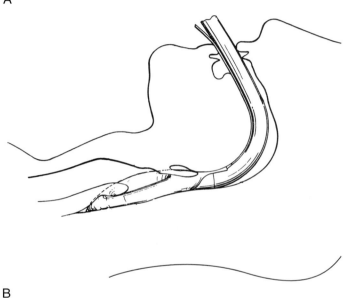

B

FIGURE 44–8   A, The laryngeal mask airway (LMA). **B,** The LMA is placed above the glottis and a seal of approximately 20 cm H_2O is obtained. Muscle relaxation is not required for placement of a LMA. The LMA is routinely used in cases that do not require tracheal intubation. In experienced hands, neuromuscular blockers and the ventilator can be used. The LMA has become one of the favored devices in the difficult-to-intubate scenario. (Right panel from Brain AI: The laryngeal mask-a new concept in airway management. Br J Anaesth 1983;55:801, by permission of Oxford University Press.)

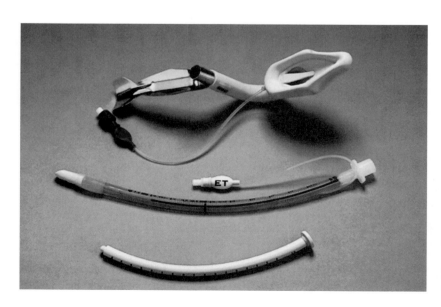

FIGURE 44–9 Several modifications of the LMA have resulted in the Fast Trach Laryngeal Mask Airway, an intubating LMA (pictured here). The endotracheal tube is placed through the LMA after it is positioned. The Fast Trach can be used as the primary intubating device or can be used as a rescue device in the difficult-to-intubate or ventilate patient.

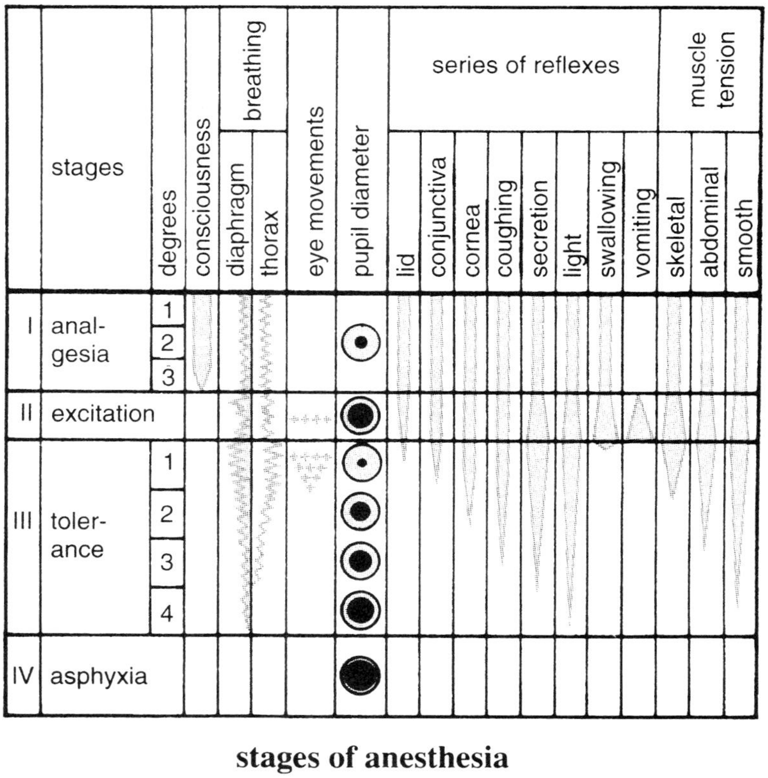

FIGURE 44–10 The stages of anesthesia. The optimal stage for the majority of surgical procedures is stage 3. (From Stedman's Medical Dictionary [26th ed]. Baltimore: Williams & Wilkins, 1995:79, with permission.)

stages of anesthesia

Bibliography

Anesthesia. *In* Dorland's Illustrated Medical Dictionary (27th ed). Philadelphia: WB Saunders, 1988:79.

Mallampati SR, Gatt SP, Gugino LD, et al: A clinical sign to predict difficult tracheal intubation: a prospective study. Can Anaesth Soc J 1985;32:429.

Morgan GE Jr, Mikhail MS, Murray MJ: Anesthesia for patients with cardiovascular disease. *In* Morgan GE Jr, Mikhail MS, Murray MJ (eds): Clinical Anesthesiology (3rd ed). New York: Lange Medical Books/McGraw-Hill, 2002:386.

Practice guidelines for management of the difficult airway: a report by the American Society of Anesthesiologists Task Force on Management of the Difficult Airway. Anesthesiology 1993;78:597.

Roizen MF: Anesthetic implications of concurrent diseases. *In* Miller RD (ed): Anesthesia (5th ed). New York: Churchill Livingstone, 2000:903.

CHAPTER 45

Sedation and Regional Anesthesia

Robert S. Weller, M.D.

▶ Pharmacology of Local Anesthetics
  Mechanism of Action
  Allergy and Toxicity
  Addition of Vasoconstrictors
▶ Sedation and Analgesia
▶ Neuraxial Block
  Spinal and Epidural Anesthesia
  Neuraxial Anesthesia and Anticoagulation
▶ Peripheral Nerve Block
  Upper Extremity Blocks
  Lower Extremity Blocks
  Local Infiltration
  Postoperative Nerve Injury
▶ Bibliography

Pharmacology of Local Anesthetics

Mechanism of Action

Understanding local anesthetics (LAs) is necessary for safe and successful regional anesthesia. LAs interfere with sodium ion transport through the membranes of conducting tissues in the body. Blocking a sufficient number of sodium channels prevents propagation of an action potential along nerve membrane and produces a "block." This property accounts for both the desirable effects of blocking efferent and afferent conduction in nerves, and the toxic effects in brain, cardiac, and vascular tissue seen with overdose. Structurally, the LAs are organic chains consisting of an aromatic compound and a substituted amine joined by either an ester or an amide link. Thus there are two primary types of LAs defined by the intermediary link and mode of metabolism: the ester group, which are hydrolyzed in the plasma, and the amide group, which are hydrolyzed in the liver. Hydrolysis is a prerequisite for renal excretion for both types.

Physicochemical properties of LAs that have clinical significance include protein binding and stereoisomerism. LAs are primarily bound by circulating α_1-acid glycoprotein, and, like most drugs, the free fraction is the active moiety for nerve block as well as toxic effects. Conditions predisposing to lowered plasma-binding proteins, such as cachexia and renal failure, may lead to higher unbound LA and greater risk of toxicity with conventional doses. The issue of stereoisomerism is relevant because a number of LAs have a chiral center and exist as a mixture of S- and R-enantiomers. The S- form appears to have greater anesthetic potency, and the R- form demonstrates greater cardiovascular toxicity. For this reason, the newest long-acting LAs, ropivacaine and levobupivacaine, are prepared as a pure S-enantiomeric form. Although the cost of the newer agents is higher, the potential for cardiovascular toxicity is lower.

Allergy and Toxicity

Allergy to LAs is uncommon, but patients occasionally describe a history of an allergic reaction to LAs after injection for a dental procedure. The history will often include tremor, palpitation, and anxiety, which suggest the reaction is actually due to epinephrine absorption. If true allergy to LAs exists, however, it is usually to a drug in the ester class. The ester LAs are hydrolyzed to *para*-aminobenzoic acid (PABA), which is a known allergen in some individuals. If a patient is known to be PABA allergic, use of an amide LA is recommended. True allergy to amide LAs is extremely rare.

Toxic reaction to LA injection can be life threatening, and knowledge of usual signs and symptoms of toxicity, as well as preparation to treat toxic reactions, is necessary to safely administer regional anesthesia. It is particularly important to know recommended dosages of LAs to use, which depend upon the site of injection, vasoconstrictors, and other factors (Table 45–1). These recommended dosages presume the LA is injected into the appropriate tissue; much smaller doses will result in a toxic reaction if intravascular injection occurs. Toxicity resulting from high plasma levels of LA is first detected by signs and symptoms of central nervous system (CNS) excitation. The patient

Table 45–1

Common local anesthetics

Name	Ester (E) or Amide (A)	Usual Concentration (%) Peripheral Block	Epidural	Spinal	Maximum Dose (mg)* Peripheral Block	Epidural	Spinal	Duration (hr)† Peripheral Block	Epidural	Spinal
Procaine	E	1–2	2	5	1000	1000	100	0.5–1	0.5–1	0.5–1
Tetracaine	E			0.5			20			2–4
Chloroprocaine	E	2	2–3		1000‡	1000‡		0.5–1	0.5–1	
Lidocaine	A	1–1.5	1.5–2	5	500‡	500‡	100	1–3	1–2	0.5–1.5
Mepivacaine	A	1–1.5	1.5–2	4	500‡	500‡	100	2–4	1.5–3	1–1.5
Bupivacaine	A	0.25–0.5	0.25–0.75	0.5–0.75	225‡	225‡	20	4–12	2–5	2–4
Levobupivacaine	A	0.25–0.5	0.5–0.75		150	150		4–12	2–5	
Ropivacaine	A	0.5	0.5–1.0		300	200		5–8	2–6	

*Dosage recommendations are those of the manufacturers and should be considered as guidelines. Variation based upon site of injection and patient age and disease must be considered.
†Duration listed is for surgical anesthesia. The duration of postoperative analgesia is significantly longer than surgical anesthesia.
‡With epinephrine.

Modified from Covino BG, Wildsmith JAW: Clinical pharmacology of local anesthetic agents. In Cousins MJ, Bridenbaugh PO (eds): Neural Blockade in Clinical Anesthesia and Management of Pain (3rd ed.), Philadelphia: Lippincott-Raven, 1998:98.

may become restless or confused, and demonstrate slurred speech. It is safest to inject LAs in small, incremental doses while maintaining verbal contact with the patient to detect these early signs of toxicity before continued injection leads to frank seizure activity with higher plasma level. Even higher plasma levels produce cardiovascular depression. These cardiovascular effects result from vasodilation, depression of cardiac contractility, and arrhythmias. Lethal ventricular fibrillation, resistant to prolonged resuscitative efforts, has most often occurred with intravascular injection of the long-acting LA bupivacaine. This complication spurred the development of ropivacaine and levobupivacaine, which appear to have lower potential for cardiac toxicity than does bupivacaine. Any LA, however, can produce cardiovascular collapse at a high plasma level, so emphasis is placed on incremental injection, frequent aspiration for blood, and constant monitoring of the patient. In addition, the practitioner should be prepared with drugs and equipment to immediately provide ventilatory and cardiovascular support should a toxic reaction occur.

Addition of Vasoconstrictors

Vasoconstrictors such as epinephrine are often added to LAs to reduce vascular uptake of the LA, thereby reducing the plasma level as well as prolonging the duration of the block. In addition, the epinephrine serves as an intravascular marker at the time of LA injection, such that tachycardia should prompt adjustment of the needle position. The usual concentration of epinephrine is 1:200,000, which has been shown to lower the level of nearly all LAs

injected for peripheral nerve block. Higher concentrations are often used for head and neck injection, but the total dose of epinephrine must be considered because, as noted above, cardiovascular side effects of epinephrine may occur, such as increased heart rate and blood pressure.

Sedation and Analgesia

Patients often receive sedative and analgesic medications for painful procedures such as endoscopy or reduction of orthopedic injuries. Hospitals are required to develop guidelines and credentialing mechanisms for nonanesthesiologists to administer such medications because of the recognition in the 1980s of adverse respiratory events resulting from inappropriate sedative techniques. The American Society of Anesthesiologists has defined a continuum of consciousness, from light sedation to general anesthesia, which is achieved by the administration of sedative and analgesic drugs (Table 45-2). Moderate sedation and analgesia, formerly known as *conscious sedation*, is defined as a state in which a patient is sedate, but is expected to maintain and protect his or her airway and not require ventilatory or circulatory support. This is distinguished from deep sedation and analgesia in which the patient may require intervention for adequate ventilation and protection of the airway from secretions. Patients at particular risk for complications include very old or young patients, patients with morbid obesity or sleep apnea, patients with severe cardiovascular or pulmonary disease, and uncooperative patients. Consultation with an anesthesiologist is recommended before attempting sedation in these individuals.

Table 45–2
Continuum of depth of sedation

	Minimal Sedation (Anxiolysis)	Moderate Sedation/Analgesia "Conscious Sedation"	Deep Sedation/ Analgesia	General Anesthesia
Responsiveness	Normal response to verbal stimulation	Purposeful response to verbal or tactile stimulation*	Purposeful response to repeated or painful stimulation*	No response to painful stimulation
Airway	Unaffected	No intervention required	Intervention may be required	Intervention often required
Spontaneous ventilation	Unaffected	Adequate	May be inadequate	Frequently inadequate
Cardiovascular function	Unaffected	Usually maintained	Usually maintained	May be impaired

*Reflex withdrawal from a painful stimulus is NOT considered a purposeful response.
Modified from the American Society of Anesthesiologists' Continuum of Depth of Sedation: Definition of General Anesthesia and Levels of Sedation/Analgesia. Approved by House of Delegates, October 13, 1999. A copy of the full text can be obtained from ASA, 520 N. Northwest Highway, Park Ridge, Illinois 60068-2573. Available at www.asahq.org/Standards/20.htm

The guidelines for sedation and analgesia generally require preprocedure evaluation and consent, and postprocedure observation until the patient is no longer at risk. A second individual other than the physician performing the procedure will monitor the patient, administer sedative medication, and record vital signs throughout the procedure. Because the most likely complication of sedation is respiratory depression, monitoring of ventilation as well as oxygenation is routine. Pulse oximetry is frequently recommended as an essential monitor, but the pulse oximeter alone is not sufficient to guarantee safety of the patient. Monitoring level of consciousness with response to verbal stimuli is routine, as is regular recording of pulse and blood pressure. Oxygen, suction, a self-inflating resuscitation bag, and other emergency equipment should be immediately available to treat complications.

The agents most often used to provide sedation and analgesia, antagonist drugs, and common dosages are shown in Table 45–3. Sedative-hypnotics such as benzodiazepines are used for sedation, anxiolysis, and amnesia and provide no analgesia. Narcotic medications are used for analgesia and provide modest sedation without amnesia. Benzodiazepines or narcotics each produce dose-related respiratory depression, but synergistic and profound respiratory depression results when drugs from both classes are combined. Most patients receiving the combination will become hypoxemic unless breathing supplemental oxygen. Specific antagonists for both narcotic analgesics (naloxone) and benzodiazepines (flumazenil) are available, but may also produce side effects. Prompt reversal of the sedative state may result in hypertension and tachycardia, and the short duration of the antagonists and potential for resedation mandate observation postreversal. Ketamine is a unique drug that produces both analgesia and amnesia, but may be associated with delirium and has a steep dose-response curve such that small incremental doses may rapidly produce deep sedation or anesthesia. In addition, recovery may be prolonged.

Neuraxial Block

Spinal and Epidural Anesthesia

Spinal and epidural anesthesia, collectively known as neuraxial block, employs LAs to block spinal nerves within the vertebral column, resulting in highly reliable surgical anesthesia. Spinal anesthesia is produced by injecting very low doses of LA (e.g., 50 mg lidocaine) via lumbar puncture into the cerebrospinal fluid (CSF) below the termination of the spinal cord (Fig. 45–1A). The LA diffuses in the CSF and produces dense anesthesia extending cephalad from the sacral dermatomes to as high as the lower cervical dermatomes. A single dose of LA through a fine-gauge (22- to 29-gauge) needle is usually injected, which results in a finite duration of anesthesia, but catheters can be placed in the subarachnoid space for prolonged anesthesia. Spinal anesthesia is usually chosen for procedures performed in the dermatomes at or below the midabdomen. Spinal LA blocks somatic and visceral sensory afferent nerves, as well as efferent motor and autonomic (sympathetic) fibers. Sensory anesthesia, muscle relaxation, and sympathetic block are the result of this

Table 45–3
Medications and intravenous dosages for "conscious sedation"

Medication Name	Class	Therapeutic Effect	Dose (Adult)	Interval (min)	Maximum Dose
Agonists					
Diazepam (Valium)	Benzodiazepine	Amnesia/anxiolysis	0.5–2 mg	5	10 mg
Midazolam (Versed)	Benzodiazepine	Amnesia/anxiolysis	0.5–1 mg	5	5 mg
Fentanyl (Sublimaze)	Opioid	Analgesia	25–50 µg	5	100–150 µg
Morphine	Opioid	Analgesia	1–2 mg	5	10 mg
Meperidine (Demerol)	Opioid	Analgesia	12.5–25 mg	5	100 mg
Antagonists					
Flumazenil (Romazicon)	Benzodiazepine antagonist	Reversal of benzodiazepine	0.2 mg	1–2	1.0 mg
Naloxone (Narcan)	Opioid antagonist	Reversal of opioid	0.1–0.4 mg	2–3	2.0 mg

Modified from Adult Medication Dosages (Department of Nursing Policy and Procedures Bulletin No. 158). Winston-Salem: North Carolina Baptist Hospital, 1999.

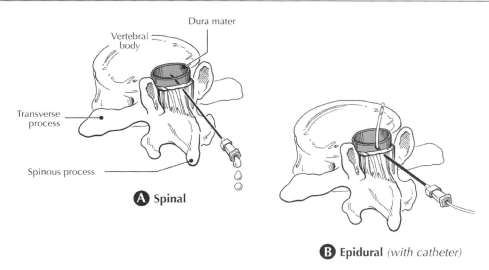

Dura mater

Vertebral body

Transverse process

Spinous process

A Spinal

B Epidural *(with catheter)*

FIGURE 45–1 Anatomy of the lumbar spine and needle placement for spinal anesthesia (**A**) and epidural anesthesia with catheter (**B**). (Modified from Gordh T: Spinal anesthesia. *In* Eriksson E [ed]: Illustrated Handbook in Local Anaesthesia. London: Edward Arnold, 1979:120. Reproduced by permission of Hodder Arnold.)

blockade and produce numerous advantages and disadvantages. Benefits of spinal compared to general anesthesia include reduction of blood loss, reduction of deep vein thrombosis, maintenance of protective airway reflexes and avoidance of an endotracheal tube, and gradual offset of anesthesia/analgesia. Disadvantages include potential failure or inadequate duration, post–lumbar puncture headache (minimal with fine needles), urinary retention, and exaggerated hypotension or intolerance of hemorrhage.

Epidural anesthesia is produced by injection of LA into the epidural space outside the dura mater (Fig. 45–1B). An epidural injection requires significantly more LA in both volume and dose than a spinal injection, but the injection can be made anywhere from the cervical epidural space to the sacral hiatus (caudal anesthesia). The spinal nerves are blocked most intensely at the site of injection, and less intensely both above and below that site; the block is therefore more "segmental" than spinal anesthesia. An injection, for example, at the T10 intervertebral level will provide the greatest anesthesia for midabdominal procedures, and much less or no anesthesia at the sacral roots. Compared to spinal anesthesia, epidural anesthesia is often performed through a catheter introduced into the epidural space through a large (16- to 18-gauge) needle (Fig. 45–1B). The catheter provides flexibility for prolonged anesthesia as well as prolonged analgesia for days into the postoperative period with infusion of dilute LA/narcotic solutions. The benefits of epidural are similar to those of spinal when compared to general anesthesia, but add greater flexibility for postoperative analgesia. Disadvantages compared to spinal anesthesia include the additional potential for systemic toxicity from intravascular injection

or overdose, since larger doses of LAs are used. Accidental, unrecognized spinal puncture and injection will result in total spinal anesthesia requiring ventilatory and circulatory support. The onset of anesthesia is 10 to 15 minutes later than with spinal anesthesia, and the larger needle and catheter result in a greater frequency of back pain, greater potential for bleeding in the epidural space, and a high risk of headache should dural puncture occur. Finally, the epidural space is usually located "by feel," or a loss of resistance as the needle is advanced into the space. This is a less definitive end point than CSF appearance with spinal anesthesia, and the technique is somewhat less reliable than the spinal technique.

A relatively new technique; combined spinal-epidural (CSE), brings together some of the advantages of each technique. A lumbar epidural needle is placed, and a longer spinal needle advanced through it until CSF is aspirated. The spinal anesthetic is performed to provide reliable and rapid anesthesia, and an epidural catheter is threaded to provide extended anesthesia for surgery as well as postoperative analgesia. The CSE is most useful when a lumbar epidural catheter is indicated for postoperative use; it is generally not performed in the thoracic region.

The pulmonary and cardiovascular side effects and complications of neuraxial block are due to the blockade of efferent motor and autonomic activity. Diaphragmatic activity and inspiratory effort are usually well preserved, but abdominal muscle relaxation may reduce expiratory force and the ability to cough. Arterial and venous dilatation occur below the level of the block as a result of decreased sympathetic activity; the reduction of both preload and afterload result in modest decreases in blood pressure in a euvolemic patient. Heart rate typically is reduced, and cardiac contractility is reduced if thoracic sympathetic nerves are blocked. These effects result in decreased myocardial oxygen consumption and are advantageous in the patient with coronary artery disease as long as diastolic pressure is adequate. The vasodilation and blockade of the prothrombotic effect of surgery under general anesthesia contribute to reduced deep vein thrombosis and improved arterial graft patency. The moderate hypotension and reduced venous pressure help to reduce surgical blood loss and transfusion requirement. Severe hypotension may occur, however, in a patient with hypovolemia, fixed stroke volume, or aortic stenosis, and neuraxial block is usually avoided in these patients. Rarely, the parasympathetic predominance produced by high spinal block (which does not block the vagus, a cranial nerve) results in profound bradycardia requiring atropine or epinephrine treatment.

The usual indications for neuraxial block, then, are for patients undergoing surgical procedures below the midabdomen, and for whom the position or duration of surgery will not be uncomfortable for a sedated patient. There are particular advantages for patients with reactive airways or full stomachs and for patients with certain cardiovascular diseases as noted above. Alternatively, general anesthesia may be combined with neuraxial block to gain advantages of both. Contraindications include patient refusal, local infection at the site of spinal puncture, and systemic anticoagulation at the time of puncture because of the risk of epidural hematoma formation and neurologic injury. Controversy continues over neuraxial block in the patient prone to bacteremia because of concern for CNS infection. Many believe neuraxial block can be performed if the patient is on appropriate antibiotic coverage, but tend to avoid indwelling catheters. No study can answer the question of the relative risk of this approach because of the rarity of epidural abscess.

Neuraxial Anesthesia and Anticoagulation

The issue of epidural anesthesia and perioperative anticoagulation for prophylaxis against deep vein thrombosis is important because of the multitude of antiplatelet and anticoagulant choices available. Low-molecular-weight heparin (LMWH) was released in the United States in 1995, and within 5 years more than 50 cases of epidural hematoma with paraplegia were related to the concurrent use of epidural (and spinal) anesthesia and enoxaparin. This prompted the Food and Drug Administration to issue a letter to physicians and to include a black-boxed notice on the package information for enoxaparin warning of the danger of epidural hematoma with concurrent use of epidural anesthesia and this drug. The American Society of Regional Anesthesia reviewed relevant literature and

published recommendations for neuraxial block. In general, spinal is considered to be less traumatic than epidural anesthesia and may be performed at least 12 hours after a prophylactic dose of LMWH in the absence of other anticoagulants. Larger, therapeutic doses of LMWH mandate a delay of at least 24 hours before neuraxial block. Continuous epidural anesthesia and analgesia is poorly compatible with q12h dosing of LMWH because there is no nadir of drug effect to allow removal of the epidural catheter. Postoperative initiation of LMWH therapy should occur at least 2 hours after removal of an epidural catheter. The use of unfractionated heparin, and the use of aspirin or nonsteroidal anti-inflammatory drugs, are not considered to be contraindications to neuraxial blockade. With newer, more potent and long-acting antiplatelet drugs, it is recommended that neuraxial block be avoided within 7 days of clopidogrel, and within 14 days of tielopidine administration.

Traumatic neuraxial block, where blood is encountered with needle or catheter placement, requires higher surveillance in the postoperative period as well as the use of postoperative infusions that will not mask neurologic deficits. Epidural hematoma may present as back pain or neurologic deficit without pain, and, if it is not diagnosed and treated within 8 to 12 hours, complete neurologic recovery is unlikely. The best test to diagnose epidural hematoma is magnetic resonance imaging.

Peripheral Nerve Block

There is increased interest in the perioperative use of peripheral nerve block for anesthesia or postoperative analgesia. This is due, in part, to the complications and side effects of neuraxial block mentioned above, including urinary retention, nausea, or postoperative weakness, which can interfere with rehabilitation or discharge after surgery, as well as the concern for epidural hematoma following aggressive perioperative anticoagulation. Peripheral nerve block with long-acting LAs or even perineural catheters can provide many hours or days of analgesia, avoidance of systemic narcotics and their side effects, and minimal interference with rehabilitation. The development of nerve localization techniques and equipment, improved education of anesthesiologists and surgeons in this area, and research in the field of long-acting LAs will promote accelerating growth in this field.

Upper Extremity Blocks

Upper extremity nerve blocks have been used for over a century, and, with the exception of intravenous regional anesthesia (IVRA) or Bier block, involve injection of LA adjacent to the brachial plexus or specific peripheral nerves to produce anesthesia. The most common LAs employed are 1% to 1.25% lidocaine or mepivacaine with epinephrine for 2- to 4-hour duration of surgical block. Longer blockade (but slower onset) is achieved with 0.5% bupivacaine, levobupivacaine, or ropivacaine with epinephrine, which provide 4 to 12 hours of surgical block. It should be noted that the duration of postoperative analgesia is significantly longer than the duration of surgical block. The upper extremity is innervated almost entirely by the brachial plexus, derived from nerve roots C5 to T1. In addition, the cervical plexus innervates the skin over the shoulder, and the intercostobrachial nerve (T1-T2) innervates the inner aspect of the arm. These two areas may require separate injection for complete surgical anesthesia. This section reviews IVRA, brachial blocks above the clavicle, and blocks below the clavicle.

The technique of IVRA is simple and highly successful. An intravenous catheter is placed in the hand, a tourniquet (usually a double cuff) is applied to the arm, the limb is exsanguinated by elevation and wrapping with an elastic bandage, and the proximal tourniquet is inflated well above arterial pressure. The bandage is removed and a dilute LA solution, usually 40 to 50 mL of 0.5% lidocaine, is injected into the catheter. The LA gains access to nerves through the blood vessels supplying those nerves, and anesthesia occurs in 10 to 15 minutes and remains as long as the tourniquet is inflated. Tolerance of tourniquet pain is the limiting factor for duration, although a double-cuff technique allows for inflation of the more distal tourniquet on a part of the arm that is anesthetized and 1 hour of

surgical anesthesia may readily be achieved. Inadequate exsanguination or incomplete arterial occlusion results in venous congestion, dilution of the LA, and inadequate block. High systemic levels of lidocaine and toxicity can occur from early (<15 minutes) or accidental tourniquet deflation. Finally, anesthesia rapidly resolves after tourniquet deflation, and alternative analgesic approaches such as local infiltration or systemic analgesics should be administered prior to this.

Brachial plexus blocks above the clavicle include interscalene (ISB) and supraclavicular (SCB) blocks (Fig. 45–2A and B). The ISB is performed at the level of the C6 transverse process, and 30 mL of LA is injected between the fascia of the anterior and middle scalene muscles after identification of the C5-C6 nerve roots. Rapid anesthesia of the superficial cervical plexus and upper roots of the brachial plexus ensues, so the technique is particularly well suited for shoulder procedures. Side effects include 100% incidence of ipsilateral phrenic block, Horner's syndrome, and occasional block of the recurrent laryngeal nerve and hoarseness. Complications include intravascular injection with immediate convulsion, epidural or spinal injection, and pneumothorax. The latter two should not occur with proper technique. There are many techniques of SCB, but all result in injection of approximately 30 mL of LA adjacent to the three trunks of the brachial plexus at the point where the trunks pass over the first rib. Because the plexus is very compact at this site, anesthesia of the entire plexus is likely with a relatively small dose of LA.

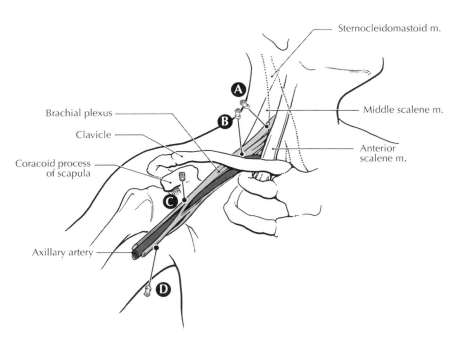

FIGURE 45–2 Four sites for brachial plexus block: interscalene (**A**), supraclavicular (**B**), infraclavicular (**C**), and axillary (**D**). (Modified from Murphy TM: Nerve blocks. *In* Miller RD [ed]: Anesthesia [2nd ed]. New York: Churchill Livingstone, 1986:1025.)

The intercostobrachial nerve (upper, inner arm) and cervical plexus are spared, and require separate injection if anesthesia is needed in these distributions. Side effects include a 60% incidence of phrenic block and occasional Horner's syndrome and recurrent laryngeal block. Pneumothorax is more likely (from 0.5% to 6%) with SCB than any other brachial block, and must be considered if the SCB is used for an outpatient. Catheters can be placed with proper equipment at the ISB or SCB site to provide prolonged postoperative analgesia.

Brachial plexus blocks below the clavicle include infraclavicular (IFCB) and axillary (AXB) blocks (Fig. 45–2C and D) and peripheral blocks at the elbow, wrist, and digits (Figs. 45–3 and 45–4). The side effects or complications of phrenic block, recurrent laryngeal nerve block, and pneumothorax do not occur with these approaches, so they are well tolerated by patients with pulmonary disease. These blocks are most often employed for procedures on the elbow, forearm, and hand. The IFCB is performed by locating the brachial plexus as it passes inferior to the coracoid process of the scapula. The appropriate volume (40 mL) of LA is injected at the level of the cords of the brachial plexus, and the axillary nerve and musculocutaneous nerve are more frequently blocked than with the AXB. Side effects and complications include more pain than with AXB because the needle must traverse the

pectoral muscles, and vascular puncture at a site that does not allow for easy compression. The needle path is outside the thorax, and pneumothorax should not occur with proper technique. There are many techniques for performing AXB, but the objective is to inject LA into the axilla where the median, radial, and ulnar nerves closely surround the axillary artery. Typically 40 mL of LA is required, and many have found that injection at multiple sites rather than a single site results in higher frequency of complete anesthesia. The musculocutaneous nerve is distant from the brachial plexus in the axilla and requires separate injection in the body of the coracobrachialis muscle if needed for the surgical site. The axillary nerve is rarely blocked by AXB. Side effects and complications include vascular puncture and toxicity or hematoma formation, but compression is readily achieved here.

The nerves of the brachial plexus have widely diverged at the elbow and wrist, and require separate injection for anesthesia in their territories. These nerves may be blocked to supplement an incomplete proximal block or to provide prolonged postoperative analgesia after IVRA, for example, but the total dose of LA must be considered to avoid toxicity. The median nerve is located just medial to the brachial artery pulse, 2 to 3 cm proximal to the elbow flexion crease, and the radial nerve is located as it courses around the lateral supracondylar ridge of the

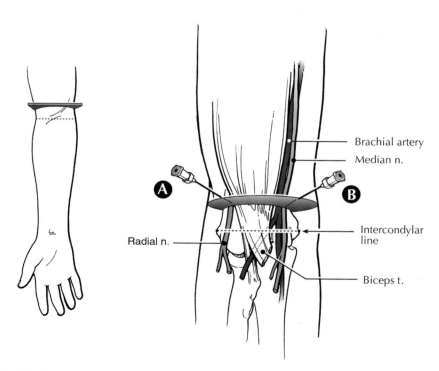

FIGURE 45–3 Peripheral nerve block at the elbow. Technique for radial (**A**) and median (**B**) nerve blocks. (Modified from Brown DL, Bridenbaugh LD: The upper extremity: somatic block. *In* Cousins M, Bridenbaugh P [eds]: Neural Blockade in Clinical Anesthesia and Management of Pain [3rd ed]. Philadelphia: Lippincott–Raven, 1998:364.)

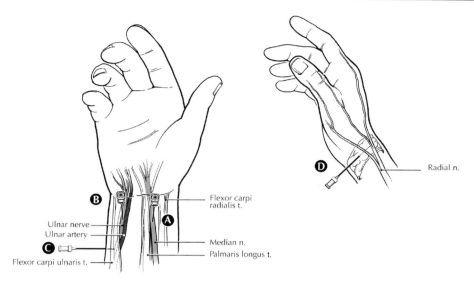

FIGURE 45–4 Peripheral nerve block at the wrist. Technique for median (**A**) and ulnar (**B**) block, with alternative approach to the ulnar block (**C**). Subcutaneous injection for radial block (**D**). (Modified from Wedel DJ: Nerve blocks. *In* Miller RD [ed]: Anesthesia [2nd ed]. New York: Churchill Livingstone, 1986:1528; and Löfström B: Nerve block at the wrist. *In* Eriksson E [eds]: Illustrated Handbook in Local Anaesthesia. London: Edward Arnold, 1979:92. Reproduced by permission of Hodder Arnold.)

humerus 3 to 4 cm proximal to the elbow crease. Each is blocked with 5 to 10 mL of LA (Fig. 45–4). Many avoid block of the ulnar nerve at the elbow because the tight fascial tunnel predisposes the nerve to compression from small volumes of LA, and the sensory blockade of the ulnar side of the hand is identical to that achieved by wrist block. Wrist block of the three peripheral nerves is performed with 3 to 5 mL of LA per nerve, as shown in Figure 45–4. Finally, digital block can be performed for individual fingers with non–epinephrine-containing LA just distal to the metacarpophalangeal joint. Complications of distal blockade include vascular puncture and high compartment pressure from excessive volume of LA.

Lower Extremity Blocks

Lower extremity (LE) peripheral nerve blocks are increasingly used because they provide an alternative to neuraxial block's side effects of hypotension, bilateral weakness, and urinary retention. They may be more compatible with modest degrees of anticoagulation. The LE blocks provide prolonged analgesia and less hypotension than neuraxial block because the sympathetic block occurs in only one LE. Disadvantages compared to neuraxial block include greater complexity and potential discomfort with LE block, larger LA volume and dose required, and greater difficulty reliably placing and securing catheters for postoperative infusion. Thorough knowledge of the neuroanatomy and use of a peripheral nerve stimulator enhance the success

of LE block. In addition, the use of a tourniquet must be considered in planning the level of a block, because a distal block may provide excellent surgical anesthesia, but tourniquet ischemia will not be tolerated by the patient. The innervation of the LE consists of nerves of the lumbar plexus: the femoral, lateral femoral cutaneous (LFCN), and obturator nerves responsible for muscular and sensory innervation of the anterior and medial thigh and knee, and cutaneous sensation of the anteromedial leg (saphenous nerve). All other innervation is through the sciatic nerve, which derives from the lumbosacral plexus and is made up of the fibular (peroneal) and tibial nerves. The sciatic (with the posterior femoral cutaneous nerve) provides sensory and muscular innervation of the posterior thigh and all structures below the knee except for the cutaneous sensation of the anteromedial leg. The LAs used are the same as those for brachial plexus blockade, and typical durations are shown in Table 45–1.

Lumbar plexus block (LPB) is performed from a posterior approach with a translumbar, paravertebral needle placed to stimulate the plexus (Fig. 45–5). A volume of 25 to 30 mL of LA, incrementally dosed, provides adequate block. Complications include intravascular injection or hematoma, and epidural spread of LA with resultant epidural, bilateral anesthesia. An anterior approach to LPB is described at the groin, with placement of the needle into the femoral nerve sheath and injection of 25 to 30 mL of LA (Fig. 45–6). This volume may result in proximal spread sufficient to anesthetize the LFCN and obturator

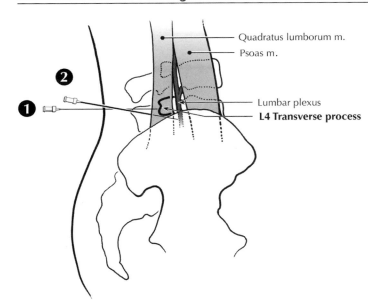

FIGURE 45–5 Paravertebral lumbar plexus block viewed in sagittal section. The needle is placed 5 cm from the midline at the level of the L4 vertebra. After contact with the transverse process (*1*), the needle is passed inferior and 1 to 2 cm beyond the process (*2*) to stimulate the branches of the lumbar plexus between the quadratus lumborum and psoas muscles. (Modified from Murphy TM: Nerve blocks. *In* Miller RD [ed]: Anesthesia [2nd ed]. New York: Churchill Livingstone, 1986:1038.)

nerves, but will not reliably do so. Catheters may be placed at either site to provide postoperative analgesia and are particularly useful for procedures on the knee.

The sciatic nerve block has been refined with at least seven different approaches or levels of block. The surgical requirements and ability to position a patient in the lateral position determine which approach is chosen. One or both halves of the nerve are identified, and 20 to 40 mL of LA injected to achieve blockade. The classic approach deep to the gluteal muscles is easily made at the same time as posterior LPB (Fig. 45–7), and a more distal approach in the popliteal fossa is popular when anesthesia of the hamstring muscles is not desired. Complications include intravascular injection or hematoma formation. Catheters may be placed adjacent to the sciatic nerve, but dislodgement is more common than with epidural catheters. Catheters for postoperative analgesia may be placed by the surgeon in the surgical field, and

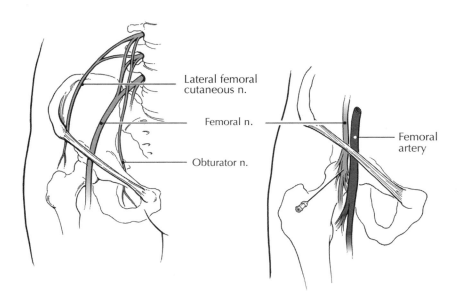

FIGURE 45–6 Nerve supply of the anterior thigh and technique for blockade. Terminal branches of the lumbar plexus include the femoral, lateral femoral cutaneous, and obturator nerves. These nerves can be located and blocked individually distal to the inguinal ligament, or by a single large-volume injection into the femoral sheath located 1 cm lateral to the femoral artery pulsation. (Modified from Murphy TM: Nerve blocks. *In* Miller RD [ed]: Anesthesia [2nd ed]. New York: Churchill Livingstone, 1986:1039.)

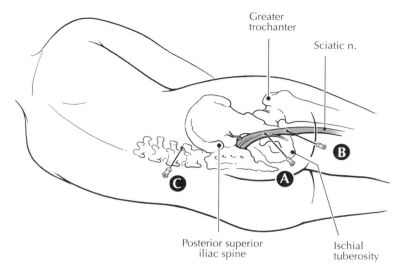

FIGURE 45–7 Anatomy and technique for blockade of the sciatic nerve and lumbar plexus. **A,** The landmarks for sciatic block include the posterior superior iliac spine and the greater trochanter, and the nerve is located 4 to 5 cm caudad to the midpoint of a line connecting these landmarks. **B,** A second, more distal site for sciatic block is shown at the midpoint of a line connecting the ischial tuberosity and greater trochanter. **C,** The lumbar plexus block is performed through a needle inserted 5 cm from the midline on the intercristal line and 1 to 2 cm inferior and deep to the transverse process of the L4 vertebra. (Modified from Murphy TM: Nerve blocks. *In* Miller RD [ed]: Anesthesia [2nd ed]. New York: Churchill Livingstone, 1986:1036.)

exteriorized through a separate needle puncture. This has been successful for amputations (for both lower and upper extremities) when the nerves are directly visualized, and there is suggestion that phantom-limb pain is reduced by postoperative infusion.

Finally, ankle block is a reliable technique that can be used as sole anesthetic or for postoperative analgesia for procedures on the foot. The nerves to the foot diverge below the knee, and five separate nerve branches must be blocked for complete anesthesia, as shown in Figure 45–8. The entire ankle block requires 20 to 25 mL of LA, and care should be taken in patients with vascular insufficiency to avoid a complete ring of LA around the ankle, which could impede venous outflow and lead to ischemia. If cellulitis involves the ankle, a more proximal block would be advisable.

Local Infiltration

One of the most common and simplest forms of regional anesthesia is the injection of LA in and around the site of surgery, also known as local infiltration. This can be performed as the sole anesthetic, or as an adjunct to provide postoperative analgesia. Common concentrations of LA and dosage limitations are the same as those used for peripheral nerve block (see Table 45–1), and care must be taken to avoid direct intravascular injection. Intradermal and immediate subcutaneous injection is most effective; injection of LA into the thick adipose layer

does not provide equally effective cutaneous anesthesia. Finally, mention must be made of subcutaneous injection of large doses of highly diluted lidocaine solutions (0.05% to 0.1%) with epinephrine for liposuction. Healthy patients have been given five to eight times the standard "maximum" dose of lidocaine at this dilution with nontoxic plasma levels. Deaths have also occurred from liposuction, however, and some were believed to be due to LA toxicity.

Postoperative Nerve Injury

A discussion of regional anesthesia and peripheral nerve block would be incomplete without mention of nerve injury and postoperative paresthesia or weakness. Postoperative transient paresthesia sensation may occur in as many as 1% to 2% of patients after peripheral block, but usually resolves in a few days. More prolonged complaints, or those associated with motor weakness, occur at a rate of 0.02%. Unfortunately, many factors can contribute to postoperative nerve injury, such as stretch resulting from positioning, surgical trauma, and tourniquet injury, in addition to needle trauma during blockade. Patients with preexisting vasculitis, such as diabetics, may be more susceptible to intraoperative nerve injury. Significant nerve dysfunction that persists after surgery should trigger neurology consultation and study. This will help characterize the type and site of injury, and provide prognostic information and follow-up for the patient.

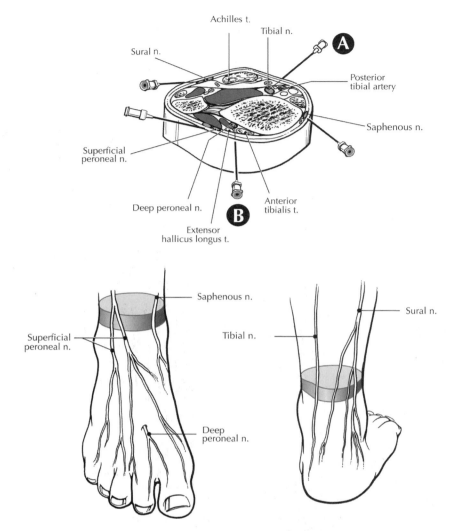

FIGURE 45–8 Anatomy and technique for ankle block. The injection sites for the tibial (**A**) and deep peroneal (**B**) nerves are deep to the fascia and close to the arteries supplying the foot. The three additional nerves (saphenous, sural, and superficial peroneal) are blocked by subcutaneous injection. (Modified from Bridenbaugh PO, Wedel DJ: The lower extremity: somatic blockade. *In* Cousins M, Bridenbaugh P [eds]: Neural Blockade in Clinical Anesthesia and Management of Pain [3rd ed]. Philadelphia: Lippincott–Raven, 1998:388.)

Bibliography

Albright GA: Cardiac arrest following regional anesthesia with etidocaine or bupivacaine. Anesthesiology 1979;51:285.

Auroy Y, Narchi P, Messiah A, et al: Serious complications related to regional anesthesia: results of a prospective survey in France. Anesthesiology 1997;87:479.

Bailey PL, Pace NL, Ashburn MA, et al: Frequent hypoxemia and apnea after sedation with midazolam and fentanyl. Anesthesiology 1990;73:826.

Caplan RA, Ward RJ, Posner K, et al: Unexpected cardiac arrest during spinal anesthesia: a closed claims analysis of predisposing factors. Anesthesiology 1988;68:5.

Daneshmend TK, Bell GD, Logan RF: Sedation for upper gastrointestinal endoscopy: results of a nationwide survey. Gut 1991;32:12.

De Visme V, Picart F, Le Jouan R, et al: Combined lumbar and sacral plexus block compared with plain bupivacaine spinal anesthesia for hip fractures in the elderly. Reg Anesth Pain Med 2000;25:158.

Fisher A, Meller Y: Continuous postoperative regional anesthesia by nerve sheath block for amputation surgery—a pilot study. Anesth Analg 1991;72:300.

Horlocker TI, Wedel DJ: Neuraxial block and low-molecular-weight heparin: balancing perioperative analgesia and thromboprophylaxis. Reg Anesth Pain Med 1998;23 (3 Suppl 2):164.

Horlocker TI, Wedel DJ: Neurologic complications of spinal and epidural anesthesia. Reg Anesth Pain Med 2000;25:83.

Klein JA: Tumescent technique for regional anesthesia permits lidocaine doses of 35 mg/kg for liposuction. J Dermatol Surg Oncol 1990;16:248.

Rao RB, Ely SF, Hoffman RS: Deaths related to liposuction. N Engl J Med 1999;340:1471.

Rodgers A, Walker N, Schug S, et al: Reduction of postoperative mortality and morbidity with epidural or spinal anaesthesia: results from overview of randomised trials. BMJ 2000; 321:1.

Tuman, KJ, McCarthy RJ, March RJ, et al: Effects of epidural anesthesia and analgesia on coagulation and outcome after major vascular surgery. Anesth Analg 1991;73:696.

PART X

Oncology

CHAPTER 46

Principles of Tumor Biology

Herbert Chen, M.D. and John E. Niederhuber, M.D.

The term *cancer* embraces a group of diseases characterized by uncontrolled growth and spread of normal cells that have become transformed through a series of genetic changes. It affects both young and old, and people of all races and ethnicities. The National Cancer Institute estimates that approximately 8.4 million Americans alive today have a history of cancer. Approximately 1,284,900 new cases of cancer were diagnosed in the year 2002. About half a million Americans die of cancer each year, making it the second leading cause of death in the United States, exceeded only by heart disease. In other words, one out of every four deaths in the United States is due to cancer. The leading sites of new cancer cases and deaths in the year 2000 are shown in Table 46–1. Lung cancer remains the most common cause of cancer deaths, while prostate cancer and breast cancer are the most common malignancies present in males and females, respectively. In this chapter, we review the process by which normal cells become transformed to a cancer phenotype, and progress through stages of local growth, invasion, and metastasis.

Tumorigenesis

Tumor is a term frequently used to describe an abnormal growth. Often the words *tumor* and *neoplasm* are used interchangeably. A tumor, however, can be either benign or malignant. Malignancy denotes uncontrolled growth with the potential for dissemination of cancer cells from the primary lesion to distant sites in the body. In general, the use of the term *cancer* encompasses the stages of the malignant process.

Characteristics of Malignant Cells

Cancer cells possess unique biologic properties that distinguish them from nonmalignant cells, collectively referred to as the transformed phenotype. In tissue culture, transformed cells have the unlimited ability to proliferate, reflecting the loss of the normal contact inhibition mechanisms that regulate cellular growth. They can grow in an anchorage-independent fashion, representing the loss of the normal requirements for cell attachments to the extracellular matrix. Transformed cells also have the ability to grow in low concentrations of serum, representing the acquired trait of synthesis of autocrine growth factors.

As described by the unicellular origin theory, tumors are thought to arise from a single transformed cell. Transformed cells, however, can become tumorigenic (malignant or cancerous) or can be nontumorigenic. All malignant cells possess the ability to form tumors after inoculation into immunocompromised mice. Nontumorigenic cells lack the ability to form tumors in vivo. The process by which transformed cells become cancerous is termed *carcinogenesis* (the forming of cancer). Carcinogenesis is a complex process consisting of three distinct stages—initiation, promotion, and progression—and is thought to be the result of the accumulation of genetic modifications. In order to undergo malignant transformation, a series of changes must occur in the mechanisms governing normal cellular differentiation and growth at each of these three stages. When cells accumulate one or more critical genetic alterations in these cellular

Table 46–1
2000 estimates of the five leading sites of new cancer cases and deaths

Cancer Cases by Site and Sex		Cancer Deaths by Site and Sex	
Men	**Women**	**Men**	**Women**
Prostate (180,400)	Breast (182,000)	Lung (89,300)	Lung (67,600)
Lung (89,500)	Lung (74,600)	Prostate (27,800)	Breast (28,500)
Colorectal (63,600)	Colorectal (66,600)	Colorectal (27,800)	Colorectal (28,500)
Urinary bladder (38,300)	Uterus (36,100)	Pancreas (13,700)	Pancreas (14,500)
Melanoma (27,300)	Ovary (23,100)	Lymphoma (13,700)	Ovary (14,000)

Data from American Cancer Society: Cancer Facts and Figures 2000. New York: American Cancer Society, 2000.

pathways, they may undergo malignant transformation. This process can occur because of changes caused by direct interaction of environmental toxins on cells, as well as by inherited and acquired genetic alterations that occur by chance during DNA replication and cell division. The most well-known genetic model is that proposed by Vogelstein for the development of colorectal cancer. In Vogelstein's model, the effects of oncogene activation and tumor suppressor gene loss are thought to be a multistep process leading to colorectal tumor formation and subsequent metastasis (Fig. 46–1). Because of these progressive genetic changes, the phenotype of cancerous cells can be characterized by alterations in nuclear and cellular morphology. Often cancerous cells possess chromosomal aberrations, including rearrangements, losses of portions of the chromosome, trisomy, and aneuploidy. There may also be presence of increased mitoses or other nuclear abnormalities.

Risk Factors for Cancer

The malignant transformation of a cell leading to tumor formation is a complex, sequential process. Any human being is at risk of developing cancer. Most individuals who develop cancer do so later in life. Over 80% of all cancers

are diagnosed at the age of 55 or older. In the United States, men have a 1 in 2 lifetime risk of developing a cancer, while women have a lifetime risk of 1 in 3. Often the risk of cancer is defined as the relative risk. This compares the risk of developing cancers in persons with a certain exposure or trait to the risk in people who do not have this exposure or trait. Risk can be categorized as environmental, such as smoking, or genetic, such as having a family history of breast cancer. Risk factors include environmental exposure, such as physical, chemical, or viral carcinogens causing genetic alterations in cells of a specific tissue. In addition, risks factors can be inherited, such as activated oncogenes or inherited mutations in tumor suppressor genes.

Physical carcinogens

Physical carcinogens include ionizing radiation, ultraviolet light, foreign bodies, hypertrophied scarring of burn, and other physical insults to tissue. These agents often cause damage and changes in the cellular DNA, leading to induction of cellular proliferation in response to the injury. One example of this process is the occurrence of squamous cell cancers within Marjolin's ulcers in patients with longstanding skin wounds. Patients with inflammatory disease of the bowel often are at risk for adenocarcinomas of the

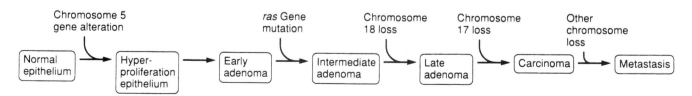

FIGURE 46–1 A model of colorectal tumorigenesis proven by Vogelstein. Colorectal tumors are thought to arise from mutational activation of oncogenes with inactivation of tumor suppressor genes. It is thought that at least five genes are required for full malignant transformation. It is the total accumulation of changes, rather than the sequence, that is important. (Adapted from Fearon ER, Vogelstein B: A genetic model for colorectal tumorigenesis. Cell 1990;61:769, with permission from Elsevier.)

gastrointestinal (GI) tract. Exposure to asbestos is a risk factor for mesothelioma and lung cancer. Ultraviolet light induces the formation of skin tumors such as melanoma and squamous cell carcinomas. In addition, exposure to high-frequency ionizing radiation is a significant risk factor for thyroid carcinoma. Virtually any part of the body can be affected by ionizing radiation, especially the bone marrow and thyroid gland.

Chemical carcinogens

Chemical carcinogens cause tumor formation in a similar manner, damaging tissue and causing a corresponding inflammatory response. Chemical carcinogens include benzene, vinyl chloride, aflatoxin, chloroform, formaldehyde, bicyclohydrocarbone, nitrosamines, and heavy metals such as nickel, cadmium, chromium, arsenic, and lead, and others. The most common chemical carcinogens are cigarette smoke and alcohol. The American Cancer Society estimates that approximately 170,000 cancer deaths can be attributed to tobacco while almost 20,000 cancer deaths can be attributed to alcohol.

DNA damage repair

As mentioned above, both physical and chemical agents can cause cellular DNA damage. Furthermore, spontaneous DNA damage can occur during normal cellular processes such as DNA replication or rearrangement. Normal cells possess the ability to repair these acquired defects in their DNA. Without repair, damaged DNA sites can be converted to permanent mutations during cellular DNA replication. Therefore, cells that lack one or more of these repair processes are at a significant risk for DNA damage leading to malignant transformation. Listed in Table 46–2 are familial cancer syndromes associated with an inherited defect in DNA repair mechanisms.

Viruses

Viruses have clearly been shown to induce tumor formation in humans. Hepatitis B infection can lead to development of hepatocellular cancer. Strains of human papillomaviruses can cause genital warts as well as cervical cancer. Human immunodeficiency virus is associated with a high incidence of Kaposi's sarcoma. Epstein-Barr virus has been implicated as a cause of Burkitt's lymphoma and nasopharyngeal carcinoma. Infection with human T-cell leukemia virus can lead to sarcomas, leukemia, and lymphoid tumors.

Oncogenes

Oncogenes are genes that, when expressed, cause malignant transformation of cells in vitro and tumor formation in vivo.

Table 46–2
Familial cancer syndromes

Cancer Syndrome	Gene	Malignancy
Loss of function of a DNA repair gene		
Ataxia-telangiectasia	ATM	Lymphoma
Xeroderma pigmentosum	XPB, XPD, XPA	Skin cancer
Hereditary nonpolyposis colorectal cancer	MSH2, MSH6, MLH1, PMS1, PMS2	Colorectal, gastric, endometrial cancer
Loss of function of a tumor suppressor gene		
Adenomatous polyposis coli	APC	Colon cancer, desmoid tumors, polyp
Familial breast cancer	BRCA1, BRCA2	Breast, ovarian cancer
Hereditary papillary renal cancer	MET	Renal cancer
Li-Fraumeni syndrome	TP53	Sarcoma, breast, brain cancer
Von Hippel-Lindau disease	VHL	Renal cell, adrenal pheochromocytoma
Retinoblastoma	RB1	Retinoblastoma, osteosarcoma
Neurofibromatosis type 1	NF1	Neurofibromas, sarcomas, gliomas
Neurofibromatosis type 2	NF2	Schwannomas, meningiomas
Wilms' tumor	WT1	Nephroblastoma
Gain of function, activation of a proto-oncogene		
Multiple endocrine neoplasia	RET	Medullary thyroid cancer

Data from Dove WF: Genes and cancer: risk determinants and agents of change. In Abeloff MD, Armitage JO, Litcher AS, et al (eds): Clinical Oncology. New York: Churchill-Livingstone, 2000:60.

An understanding of oncogenes came from the discovery of these sequences within the genome of RNA retroviruses. These oncogenes are thought to originate from normal cellular genes called proto-oncogenes, which are "accidentally" incorporated into the viral gene during recombination events between RNA viruses and host DNA. During this transduction, the normal gene can be mutated or rearranged. Proto-oncogenes generally serve a critical function within the cell (Table 46–3). Therefore, they are ideal candidates for mutation, which would alter gene expression, resulting in abnormal cellular growth. The altered form of the proto-oncogene, which becomes integrated in the viral genome, codes for an abnormal or mutant form of the gene's protein. Expression of the mutant protein then leads to malignant transformation of the cell. Oncogenes are designated by the three-letter names representing the tumors induced by the gene or the cell line from which the oncogene was isolated. They can be preceded by the letter "v," implying the oncogene originated from a virus, or "c," indicating the oncogene came from host cellular DNA. Therefore, infection with retroviruses containing oncogenes can lead to malignant transformation, and similarly, mutations in normal cellular proto-oncogenes can result in cancerous changes without viral infection.

For instance, one proto-oncogene is the *ras* gene. The *ras* gene is responsible for transmitting extracellular signals from the cell surface, through a signal transduction pathway, to the nucleus, resulting in changes in cellular growth and differentiation. *Ras* is normally intermittently

Table 46–3
Common oncogenes activated in tumors

Oncogene	Tumor	Original Function of Proto-oncogene
N-*myc*	Neuroblastoma	Transcription factor
L-*myc*	Lung carcinoma	Transcription factor
v-*fos*	Osteosarcoma	Transcription factor
v-*jun*	Sarcoma	Transcription factor
v-*ski*	Carcinoma	Transcription factor
v-*rel*	Leukemia	Transcription factor
v-*sis*	Glioma	Platelet-derived growth factor
INT2	Breast cancer	Fibroblast growth factor family member
EGFR	Squamous cell cancer	Tyrosine protein kinase
v-*fms*	Sarcoma	Tyrosine protein kinase
v-*kit*	Sarcoma	Tyrosine protein kinase
v-*ros*	Sarcoma	Tyrosine protein kinase
MET	Sarcoma	Tyrosine protein kinase
TRK	Colon carcinoma	Tyrosine protein kinase
NEU	Neuroblastoma	Tyrosine protein kinase
v-*src*	Sarcoma	Tyrosine protein kinase
BCR/ABL	CML	Tyrosine protein kinase
K-*ras*	Colon, lung, pancreas adenocarcinoma	GTPase
N-*ras*	AML	GTPase
H-*ras*	Carcinoma, melanoma	GTPase
GSP	Thyroid cancer	G protein
GIP	Ovarian, adrenal carcinoma	G protein
v-*mos*	Sarcoma	Serine/threonine protein kinase
v-*raf*	Sarcoma	Serine/threonine protein kinase
PIM1	T-cell lymphoma	Serine/threonine protein kinase

AML, acute myelogenous leukemia; CML, chronic myelogenous leukemia.
Data from Park M: Oncogenes. In Vogelstein B, Kinzler KW (eds): The Genetic Basis of Human Cancer. New York: McGraw-Hill, 1998:205, with permission.

activated when growth factor receptors have been triggered at the cell surface. However, point mutations in the Ras protein lead to constitutive activation of the protein. These mutations have been shown to be highly prevalent in human cancers. For example, 50% of colonic and 85% of pancreatic adenocarcinomas harbor *ras* mutations. Another well-studied proto-oncogene is *RET*. Mutational activation of the *RET* proto-oncogene in thyroid tissue has been shown to cause medullary thyroid cancer. Furthermore, germline mutations in the *RET* gene have been shown to result in inherited forms of medullary thyroid cancer (see Table 46–2). In addition to viral transduction and point mutation, oncogenes can be activated by other methods. Chromosomal translocation occurs in patients with chronic myelogenous leukemia. In this disease, the proto-oncogene c-*abl* is translocated from chromosome nine to the *BRCA1* locus on chromosome 22. In other cases an oncogene can be amplified, or increased in copy number. The N-*myc* oncogene is often amplified in lung tumors. This amplification leads to increase expression of the oncogene. Examples of proto-oncogenes are shown in Table 46–3.

Tumor suppressor genes

As opposed to activation of a particular oncogene causing initiation of tumorigenesis, certain genes are thought to inhibit tumor formation. These genes have been named tumor suppressor genes, and in normal cells are thought to oppose the actions of oncogenes. Much of our understanding of tumor suppressor genes came from studies by Knudsen on retinoblastoma. Knudsen observed that 40% of patients with retinoblastoma developed multiple tumors at younger ages and often had a family history of retinoblastoma, suggesting an inherited pattern. However, not all family members developed cancer. In contrast, the other 60% of patients with retinoblastoma usually had single tumors that develop at a much older age. Based on these observations, Knudsen proposed a theory that could explain the development of retinoblastoma in both groups of patients, termed the "two-hit hypothesis." He proposed that two distinct mutagenic events were necessary for tumor development. Normally, a cell would contain two functional copies of a tumor suppressor gene, in this case the retinoblastoma (*RB*) gene. In order for tumorigenesis to occur, both copies would have to be mutated, leading to an ineffective protein. In the inherited form of retinoblastoma, Knudsen hypothesized that these patients had one mutation present in the germline and therefore in all cells within the body. A second mutation occurring in the retinoblasts would lead to retinoblastoma. The frequency of cancer in this group of patients with the inherited gene defect was dependent on frequency of the second mutation. In the second group of patients, without an inherited defect, both normal copies of the *RB* gene must be mutated.

Other familiar cancers caused by mutations in tumor suppressor genes are shown in Table 46–2.

Tumor Proliferation

Fraction of Tumor in Growth Phase

A tumor is made up of many heterogeneous cell types, including fibroblasts, lymphocytes, macrophages, normal epithelial cells, and cancerous cells. Only a certain fraction of the tumor is growing at any one time. The fraction of tumor growth can vary from 3% to 25% in several different tumors. The theoretical growth curve for human tumors is shown in Figure 46–2. Tumors often have a phase of exponential tumor growth prior to clinical detection. The fraction of the tumor growing can be as high as 40% during this phase. Tumor proliferation depends on several key elements, including the fraction of cells cycling, the duration of the cell cycle, and the number of cells dying.

Cell Cycle

The cell cycle is defined as a sequence of events involving growth and division of a parental cell into two daughter cells with identical chromosomal composition. The cell cycle is divided into four sequential phases: G_1 (gap 1), S (DNA synthesis), G_2 (gap 2), and M (mitosis/meiosis). A G_0 phase (rest or quiescent state) has been described for cells not actively proliferating but capable of undergoing cellular division after an appropriate signal. G_1 is the variable growth phase between the completion of cell division and the start of DNA synthesis (the S phase). During the

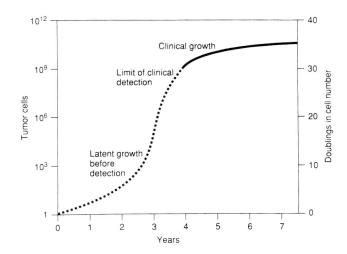

FIGURE 46–2 A theoretical growth curve for human tumors. (From Tannock IF: Principles of cell proliferation: cell kinetics. *In* DeVita VT, Hellman S, Rosenberg SA [eds]: Cancer: Principles and Practice of Oncology [3rd ed]. Philadelphia: JB Lippincott, 1989:703.)

S phase, after DNA synthesis occurs, the cells have two diploid sets of chromosomes. The S phase is followed by a second gap phase, G_2, when further cellular growth occurs. Duplication of cellular organelles and other machinery is completed during this phase. Finally, the process of mitosis occurs whereby a single cell splits into two identical daughter cells.

The fraction of cells cycling is the proportion of the total cell number going through the cell cycle (replicating) at a point in time (cells not in G_0). Therefore, cells residing in G_1, S, G_2, or M are those that are in the proliferative or growth fraction, and are the fraction of the cells that are cycling. The remaining cells in the G_0 phase are in the nonproliferative fraction. The fraction of cells in each compartment can be measured by DNA flow cytometry. The duration of the cell cycle is similar for most tumors, ranging from 2 to 4.5 days.

Regulation of the cell cycle occurs at multiple levels. Cell cycle progression is controlled by regulatory proteins called cyclins and cyclin-dependent kinases, or cdks, which through association with one another form active complexes. Changes in these complexes, often by cyclin phosphorylation and/or inhibition by molecules called cyclin kinase inhibitors, are responsible for allowing cells to progress from one cell cycle phase to another. In addition to regulation by cdks, other factors also ensure that DNA replication and chromosomal segregation have taken place in an orderly programmed fashion. These checkpoints for DNA integrity generally occur between G_1 and S phase and between G_2 and M phase. If cellular DNA damage has occurred and has not been repaired, these checkpoints will not allow the cell to continue through the cycle, resulting in cell cycle arrest. Mutation or absence of any of these regulatory molecules is one mechanism by which cancer cells evade cell cycle control and can thus proliferate in an uncontrolled manner.

Cell Death

Another determinate of tumor growth is cell death. After every cell cycle, a fraction of cells undergo cell death. For some normal tissues, the high cellular proliferation occurring in normal bone marrow and in the cells lining the GI tract is balanced with a high cell loss in these tissues. Cell loss in these normal tissues primarily occurs via a genetically regulated process of programmed cell death known as apoptosis. During this essential, strictly regulated phenomenon, cells undergo autodigestion without an associated inflammatory response. In most instances, however, the amount of cell death does not compensate for the increased growth.

Apoptosis occurs in all organs and is also an important component of tumor progression. Cells that fail to undergo apoptosis are responsible for several pathologic processes, including cancer, autoimmune disease, and viral infection. Cells with damaged DNA are normally eliminated by the apoptotic process. Cells that are unable to undergo apoptosis in response to DNA damage survive longer and are more apt to develop genetic mutations and progress to a cancerous phenotype.

During the progressive growth of a tumor, cell death occurs as a result of apoptosis and by cell necrosis. In contrast to apoptosis, cell necrosis occurs secondary to a lack of blood supply and nutrient, and is usually associated with a proinflammatory response. Cell necrosis can also result from host responses (antitumor immune response), lack of needed growth factors, and therapy given to the patient.

Tumor Doubling Time

The measurement of tumor growth is often termed the *tumor doubling time*. This is defined as the amount of time taken to increase the tumor volume by twofold. On average, solid tumor will have undergone 30 doublings to reach 1 cm in diameter. Starting from a single tumor cell, after 30 doublings, the tumor will have approximately 10^9 cells. After 10 more doublings, the cell mass will have reached approximately 1 kg or 10^{12} cells, which is generally the maximal amount of tumor mass compatible with life.

Metastasis

What distinguishes malignant from benign tumors is the ability to invade extensively into surrounding tissue(s) and to disseminate throughout the body. Like the formation of the tumor itself, the process of metastasis is a series of sequential steps. The major steps of metastasis formation have been eloquently defined by I. Fidler (illustrated in Figure 46–3):

1. Transformation of normal cells into tumor cells and growth after the initial transforming event

2. Extensive vascularization with the secretion of angiogenesis factors

3. Local invasion of the host stroma by tumor cells that are genetically programmed for entrance into lymphatic or vascular channels

4. Detachment and embolization of single or multiple tumor cells into the circulation

5. The tumor cell surviving in the circulation

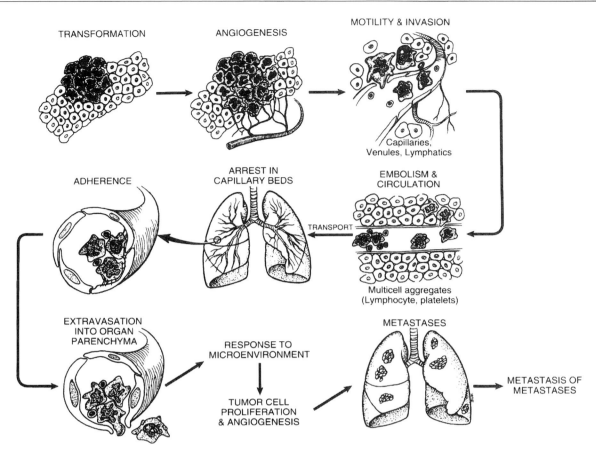

FIGURE 46–3 A model of tumor metastases proposed by I. Fidler. (From Fidler IJ: Molecular biology of cancer: invasion and metastases. *In* DeVita VT, Hellman S, Rosenberg SA [eds]: Cancer: Principles and Practice of Oncology [5th ed]. Philadelphia: JB Lippincott, 1997:136.)

6. The tumor cell arresting in the capillary beds of distant organs by adhering to the capillary epithelium

7. Invasion into the distant organ

8. Proliferation as a metastatic implant within the distant organ

Expansion of the primary tumor beyond 1 mm depends on development of a new blood supply. This process has been termed *angiogenesis*. Multiple molecules have been implicated in the cascade of cellular signals required for new vessel formation. These factors include vascular epithelial growth factor, interleukin-8, angiogenin, epidermal growth factor, platelet-derived epithelial cell growth factor, transforming growth factor-α and -β, and tumor necrosis factor. The extent of angiogenesis is a balance between factors that stimulate and inhibit new blood vessel formation. After creating a new blood supply, the tumor cells must have the ability to penetrate the stromal tissue,

including the basement membrane, to enter the vascular system and/or lymphatics. Tumor cells must possess the necessary genetically programmed protein molecules and signal pathways for motility as well the ability to disassociate from one another. In epithelial tumors, the cell-to-cell contact is often due to expression of E-cadherin, a cell surface glycoprotein. Reduced levels of E-cadherin have been found in higher grade carcinomas as well as metastatic lesions. For example, in islet cell tumors, the loss of E-cadherin has been shown to correspond with formation of liver metastasis. Other key cell surface proteins also play a key role in metastasis, such as integrins, catenins, laminins, and lectins.

Tumors normally disseminate through lymphatic and/or hematogenous routes. Regional lymph nodes are thought to play a role in tumor containment, serving as a barrier to cell dissemination. After tumor invasion to lymphatics, cells can easily be transported along the lymphatics, and drain first to local regional lymph nodes and then to distant ones. The presence of tumor in lymph nodes is an important criterion for staging. Often, lymphadenectomies are employed in certain tumors for prognostic as well as therapeutic reasons. In contrast to lymphatic metastasis, with hematogenesis metastasis, tumor cells must survive in the circulation and have the ability to adhere to capillaries in the distant organs. Several studies have shown that most tumor cells that enter the blood stream are eliminated rapidly. Tumor cells often survive in the circulation by self-aggregation or adherence to blood-borne structures such as platelets. Attachment of tumor cells to capillaries in the distant organ could be due to the adherence of platelets to damaged epithelium, providing an entry site for tumor cells. The final step of metastasis is tumor cell proliferation in the distant organ. The most common organs of metastasis include the lung and the liver. The liver is known to produce many growth factors that stimulate the proliferation of many tumors. For example, neuroendocrine tumors frequently metastasize to the liver. Insulin-like growth factor is synthesized in the liver and has been shown to stimulate growth of these tumors in vitro.

Clinical Treatment

Screening

The treatment of cancer begins with diagnosis. Generally, the earlier the diagnosis is made the more treatable the malignancy. However, screening all patients for every type of tumor would be impractical as well as expensive. Thus cancer screening targets individuals who are at risk for developing cancer. These individuals include patients with a family history of breast, colon, or thyroid cancer. In addition, routine mammographic and endoscopic surveillance are used to screen for breast and colon cancer. However, the majority of individuals with cancer present with distinct lesions causing symptomatology or are diagnosed incidentally when an imaging technique is used for another reason.

Tumor markers

In addition to imaging modalities, some tumors produce proteins that can be detected in the patient's serum. These proteins are called tumor markers. The first tumor marker identified was the enzyme acid phosphatase, found in 1938 in patients with metastatic prostate carcinoma. A common tumor marker, carcinoembryonic antigen, was shown in 1965 to be elevated in a percentage of colon cancers. Tumor markers can range from tumor antigens to enzymes/hormones produced by the tumor. A variety of tumor markers routinely used in practice are shown in Table 46–4. Tumor markers are frequently elevated in patients with the corresponding tumor. Serum levels of a marker can be used for monitoring response to therapy and for detecting tumor recurrence.

Needle biopsy

Needle biopsies are most often performed in an office setting under local anesthesia. Most commonly, biopsies are performed either as fine-needle aspiration (FNA) or large-needle cutting biopsies (such as true-cut needles). With FNA, the diagnosis of cancer is achieved by the detection of abnormal cellular or nuclear features seen in individual cells. In addition, immunohistochemistry and flow cytometry can be used to check for expression of any tumor antigens and/or markers. However, FNA is limited because frequently the diagnosis of cancer depends on the presence of structural tissue abnormalities such as formation of tissue structures (ducts) by abnormal cells, invasion through basement membranes, and invasion of blood vessels, nerves, or other structures. In these cases, large-needle cutting biopsies can be used to obtain a core fragment of tissue that allows the histologic diagnosis of cancer.

Staging

After making the diagnosis of cancer, staging is required. Staging is the process of describing the extent of the disease, or how far the cancer has spread from its site of origin. It is essential for determining prognosis as well as for deciding on the appropriate therapy. Staging is based on several factors, including factors related to the primary tumor itself (size, location, and involvement of adjacent organs), the degree of lymph node involvement, and the presence of distant metastasis. The most common system used is the TNM staging system. The "T" status is determined by the tumor size and location and often the presence of local invasion. For certain tumors, such as sarcomas, the histologic grade of the tumor also plays a role in the T status. The "N" status denotes either the absence or presence of regional lymph node involvement by the tumor. The "M" status refers to the absence or presence of distant metastasis. Once the T, N, and M statuses are determined, an overall cancer stage of I, II, III, or IV is assigned (with stage I being early cancer and stage IV being advanced cancer). Staging procedures may include lymph node sampling, sentinel lymph node mapping and biopsy, anatomic imaging techniques such as computed tomography (CT) scanning and magnetic resonance imaging, and functional imaging by positron emission tomography, as well as other noninvasive methods including nuclear scans and ultrasound.

Therapy

The future of cancer care rests on the appropriate integration of all available therapeutic modalities, including surgery, radiotherapy, chemotherapy, hormonal therapy,

Table 46-4
Tumor markers

Marker	Normal Value	Tumors	Conditions Causing False Positives
Carcinoembryonic antigen	<2.5 ng/mL	Colorectal, pancreas, breast, lung, gastric, medullary thyroid	Hepatitis, cirrhosis, jaundice, COPD, ulcers, IBD, renal failure
α-Fetoprotein	<40 ng/mL	Hepatoma, testicular	Hepatitis, cirrhosis, pregnancy, IBD
β-Human chorionic gonadotropin	<3 U/mL	Testicular, trophoblastic gestational tumors	Pregnancy
Prostate-specific antigen	<2.5 ng/mL	Prostate	Benign prostatic hypertrophy
Tissue polypeptide antigen	<100 U/L	Breast, gynecologic	None
CA-15-3	<22 U/mL	Breast	Hepatitis, cirrhosis, benign breast disease
CA-19-9	<35 U/mL	Colorectal, biliary, pancreas, gastric	Hepatitis, cirrhosis, cholangitis, cholestasis
CA-50	<17 U/mL	Colorectal, pancreas, gastric	Pancreatitis, cirrhosis, IBD, cholangitis
CA-242	<20 U/mL	Colorectal, pancreas, gastric	Pancreatitis, cirrhosis, IBD, cholangitis
CA-125	<35 U/mL	Ovarian	Pregnancy, endometriosis, PID, renal failure, menstruation
Neuron-specific enolase	<13 ng/mL	Neuroendocrine, small cell lung, medullary thyroid, carcinoid, islet cell	None
Prostatic acid phosphatase	<0.8 U/L	Prostatic	Benign prostatic hypertrophy, dermatologic disorders
CYFRA-21-1	<3.3 ng/mL	Non–small cell lung	Benign lung disorders

COPD, chronic obstructive pulmonary disease; IBD, inflammatory bowel disease; PID, pelvic inflammatory disease.
Data from Norton JA, Fraker DL: Tumor markers. In Sabiston DC, Lyerly HK (eds): Textbook of Surgery. Philadelphia: WB Saunders, 1997:494.

and biologic therapy. It is rare that any cancer can be cured with one modality alone. Surgery and radiotherapy are often used to achieve local tumor control. Surgery offers the advantage of removing the bulk of the tumor mass, but can be limited by the inability to obtain clear margins, or the presence of microscopic disease near the primary site and in distant organs. Radiotherapy frequently can achieve microscopic tumor control of the primary tumor site following resection. Chemotherapy is utilized primarily to treat the possible existence of occult systemic disease or measurable recurrent nonresectable metastases. Several studies have shown that tumor cells can be detected in the blood stream of individuals bearing a primary tumor and prior to the development of clinically detectable metastases. In theory, these tumor cells outside the local area of the primary tumor can be effectively treated with chemotherapy, hormonal therapy, or biologic therapy. A discussion of the specific treatments for certain tumors is beyond the scope of this chapter. However, we briefly review the concepts of oncologic surgery, radiation therapy, chemotherapy, and biologic therapy.

Surgery

Since the time of William S. Halsted, surgery has been recognized as the mainstay of cancer therapies. When Halsted developed the radical mastectomy, it was the only potentially curative treatment for patients with breast carcinoma. However, with our rapidly expanding knowledge of tumor progression and metastases, we have come to realize that, at the time of cancer diagnosis, almost 70% of solid tumors have already spread systemically. Therefore, in these cases, surgery alone is rarely curative. Today, surgical oncologists must have an understanding of all of the cancer treatment modalities to effectively integrate and coordinate the care of cancer patients. Surgeons will certainly be involved in treating patients with resectable tumors. They are also called upon to manage surgical emergencies that occur in cancer patients with advanced disease, including bowel perforation, bowel obstruction, GI bleeding, and sepsis. In addition, surgery is more and more frequently utilized in the treatment of metastatic disease, especially in cases of isolated malignant lesions within the liver and lung. However, surgeons are now becoming more involved in the delivery of chemotherapy through placement of central venous catheters and implantation of drug delivery pumps. Furthermore, surgeons have been at the forefront of the development of nonsurgical treatment of metastatic disease, such as local ablative therapies within the liver, and the experimental development and testing of biologic therapies. They are also involved extensively in screening and increasingly are the source of prevention efforts for patients at increased risks for developing cancer. Thus the surgical oncologist continues to have an essential role in the management of cancer patients.

Chemotherapy

Most active chemotherapeutic agents are designed to inhibit cellular processes occurring during the S or M phase of the cell cycle. Thus these drugs are generally more effective in actively dividing cells, which spend a larger proportion of their cell life in these two phases of the cell cycle, than they are in slowly dividing cells. Because cytotoxic drugs are not selective for cancerous cells, chemotherapeutic agents also affect rapidly proliferating normal tissues, such as bone marrow and GI epithelial cells. In designing potential drugs, tumor kill efficacy must be balanced with toxicity. To achieve this balance, chemotherapeutic regimens often utilize multiple drugs with different mechanisms of action. Single agents rarely cure cancer. In addition, tumor cells can often develop resistance to single agents. Thus combination chemotherapy is the standard treatment for many widespread tumors.

As mentioned before, chemotherapy, given in proximity to surgery and radiation, is delivered to eradicate occult systemic disease and is called adjuvant treatment. Chemotherapy administered before local therapy is often referred to as neoadjuvant or primary therapy. In theory, neoadjuvant treatment reduces the primary lesion and allows for a more successful surgical resection. It might also treat micrometastatic disease that may be present at the time of surgery. An advantage of neoadjuvant therapy is that it provides earlier exposure to chemotherapy drugs for patients at higher risk of harboring micrometastases. Furthermore, an observed response in primary tumors provides in vivo evidence of antitumor activity of the drug. The main disadvantage of neoadjuvant therapy is that it may preclude accurate tumor staging. Chemotherapy can be administered intravenously, which is the most common route; however, some chemotherapy is administered orally. Occasionally chemotherapy is given intra-arterially, for example, to the liver, head, neck, pelvis, or limbs.

Radiation therapy

Radiation therapy delivers ionizing radiation energy to tumor tissue. The amount of radiation is quantified in units called rads. One hundred rads equals 1 J/kg, which is the clinical description of the amount of energy absorbed per unit mass. Radiation is usually dosed as grays (Gy) with 1 Gy = 100 rads. Radiation kills tumor cells in two ways. It kills cells directly by causing breaks in chromosomal DNA, rendering it incapable of replication, or more commonly, indirectly by generating oxygen free radicals through the interaction of the ionized radiation with water. These free radicals cause damage to DNA and other essential intracellular structures. Thus radiation therapy depends on adequate oxygen delivery to the irradiated tissue. Radiation therapy is similar to chemotherapy in that it does not discriminate between normal and neoplastic tissue. Highly proliferative normal tissues, such as skin, GI epithelium, and bone marrow, are at risk from radiation exposure. Therefore, the benefit of radiation must be weighed as a balance between the killing of normal versus neoplastic tissue.

Radiotherapy is most often fractionated. Fractionization is the process by which the total dose of radiation is given in a series of small doses rather than a large single dose. Multifractionated regimens have several advantages. Normal tissue is spared because it is allowed to recover from radiation damage in between treatments. In addition, this recovery period allows reoxygenation of tissues and therefore allows delivery of oxygen to the tumor. As previously mentioned, tumor killing by ionizing radiation is highly dependent on development in the targeted tissue of oxygen free radicals. Radiation can be delivered in several ways. External beam radiation is the most common, but brachytherapy through operatively placed catheters is another method that allows localization to deep tissues. The delivery of radiation has been greatly enhanced by the ability of CT scanning to generate precise images of the target and the availability of sophisticated software developed to accurately plan the field and the delivery technique to be employed.

Biologic therapy

The field of biologic therapy continues to evolve because of the growing knowledge of the role of the immune system in cancer surveillance and containment. Biologic therapy produces antitumor activity through the action of natural host defense mechanisms augmented by the administration of immune-enhancing drugs. The host immune response to tumors includes the antibodies and natural killer cells that are present in the circulatory system, and cytotoxic T lymphocytes and macrophages, which provide immune defenses at the local tissue level. Modern methods of biologic therapy have focused on ways of improving the response of cytotoxic T cells (tumor-infiltrating lymphocytes) as well as activated natural killer cells to respond to tumors.

The naturally occurring cytokines known as interferon-α, -β, and -γ have been utilized over the last 30 years in the treatment of several solid organ malignancies, including renal cell carcinoma and endocrine tumors. Interleukins are produced by leukocytes and have several immune system–enhancing activities. There are over 12 well-studied interleukins. The most well-studied, interleukin-2, has been approved for use by the Food and Drug Administration, and has been shown to provide long-term responses in patients with renal cell carcinoma and melanoma. Another method to stimulate the immune system other than cytokine administration is through tumor cell vaccines. In this approach, cancer patients are immunized against tumor-associated antigens in order elicit an antibody response against tumors that possess these antigens. Ongoing vaccine protocols are being evaluated for melanoma, colon cancer, renal cell carcinoma, and ovarian carcinoma. Lastly, another approach is gene therapy. Common techniques involve transfer of cytokine genes into irradiation tumor cells. These cells are then introduced into the patient and stimulate an immune response.

Outcomes

The response to therapy can be classified as a complete response (total disappearance of all measurable malignant lesions), a partial response (a 50% reduction in measurable disease), stable disease, or no response. Sometimes the disease remains stable with no new disease, decreases somewhat, and/or shows only decreases in tumor serum markers. Responses or stabilization of disease correlate significantly with improved quality of life for cancer patients.

The true measure of the success of a cancer treatment, however, is survival. Survival can be described as either disease-free survival or overall survival. *Disease-free* survival is the time that the patient is alive after a complete response to cancer therapy without any signs of tumor recurrence. *Overall* survival is the time from tumor diagnosis to the patient's death regardless of the status of the tumor. Five-year survival rates are commonly used to monitor progress in the treatment of various cancers. The *relative* 5-year survival rate refers to the survival rate for an observed number of cancer patients during a 5-year interval compared to the survival rate for a group of patients who are similar with respect to age, gender, race, and other factors such as the incidence of heart disease and accidents. While these rates provide some indication about the average survival experience of cancer patients in a given population, they are less informative when used to predict individual prognosis.

For instance, the 5-year survival rate is based on patients who were treated at least 5 years ago and does not represent the most recent advances in treatment. Second, information about the treatment, diagnosis, and other factors that influence outcome is now being taken into consideration in the estimation of survival rate. For many tumors, recurrences can develop many years following initial treatment of the primary tumor. More realistic follow-up statistics are frequently based on a 10-year period. The 5-year survival rate for all cancers combined is about 60%.

Summary

The field of tumor biology is constantly changing. With the advancement of molecular biology and other diagnostic and therapeutic clinical treatments, the treatment of cancer is increasingly becoming a multidisciplinary endeavor.

Acknowledgments

We would like to thank Tara Breslin, M.D., and Greg Kennedy, M.D., for their helpful suggestions and review of the manuscript.

Bibliography

Bos JL, Fearon ER, Hamilton SR, et al: Prevalence of *ras* gene mutations in human colorectal cancers. Nature 1987;327:293.

Fidler IJ: Critical determinants of cancer metastasis: rationale for therapy. Cancer Chemother Pharmacol 1999;43(Suppl):S3.

Fidler IJ: Angiogenesis and cancer metastasis. Cancer J Sci Am 2000;6(Suppl 2):S134.

Knudson AG: Hereditary cancer: two hits revisited. J Cancer Res Clin Oncol 1996;122:135.

Moley JF, Lairmore TC, Phay JE: Hereditary endocrinopathies. Curr Probl Surg 1999;36:653.

O'Reilly MS, Holmgren L, Shing Y, et al: Angiostatin: a novel angiogenesis inhibitor that mediates the suppression of metastases by a Lewis lung carcinoma [see comments]. Cell 1994;79:315.

Perl AK, Wilgenbus P, Dahl U, et al: A causal role for E-cadherin in the transition from adenoma to carcinoma. Nature 1998;392:190.

Rodenhuis S: *ras* and human tumors. Semin Cancer Biol 1992;3:241.

Singer AL, Nakeeb A: Needle biopsies. *In* Chen H, Sonnenday CJ (eds): Manual of Common Bedside Procedures. Baltimore: Lippincott Williams & Wilkins, 2000:303.

CHAPTER 47

Cancer Therapy Alternatives

Suzanne E. Patton, M.D., Ph.D. and Frank M. Torti, M.D., M.P.H.

Chemotherapy

History

Surgical resection alone, even with radiation therapy to control local spread, is insufficient to cure many malignancies, which may have already spread to distant sites at the time of diagnosis. The need for systemic treatment of cancer has been recognized since the early 1900s. Paul Ehrlich originally coined the term *chemotherapy* in developing antibiotics in rodent model systems to treat infectious diseases. George Clowes of Roswell Park Memorial Institute in Buffalo, NY, then applied the term to screening potential anticancer drugs in transplanted tumor-bearing rodent models. However, the first effective chemotherapeutic agents were stumbled upon almost by accident, when it was discovered that the chemical warfare agent mustard gas, used in both world wars, caused bone marrow and lymphoid hypoplasia in military seamen. This observation led physicians at Yale University to treat humans with hematologic neoplasms, such as lymphomas, with nitrogen mustard. The dramatic regression of a mediastinal mass in a patient with Hodgkin's disease constituted the first successful demonstration of systemic anticancer therapy.

Soon thereafter, Sidney Farber reported that folic acid had a proliferative effect on childhood lymphoblastic leukemia. This sparked the scientists at American Cyanamid to develop antifolates, such as aminopterin and methotrexate, which had marked but transient responses in acute lymphoblastic leukemia (ALL). In 1951, Hitchings, Elion, and colleagues at Burroughs-Wellcome developed the purine analogs 6-thioguanine (6-TP) and 6-mercaptopurine (6-MP), and corticosteroids subsequently were shown to have activity in leukemia and lymphoma. Later in the 1950s, while evaluating natural products for the treatment of diabetes, scientists at Eli Lilly found that vinca alkaloids had antimitotic activity useful in killing rapidly dividing cancer cells. Other classes of chemotherapeutic agents from natural products followed, including mitomycin C, bleomycin, the anthracyclines, and more recently the taxanes and camptothecins.

Hopes soared in the 1960s, with the cure of many childhood leukemias and Hodgkin's disease. However, apart from testicular cancer, most solid tumors were disappointingly refractory to cure with chemotherapy. This was true even in cases in which the tumor had been completely resected, leaving a very small residual tumor burden. It turned out that nearly 90% of all drug cures occur in just 10% of all cancer types. This observation led to the investigation of intrinsic and acquired mechanisms of resistance. During the 1980s, the multidrug resistance (*MDR1*) gene was identified. It encodes the 170-kD P-glycoprotein, a cellular membrane pump that rapidly extrudes natural-product anticancer drugs, including the anthracyclines, taxanes, vinca alkaloids, and some antifolate drugs, from the cancer cells before they can exert their damaging effects. The enigma was, however, that normal tissues with rapid turnover, such as bone marrow and gastrointestinal (GI) mucosa, never develop multidrug resistance. This is now explained by the relative preservation of the cell cycle checkpoint and apoptosis in normal host tissues.

In order to attack cancer cells selectively, it is necessary to exploit the differences they have acquired from their normal progenitors. However, these invaders are much more similar to the host cells than are bacterial invaders. Hence there is potential for more toxicity to normal cells with anticancer chemotherapy than with antibacterial chemotherapy. One major difference between cancer cells and normal cells, appreciated early, was that some cancer cells divide more frequently than their normal counterparts. The cyclic process of cell division, including DNA uncoiling from chromosomes and copying from precursors, followed by segregation of the duplicate chromatids via the mitotic spindle, and finally cell division, has provided many essential functions that can be targeted for disruption. Other essential properties of malignant cells that have spawned new classes of anticancer therapies include invasiveness across tissue planes, metastasis to distant sites via the blood stream and lymphatics, ability to attract blood vessel ingrowth to feed growing tumors, ability to escape immune surveillance, and loss of terminal differentiation toward apoptosis.

Chemotherapeutic Agents

Alkylating Agents

The alkylating agents are metabolically activated to form reactive intermediates (potent electrophiles) capable of forming covalent bonds with DNA bases on one or both strands of the double helix, often forming intra- or interstrand cross-links. They attack and add alkyl groups at negatively charged oxygen, nitrogen, phosphorus, and sulfur atoms, especially N-7 guanine, O-6 guanine, and N-3 cytosine on DNA and RNA, interfering with DNA base pairing, transcription, and replication. They exert these effects throughout the cell cycle, and thus are cell cycle independent. However, major problems occur when the cell tries to copy its DNA preparatory to mitosis. Thus nondividing cell types are less vulnerable. Nonlethal mutations can result, some of which are carcinogenic themselves, posing a risk of secondary malignancies. The subclasses

differ in their degree and types of toxicities, clinical pharmacology, applications, and mechanisms of resistance.

Nitrogen mustards

Mechlorethamine

Cyclophosphamide (Cytoxan)

Ifosfamide

Melphalan (Alkeran)

Chlorambucil (Leukeran)

Nitrosoureas

CCNU

BCNU

Methyl-CCNU

Streptozotocin

Triazines

Dacarbazine (DTIC)

Procarbazine

Temozolamide

Aziridines

Thiotepa

Mitomycin C

Bioreductive alkylating agents

Tirapazamine

Platinum Complexes

The discovery of antitumor activity for the platinum compounds was based on the serendipitous finding by B. Rosenberg and colleagues in the 1960s that the delivery of alternating current through a set of platinum electrodes inhibited bacterial culture growth, not directly by the electromagnetic field, but by the chemical electrolysis products from the electrodes. A subsequent series of experiments revealed that the active species was the *cis* isomer of diaminodichloroplatinum (*cisplatin*). Steric conformation is important because the *trans* isomer has no clinical activity. High concentrations of chloride in plasma (100 nM) maintain cisplatin in the uncharged form, while in the cytoplasm low concentrations (4 mM) favor replacement of the chloride atom by a water molecule (aquation), resulting in a highly reactive species. These molecules bind to the N-7 positions of guanine and adenine to produce DNA and RNA cross-links, either intrastrand (>90%) or interstrand (<5%). Cisplatin is nephrotoxic, ototoxic, and neurotoxic, as well as being extremely emetogenic and causing alopecia and hypomagnesemia.

In contrast, *carboplatin* is more myelosuppressive and less emetogenic than cisplatin, with minimal nephrotoxicity, ototoxicity, and neurotoxicity. It can be substituted for cisplatin in many cases, the notable exception being testicular cancer. Even this exception might not hold up if carboplatin were dosed based on the now widely accepted "area under the concentration-time curve," based on creatinine clearance. Doses some 30% higher than would be calculated based on body surface area may now be used safely. These agents have a broad spectrum of clinical antitumor activity, including small cell lung cancer (SCLC) and non–small cell lung cancer (NSCLC), head and neck cancer, ovarian cancer, urothelial malignancies, and lymphomas. Both are cleared by renal excretion.

Oxaliplatin is a third-generation platinum compound with activity in colorectal cancer both as a single agent (10% to 18% response rate) and in synergy with 5-fluorouracil (5-FU)/leucovorin (30% to 40% response rate). It forms adducts with DNA that are more cytotoxic than those of cisplatin or carboplatin, and lacks cross-resistance with the first two members of this class. Reversible sensory neuropathy enhanced by exposure to cold temperatures is dose limiting and cumulative, affecting all patients who receive more than 540 mg/m^2 over four cycles or more. Patients also can have laryngopharyngeal dysesthesia, leading to dysphagia and allergic reactions, as well as nausea, vomiting, and diarrhea, but with only mild myelosuppression, minimal ototoxicity, and no nephrotoxicity.

Antimetabolites

Folate antagonists

Antifolates act by blocking steps in the intermediary metabolism of thymidine. *Aminopterin* was the first member of the class. It induced remissions in childhood acute leukemia in the 1940s. Methotrexate and 5-FU are now the two most widely used members of this class. In addition

to treating a wide spectrum of malignancies, antifolates also have been used to treat a variety of rheumatologic disorders, graft-versus-host disease, parasitic infections associated with the acquired immunodeficiency syndrome (AIDS), and other bacterial and plasmodial pathogens.

Methotrexate is a tight-binding inhibitor of dihydrofolate reductase. Its action results in the depletion of reduced folates, which serve as one-carbon carriers used by thymidylate synthase to convert deoxyuridine monophosphate (dUMP) to deoxythymidine monophosphate. The resulting depletion of deoxythymidine triphosphate interferes with cellular DNA repair functions. The excess dUMP leads to formation of deoxyuridine triphosphate, which then is misincorporated into DNA, interfering with DNA chain elongation and leading to further DNA fragmentation, when uracil DNA glycosylase attempts excision repair of the DNA. Thus its cytotoxic effect occurs primarily during the S phase of the cell cycle. Methotrexate has a documented broad spectrum of activity against leukemia, breast cancer, colorectal cancer, gastric cancer, head and neck cancer, lymphoma, osteogenic sarcoma, urothelial cancer, and choriocarcinoma. It has been included in many combination chemotherapy regimens with acronyms such as CMF, FAMtx, M-VAC, CMV, AFM, MIME, m-BACOD, MACOP-B, and PRO-MACE-Cyta-BOM. It distributes into and exits slowly from third-space fluid collections, such as pleural effusions and ascites. This prolongs the terminal half-life of the drug and can be equivalent to giving much higher than intended doses, with unpredictably higher attendant toxicities. Consequently, it is best to avoid using this agent in patients with ascites, pleural effusions, or other third-space fluid collections. Methotrexate is one of the few chemotherapy drugs sufficiently safe and effective for intrathecal administration, either via serial lumbar punctures or via an Ommaya reservoir, for meningeal carcinomatosis or leukemia. High-dose methotrexate is used in the treatment of osteogenic sarcomas and high-grade lymphomas or acute leukemias. This involves giving an otherwise lethal dose, followed by leucovorin rescue with vigorous intravenous hydration and urinary alkalinization to increase drug solubility, along with plasma drug level monitoring. Doses of greater than 100 mg/m^2 usually are followed by leucovorin rescue. The primary toxic effects of methotrexate are myelosuppression and GI mucositis. Hepatotoxicity, nephrotoxicity, and pulmonary toxicity also can occur.

Another lesser known analog is *trimetrexate*. It has a shorter intracellular half-life and, unlike methotrexate, is a substrate for P-glycoprotein, with consequent cross-resistance to a host of other natural products. It has a single-agent response rate of 26% in head and neck cancers, 19% in lung cancers, and, in combination with 5-FU/leucovorin, 30% to 35% in untreated metastatic colorectal cancer.

5-Fluorouracil easily enters cells via their facilitated uracil transport mechanism and then is converted to 5-fluoro-2′-deoxyuridine (FUdR) by thymidine phosphorylase. Subsequent phosphorylation of the drug by thymidine kinase gives rise to 5-fluorodeoxyuridine monophosphate (FdUMP), which covalently binds to and inhibits thymidylate synthase. This depletes deoxythymidine triphosphate (dTTP) and interferes with DNA synthesis and repair. The genotoxic stress resulting from thymidylate synthetase inhibition may activate programmed cell death (apoptosis), reflected in the classic DNA laddering response. Additionally, 5-fluorodeoxyuridine triphosphate is incorporated into DNA and fluorouridine triphosphate into RNA. 5-Fluorouracil is used to treat a variety of malignancies, including breast and all GI malignancies from mouth to anus: head and neck, esophageal, gastric, small bowel, pancreatic, colon, and anal. The major toxicities of 5-FU are schedule dependent and consist of stomatitis and diarrhea, when it is given as a continuous infusion, and myelosuppression, when it is given as a bolus 5 days a month. There are very few side effects when it is given as a weekly bolus. The painful hand-foot syndrome (palmar-plantar erythrodysesthesia) is a subacute toxicity of continuous infusion at high doses. 5-Fluorouracil also can cause photosensitivity of the skin and eyes; dermatitis; hyperpigmentation of hands, nails, and arm veins; conjunctivitis; tear duct stenosis; central nervous system toxicity; and coronary vasospasm. The 3% to 5% of adult cancer patients with congenital autosomal recessive deficiency of the catabolizing enzyme dihydropyrimidine dehydrogenase (DPD) may experience markedly exaggerated and even life-threatening or fatal toxicities without prior warning. Direct intrahepatic administration of the active metabolite FUdR (floxuridine) as adjuvant treatment after hepatic metastectomy can be complicated by cholestatic jaundice and biliary sclerosis.

Whereas leucovorin (folinic acid) antagonizes the effects of methotrexate to rescue normal tissues selectively from that drug's toxicity, it is used for the opposite purpose when given in conjunction with 5-FU. That is, it prolongs the effective half-life of 5-FU when given on a bolus schedule. *Capecitabine* (Xeloda) is an oral equivalent of continuous-infusion 5-FU. It is absorbed intact through the intestinal mucosa. It then undergoes metabolic activation in the liver to 5′-deoxy-5-fluorocytidine by a carboxylesterase, and then to 5′-deoxy-5-fluorouridine by cytidine deaminase. It is further activated by thymidine phosphorylase at the tumor site. Like continuous-infusion 5-FU, it appears to have a similar toxicity profile and better response rates than bolus 5-FU/leucovorin, with considerably easier administration, and is active in metastatic breast cancer and colorectal cancer.

Pemetrexed (Alimta) is a new investigational multitargeted antifolate due to come on the market near the end of 2003 with activity against mesothelioma in combination with cisplatin and against non-small cell lung cancer in combination with several other drugs active against that malignancy.

Deoxycytidine analogs

Cytarabine (1-β-D-arabinosylfuranosylcytosine, or ara-C) is a natural product of the sponge *Cryptothethya crypta*. It is one of the most important drugs used in the standard induction therapy for acute myelogenous leukemia (AML), and in higher dose for consolidation thereof. It also has activity in other hematologic malignancies, such as chronic myelogenous leukemia (CML), ALL, and non-Hodgkin's lymphoma (NHL), but interestingly not in solid tumors. It inhibits DNA synthesis and repair, as well as ribonucleotide reductase. It is activated by deoxycytidine kinase to ara-CTP, which is in turn incorporated into DNA and RNA. It also inhibits DNA synthesis (polymerase alpha) and repair (polymerase beta) and ribonucleotide reductase. Like methotrexate, it is another of the handful of chemotherapeutic agents that can be given intrathecally for meningeal involvement, occasionally producing transient fever, seizures, or altered mental status. However, it crosses the blood-brain barrier better than methotrexate. Myelosuppression and GI toxicity are the primary toxicities with standard induction doses and are even more profound at higher doses. High-dose Ara-C can be associated with toxicity that persists in up to 30% of affected individuals despite discontinuation of therapy. Other side effects include pulmonary edema, conjunctivitis, painful hand-foot syndrome, and neutrophilic eccrine hydradenitis.

Gemcitabine (2′,2′-difluorodeoxycytidine; Gemzar) inhibits DNA synthesis/repair and ribonucleotide reductase, with incorporation of difluorodeoxycytidine triphosphate into DNA and RNA. The drug is cell cycle specific, blocking at the G_1/S interface. Despite its similar structure and mechanism of action, gemcitabine differs from cytarabine in having a broader and very different tumor spectrum. It targets many solid tumors, including pancreatic cancer, NSCLC, bladder cancer, and breast cancer. It is generally given at doses of 800 to 1250 mg/m^2 weekly for 2 to 3 weeks followed by 1 week off. It was initially approved for pancreatic cancer largely for its ability to improve quality of life. Its primary dose-limiting toxicity is myelosuppression, especially thrombocytopenia, but it can cause mild nausea, fever without infection, dyspnea (23%), and rarely hemolytic uremic syndrome, parenchymal pneumonitis, noncardiogenic pulmonary edema, or even acute respiratory distress syndrome (ARDS). Alopecia is uncommon. It is a strong radiosensitizer, requiring much lower doses in combination with radiation.

Purine analogs

6-Mercaptopurine and *6-thioguanine* were synthesized nearly 45 years ago by Hitchings and Elion, who received the Nobel Prize in 1988. They are both administered orally. 6-Mercaptopurine is metabolically activated by hypoxanthine-guanine phosphoribosyltransferase (HGPRT) to 6-MP–ribose phosphate, which inhibits purine synthesis and is useful for remission induction and maintenance therapy of ALL. Allopurinol inhibits xanthine oxidase (XO), which is one of the major detoxification routes for 6-MP. Thus it should be avoided or the 6-MP dose reduced in its presence. The other major detoxification route is by the enzyme thiopurine methyltransferase. There is a pharmacogenetic syndrome in which this enzyme is congenitally absent. Patients with this syndrome may experience severe myelosuppression and GI toxicity, usually with no prior warning, as with DPD (dihydropyrimidine dehydrogenase) deficiency and 5-FU. 6-Mercaptopurine is one metabolic step away from azathioprine and can be used for immunosuppression at doses of 100 mg/day. Chronic use predisposes to bacterial, parasitic, and opportunistic infections. 6-Thioguanine is activated by HGPRT and phosphorylation, causing thiopurine nucleotide analogs to be incorporated into DNA and RNA. These fraudulent nucleotides contribute to DNA-RNA strand breaks. 6-Thioguanine is active in remission induction and maintenance therapy for AML. In contrast to 6-MP, 6-TG is not a direct substrate for XO. It is initially deactivated to 6-thioxanthine by guanine deaminase and then to 6-thiouric acid by XO; thus no dose reduction is required in the presence of allopurinol.

Fludarabine was synthesized in a rational search for active analogs of cytarabine. It enters cells by nucleoside-specific membrane transport and, is phosphorylated to 2-fluoro-ara-AMP and then to 2-fluoro-ara-ATP, which is incorporated into DNA and RNA. It also directly inhibits DNA polymerases involved in DNA synthesis and repair and induces apoptosis. It has activity against lymphoid malignancies, including chronic lymphocytic leukemia (CLL), for which it is the most active single agent, Waldenström's macroglobulinemia, and low-grade NHL, with response rates in the range of 50% to 70%, largely because of its ability to induce apoptosis in indolent malignant cells. It is myelosuppressive, with neutropenia predominating. It is also immunosuppressive, increasing the risk of opportunistic infections. Trimethoprim-sulfamethoxazole (Bactrim) prophylaxis for *Pneumocystis carinii* pneumonia is recommended. Central nervous system toxicity has been observed only with doses higher than currently routinely used. Nausea, vomiting, diarrhea, mild transaminitis, and self-limited somnolence and fatigue can be observed.

Cladribine (2-chloro-2′-deoxyadenosine [2-CdA]) likewise is resistant to adenosine deaminase and also inhibits DNA synthesis and ribonucleotide reductase, as well as being incorporated into DNA and RNA. It also induces apoptosis and is unique among traditional antimetabolites in being active against both dividing and resting cells. It is highly effective against hairy cell leukemia and also is used clinically for CLL, low-grade NHL, and cutaneous T-cell lymphoma (mycosis fungoides). Its toxicities include myelosuppression with profound neutropenia and cumulative thrombocytopenia as well as fevers from pyrogenic cytokine release by dying hairy cells. 2-CdA affects both T and B cells equally, with T-cell recovery in 6 to 12 months but B-cell lymphopenia continuing beyond 2 years. There is no nausea, alopecia, nephrotoxicity, hepatotoxicity, pulmonary or cardiac toxicity, or neurotoxicity at conventional doses.

Pentostatin (Deoxycoformycin) is the least myelosuppressive of the three purine analogs with a similar spectrum of activity. It has recently been combined with cyclophosphamide and Rituximab for the treatment of chronic lymphocytic leukemia.

Topoisomerase I Inhibitors

Topoisomerase I binds preferentially to duplex DNA but cleaves only one strand, binding the sticky ends to tyrosines on the enzyme. Through a swivel mechanism, the unbroken DNA strand then passes through the nicked strand, releasing torsional strain. The camptothecins are derived from the bark and wood of the Chinese *Camptotheca acuminata* tree. The two clinically useful members of this class (*topotecan* and *irinotecan*) contain a pentocyclic lactone ring that is essential for activity. Topotecan is useful against SCLC and ovarian cancer, but has no activity against colorectal or pancreatic cancer. Irinotecan (CPT-11; Camptosar), in contrast, has a broader spectrum of activity. It is active against colorectal, gastric, and pancreatic cancer as well as NSCLC and SCLC, cervical and ovarian cancer, and lymphoma. The major toxicity associated with irinotecan is diarrhea, both early, which may require atropine during the infusion, and delayed, which may require prolonged use of loperamide. Myelosuppression occurs with both members of this class.

Topoisomerase II Inhibitors

Topoisomerase II normally functions by binding to duplex DNA and sequentially cleaving the two complementary strands four base pairs apart, covalently linking the split ends to pairs of tyrosine groups in each half of the enzyme. A second double-stranded segment of DNA then is passed through the break in the first segment, in a magnesium- and ATP-dependent manner, followed by re-ligation of the original DNA segment, producing net DNA uncoiling. Topoisomerase II inhibitors prevent re-ligation of the cleaved DNA by the enzymatic protein, leaving the DNA held together by protein.

Epipodophyllotoxins

Although extracts of *Podophyllum peltatum* (May apple) had been used for over a century by natives of the Himalayas and the Americas as cathartics and antihelmintics, it was not until 1942, when the curative effect of podophyllin on condylomata acuminata was discovered, that derivatives began to be synthesized and systematically tested. *Etoposide* (VP-16) was introduced in 1973 and quickly approved as efficacious against SCLC and lymphoma and testicular tumors in 1983. Its cousin *teniposide* (VM-26) was introduced in 1967 and approved in 1993 in combination for refractory ALL. Both drugs modify the topologic state of DNA by inhibiting topoisomerase II. Etoposide's dose-limiting toxicity is myelosuppression. It also should be noted that etoposide has a significant risk of inducing secondary leukemias, often within 5 years of treatment, possibly more likely with cumulative doses over 2 to 3 g/m^2. Gastrointestinal toxicity is relatively mild at submyeloablative doses, but may be more prominent when the drug is given by the oral route. Mild, easily controlled infusional hypotension can occur from vasomotor effects.

Anthracyclines

The first anthracyclines, *doxorubicin* and *daunorubicin*, which have been in clinical use since the 1960s, were produced by the fungus *Streptomyces*. Hence they were initially classed as antitumor antibiotics. However, they are now classified by mechanism of action, along with the new anthracyclines, *epirubicin*, *mitoxantrone*, and *idarubicin*. Like the other topoisomerase II inhibitors, anthracyclines induce formation of covalent topoisomerase-DNA complexes and prevent the enzyme from re-ligating the DNA after the other strand passes through. Additionally, these agents intercalate their planar four-ring structure into the DNA ladder between two adjacent base pairs, causing single- and double-strand breaks. They also delocalize electrons well, and thus can undergo chemical reduction, often catalyzed by iron, to form oxygen free radicals causing oxidative damage to proteins and DNA. Of these three mechanisms, topoisomerase II inhibition is the most important. Doxorubicin (Adriamycin) is active in a host of solid tumors, including breast, ovarian, thyroid, NSCLC, SCLC, soft tissue sarcomas (including Kaposi's sarcoma), and Hodgkin's lymphoma and NHL. Epirubicin and mitoxantrone also seem to be primarily active in the solid tumors. In contrast, daunorubicin and idarubicin are active primarily in leukemias (ALL and AML). Resistance can develop by several routes, including mutations in topoisomerase II or increased levels of glutathione-mediated detoxification enzymes, but the primary resistance mechanism is extrusion from cells by the *MDR1* (multi-drug resistance gene 1) protein product, P170 glycoprotein. In this mechanism, Adriamycin is cross-resistant with other natural-product chemotherapy drugs. Doxil (liposomal doxorubicin) carries a possible slight

attenuation of all the traditional side effects of doxorubicin; all cautions associated with that drug still apply.

Several forms of significant toxicity are associated with these drugs. The most unique and concerning is their cardiotoxicity. The heart is very rich in iron (hemoglobin and myoglobin), with low levels of catalase. Adriamycin itself inactivates glutathione peroxidase. The risk of cardiotoxicity goes up with age over 70 or prior cardiac disease or radiation exposure to the mediastinum. The ejection fraction should be at least 50% prior to initiating treatment and checked fairly frequently once total cumulative doses exceed 350 mg/m^2. The risk goes up significantly once the cumulative dose reaches 450 to 500 mg/m^2. Mitoxantrone, idarubicin, and Doxil are less cardiotoxic. Also, epirubicin is cardiotoxic, and 900 mg/m^2 is the cumulative dose above which concern increases. Adriamycin is also an extreme vesicant that can cause severe local injury if it leaks out of the vasculature. Hence, administration by a central line, such as a Port-A-Cath, is an important safety measure. The dose-limiting acute toxicity is myelosuppression. It also causes alopecia and "radiation recall," characterized by erythematous skin rash in radiation fields even many years after radiation.

Dactinomycin is a planar tricyclic ring isolated from the fungus *Streptomyces parvulus* that is highly effective in Wilms' tumor, Ewing's sarcoma, embryonal rhabdosarcoma, gestational choriocarcinoma, testicular cancer, Kaposi's sarcoma, and lymphoma. It intercalates into DNA and binds to deoxyguanosine, blocking the ability of DNA to act as a template for DNA and RNA synthesis. It also can cause topoisomerase-mediated single-strand breaks in DNA. Its dose-limiting toxicity is myelosuppression in the form of neutropenia and thrombocytopenia. It is also a vesicant that can cause severe nausea and vomiting and stomatitis. Additionally, it is a radiation sensitizer, enhancing skin and GI toxicity when administered concurrently with radiation. It also enhances late radiation-mediated lung and liver damage because it blocks repair of radiation-mediated DNA damage.

Mitotic Spindle Poisons

Vinca alkaloids

The vinca alkaloids are natural products obtained from the periwinkle plant. They bind to specific sites on tubulin, preventing polymerization of tubulin dimers and thus inhibiting microtubule formation. This interferes with mitotic spindle formation, arresting cell division in metaphase, and with maintenance of the long axons of peripheral nerves, causing predominantly sensory neuropathy.

Vinblastine (Velban) is used clinically for germ cell tumors, lung cancer, esophageal cancer, and Hodgkin's lymphoma (in the ABVD regimen). It only rarely causes peripheral neuropathy, but can cause alopecia.

Vincristine (Oncovin) is used in pediatric and adult ALL, Hodgkin's lymphoma and NHL, and pediatric Wilms' tumor, Ewing's sarcoma, neuroblastoma, and rhabdomyosarcoma. It is also commonly used for multiple myeloma (in the VAD regimen) and as an immunosuppressant in immune thrombocytopenic purpura. It should never be administered intrathecally because this causes fatal ascending paralysis. Although the bolus dose is generally given as 1.4 mg/m^2, it is also usually capped at a maximum of 2 mg. Autonomic toxicity with severe constipation can occur.

Vinorelbine (Navelbine) is a semisynthetic analog of vinblastine, which is Food and Drug Administration (FDA) approved for NSCLC and also useful for breast cancer, head and neck cancer, and Hodgkin's lymphoma. It has the same mechanism of action, but affects axonal microtubules to a much lesser degree. The intravenous dose is usually 25 to 30 mg/m^2/wk.

Vinblastine and vinorelbine are myelosuppressive, with neutropenia predominating and dose limiting. All three of these drugs are potent vesicants for which central intravenous access is desirable for safety. None of these drugs causes significant nausea and vomiting.

Taxanes

Paclitaxel (Taxol) was first extracted from the bark of the Pacific yew tree, *Taxus brevifolia*, in 1963. A 15-membered ring structure with an ester side chain was identified in 1971 as the active agent, but difficulties in mass producing it, coupled with its poor aqueous solubility, delayed clinical trials several more years. It acts as a microtubule stabilizer, binding to β-tubulin, enhancing its polymerization, and then freezing the microtubules in the polymerized state, preventing dissolution of the spindle apparatus during mitosis. It is cross-resistant to the vincas, Adriamycin, and etoposide with respect to *MDR1* phenotype and P-glycoprotein. The toxicities include total alopecia, peripheral neuropathy, and generally mild myelosuppression, especially with shorter infusion times. Also, an acute anaphylactoid hypersensitivity reaction that may occur within the first 2 to 10 minutes of infusion, probably related to the Cremophor vehicle. Accordingly, patients generally are premedicated with dexamethasone, 20 mg 12 and 6 hours before treatment; diphenhydramine, 50 mg IV; and a histamine$_2$ antagonist, such as ranitidine, 50 mg IV, along with a serotonin receptor antagonist. Sinus bradycardia and Mobitz types I and II block have been observed. Ventricular arrhythmias are rare. It has a broad spectrum of clinical uses, including breast cancer, ovarian cancer, Kaposi's sarcoma, NSCLC, bladder cancer, testicular cancer, and head and neck cancer.

Docetaxel (Taxotere) is derived semisynthetically from the European yew tree and shares the same mechanism of action as paclitaxel. Hypersensitivity reactions can occur, and require a less intense premedication regimen, usually with dexamethasone alone given 8 mg PO bid for five

doses, beginning 24 hours prior to treatment. Docetaxel is slightly less neurotoxic, but slightly more myelosuppressive. It also damages finger nails with prolonged use and occasionally causes mild third spacing of bodily fluids.

Antitumor Antibiotics

Bleomycin is a small (1500-Da) peptide isolated from the fungus *Streptomyces verticillus*. It has a DNA-binding region at one end of the peptide and an iron-binding region at the other end. Its mechanism of action begins when it complexes with oxidized iron, enabling it to catalyze reduction of O$_2$ to superoxide and hydroxyl radicals, producing single- and double-stranded DNA strand breaks. It can be administered intramuscularly, subcutaneously, or intravenously with equal efficacy. It also can be delivered into the pleural or peritoneal space to control malignant effusions. It is not myelosuppressive. The major serious toxicity of bleomycin is pulmonary oxygen toxicity mediated by oxygen radical formation, and hence exacerbated by high oxygen flow rates (which should be avoided during surgery), prior pulmonary or mediastinal radiation, age greater than 70, and underlying lung disease. Pulmonary function tests (forced vital capacity and diffusion capacity of the lung for carbon monoxide) should be obtained at baseline and prior to each cycle. If either declines 10% to 15%, the drug should be stopped to avoid devastating pulmonary consequences. Skin erythema, induration, desquamation, and hyperpigmentation also can occur. Bleomycin is used for Hodgkin's disease in the ABVD regimen and for testicular cancer in the BEP regimen.

Homoharringtonine (HUT) is derived from the Chinese evergreen tree, *Cephalotaxus fortunei*. It inhibits protein synthesis, with degradation of polyribosomes and inhibition of peptide bond formation, and also may block the cell cycle at the G$_1$/S and G$_2$/M phase transitions. It is useful in chronic-phase CML, alone or combined with ara-C or interferon. It has minimal nonhematologic toxicities.

L-*Asparaginase* (L-Spar) catalyzes the conversion of asparagine to aspartic acid and ammonia, thus depleting the extracellular pool of this amino acid. Most normal cells can induce asparagine synthase to compensate, but many lymphoid malignancies cannot, hence the selectivity. It is a bacterial enzyme, generally produced from *Escherichia coli*, but a preparation from *Erwinia* also is available for patients who develop hypersensitivity to the *E. coli*–derived agent. It is used for ALL.

Bisphosphonates

Pamidronate (Aredia) strengthens bones and decreases bone pain at sites of bone metastases by inhibiting bone destruction by osteoclast activity. It also prevents and treats hypercalcemia of malignancy and is delivered as a dose of 60 to 90 mg by intravenous infusion over at least 2 hours in the outpatient setting every 3 to 4 weeks.

Zoledronic acid (Zometa) is a high-potency bisphosphonate, with a 4-mg dose being about as effective as 90 mg of pamidronate in a recent randomized study of 280 patients with multiple myeloma or metastatic breast cancer. It is more convenient because it is delivered in a 5-minute intravenous infusion. Additionally, zoledronic acid at 4 mg reduced skeletal-related events in prostate cancer patients with bone metastases.

Texaphyrins

Texaphyrins are a new class of ring-shaped anticancer drugs adapted from porphyrins. *Motexafin gadolinium* (Xcytrin) consists of a molecule of the well-known magnetic resonance imaging (MRI) contrast molecule gadolinium inserted into the center of the motexafin ring, making the agent visible on MRI. In a preliminary report of an ongoing Phase III trial presented at the 2003 meeting of the American Society for Therapeutic Radiology and Oncology by Dr. Minesh Mehta, brain tumor volume was reduced in 65% to 70% of the small cohort of evaluable patients, comparable to the prior Phase II data. The mechanism is based on selective uptake by cancer cells, followed by induction of futile redox cycling, depriving the cell of glucose and inducing cell death or at least substantially compromising the ability of tumor cells to repair radiation-induced damage. The drug is well tolerated, with only minor reversible side effects, such as temporary changes in skin and urine color, nausea, hypertension, and hepatic transaminase elevations. In patients with an average of 12 brain metastases, injection of motexafin gadolinium followed by standard whole-brain radiation for 10 days resulted in 81% median reduction of tumor volume with 45% improvement in neurocognitive function. It is being tested in combination with other redox active drugs, such as doxorubicin and bleomycin for possible synergy.

Hyperthermia

Peritoneal carcinomatosis is a common and lethal complication of GI and ovarian cancers. It also causes a great deal of morbidity from intestinal and ureteral obstruction in the process. Intravenous chemotherapy has had little impact on the natural history of this entity, perhaps because of the peritoneum-plasma barrier that limits the resorption of high-molecular-weight and hydrophilic drugs such as mitomycin-C and cisplatin. Recently, extensive cytoreductive surgery, with complete removal of all macroscopic tumor leaving an aggregate residual of less than 1 cm, combined with intraperitoneal heated chemotherapy (IPHC) has produced good palliation with increased long-term survival. The hyperthermia helps overcome the

problems with depth of tumor penetration, activates the drugs faster, and inhibits DNA repair. The indications include GI cancer with perforation, positive peritoneal cytology, or peritoneal carcinomatosis; peritoneal sarcomatosis; mesothelioma from ovarian cancer; pseudomyxoma peritonei; or palliation of malignant ascites. A peritoneal cancer index is used to estimate the likelihood that complete cytoreduction will be achievable.

The procedure can be performed by either open-abdomen or closed-abdomen technique. In the open-abdomen technique, a self-retaining Thompson retractor is positioned to hold open the laparotomy incision. Three drains are placed, under the right hemidiaphragm, behind the spleen, and in the pelvis. They are connected with the extracorporeal circuit during the procedure and left in place postoperatively until all drainage subsides. In the closed-abdomen technique, four silicone catheters are placed through the abdominal wall into the cavity after cytoreduction but prior to closure. They are placed in the right and left subphrenic cavities and in deep and superficial pelvic sites. Continuous peritoneal temperature monitoring is facilitated by two thermocouples, one in the abdominal cavity and the other in a subperitoneal site. After abdominal skin closure, the catheters are connected to the extracorporeal circuit, through which a preheated solution is pumped. Once the temperature reaches 42.5°C, the chemotherapy drugs are injected into the circuit inflow. Postoperatively, all patients receive albumin, 10 to 20 g/day IV for 1 week, and fresh frozen plasma 250 mL daily for 3 days, as well as vigorous hydration and renal-dose dopamine to protect the kidneys from cisplatin.

In a study of 41 patients with gastric peritoneal carcinomatosis using cisplatin and mitomycin-C combined with cytoreductive surgery, with complete resection in only 7, the median overall survival was 14.6 months, with a 3-year survival of 28.5%. In a nonrandomized study of 48 patients who underwent aggressive cytoreduction and mitomycin IPHC alone, the 3-year survival rate was 41.5% versus 0% in 18 historical controls.

Hormone Manipulation

Many hormonal agents are used in the treatment of cancer. They are used primarily in the sex hormone–responsive cancers such as breast, prostate, and endometrial carcinomas. The corticosteroids, however, are used both as antitumor drugs for lymphoid malignancies and as a premedication for chemotherapy-induced nausea or to treat tumor encroachment edema in a variety of malignancies.

Luteinizing hormone–releasing hormone (LHRH) peptide analogs, which possess partial agonist activity, have been used extensively in the treatment of prostate cancer. The commercially available agents leuprolide (Lupron) and goserelin (Zoladex) have both agonistic and antagonistic activity. They initially cause a transient increase in luteinizing hormone (LH) and follicle-stimulating hormone (FSH) production over about 2 weeks, followed by an even more profound decline over about 3 months. Serum testosterone levels consequently decrease to castrate levels and stay there, effectively producing a medical orchiectomy for as long as the drug is present to maintain it. It is usually continued until the initiation of hospice care, even in the face of rising prostate-specific antigen (PSA) levels. This is because it is believed that only some of the prostate cancer cell clones have acquired a mutation conferring resistance. The rest are still being controlled by the LHRH agonist but would grow and exacerbate the tumor burden, if the drug were stopped prematurely. Depot formulations permitting administration monthly or every 3 to 4 months are available. In patients with significant bony metastases, there is a concern that isolated initiation of LHRH agonists may cause a "flare" in the disease and resultant bone pain in the first 2 weeks. This can be ameliorated by concomitant administration of antiandrogens to block the effect of any extra circulating testosterone at the end-organ receptor level. The nonsteroidal antiandrogens flutamide (Eulexin) and bicalutamide (Casodex) are competitive inhibitors of testosterone at the androgen receptor. They have been used in four clinical settings: (1) as part of combined androgen blockade in conjunction with surgical or chemical castration, (2) as salvage monotherapy, (3) as initial monotherapy without castration, and (4) by their absence in the form of antiandrogen withdrawal after combined androgen blockade.

Diethylstilbestrol (DES) is an estrogenic agent that inhibits LHRH production by the hypothalamus and LH production by the pituitary, thus reducing serum levels of testosterone. Additionally, the presence of estrogen receptors on the prostate epithelium suggests that there also may be a direct cytoxic effect. In the Veterans Administration randomized trial of DES, 5 mg/day, versus orchiectomy versus both, the overall survival was the same across the board, but the cancer-specific mortality was lower in the DES-treated groups, but was offset by the increased cardiovascular mortality of DES.

Tamoxifen is a selective estrogen receptor modulator. The most prominent toxicity is hot flushes in 50% of women, which can be ameliorated by concurrent use of very-low-dose megestrol. The most deleterious side effect of tamoxifen is a threefold increase in the risk of endometrial cancer over the general population. It is not yet known whether progestins can ameliorate this as they do for estrogen. Beneficial estrogenic effects include a decrease in total cholesterol and possibly heart disease and preservation of bone density in postmenopausal women only. It may deplete bone density in premenopausal women, because of its partial competitive inhibition of the abundant native

estrogen. A few patients complain of vaginal dryness/dyspareunia. Tamoxifen may predispose to thromboembolic phenomena, particularly in conjunction with chemotherapy. It should not be given concurrently with chemotherapy for efficacy reasons as well. *Toremifene* is thought to be a pure anti-estrogen, similar to tamoxifen, and is available in the United States for metastatic breast cancer. A randomized comparison in metastatic breast cancer has suggested that tamoxifen and toremifene have similar efficacy and toxicity and are cross-resistant. *Raloxifene* (Evista) is an estrogen agonist and antagonist (partial agonist) that appeared less promising than tamoxifen in early development as an anti–breast cancer agent. It has an established role, based on large placebo-controlled trials, in retarding osteoporosis in women who are at risk. It also appeared to reduce the risk of developing breast cancer in these women without inducing endometrial cancer, though it still causes hot flushes. A large randomized breast cancer chemoprevention trial comparing it to tamoxifen in high-risk postmenopausal women is underway and results are not yet available.

Megestrol (Megace) and medroxyprogesterone acetate (its European cousin) are progestins of similar use differing only in a double bond. Megestrol was one of the earliest second-line hormonal agents used in metastatic breast cancer at a daily dose of 160 mg. This dose also has been used occasionally to treat prostate cancer, with a low response rate. Megestrol also has been used to treat hormonally responsive endometrial cancer, at a dose of 320 mg/day, and to treat anorexia, with a linear dose-response relationship up to 800 mg/day. It may cause impotence in men and withdrawal uterine bleeding in women. It also suppresses the pituitary-adrenal axis, usually subclinically.

Aminoglutethimide was the first aromatase inhibitor used clinically. Unfortunately, it produced a medical adrenalectomy, which, although effective (32% response rate in metastatic breast cancer), was too toxic for routine use as well as cumbersome in requiring coadministration of hydrocortisone. The second-generation aromatase inhibitors have now all but replaced Megace as first choice in the second-line treatment of breast cancer. *Anastrozole* (Arimidex) is an aromatase inhibitor 200 times more potent than aminoglutethimide. It inhibits conversion of androgens to estrogens with no effect on the adrenal glands. *Letrozole* (Femara) is an aromatase inhibitor 180 times more potent than aminoglutethimide. Both are more efficacious than Megace in the second-line setting for metastatic breast cancer. *Aromasin* (Exemestane) is the newest aromatase inhibitor.

Octreotide is an 8-amino-acid analog of the 14-amino-acid peptide somatostatin. It is useful in the treatment of carcinoid syndrome and other hormonal excess syndromes associated with some pancreatic islet cell cancers. Symptomatic response rates are high and long lasting. Occasionally, antitumor responses are seen as well.

It can be administered intravenously or subcutaneously three times a day or in a monthly depot form (Lanreotide). It also appears to be able to alleviate severe therapy-related diarrhea caused by 5-FU and irinotecan.

Immunotherapy

Monoclonal Antibodies

Rituxumab (Rituxan) is a monoclonal antibody to Bcl-2 (CD 20) pioneered in low-grade follicular lymphoma; it is now know to have activity in any Bcl-2–expressing lymphoproliferative disease. It was shown in a recent trial overseas to improve the outcome of patients with diffuse large cell lymphoma when combined with a CHOP regimen over the gold standard CHOP alone. This awaits confirmation by the North American Intergroup trial. Rituximab is also active in the treatment of B-cell CLL and Waldenström's macroglobulinemia.

Two similar radiolabeled monoclonal antibodies that have been recently FDA-approved are ^{131}I-tositumomab (Bexxar) and ^{90}Y-ibritumomab (Zevulin). Bexxar is an ^{131}I-labeled monoclonal antibody to Bcl-2 that has shown a 35% complete remission (CR) rate in relapsed or transformed NHL overall, with a CR rate as high as 58% in previously untreated patients. Zevulin is an yttrium-90–labeled monoclonal antibody to Bcl-2, with a 67% response rate in a recent Phase I/II trial in relapsed/refractory NHL, with median time to progression exceeding 1 year. The most serious toxicities were hematologic, with 61% grade 3-4 neutropenia and 8% febrile. Two thirds had grade 3-4 thrombocytopenia and 18% grade 3-4 anemia. All hematologic toxicities were transient over less than 2 weeks. Additionally, 15% had cardiotoxicity, 14% had arthralgia/myalgia, 19% experienced neurotoxicity, and 30% had upper respiratory symptoms.

Gemtuzumab ozagamicin (Mylotarg), a monoclonal antibody to CD 33, has been conjugated to calicheamycin for outpatient treatment of CD33-positive AML in first relapse. It appears to be less toxic than conventional chemotherapy in this setting, permitting more days to be spent as an outpatient.

Alemtuzumab (Campath-1H) is a humanized monoclonal antibody to the CD52 antigen on B and T cells, but not on bone marrow progenitors cells. It was developed at Cambridge University in England (Campath stands for Cambridge Pathology), and acts by lysing leukemia cells expressing the CD52 antigen. It had a 33% response rate in a Phase II trial of 93 patients and in a smaller Phase II trial of 24 patients with CLL refractory to fludarabine. Unfortunately, this is a very toxic drug, with 67% of patients experiencing serious infusional, infectious, or hematologic events. Of the 90% of patients experiencing

infusional toxicity, 13% were grade 3-4. Additionally, 47% had grade 3-4 anemia and 24% had grade 3 and 55% grade 4 neutropenia, with a significant toxic death rate of up to 15%.

Trastuzumab (Herceptin) is a humanized monoclonal antibody to the human epidermal growth factor receptor-2 (HER2)-*neu* growth factor receptor. It was discovered when researchers screened human DNA for sequences similar to a known rat neuroblastoma oncogene called *neu*. HER2 is a cell membrane–spanning growth factor receptor with tyrosine kinase activity on the inner membrane surface that serves to activate the *ras* signaling pathway that transmits instructions for cell proliferation to the cell nucleus. Cancer cells may overexpress the HER2 receptor, leading to increased cell division, increased tumor growth rate, and transformation to the malignant phenotype. Approximately 25% to 30% of breast cancers overexpress HER2, and these patients have more aggressive disease, decreased overall survival time, and a higher probability of tumor recurrence. HER2 overexpression has also been reported in many other solid tumors, including ovarian cancer, gastric cancer, colon cancer, lung cancer, salivary gland cancer, pancreatic cancer, and prostate cancer. Herceptin downregulates HER2 receptor expression, inhibits proliferation, and enhances antibody-dependent cellular cytotoxicity. Herceptin is given as a loading dose of 4 mg/kg IV, followed by 2 mg/kg IV weekly. It is quite safe and effective when combined with weekly paclitaxel (11% cardiotoxicity), with an increase in median time to progression from 2.5 to 6.7 months. When combined with Adriamycin and cyclophosphamide chemotherapy, however, the cardiotoxicity of both Herceptin (7%) and Adriamycin (7%) act synergistically (28%). Accordingly, this combination is not recommended. Easily managed infusion-associated symptoms are experienced by 40% of patients, primarily during the first infusion, consisting of fevers and chills and occasionally nausea, vomiting, and pain at the tumor site. The addition of Herceptin to paclitaxel significantly increased the overall response rate from 15% to 38%, with median duration of response up from 4.3 to 8.3 months and 1-year survival up from 61% with paclitaxel alone to 73% with Herceptin plus paclitaxel.

Cetuximab (Erbitux; IMC-C225) is a chimerized monoclonal antibody to the epidermal growth factor receptor. It should be available for colorectal cancer by early 2004, with skin rash correlating with objective response and median survival, as with small molecule inhibitors of EGFR (Iressa, Tarceva).

Bevacizumab (Avastin, rHuMoAb VEGF) is a humanized monoclonal antibody against the vascular endothelial growth factor receptor (VEGF-R). It is designed to inhibit angiogenesis triggered by tumoral release of VEGF. This is because increased vascularization is essential to permit tumor growth beyond about 1 cm, secondary to limited nutrient diffusion distance. Life-threatening hemorrhages have occurred with large central tumors, particularly squamous cell lung cancer. It also has shown promise in metastatic colorectal cancer and should be on the market by late 2003 or early 2004.

Vaccines

The rationale for anticancer vaccine therapy is harnessing the immune system to perform its intended function of providing defense against invaders; in this case the "invaders" are from within and need to be recognized as no longer "self." This approach was pioneered in melanoma for a couple of reasons. First, there was a great need to find another approach to attack this aggressive and pervasively metastatic tumor that is unresponsive to traditional cytotoxic chemotherapy. Second, there are several lines of evidence indicating that the immune system already targets melanomas more noticeably than most other malignancies. Spontaneous partial or complete regressions have been observed, sometimes manifesting as dark, heaped-up rings with flat amelanotic centers. As many as 15% of all melanomas are diagnosed as nodal or distant metastatic lesions with unknown primary tumors. Also, blood from melanoma patients has revealed antibodies against tumor antigens and cytotoxic T lymphocytes capable of destroying melanoma cells in vitro.

Vaccines can be either polyvalent (against multiple antigens) or univalent (against a single antigen). Polyvalent vaccines can be made from living whole melanoma cells, which have been irradiated so as not to propagate, or from cell lysates or partially purified antigens. Whole cells provide direct antigen presentation to T cells, with multiple relevant highly immunogenic antigens, but are difficult to characterize and reproduce, and may also induce immunosuppressive factors. They may be allogeneic, from multiple melanoma cell lines.

An example is *CancerVax*, developed at the John Wayne Cancer Institute (Santa Monica, CA). It is derived from three irradiated melanoma cell lines, and is administered intradermally biweekly for 12 weeks with bacille Calmette-Guérin (BCG) with the first two injections, then monthly for 1 year, then every 2 to 3 months indefinitely for maintenance. The toxicity consists of mild flulike symptoms and local skin inflammation, attributable to the adjuvant BCG. It has proved quite effective in Phase II trials, with median survival increased from 7.5 to 23 months in one study of stage IV patients, and 5-year survival of completely metastectomized patients up from 13% to 40% in another. A Phase III trial in metastatic melanoma is underway.

Polyvalent vaccines may also be autologous, but they require a large amount of tumor (5 g) from the patient, precluding their use in early-stage or low-tumor-burden advanced disease. Additionally, the fact that such a tumor

has persisted to such a large tumor burden suggests that it may have modified its antigens to be less immunogenic. In order to counteract this, it is best to modify autologous vaccines with a hapten, such as dinitrophenyl.

Disruption of whole melanoma cells may enhance antigen presentation. This can be accomplished with vaccinia virus (*vaccinia melanoma oncolysate* [VMO]) or mechanically (*Melacine*). VMO was constructed by infecting four melanoma cell lines with live vaccinia virus. Although the Phase II trial showed a significantly prolonged disease-free survival, the Phase III trial randomizing to that or vaccinia virus alone showed no significant difference, except in retrospective subgroup analysis. This could be because treatment was discontinued after 1 year, without long-term maintenance. Another type of vaccine, the *shed-antigen vaccine*, attempts to balance the advantages and disadvantages of the polyvalent and univalent approaches by minimizing irrelevant cellular material while enhancing the number of different tumor antigens presented over the purified univalent antigen preparations. It is a mixture of cell-surface antigens shed by melanoma cells into culture medium, given intradermally every 3 weeks for 2 months, then every month for 3 months, and then at fixed intervals over 5 years or until progression. In Phase II trials of stage IV melanoma, the median overall survival was 31 months versus 7.6 months for historical controls. A recently completed Phase III randomized trial in stage III melanoma of shed-antigen vaccine versus placebo albumin vaccine yielded a median recurrence-free survival of 18.6 months versus 7.1 months in placebo patients.

Biotherapy

Biologic Response Modifiers

The interferons and interleukin-2 (IL-2) provide a selective means of stimulating the immune system to recognize cancer cells as nonself invaders that should be destroyed. The interferons are a family of proteins produced by cells of the immune system in response to viral infection or other foreign stimuli, such as double-stranded RNA, mitogens, and antigens. They "interfere" with subsequent viral challenge and have immunomodulatory and antiproliferative effects. *Interferon-α* is a cytokine derived from lymphocytes and has antitumor activity against hairy cell leukemia, chronic myelogenous leukemia, cutaneous T-cell lymphoma, renal cell cancer, melanoma, superficial bladder cancer, cervical intraepithelial neoplasia, malignant neuroendocrine tumors, multiple myeloma, and Kaposi's sarcoma. The side effects of interferon therapy include flulike symptoms, rashes, chronic fatigue, gastrointestinal or neurologic complaints, and hepatic dysfunction.

Interleukin-2 is now commonly used for the treatment of metastatic melanoma and renal cell cancer. While it has no direct cytotoxic effect on cancer cells, it does stimulate the immune system to eliminate them. In the National Cancer Institute's study on 182 melanoma patients and 227 renal cancer patients treated with a high-dose bolus (720,000 IU/kg) every 8 hours, the overall response rates (CR + partial remission [PR]) were 15% for melanoma and 19% for renal cancer. Outpatient low-dose (9 to 18 million IU subcu qd) therapy is being evaluated with increasing frequency as a means to decrease toxicity while maintaining clinical efficacy. The major side effects of IL-2 include the flulike symptoms of fevers, chills, myalgias, arthralgias, and nasal stuffiness, similar to the side effects of interferon, starting 4 to 6 hours after therapy begins. However, other unique side effects include capillary leak syndrome, which may require pressor support in an intensive care unit; severe pruritus, secondary to eosinophilia; nausea, vomiting, diarrhea, and anorexia; painful raised welts at injection sites; ARDS; renal insufficiency; and transient hepatic insufficiency. Unfortunately, concomitant use of corticosteroids to ameliorate the side effects may reduce the efficacy.

Cytokine Receptor Inhibitors

Denileukin diftitox (DAB389IL-2; ONTAK) is a recombinant fusion toxin in which the receptor-binding domain of native diphtheria toxin is replaced by sequences encoding the IL-2 gene. It delivers the catalytic domain of diphtheria toxin to lymphocytes expressing the IL-2 receptor, including cutaneous T-cell lymphoma (CTCL), NHL, and Hodgkin's disease. It requires premedication with acetaminophen (Tylenol), diphenhydramine (Benadryl), and corticosteroids to counteract acute hypersensitivity reactions and capillary leak syndrome. Steroids do not compromise the efficacy. It had a 60% response rate in a small trial in CTCL.

Signal Transduction Inhibitor Targeted Therapies

Imatinib (ST1571, Gleevec) is an Abl protein-tyrosine kinase inhibitor that inhibits signal transduction mediated by c-*kit* (stem cell factor receptor) and α and β platelet-derived growth factor (PDGF) receptors. It selectively inhibits PDGF- and stem cell factor–mediated cellular signaling, including ligand-stimulated receptor autophosphorylation, inositol phosphate formation, and mitogen-activated protein kinase activation and proliferation. It is effective in Philadelphia chromosome–positive CML at a dose of 400 mg PO qd, with a 90% complete hematologic response rate and a 37% major cytogenetic response rate (13% CR and 23% PR) with 3 months of treatment, and 56% major cytogenetic response (28% CR) with 6 months of treatment. It is also quite effective in metastatic gastrointestinal stromal tumors (GIST)

that have been documented to express c-*kit* as surface CD-117 dosed at 600 mg po qd.

Gefitinib (Iressa, ZD1839) is an epidermal growth factor receptor tyrosine kinase inhibitor recently approved for third line treatment of non-small cell lung cancer. Its major toxicity is an acneiform rash which seems to correlate with efficacy and mild diarrhea.

Erlotinib (Tarceva, OSI-774) is an investigational epidermal growth factor receptor tyrosine kinase inhibitor with similar effects and side effects to Iressa.

Bryostatin-1 (NSC 339555) is an investigational macrocyclic lactone, originally isolated from the murine animal *Bugula neritina*, that inhibits protein kinase C and has both activity against a variety of cancers and immunomodulatory activity. It has been shown to act synergistically with several cytotoxic agents, including paclitaxel, in a sequence-dependent manner. The dose-limiting toxicities in Phase I studies in combination with weekly paclitaxel were dysrhythmia, neutropenia, and myalgia.

Farnesyltransferase inhibitors represent another investigational pharmacologic approach to signal transduction inhibition, specifically targeting the *ras* intracellular signal transduction pathway. They were originally designed to target tumors with a mutated *ras* oncogene. It has subsequently become evident that many other tumors signal through the *ras* pathway as a result of upregulated growth factor receptor tyrosine kinases, autocrine loops at the cell surface level, increased growth factors, and the like. *Ras* mutations result in conformational changes that constitutively activate *ras*, continuously sending the same proliferative signal downstream via the mitogen-activated protein kinase pathway to the cell nucleus. Farnesylation is the enzyme-mediated process of addition of a 15-carbon lipid moiety to make the Ras protein sufficiently lipophilic to bind to the cell membrane in close proximity to the receptor tyrosine kinase to permit GTP activation of *ras*. A Phase II trial of *Tipifarnib* (Zarnestra; Ri 15777) conducted in 41 advanced breast cancer patients who were not candidates for endocrine therapy, reported at the 23rd Annual San Antonio Breast Cancer Symposium, showed 10% PR and 15% minor response with about 25% having no change, with responses lasting 4 to 12 months. Hematologic toxicity was dose limiting, with grade 3-4 neutropenia in 43% at 300 mg/day. Additionally, 15% had peripheral neuropathy after 3 to 4 months of therapy, which was subsequently eliminated by changing the dosing schedule to 3 weeks on and 1 week off. Tipifarnib has also shown activity in chronic myelogenous leukemia, acute myeloid leukemia and myelodysplasia.

Antiangiogenesis Agents

Thalidomide has recently reemerged from its long banishment from the pharmacopoeia, as a result of its teratogenic effects, for a limited indication to treat leprosy.

However, data are mounting indicating its effectiveness as an anti-angiogenesis inhibitor, limiting blood supply recruitment by tumors. It inhibits tumor necrosis factor-α, which is important in the pathogenesis of plasma cell dyscrasias and possibly amyloidosis. It has other effects as well, including reducing T-helper and relatively increasing T-suppressor cells and causing oxidative/free radical damage to DNA. The latter mechanism probably plays a role in its teratogenicity. It is given in the evening because of its somnolence, in escalating doses from 200 to 800 mg, with 400 the average tolerated by most. Other dose-related toxicities include constipation, weakness, numbness, and tingling. Its use as an anticancer drug was pioneered by Dr. Bart Barlogie at the University of Arkansas in patients with refractory myeloma, three fourths of whom had had one or more prior autologous bone marrow transplants. He observed at least a 25% paraprotein reduction in 37% of patients, with 14% achieving CR. Pilot studies also showed benefit in colorectal cancer, at least in terms of counteracting the diarrhea from irinotecan when given in combination with it, and in amyloidosis when combined with corticosteroids.

Other investigational members of this class, such as *Revimid*, are likely to be more effective and less toxic (lacks sedation and teratogenicity).

Differentiation Agents

Fenretinide

Fenretinide is an investigational retinoid agent in neuroblastoma.

Arsenic trioxide

Arsenic trioxide is an FDA-designated orphan drug used for remission-induction and consolidation of the acute promyelocytic (M3) subtype of acute myeloid leukemia (AML) that is refractory to all trans-retinoid (ATRA) and anthracycline therapy or has relapsed despite such therapy. A complete response with a confirmatory bone marrow at least 30 days later, was reported in 70%. Among the 28 patients who achieved a complete response to arsenic trioxide therapy, cytogenetic response [consisting of conversion to no detection of APL chromosome rearrangement based on reverse transcriptase polymerase chain reaction (RT-PCR)] was seen in 79%.

Proteosome Inhibitors

Bortezomib (Velcade) is the first member of a new class of anti-cancer drugs shown to be active in relapsed multiple myeloma that is refractory to conventional chemotherapy. The proteosome is a multi-enzyme complex present in all cells that degrades cell-cycle regulatory proteins and causes proteolysis of IkappaB. This in turn activates NFkappaB, up-regulating the transcription of proteins promoting cell survival and growth and reducing susceptibility to apoptosis (programmed cell death). NFkappaB also induces drug resistance in myeloma cells and modulates the secretion of bone marrow stromal cytokines which mediate myeloma cell growth, survival, and migration.

Clinically Useful Tumor Markers

Carcinoembryonic antigen is elevated primarily in GI malignancies, but also in other adenocarcinomas, including those of the breast and lung. It is useful to follow tumor burden as a function of treatment, particularly in those colorectal tumors that produce it. It facilitates work-up for recurrence in asymptomatic patients most likely to be able to undergo a curative surgical resection (metastectomy).

Elevated serum levels of *CA-27-29* or *CA-15-3* suggest the presence of uncontrolled breast cancer. The presence of estrogen and/or progesterone receptors in breast cancer suggests a more well-differentiated and less aggressive tumor that will be likely to respond to hormonal therapies signaling through receptors, such as tamoxifen. Breast cancer HER2-*neu* overexpression suggests both a more aggressive phenotype and responsiveness to Herceptin.

Prostate-specific antigen (PSA) is the most useful serum test to suggest the diagnosis of prostate cancer and follow its response to treatment. PSA is highly specific for the prostate, and is not elevated in any other type of cancer. However, it can be elevated in benign prostatic hypertrophy.

Substantial elevation of serum β-*human chorionic gonadotropin* (hCG) suggests either a germ cell tumor or choriocarcinoma. hCG is a glycoprotein dimer produced by syncytiotrophoblasts. Its α subunit is identical to that of LH, FSH, and thyroid hormone. The β subunits of each are homologous but distinct. β-hCG can be elevated in both pure seminoma and nonseminomatous germ cell tumors.

Substantial elevation of α–*fetoprotein* suggests either a nonseminomatous germ cell tumor or hepatocellular carcinoma. It is a 70kD glycoprotein produced in the liver, GI tract, and fetal yolk sac. Its secretion in germ cell tumors is restricted to those of nonseminomatous histology, usually of embryonal cell carcinoma or endodermal sinus tumor origin.

CA-19-9 is elevated in pancreatic carcinoma and peritoneal carcinomatosis of any primary site. *CA-125* is elevated in ovarian cancer.

Lactate dehydrogenase is elevated in lung cancers and lymphomas. Monoclonal serum and urine gamma globulins (M *spikes*) and quantitative serum *immunoglobulin* G, A, or M may be elevated in multiple myeloma, with the other two uninvolved classes (D and E) quantitatively depressed. Certain B cell lymphomas may also share this phenomenon.

Bibliography

Alexander SE: Final Report of Ban Mustard Casualties. Washington, DC: Allied Forces Headquarters, Office of the Surgeon, 1944.

Baaske DM, Heinstein P: Cytotoxicity and cell cycle specificity of homoharringtonine. Antimicrob Agents Chemother 1977;12:298.

Baker WJ, Royer GL Jr, Weiss RB: Cytarabine and neurologic toxicity. J Clin Oncol 1991;9:679.

Barillari P, Ramacciato G, Manetti G, et al: Surveillance of colorectal cancer: effectiveness of early detection of intraluminal recurrences on prognosis and survival of patients treated for cure. Dis Colon Rectum 1996;39:388.

Bellone JD: Treatment of vincristine extravasation. JAMA 1981;245:343.

Berd D, Maguire HC Jr, Schuchter LM, et al: Autologous hapten-modified melanoma vaccine as postsurgical adjuvant treatment after resection of nodal metastases. J Clin Oncol 1997;15:2359.

Blackstock AW, Lesser G, Tucker R, Case D: Twice-weekly gemcitabine and concurrent thoracic radiotherapy—a Phase I/II study in patients with advanced non-small cell lung cancer [abstr 1846]. Proc Am Soc Clin Oncol 2000;19:470a.

Bonkhoff H, Fixemer T, Hunsicker I, Remberger K: Estrogen receptor expression in prostate cancer and premalignant prostatic lesions. Am J Pathol 1999;155:641.

Bosl GJ, Geller NL, Chan EY: Stage migration and the increasing proportion of complete responders in patients with advanced germ cell tumors. Cancer Res 1988;48:3524.

Brienza S, Vignoud J, Itzhaki M, Krikorian A: Oxaliplatin (L-OHP): global safety in 682 patients. Proc Am Soc Clin Oncol 1995;14:209.

Buchdunger E, Cioffi CL, Law N, et al: Abl protein-tyrosine kinase inhibitor STI571 inhibits in vitro signal transduction mediated by c-kit and platelet-derived growth factor receptors. J Pharmacol Exp Ther 2000;295:139.

Byar DP: The Veterans Administration Cooperative Urologic Research Group's studies of cancer of the prostate. Cancer 1973;32:1126.

Byrd J, Grever M, Davis B, et al: Phase I/II study of thrice weekly rituximab in chronic lymphocytic leukemia/small lymphocytic lymphoma: a feasible and active regimen [abstr 3114]. Blood 1999;94:704a.

Byrd JC, White CA, Link B, et al: Rituximab therapy in Waldenstrom's macroglobulinemia: preliminary evidence of clinical activity. Ann Oncol 1999;10:1525.

Bystryn JC, Oratz R, Roses D, et al: Relation between immune response to melanoma vaccine immunization and clinical outcome in stage II malignant melanoma. Cancer 1992;69:1157.

Bystryn J, Oratz R, Shapiro RL, et al: Phase 3, double-blind, trial of a shed, polyvalent, melanoma vaccine in stage III melanoma [abstr 1673]. Proc Am Soc Clin Oncol 1998; 17:434a.

Calvert AH, Newell DR, Gumbrell LA, et al: Carboplatin dosage: prospective evaluation of a simple formula based on renal function. J Clin Oncol 1989;7:1748.

Canman CE, Tang HY, Normolle DP, et al: Variations in patterns of DNA damage induced in human colorectal tumor cells by 5-fluorodeoxyuridine: implications for mechanisms of resistance and cytotoxicity. Proc Natl Acad Sci U S A 1992;89:10474.

Carter P, Presta L, Gorman CM, et al: Humanization of an anti-p185HER2 antibody for human cancer therapy. Proc Natl Acad Sci U S A 1992;89:4285.

Cascinu S, Fedeli A, Fedeli SL, Catalano G: Octreotide versus loperamide in the treatment of fluorouracil-induced diarrhea: a randomized trial. J Clin Oncol 1993;11:148.

Chabner BA: Cytidine analogs. In Chabner BA, Longo DL (eds): Cancer Chemotherapy and Biotherapy: Principles and Practice (2nd ed). Philadelphia: Lippincott–Raven, 1996:213.

Chabner BA, Stoler RG, Hande K, et al: Methotrexate disposition in humans: case studies in ovarian cancer and following high-dose infusion. Drug Metab Rev 1978;8:107.

Chaudhary PM, Roninson IB: Expression and activity of P-glycoprotein, a multidrug efflux pump, in human hematopoietic stem cells. Cell 1992;66:85.

Chen AY, Liu LF: DNA topoisomerases: essential enzymes and lethal targets. Annu Rev Pharmacol Toxicol 1994;34:191.

Christie NT, Drake S, Meyn RE, Nelson JA: 6-Thioguanine-induced DNA damage as a determinant of cytotoxicity in cultured Chinese hamster ovary cells. Cancer Res 1984;44:3665.

Chu E, Allegra CJ: Antifolates. In Chabner BA, Longo DL (eds): Cancer Chemotherapy and Biotherapy: Principles and Practice (2nd ed). Philadelphia: Lippincott–Raven, 1996:109.

Chun HG, Leyland-Jones B, Cheson BD: Fludarabine phosphate: a synthetic purine antimetabolite with significant activity against lymphoid malignancies. J Clin Oncol 1991;9:175.

Cormier JN, Patel SR, Pisters PW: Gastrointestinal stromal tumor: rationale for surgical adjuvant trials with imatinib. Curr Oncol Rep 2002;4:504.

Cortes J, Albitar M, Thomas D, et al: Efficacy of the farnesyltransferase inhibitor R115777 in chronic myeloid leukemia and other hematologic malignancies. Blood 2003; 100;1692.

DeVita VT Jr: The evolution of therapeutic research in cancer. N Engl J Med 1978;298:907.

DeVita VT Jr: The influence of information on drug resistance on protocol design: the Harry Kaplan Memorial Lecture given at the Fourth International Conference on Malignant Lymphoma, June 6–9, 1990, Lugano, Switzerland. Ann Oncol 1991;2:93.

DeVore RF, Fehrenbacher L, Herbst RS, et al: A randomized phase II trial comparing rhumab VEGF (recombinant humanized monoclonal antibody to vascular endothelial growth factor) plus carboplatin/paclitaxel (CP) to CP alone in patients with stage IIIB/IV NSCLC. Proc Am Soc Clin Oncol 2000;19:485a.

Dighiero G: Adverse and beneficial immunological effects of purine nucleotide analogues. Hematol Cell Ther 1996;38(Suppl 2):575.

Dukes M, Edwards PN, Large M, et al: The preclinical pharmacology of "Arimidex" (anastrozole; ZD1033)—a potent, selective aromatase inhibitor. J Steroid Biochem Mol Biol 1996;58:439.

Farber S, Diamond LK, Mercer RD, et al: Temporary remissions in acute leukemia in children produced by folic acid antagonist, 4-aminopteroylglutamic acid (aminopterin). N Engl J Med 1948;238:787.

Farber S, Selman A: Waksman Conference on Actinomycins: their potential for cancer chemotherapy. Opening remarks. Cancer Chemother Rep 1974;58:5.

Foss FM, Bacha P, Osann KE, et al: Biological correlates of acute hypersensitivity events with DAB(389)IL-2 (denileukin diftitox, ONTAK) in cutaneous T-cell lymphoma: decreased frequency and severity with steroid premedication. Clin Lymphoma 2001;1:298.

Fujimoto S, Takahashi M, Mutou T, et al: Improved mortality rate of gastric carcinoma patients with peritoneal carcinomatosis treated with intraperitoneal hyperthermic chemoperfusion combined with surgery. Cancer 1997;79:884.

Fung MC, Storniolo AM, Nguyen B, et al: A review of hemolytic uremic syndrome in patients treated with gemcitabine therapy. Cancer 1999;85:2023.

Goodman LS, Wintrobe MM, Dameshek W, et al: Landmark article Sept. 21, 1946: Nitrogen mustard therapy: use of methyl-bis(beta-chloroethyl)amine hydrochloride and tris(beta-chloroethyl)amine hydrochloride for Hodgkin's disease, lymphosarcoma, leukemia and certain allied and miscellaneous disorders. By Louis S. Goodman, Maxwell M. Wintrobe, William Dameshek, Morton J. Goodman, Alfred Gilman and Margaret T. McLennan. JAMA 1984;251:2255.

Goulian M, Bleile B, Tseng BY: Methotrexate-induced misincorporation of uracil into DNA. Proc Natl Acad Sci U S A 1980;77:1956.

Hande KR, Garrow GC: Purine metabolites. In Chabner BA, Longo DL (eds): Cancer Chemotherapy and Biotherapy: Principles and Practice (2nd ed). Philadelphia: Lippincott–Raven, 1996:235.

Haskell CM, Canellos GP: L-asparaginase resistance in human leukemia—asparaginase synthetase. Biochem Pharmacol 1969;18:2578.

Hayes DF, Van Zyl JA, Hacking A, et al: Randomized comparison of tamoxifen and two separate doses of toremifene in postmenopausal patients with metastatic breast cancer. J Clin Oncol 1995;13:2556.

Hetzel DJ, Wilson TO, Keeney GL, et al: HER-2/neu expression: a major prognostic factor in endometrial cancer. Gynecol Oncol 1992;47:179.

Hochster HS, Kim KM, Green MD, et al: Activity of fludarabine in previously treated non-Hodgkin's low-grade lymphoma: results of an Eastern Cooperative Oncology Group study. J Clin Oncol 1992;10:28.

Holzmann K, Welter C, Klein V, et al: Tumor-specific methylation patterns of erbB2 (HER2/neu) sequences in gastro-intestinal cancer. Anticancer Res 1992;12:1013.

Hornung RL, Pearson JW, Beckwith M, Longo DL: Preclinical evaluation of bryostatin as an anticancer agent against several murine tumor cell lines: in vitro versus in vivo activity. Cancer Res 1992;52:101.

Horwich A, Sleijfer DT, Fossa SD, et al: Randomized trial of bleomycin, etoposide, and cisplatin compared with bleomycin, etoposide and carboplatin in good-prognosis metastatic nonseminomatous germ cell cancer: a Multiinstitutional Medical Research Council/European Organization for Research and Treatment of Cancer Trial. J Clin Oncol 1997;15:1844.

Hsueh EC, Nizze A, Essner R, et al: Adjuvant immunotherapy with polyvalent melanoma cell vaccine (PMVC) prolongs survival after complete resection of distant melanoma metastases [abstr 1772]. Proc Am Soc Clin Oncol 1997;16:492a.

Huang MT: Harringtonine, an inhibitor of initiation of protein biosynthesis. Mol Pharmacol 1975;11:511.

Hurwitz H, Fehrenbacher I, et al: Bevacizumab (a monoclonal antibody to vascular endothelial growth factor) prolongs survival in first-line colorectal cancer (CRC): results of a phase II trial of bevacizumab in combination with bolus IFL (irinotecan, 5-fluorouracil, leucovorin) as first-line therapy in subjects with metastatic CRC. Proc Am Soc Clin Oncol 2003;22.

Hussein MA (ed): Reports from ASCO 2000: research on thalidomide in solid tumors, hematologic malignancies, and supportive care. Oncology (Huntingt) 2000; 14(11 Suppl 12):9.

Hynes NE, Stern DF: The biology of erbB-2/neu/HER-2 and its role in cancer. Biochim Biophys Acta 1994;1198:165.

Jacquet P, Sugarbaker PH: Peritoneal-plasma barrier. In Sugarbaker PH (ed): Peritoneal Carcinomatosis: Principles of Management. Boston: Kluwer Academic Publishers, 1966:S3.

Jordan MA, Thrower D, Wilson L: Mechanism of inhibition of cell proliferation by Vinca alkaloids. Cancer Res 1991;51:2212.

Kaubisch A, Kehsen DP, Saltz L, et al: A Phase I trial of weekly sequential bryostatin- I (BRYO) and paclitaxel in patients with advanced solid tumors. Proc Am Soc Clin Oncol 1999;18:639.

Keating MJ, Byrd J, Rai K, et al: Multicenter study of Campath-IH in patients with chronic lymphocytic leukemia (B-CLL) refractory to fludarabine [abstr 3118]. Blood 1999;94:705a.

Kern JA, Torney L, Weiner D, et al: Inhibition of human lung cancer cell line growth by an anti-p185HER2 antibody. Am J Respir Cell Mol Biol 1993;9:448.

Koutcher JA, Matel C, Zakian K, et al: In vivo metabolic and tumor growth delay studies with paclitaxel and bryostatin 1, a PKC inhibitor, are sequence dependent. Proc Am Assoc Cancer Res 1998;39:l9la.

Labrie F, Dupont A, Belanger A, Lachance R: Flutamide eliminates the risk of disease flare in prostatic cancer patients treated with a luteinizing hormone-releasing hormone agonist. J Urol 1987;138:804.

Lancet JE, Karp JE, Gotlib J, et al: Zarnestra (R115777) in previously untreated poor-risk AML and MDS: preliminary results of a phase II trial. Blood 2002;100:560a.

Leonard JP, Zelenetz AD, Vose JM, et al: Iodine 131 tositumomab for patients with low-grade or transformed low-grade NEIL: complete response data [abstr 3148]. Blood 2000;96:728a.

Liu Y, Tohnya TM, et al: Phase I study of CC-5013 (Revimid), a thalidomide derivative, in patients with refractory metastatic cancer. Proc Am Soc Clin Oncol 2003;22:231a.

Loprinzi CL, Michalak IC, Quella SK, et al: Megestrol acetate for the prevention of hot flashes. N Engl J Med 1994;331:347.

Love RR, Weibe DA, Newcomb PA, et al: Effects of tamoxifen on cardiovascular risk factors in postmenopausal women. Ann Intern Med 1991;115:860.

Magda D, Lepp C, et al: The redox mediator motexafin gadolinium (MGd) enhances the activity of several chemotherapy drugs. Proc Am Soc Clin Oncol 2003;22:229a.

Marchall EK Jr: Historical perspectives in chemotherapy. Adv Chemother 1964;1:1.

Mathews V, Balasubramanian P, Shaji RV, et al: Arsenic trioxide in the treatment of newly diagnosed acute promyelocytic leukemia: a single center experience. Am J Hematol (United States) 2002;70:292.

McDonald CC, Stewart HJ for the Scottish Breast Cancer Committee: Fatal myocardial infarction in the Scottish adjuvant tamoxifen trial. BMJ 1991;303:435.

McLaughlin P, Grillo-Lopez AJ, Link BK, et al: Rituximab chimeric anti-CD20 monoclonal antibody therapy for relapsed indolent lymphoma: half of patients respond to a four-dose treatment program. J Clin Oncol 1998;16:2825.

Montgomery JA, Hewson K: Nucleosides of 2-fluoroadenine. J Med Chem 1969;12:498.

Morton DL, Malmgren RA, Holmes EC, Ketcham AS: Demonstration of antibodies against melanoma by immunofluorescence. Surgery 1968;64:233.

Morton DL, Nizze A, Hoon DSB, et al: Improved survival of advanced stage IV melanoma following active immunotherapy: correlation with immune response to melanoma vaccine [abstract]. Proc Am Soc Clin Oncol 1993;12:391a.

Morton DL, Wanek L, Nizze JA, et al: Improved long-term survival after lymphadenectomy of melanoma metastatic to regional nodes: analysis of prognostic factors in 1134 patients from the John Wayne Cancer Clinic. Ann Surg 1991;214:491.

Mukherji B, Chakraborty NG, Sivanandham M: T-cell clones that react against autologous human tumors. Immunol Rev 1990;116:33.

O'Brien S, Kantarjian H, Koller C, et al: Sequential homoharringtonine and interferon-alpha in the treatment of early chronic phase chronic myelogenous leukemia. Blood 1999;93:4149.

Pavlakis N, Bell DR, Millward MJ, Levi JA: Fatal pulmonary toxicity resulting from treatment with gemcitabine. Cancer 1997;80:286.

Pegram MD, Daly D, Wirth C, et al: Antibody dependent cell-mediated cytotoxicity in breast cancer patients in Phase III clinical trials of a humanized anti-HER2 antibody [abstract]. Proc Am Assoc Cancer Res 1997;38:602.

Peiper M, Goedegebuure PS, Linehan DC, et al: The HER2/neu-derived peptide p654-662 is a tumor-associated antigen in human pancreatic cancer recognized by cytotoxic T lymphocytes. Eur J Immunol 1994;27:1115.

Pietra N, Sarli L, Costi R, et al: Role of follow-up in management of local recurrences of colorectal cancer: a prospective, randomized study. Dis Colon Rectum 1998;41:1127.

Powles TJ, Hickish TF, Kanis JA, Ashley S: Tamoxifen preserves bone mineral density in postmenopausal women but causes loss of bone density in premenopausal women [abstract]. Proc Am Soc Clin Oncol 1995;14:165.

Press MF, Pike MC, Hung G, et al: Amplification and overexpression of HER-2/neu in carcinomas of the salivary gland: correlation with poor prognosis. Cancer Res 1994;54:5675.

Punt CJA, Keiser HI, Douma J, et al: Multicenter randomized trial of 5-fluorouracil (5FU) and leucovorin (LV) with or without trimetrexate (TMTX) as a first line treatment in patients with advanced colorectal cancer (ACC). Proc Am Soc Clin Oncol 1999;18:262.

Rai K, Mercier RI, Cooper MR, et al: Campath-IH is an effective salvage therapy for fludarabine failing CLL patients: results of a Phase II trial [abstr 703]. Blood 2000;96:163a.

Rai KR, Peterson B, Kohitz I, et al: Fludarabine induces high complete remission rate in previously untreated patients with active chronic lymphocytic leukemia (CLL): a randomized inter-group study. Blood 1995;86(Suppl I):607.

Richardson PG, Barlogie B, Berenson J, et al: A Phase 2 study of bortezomib in relapsed, refractory myeloma. N Engl J Med 2003;348:2609.

Ridge SA, Sludden J, Wei X, et al: Dihydropyrimidine dehydrogenase pharmacogenetics in patients with colorectal cancer. Br J Cancer 1998;77:497.

Rosenberg B, VanCamp L, Trosko I, Mansour VH: Platinum compounds: a new class of potent antitumour agents. Nature 1969;222:385.

Rosenberg SA, Yang JC, White DE, Steinberg SM: Durability of complete responses in patients with metastatic cancer treated with high-dose interleukin-2: identification of the antigens mediating response. Ann Surg 1998;228:307.

Ross JS, Sheehan CE, Hayner-Buchan AM, et al: Prognostic significance of HER2/neu gene amplification status by fluorescence in situ hybridization of prostate carcinoma. Cancer 1997;79:2162.

Ross WE, Bradley MO: DNA double-stranded breaks in mammalian cells after exposure to intercalating agents. Biochim Biophys Acta 1981;654:129.

Rowinsky EK, Donehower RC: Paclitaxel (Taxol). N Engl J Med 1995;332:1004.

Saad F, Gleason DM, Murray R, et al: A randomized, placebo-controlled trial of zoledronic acid in patients with hormone-refractory metastatic prostate carcinoma. J Natl Cancer Inst 2002;94:1458.

Saltz L, Rubin M, Hochster H, et al: Cetuximab (IMC-C225) plus Irinotecan is active in CPT-11-refractory colorectal cancer that expresses epidermal growth factor receptor. Proc Am Soc Clin Oncol 2001;20:3a.

Sandler AB: Clin Lung Cancer 2003;5:S22.

Santi DV, McHenry CS, Raines RT, Ivanetich KM: Kinetics and thermodynamics of the interaction of 5-fluoro-2′-deoxyuridylate and thymidylate synthase. Biochemistry 1987;26:8606.

Scagliotti G, Kortsik C, et al: Phase II randomized study of Pemetrexed and carboplatin or oxaliplatin, as front-line chemotherapy in patients with locally advanced or metastatic non-small cell lung cancer. Proc Am Soc Clin Oncol 2003;22:625a.

Slamon DJ, Clark GM, Wong SG, et al: Human breast cancer: correlation of relapse and survival with amplification of the HER-2/neu oncogene. Science 1987;235:177.

Slamon DJ, Godolphin W, Jones LA, et al: Studies of the HER-2/neu proto-oncogene in human breast and ovarian cancer. Science 1989;244:707.

Smith PJ, Soues S: Multilevel therapeutic targeting by topoisomerase inhibitors. Br J Cancer 1994;23:S47.

Stahelin HF, von Wartburg A: The chemical and biological route from podophyllotoxin glucoside to etoposide: ninth Cain memorial award lecture. Cancer Res 1991;51:5.

Stenbygaard LE, Herrstedt J, Thomsen JF, et al: Toremifene and tamoxifen in advanced breast cancer—a double-blind cross-over trial. Breast Cancer Res Treat 1993;25:57.

Sugarbaker PH: Management of Peritoneal Surface Malignancy Using Intraperitoneal Chemotherapy and Cytoreductive Surgery: A Manual. Grand Rapids, MI: The Ludann Company, 1998.

Sugarbaker PH, Averbach AM, Jacquet P, et al: A simplified approach to hyperthermic intraoperative intraperitoneal chemotherapy (HIIC) using a self retaining retractor. Cancer Treat Res 1996;82:415.

Symanowski JT, Rusthoven J, et al: Multiple regression analysis of prognostic variables for survival from the phase III study of

Pemetrexed and cisplatin vs cisplatin in malignant pleural mesothelioma. Proc Am Soc Clin Oncol 2003;22:647a.

Thomas JP, Ramanathan RK, Wilding G, et al: A phase I study of motexafin gadolinium (MGd) in combination with doxorubicin (Dox). Proc Am Soc Clin Oncol 2003;22:227a.

Trenn G, Pettit GR, Takayama H, et al: Immunomodulating properties of a novel series of protein kinase C activators: the bryostatins. J Immunol 1988;140:433.

Vaitukaitis JL: Human chorionic gonadotropin as a tumor marker. Ann Clin Lab Sci 1974;4:276.

Vose JM, Wall RL, Saleh M, et al: Multicenter Phase II study of iodine-131 tositumomab for chemotherapy-relapsed/refractory low-grade and transformed low-grade B-cell non-Hodgkin's lymphomas. J Clin Oncol 2000;18:1316.

Wallack MK, Sivanandham M, Balch CM, et al: Surgical adjuvant active specific immunotherapy for patients with stage III melanoma: the final analysis of data from a Phase III, randomized, double-blind, multicenter vaccinia melanoma oncolysate trial. J Am Coll Surg 1998;187:69.

Ward RI, Morgan G, Dalley D, Kelly PJ: Tamoxifen reduces bone turnover and prevents lumbar spine and proximal femoral bone loss in early postmenopausal women. Bone Miner 1993;22:87.

Weiss MA, Lamanna N, Maslak PG, et al: Pentostatin, cyclophosphamide and rituximab (PCR therapy): A new active regimen for previously treated patients with chronic lymphocytic leukemia (CLL). Proc Am Soc Clin Oncol 2003;22:580a.

Wigley DB: Structure and mechanism of DNA topoisomerases. Annu Rev Biophys Biomed Struct 1995;24:185.

Wilkowski R, Heinemann V, Rau H: Radiochemotherapy including gemcitabine and 5-fluorouracil for treatment of locally advanced pancreatic cancer [abstr 1078]. Proc Am Soc Clin Oncol 2000;19:276a.

Williams DP, Parker K, Bacha P, et al: Diphtheria toxin receptor binding domain substitution with interleukin-2: genetic construction and properties of a diphtheria toxin-related interleukin-2 fusion protein. Protein Eng 1987;1:493.

Witzig TE, White CA, Wiseman GA, et al: Phase I/II trial of IDEC-Y2B8 radioimmunotherapy for treatment of relapsed or refractory CD20(+) B-cell non-Hodgkin's lymphoma. J Clin Oncol 1999;7:3793.

Yonemura Y, Fujimura T, Fushida S, et al: Hyperthermo-chemotherapy combined with cytoreductive surgery for the treatment of gastric cancer with peritoneal dissemination. World J Surg 1991;15:530.

Yonemura Y, Ninomiya I, Yamaguchi A, et al: Evaluation of immunoreactivity for erbB-2 protein as a marker of poor short-term prognosis in gastric cancer. Cancer Res 1991;51:1034.

CHAPTER 48

Radiation Therapy and Radiation Injury

T. William Huang, M.D., Ph.D., Suzanne M. Russo, M.D., Volker W. Stieber, M.D.,
Costas Koumenis, Ph.D., Allan F. deGuzman, Ph.D., and Edward G. Shaw, M.D.

Radiation therapy (RT) has come a long way since the initial discovery of x-rays by Roentgen in 1895. Significant technical advances in computers, imaging, and radiation treatment planning and delivery along with improved knowledge of clinical oncology, radiation physics, and radiobiology have made radiation therapy the definitive, often organ-preserving local treatment of choice with a high likelihood of cure for many cancers such as prostate, anal, and early-stage glottic laryngeal cancers. Radiation therapy is also an integral part of the multimodality treatment of breast, lung, rectal, and other types of cancer. In recent years, its utility has expanded to treatment of benign diseases such as arteriovenous malformations and coronary artery in-stent restenosis.

Radiation therapy has several unique characteristics that make it a good complementary or alternative treatment to surgery. In contrast to surgery, it is noninvasive and can eradicate tumors in a broader area and in surgically inaccessible locations. It can also eliminate microscopic residual disease in the surgical bed. These factors combine to improve the local control of cancers when radiation is used in a postoperative setting. When delivered preoperatively, radiation therapy can make marginally resectable or unresectable tumors, such as locally advanced rectal adenocarcinoma or soft-tissue sarcoma, more resectable. Preoperative irradiation can also reduce the risk of intraoperative spread of viable tumor cells or rupture of tumors such as large Wilms' tumors. For patients with significant local symptoms arising from their cancer, radiation therapy is frequently the most effective palliative measure and is often used to treat "oncologic emergencies" such as malignant epidural spinal cord compression, upper airway or vascular obstruction, and brain metastases.

A good understanding of radiation therapy in terms of its uses, mechanisms, and toxicity is important for any surgical practice in several key ways. First, a surgeon is often the first physician to see a patient who may need radiation therapy to achieve the best possible clinical outcome in terms of local control, survival, and quality of life. A surgeon needs to know the indications for preoperative, intraoperative, postoperative, and definitive radiation therapy to counsel the patient appropriately and to make a referral to a radiation oncologist in a timely fashion. Second, proper timing of surgery before or after radiation therapy is essential to minimize perioperative wound complications and the risk of local recurrence. If postoperative radiation therapy is planned, surgical procedures, such as the use of an absorbable mesh sling to move small bowel away from the pelvic radiation fields in a patient with rectal cancer, should be considered to minimize the risk of radiation-induced toxicity. Surgical clips should be placed in the tumor bed to help plan postoperative radiation therapy. To make the proper diagnosis and manage the situation appropriately, the surgeon must recognize radiation-related toxicity and complications. Finally, a surgeon and other medical personnel may be exposed to radiation when intraoperative radiation therapy or brachytherapy is used. Hence, one must be familiar with radiation safety and the risks of occupational radiation exposure to avoid exceeding the recommended radiation exposure limits and having an irrational fear of radiation.

This chapter outlines the basics of radiation physics, radiation biology, treatment techniques, clinical uses, radiation-related acute and long-term toxicity, and radiation safety. For additional details, the interested reader may refer to standard textbooks of radiation physics, radiobiology, and radiation oncology.

Radiation Physics and Techniques

Basic Radiation Physics

A basic knowledge of radiation physics is necessary to understand the potential benefits and limitations of radiation treatment. The most common types of radiation for clinical use are high-energy x-rays, gamma rays, and electrons. High-energy x-rays and electrons are produced by linear accelerators. Gamma rays are electromagnetic radiation physically equivalent to x-rays with a wavelength of approximately 10^{-12} meter, but they originate from the decay of radioisotopes such as ^{60}Co in cobalt-60 teletherapy machines and the Leksell Gamma Knife (Elekta Instruments), a device used for intracranial stereotactic radiosurgery. The x-rays and gamma rays, also referred to as photons, are massless and are able to penetrate tissue to reach deep-seated targets when applied at megavoltage energies.

In contrast, electrons have a definite mass and a negative charge and thus have much more limited penetration into tissue than photons of the same energy. A useful analogy is the differing results when one is hit by a fast baseball versus a bullet traveling with the same kinetic energy. This depth-dose characteristic of electrons is advantageous when the target is on the surface or at a shallow depth with an underlying critical organ, such as the cervical spinal cord. Typical examples are the use of electrons as a definitive treatment for skin cancer and as a radiation "boost" to a breast lumpectomy cavity and cervical lymph nodes in patients with head and neck cancer. Electrons deposit a significant radiation dose to the skin and are often used in conjunction with photons. Electrons originating from a radioisotope, such as ^{32}P, are referred to as beta rays. Electrons comprise the most common type of particle-beam radiation used clinically. Other types of particle-beam radiation (e.g., protons and neutrons) are available only at a small number of facilities because of their limited application, highly complex and costly production, and potentially greater toxicity, although they may have greater efficacy in some settings.

High-energy x-rays and gamma rays are classified as ionizing radiation, which means there is sufficient energy to cause ejection of orbital electrons when they travel through matter. Photons interact with matter in two major ways. Diagnostic x-rays, with energy typically in the range of 25,000 to 125,000 electron volts (25 to 125 keV), interact with matter primarily through the photoelectric effect. This is a type of photon–matter interaction whereby the energy of the photon causes ejection of a tightly bound orbital electron from the target, and the energy of the incident photon is completely transferred to the ejected electron. The absorption of energy by the photoelectric effect varies with the cube of the atomic number (Z) of the absorbing material. This is why bone, with a high content of calcium, is well visualized on a diagnostic radiograph. However the Z-dependent absorption makes kilovoltage x-rays a poor choice for therapy. Normal bone inevitably receives a much higher dose than would a soft tissue target.

At higher energies, in the range of 1 million to 20 million electron volts (1 to 20 MeV), x-rays and gamma rays interact with matter primarily through the Compton effect. Compton interactions involve scattering of photons by the loosely bound outer orbital electrons. The incident x-rays do not give up all of their energy to a single electron. As a result, energy deposition by the Compton effect does not depend on the atomic number of matter but only on their electron density. Radiation of this energy is useful for therapy because there is no significant energy-deposition differential between bone and soft tissue.

In contrast to photons (x-rays and gamma rays), charged particles such as protons and electrons interact with matter predominantly by ionization and excitation of atoms. Ionization occurs when charged particles have sufficient energy to strip orbital electrons from atoms. If the energy of the charged particles is less than the binding energy of the orbital electrons, the orbital electrons are displaced from their stable orbit but then return to the orbit. This is called excitation. Heavy charged particles such as protons and alpha particles lose energy slowly in soft tissue at first but then deposit a large portion of their energy as a dose at the end of their track, a phenomenon referred to as the Bragg peak. Because of the Bragg peak, heavy charged particles are clinically useful for treating deep targets surrounded by critical, sensitive organs such as skull-base chordomas, which lie adjacent to the lower brainstem and upper cervical spinal cord. Electrons, owing to their light mass, are easily scattered and do not produce a Bragg peak. High-energy neutrons, which are uncharged, interact with tissue principally by recoiling the protons found in hydrogen. Therefore, neutrons deposit more dose in fat, which has a high content of hydrogen. Neutrons are used clinically to treat large, unresectable, "radioresistant" tumors such as bone and soft tissue sarcomas and adenoid cystic carcinomas of the head and neck.

As a result of the interactions of photons and particles with matter, radiation loses energy and becomes attenuated as it travels through tissue. The degree of attenuation depends on the type of radiation, its energy, and the density and composition of the matter through which it is passing. The radiation dose also depends on the inverse-square law, which states that the intensity of a radiation beam at a given point is inversely proportional to the square of the distance from its source. An analogy is the intensity of a light bulb, which would only be one fourth as bright at 2 meters as it is at 1 meter. The inverse square law is especially important for radiation safety and for proper use of brachytherapy (radioactive implants).

The radiation absorbed dose, formerly in units of "rads," is now measured in the SI units of Gray (Gy), where 1 Gy is equivalent to 1 joule/kg, 100 rad, or 100 centigray (cGy). Typical total radiation doses when treating cancer are 50 to 70 Gy or 5000 to 7000 cGy. The units Gy and cGy are preferred to the old term "rad" because the latter measure did not comply with international metric system standards.

Radiation Techniques

Radiation therapy delivery systems

Teletherapy and brachytherapy are two basic ways to deliver therapeutic radiation. Teletherapy, also referred to as external-beam radiation therapy, means treatment at a long distance. The distance between the source of radiation and the target is usually 80 to 120 cm but may be much longer in some treatment setups such as total body irradiation. Brachytherapy, in contrast, means treatment at a short distance and employs the use of radioactive materials implanted within or close to the target. Teletherapy is the more commonly used modality and is discussed first.

Before 1950 teletherapy machines could produce only x-rays of slightly higher energy (250 keV) than those from diagnostic machines. Use of these "orthovoltage" machines often resulted in substantial patient morbidity because the x-rays they produce have a poor penetrating power and deposit their maximum dose within the first few millimeters of tissue. For example, a tumor at 10 cm depth may receive only about 40% of the surface or entrance dose. This results in an excessive skin dose, leading to skin breakdown and subsequent subcutaneous fibrosis. Thus, the total dose that could be delivered to a deep-seated tumor was significantly limited. Moreover, orthovoltage x-rays deposit a significantly larger dose in high-Z tissues (e.g., bone) through photoelectric interactions. Presently, the main utility of orthovoltage machines is in the treatment of cutaneous squamous cell carcinomas and basal cell carcinomas.

The morbidity associated with radiation therapy was markedly reduced by the development of therapy machines capable of producing megavoltage x-rays or gamma rays (1 million electron volts or more) because of their "skin-sparing" effect. The degree of skin sparing is related to Dmax, the depth of maximal radiation dose deposited in tissue from a single radiation beam. Dmax increases with the increasing energy of x-rays, from 5 mm for a 1 MeV beam to more than 3 cm for a 20 MeV beam. For orthovoltage, Dmax is less than 100 μm.

The cobalt-60 machine, first available during the 1950s, is the first megavoltage treatment machine that became widely used clinically, ushering in the modern era of therapeutic radiology (i.e., radiation oncology). ^{60}Co emits gamma rays at 1.25 MeV and has a half-life of 5.26 years. Because ^{60}Co emission is in the megavoltage range, the differential absorption by bone ceases to be a problem, modest skin sparing is achieved, and the dose at a deep depth is greatly improved over that achieved with orthovoltage units. These three improvements have allowed clinicians to employ tumor doses that are considerably increased over historical values. Cobalt-60 units are still popular in Third World countries because of their relative low cost and simplicity, but they are being phased out in the United States because of their low energy and radiation safety concerns with the maintenance and disposal of ^{60}Co sources.

The workhorse in radiation therapy today is the linear accelerator, or "linac," because of its versatility. A typical linac is capable of producing x-rays at 4 to 20 MeV and electrons from 6 to 21 MeV. It produces high-energy x-rays and electrons by accelerating electrons from an electron gun in a linear accelerator tube. The electrons gain energy as they "surf" down the tube (wave guide) in a strong electromagnetic field of microwaves generated by a magnetron or klystron. These electrons can be used for treatment after they go through a beam transport system. To obtain x-rays, the accelerated electrons are made to strike a high-Z target, such as tungsten. Collision between a high-speed electron and a tungsten nucleus results in loss of energy of the electron. This energy loss is transformed into heat and bremsstrahlung x-rays. These x-rays exit from the linac's treatment head and go through a system of collimators, which can be adjusted to determine the size of the radiation fields. The radiation fields can be further shaped by the use of a custom block composed of a lead-equivalent alloy called Cerrobend. More advanced linacs use multileaf collimators for field shaping. The angle of the beam is controlled by rotating the linac about a horizontal axis (Fig. 48–1).

Photons produced by linear accelerators have better skin-sparing qualities than those from cobalt-60 machines and a higher dose at depth. In addition, a radiation beam from a linear accelerator has a sharper field "edge," or penumbra, than a beam generated by ^{60}Co. This makes more precise tumor targeting possible. In additional to conventional radiation therapy, a modern linac, when properly adapted, is capable of delivering three-dimensional

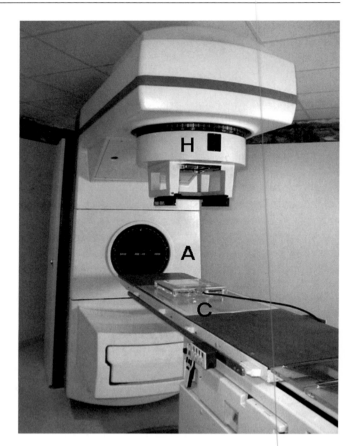

FIGURE 48–1 Linear accelerator. Radiation exits from the treatment head *(H)* and is directed toward the couch *(C)*, where a patient typically lies. The direction of the radiation can be changed by rotating the linac about its horizontal axis *(A)*.

conformal therapy, intensity-modulated radiation therapy, intraoperative radiation therapy, and stereotactic radiosurgery—additional ways of delivering more precise radiation doses.

Heavy particle machines for clinical use are available in a limited number of locations around the world because they are much larger, more complex, and more costly than standard linacs. The most common heavy particles currently used for therapy are neutrons and protons. Neutrons are produced most commonly by accelerating protons or deuterons in a cyclotron and allowing them to strike a beryllium target. High energy, or "fast," neutrons (15 to 50 MeV) have the chief advantage of having a high linear energy transfer (LET), a measure of the amount of energy deposited per unit length of travel in tissue. For example, 19 MeV neutrons have a LET of approximately 15 keV/mm, compared to 0.3 keV/mm for 6 MeV x-rays. The high LET of neutrons increases their relative biologic effectiveness (RBE) compared to that of photons. Improved local control with use of neutron therapy has been observed for tumors such as unresectable or recurrent salivary gland cancers and unresectable sarcomas. Therapeutic protons are produced in cyclotrons or synchrotrons and typically have an energy of 150 to 250 MeV. They have a characteristic Bragg peak, which is used to achieve a conformal dose distribution. Protons are currently used for tumors such as prostate cancers, uveal melanomas, and skull-base tumors such as chordomas and sarcomas.

Brachytherapy owes its start to the Curies when they discovered radium in 1898. Radium is the first radioisotope used to treat cancers. It can, for instance, be placed in a hollow applicator and inserted into a cavity such as the vagina to treat cervical cancer. This technique is called intracavitary brachytherapy. Radium-filled needles can also be inserted directly into a tumor, a technique termed interstitial brachytherapy. Presently, safer radioactive isotopes have replaced radium for this use. Cesium (^{137}Cs), with an energy of 0.661 MeV and half-life of 30 years, is commonly utilized for intracavitary brachytherapy of gynecologic malignancies. Iridium (^{192}Ir), with an energy of 0.35 MeV and half-life of 74 days, is the most popular radioisotope for interstitial brachytherapy owing to its smaller physical size. Interstitial ^{192}Ir brachytherapy is typically used to treat soft tissue sarcomas and for endobronchial, endobiliary, and endovascular brachytherapy.

To protect operating room personnel from irradiation, temporary brachytherapy using radioisotopes such as ^{137}Cs and ^{192}Ir is often done using an afterloading technique. Here, hollow applicators or catheters are placed in the desired locations and secured in place in the operating room or special procedure room (Fig. 48–2). For conventional low-dose-rate (LDR) brachytherapy (dose rate 40 to 200 cGy per hour),

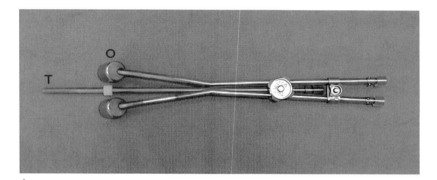

A

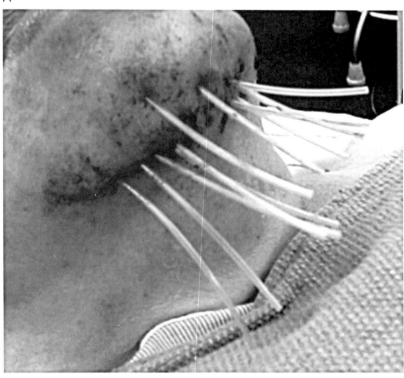

B

FIGURE 48–2 Brachytherapy afterloading implant devices. **A,** Fletcher-Suit applicator for low-dose-rate intracavitary brachytherapy used to treat cervical cancer. When properly placed, the tip of the tandem *(T)* is in the intrauterine cavity near the fundus. The ovoids *(O)* are placed on the right and left sides of the cervix. The applicator is hollow, allowing insertion of ^{137}Cs sources. **B,** Interstitial brachytherapy catheters implanted in the floor of mouth. ^{192}Ir sources are inserted postoperatively into these afterloading catheters.

radioisotopes are typically loaded manually after the patient has been properly shielded in a private room. The patient is then treated continuously for 1 to 6 days. Short-half-life and low-energy radioisotopes may be used for permanent interstitial brachytherapy. A typical example is a prostate implant with iodine-125 seeds, which have an energy of 0.028 MeV and a half-life of 60 days. Because of their relatively low energy, they do not require heavy shielding and can be inserted directly into the prostate in the operating room. The patient may be discharged home after the procedure with the radiation exposure to the general public maintained within safe limits.

As a consequence of the inverse-square law, a large dose may be delivered directly to the target with brachy-therapy, sparing critical organs. However, proper placement of radioactive implants is critical to achieve the desired dose distribution. Compared to external beam radiation therapy, the dose distribution achieved with brachytherapy is significantly less homogeneous, and the size of the target that can be adequately treated is much smaller. For these reasons, brachytherapy is more often used as a "boost," combined with external beam radiation therapy.

Gaining in popularity in recent years is high-dose-rate (HDR) brachytherapy, which typically uses a high-activity ^{192}Ir source with approximately 10 Ci of activity. It is capable of achieving a dose rate of more than 12 Gy (1200 cGy) per hour, which is the definition of HDR brachytherapy (ICRU, 1985). HDR brachytherapy reduces the treatment time to a few minutes and avoids the need for prolonged bed rest during brachytherapy. However, it requires a heavily shielded treatment room and an HDR remote afterloader, a device that transports the radioactive source from a shielded container to the applicator(s) via one or more catheters. A computer console outside the treatment room controls the afterloader. By controlling the dwell times of the radioactive source at various positions within the applicator(s), the dose distribution can be more easily optimized than with LDR brachytherapy. However, because of its high dose rate, HDR brachytherapy is usually fractionated, meaning that two or more treatments (usually two to five) are given with a smaller dose per fraction (usually 400 to 1000 cGy) to keep the normal-tissue toxicity within safe limits.

Radiation treatment planning

To optimize the therapeutic ratio of radiation therapy, the dose delivered to the target must be maximized and the dose received by surrounding normal tissues minimized. This can be accomplished by controlling the field size, field shape, beam arrangement, type of radiation, energy, and other technical factors. The process of calculating the radiation dose distribution is referred to as dosimetry. Optimizing this parameter requires the use of computer-based treatment planning systems, which range in sophistication from conventional two-dimensional planning systems to three-dimensional planning systems and specific planning systems for intensity-modulated radiation therapy, stereotactic radiosurgery, and brachytherapy.

CONVENTIONAL TWO-DIMENSIONAL PLANNING. The first step in conventional two-dimensional (2D) planning is simulation on a simulator. A simulator is a specialized diagnostic-quality x-ray machine that is able to reproduce the setup of a therapy machine such as a linac. The patient is placed in the treatment position, which is usually supine or prone. Patient-immobilization devices may be used to make the daily setup more reproducible. The size and location of the radiation treatment fields and the beam angles are set under fluoroscopic guidance. With the aid of a laser alignment system, alignment points (used for daily positioning on the therapy machine) are marked on the patient. Diagnostic x-ray films called simulation, or "sim," films are obtained. The shape of the radiation fields can be customized by outlining the areas to be blocked on sim films (Fig. 48–3A). Custom-shaped radiation fields using Cerrobend blocks or multileaf collimators are now used routinely.

Typically, one to four radiation fields, or portals, are utilized, and they combine to form the treatment volume (TV). The TV is determined by the planning target volume (PTV) and the penumbra of the radiation beam. The penumbra is the region at the edge of the radiation field where the dose decreases rapidly from 90% to 50% of the central-axis dose. The size of the penumbra varies with the energy of the radiation beam and type of therapy machine. For example, the penumbra is approximately 1.5 cm for a cobalt-60 machine and 0.7 cm for an 18 MeV x-ray beam. The PTV encompasses the gross tumor or target volume (GTV), the clinical target volume (CTV), and an additional margin for daily setup errors and target movements (ICRU, 2000) (Fig. 48–4). The GTV is defined as the area of the clinically evident disease, such as a lung mass seen on diagnostic computed tomography (CT) or plain radiography. The CTV includes the GTV and areas at high risk of microscopic spread, such as ipsilateral hilar and mediastinal nodal regions for lung cancer. The thickness or a contour of the body in the area of interest is obtained manually or with a CT slice, and computerized 2D dosimetry is then performed in a limited number of planes.

This conventional, or 2D, approach to treatment planning is limiting in several ways. First, targeting is less precise. Second, even if the CTV is identified correctly on a chest x-ray film acquired in the anteroposterior (AP) direction, for example, this information cannot be used to design a beam oriented in another direction, such as an oblique beam. Third, 2D planning does not allow volumetric calculations of the dose delivered to the target or critical surrounding tissues. This point is important because dose–volume data are used to predict radiation injury of the lung and other organs. Despite the limitations of conventional treatment planning, however, it is quick, efficient, and adequate for most clinical situations, such as postlumpectomy breast irradiation and pelvic irradiation for gynecologic malignancies.

THREE-DIMENSIONAL TREATMENT PLANNING. Three-dimensional (3D) treatment planning systems allow one to build and manipulate 3D patient models and to

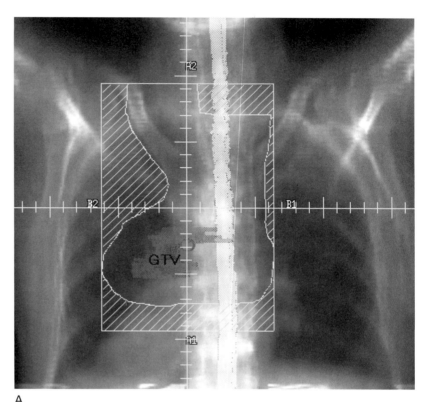

A

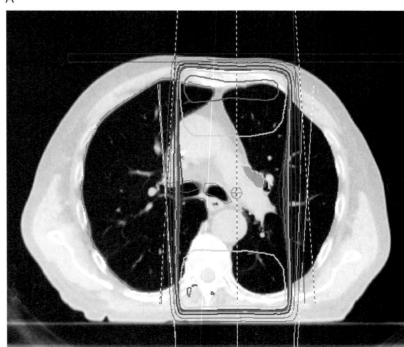

FIGURE 48–3 Images generated from a three-dimensional treatment planning system. **A,** Digitally reconstructed radiograph (DRR) of a simulation film illustrating a typical radiation portal for non-small-cell lung cancer. The gross tumor volume (GTV) and blocks are outlined. **B,** Corresponding radiation dose distribution or gradient in a horizontal plane at the level of the GTV.

Figure continued on following page   B

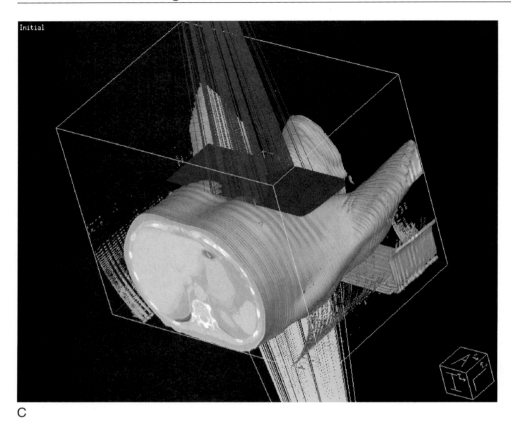

C

design and display entire 3D treatment plans. These systems became routinely available during the mid-1990s and are still undergoing refinement. They require specially adapted CT or magnetic resonance imaging (MRI) scanners. Patients are placed in the treatment position with radiopaque

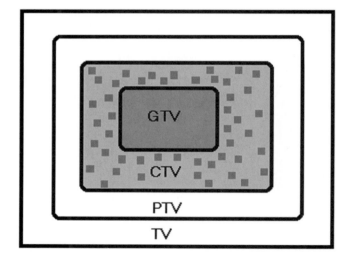

FIGURE 48–4 Radiation treatment volume (TV) or portal that emcompasses the gross tumor or target volume (GTV), clinical target volume (CTV), and planning target volume (PTV).

reference or fiducial markers. The region of interest is scanned, and the images are transferred to a 3D treatment-planning computer. The GTV, CTV, PTV, and critical organs are outlined, or "contoured," by the radiation oncologist. The dose distribution of various plans using different beam arrangements may then be evaluated. The general goal is to deliver at least 95% of the prescribed dose to the PTV while minimizing or not exceeding the tolerance dose of critical organs. To make alterations to the plan interactively, a treatment plan may be viewed on a succession of CT or MRI slices, a reconstructed 3D image, or a digitally reconstructed radiograph. Figure 48–3 shows images from one such system. State-of-the-art treatment planning systems also allow data from multiple imaging studies to be utilized in the planning process so positron emission tomography (PET) scans, for example, can be used to help define the GTV. In addition, such systems allow one to modulate the incident radiation beams to ensure a uniform tumor dose and the lowest possible dose to surrounding dose-critical tissue. Because of more accurate targeting, smaller and more conformal radiation fields may be used.

Computed tomography- or MRI-based 3D treatment planning, combined with improved patient immobilization, allows accurate delivery of 3D conformal therapy. 3D conformal therapy is now used routinely for central nervous system (CNS) tumors and prostate cancer and is gaining popularity for other sites. Several centers have begun exploiting this approach to escalate radiation doses above the traditional levels for selected tumor types (e.g., brain, prostate, and lung cancers). In recent years, with the increased sophistication of 3D treatment planning systems and linear accelerators, intensity-modulated radiation therapy (IMRT) has evolved from 3D conformal therapy. IMRT typically uses multileaf collimators to modulate the intensity of each radiation beam. The intensity may be modulated dynamically, with the collimator leaves moving while the beam is on. Simpler systems may use a static mode; here multileaf collimators are set, or shaped blocks are placed, before the beam is turned on. Usually seven or more beams are used to achieve a highly conformal dose distribution. New IMRT treatment planning systems are also capable of "inverse treatment planning."

To start the inverse planning process, a radiation oncologist first outlines the PTV and critical organs. The minimal target dose and maximal dose to critical organs are then set, along with priorities and allowable deviations. The treatment planning computer then determines the best beam arrangements and collimator leaf settings to achieve a conformal dose distribution and maintain the required dose levels. Compared to conventional 3D conformal therapy, IMRT is better at reducing the dose to critical organs. For example, for head and neck cancer, IMRT may reduce the risk of xerostomia by sparing more of the salivary glands from high doses of radiation. IMRT is also being used to treat prostate cancers, CNS tumors, and skull-base tumors.

Perhaps the ultimate form of 3D conformal therapy is stereotactic radiosurgery (SRS). The term "radiosurgery" was first coined in 1951 by a Swedish neurosurgeon, Lars Leksell. To treat small, surgically inaccessible brain tumors, he developed the Gamma Knife. The most current version of the Gamma Knife has 201 ^{60}Co sources arranged in a helmet-like array, into which the patient's head is positioned. The 201 "pencil beams" converge on a single point in 3D space, creating a spherical "cloud" of radiation dose. Multiple spheres of the radiation dose are combined in a sphere-packing algorithm to conformally irradiate small intracranial targets, resulting in a high dose of radiation to a small volume with a steep dose drop-off away from it, sparing the surrounding normal brain. The accuracy of the Gamma Knife is within 0.1 mm. Its precision requires high-resolution imaging and placement of a modified stereotactic head frame, which is fixed to the patient's skull. The stereotactic frame serves as an immobilization device as well as a reference system for the images used during the treatment-planning process. Once the head frame is in place, the patient is scanned, usually with MRI. For arteriovenous malformations (AVMs), angiography

is also performed. Because of the accuracy of the Gamma Knife, a single large fraction of radiation typically ranging from 12 to 24 Gy may be delivered with a high degree of efficacy and an acceptable risk of neurotoxicity. Presently, use of the Gamma Knife is limited to intracranial and skull-based targets with a size of approximately 3 to 4 cm or less.

Linac-based SRS systems such as the X-Knife are used more often in centers with a small volume of radiosurgery-eligible patients. Standard linacs are adapted with special collimators, or "cones," that produce beams of radiation with a diameter of up to 4 cm, which is generally the size limit for targets. Rigid immobilization with a stereotactic frame and combined CT/MRI-based 3D treatment planning are also done. The target is treated with multiple radiation arcs that converge to result in a spherical volume of high radiation dose. The accuracy of the linac-based SRS is within 0.5 mm or less. Presently, appropriate candidates for Gamma Knife and linac-based SRS include patients with malignant gliomas, brain metastases (especially if recurrent after prior conventionally fractionated radiation), AVMs, acoustic neuromas, trigeminal neuralgia, pituitary adenomas, and meningiomas.

Radiation Biology

Basic Principles

The most important target molecule for radiation is DNA. High-LET or densely ionizing radiation such as fast neutrons causes direct DNA damage by strand breakage. With x-rays and gamma rays, however, the predominant mechanism of DNA injury is indirect via interaction with water and oxygen molecules to form free hydroxyl radicals, which in turn cause DNA damage. Oxygen is an important element in cell injury by photons because it interacts with free radicals to produce organic peroxides, which inflict additional DNA damage. The degree to which oxygen enhances the cytotoxicity of radiation is described by the oxygen enhancement ratio (OER). The OER is the ratio of doses without and with oxygen that produce the same biologic effect. The OER is 3.0 for photons and decreases as the LET increases. For high-energy, or fast, neutrons, the OER is 1.6. Therefore, fast neutrons have an advantage over photons for treatment of large necrotic tumors, which are hypoxic centrally. The effectiveness of radiation to achieve a given biologic response is denoted by the relative biologic effectiveness (RBE). The RBE is the ratio of the dose of the reference radiation (usually 250 KeV x-rays) to the dose of the radiation of interest needed to produce the same biologic response. The RBE increases as the LET increases. The RBE for 6 MV x-rays is 0.8, and it is 1.0 to 2.0 for fast neutrons.

After a dose of radiation that produces a lethal injury to the DNA, dividing cells undergo reproductive death (i.e., the cells are unable to produce viable progeny cells). In addition, radiation induces apoptosis or programmed cell death but to a lesser degree. The radiation sensitivity of cells can be estimated by the clonogenic cell survival assay, which entails generating a cell survival curve (Fig. 48–5). Because radiation injury is a combination of reversible and irreversible DNA damage, the cell survival curve after exposure to photons has a complex shape. It is initially linear with a shallow slope followed by a shoulder in the low-dose range. At higher doses it bends, and the slope becomes steeper; and at even higher doses the curve becomes linear again. The experimental data are best fitted to a mathematic model utilizing a linear-quadratic equation, known as the α/β model, where survival fraction $= e^{-(\alpha\bullet Dose)-(\beta\bullet Dose2)}$. This model illustrates that there are two components of cell killing: one proportional to the dose ($\alpha\bullet Dose$) and the other proportional to the dose squared ($\beta\bullet Dose^2$). For the so-called early-responding or rapidly proliferating cells such as intestinal epithelial cells and most tumor cells, the survival curve has a steep initial slope and less noticeable shoulder (Fig. 48–5, curve B). Their α/β ratio in general is approximately 10 Gy. For late-responding, slowly dividing, nonproliferating cells such as myocytes, which have more capacity to repair sublethal radiation injury at low doses, the survival curve has a shallow initial slope. At high doses, however, the survival curve becomes steep (Fig. 48–5, curve A). The α/β ratio for late-responding tissues is approximately 1.5 to 3.0 Gy. Because of this characteristic, external beam radiation therapy is usually fractionated (given in multiple small doses)

to optimize the therapeutic ratio (i.e., high efficacy with low toxicity). For conventionally fractionated radiation, one treatment or fraction is given per day, 5 days per week, at 180 to 200 cGy per fraction.

To decrease normal tissue toxicity, smaller doses per fraction may be given two or three times per day while maintaining a comparable overall treatment time. This approach is called hyperfractionation. The multiple fractions during a given day are separated by at least 6 hours, which is considered the minimal amount of time needed for normal tissues to repair sublethal damage. However, to increase tumor cell kill, the biologically effective dose of radiation (BED) to the tumor must be increased. The BED can be estimated by the equation

$$BED = nd[1 + d/(\alpha/\beta)]$$

where n is the number of fractions, and d is the dose per fraction (in Gy). This equation is based on the linear-quadratic model. If the overall treatment time is significantly shortened in a hyperfractionated regimen by increasing the dose per fraction, it is referred to as *accelerated hyperfractionation*. Variations of accelerated hyperfractionation have been shown to improve local tumor control in locally advanced head and neck cancers and small cell lung cancers.

When radiation therapy is given once daily but the fraction size is significantly larger (300 to 1000 cGy), it is referred to as a *hypofractionated regimen*. Hypofractionation is used when acute and long-term toxicity is less of a concern, such as in the case of palliation of metastatic disease. It is also used in radiation-resistant tumors, such as melanoma.

Tumor control using radiation is dependent on treatment factors such as total dose, fractionation, overall treatment time, RBE, and the LET of the radiation. Also crucial are tumor and host factors. The most important is tumor size or volume. As the tumor volume increases, the total dose needed to achieve local tumor control increases dramatically. This has been demonstrated for head and neck squamous cell carcinomas. It points to the pivotal role a surgeon has when treating many tumor types to achieve complete resection with negative margins. Gross residual disease after resection adversely affects local control for essentially all solid tumors. In general, based on data from patients with breast cancer or squamous cell carcinoma of the head and neck, 45 to 50 Gy produces a 90% control rate for clinically occult or subclinical microscopic disease. Pathologically evident microscopic disease (e.g., microscopically positive surgical margins) requires 55 to 65 Gy for control, and gross disease may need 70 to 80 Gy or higher doses for adequate control. Because radiation-induced toxicity depends on the dose as well as the volume of radiation, radiation therapy is usually given with a "shrinking-field" technique: The initial large

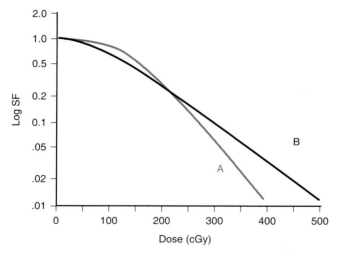

FIGURE 48–5 Cell survival curves after exposure to a single fraction of radiation. The survival fraction (SF) on a logarithmic scale is plotted against the radiation dose. Curve *A* is typical for late-responding cells and curve *B* for early-responding and most tumor cells.

fields are treated with 45 to 50 Gy, followed by one or more "boost" doses with smaller fields to provide a higher dose to the area with the highest tumor burden.

Tumor control is also affected by the intrinsic radiation sensitivity of the tumor cell type being treated. For example, lymphomas and seminomas are highly radiation-sensitive and require only modest doses (e.g., 25 to 40 Gy) to obtain good local control. Radiation-sensitive tumors such as lymphomas rarely require surgical resection, even when bulky. The primary role of the surgeon in these cases is to establish a tissue diagnosis.

Four additional tumor and host factors that influence tumor control after irradiation are called the "4 R's" of radiobiology: repair, repopulation, reoxygenation, and reassortment of tumor cells. An increased ability to repair sublethal radiation injury to the DNA and the repopulation of tumor cells would decrease the effectiveness of the irradiation. Rapid repopulation for fast-growing tumors is an important rationale for the use of accelerated hyperfractionation. Repopulation is also a reason that prolongation of the time span over which a course of radiation therapy is completed adversely affects local control of many tumors, such as cervical cancer. Reoxygenation and reassortment of tumor cells after a dose of radiation improve the effectiveness of subsequent radiation fractions. Reoxygenation of a tumor after irradiation occurs as the outer, well oxygenated cells die and are removed. The previously centrally necrotic inner cells then become better oxygenated, making them more radiosensitive. The importance of oxygenation has been indirectly shown by the observation that anemia is an adverse factor in local control of cervical cancers treated with radiation. Transfusions to a hemoglobin level of 12 mg/dl or higher can improve the outcome of radiation therapy. Reassortment of tumor cells out of radioresistant phases of the cell cycle (G_1-S) into more radiation-sensitive phases (G_2-M) occurs with conventionally fractionated radiation and other radiation techniques such as low-dose-rate brachytherapy. Lack of reoxygenation and reassortment is a theoretical disadvantage of single-fraction radiation therapy such as stereotactic radiosurgery, where target cells may be hypoxic or in the radiation-resistant phases (G_0/G_1-S) during radiation exposure.

Radiosensitizers and Radioprotectors

Radiosensitizers enhance the cytotoxic effects of radiation therapy and are beneficial in cases of locally advanced malignancies treated by definitive radiation therapy. The most commonly used agents with radiosensitizing effects are cytotoxic chemotherapeutic drugs such as cisplatin, 5-fluoruracil (5-FU), and mitomycin C, which are given currently with radiation therapy. In addition to having cytotoxic effects, they also inhibit repair of

radiation-induced DNA damage. Mitomycin C is cytotoxic for hypoxic cells and has been found to be particularly active when combined with concurrent radiation therapy for anal squamous cell carcinomas. Concurrent cisplatin and 5-FU-based chemotherapy with radiation therapy has also been shown to improve outcome in subsets of patients with cervical, nasopharyngeal, lung, pancreatic, or esophageal cancers.

For most noncytotoxic radiosensitizers, no clear benefit has been shown in clinical trials. Examples are nitroimidazole hypoxic cell radiosensitizers (e.g., etanidazole) and halogenated pyrimidine analogs (e.g., bromodeoxyuridine). RSR13, which is an allosteric modifier of hemoglobin that increases oxygen release in tissues, has shown promise as a radiosensitizer in Phase II trials for patients with brain metastases. Gadolinium texaphyrin, a porphyrin-like molecule, may also have radiosensitizing properties.

Most of the current radioprotectors are free-radical scavengers. The best known is a sulfhydryl compound, WR-2721, also known as amifostine. It is activated by alkaline phosphatase, which is present at higher levels in normal tissues than in tumor cells. Consequently, it offers more radioprotection to normal tissues than to tumors. For radiation therapy it is most commonly used to treat head and neck cancers to reduce the severity of acute mucositis and chronic xerostomia.

Clinical Uses

The clinical indications for radiation therapy are numerous, and a synopsis is presented according to sites relevant to surgical specialties. There are also several general relative contraindications for radiation therapy. First, if a site has been previously irradiated, additional curative doses of radiation are usually not feasible. However, the prior total dose of radiation, the time elapsed since the earlier irradiation, the critical organs at risk, and their tolerance doses should all be taken into consideration before a joint decision can be made by the surgeon and radiation oncologist regarding repeat irradiation. Patients with some autoimmune diseases, particularly active lupus or scleroderma, have an increased risk of normal tissue toxicity and are generally not considered good candidates for radiation therapy. Because of the teratogenic effects and significant risk of intrauterine and neonatal mortality, radiation therapy is usually contraindicated in pregnant women as well.

Lung Cancer

Early-stage (stages I and II) non-small-cell lung cancer is managed by surgical resection. If surgical margins are close or positive, postoperative radiation therapy to 55 to 60 Gy is given to decrease the risk of recurrence.

For surgically inoperable early-stage disease, definitive radiation therapy to a high dose (66 to 70 Gy) may be given.

For locally advanced non-small-cell lung cancer (stage III), definitive radiation therapy to 60 Gy or more with concurrent chemotherapy is used for patients with a good performance status (Karnofsky performance status of 70 or better) and minimal weight loss (less than 5% to 10%). The 3-year survival may be 24% for this group of patients. Those with poor performance status are better treated with radiation therapy alone. Subsets of stage IIIA disease may be resected followed by postoperative radiation therapy. The Lung Cancer Study Group has demonstrated that postoperative irradiation decreases the local recurrence from 35% to 3% in those with stage II and III disease, but overall survival is not improved. Preoperative radiation therapy using 40 to 50 Gy in conjunction with chemotherapy followed by resection may also be considered for disease that is marginally resectable.

Breast Cancer

Ductal carcinoma in situ

Standard treatment for ductal carcinoma in situ (DCIS) consists of lumpectomy with negative surgical margins followed by whole-breast irradiation. Postoperative radiation therapy has been shown in a Phase III trial to decrease ipsilateral breast recurrence of DCIS and invasive cancers to 8.2% and 3.4%, respectively, from 13.4%, compared to surgery alone at 8 years. A typical radiation dose is 50 Gy given over 5 weeks. A 10- to 15-Gy boost is added for close margins (1 mm or less). The benefit of tamoxifen in addition to radiation therapy has also been demonstrated. Small (1 to 2 cm), unicentric, low grade DCIS may be observed after resection with a margin of 1 cm or wider based on retrospective data. Women with diffuse abnormal micro-calcifications on mammography with biopsy positive for DCIS should be considered for mastectomy. Patients with contraindications for radiation therapy such as prior chest irradiation, active lupus, scleroderma, or pregnancy should also be considered for mastectomy or close surveillance after lumpectomy for DCIS.

Infiltrating ductal and lobular carcinomas

Most women with early-stage breast cancer (stages I to II) are candidates for breast-conserving therapy (BCT), which consists of lumpectomy with negative surgical margins followed by whole-breast irradiation to 50 Gy and a 10- to 15-Gy boost to the lumpectomy cavity. BCT for early-stage breast cancer has been demonstrated by several randomized trials to be equivalent to modified radical mastectomy in terms of local control and survival. The cosmetic outcome is generally excellent. Patients who have adverse risk factors that would increase their risk of local recurrence or poor

cosmetic outcome are not appropriate candidates for BCT. They include women with multicentric disease, persistent positive margins despite two or more reexcisions, and small breast size relative to the primary tumor. Patients with contraindications to radiation therapy are also not good candidates for BCT. Radiotherapy to the breast should be started within 6 weeks after surgery if chemotherapy is not given and within 16 weeks if chemotherapy is given first. Patients with a delay in radiation therapy for more than 16 weeks have an increased risk of local recurrence.

For those who have undergone a modified radical mastectomy for early-stage breast cancer, postmastectomy radiation therapy to 50 Gy followed by a 10- to 15-Gy boost to the mastectomy scar should be given for positive or close margins. Other indications for postmastectomy radiation therapy include four or more positive axillary lymph nodes, extracapsular nodal extension, and nodes larger than 2.5 cm. Two randomized trials have shown significantly improved survival after postoperative radiation therapy to the chest wall and nodal areas after mastectomy.

Unresectable and marginally resectable locally advanced breast cancers (T4, large T3, or N2) are best treated by neoadjuvant chemotherapy, modified radical mastectomy, and postoperative radiation therapy to the chest wall and regional nodes to the doses noted in the prior paragraph. If the disease progresses on neoadjuvant chemotherapy or remains unresectable despite chemotherapy, preoperative radiation therapy to 50 Gy should be considered. For patients who have a chest wall recurrence after mastectomy, resection followed by irradiation of the chest wall, usually with regional nodal irradiation, is recommended to reduce the risk of local and regional nodal recurrence if no prior radiation therapy has been given.

Prostate Cancer

For localized adenocarcinoma of the prostate, radiation treatment options are numerous. For patients with favorable prognostic factors, including T1 to T2a disease, a prostate-specific antigen (PSA) level of 10 ng/mL or less, and a Gleason score of 6 or less, conventional external beam radiation to 70 Gy or permanent prostate seed implants with ^{125}I offer biochemical control comparable to that achieved with radical prostatectomy. For those with intermediate prognostic factors (T2b, PSA 10 to 20, ng/mL, Gleason score 7 or higher), 3D conformal therapy to a higher total dose (80 Gy) or external beam radiation therapy to the pelvis (45 to 50 Gy) with a prostate implant as a boost produce better biochemical control than conventional external beam therapy alone. For locally advanced prostate cancer (T3 to T4), external beam irradiation with long-term hormonal therapy (2 to 3 years) has been shown to improve survival. Compared to radical prostatectomy, radiation therapy has a lower risk of impotence and negligible risk of urinary incontinence. However, patients have about a 10% incidence of grade 2 long-term gastrointestinal side effects such as proctitis.

Patients who have positive margins after a radical prostatectomy should be considered for postoperative external beam irradiation to the surgical bed, especially when the disease is high grade or there is a persistently elevated PSA level in the absence of clinically evident metastases. Similarly, patients with a local recurrence after prostatectomy are candidates for radiation therapy to the area of recurrence.

Testicular Cancer

Seminoma is a radiosensitive, chemosensitive tumor. Prophylactic radiation therapy to the paraaortic lymph nodes with or without inclusion of the ipsilateral upper pelvic lymph nodes to 25 Gy is recommended for stage I seminoma (tumor confined to the testis) after radical inguinal orchiectomy. With proper radiation technique including testicular shielding, permanent sterility is uncommon. For reliable patients with small, well differentiated, stage I seminomas, close surveillance after a radical inguinal orchiectomy with negative margins may be done. These patients have an approximately 15% risk of regional recurrence, mostly to the paraaortic lymph nodes. For those with stage II seminoma (metastasis to abdominal paraaortic lymph nodes), radiation therapy to paraaortic lymph nodes and the ipsilateral pelvis to 25 Gy followed by a 10 Gy boost to the paraaortic adenopathy offers an 89% probability of definitive control if the paraaortic disease is 5 cm or less (Warde et al., 1998). However, for larger tumors and stage III seminomas, chemotherapy is recommended.

Bladder Cancer

External-beam radiation therapy for localized, muscle-invasive transitional cell carcinoma of the bladder is indicated for patients who are not surgical candidates. Radiation therapy is delivered to the lower pelvis to 45 to 50 Gy followed by a 15- to 25-Gy boost to the bladder tumor. Local control is improved if chemotherapy is added. Concurrent chemotherapy and radiation therapy are presently being used as bladder-preserving treatment for localized muscle-invasive transitional cell carcinoma. After maximal transurethral resection of a bladder tumor, cisplatin-based chemotherapy and radiation therapy to the lower pelvis to a dose of 45 Gy are given. Repeat cystoscopy is then done. If there is a complete clinical response, the patient is given additional chemotherapy and radiation therapy to bring the total dose to 70 Gy. The bladder preservation rate is approximately 45% with an overall survival of 62% at 4 years.

Kidney Cancer

Radiation therapy has a limited role in the treatment of renal cell cancer. Postoperative radiation therapy to the kidney bed and regional lymph nodes to 45 to 50 Gy after radical nephrectomy should be considered for T3 and T4 disease to improve local control. Preoperative irradiation may also improve the resectability of locally advanced disease. Similarly, postoperative radiation therapy for T3 and T4 transitional cell carcinoma of the renal pelvis and ureter improves their local control. Positive margins and/or residual nodal disease are other indications for postoperative radiation therapy.

Mid and Distal Esophageal Cancers

For resectable localized thoracic and distal esophageal carcinomas, preoperative cisplatin-based chemotherapy and radiation therapy (40 to 45 Gy) followed by resection may improve the overall survival compared to surgery alone. This has been demonstrated in adenocarcinomas by a randomized study. Postoperative radiation therapy is indicated for those with positive margins and lymph node metastases. Although local control is improved in this setting, no clear survival benefit has been associated with postoperative radiation therapy.

For those who are not surgical candidates, definitive radiation therapy to 50 Gy or more with concurrent cisplatin-based chemotherapy cures approximately 26% of patients. Those with poor performance status are better treated with radiation therapy alone. Radiotherapy alone is also an effective palliative treatment for dysphagia in stage IV disease.

Stomach Cancer

Adjuvant postoperative irradiation to 45 to 50 Gy with concurrent 5-FU and leucovorin has been shown to improve the survival of patients with resectable adenocarcinoma of the stomach and gastroesophageal junction. For an unresectable gastric carcinoma, chemotherapy and radiation therapy also produce better survival than does supportive care alone.

Pancreatic Cancer

Similar to gastric carcinoma, adjuvant postoperative radiation therapy to 45 to 50 Gy with concurrent 5-FU has been shown to improve survival after resection of a pancreatic adenocarcinoma compared to surgery alone. Intraoperative electron-beam therapy as a boost to conventional external beam radiation therapy should also be considered for select patients with small unresectable pancreatic cancers, although local control rather than survival is improved in this setting. For unresectable pancreatic cancer, combined chemotherapy and external-beam radiation therapy prolong the median survival compared to irradiation alone.

Colorectal Cancer

Postoperative radiation therapy with concurrent continuous infusion of 5-FU and leucovorin is generally indicated for resected T3, T4 and node positive adenocarcinomas of the rectum. It has been shown to decrease the rate of local recurrence. Preoperative radiation therapy and chemotherapy followed by resection comprise an alternative approach and should be considered when the disease is marginally resectable. One large randomized trial has shown a survival advantage of preoperative radiation therapy. Intraoperative radiation therapy with electrons or brachytherapy to areas of unresectable residual disease should be considered. Postoperative radiation therapy is indicated for T4 colon cancers with extension to the retroperitoneal space or adjacent organs to decrease the risk of local recurrence.

Anal Canal Cancer

Squamous cell carcinoma of the anal canal is more sensitive to irradiation and chemotherapy than adenocarcinoma of the gastrointestinal tract. Most patients with localized anal cancers with an intact anal sphincter achieve a complete clinical tumor response and have a 70% chance of retaining a functional sphincter after definitive radiation therapy to 50 to 60 Gy with concurrent mitomycin C and 5-FU chemotherapy.

Cervical Cancer

For nonbulky (4 cm or less) stage I or IIA cervical squamous cell carcinoma and adenocarcinoma, external beam radiation therapy to the pelvis (45 to 50 Gy) followed by one or two intracavitary brachytherapy implants produces results in terms of local control and survival comparable to those of radical hysterectomy. However, radiation therapy induces ovarian failure in premenopausal women and causes vaginal dryness and stenosis. Thus, surgery is preferred for nonbulky stage I or IIA cervical cancer, reserving radiation therapy for older, postmenopausal women. For bulky stage IB or IIA or more advanced localized cervical cancers, definitive radiation therapy (external beam pelvic irradiation plus brachytherapy) with concurrent cisplatin-based chemotherapy is the treatment of choice.

Postoperative pelvic irradiation with concurrent cisplatin-based chemotherapy is indicated when surgical margins are positive or when lymph node metastases are present. A randomized trial, GOG 92, showed that the rate of overall recurrence decreased to 15% with postoperative radiation therapy of 46.0 to 50.4 Gy compared to 28% after radical hysterectomy alone for stage IB disease with unfavorable pathologic features (i.e., capillary-lymphatic space invasion with deep-third wall penetration; invasion into the middle third and tumor size 2 cm or larger; superficial invasion and size larger than 5 cm; or no angiolymphatic invasion, middle- or deep-third invasion, and size 4 cm or larger). In a SWOG Phase III trial, overall survival at 4 years was improved from 71% to 81% after postoperative concurrent pelvic irradiation and cisplatin plus fluorouracil compared to postoperative irradiation alone for stage IA2 to IIA disease with pelvic lymph node metastases, positive surgical margins, or microscopic involvement of the parametrium.

Endometrial Cancer

For localized, resectable endometrial cancers, the standard treatment is surgical staging including total abdominal hysterectomy and bilateral salpingo-oophorectomy (TAH/BSO). The use of postoperative irradiation to the pelvis and/or vaginal cuff depends on the stage and grade of the disease. Brachytherapy alone to treat the vaginal cuff can be utilized for grade 3/stage IA, grade 1 to 3/stage IB with less than one third myometrial invasion, and grade 1/stage IB with myometrial invasion to the middle third. The usual dose for low-dose-rate brachytherapy to the vaginal cuff is 60 Gy to the vaginal mucosa. For more advanced stage 1 disease, external beam radiation therapy (45 to 50 Gy) to the pelvis is recommended because the risk of pelvic nodal metastasis is increased. For stage II disease with myometrial invasion, pelvic irradiation (45 to 50 Gy) followed by a vaginal cuff boost (20 Gy LDR) with intracavitary brachytherapy is indicated.

If peritoneal cytology is positive and minimal residual disease remains, whole-abdomen radiation therapy to 30 Gy with a boost to the pelvis to 45 to 50 Gy is a treatment option. When paraaortic lymph nodes are involved, extended-field radiation therapy (pelvis and paraaortic area) should be considered. Definitive treatment with external-beam pelvic irradiation and intracavitary brachytherapy is recommended for medically inoperable localized endometrial carcinoma, although survival rates are significantly lower than if surgical resection could be performed.

Ovarian Cancer

Whole-abdomen radiation therapy (WART) to 30 Gy with a boost to the pelvis to 45 Gy is one treatment option for stage I/II ovarian adenocarcinomas with an intermediate risk of recurrence after TAH/BSO and surgical staging. Alternatively, chemotherapy with carboplatin and taxol is used. Intraperitoneal ^{32}P liquid brachytherapy may also be given in select patients. The intermediate risk group includes stage I/grades 2 and 3 disease; completely resected stage II/grade 1 to 3 disease; stage II/grades 1 and 2, with residual disease less than 2 cm in size; and stage III/grade 1, with residual disease less than 2 cm. More advanced ovarian carcinomas and residual disease of more than 2 cm are better treated with chemotherapy. WART can also be used as a salvage therapy for patients who have failed if they have peritoneal disease only and minimal residual disease after optimal surgical debulking.

Vaginal Cancer

Localized vaginal cancer is most often managed by definitive radiation therapy because of the significant morbidity associated with radical vaginectomy. External-beam radiation therapy to the pelvis (45 to 50 Gy) is followed by intracavitary brachytherapy with a vaginal cylinder as a boost (20 to 30 Gy LDR) if the gross disease is 0.5 cm or less in thickness. Thicker lesions require interstitial brachytherapy. Inguinal lymph nodes are also irradiated prophylactically in women with lesions in the lower third of the vagina.

Vulvar Cancer

Early-stage vulvar carcinomas are managed by modified radical vulvectomy and inguinal lymph node dissection. Patients with clinically negative inguinal lymph nodes may be treated with inguinal irradiation, which provides results comparable to those achieved with nodal dissection. Adjuvant postoperative radiation therapy to the vulva, pelvis, and inguinal nodes is indicated for surgical margins less than 8 mm, capillary-lymphatic space invasion, thickness greater than 5 mm, and positive inguinal nodes. Postoperative irradiation is also needed for patients with two or more positive inguinal nodes and/or fixed or ulcerated groin nodes.

Definitive radiation therapy with or without concurrent chemotherapy may be used for medically inoperable or unresectable squamous cell carcinoma of the vulva. Preoperative external beam radiation therapy (45 to 50 Gy) to the vulva and pelvis/inguinal lymph nodes with concurrent cisplatin-based chemotherapy may be used to render locally advanced vulvar cancer more resectable. A complete response rate of 46% after preoperative chemotherapy and radiation therapy has been reported.

Brain Tumors

For benign brain tumors such as meningiomas, craniopharyngiomas, and pituitary adenomas and for low grade gliomas, radiation therapy to 45 to 54 Gy is indicated after partial or subtotal resection and for unresectable and recurrent disease to prolong the disease-free survival and in some cases achieve a cure. For high grade gliomas (e.g., glioblastoma multiforme), radiation therapy to 60 Gy or more is used in conjunction with BCNU chemotherapy, although the 2-year survival rate is only 10%. Cranial plus spinal irradiation to 36 Gy with an additional boost of 18 to 20 Gy to the primary tumor is employed for high grade malignant brain tumors with a propensity for leptomeningeal dissemination, such as medulloblastomas, primitive neuroectodermal tumors, and ependymoblastomas. Stereotactic radiosurgery may be used for selected primary brain tumors measuring 3 to 4 cm or less in diameter. As discussed previously, this is usually in the setting of local progression following previous external beam irradiation.

Head and Neck Cancers

In general, T1 and T2 squamous cell carcinomas of the head and neck may be managed by definitive radiation therapy or surgery. Irradiation is preferred when surgery (e.g., total laryngectomy or total glossectomy) causes significant functional morbidity. For example, for T1 and T2 squamous cell carcinomas of the glottic larynx, radiation therapy alone results in a 75% to 90% rate of local control. Another example is nasopharyngeal carcinoma, which is a chemosensitive and radiosensitive disease. It is treated with concurrent chemotherapy and irradiation with a local control rate of 65% even for locally advanced disease.

Interstitial brachytherapy as a boost is an important component of radiation therapy for squamous cell carcinoma of the oral tongue and floor of the mouth. Brachytherapy enables a high dose of radiation to be delivered to the primary tumor without exceeding the tolerance dose of the mandible, which is approximately 70 Gy. Electron therapy with an intraoral cone as a boost is an alternative option for oral cavity squamous cell carcinoma. Interstitial brachytherapy and intraoral electron therapy are contraindicated if gross disease abuts or involves the mandible because of the significant risk of osteoradionecrosis of the mandible.

Optimal control of locally advanced head and neck squamous cell carcinomas (T3 and T4) generally requires combined surgery and radiation therapy. A Radiation Therapy Oncology Group (RTOG) randomized study has demonstrated that postoperative radiation therapy was associated with fewer postoperative complications and better local control than preoperative radiation therapy. Because of the relative decrease in oxygenation of postoperative surgical beds, a postoperative dose of at least 60 Gy is recommended. Higher doses are needed for positive margins or extracapsular nodal disease. In general, postoperative radiation therapy is indicated for close or positive surgical margins, perineural invasion, lymphovascular invasion, locally advanced disease, or the presence of two or more positive neck nodes.

Larynx-preserving therapy with induction cisplatin-based chemotherapy followed by radiation therapy may be feasible in a subset of patients with locally advanced laryngeal or hypopharyngeal carcinomas who have a partial or complete response to induction chemotherapy. A Veterans Administration study for T3 and T4 glottic squamous cell carcinomas showed that induction cisplatin and 5-FU for three cycles followed by radiation therapy in responders resulted in a larynx preservation rate of 64%.

Locally advanced head and neck cancers may also be treated with hyperfractionated radiation therapy (e.g., 120 cGy per fraction, twice daily, to 81.6 Gy over 7 weeks) or accelerated hyperfractionated radiation therapy with concomitant boost (180 cGy per fraction per day and 150 cGy per fraction per day to a boost field as a second daily treatment for the last 12 treatment days to 72 Gy over 6 weeks). Both approaches have been shown in a randomized study to improve local control compared to conventionally fractionated radiation therapy. Addition of concurrent cisplatin-based chemotherapy may further enhance local control and survival compared to irradiation alone. Acute mucositis is often severe in patients undergoing concurrent chemotherapy and irradiation. Nutritional support via a nasogastric or gastrostomy tube is beneficial for maintaining adequate nutrition and hydration in these patients.

Salivary Gland Cancer

The treatment of choice for salivary gland cancers is complete resection followed by radiation therapy for high-grade carcinomas, positive or close margins, locally advanced stage, and involvement of the facial nerve. Neutron therapy should be considered for unresectable or recurrent disease.

Thyroid Cancer

External-beam radiation therapy is rarely used for papillary or follicular thyroid cancers but is indicated for postoperative or definitive treatment of anaplastic thyroid carcinomas. Palliative external-beam radiation therapy should be considered for bone metastases, malignant spinal cord compression, superior vena cava syndrome, and brain metastases from thyroid cancers. In addition, patients who present with thyroid cancers with poor ^{131}I uptake and recurrent disease after the maximal dose of ^{131}I (approximately 800 to 1000 mCi) may respond to external beam radiation therapy.

Soft-Tissue Sarcomas

Presently, amputations are required for only 5% of soft-tissue sarcomas of the extremities in cases when neurovascular function of the limb has already been lost. "Limb-preserving"

treatment is recommended to preserve the function of a limb. It consists of wide local excision followed by external beam radiation therapy to 60 to 70 Gy or adjuvant interstitial brachytherapy to 45 Gy. Small (T1), low grade sarcomas may not require postoperative radiation therapy if surgical margins are wider than 1 to 2 cm. For those with gross residual disease, intraoperative placement of brachytherapy afterloading catheters should be considered so brachytherapy can be used as a boost followed by external beam radiation therapy. Another approach in this situation is the use of intraoperative electrons.

Preoperative radiation therapy to 50 Gy is indicated to make a marginally resectable sarcoma more resectable and to spare an intact neurovascular bundle when there is disease abutting it. When the sarcoma is located in the proximal thigh or the pelvic girdle in a patient who desires preservation of fertility, preoperative radiation therapy is advantageous because the radiation fields are generally smaller than postoperative fields. When surgical margins are close or positive, an additional radiation boost with brachytherapy or postoperative external beam radiation therapy to 16 to 20 Gy is recommended.

For retroperitoneal soft-tissue sarcomas, wide local excision is rarely achievable. Postoperative radiation therapy to 45 Gy followed by a carefully planned boost of 540 cGy or higher is recommended. If a needle biopsy can establish a diagnosis preoperatively, radiation therapy to 45 Gy prior to definitive resection should be considered. Preoperative radiation therapy has the advantage of having smaller fields, thereby decreasing the risk of normal tissue toxicity. In addition, the primary tumor may become more resectable after preoperative radiation therapy, after which a further boost of 15 to 20 Gy via intraoperative electrons or interstitial brachytherapy may be given.

Skin Cancer

Definitive radiation therapy for basal cell and squamous cell carcinomas of the skin is preferred when surgical excision would produce an inferior cosmetic outcome. For this reason, radiation therapy is recommended for lesions of the nasolabial sulcus, the midline of the face, the eyelids, nose, lip, skin of the auricle, and the commissure of the mouth. For T1 and T2 lesions, local control is approximately 90% after radiation therapy. Surgery is indicated for lesions arising from thermal burns, chronic radiation dermatitis, or atrophic or aged skin. Surgical excision is also recommended for patients with infected tumors in the pinna of the ear with chondritis, large lesions requiring plastic surgery, or bone invasion.

For melanomas, postoperative radiation therapy is indicated when there are positive margins, four or more positive nodes, matted lymph nodes, or extracapsular extension. A hypofractionated regimen of 30 to 36 Gy over five or six fractions is used, provided that critical normal tissues such as the brain or spinal cord are not in the field. Otherwise, conventional fractionation to 50 to 60 Gy is utilized.

Pediatric Tumors

Because of the exquisite radiosensitivity of developing organs and tissues of young children, radiation therapy, when necessary, is given at a reduced dose. In children under 2 years of age, chemotherapy may be given to slow clinical progression so radiation therapy can be delayed. Indications for irradiation of pediatric malignancies encountered in a surgical practice are discussed briefly below. Because of the relative rarity of pediatric malignancies, enrollment in clinical trials is advised.

For resectable Ewing's sarcomas, preoperative chemotherapy is given prior to wide local excision. Postoperative radiation therapy is recommended for those with positive or close margins. A dose of 45 Gy to the pretreatment gross tumor volume (GTV), followed by a boost to a total dose of 50.4 Gy for microscopic residual disease and 55.8 Gy for gross residual disease is prescribed. Sites of metastatic disease are also treated with radiation. For osteogenic sarcomas, the role of radiation therapy is limited to palliation of metastatic disease and transient local control of unresectable disease after chemotherapy. Neutron therapy is also a consideration for unresectable osteogenic sarcomas.

The treatment of rhabdomyosarcomas varies by site, histology, stage, and grouping. In general, initial resection is followed by chemotherapy. Radiation therapy is indicated for positive margins, gross residual disease, unfavorable histology (alveolar and undifferentiated), and lymph node involvement. Radiation therapy may be withheld if there is a complete pathologic response documented by a second-look surgery after chemotherapy. Radiation therapy to a dose of 40 to 55 Gy is given to patients with unresectable disease after several cycles of chemotherapy.

For Wilms' tumors, as per the guidelines of the National Wilms' Tumor Study, postoperative radiation therapy is not needed for stage 1 or 2 disease; the exception is stage 2 Wilms' tumor with anaplastic histology. Low dose radiation (10 Gy) with a 10 Gy boost for residual disease more than 3 cm in size, is given postoperatively for stage 3 and 4 Wilms' tumors with favorable histology and stage 2 to 4 tumors with anaplastic histology. Radiation therapy should be started within 10 days after surgery. Preoperative radiation therapy should be considered for bulky disease with a high risk of intraoperative spill.

Completely resected neuroblastomas with favorable biologic features do not require adjuvant radiation therapy. For children older than 1 year of age, chemotherapy and radiation therapy are indicated for unresectable or

incompletely resected disease and lymph node metastases. The usual doses are 14.4 to 25.0 Gy for children 1 to 3 years of age and 30 to 36 Gy or more for older children.

Ocular Neoplasms

To preserve vision, small uveal melanomas (15 mm or less in diameter and 10 mm or less in thickness) may be treated with definitive radiation therapy using eye plaque brachytherapy with ^{125}I seeds. Enucleation is recommended for larger lesions and when there is no useful vision remaining. Similarly for retinoblastomas, definitive treatment with external beam radiation therapy to 45 Gy or eye plaque brachytherapy is highly effective for local control and for preserving vision in the presence of small lesions (10 disk diameter or less and posterior to the equator). Bulky retinoblastomas involving more than half of the retina should be treated by enucleation.

Palliation

A significant portion of a radiation oncology practice involves palliation of the symptoms produced by malignant disease. Indications include painful bone metastases; bone metastases in a weight-bearing bone; brain metastases; spinal cord compression; bleeding secondary to cervical, bladder, lung, or gastric cancers; obstructive jaundice; symptomatic airway compression; dysphagia secondary to esophageal cancer or extrinsic compression from mediastinal metastases; and symptomatic soft-tissue or visceral metastases. Conventional external beam radiation therapy with a hypofractionated regimen such as 30 Gy in 10 fractions is usually used. Brachytherapy such as endobronchial, intrabiliary, intraesophageal, or intravaginal implants may be used for select cases. Stereotactic radiosurgery using the Gamma Knife or a linac is indicated for brain metastases that have progressed despite whole-brain irradiation and in selected cases of newly diagnosed brain metastases (three or fewer brain metastases measuring 3 to 4 cm or less in diameter and controlled or absent primary and extracranial metastatic disease). The usual radiosurgical dose is 15 to 24 Gy in one fraction.

For malignant spinal cord compression and brain metastases with moderate to severe vasogenic edema, urgent treatment with corticosteroids and radiation therapy is essential to reverse or stabilize any neurologic deficits. Patients with spinal cord compression who deteriorate neurologically while undergoing radiation therapy should be considered for emergency surgical decompression. For metastases in weight-bearing bones such as the femur or spine, surgical stabilization should be considered if the structural integrity is in doubt. After surgical excision of a brain metastasis or surgical intervention for a pathologic fracture, postoperative radiation therapy is usually recommended with 30 Gy in 10 fractions or a more protracted regimen of 40 to 50 Gy in 20 to 25 fractions in favorable patients.

In general, multiple lesions consistent with metastases on imaging studies in a patient with known cancer do not require a biopsy. However, in the case of a solitary metastasis in a patient without a history of cancer or with a long disease-free interval after initial treatment, biopsy is recommended when feasible.

Nonneoplastic Diseases

Radiation has an inhibitory effect on the proliferation of fibroblasts and endothelial cells after an injury. Therefore, when given within 1 to 3 days after an operation, low-dose radiation can prevent the development of keloids that are unresponsive to steroid injections (12 Gy in three fractions), heterotopic bone formation after joint surgery (700 to 800 cGy in one fraction), and in-stent restenosis after coronary angioplasty (18 to 23 Gy with endovascular brachytherapy).

Several benign eye diseases are responsive to radiation therapy. Beta radiation with a strontium-90 applicator started during the immediate postoperative period after resection of pterygium reduces the risk of recurrence. External beam radiation therapy to 20 Gy over 10 fractions to the posterior orbit is used for exophthalmos and diplopia secondary to Graves' disease that is refractory to steroid therapy. External beam radiation therapy to 1440 cGy can also stabilize vision for patients with the exudative type of age-related macular degeneration.

Radiation therapy also has a potent immunosuppressive effect via inhibition of T-helper cells and other types of lymphocytes and monocytes. For patients who have failed conventional immunosuppressive therapy after organ transplantation, total lymphoid irradiation is an option for treating allograft rejection.

Radiation therapy at high doses can obliterate small blood vessels. For this reason, surgically inaccessible small arteriovenous malformations in the brain are amenable to stereotactic radiosurgery. A dose of 16 to 25 Gy in a single fraction is typically given.

Radiation Injury and Toxicity

After exposure of normal tissue to radiation therapy, there is a variable degree of acute inflammatory response with increased local blood flow and increased capillary permeability. This is the rationale for pretreating patients who have malignant spinal cord compression with steroids prior to starting radiation therapy (to prevent any worsening of vasogenic edema). Late damage is manifested as fibrosis, loss of parenchymal cells, and occlusion of the microvasculature. Radiation-related toxicity varies with the treatment site, total dose delivered, fractionation schedule, volume of normal tissues or organs irradiated, and use of chemotherapy.

Tolerance dose data for applying radiation to partial or whole organs have been compiled. The tolerance dose can be described in terms of $TD_{5/5}$ and $TD_{50/5}$, which are the doses that would produce a 5% and 50% incidence of complications, respectively, at 5 years. With evolving radiation techniques such as 3D conformal therapy and stereotactic radiosurgery, the concept of dose tolerance of normal tissues is undergoing a reevaluation.

Radiation-induced injury to normal tissues is also influenced by biologic predisposition. Individuals with ataxia-telangiectasia are extremely sensitive to radiation. Patients with diabetes, multiple sclerosis, scleroderma, lupus, and other autoimmune diseases may have a higher risk of radiation-induced normal tissue toxicity. Moreover, developing organs and tissues in children have a lower threshold for significant radiation injury. Severe toxicity is defined as serious (grade 3), life-threatening (grade 4), or fatal (grade 5) according to published criteria. Acute toxicity usually occurs within 90 days and is often self-limited, whereas late toxicity is usually related to irreversible tissue damage. Its onset may occur 3 to 18 months or longer after the end of treatment. Various types of acute and late toxicity to major organs may be encountered in a surgical practice. Their management is described below according to site.

Skin/Soft Tissue/Surgical Wounds

With normal wound healing after primary surgical closure, fibroblasts proliferate during the first 10 days with collagen formation and increased tensile strength. Thus, conventionally fractionated radiation therapy encompassing surgical wounds starting approximately 2 weeks postoperatively does not adversely affect wound healing to a significant degree. This has been shown by a study that reported increased wound complications only if brachytherapy was given before postoperative day 6 for soft-tissue sarcomas. For routine cases of postoperative external beam therapy, most surgeons and radiation oncologists wait 2 to 4 weeks until the skin incision is well healed and sutures or staples are removed.

If preoperative radiation therapy is applied, skin and soft tissues require approximately 2 weeks for the acute reaction to subside and for adequate healing of the radiation injury before surgery can be performed without a significantly increased risk of wound complications. This is not a rigid guideline, however, because it has been shown that surgery for rectal cancer can be done within a week after completing radiation therapy, with an acceptable incidence of significant wound complications. Waiting too long before performing surgery is problematic as well because the onset of fibrosis starts approximately 6 weeks after completion of radiation therapy and because of concerns about tumor repopulation. For rectal cancers, allowing 4 weeks for tumor down-staging and recovery from radiation-related toxicity is a reasonable compromise.

Significant acute skin reaction is an expected side effect of radiation therapy when skin is a part of the target, such as with skin cancers. A significant skin reaction is also common when the target is superficial, such as with breast cancer, head and neck cancer, or vulvar cancer. A mild skin reaction typically presents within the first week as mild erythema. At higher doses, dry desquamation occurs after 2 to 3 weeks of daily radiation treatment. With continued irradiation, erythema increases along with epilation and dysfunction of the sweat glands. Higher doses lead to moist desquamation, where there is loss of epidermis and oozing of serous fluid from denuded areas. Epidermis regenerates from the periphery and hair follicles. Full-thickness skin necrosis is rare.

Skin care during radiation therapy consists of avoidance of further injury from other sources, such as sun exposure, tight-fitting clothing, trauma, shaving, and infection. Cosmetics and alcohol-containing skin products should be avoided. Moist desquamation is managed by applying hydrogel wound dressings or 1% gentian violet. The presence of infection may require Silvadene cream, antibiotic ointment, or systemic antibiotics.

Common late radiation-induced skin reactions are thinning of skin with telangiectasia and mild subcutaneous induration. Severe late injury is uncommon and includes chronic ulceration of severely atrophic skin and woody subcutaneous fibrosis.

Lung

Radiation therapy for lung cancer, esophageal cancer, breast cancer, and other targets in the chest, supraclavicular areas, and upper abdomen encompasses variable amounts of lung tissue in the radiation portals. Target cells for radiation-induced pulmonary toxicity are the type II alveolar cells. Their injury results in early surfactant release into alveoli; this may manifest clinically as radiation pneumonitis, which usually occurs 1 to 3 months after irradiation alone. Patients typically present with low grade fever, cough, and pleuritic chest pain. A chest radiograph typically shows pneumonitis geometrically reproducing the shape of the radiation treatment fields. The fibrotic phase begins at 3 to 6 months with sclerosis of the alveolar walls, extensive endothelial damage with loss and replacement of capillaries, and fibrosis with loss of function. Symptoms are generally minimal if fibrosis is limited to less than 50% of one lung.

The TD_5 for radiation-induced pneumonitis is 8 Gy after a single fraction to the entire lung. For radiation therapy using conventional fractionation to a limited lung volume (< 30%), the TD_5 is 45 to 50 Gy. A recent analysis of patients with non-small-cell lung cancer treated with radiation therapy suggests that the volume of lung that receives more than 20 Gy, the so-called V_{20}, is the best predictor of radiation pneumonitis. The risk of grade 3 or worse radiation pneumonitis is 19% when the V_{20} exceeds 37% versus 0% to 2% for smaller volumes. The mainstay of treatment for acute radiation pneumonitis is high-dose steroids, usually 60 to 80 mg prednisone daily, along with supportive care such as supplemental oxygen if necessary. A dramatic improvement within 24 to 48 hours is often seen.

Heart

Acute radiation-induced cardiac toxicity such as acute pericarditis is unusual. However, coronary artery disease as a late complication of radiation therapy for breast cancers and mediastinal lymphomas is a significant concern. It occurs after conventionally fractionated doses of 24 Gy or higher and frequently involves the proximal portion of the arteries, especially the left anterior descending artery. In long-term survivors of Hodgkin's disease, there is an increased relative risk for coronary artery disease (three times that of the normal control population). For patients who have undergone radiation therapy during childhood, especially women, the relative risk increases to 40%. Other uncommon late manifestations of cardiac injury include chronic pericarditis, cardiomyopathy, valvular heart disease, and conduction abnormalities.

Liver

A small portion of the liver is frequently irradiated during treatment of cancers such as gastric and pancreatic adenocarcinomas and lung cancers in the right lower lobe. It is well tolerated, and patients are usually asymptomatic. One third to one half of the liver volume can receive 40 Gy safely, but radiation to the entire liver is poorly tolerated with a TD_5 of 20 to 30 Gy. The acute clinical period tends to be relatively silent. After high doses to the entire liver, dilatation and congestion of sinusoids, atrophy of hepatocytes, and venoocclusive lesions appear at 2 to 6 months. Ascites develops and is usually accompanied by hepatomegaly and painful jaundice. There is no effective treatment for venoocclusive disease of the liver. Supportive therapy is given, and liver transplant may be performed in selected patients.

Kidneys

Like the liver, the kidneys are highly radiation-sensitive. The TD_5 for renal failure is 20 Gy when both kidneys are irradiated. After radiation injury, there is an initial increase in the glomerular filtration (GFR) and renal plasma flow due to glomerular vasodilatation and permeability.

The GFR later decreases as tuft scarring occurs. Pathologically, vascular changes occur first with glomerulosclerosis followed by tubular atrophy, usually involving the cortical tubules.

Symptoms of acute radiation nephropathy usually appear at 6 to 12 months, and chronic radiation nephropathy and hypertension may develop at 18 months. Management includes a low-protein diet and fluid and salt restrictions. Dialysis and renal transplantation should be considered for end-stage renal disease in long-term survivors free of recurrent cancer.

Esophagus

Esophagitis is a frequent side effect during radiation therapy of lung and esophageal cancers. Patients present with dysphagia and odynophagia. Acute esophagitis is treated with a cocktail of viscous lidocaine, antacids, diphenhydramine, and analgesics. Chronic dysphagia may also occur at 3 to 6 months. It is due to peristalsis dysfunction often caused by muscle damage leading to fibrosis and stricture formation. Another complication after high-dose radiation to the esophagus, particularly after intraluminal brachytherapy, is esophageal ulceration, which occurs most frequently at the gastroesophageal junction. Pseudodiverticula, sinus tracts, and fistula formation are also possible.

The TD_5 for strictures or ulceration is 60 Gy if one third of the esophagus is irradiated and 55 Gy when the whole esophagus is treated. Pathologically, acute injury leads to mucosal denudation followed by regenerating foci of epithelium within 7 to 14 days. Focal necrosis of the muscularis mucosa and deep muscles may occur.

Stomach

Exposure of the stomach to radiation leads to variable degrees of nausea, vomiting, and gastritis. Pretreatment with antiemetics and the use of H_2-blockers are helpful for preventing significant acute side effects. After 40 to 50 Gy to the stomach, acute gastritis develops in 20%. Late toxicity includes ulcer formation and development of an atrophic, contracted stomach. The incidence of gastric ulcer is 15% after 50 Gy or more. The risk of a perforated ulcer is 6% after 40 to 50 Gy and 10% after 50 to 60 Gy.

Small Intestine

Acutely after radiation injury, there is mucosal cell loss during the first 48 hours, with shortening of the crypts and villi. Subsequently, the villi show progressive denudation, resulting in a loss of protein and electrolytes. Clinically, patients develop increased stool frequency and diarrhea secondary to malabsorption of fat and hypermotility. Antidiarrheal agents and a low-residue diet are helpful for controlling radiation-induced diarrhea. The main feature of late toxicity at 6 months to 2 years is progressive endarteritis. This may lead to ulceration and infarction necrosis with acute occlusion of supplying vessels. Fibrosis and stricture may also occur if there is gradual narrowing of the vasculature. There is a 4% risk of small bowel obstruction after postoperative irradiation to a dose of 27.5 Gy to the entire abdomen and 45.0 Gy to the pelvis for ovarian cancer. Special precaution is needed when operating on irradiated small bowel because manipulation and freeing of adhesions may interfere with a tenuous blood supply, leading to infarctions and fistula formation. The TD_5 for small bowel injury is 50 Gy, but the risk of injury increases to 15% to 25% after 55 Gy.

Rectum

Acute proctitis, which presents as an increased frequency of bowel movements with tenesmus, is a common side effect of radiation therapy for prostate and cervical cancers. Severe chronic proctitis with painless bleeding, segmental colitis, and rectal strictures is uncommon. Its incidence after external-beam pelvic irradiation and brachytherapy for cervical cancer is less than 4% with doses of 80 Gy or less, 7% to 8% for 80 to 95 Gy, and 13% for 95 Gy or more. After radiation therapy for prostate cancer, the incidence of severe proctitis in patients with prostate cancer is 5% for doses of 65 to 70 Gy using conventional treatment planning and less with more conformal 3D techniques. Mild to moderate symptomatic proctitis may be treated with steroid-containing enemas (e.g., hydrocortisone retention enema). Severe proctitis may require surgical intervention.

Bladder

Cystitis with dysuria develops during the course of pelvic irradiation. When severe, it can be treated with medications such as phenazopyridine. When severe cystitis occurs, urinalysis and urine culture should be undertaken to exclude a urinary tract infection. When a limited volume of bladder is irradiated, the incidence of moderate to severe toxicity is approximately 5% after 75 Gy.

Brain

The radiation-sensitive cells in the CNS are proliferating cells such as oligodendrocytes, endothelial cells, and astrocytes. Acutely, inflammation and increased permeability of capillaries develop, producing vasogenic edema. This can result in increased intracranial pressure with headaches and nausea. Maintaining patients on corticosteroids while they undergo large-field radiation to the brain is effective in controlling edema.

Late findings include regions of demyelination, proliferative and degenerative changes in glial cells, and vascular occlusive changes. Clinical side effects include impaired of short-term memory and concentration. When the radiation injury is severe, frank radiation-induced brain necrosis may develop, usually 9 to 18 months after radiation. Imaging with CT or MRI scans reveals a contrast-enhancing mass lesion often with surrounding edema. Positron emission tomography (PET) or MR spectroscopy is helpful for distinguishing necrosis from tumor recurrence. Corticosteroids are the mainstay of treatment, although surgical debulking may be needed for severe symptoms refractory to corticosteroids. Radiation necrosis occurs in 1% to 5% of patients after 55 to 60 Gy with conventional fractionation.

Spinal Cord

The spinal cord is often in the irradiated volume when treating lung cancers, head and neck cancers, and upper gastrointestinal malignancies. Significant injury is rare when the cord dose is limited to 45 Gy with conventional fractionation, which has a risk of myelopathy of less than 1%. The TD_5 is approximately 57 Gy.

Radiation to the spinal cord may also produce a mild degree of vasogenic edema acutely. It is even more important for patients with malignant spinal cord compression to be pretreated with, and be maintained on, corticosteroids while undergoing radiation therapy to the spine.

Two to six months after radiation to the spinal cord, there may be transient, reversible demyelination that produces tingling sensations and shooting pains, especially with flexion of the neck (Lhermitte's sign). If irreversible spinal cord injury has occurred, symptoms of myelopathy start approximately 6 months after irradiation has been completed.

Head and Neck

The head and neck area contains many radiosensitive structures that require special care to minimize radiation-induced toxicity. The risk of osteoradionecrosis of the mandible is increased with doses above 70 Gy in the presence of poor dental hygiene. To minimize its risk when the mandible is in the radiation field, patients should undergo a dental evaluation and any necessary dental extractions prior to beginning a course of high-dose radiation therapy. After dental extractions, adequate healing for 1 to 2 weeks is recommended before treatment begins. During and after the course of radiation therapy, topical fluoride using a custom-fit fluoride tray should be used daily. When osteoradionecrosis does occur, it is treated by surgical débridement. Hyperbaric oxygen may be used to promote healing.

Mucositis develops after approximately 2 weeks of irradiation and is treated with "miracle mouth wash" (viscous lidocaine, antacid, and Benadryl mixture). These patients are prone to develop thrush, and prophylactic antifungal drugs may be given to patients with severe mucositis. Laryngeal edema may occur acutely and is treated with corticosteroids. Xerostomia is a common chronic side effect of head and neck irradiation after the major salivary glands have been exposed to more than 30 Gy. Pilocarpine may be given during the course of radiation therapy to reduce the severity of xerostomia; and may also be used on a long-term basis. More recently, intravenous amifostine, a radioprotectant of normal tissue, is being used during the course of radiation therapy to minimize mucositis and xerostomia.

Radiation therapy for nasopharyngeal, paranasal sinus, and orbital neoplasms may produce a variety of late effects in orbital structures. One third of patients develop cataracts after 12 Gy. The tolerance dose for lacrimal glands is 35 to 40 Gy. Dry eye syndrome is treated symptomatically with artificial tears. The tolerance doses for the retina and optic nerves are 50 and 60 Gy, respectively, when fraction sizes are kept below 1.9 Gy per day.

Radiation-Related Carcinogenesis

The development of radiation-related malignancies is a concern for radiation therapy patients and for those with occupational or accidental exposure to radiation from various sources. Radiation carcinogenesis is described as a stochastic effect, which means that there is no threshold under which the probability of carcinogenesis is zero. However, the probability of developing cancer increases with increasing radiation dose. According to the atom bomb experience at Hiroshima and Nagasaki, there is a latency period between radiation exposure and cancer formation: 5 to 7 years for leukemias and 10 or more years for solid tumors. For the working population, the risk of carcinogenesis is 8% per sievert (equivalent to 1 Gy) for high doses and high dose rates and 4% per sievert for low doses and low dose rates.

The risk of developing second malignancies in irradiated areas is increased in young patients. However, it is not always clear whether they develop second cancers because of their radiation exposure or because of a genetic predisposition to neoplasm. For example, in men with testicular seminomas, the risk of developing a second non-germ-cell tumor at 15 years is 7.6% after irradiation. The risk is 9.3% without chemotherapy or radiation therapy. Because young patients are at increased risk of developing second cancers after radiation therapy, early screening and increased surveillance are necessary. For example, young women who have undergone mantle irradiation for mediastinal lymphomas should undergo screening mammography at least 10 years earlier than the general population (i.e., at age 30 years).

Hereditary Effects of Irradiation

Another concern after occupational, accidental, or therapeutic exposure to radiation is the development of birth defects in offspring due to mutations in germ cells. Based on the Japanese atomic bomb data, the average doubling dose for genetic mutations is 1.58 sievert. The doubling dose is the dose required to double the spontaneous mutation incidence, which is approximately 1% to 6%. After radiation therapy or significant occupational exposure, contraception for approximately 6 months is advised.

Temporary sterility in men may occur after 15 cGy to the testis. Permanent sterility develops after 350 to 600 cGy in men and after 250 to 600 cGy to the ovaries in women.

Pregnancy and Effects on the Embryo and Fetus

A developing embryo or fetus is extremely sensitive to radiation therapy. During the preimplantation stage (1 to 9 days after conception), direct exposure results in death of the embryo and spontaneous abortion. During early organogenesis (10 days to 6 weeks) there is severe intrauterine growth retardation, but recovery occurs after birth. The risk of teratogenesis or congenital malformations is the highest during this phase. Irradiation during the fetal period leads to permanent growth retardation. Based on the Japanese atomic bomb data, irradiation with a dose as low as 10 to 19 cGy in utero before 8 weeks' gestation results in microcephaly. Mental retardation develops when exposure occurs primarily at 8 to 15 weeks, with a risk coefficient of 0.4 per Gy. The risk of developing childhood cancer is also increased by a factor of 1.5 to 2.0. Termination of pregnancy is recommended if an embryo receives 10 cGy or more during the first 26 weeks to avoid having a baby with severe birth defects.

Radiation Safety and Protection

In addition to proper shielding, important factors involved in minimizing occupational radiation exposure are distance and time. Based on the inverse-square law, radiation intensity decreases to one fourth as the distance from the source doubles. Thus, when handling radioactive sources for low-dose-rate brachytherapy, for example, one should use long instruments to manipulate sources and keep the sources as far away from the operator's body as possible. The amount of time used to handle the sources should be kept to a minimum.

Table 48–1	
NCRP recommended dose limits	
Exposure	**Effective Dose Limits**
Occupational	
Cumulative	10 mSv × age in years
Annual	50 mSv per year
Lens of eye	150 mSv per year
Skin, hands, and feet	500 mSv per year
Embryo/fetus	5 mSv total and 0.5 mSv per month
Public	
Continuous or frequent	1 mSv per year
Infrequent	5 mSv per year
Lens, skin, and extremities	50 mSv per year

NCRP, National Council on Radiation Protection and Measurement. From NCRP: recommendations on limits for exposure to ionizing radiation (no. 116). Bethesda, MD: National Council on Radiation Protection and Measurement, 1993.

Individuals who have routine occupational exposure to radiation should wear an x-ray film badge on their trunk. Additional badges are worn over the abdomen for pregnant women and on a finger for those manually manipulating radioactive sources. The level of exposure is monitored by the radiation safety officers, whose responsibility is to ensure that workers and the public are not exceeding recommended dose limits (Table 48–1). These limits are based on the ALARA principle (as low as reasonably achievable), balancing the health risks of radiation exposure, the benefits of using radiation, and economic constraints. The dose limits do not include the radiation exposure due to medical necessity for that individual.

Exposure to radiation in radiation safety is measured in sievert (Sv), which is the product of the absorbed dose (gray) and the quality factor. For x-rays and gamma rays, the quality factor is 1, and so 1 Gy is equal to 1 Sv. The older, non-SI unit is rem, and 1 rem is equal to 10 mSV. For the purpose of comparison, the total annual dose to the bronchial epithelium from natural background radiation including radon is about 25 mSv.

Future Directions

Radiation therapy is a continuously evolving discipline, with its efficacy increasing and its toxicity decreasing as imaging techniques, computers, dosimetry, treatment planning, and radiation production and delivery continue to improve. Better target localization will be realized from advances in functional or biologically based imaging techniques such as PET and MR spectroscopy and their fusion with anatomically based imaging studies such as CT and MRI.

Future radiation therapy simulators may be based on new imaging techniques that are linked directly with treatment planning systems. Highly conformal intensity-modulated radiation therapy may then be undertaken to deliver a large dose to the area with the greatest tumor burden and a low dose to areas with minimal tumor burden.

The accuracy of future treatment planning systems will increase as better computers allow the use of more precise dosimetry modeling systems. The current gold standard is the Monte Carlo system, a computer modeling program that simulates the trajectories of individual photons and particles as they travel through matter and calculates the resulting dose distribution.

Future radiation therapy machines will be more intelligent; be able to track body, organ, and target movements; and hence make automatic adjustments. Inroads have already been made in this direction with the development of the CyberKnife, which is a compact linear accelerator mounted on a robotic arm; it is used for cranial and extracranial stereotactic radiosurgery. More portable and compact linacs are also being developed to make intraoperative radiation therapy easier and more widely available. An example of an early-generation machine of this type is the Mobetron, a portable linac capable of producing 4 to 12 MeV electrons. It is designed to be used in an operating suite and can be transported between operating rooms.

Ultimately, advances in oncology depend on a better understanding of tumor biology, which is a prerequisite to the development of specific molecular targeting using gene therapy, antibodies, toxins, and other novel techniques. Treatments based on this approach ideally will have high tumoricidal activity both locally and systemically with low toxicity. It is unlikely, however, that molecularly targeted therapies will replace surgery, radiation therapy, and chemotherapy. Rather, the cure for cancer will more likely be a combination of traditional and targeted therapies.

Bibliography

Al-Sarraf M, LeBlanc M, Shanker PG, et al: Chemoradiotherapy versus radiotherapy in patients with advanced nasopharyngeal cancer: phase III randomized intergroup study 0099. J Clin Oncol 1998;16:1310.

Bolla M, Gonzalez D, Warde P, et al: Improved survival in patients with locally advanced prostate cancer treated with radiotherapy and goserelin. N Engl J Med 1997;337:295.

Brizel DM, Albers ME, Fisher SR, et al: Hyperfractionated irradiation with or without concurrent chemotherapy for locally advanced head and neck cancer. N Engl J Med 1998;338:1798.

Brookland RK, Richter MP: The postoperative irradiation of transitional cell carcinoma of the renal pelvis and ureter. J Urol 1985;133:952.

Byhardt RW, Martin L, Pajak TF, et al: The influence of field size and other treatment factors on pulmonary toxicity following hyperfractionated irradiation for inoperable non-small cell lung cancer (NSCLC)—analysis of a Radiation Therapy Oncology Group (RTOG) protocol. Int J Radiat Oncol Biol Phys 1993;27:537.

Calais G, Alfonsi M, Bardet E, et al: Radiation alone versus RT with concomitant chemotherapy in stages III and IV oropharynx carcinoma: final results of the 94-01 GORTEC randomized study. Int J Radiat Oncol Biol Phys 2001;51(Suppl)1:1.

Cassady JR: Clinical radiation nephropathy. Int J Radiat Oncol Biol Phys 1995;31:1249.

Castleberry RP, Kun LE, Shuster JJ, et al: Radiotherapy improves the outlook for patients older than 1 year with Pediatric Oncology Group stage C neuroblastoma. J Clin Oncol 1991;9:789.

Coia LR, Myerson RJ, Tepper JE: Late effects of radiation therapy on the gastrointestinal tract. Int J Radiat Oncol Biol Phys 1995;31:1213.

Cooper JS, Guo MD, Herskovic A, et al: Chemoradiotherapy of locally advanced esophageal cancer: long-term follow-up of a prospective randomized trial (RTOG 85-01): Radiation Therapy Oncology Group. JAMA 1999;281:1623.

Cox JD (ed): Moss' Radiation Oncology: Rationale, Technique, Results (7th ed). St. Louis: Mosby, 1994.

Crist WM, Garnsey L, Beltangady MS, et al: The Third Intergroup Rhabdomyosarcoma Study. J Clin Oncol 1995;13:610.

D'Amico A, Whittington R, Malkowicz B, et al: Biochemical outcome after radical prostatectomy, external beam radiation therapy, or interstitial radiation therapy for clinically localized prostate cancer. JAMA 1998;280:969.

Dembo AJ: Abdominopelvic radiotherapy in ovarian cancer: a 10-year experience, Cancer 1985;55:2285.

Department of Veterans Affairs Laryngeal Cancer Study Group: Induction chemotherapy plus radiation compared with surgery plus radiation in patients with advanced laryngeal cancer. N Engl J Med 1991;324:1685.

Dillman, RO, Herndon, J, Seagren, SL, et al: Improved survival in stage III non-small-cell lung cancer: 7-year follow-up CALGB 8433 trial. J Natl Cancer Inst 1996;88:1210.

Dunsmore LD, LoPonte MA, Dunsmore RA: Radiation-induced coronary artery disease. J Am Coll Cardiol 1986;8:239.

Eisbruch A, Perez CA, Roessler E, et al: Adjuvant irradiation after prostatectomy for carcinoma of prostate with positive surgical margins. Cancer 1994;73:884.

Emami B, Lyman J, Brown A, et al: Tolerance of normal tissue to therapeutic irradiation. Int J Radiat Oncol Biol Phys 1991;21:109.

Eschwege F, Sancho-Garnier H, Chassagne D, et al: Results of a European randomized trial of etanidazole combined with radiotherapy in head and neck carcinomas. Int J Radiat Oncol Biol Phys 1997;39:275.

Fisher B, Anderson S, Redmond CK, et al: Reanalysis and results after 12 years of follow-up in a randomized clinical trial comparing total mastectomy with lumpectomy with or without irradiation in the treatment of breast cancer. N Engl J Med 1995;333:1456.

Fisher B, Dignam J, Wolmark N, et al: Lumpectomy and radiation therapy for the treatment of intraductal breast cancer: findings from National Surgical Adjuvant Breast and Bowel Project B-17. J Clin Oncol 1998;16;441.

Fisher B, Dignam J, Wolmark N, et al: Tamoxifen in treatment of intraductal breast cancer: National Surgical Adjuvant Breast and Bowel Project B-24 randomised controlled trial. Lancet 1999;12:1993.

Fisher B, Wolmark N, Rockette H, et al: Postoperative adjuvant chemotherapy or radiation therapy for rectal cancer: results from NSABP protocol R-01. J Natl Cancer Inst 1988;80:21.

Flam M, John M, Pajak TF, et al: Role of mitomycin in combination with fluorouracil and radiotherapy, and of salvage chemoradiation in the definitive nonsurgical treatment of epidermoid carcinoma of the anal canal: results of a phase III randomized intergroup study. J Clin Oncol 1996;14:2527.

Fletcher GH: Local results of irradiation in the primary management of localized breast cancer. Cancer 1972;29:545.

Fletcher GH: Clinical dose-response curve of human malignant epithelial tumors. Br J Radiol 1973;46:1.

Fu KK, Pajak TF, Trotti A, et al: A Radiation Therapy Oncology Group (RTOG) phase III randomized study to compare hyperfractionation and two variants of accelerated fractionation to standard fractionation radiotherapy for head and neck squamous cell carcinomas: first report of RTOG 9003. Int J Radiat Oncol Biol Phys 2000;48:7.

Fyles AW, Dembo AJ, Bush RS, et al: Analysis of complications in patients treated with abdominopelvic radiation therapy for ovarian carcinoma. Int J Radiat Oncol Biol Phys 1992;22:847.

GITSG (Gastrointestinal Tumor Study Group): Further evidence of effective adjuvant combined radiation and chemotherapy following curative resection of pancreatic cancer. Cancer 1987;59:2006.

GITSG: Radiation therapy combined with adriamycin or 5 fluorouracil for the treatment of locally unresectable pancreatic carcinoma. Cancer 1985;56:2563.

Graham MV: Normal tissue complication probability for the esophagus and lung. Presented at the 3rd International Symposium: 3D-Radiation Treatment Planning and Conformal Therapy, Chapel Hill, NC, September 1998.

Grogan M, Thomas GM, Melamed I, et al: The importance of hemoglobin levels during radiotherapy for carcinoma of the cervix. Cancer 1999;86:1528.

Gunderson LL, Tepper JE (eds): Clinical Radiation Oncology. New York: Churchill Livingstone, 2000.

Hall EJ: Radiobiology for the Radiologist (4th ed). Philadelphia: JB Lippincott, 1994.

Hanks GE, Lee WR, Hanlon AL, et al: Conformal technique dose escalation for prostate cancer: chemical evidence of improved cancer control with higher doses in patients with pretreatment PSA ≥ 10 ng/ml. Int J Radiat Oncol Biol Phys 1996;35:861.

Hanks GE, Peters T, Owen J: Seminoma of the testis: long-term beneficial and deleterious results of radiation. Int J Radiat Oncol Biol Phys 1992;24:1913.

Homesley HD, Bundy BN, Sedlis A, et al: Radiation therapy versus pelvic node resection for carcinoma of the vulva with positive groin nodes. J Am Coll Obstet Gynecol 1986;68:733.

ICRP (International Commission on Radiological Protection): Recommendations. Annals of the ICRP, Publication 60. Oxford: Pergamon Press, 1990.

ICRU (International Commission on Radiation Units and Measurements): Dose and Volume Specification for Reporting Intracavitary Therapy in Gynecology. Report No. 38. Bethesda, MD: ICRU, 1985.

ICRU: Prescribing, Recording, and Reporting Photon Beam Therapy. ICRU Report No. 50. Bethesda, MD: ICRU, 1993.

Khan FM: The Physics of Radiation Therapy (2nd ed). Baltimore: Williams & Wilkins, 1994.

Khanfir K, Alzieu L, Terrier P, et al: Does adjuvant radiation therapy increase loco-regional control after optimal resection for soft-tissue sarcoma of the extremities [abstract]? Proc ASTRO 2000;205.

Kinsella TJ, Sindelar WF, Lack E, et al: Preliminary results of a randomized study of adjuvant radiation therapy in resectable adult retroperitoneal soft tissue sarcomas. J Clin Oncol 1988;6:18.

Koh WJ, Laramore G, Griffin T, et al: Fast neutron radiation for inoperable and recurrent salivary gland cancers. Am J Clin Oncol 1989;12:316.

Kramer A, Gelber RD, Snow JB, et al: Combined radiation therapy and surgery in the management of head and neck cancer: final report of study 73-03 of the Radiation Therapy Oncology Group. Head Neck Surg 1987;10:19.

Lanciano RM, Pajak TF, Martz K, et al: The influence of treatment time on outcome for squamous cell cancer of the uterine cervix treated with radiation: a patterns of care study. Int J Radiat Oncol Biol Phys 1993;25:391.

Lawrence TS, Robertson JM, Anscher MS, et al: Hepatic toxicity resulting from cancer treatment. Int J Radiat Oncol Biol Phys 1995;31:1237.

Lefebvre J, Chevalier D, Luboinski B, et al: Larynx preservation in pyriform sinus cancer: preliminary results of a European Organization for Research and Treatment of Cancer phase III trial. J Natl Cancer Inst 1996;88:890.

Lemerle J, Voute PA, Tournade MF, et al: Preoperative versus postoperative radiotherapy, single versus multiple courses of actinomycin D in the treatment of Wilms' tumor. Cancer 1976;38:647.

Lung Cancer Study Group: Effects of postoperative mediastinal radiation on completely resected stage II and stage III epidermoid cancer of the lung. N Engl J Med 1986;315:1377.

MacDonald J, Smalley S, Benedetti J, et al: Chemoradiotherapy after surgery compared with surgery alone for adenocarcinoma of the stomach or gastroesophageal junction. N Engl J Med 2001;345:725.

Marks JE, Davis C, Gottsman V, et al: The effects of radiation on parotid salivary function. Int J Radiat Oncol Biol Phys 1981;7:1013.

McDonald S, Rubin P, Phillips TL, Marks LB: Injury to the lung from cancer therapy: clinical syndromes, measurable endpoints, and potential scoring systems. Int J Radiat Oncol Biol Phys 1995;31:1187.

Mendahall WM, Can Cise WS, Bova FJ, et al: Analysis of time-dose factors in squamous cell carcinoma of the oral tongue and floor of mouth treated with radiation therapy alone. Int J Radiat Oncol Biol Phys 1981;7:1005.

Moore DH, Thomas GM, Montana GS, et al: Preoperative chemoradiation for advanced vulvar cancer: a phase II study of the GOG. Int J Radiat Oncol Biol Phys 1998;42:79.

Morris M, Eifel P, Lu J, et al: Pelvic radiation with concurrent chemotherapy compared with pelvic and para-aortic radiation for high-risk cervical cancer. N Engl J Med 1999;340:1137.

National Council on Radiation Protection and Measurement (NCRP): Recommendations on Limits for Exposure to Ionizing Radiation. NCRP Report No. 116. Bethesda, MD: NCRP, 1993.

Overgaard M, Hansen PS, Overgaard J, et al: Postoperative radiotherapy in high-risk premenopausal women with breast cancer who receive adjuvant chemotherapy. N Engl J Med 1997;337:949.

Parsons JT, Bova FJ, Fitzgerald CR, et al: Radiation optic neuropathy after megavoltage external beam irradiation: analysis of time-dose factors. Int J Radiat Oncol Biol Phys 1994;30:755.

Parsons JT, Fitzgerald CR, Hood CI, et al: The effects of irradiation on the eye and optic nerve. Int J Radiat Oncol Biol Phys 1983;9:609.

Perez CA, Brady LW (eds): Principles and Practice of Radiation Oncology (3rd ed). Philadelphia: Lippincott-Raven, 1998.

Perez CA, Breaux S, Bedwinek JM, et al: Radiation therapy alone in treatment of carcinoma of the uterine cervix. II. Analysis of complications. Cancer 1984;54:235.

Perez CA, Fields JN, Fracasso PM, et al. Management of locally advanced carcinoma of the breast. II. Inflammatory. Cancer 1994;74:466.

Perez CA, Fox S, Lockett MA, et al: Impact of dose in outcome of irradiation alone in carcinoma of the uterine cervix: analysis of two different methods. Int J Radiat Oncol Biol Phys 1991;21:885.

Perez CA, Graham ML, Taylor ME, et al: Management of locally advanced carcinoma of the breast. I. Non-inflammatory. Cancer 1994;74:453.

Petereit DG, Mehta MP, Buchler DA, et al: Inguinofemoral radiation of N0,N1 vulvar cancer may be equivalent to lymphadenectomy if proper radiation technique is used. Int J Radiat Oncol Biol Phys 1993;27:963.

Peters WA, Liu PY, Barrett RJ, et al. Concurrent chemotherapy and pelvic radiation therapy compared with pelvic radiation therapy alone as adjuvant therapy after radical surgery in high-risk early-stage cancer of the cervix. J Clin Oncol 2000;18:1606.

Pisters WT, Harrison LB, Leung DH, et al: Long-term results of a prospective randomized trial of adjuvant brachytherapy in soft tissue sarcoma. J Clin Oncol 1996;14:859.

Prados M, Scott C, Sandler H, et al: A phase 3 randomized study of radiotherapy plus procarbazine, CCNU, and vincristine (PCV) with or without BUdR for the treatment of anaplastic astrocytoma: a preliminary report of RTOG 9404. Int J Radiat Oncol Biol Phys 1999;45:1109.

Ragaz J, Jackson SM, Le N, et al: Adjuvant radiotherapy and chemotherapy in node-positive premenopausal women with breast cancer. N Engl J Med 1997;337:956.

Recht A, Come SE, Henderson IC, et al: Sequencing of chemotherapy and radiation therapy after conservative surgery for early stage breast cancer. N Engl J Med 1996;334:1356.

Roldan GE, Gunderson LL, Nagorney DM, et al: External beam versus intraoperative and external beam irradiation for locally advanced pancreatic cancer. Cancer 1988;61:1110.

Rosenman JG, Miller EP, Tracton G, et al: Image registration: an essential part of radiation therapy treatment planning. Int J Radiat Oncol Biol Phys 1998;40:197.

Rosenthal DI, Nurenberg P, Becerra CR, et al: A phase I single-dose trial of gadolinium texaphyrin (Gd-Tex), a tumor selective radiation sensitizer detectable by magnetic resonance imaging. Clin Cancer Res 1999;5:739.

Rubin P: The law and order of radiation sensitivity, absolute vs relative: radiation tolerance of normal tissues. Front Radiat Ther Oncol 1989;23:7–40.

Russell LB, Russell WL: An analysis of the changing radiation response of the developing mouse embryo. J Cell Physiol 1954;43:103.

Schein PS, Novak J: A comparison of combination chemotherapy and combined modality therapy for locally advanced gastric carcinoma. Cancer 1982;49:1771.

Schull WJ, Otake M, Neal JV: Genetic effects of the atomic bomb: a reappraisal. Science 1981;213:1220.

Schultheiss TE, Kun LE, Ang KK, et al: Radiation response of the central nervous system. Int J Radiat Oncol Biol Phys 1995;31:1093.

Sedlis A, Bundy BN, Rotman MZ, et al: A randomized trial of pelvic radiation therapy versus no further therapy in selected patients with stage IB carcinoma of the cervix after radical hysterectomy and pelvic lymphadenectomy: a GOG study. Gynecol Oncol 1999;73:177.

Shaw E: Central nervous system tumors—overview. In Gunderson LL, Tepper JE (eds): Clinical Radiation Oncology. New York: Churchill Livingstone, 2000:314.

Shaw E, Scott C, Stea B, et al: RSR13 plus cranial radiation therapy improves survival in patients with brain metastases compared to the RTOG recursive partitioning analysis brain metastases database [abstract]. Proc ASTRO 2000;183.

Silverstein MJ, Lagios MD, Groshen S, et al: The influence of margin width on local control of ductal carcinoma in situ of the breast. N Engl J Med 1999;340:1455.

Stein M, Kuten A, Halperin J, et al: The value of postoperative irradiation in renal cell cancer. Radiother Oncol 1992;24:41.

Stewart JR, Fajardo LF, Gillette SM, et al: Radiation-induced heart disease: an update. Prog Cardiovasc Dis 1984;27:173.

Swedish Rectal Cancer Trial: Improved survival with preoperative radiotherapy in resectable rectal cancer. N Engl J Med 1997;336:980.

Tester W, Caplan R, Heaney J, et al: Neoadjuvant combined modality program with selective organ preservation for invasive bladder cancer: results of RTOG phase II trial 8802. J Clin Oncol 1996;14:119.

Tewfik HH, Buchsbaum HJ, Latourette HB, et al: Para-aortic lymph node irradiation in carcinoma of the cervix after exploratory laparotomy and biopsy-proven positive aortic nodes. Int J Radiat Oncol Biol Phys 1982;8:13.

Thomas PRM: Ewing's sarcoma. *In* Perez CA, Brady LW (eds): Principles and Practice of Radiation Oncology (3rd ed). Philadelphia: Lippincott-Raven, 1998:2038.

Thomas PRM: Wilms' tumor. *In* Perez CA, Brady LW (eds): Principles and Practice of Radiation Oncology (3rd ed). Philadelphia: Lippincott-Raven, 1998:2107.

Trog D, Bank P, Wendt TG, et al: Daily amifostine given concomitantly to chemoradiation in head and neck cancer: a pilot study. Strahlenther Onkol 1999;175:444.

Turrisi AT, Kim K, Blum R, et al: Twice-daily compared with once-daily thoracic radiotherapy in limited small-cell lung cancer treated concurrently with cisplatin and etoposide, N Engl J Med 1999;340:265.

Van den Brenk HAA: Results of prophylactic postoperative irradiation in 1300 cases of pterygium. AJR Am J Roentgenol 1968;103:723.

Van der Werf-Messing B, van der Heul RO, Ledeboer RCH: Renal cell carcinoma trial. Cancer Clin Trials 1978;1:13.

Walsh TN, Noonan N, Hollywood D, et al: A comparison of mutimodal therapy and surgery for esophageal adenocarcinoma. N Engl J Med 1996;335:462.

Wanderas EF, Fossa SD, Tretli S: Risk of subsequent non-germ cell cancer after treatment of germ cell cancer in 2006 Norwegian male patients. Eur J Cancer 1997;2:253.

Wang CC: Radiotherapeutic management and results of T1N0, T2N0 carcinoma of the oral tongue: evaluation of boost techniques. Int J Radiat Oncol Biol Phys 1989;17:287.

Warde P, Gospodarowicz M, Panzarella T, et al: Management of stage II seminoma. J Clin Oncol 1998;16:290.

Warde PR, Gospodarowicz MK, Goodman PJ, et al: Results of a policy of surveillance in stage I testicular seminoma. Int J Radiat Oncol Biol Phys 1993;27:11.

Willett CG, Fung CY, Kaufman DS, et al: Postoperative radiation therapy for high-risk colon carcinoma. J Clin Oncol 1993;11:1112.

Wolmark N, Wieand HS, Hyams DM, et al: Randomized trial of postoperative adjuvant chemotherapy with or without radiotherapy for carcinoma of the rectum: NSABP R-02. J Natl Cancer Inst 2000;92:388.

Yang JC, Chang AE, Baker AR, et al: Randomized prospective study of the benefit of adjuvant radiation therapy in the treatment of soft tissue sarcomas of the extremity. J Clin Oncol 1998;16:197.

Zeitlin SI, Sherman J, Raboy A, et al: High dose combination radiotherapy for the treatment of localized prostate cancer. J Urol 1998;160:91.

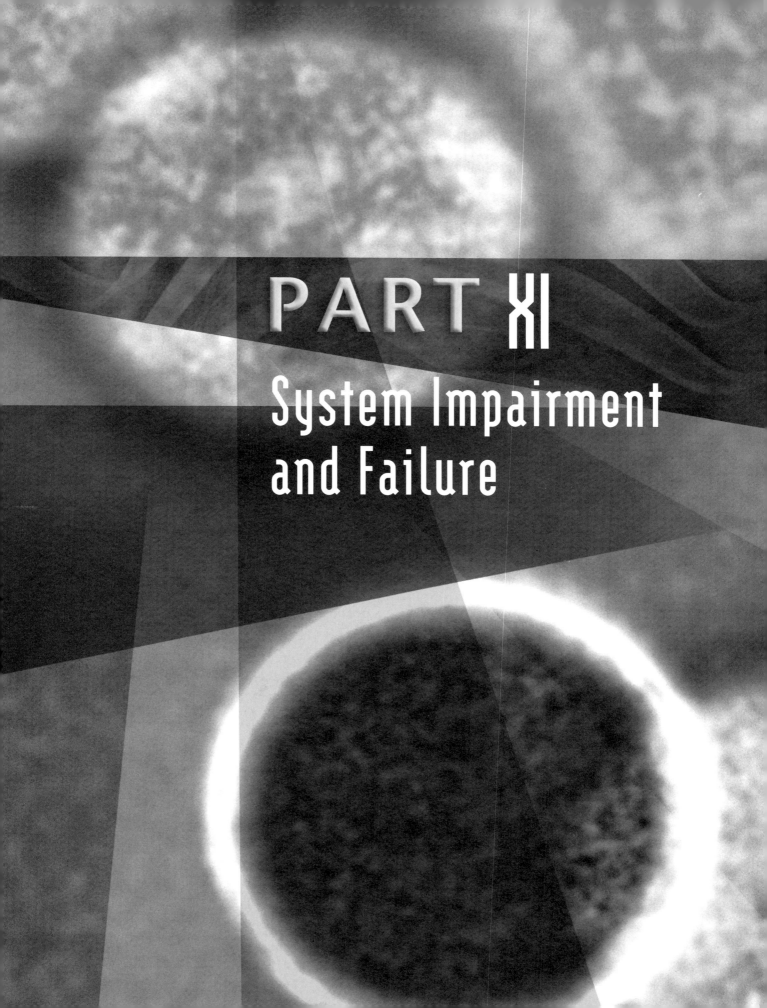

PART XI
System Impairment and Failure

CHAPTER 49

Central Nervous System Impairment, Seizure, Coma, and Death

Alex B. Valadka, M.D., F.A.C.S.

Neurologic Assessment

An accurate neurologic examination is essential to identify the existence and severity of central nervous system (CNS) impairment and to serve as a baseline against which to gauge subsequent improvement or deterioration. Such an examination may be compromised, however, by confounding factors such as drug intoxication, pharmacologic paralysis and sedation, inadequate cerebral blood flow (CBF) during hemorrhagic shock, the presence of an endotracheal tube that prohibits assessment of speech, and the like. Such limiting factors must be noted in the documentation of the neurologic examination.

Glasgow Coma Scale

The Glasgow Coma Scale (GCS) (Table 49–1) is probably the most widely used scoring system for assessing coma and impaired consciousness. The GCS scores a patient's motor function, verbal function, and eye opening. Although scores for each component are summed to produce a single GCS score, listing the score for each category separately avoids ambiguity if a certain category cannot be assessed (e.g., the verbal score in intubated patients or the eye opening score in patients with eyes swollen shut).

Pupillary Examination

Other aspects of the neurologic examination besides those included in the GCS are important. Pupillary size,

Table 49–1
Glasgow coma scale

Score	Component of Exam
	Motor
6	Obeys commands
5	Localizes stimulus
4	Withdraws from stimulus
3	Flexes arm
2	Extends arm
1	No response
	Verbal
5	Oriented
4	Confused
3	Recognizable words/phrases
2	Makes sounds
1	No response
	Eye Opening
4	Spontaneously
3	To voice
2	To pain
1	Remain closed

symmetry, and reactivity to bright light must be assessed. A pupil that is unilaterally dilated and nonreactive suggests the presence of transtentorial herniation. As it is forced through the tentorial incisura, the uncus, located at the medial part of the temporal lobe, compresses the third cranial nerve. Because the nerve fibers that mediate pupillary constriction lie on the surface of the third nerve, external compression inactivates these fibers first, leading to unopposed dilatory input to the pupil. Ischemia of the midbrain, in which are located the cranial nerve nuclei that modulate pupillary constriction, also may play a role. Finally, direct ocular trauma may cause pupillary dilatation even when no life-threatening intracranial emergency exists.

Systemic/Environmental Examination

A careful systemic assessment may yield important clues to the etiology of CNS impairment. Obvious signs of injury to the scalp and face suggest trauma as the cause; atrial fibrillation suggests possible cerebral embolism; and diffuse petechial rash in a febrile patient may suggest meningitis or other infectious disease that requires appropriate precautions to be followed in the emergency center. Inspection of the patient's surroundings by prehospital

providers also may yield clues, such as bottles of pills suggesting accidental or intentional medication overdose.

Computed Tomography Scanning

Although a large body of classic neurologic literature attempts to correlate specific physical findings (respiratory pattern, cardiac and blood pressure changes, pupillary exam, motor responses, etc.) with depth of coma and with its neuroanatomic basis, such educated guesswork is far less precise than imaging studies such as cerebral computed tomography (CT) scans. CT scanning is the imaging modality of choice for cerebral emergencies. A CT scan is quite useful for differentiating structural from functional causes of CNS impairment, and especially for identifying surgical emergencies.

General Clinical Support for CNS-Impaired Patients

Importance of Secondary Insults

After traumatic injury, the brain becomes exquisitely vulnerable to subsequent deviations from normal homeostasis. Even brief episodes of hypoxia, hypotension, or other abnormalities that normally would be well tolerated can worsen outcome significantly. Such deleterious events are called "secondary insults" to distinguish them from the primary damage caused directly by the traumatic event. Secondary insults also may be important in worsening the outcome from other types of CNS insults.

Basic Physiologic Support

The goal of clinical support of patients with acute CNS disturbances is to prevent secondary insults and, when they occur, to identify and to reverse them as rapidly as possible. As with any type of resuscitation, treatment begins with the ABCs (airway, breathing, and circulation). The physician should have a low threshold for instituting interventions to support ventilation and blood pressure. Endotracheal intubation and mechanical ventilation may be necessary. Control of blood pressure may require either pressors or antihypertensive agents. Samples of blood and urine should be sent for basic metabolic tests to identify any abnormalities that require prompt intervention, and other specific diagnostic studies may be indicated, depending upon the specific circumstances (Box 49–1). Interventions unique to patients with CNS impairments may include monitoring of intracranial pressure (ICP) or aggressive measures to terminate seizures. Because acute CNS impairments may require days or even weeks to

General Evaluation of Cerebral Impairment

- Check blood pressure, pulse, respirations, temperature
- Thorough general examination
- Careful neurologic examination
- Imaging: computed tomography scan acutely; magnetic resonance imaging, cerebral angiography, etc. also may be needed
- Electrolytes: Na, K, Cl, CO_2, Mg, Ca, PO_4
- Glucose
- Blood urea nitrogen, creatinine
- Complete blood count: hemoglobin, hematocrit, white blood cell count, platelet count
- Arterial blood gas analysis
- Liver function tests: prothrombin time, partial thromboplastin time, aspartate transaminase, alanine transaminase, γ-glutamyl transpeptidase
- Thyroid function panel; cortisol; other endocrine tests
- Human immunodeficiency virus titers
- Rapid plasma reagent
- Folate and vitamin B_{12} levels
- Urinalysis
- Urine pregnancy test in females of child-bearing age
- Toxicology screen for drugs of abuse (including alcohol)
- Serum levels of known medications
- Chest radiograph
- Electrocardiogram
- Lumbar puncture

resolve, supportive measures may be necessary for a prolonged period.

Increased ICP: Acute and Chronic

Acute

The intradural space may be divided broadly into three compartments: brain (80% of space), intravascular blood (10%), and cerebrospinal fluid (CSF) (10%). The Monro-Kellie doctrine states that, because the intracranial volume is fixed by the rigid walls of the skull, an increase in volume of one of these compartments (or addition of another component, such as a tumor or hematoma) requires compensatory decreases in the volumes of the other compartments

if ICP is to remain constant. A gradual increase in the volume of one of the intracranial compartments is generally tolerated much better than a rapid change. For example, slow growth of a brain tumor may be tolerated well for long periods because of progressive compensatory decreases in volumes of CSF and, to a lesser extent, of venous blood. Intracranial hypertension may result from a sudden increase in volume of one of the intracranial compartments (e.g., acute hydrocephalus, cerebral edema) or from progression of chronic processes beyond the limits of compensation.

Common causes of acute intracranial hypertension include hemorrhage (subdural, epidural, and/or intracerebral); cerebral contusion; neoplasm; abscess; diffuse cerebral edema; large infarction; superior sagittal sinus thrombosis; metabolic disorders such as hepatic encephalopathy and Reye's syndrome; and encephalitis, meningitis, and other diffuse infections. Obstruction of CSF flow or impairment of normal CSF resorption also may cause acute elevations of ICP. Overproduction of CSF is a rare cause, occurring only when choroid plexus tumors (which are uncommon) are seen.

Chronic

Many of the same processes that cause acute intracranial hypertension also can cause chronic elevations of ICP if their course is more protracted. Examples include undiagnosed tumor, chronic meningitis, and chronic subdural hematoma. Hydrocephalus from impaired resorption of CSF through the arachnoid granulations into the cerebral venous sinuses is another common cause. Such impairment may result from intracranial hemorrhage, meningitis, dural venous sinus thrombosis, or other causes. Benign intracranial hypertension, or pseudotumor cerebri, also must be considered in the differential diagnosis of chronically elevated ICP.

Treatment

Treatment of intracranial hypertension is directed at the cause. Mass lesions such as hematomas, contusions, and tumors may be removed surgically. Sedation and pharmacologic paralysis may be helpful if a patient is agitated and constantly straining, with resultant increases in ICP.

CSF may be diverted via an externally draining catheter inserted into the ventricles of the brain. After patients have stabilized, those who require permanent CSF diversion can undergo insertion of a shunt that drains into the peritoneal cavity, the right atrium, or another body cavity. Parenchymal brain edema may respond to mannitol or other osmotic diuretics that pull water from the brain into the vasculature. Mannitol also causes a decrease in diameter of cerebral resistance vessels because it effects a decrease in blood viscosity. At a lower viscosity, constant flow may be obtained through a narrower vessel, and the corresponding decrease in cerebral blood volume, although relatively slight, often is associated with a significant reduction in ICP.

Hyperventilation also may reduce vascular diameter, but prophylactic long-term hyperventilation of head-injured patients in an attempt to prevent intracranial hypertension adversely affects outcome, perhaps because the vascular narrowing reduces CBF below critical levels and because loss of bicarbonate buffer in the CSF diminishes the ability of the brain to compensate for lactic acidosis produced by ischemia.

Pentobarbital-induced coma lowers cerebral metabolic requirements and is often useful in treating intracranial hypertension that is refractory to other therapies, especially in patients with a greater likelihood of good recovery. Hypothermia was not beneficial in a multicenter trial that investigated its utility in traumatic brain injury. Decompressive craniectomy, in which part of the skull is removed to give edematous brain room to swell, has seen a resurgence of interest over the past decade, but careful investigation of its usefulness has not yet been done.

Coma: Pathophysiology and Differentiation

Coma has been defined in many ways, but the essential aspect of all these definitions is an impairment of self-awareness that prohibits conscious interaction with the outside world. The alteration of consciousness often is accompanied by a disturbance in normal arousal mechanisms. Patients appear to be asleep, but without the ability to awaken. This clinical picture encompasses a broad spectrum, from patients who are nearly dead to those who seem on the verge of speaking and obeying commands. Inability to obey simple one-step commands, such as to hold up two fingers, is a simple yet very useful bedside definition of coma.

The anatomically indistinct reticular activating system (RAS) in the upper brainstem and lower diencephalon sends diffuse projections to the cerebral cortex. Focal damage in this area, such as infarction or hematoma, may result in coma by interrupting these pathways. Larger mass lesions such as tumors, hematomas, or large infarctions may interfere with the RAS via displacement or compression. Large masses also may cause increased ICP that diffusely affects the entire brain, as can hydrocephalus or other causes of high ICP. Widespread bilateral cortical destruction from trauma, anoxia, or other causes may result in coma. Finally, many extracerebral metabolic abnormalities can cause coma in the absence of structural changes to the brain.

Some of the more common causes of coma are summarized in Box 49–2. Regardless of etiology, all coma

---

Box 49–2
Causes of Coma

Mass lesions
- Hematoma
- Tumor
- Large infarction
- Cerebral abscess
- Brainstem/diencephalic infarction

Diffuse or metabolic processes
Cerebral
- Traumatic brain injury
- Encephalitis
- Meningitis
- Cerebral metabolic disorders
- Seizure/postictal state
- Demyelinating disease
- Subarachnoid hemorrhage

Extracerebral
- Intoxication/medication overdose
- Renal failure
- Hepatic failure
- Sepsis
- Anoxia
- Hypoglycemia
- Hypothermia
- Shock
- Hypothyroidism
- Other

Functional
- Malingering
- Conversion reaction (hysteria)
- Depression/catatonia

---

states must be considered to be an emergency. Because the body's adaptive responses to stress attempt to preserve CNS function above almost all other functions, coma does not usually occur unless an insult has been overwhelming or until physiologic reserves have been exhausted.

The most urgent differentiation of the etiology of coma is whether it is caused by a structural lesion that requires immediate surgical intervention. Accordingly, preparations for an immediate CT scan of the brain should begin while specimens for laboratory analysis are being collected (see Box 49–1).

Seizure

A seizure may be defined as a sudden, excessive, uncontrolled burst of electrical activity within the brain. Seizures may be broadly classified as partial or generalized (Box 49–3).

As with coma, the etiologies of seizures are numerous. Both diffuse processes and focal structural lesions may cause seizures, and the etiology may be systemic as well as within the CNS. The new onset of a focal seizure is highly suggestive of the existence of a structural lesion.

The main goals of supportive care for a patient who is actively seizing are to support airway, breathing, and circulation while simultaneously preventing the patient from injuring himself or herself. Turning the patient onto his or her side may prevent aspiration, as can suctioning oral secretions. Many observers feel the need to place a padded tongue depressor or other object into the mouth to prevent the patient from biting his or her tongue. Such a maneuver may be of benefit, but care must be taken not to interfere with the airway, not to allow the tongue depressor to be aspirated, and not to cause vomiting by stimulating the gag reflex.

Neurologic and radiologic assessment of seizures is similar to that described for coma. However, an additional confounding variable in patients who have seized is the postictal state. After a seizure, the affected part of the brain may undergo a period of depressed metabolic activity, possibly as a result of depletion of glucose by seizing neurons, with consequent accumulation of lactic acid. Depending upon the type of seizure, this phenomenon may cause a depressed level of consciousness or paralysis ("Todd's paralysis") of specific limbs. When it occurs, the postictal state usually resolves within minutes, but rarely it may persist beyond 24 hours. Because a postictal state can mask the existence of significant underlying neurologic dysfunction, it is important to proceed with a complete assessment, including thorough physical examination, imaging with cerebral magnetic resonance or CT scanning both without and with intravenous contrast, and clinical chemistries.

Patients may require long-term treatment with anticonvulsants. Decisions about whether to start and when to stop anticonvulsants depend upon many factors, including an honest evaluation of patient compliance. New anticonvulsants become available for commercial use on a regular basis. The choice of the optimal agent for a given patient depends, among other things, on the type of seizures the patient has and on the patient's tolerance of various side effects. Surgical treatment may play a role in some cases.

Treatment of Status Epilepticus

Status epilepticus commonly is defined as seizure activity lasting more than 30 minutes in duration or as two or more generalized tonic-clonic seizures without return to normal consciousness between the events. Other authorities shorten the time interval required for diagnosis of status epilepticus to 10 or 15 minutes. Status epilepticus is an emergency that can produce permanent brain damage or even death if the seizure activity is not aborted promptly.

Box 49–4 depicts a standard treatment strategy for status epilepticus. Endotracheal intubation may be required for airway and ventilatory support during prolonged seizures. Because long-acting paralytic agents used for intubation make it impossible to determine when a seizure has stopped, short-acting agents should be considered whenever possible.

Febrile Seizures

Febrile seizures may occur during the first 6 years of life. Most commonly, a single generalized seizure occurs during the rise or peak of temperature during a febrile illness. Simple febrile seizures seem to have little long-term significance. Of greater concern are complex febrile seizures, defined as those that (1) are greater than 15 minutes in duration, (2) have focal features, or (3) are multiple (i.e., more than one seizure during the same febrile episode). Children with complex febrile seizures have a significantly greater likelihood of having seizures (not induced by fever)

Box 49–3
Classification of Seizures

Partial
Simple
- Motor
- Sensory
- Autonomic
- Psychic

Complex
Partial with secondary generalization

Generalized
Tonic/clonic/tonic-clonic (grand mal)
Absence (petit mal)
Atonic
Lennox-Gastaut syndrome
Juvenile myoclonic epilepsy
Infantile spasms

Psychogenic

Box 49–4

Approach to Treatment of Status Epilepticus

- Provide supplemental oxygen, suction oral secretions as needed, consider turning patient to side to minimize aspiration, consider intubation.
- Monitor blood pressure and oxygen saturation.
- Establish intravenous access.
- Check fingerstick glucose; if not available, consider 25–50 mL D_{50} IV after bolus of 50–100 mg thiamine IV.
- Prevent patient from hurting self (pad bed rails, etc.)
- Give lorazepam (Ativan) 0.1 mg/kg (up to 4 mg total) IV over 2 min; repeat after 5 min if still seizing (alternative: diazepam [Valium] 0.2 mg/kg [up to 10 mg] repeated if needed after 5 min).
- While above is taking place, begin loading with phenytoin (Dilantin) 20 mg/kg at < 50 mg/min; monitor blood pressure (BP) and electrocardiogram; must use normal saline (no dextrose). If using fosphenytoin: give up to 150 mg of phenytoin equivalents/min. (If patient is already on phenytoin and level is not known, give bolus with 500 mg phenytoin IV at < 50 mg/min.)
- *If seizures continue*: give phenobarbital 20 mg/kg IV at < 100 mg/min until seizures stop; watch for hypotension.
- *If seizures continue*: intubate patient and induce general anesthesia with pentobarbital 15 mg/kg IV at 25 mg/min (watch BP: may need fluids and dopamine or other pressors.) Maintain at 1 mg/kg/hr and increase for breakthrough seizures or, if monitoring electroencephalogram (EEG), for increased EEG activity beyond burst suppression.
- *If seizures continue*: consider midazolam (Versed) drip or inhalational anesthetics.

---

later in life. In such cases, the fever may have unmasked a pre-existing structural brain lesion or may herald the onset of meningitis, encephalitis, or other CNS infection.

Dementia

The word *dementia* most commonly refers to a decline in level of function of mental faculties, especially memory and cognition, with a normal level of alertness. Among the most common causes of dementia are progressive degenerative processes such as Alzheimer's disease or repeated cerebral ischemic episodes (Box 49–5). Evaluation for other causes (such as depression, metabolic or nutritional abnormalities, chronic infections, large benign brain tumors, etc.) may reveal a disease process that is readily treatable.

As with coma and seizures, the evaluation of dementia begins with a careful history, detailed physical examination, and appropriate imaging and laboratory studies (see Box 49–1). Neuropsychological testing may be important in helping to define the severity of the dementia. Cholinesterase inhibitors may provide mild symptomatic improvement or stabilization of cognitive function in patients with mild to moderate Alzheimer's disease, at least temporarily.

Delirium

The term *delirium* commonly is used to refer to an acute state of marked confusion and restlessness. As with

dementia, delirium is a symptom; treatment requires identification of the underlying etiology. Alcohol withdrawal is a common cause, as are serious systemic illnesses such as sepsis, shock, uremic encephalopathy, hepatic encephalopathy, hypoxia, hypoglycemia, and the like.

Delirium is characterized by an altered sensorium with heightened awareness of sensory stimuli and misperception of these stimuli, often contributing to illusions (misinterpretation of sensory stimuli), hallucinations (apparent perception of unreal sensory stimuli), and inability to tell where reality ends and where vivid dreams begin. Associated features may include insomnia, seizures, and extreme emotional lability. Such patients are often paranoid, loud, and disruptive.

As with other causes of acute CNS impairment, treatment is directed simultaneously at two goals: support of patients in the acute phase and investigation of the cause of the delirium. Antipsychotics such as haloperidol are often helpful for controlling symptoms. However, these agents can lower the seizure threshold, which may limit their effectiveness in conditions such as alcohol withdrawal. Benzodiazepines are the most commonly used treatment for alcohol withdrawal syndrome.

The occurrence of postoperative confusion is worrisome for physicians and patients alike. Most literature in the field of postoperative confusional states focuses on elderly patients. Predisposing factors seem to include older age, pre-existent cognitive impairment, and pre-existing cerebral disease, especially cerebrovascular. Many causes must be considered, such as slow metabolism of anesthetic

Some Common Causes of Dementia

Cerebral

Chronic cerebral degenerative diseases

- Alzheimer's disease
- Parkinson's disease
- Huntington's chorea

Cerebrovascular diseases

- Multi-infarct dementia
- Atherosclerosis (chronic diabetes, hypertension)
- Vasculitis

Mass lesions

- Tumor
- Chronic subdural hematoma

Trauma

Hydrocephalus

Systemic

Chronic medication overdose

Infectious diseases

- Acquired immunodeficiency syndrome
- Syphilis
- Creutzfeldt-Jakob disease
- Chronic meningoencephalitis
  - Cryptococcus
  - Tuberculosis
  - Meningeal carcinomatosis

Alcoholism

Endocrine disorders

- Pituitary disease
- Thyroid disease
- Adrenal disease

Poisoning, e.g., heavy metals (lead, mercury, arsenic)

Nutritional: thiamine, B_{12}, folate deficiencies

Wilson's disease

Psychiatric disease

Depression

Schizophrenia

Malingering

Conversion reaction

agents; metabolic disturbances, including hyponatremia, hypoxia, and hypoglycemia; withdrawal from alcohol or other drugs; and injury to the brain from intraoperative ischemia, intracranial hemorrhage, and the like.

Prognostic Implications of Cerebral Impairments

It must be remembered that coma, seizures, and dementia are not specific diseases with well-defined outcomes. Instead, they are only symptoms, and the prognosis of these conditions depends upon the extent of the underlying disease that produced the symptoms. A single febrile seizure may have little long-term significance; at the other extreme, a trauma patient with a postresuscitation GCS score of 3 has a likelihood of dying that exceeds 75% and a likelihood of good recovery or moderate disability of only 7%.

The importance of providing necessary support (intubation, oxygenation, blood pressure, etc.) during the acute period of even reversible CNS impairments cannot be overstated. Lack of such support—even if needed for only a few minutes—may be the difference between excellent and poor or even fatal outcomes.

Perhaps the crudest measure of outcome is mortality. A 1982 study of 500 patients with coma of unknown etiology (excluding known causes such as traumatic brain injury and poisonings) reported 76% mortality at 1 month and 88% mortality at 1 year. Advances in intensive care and long-term management in the years since these data were collected may have lowered those figures somewhat for patients seen nowadays. Delirium also is associated with an increase in mortality in the months following diagnosis, presumably because of the frequency with which delirium occurs in patients with advanced chronic illnesses. Delirium tremens has been reported to have a mortality rate of 5% to 10%.

One widely used tool for measuring outcome is the Glasgow Outcome Scale (GOS) (Table 49–2). The GOS often is modified according to the type of data sought. The simplest modification divides outcomes into two groups. Good recovery and moderate disability are considered to be "good" outcomes; the other three categories (severe disability, persistent vegetative state, and death) are considered to be "poor" outcomes. Another modification addresses concerns that even patients with good recovery on the GOS can have serious psychological deficits. Expanding the GOS into the eight-level extended GOS addresses some of these issues. More importantly, however, detailed neuropsychological evaluation may be needed for an accurate assessment of the deficits that may be present even in patients who score well on more generalized outcome scales.

Persistent Vegetative State

Up to this point, coma has been discussed as an acute, reversible phenomenon. Such is not always the case.

Table 49–2
Glasgow outcome scale

Score	Category	Description
5	Good Recovery (GR)	Able to live and work independently despite minor disabilities.
4	Moderate Disability (MD)	Able to live independently despite disabilities. Can use public transportation, work with assistance/supervision, etc.
3	Severe Disability (SD)	Conscious but dependent upon others for self-care. Often institutionalized.
2	Persistent Vegetative State (PVS)	Not conscious, but may appear "awake."
1	Death (D)	Self-explanatory.

Although most patients with acute CNS impairment either begin to exhibit some sort of recovery or progress to death, a few patients sustain profound and permanent impairment of consciousness. Within a few weeks, they enter a state in which the eyes may be spontaneously open, sleep/wake cycles are evident, and visual tracking of objects that move in front of them may be seen. However, they still do not follow simple commands or engage in interpersonal interaction. There is no evidence of awareness of self or environment. This condition is termed the *persistent vegetative state*. The frequency with which it occurs has increased as modern biomedical technology has succeeded in preventing death in many patients who previously would have expired. However, although their life has been preserved, these patients survive only in the vegetative state.

Brain Death: Definition and Evaluation

Throughout history, death has been understood to occur when the heart stops beating. For almost half a century, however, it has been recognized that technology is capable of supporting cardiac and respiratory function even after the brain has ceased to function. This situation has been termed *brain death*. Although this term has an intuitively obvious meaning, family members of patients sometimes misconstrue it as describing some sort of qualified death— that a person who is "brain dead" is not really dead. Health care providers must be careful not to create such misunderstandings and to correct them when they exist.

Before a reliable examination can be carried out, the physician must be certain that no confounding factors are present (e.g., hypothermia, neuromuscular blocking drugs, high doses of barbiturates or other drugs that can profoundly depress brain function). It is also helpful to verify that the cause of the brain injury was consistent with the severity and irreversibility of the patient's condition.

Careful neurologic examination then is performed to look for any signs of brain or brainstem function, however slight or subtle they may be. Neurologically devastated patients sometimes demonstrate minimal signs of cerebral function, such as weak spontaneous respiratory effort or gag reflex.

Depending upon hospital policies, a single neurologic examination may be sufficient to declare a patient dead. A minimum observation period of 2 hours, 6 hours, or some similar interval sometimes is advocated as a further safeguard against the premature declaration of death, although the evidentiary basis of such requirements is not clear. An observation period may be especially warranted for cases of diffuse cerebral injury, such as that following cardiac arrest, as opposed to cases of massive brain destruction from trauma or spontaneous intracranial hemorrhage. Similarly, extra caution may be exercised when the cause of the neurologic dysfunction is not readily apparent or when intoxication may be a factor. For neonates and young infants, an extended observation period of several days may be recommended.

Various studies also may be performed to confirm the clinical suspicion of brain death. An apnea test is based upon the absence of respiratory drive when medullary centers no longer initiate breathing in response to hypercapnia. In this test, patients are placed on 100% inspired oxygen, but no spontaneous respirations are given. Some clinicians choose to supplement a closed respiratory circuit with additional instillation of maximally flowing oxygen directly into the trachea, such as via a suction catheter in which the side hole has been occluded with tape. In the absence of ventilation, carbon dioxide accumulates, but aerobic metabolism is sustained because of continued oxygen administration. Monitoring of peripheral oxygen saturation via pulse oximetry is helpful. The test is aborted if the patient demonstrates any cardiopulmonary instability. Arterial blood gas measurements are obtained after approximately 10 minutes and, if necessary, every few minutes thereafter. If the arterial partial pressure of carbon dioxide reaches 60 mm Hg without any evidence of respiratory effort by the patient, the results of the apnea test are considered to be consistent with the diagnosis of brain death.

Other confirmatory tests require more specialized equipment. An electroencephalogram may be performed to assess for electrocerebral silence, or lack of cerebral electrical activity, which is consistent with brain death. Special techniques are used to increase the sensitivity of such studies, and background electrical activity from medical equipment and other sources may cause enough artifact to render the study nondiagnostic. Other tests rely upon proof of absence of CBF. Conventional cerebral angiography may be used for this purpose, but it requires patient transport, is rather invasive, and requires considerable radiologist time to perform the study. Radionuclide brain scanning is more useful for this purpose. Portable scintillation cameras are available that permit these studies to be performed in the intensive care unit, eliminating the need to transport patients to other parts of the hospital.

It should be emphasized that brain death is determined by careful clinical examination. A major impetus to obtain confirmatory studies promptly (as opposed to performing a repeat examination several hours later) is to expedite the declaration of brain death so that organ donation may be discussed with family members before a patient suffers hemodynamic collapse. Most supportive studies cannot be used by themselves to make the diagnosis of brain death. It is for this reason that the results of such studies often are reported using terms such as "consistent with" or "compatible with," instead of "diagnostic of," a diagnosis of brain death.

Spinal Cord Injury

Spinal cord injury (SCI) must be distinguished from spinal column injury. Cord injury is characterized by some type of neurologic deficit, whereas spinal column injury is injury to the bones or ligaments of the spine. A major tenet of trauma care is to assume that every patient has a spinal column injury until proven otherwise. Such an approach prevents creation of neurologic deficits in intact patients with not-yet-diagnosed spinal column injuries by manipulation of their unstable spines in such a manner that cord injury is produced.

As with most types of trauma, SCI occurs most commonly in young males. Motor vehicle accidents, falls, and assaults are the most common causes. More than half of all cases occur in the cervical spine, about a third affect the thoracic spine, and the remainder occur in the lumbar spine.

About half of all cord injuries are incomplete, meaning that patients retain at least some motor or sensory function below the level of injury, sometimes even as slight as "sacral sparing," or preservation of perineal sensation and reflexes. Complete injuries have no such function below the level of the lesion. Immediately after injury, the spinal cord may exhibit so-called spinal shock, with no function below the level of the lesion. Accurate long-term prognostication is not possible while spinal shock is present. Return of the bulbocavernosus reflex (most commonly tested by checking for anal sphincter contraction while squeezing the glans penis or by feeling

Table 49–3
ASIA/IMSOP motor scale

ASIA/IMSOP Motor Scoring System

Right Score	Segment	Muscle	Motion	Left Score
0, 1, 2, 3, 4, 5	C5	Deltoid or biceps	Abduct arm or flex forearm	0, 1, 2, 3, 4, 5
0, 1, 2, 3, 4, 5	C6	Wrist extensors	Wrist extension	0, 1, 2, 3, 4, 5
0, 1, 2, 3, 4, 5	C7	Triceps	Elbow extension	0, 1, 2, 3, 4, 5
0, 1, 2, 3, 4, 5	C8	Flexor digitorum profundus	Grip	0, 1, 2, 3, 4, 5
0, 1, 2, 3, 4, 5	T1	Hand intrinsics	Abduct fifth finger	0, 1, 2, 3, 4, 5
0, 1, 2, 3, 4, 5	L2	Iliopsoas	Flex thigh	0, 1, 2, 3, 4, 5
0, 1, 2, 3, 4, 5	L3	Quadriceps	Extend knee	0, 1, 2, 3, 4, 5
0, 1, 2, 3, 4, 5	L4	Tibialis anterior	Dorsiflex foot	0, 1, 2, 3, 4, 5
0, 1, 2, 3, 4, 5	L5	Extensor hallucis longus	Extend big toe	0, 1, 2, 3, 4, 5
0, 1, 2, 3, 4, 5	S1	Gastrocnemius	Plantarflex foot	0, 1, 2, 3, 4, 5

← TOTAL SCORE FOR EACH SIDE (range 0–50) →
TOTAL SCORE FOR BOTH SIDES (range 0–100):

Table 49–4
Grading of motor strength

Score	Description
0	No evidence of contraction
1	Trace movement
2	Movement with gravity eliminated
3	Movement against gravity
4	Movement against resistance (often qualified as 4−, 4, or 4+)
5	Normal strength

for muscular contraction in the floor of the pelvis while gently tugging on a Foley catheter) signifies resolution of spinal shock.

Various classification schemes have been created to describe the degree of impairment after SCI, but the American Spinal Injury Association/International Medical Society of Paraplegia (ASIA/IMSOP) scale (the motor scoring for which is summarized in Table 49–3) has become the most widely recommended international standard. On this scale, motor strength in individual muscle groups is graded on the Medical Research Council of Great Britain grading scale of 0 to 5 (Table 49–4). In addition, sensation is tested by both pinprick and light touch in 28 dermatomes (C2 through C8, T1 through T12, L1 through L5, and S1 through S4) on each side of the body. Scoring is 2 if normal, 1 if impaired, and 0 if absent. The maximum possible score is 112 (56 on each side) for both pinprick and light touch.

Traction may be needed immediately after injury to restore proper alignment to the spine. Surgery may be required to fuse unstable injuries in order to prevent additional cord damage and possible future deformities. More importantly, intervention also may be needed to decompress the spinal cord if it is compressed by bone fragments, herniated disks, or other lesions. Such treatment usually is performed promptly, but solid evidence to support this practice has been difficult to gather.

Survival after SCI depends upon the severity of associated injuries. Isolated SCI has a mortality rate of 5% to 7% after 1 year, and 77% of patients who survive the first day and 87% of those who survive at least 1 year after injury live at least 10 years. Patients with incomplete injuries probably will experience at least some improvement in function, but those with complete injuries are unlikely to do so. Likewise, younger patients are more likely to improve than older patients.

Bibliography

Burney RE, Maio RF, Maynard F, et al: Incidence, characteristics, and outcome of spinal cord injury at trauma centers in North America. Arch Surg 1993;128:596.

Chesnut RM, Marshall LF, Klauber MR, et al: The role of secondary brain injury in determining outcome from severe head injury. J Trauma 1993;34:216.

Clifton GL, Miller ER, Choi SC, et al: Lack of effect of induction of hypothermia after acute brain injury. N Engl J Med 2001; 344:556.

Committee on Trauma of the American College of Surgeons: Advanced Trauma Life Support Student Manual (6th ed). Chicago: American College of Surgeons, 1997.

Cormio M, Gopinath SP, Valadka A, et al: Cerebral hemodynamic effects of pentobarbital coma in head-injured patients. J Neurotrauma 1999;16:927.

Duppils GS, Wikblad K: Acute confusional states in patients undergoing hip surgery: a prospective observation study. Gerontology 2000;46:36.

Eisenberg HM, Frankowski RF, Contant CF, et al: High-dose barbiturate control of elevated intracranial pressure in patients with severe head injury. J Neurosurg 1988;69:15.

Fehlings MG, Tator CH: An evidence-based review of decompressive surgery in acute spinal cord injury: rationale, indications, and timing based on experimental and clinical studies. J Neurosurg 1999;91(1 Suppl):1.

Griffin MR, O'Fallon WM, Opitz JL, et al: Mortality, survival and prevalence: traumatic spinal cord injury in Olmsted County, Minnesota, 1935–1981. J Chronic Dis 1985;38:643.

Jenkins LW, Moszynski K, Lyeth BG, et al: Increased vulnerability of the mildly traumatized rat brain to cerebral ischemia: the use of controlled secondary ischemia as a research tool to identify common or different mechanisms contributing to mechanical and ischemic brain injury. Brain Res 1989;477:211.

Jennett B, Bond M: Assessment of outcome after severe brain damage. Lancet 1975;1:480.

Jennett B, Snoek J, Bond MR, et al: Disability after severe head injury: observations on the use of the Glasgow Outcome Scale. J Neurol Neurosurg Psychiatry 1981;44:285.

Marshall LF, Gautille T, Klauber MR, et al: The outcome of severe closed head injury. J Neurosurg 1991;75:S28.

Medical Research Council: Aids to the Examination of the Peripheral Nervous System. London: Her Majesty's Stationery Office, 1976.

Muizelaar JP, Marmarou A, Ward JD, et al: Adverse effects of prolonged hyperventilation in patients with severe head injury: a randomized clinical trial. J Neurosurg 1991;75:731.

Muizelaar JP, Wei EP, Kontos HA, et al: Mannitol causes compensatory cerebral vasoconstriction and vasodilation in response to blood viscosity changes. J Neurosurg 1983;59:822.

Plum F, Posner JB: The Diagnosis of Stupor and Coma (3rd ed). Philadelphia: FA Davis, 1982.

Ritter AM, Muizelaar JP, Barnes T, et al: Brain stem blood flow, pupillary response, and outcome in patients with severe head injuries. Neurosurgery 1999;44:941.

Tator CH: Classification of spinal cord injury based on initial presentation. *In* Narayan RK, Wilberger JE, Povlishock JT (eds): Neurotrauma. New York: McGraw-Hill, 1996:1059.

Teasdale G, Jennett B: Assessment of coma and impaired consciousness: a practical scale. Lancet 1974;2:81.

Treatment of convulsive status epilepticus: recommendations of the Epilepsy Foundation of America's Working Group on Status Epilepticus. JAMA 1993;270:854.

Verity CM, Golding J: Risk of epilepsy after febrile convulsions: a national cohort study. BMJ 1991;303:1373.

CHAPTER 50

Gastrointestinal Failure and Liver Failure

Robert A. Cowles, M.D. and
Frederic E. Eckhauser, M.D.

Adequate gastrointestinal and liver function is of vital importance to the organism. The gastrointestinal tract is responsible for the processing and absorption of nutrients that provide energy and of molecules that are critical for building or repairing tissues. The liver is crucial for survival because it is responsible for glucose homeostasis, removal of blood-borne toxins produced by the gastrointestinal tract, excretion of bilirubin, and production of plasma proteins such as albumin and clotting factors.

Alterations in gastrointestinal and liver function occur commonly and often complicate surgical diseases. The severity of the alterations may vary from an inconvenience to a major management problem for the surgeon caring for these patients. This chapter reviews several aspects of gastrointestinal and liver failure with emphasis on proper evaluation and treatment of these conditions in surgical patients.

Gastrointestinal Failure

Gastrointestinal Motility Disorders

Gastric dysmotility

Abnormal motility of the upper gastrointestinal tract can result from a variety of conditions. Gastric dysmotility, or gastroparesis, is most commonly due to long-standing diabetes mellitus. Other common etiologies include previous stomach surgery, drugs, and connective tissue disorders. In nearly 25% of these patients, no etiology is identified.

DEFINITION OF GASTROPARESIS. Gastroparesis is defined as delayed gastric emptying resulting from poor gastric motility in the absence of a mechanical obstruction. It is thus a functional disorder.

SYMPTOMS. Nausea, vomiting, and early postprandial satiety are the most common symptoms of gastroparesis. Other symptoms can include heartburn and postprandial abdominal pain. Symptoms are generally more distressing after solid rather than liquid meals because gastric emptying of solids is more severely affected.

WORKUP.
History. First, a careful history should be elicited to determine the presence or absence of risk factors for gastroparesis. A history of long-standing type 1 diabetes mellitus is an important clue to the underlying etiology in many patients. Some patients may recall a viral syndrome prior to presentation, suggesting an infectious etiology that is generally reversible. Prior operations on the upper gastrointestinal tract, such as vagotomy, fundoplication,

gastric resection, pylorus-preserving pancreaticoduodenectomy, and esophagectomy, are also important to document because they have been found to place patients at higher risk for gastroparesis. Each patient's medication list should be reviewed in detail, and all medications that have the potential to exacerbate gastroparesis should be discontinued. Commonly prescribed drugs that have been associated with gastroparesis include aluminum hydroxide antacids, calcium channel blockers, diphenhydramine, lithium, omeprazole, opiates, phenothiazines, sucralfate, and tricyclic antidepressants. Frequently abused substances such as ethanol, tetrahydrocannabinol, and tobacco also have been associated with gastroparesis. If the patient complains of refractory vomiting and is unable to maintain adequate hydration, immediate consideration should be made for hospital admission, volume resuscitation, bowel rest, and possible nasogastric suction.

Physical examination. A physical examination should be performed routinely to evaluate possible signs of systemic disease. Generalized peripheral neuropathy can suggest the presence of diabetic gastroparesis, while adenopathy, an abdominal mass, and poor nutritional status may suggest an occult malignancy predisposing to delayed gastric emptying. Careful abdominal examination may reveal tympany and tenderness in the epigastrium. If the stomach is fluid filled, a succussion splash may be elicited by moving the patient's abdomen from side to side. The patient's volume status should be ascertained. Hypotension, tachycardia, dry mucous membranes, and poor skin turgor are all signs of significant hypovolemia and warrant aggressive therapy.

Laboratory studies. Electrolyte abnormalities can be severe after periods of intractable vomiting caused by gastroparesis. With severe dehydration, blood urea nitrogen (BUN) and creatinine may be elevated, suggesting renal dysfunction resulting from hypovolemia. Nutritional parameters such as lymphocyte count, prealbumin, albumin, and total protein may be used to evaluate the patient's overall nutritional status.

Imaging studies. In patients who present with symptoms of nausea, vomiting, postprandial abdominal pain, and abdominal distention, the first study should be upright and supine radiographs of the abdomen to evaluate the bowel gas pattern. If these radiographs exclude small bowel and colonic obstruction, an upper gastrointestinal barium study or an upper endoscopy should be performed. The presence of a markedly dilated stomach with absent or weak contractions and retained food with no evidence of mechanical gastric outlet obstruction implies the presence of functional gastric dysmotility. The most helpful study for evaluating gastric dysmotility is the gastric solid-phase emptying study. During this study, the movement of a radiolabeled meal is followed as it exits the stomach and an emptying time for the radioactive tracer is measured.

MEDICAL THERAPY. Initial therapy for gastroparesis is aimed at avoiding factors that exacerbate gastric dysmotility. Medications that inhibit gastric emptying should be discontinued if possible, ethanol and tobacco use should be discouraged, hyperglycemia should be corrected, and patients should be encouraged to eat small, frequent liquid meals because emptying of solids is generally more severely affected.

Several prokinetic medications have been shown to accelerate gastric emptying. Cisapride, which acts on serotonin signaling systems and gastrointestinal smooth muscle, has gained much support as the agent of choice in treating delayed gastric emptying. Currently, the use of cisapride is limited by its potential side effects on myocardial conduction. Metoclopramide and a similar drug, domperidone, which act upon serotonin and dopaminergic systems, are commonly used and have been shown to increase motility of the upper gastrointestinal tract in many conditions. The antibiotic erythromycin also has been shown to exhibit promotility effects on the gastrointestinal tract. The mechanism of erythromycin action involves binding to and stimulation of endogenous motilin receptors present in gastrointestinal smooth muscle and myenteric neural systems.

SURGICAL THERAPY. Surgical therapy for gastroparesis should be considered the option of last resort except in selected patients with postoperative gastroparesis. Patients with advanced diabetic gastroparesis can be offered feeding jejunostomy with or without placement of a gastrostomy for decompression of the nonfunctioning stomach. This approach can provide patients with adequate access for enteral nutrition and also allow for gastric drainage during disease exacerbations. Recent reports of surgically placed gastric pacemakers suggest that this technique may be helpful in the treatment of chronic gastroparesis. Gastric resection or gastrojejunostomy should be avoided because these procedures often fail to improve symptoms.

Small bowel dysmotility

Small bowel dysmotility, also known as chronic intestinal pseudo-obstruction, is unusual and less common than isolated gastric or colonic dysmotility syndromes. Common etiologies include scleroderma, myxedema, amyloidosis, and long-standing diabetes mellitus. Each of these etiologies affects the neural and/or muscular layers of the bowel wall, causing ineffective intestinal contraction resulting in prolonged intestinal transit time. Patients with small bowel dysmotility present with chronic nausea, vomiting, pain, and abdominal distention. Affected patients are often malnourished and underweight. Abdominal radiographs show dilated, atonic small bowel with no obvious obstruction and significantly prolonged transit times.

Patients with small bowel dysmotility are difficulty to treat. Prokinetic agents, as detailed for gastric dysmotility above, may be used initially, and total parenteral nutrition (TPN) is often necessary. Surgical resection of the small bowel or bypass is not recommended because no significant benefit can be expected.

Colonic inertia and colonic pseudo-obstruction

Colonic motility disorders are commonly seen in surgical patients. Colonic inertia often presents as a chronic complaint, whereas colonic pseudo-obstruction can be seen in either the acute or the chronic setting. The hallmark of both conditions is poor prograde colonic motility causing abdominal discomfort or distention. Each is a specific form of constipation and can result from multiple etiologies.

COLONIC INERTIA. Colonic inertia is a diagnosis of exclusion. It is most often seen in young women and its underlying cause is not known. Patients who present with constipation (fewer than three bowel movements per week) should be evaluated first for common causes. The patient's dietary habits, stooling pattern, and underlying medical conditions should be reviewed and modified or treated. Young children and patients with a history of chronic constipation since childhood should have a rectal biopsy performed to rule out Hirschsprung's disease. Additionally, structural abnormalities should be ruled out with either a contrast enema or colonoscopy. When preliminary studies are negative, an initial trial of medical therapy aimed at increasing dietary fiber and water intake should be instituted. If no significant clinical response is noted, colonic motility and pelvic floor function should be studied. Colonic transit time can be measured using radiopaque markers that are ingested and followed with sequential abdominal radiographs as they progress through the colon. Normal colonic transit time from cecum to rectum is approximately 35 hours. Transit times greater than 72 hours are considered abnormal. Pelvic floor muscle function also can be evaluated with defacography and anorectal manometry.

Once a diagnosis of colonic inertia has been made, appropriate therapy can be recommended. Patients may elect to pursue nonsurgical therapies centered on stool softeners, enemas, a high-fiber diet, and sometimes cathartics. When surgical therapy is desired, young patients are excellent candidates for total abdominal colectomy (TAC) with ileorectal anastomosis. TAC with ileorectal anastomosis is associated with a success rate of 90% or better in this selected patient population. In special situations, other operations such as TAC with ileostomy or total proctocolectomy with ileoanal

J-pouch anastomosis may be appropriate depending on the specific situation.

COLONIC PSEUDO-OBSTRUCTION. Colonic pseudo-obstruction, also referred to as Ogilvie's syndrome, is a functional obstruction of the colon associated with colonic dilation and decreased stool and flatus output with no demonstrable mechanical obstruction. This condition commonly affects older patients and often is seen in chronically ill patients, especially following surgery. Individuals undergoing cardiac, orthopedic, and neurosurgical procedures are at particularly high risk for developing this condition.

Patients with increasing abdominal distention, little or no pain, and rare passage of flatus and stool should undergo further evaluation. Plain abdominal radiographs should be obtained to measure cecal diameter. Cecal diameter is considered to be important for assessing for the presence and severity of Ogilvie's syndrome. Although a cecal diameter of 12 cm is considered to represent a "dangerous" level of dilation, there is no consensus on the exact threshold that should be used. Most authorities believe that, when the cecum reaches 9 to 10 cm, therapy should be instituted. Initially, several simple maneuvers can benefit the patient who may be developing Ogilvie's syndrome. All electrolytes, especially potassium, should be normalized and narcotics minimized or completely stopped if possible. Second, a nasogastric tube and possibly a rectal tube should be placed to aid in elimination of intraluminal gases and swallowed air. Some authors also recommend frequent changes in patient positioning to aid in movement of gases. Gentle enemas may be used to try to stimulate colonic contraction. If these measures fail to produce improvement, a colonoscopy with decompression should be considered and repeated if necessary. Recently, the acetylcholinesterase inhibitor neostigmine has received attention as an efficacious and noninvasive treatment for Ogilvie's syndrome. Several studies have reported a high rate of successful colonic decompression using neostigmine. It is important to note that its use requires cardiac monitoring and may be contraindicated in patients with known cardiac disease.

The most feared complication of Ogilvie's syndrome is cecal necrosis and perforation. Perforation has been estimated to occur in 3% of cases. When this occurs, mortality may be as high as 50%. Surgery for Ogilvie's syndrome should be limited to patients who fail aggressive nonoperative therapy, to patients with impending cecal necrosis or perforation, and to patients with obvious peritonitis. Operative therapy should be individualized. Cecal necrosis can be treated by resection with anastomosis or with ileostomy. Uncomplicated Ogilvie's syndrome may be treated by cecostomy or resection.

Malabsorption Syndromes

Short bowel syndrome

Short bowel syndrome (SBS) is a condition that results from inadequate intestinal surface area. In the past, it was defined as resection or loss of 40% to 50% of the small intestine resulting in malabsorption. Currently, SBS is defined as the symptom complex observed in patients with less than 200 cm of small bowel. This definition, which is based solely on the remaining length of intestine, cannot be used for all patients. For example, patients with primary small bowel disease (e.g., Crohn's disease) may have poorly functioning remaining intestine and may develop SBS even following a limited dissection.

The major causes of SBS differ in adults and children and are listed in Table 50–1. Whereas the majority of children develop SBS secondary to congenital abnormalities or diseases encountered in the perinatal period, adults often develop SBS from acquired conditions. The major anatomic factors that appear to influence the development of SBS include the extent of bowel resection, the presence or absence of the ileocecal valve, the presence or absence of an end ostomy, and the health of the remaining intestinal segment(s).

Clinical findings in patients with SBS are varied and can be minor or severe. Malabsorption of nutrients is the hallmark of this syndrome. Poor nutrient absorption results in diarrhea with loss of fluids and electrolytes from the gastrointestinal tract. This can result in severe malnutrition and dehydration. Diarrhea appears to be the result of both malabsorption and accelerated or rapid transit time.

Medical management of patients with SBS begins at the time of diagnosis. Because SBS is often the result of operative intestinal resection, therapy should begin immediately following operation. TPN has become one of the primary therapies in SBS and should be instituted during the postoperative period. Patients with SBS are often discharged home with TPN as their main form of nutrition. In the acute setting, diarrhea is avoided by limiting oral intake. As the patient's condition improves, the intestine is capable of adaptation and therefore an oral diet can be cautiously started. Calories and fluid can be advanced slowly over several weeks. Diarrhea may occur at this point and can be controlled with a variety of antidiarrheal medications. As oral caloric intake increases, TPN should be weaned and discontinued if possible. When some TPN supplementation is absolutely necessary, it may be given primarily at night or on certain days to provide the necessary extra calories. Despite the institution of appropriate therapy, some patients remain on chronic TPN. It has been suggested that adults with less than 100 cm of small intestine, an absent ileocecal valve, and a small bowel end ostomy are at highest risk of requiring long-term TPN therapy. Once TPN has been necessary for 2 years' time, it is likely to be required permanently.

Surgical therapy for SBS is aimed at increasing intestinal absorption. Surgical procedures can either improve absorptive function of existing intestine or increase intestinal surface area. The commonly performed operations for SBS are listed in Box 50–1. Children undergo operative therapy more commonly than adults. This may be related to their overall longer expected lifespan and general lack of underlying disease. Each patient's condition and degree of intestinal dysfunction should be ascertained and the appropriate surgical procedure chosen. Patients with dilated bowel are candidates for intestinal tapering or stricturoplasty. Those with rapid transit time may require creation of an artificial valve or placement of an antiperistaltic

Table 50–1
Causes of short bowel syndrome in adults and children

Adults	Children
Mesenteric infarction	Necrotizing enterocolitis
Radiation enteritis	Midgut volvulus
Crohn's disease	Intestinal atresia
Volvulus	Gastroschisis
Trauma	
Tumors	

Data from Wilmore DW, Robinson MK: Short bowel syndrome. World J Surg 2000;24:1486; © Springer-Verlag Thompson JS, Langnas AN, Pinch LW: Surgical approach to short-bowel syndrome: experience in a population of 160 patients. Ann Surg 1995;222:600; Mesing B, Crenn P, Beau P, et al: Long-term survival and parenteral nutrition dependence in adult patients with the short bowel syndrome. Gastroenterology 1999;117:1042; and Webber TR: Isoperistaltic bowel lengthening for short bowel syndrome in children. Am J Surg 1999;178:600. Copyright 1999, with permission from Excerpta Medica Inc.

Box 50–1
Surgical Procedures for Short Bowel Syndrome

- Intestinal tapering
- Stricturoplasty
- Intestinal valve
- Antiperistaltic segment
- Bianchi procedures (intestinal lengthening and tapering)
- Transplantation (intestine alone, liver-intestine, multivisceral)

segment, although, in one series, the result of these procedures was disappointing. Patients with dilated bowel and very short remaining intestinal length may undergo an intestinal tapering and lengthening procedure as described by Bianchi in 1980. Overall, the results of surgery for SBS are encouraging, with almost 70% of patients becoming independent of TPN. Finally, after long-term TPN, some patients developed TPN-induced liver failure or severe TPN-related complications and become candidates for liver-intestine or intestine transplantation. These therapies are relatively new, are performed only in a few specialized centers, and have been associated with a substantial mortality.

Diarrhea

About 7 to 10 L of fluid is secreted into the gastrointestinal tract per day. The stomach, pancreas, liver, and small bowel are the major contributors to this volume. Of these 10 L, the small bowel reabsorbs approximately 8.5 L, with the remaining 1.5 L entering the colon. By the time stool is evacuated, only 150 mL of water is finally excreted. Diarrhea is considered to be present when more than 250 mL of water is excreted in stool per day.

Diarrhea is common and often multifactorial. Its causes can be categorized as either secretory, osmotic, or mixed. An important initial step in treating patients with diarrhea is to obtain a careful history. Important questions concern the stool pattern and frequency and its variation from each patient's normal routine. Additionally, questions about associated symptoms (e.g., pain, bleeding, nausea, vomiting, fever), overall health, and recent institution of new medications (antibiotics or cardiovascular drugs) may provide important clues to the diagnosis.

Acute diarrhea in surgical patients is often related to changes in intestinal flora. Diarrhea may be a normal response as ileus resolves, especially after a full mechanical bowel preparation has been performed preoperatively. This is normal and self-limited. Persistent diarrhea is more worrisome and should be fully evaluated. This section addresses the evaluation and treatment of acute diarrhea, often caused by either infection or medications, that is commonly seen in surgical patients.

Clostridium difficile–*associated diarrhea*

A history of antibiotic use within a 1- to 2-month period prior to surgery, even if only one preoperative dose was given, is important and may suggest the possibility of *C. difficile* infection. It has been estimated that 25% of antibiotic-associated diarrhea is due to *C. difficile* infection or colonization. In the remainder of cases of antibiotic-associated diarrhea, an offending organism is not identified, the clinical course is mild and self-limited, and cure is achieved by discontinuation of the causative antibiotic.

Classically, clindamycin therapy has been implicated as a major cause of *C. difficile*–associated diarrhea and *C. difficile* colitis, although, because of their widespread use, other commonly used antibiotics (penicillins and cephalosporins) have been associated with a large number of cases.

When evaluating patients with possible *C. difficile* colitis, it is important to maintain a high index of suspicion. The patient should be examined and a careful abdominal and rectal exam performed. Measures of electrolytes, BUN, and creatinine and a complete blood count should be obtained to look for acidosis, leukocytosis, and renal dysfunction. A stool sample should be collected and evaluated for fecal leukocytes as well as for the presence of *C. difficile* toxins. If the diagnosis is confirmed or if suspicion is high for the presence of *C. difficile*–associated diarrhea, treatment with antibiotics may be begun. First, the offending antibiotic should be discontinued if possible. The first-line drug for the treatment of *C. difficile* infection is oral metronidazole (250 mg qid). It can provide clinical improvement within 72 hours and can be expected to cure 95% of patients after 10 days of therapy. An alternative to metronidazole is oral vancomycin (125 mg qid). This can be used either when patients cannot tolerate metronidazole or when therapy with metronidazole is ineffective. If severe ileus prevents oral antibiotic therapy, parenteral metronidazole is effective because it is excreted into the gastrointestinal tract via the biliary system. Parenteral vancomycin is not effective and not recommended because it is not excreted into the gut.

In its most severe form, *C. difficile* infection can present as a fulminant colitis and constitutes a surgical emergency. Clinical findings include severe systemic toxicity, acute peritonitis, marked leukocytosis, and often an abnormal abdominal radiograph with either megacolon, "thumbprinting," or obvious pneumoperitoneum. If a diagnosis of *C. difficile* colitis is entertained, sigmoidoscopy may be used as a diagnostic tool to look for pseudomembranes. In this case, resuscitation should be prompt and surgery can be lifesaving. A subtotal colectomy with end ileostomy has been recommended as the procedure of choice for patients presenting with severe, fulminant *C. difficile* colitis.

Liver Failure

Basic liver physiology and function have been described in earlier sections of this text. This section outlines the common etiologies leading to hepatic dysfunction and discusses the management of specific problems encountered in patients with liver failure. For the purposes of this discussion, *cirrhosis* is used synonymously with *liver failure*, and specific issues regarding acute liver failure without cirrhosis are discussed at the end of the chapter.

Etiologies and Diagnosis

The term *liver failure* implies that the liver has been injured to an extent that it cannot perform its necessary functions within the body. The causes of this injury are multiple, with alcohol abuse, viral hepatitis, and ingestion of toxic substances being responsible for the majority of cases in the Western world.

Patients may present with a variety of findings such as jaundice, ascites, abnormal liver enzymes, coagulopathy, or even severe upper gastrointestinal bleeding from esophageal varices. When liver failure (i.e., cirrhosis) is suspected, a careful history and physical examination should be obtained. A history of viral hepatitis, blood transfusions, alcoholism, and intravenous drug abuse should be sought in an attempt to delineate the etiology. Clinical manifestations suggestive of portal hypertension, such as an abdominal fluid wave, periumbilical caput medusae, and enlarged hemorrhoids, should be documented. Additional physical findings suggestive of advanced liver disease may include palmar erythema, gynecomastia, spider angiomata, testicular atrophy, and muscle wasting. A variety of laboratory studies can help evaluate liver function and have been used to assess hepatic reserve. Serum albumin and coagulation parameters provide an estimate of the liver's protein synthetic ability. Alanine (ALT) and aspartate transaminase (AST) levels indicate the degree of liver cell injury. Finally, the bilirubin level is an indirect measure of the liver's conjugation capacity.

When the patient has been fully evaluated, the physician often has made the clinical diagnosis of cirrhosis and may begin to treat the patient empirically. It must be remembered, however, that the diagnosis of cirrhosis can only be made by histologic confirmation from either a percutaneous or an open liver biopsy specimen. Histologic findings such as bridging fibrosis with regenerating nodules and varying degrees of inflammation are diagnostic of cirrhosis. Occasionally, a percutaneous biopsy can sample a large regenerating nodule and therefore may not show the characteristic fibrosis necessary to establish a diagnosis of cirrhosis. In this case, a repeat biopsy may be necessary when suspicion is high.

Assessment of Hepatic Failure

A true assessment of hepatic function is difficult to obtain, but an estimate can and should be made when treating patients with significant liver disease. The tests and scoring systems described below are not perfect but allow for reasonable estimates of the severity of liver dysfunction.

Tests of hepatic function

The name given to the standard tests of hepatic function — "liver function tests" (LFTs) — is unfortunately a misnomer.

In most laboratories, LFTs include serum albumin, total protein, transaminases (AST, ALT), alkaline phosphatase, lactate dehydrogenase, and bilirubin levels. Of these, the transaminases, alkaline phosphatase, and lactate dehydrogenase do not actually measure hepatic function or injury to other cells. Additionally, it is well known that the liver can lose 75% of its cell mass before significant dysfunction is noticeable and before standard laboratories become abnormal. These facts therefore make the routine LFTs poor measures of hepatic function when used alone.

Because of the nonspecific nature of standard laboratory tests, several more direct tests of liver function have been developed but are not widely utilized. The aminopyrine breath test, caffeine clearance test, galactose elimination test, indocyanine green clearance test, and monoethylglycine xylidide test are examples of these specialized tests. They estimate the metabolic capacity of the liver by measuring the elimination or metabolism of an injected substance.

Scoring systems

Because LFTs alone are of limited use in evaluating liver function, several systems have been developed to try to predict hepatic reserve in surgical patients. These systems combine the results of standard laboratory tests and clinical parameters to arrive at a better estimate of hepatic functional reserve.

The most widely cited scoring system is that proposed by Child and Turcotte in 1964. The Child-Turcotte classification gives patients a score of A, B, or C based upon serum albumin and bilirubin levels combined with clinical parameters such as nutritional status, presence of ascites, and degree of hepatic encephalopathy. A score of A signifies the presence of minor liver dysfunction and predicts a good survival after portosystemic shunt surgery. A score of C, in contrast, suggests advanced liver disease and is associated with poor outcome after portosystemic shunt surgery. Although the original Child-Turcotte classification specifically addressed the predicted outcomes after portosystemic shunt surgery, this classification system has been widely applied to all patients with liver failure as a reliable measure of hepatic reserve.

The Child-Turcotte classification was modified by Pugh in 1973. This new Child-Turcotte-Pugh classification, which includes an assessment of the patient's prothrombin time, is currently used by many surgeons and plays an important role in listing liver transplant candidates. Newer scoring systems, such as the Model for End Stage Liver Disease, are being used to predict patient outcomes after transjugular intrahepatic portosystemic shunting (TIPS).

Although most of the scoring systems noted above were designed to address the outcome of patients undergoing liver procedures or portosystemic shunt surgery, they can be applied to patients undergoing any major operative procedure. A recent study found that clinical parameters such as encephalopathy, congestive heart failure, emergency procedures, and preoperative infection as well as laboratory findings such as albumin level, bilirubin level, prothrombin time, and serum creatinine level could be correlated with outcome in patients undergoing nonhepatic surgery.

Consequences of Hepatic Failure

Portal hypertension

Portal hypertension is considered to be present when the portal vein pressure is increased above 10 mm Hg. It may result from many causes, but these can be subdivided on the basis of site of obstruction into presinusoidal, sinusoidal, or postsinusoidal. Cirrhosis caused by fibrosis and regeneration is considered to be sinusoidal and is the most common form of portal hypertension. Budd-Chiari syndrome is an example of postsinusoidal portal hypertension.

The alterations that occur secondary to high portal vein pressure vary from merely inconvenient to life threatening. With sustained portal hypertension, multiple venous collaterals form between the portal and systemic circulations. The most important of these collaterals are located along the proximal stomach and esophagus. These collaterals can become dilated and engorged with blood and are prone to profuse bleeding. When associated with significant coagulopathy, variceal hemorrhage can be fatal. Although detailed discussion of the treatment of bleeding varices is beyond the scope of this chapter, esophageal varices may be treated by a variety of methods. Acute treatment of variceal bleeding can include pharmacotherapy with intravenous somatostatin or vasopressin infusions. The patient should be volume resuscitated and undergo urgent upper endoscopy to confirm that the hemorrhage is variceal in origin. During endoscopy, either sclerotherapy or variceal banding may be performed. In the chronic setting, variceal hemorrhage may be prevented by the use of β-adrenergic receptor blockers to produce a decrease in splanchnic blood flow. Other collaterals that become dilated in portal hypertension are the hemorrhoidal veins. Like esophageal varices, these may bleed heavily and should be not ignored.

Ascites formation is another result of portal hypertension and suggests decompensated disease. The presence of ascites is due to a combination of increased sinusoidal pressure with weeping of hepatic fluid and lymph, hypoalbuminemia with low plasma oncotic pressure, and poor water and sodium handling by the kidney. Ascites accompanying liver failure is managed medically. A low-sodium diet with institution of diuretic therapy (furosemide and spironolactone) can control ascites in most patients. When ascites becomes refractory, other treatments may be useful,

including peritoneovenous shunts, TIPS, and even liver transplantation.

Hepatic encephalopathy

Hepatic encephalopathy (HE) of varying degree is estimated to complicate the course of 50% to 70% of patients with cirrhosis. The condition is reversible and is thought to be due to high blood levels of ammonia and possibly other neurologically active substances that accumulate as a result of liver dysfunction. The diagnosis is made by careful neurologic examination. In its mildest form, HE can be demonstrated only by psychometric analysis. Although implicated in the pathophysiology of HE, blood ammonia levels have not been found to correlate well with the severity of encephalopathy, and therefore the measurement of blood ammonia is generally not helpful in guiding the treatment of HE.

Because ammonia is a by-product of protein catabolism, treatment of HE begins with limiting protein intake to 0.8 to 1.0 g of protein per kilogram of body weight per day. When possible, intake of branched-chain amino acids with avoidance of aromatic amino acids can improve symptoms of HE. Pharmacotherapy generally consists of administration of the cathartic lactulose. Lactulose doses should be titrated in order to produce between two and four bowel movements per day. Liver transplantation can be performed in patients with advanced cirrhosis and HE with the expectation that, once the transplanted liver begins to function, symptoms of encephalopathy will regress.

Hepatorenal syndrome

Hepatorenal syndrome (HRS) refers to the development of renal failure in patients with underlying liver failure. It is associated with low urinary sodium concentration, normal cardiovascular hemodynamics, and no demonstrable renal lesion. Two types of HRS exist. Type I HRS is associated with rapid deterioration of renal function, whereas type II HRS is more chronic, with slowly worsening renal function.

The pathophysiology of HRS is complex and at this time is poorly understood. Most authors first recommend prevention of HRS with a combination of moderate diuretic use, careful use of large-volume paracentesis, and intensive care unit monitoring when significant volume shifts are anticipated. New therapeutic modalities such as TIPS are being developed for HRS. However, the only effective permanent treatment for this condition is liver transplantation.

Coagulopathy

Elevation in the coagulation parameters is a common finding in liver failure, along with decreased levels of coagulation factors (except factor VIII) that are made in the liver. When obstructive jaundice is present, some of these elevations are reversible with the administration of vitamin K. However, because obstructive jaundice is not present in most cases of cirrhosis, vitamin K is not useful across the board. When surgery is necessary for patients with liver failure and elevated prothrombin times, liberal use of fresh frozen plasma (FFP), cryoprecipitate, and blood is recommended.

In addition to poor production of coagulation factors, liver failure also can result in varying degrees of thrombocytopenia. Low platelet counts usually can be followed, and platelet transfusion is considered only during episodes of active bleeding or when a surgical procedure is necessary.

Acute Hepatic Failure

Acute hepatic failure (AHF) occurs within a span of days to weeks and has a much faster progression than cirrhosis associated with chronic liver disease. Hepatitis B infection constitutes the leading cause of AHF worldwide, although cases resulting from ingestion of toxic drugs or chemicals outnumber those caused by hepatitis B in some countries. Other less common causes of AHF include various types of viral hepatitis, HELLP syndrome (hemolysis, elevated liver enzymes, and low platelet count in association with pre-eclampsia), Budd-Chiari syndrome, and Wilson's disease.

Patients with AHF may present with a variety of symptoms ranging from nonspecific complaints to coma. When AHF is suspected, the patient should be monitored with frequent laboratory evaluations in an intensive care unit setting. If a specialized transplant center is available and transfer of the patient is possible, this should be considered.

The mainstay of treatment for patients with AHF is supportive. Encephalopathy should be evaluated and treated as described above. Cerebral edema appears to be seen much more commonly in the setting of AHF compared with chronic liver disease. When neurologic deterioration occurs, the patient should be intubated and sedated and kept as quiet as possible to avoid increases in intracranial pressure (ICP). An ICP monitor may be helpful in this setting if reliable neurologic exam is not possible. Supportive therapy is often all that is necessary. If liver failure progresses, arrangements should be made for liver transplantation. Support should be continued aggressively until a donor organ becomes available.

Recently, some centers have begun trials using bioartificial liver devices and extracorporeal liver-assist devices, with promising results. These alternative therapies are available only at very specialized centers and may lengthen the amount of time that patients with AHF can be supported as they await liver transplantation.

Care of the Postoperative Patient with Hepatic Dysfunction

Caring for patients with liver dysfunction requires an understanding of the pathophysiology of liver failure and portal hypertension as well as attention to detail. First, strong consideration should be given to placing the patient in the intensive care unit. This facilitates monitoring of vital signs, urine output, and serial laboratory parameters. For major abdominal procedures, abdominal girth should be measured and followed frequently. When possible, colloids such as FFP, packed red blood cells, whole blood, or salt-poor albumin should be used for volume resuscitation. The use of 0.9% NaCl or other saline-containing solutions for fluid resuscitation should be actively discouraged.

The coagulation times should be maintained as close to normal as possible with the administration of FFP, and platelet counts should be kept above or near 50,000/mm^3. Antacids or histamine$_2$-blockers are recommended to prevent gastritis, and enteral nutrition should be started as soon as possible. Perioperative antibiotics should be used to prevent bacterial peritonitis. When appropriate, preoperative medications such as diuretics to control ascites should be restarted.

Bibliography

Agarwal S, Stollman N: Gastroparesis. Resident Staff Physician 1999;45:12.

Arroyo V, Gines P, Gerbes AL, et al: Definition and diagnostic criteria of refractory ascites and hepatorenal syndrome in cirrhosis. Hepatology 1996;23:164.

Bianchi A: Intestinal loop lengthening: a technique for increasing small intestinal length. J Pediatr Surg 1980; 15:145.

Caldwell SH, Schiff ER: Laboratory investigation and percutaneous biopsy of the liver. In Turcotte JG (ed): Shackelford's Surgery of the Alimentary Tract (4th ed), Vol III. Philadelphia: WB Saunders, 1996:374.

Camilleri M, Malagelada JR, Abell TL, et al: Effect of six weeks of treatment with cisapride in gastroparesis pseudo-obstruction. Gastroenterology 1989;96:704.

Child CG, Turcotte JG: Surgery and portal hypertension. In Child CG (ed): The Liver and Portal Hypertension. Philadelphia: WB Saunders, 1964.

Cotran RS, Kumar V, Robbins SL (eds): Robbins Pathologic Basis of Disease (4th ed). Philadelphia: WB Saunders, 1989.

Forster J, Sarosiek I, Delcore R, et al: Gastric pacing is a new surgical procedure for gastroparesis. Am J Surg 2001;182:676.

Grant D: Intestinal transplantation: 1997 report of the international registry. Transplantation 1999;67:1061.

Greenberger NJ (ed): Gastrointestinal Disorders: A Pathophysiologic Approach (4th ed). Chicago: Year Book Medical Publishers, 1989.

Henderson JM, Barnes DS, Geisinger MA: Portal hypertension. Curr Probl Surg 1998;35:379.

Kelly CP, Pothoulakis C, LaMont JT: Current concepts: Clostridium difficile colitis. N Engl J Med 1994;330:257.

Laine L: Management of acute colonic pseudo-obstruction. N Engl J Med 1999;341:192.

Lin HC, Meyer JH: Disorders of gastric emptying. *In* Yanmada T (ed): Textbook of Gastroenterology. Philadelphia: JP Lippincott, 1991:1213.

Malinchoc M, Kamath PS, Gordon FD, et al: A model to predict poor survival in patients undergoing transjugular intrahepatic portosystemic shunts. Hepatology 2000; 21:864.

McClelland RN, Horton JW: Relief of acute, persistent postvagotomy atony by metoclopramide. Ann Surg 1978;188:439.

Messing B, Crenn P, Beau P, et al: Long-term survival and parenteral nutrition dependence in adult patients with the short bowel syndrome. Gastroenterology 1999;117:1043.

Mylonakis E, Ryan ET, Calderwood SB: Clostridium difficile-associated diarrhea. Arch Intern Med 2001;161:525.

Paran H, Silverberg D, Mayo A, et al: Treatment of colonic pseudo-obstruction with neostigmine. J Am Coll Surg 2000;190:315.

Pfeifer J, Agachan F, Wexner SD: Surgery for constipation. Dis Colon Rectum 1996;39:444.

Ponec RJ, Saunders MD, Kimmey MB: Neostigmine for the treatment of acute colonic pseudo-obstruction. N Engl J Med 1999;341:137.

Pugh RN, Murray-Lyon IM, Dawson JL, et al: Transection of the oesophagus for bleeding oesphageal varices. Br J Surg 1973;60:647.

Rahman T, Hodgson H: Clinical management of acute hepatic failure. Intensive Care Med 2001;27:467.

Rice HE, O'Keefe GE, Helton WS, Johansen K: Morbid prognostic factors in patients with chronic liver failure undergoing nonhepatic surgery. Arch Surg 1997;132:880.

Riordan SM, Williams R: Treatment of hepatic encephalopathy. N Engl J Med 1997;337:473.

Sachar DB, Waye JD, Lewis BS (eds): Gastroenterology for the House Officer. Baltimore: Williams & Wilkins, 1989.

Tack J, Janssens J, Vantrappen G, et al: Effect of erythromycin on gastric motility in controls and in diabetic gastroparesis. Gastroenterology 1992;103:72.

Tenofsky PL, Beamer RL, Smith RS: Ogilvie syndrome as a postoperative constipation. Arch Surg 2000;135:682.

Thompson JS, Langnas AN: Small intestinal insufficiency and the short bowel syndrome. *In* Lillemoe KD (ed): Shackelford's Surgery of the Alimentary Tract (5th ed), Vol V. Philadelphia: WB Saunders, 2002:295.

Thompson JS, Langnas AN, Pinch LW: Surgical approach to short-bowel syndrome: experience in a population of 160 patients. Ann Surg 1995;222:600.

Tiao GM, Fischer JE: Perioperative management and nutrition in patients with liver and biliary tract disease. *In* Turcotte JG (ed): Shackelford's Surgery of the Alimentary Tract (4th ed), Vol III. Philadelphia: WB Saunders, 1996:400.

Webster C, Dayton M: Results after colectomy for colonic inertia: a sixteen-year experience. Am J Surg 2001;182:639.

Wilmore DW, Robinson MK: Short bowel syndrome. World J Surg 2000;24:1486.

Wong F, Blendis L: New challenge of hepatorenal syndrome: prevention and treatment. Hepatology 2001;34:1241.

Zervos EE, Rosemurgy AS: Management of medically refractory ascites. Am J Surg 2001;181:256.

Zimmerman H, Reichen J: Hepatectomy: preoperative analysis of hepatic function and postoperative liver failure. Dig Surg 1998;15:1.

CHAPTER 51

Respiratory Insufficiency, Failure, and Support

Ravi Veeramasuneni, M.D. and Harry L. Anderson, III, M.D., F.A.C.S., F.C.C.M.

General anesthesia and surgery can adversely affect the respiratory system independently. Respiratory insufficiency may be well tolerated by healthy individuals but can have severe consequences in the elderly and in patients with a history of lung disease. Pulmonary complications are common postoperative causes of morbidity and account for approximately 25% of postoperative mortality. Because pulmonary complications can be associated with a significantly prolonged hospital stay and increased morbidity and mortality, extensive efforts have been made to identify predisposing factors for complications and to develop strategies to prevent such complications. Therefore, it is important to identify the patients at risk and take adequate measures to decrease the risks. Patients who undergo abdominal surgical procedures, thoracotomy, and cardiac surgical operations are particularly prone to complications.

Understanding the mechanisms of respiratory failure can enable the physician to identify and carry out the appropriate therapeutic interventions. Although critical care has emerged as a unique clinical discipline, it is important for all surgical specialists to be particularly aware of possible pulmonary complications and to implement the appropriate interventions to decrease their incidence. The following discussion describes the physiology of normal lung function, the risk factors for pulmonary complications, and the evaluation and correction of preoperative deficiencies. We then present several mechanisms of respiratory failure with the appearance of respiratory insufficiency during the pre-, intra- and postoperative periods, and we discuss the fundamentals of treatment with mechanical ventilation.

Fundamentals of Pulmonary Physiology

The respiratory system anatomically consists of the airways, lung, chest wall, and respiratory muscles. The oxygen in inhaled air is transported through the conducting airways to the alveoli and diffuses across the alveolar-capillary membrane, thereby entering and being carried away by capillary blood. The oxygen combines with the hemoglobin of red blood cells and is carried to the peripheral tissues, where the mitochondria utilize the oxygen for production of ATP in the electron transport chain. The CO_2 produced during this metabolic process diffuses into the capillary blood, is converted to carbonic acid and is then transported back to the lungs by dissolution in venous blood. Exchange of O_2 and CO_2 at the alveolar–capillary interface is essential for normal physiologic function of the body, and any impairment of the gas exchange at this interface results in respiratory failure.

Respiratory failure is usually diagnosed based on arterial blood gas measurements. It is usually defined as a partial pressure of oxygen in arterial blood (PaO_2) of less than 60 mmHg and/or a $PaCO_2$ of more than 46 mmHg while breathing room air. Hypoxemia is often accompanied by tachypnea, tachycardia, and hypertension. Cerebral hypoxemia can produce mental status changes ranging from mild confusion to delirium. Hypercapnia can also affect the nervous system, and patients can progress from lethargy to stupor and finally to coma.

Respiratory failure can be due to inadequate oxygenation or ventilation or a combination of the two. Therefore, it is essential to understand the differences between these two concepts.

Arterial Oxygenation

Most of the oxygen in blood is bound to hemoglobin, with less than 5% dissolved in plasma. Calculating the O_2 content (CaO_2, cc/dl) requires measuring the PaO_2, the percent of hemoglobin bound to oxygen ($\%HgbO_2$), and the hemoglobin level (Hgb, g/dl). Therefore:

$$CaO_2 = (1.34 \times Hgb \times \%HgbO_2) + (0.003 \times PaO_2)$$

The affinity of hemoglobin for oxygen can be affected by several factors. Figure 51–1 shows the nonlinear relationship of the oxygen-hemoglobin dissociation curve. Loading of hemoglobin with O_2 occurs in the upper, flat portion of the curve, whereas in the steeper portion of the curve (at lower PaO_2) hemoglobin has less affinity for O_2 and the O_2 is unloaded in the peripheral tissues. High temperatures, high $PaCO_2$, and decreasing pH promote dissociation of oxygen from hemoglobin. A decrease in PaO_2

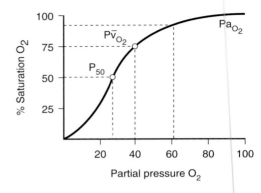

FIGURE 51–1 Hemoglobin dissociation curve. This curve shows the relationship of plasma oxygen partial pressure to the degree to which potential oxygen-carrying hemoglobin sites have oxygen attached (% saturation O_2). This nonlinear relationship accounts for most of the oxygen reserves in blood. Normally, hemoglobin is 50% saturated at a plasma PO_2 of approximately 27 mmHg. This is designated P_{50}. Normal mixed venous blood has an oxygen partial pressure (PvO_2) of 40 mmHg, and an oxyhemoglobin saturation of 75%. A PO_2 of 60 mmHg normally results in approximately 90% hemoglobin saturation. Normal arterial blood has an oxygen partial pressure (PaO_2) of 97 mmHg and an oxyhemoglobin saturation of 97%. (Adapted from Shapiro BA, Peruzzi WT: Pulmonary complications. In Civetta JM, Taylor RW, Kirby RR, [eds]. Critical Care [3rd ed]. Philadelphia: Lippincott Williams & Wilkins, 1997:924, with permission.)

to 40 mmHg is typically associated with a $\%HgbO_2$ value of less than 75% and represents a direct threat to tissue oxygenation.

The V/Q ratio is the ratio of alveolar ventilation (V or V_A) to pulmonary blood flow (Q). A normal V/Q ratio is approximately 0.8. With a pathologic shunt, a V/Q ratio much less than 1.0 describes the condition where the capillary blood flow is in excess of ventilation. Alveolar collapse due to atelectasis or alveolar flooding due to pneumonia are examples of a shunt in which the involved alveoli are bypassed by the capillary blood flow. A true shunt describes complete absence of gas exchange between capillary blood flow and alveolar gas. Examples of true shunt include congenital abnormalities such as patent ductus arteriosus or a ventricular septal defect (VSD).

Ventilation

Ventilation is the process of gas movement into and out of the respiratory system. Ventilation is composed of two components: alveolar ventilation (V_A) and dead space ventilation (V_d). Alveolar ventilation determines the rate of CO_2 removal from the blood. Dead space ventilation is that which does not participate in gas exchange. It may be comprised of the anatomic dead space, which is the volume of the conducting airways and physiologic dead space (i.e., the volume of the alveolar gas that does not diffuse across the alveolar–capillary interface). Dead space ventilation can occur in cases of destruction of the alveolar–capillary interface (e.g., emphysema) or reduced blood flow (e.g., heart failure or pulmonary embolism). Dead space ventilation is determined by the following equation

$$V_d/V_t = Pa_{CO_2} - P_E_{CO_2}/Pa_{CO_2}$$

where V_t is the tidal volume, and $P_E_{CO_2}$ is the partial pressure of exhaled CO_2. Adequate ventilation therefore requires the drive to breathe and the normal mechanics of breathing.

Pulmonary Function Testing

Pulmonary function tests are useful for diagnosing lung disease, assessing the severity of the disease, and measuring any response to therapy. Figure 51–2 shows the various lung volumes as measured by spirometry. Spirometry is used to record movement of air into and out of lungs. Measurements of flow rates during a forced expiration can help narrow the differential diagnosis of a dyspneic patient.

Lung disorders can be divided into two broad categories: obstructive disorders and restrictive disorders. With restrictive disorders, there is impaired expansion of the thoracic cavity and lung. With obstructive disorders, there is obstruction to airflow, prolonged expiration, and gas trapping.

The forced expiratory volume at 1 second (FEV_1) is the volume of air that can be expired in 1 second after a maximal inspiration. The forced vital capacity (FVC) is the volume of air that can be forcefully expired after a maximal inspiration. With restrictive disorders, both FEV_1 and FVC are reduced, so the FEV_1/FVC ratio may be normal. With obstructive disorders such as asthma, the FEV_1 is reduced more than the FVC, so the FEV_1/FVC ratio is decreased. The normal FEV_1/FVC ratio is 0.8.

Diffusion lung capacity measured using carbon monoxide (D_lCO), is a useful tool for assessing the severity of emphysema and interstitial lung diseases. A reduction in D_lCO also suggests pulmonary hypertension, vasculitis, or early/mild interstitial lung disease.

Vital capacity (VC) is the volume expired after a maximal inspiration and can be measured by simple spirometry. When the VC falls below 50% of the predicted value, CO_2 retention usually begins to occur. Secretion clearance can be impaired when the VC falls below 30 cc/kg; and progressive CO_2 retention, requiring ventilatory support, can occur when the VC falls below 10 cc/kg.

Maximum voluntary ventilation (MVV) is the volume of air that can be moved in and out of lungs in 1 minute. The MVV represents an ideal measure of overall ventilatory function.

Minute ventilation (V_E) is the total amount of air moved per minute, usually measured at rest

$$V_E = RR \times V_t$$

where RR is the respiratory rate.

Risk Factors for Pulmonary Complications

Several clinical factors, such as a history of smoking, chronic bronchitis, airflow obstruction, obesity, or a

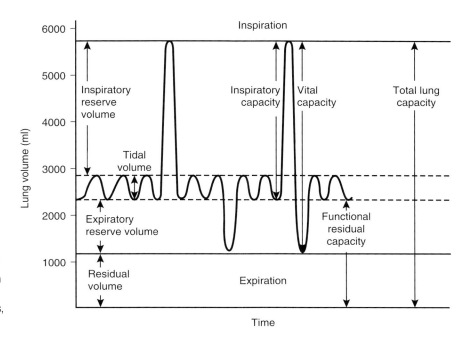

FIGURE 51–2 Spirometric measurement of lung volumes in the normal adult. (Adapted from Guyton AC, Hall JE: Textbook of Medical Physiology [10th ed]. Philadelphia: WB Saunders, 2000:437.)

Table 51–1
Risk factors for postoperative pulmonary complications

Cough

Dyspnea

Pulmonary disease

Smoking

Obesity

Abdominal or thoracic surgery

$FEV_1 < 2$ liters

MVV < 50% of predicted value

PEF < 100 L/min or < 50% of predicted value

$Paco_2 > 45$ mmHg

$Pao_2 < 50$ mmHg

FEV_1, forced expiratory volume in 1 second; MVV, maximum voluntary ventilation; PEF, peak expiratory flow rate; $Paco_2$, partial pressure of carbon dioxide in arterial blood; Pao_2, partial pressure of oxygen in arterial blood. From King MS: Preoperative evaluation. Am Fam Physician 2000;62: 387–396, with permission.

prolonged preoperative hospital stay may predict an increased frequency of pulmonary complications. Respiratory insufficiency can result from pneumonia, atelectasis, pulmonary embolism, or lobar collapse due to mucous plugging of airways. Morbidly obese patients may have undiagnosed sleep apnea or hypoventilation as well as a twofold risk of pneumonia compared to normal patients. The risk of postoperative pulmonary complications is increased two- to threefold in patients with chronic obstructive pulmonary disease (COPD). Table 51–1 summarizes some risk factors that may be predictive of postoperative pulmonary complications.

Classification of Respiratory Failure

Respiratory failure can be broadly classified into three categories: acute hypoxemic, hypercapneic, and perioperative respiratory failure. Understanding the pathophysiology of each of these types can provide useful insights to optimize ventilator support and the means to wean the patient from the ventilator. Figure 51–3 depicts features of the three forms of respiratory failure.

Hypoxic Respiratory Failure

Hypoxic respiratory failure occurs because of impaired gas exchange; it is usually associated with tachypnea and hypercapnia resulting from disease processes that cause diffuse alveolar flooding or collapse such as pneumonia, atelectasis, and pulmonary hemorrhage. Figure 51–3 depicts a flooded or collapsed alveolus, wherein an intrapulmonary shunt (Q_S/Q_T) develops, resulting in hypoxemia. In healthy individuals, hypoxemia can be defined as a PaO_2 below 80 mmHg. In critically ill patients, a PaO_2 less than 60 mmHg defines hypoxemia. In elderly individuals, normal and age-related decreases in arterial oxygen tension should be taken into account before diagnosing hypoxemia using the following formula:

$$PaO_2 = 104.2 - [0.27 \times age\ (years)]$$

Hypoxic respiratory failure may occur as a result of the following six basic pathologic processes: shunt, V/Q mismatch, low inspired FiO_2, hypoventilation, diffusion impairment, and low mixed venous O_2 content. A V/Q mismatch is the most common cause of hypoxemia.

Hypercapneic Respiratory Failure

Hypercapnia can be defined as a $PaCO_2$ of 45 mmHg or more. In a patient with severe obstruction to exhalation, respiratory rates higher than 14 breaths per minute should be avoided to allow sufficient time for exhalation. Treatable causes of hypercapneic respiratory failure include upper airway obstruction, respiratory muscle weakness, and depression of the central respiratory drive. Respiratory muscle weakness can stem from a variety of causes, including aging, malnutrition, myopathy, and metabolic disorders. Other disorders that may involve respiratory failure include disorders of peripheral nerves: Guillain-Barré syndrome, critical illness polyneuropathy, disorders of the neuromuscular junction such as myasthenia gravis, Eaton-Lambert syndrome, organophosphate poisoning, and botulism. Primary disorders of the chest wall, such as severe kyphoscoliosis, obesity, and pleural thickening, can also cause hypoventilation and increased work of breathing, leading to hypercapnic respiratory failure. Figure 51–3 depicts decreased alveolar ventilation (V_A) resulting in hypercapnia. The CO_2 level in the blood (PCO_2) is directly proportional to the rate of CO_2 production by peripheral tissues (VCO_2) and inversely proportional to the rate of CO_2 elimination by alveolar ventilation V_A. Although mild hypoxia with this form of respiratory failure can be corrected with supplemental oxygen, therapy should also be focused on correcting the underlying cause of hypoventilation and increased mechanical load.

Perioperative Respiratory Failure

Many elderly patients exhibit perioperative respiratory failure. It can involve both hypoxemia and hypercapnia. *Functional residual capacity* (FRC) is the lung volume that remains in the lung after a normal expiration, and

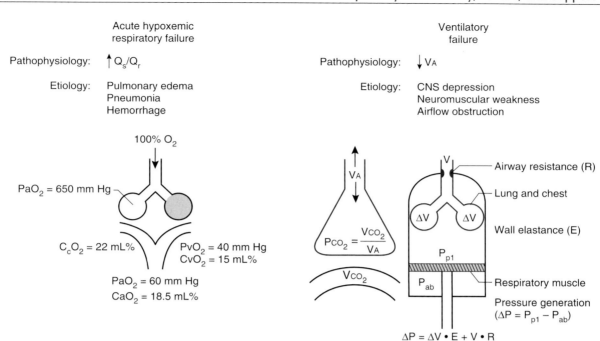

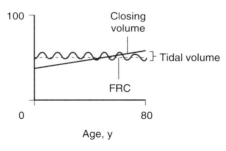

FIGURE 51–3 Classification of various forms of respiratory failure. With acute hypoxemic respiratory failure *(left)*, severe, refractory hypoxemia occurs when mixed venous blood traverses nonventilated lung units, as shown in the two-compartment model of the lung. Q_s/Q_t, intrapulmonary shunt; Cao_2, Cco_2, and Cvo_2, content of oxygen in arterial, capillary, and venous blood, respectively; Pao_2 and Pvo_2, partial pressure of oxygen in arterial and venous blood, respectively. With ventilatory failure *(center)*, gas exchange abnormalities are marked by decreasing alveolar ventilation (V_A), resulting in hypercapnea with proportional hypoxia. This diminished alveolar ventilation results from mismatch of respiratory load and neuromuscular function. CNS, central nervous system; $Paco_2$, partial pressure of CO_2 in arterial blood; Vco_2, production of CO_2 per minute; ΔV, tidal volume in liters; P_{pl}, pleural pressure; P_{ab}, abdominal pressure; V, minute ventilation. With perioperative respiratory failure *(right)*, lung volumes at which airways close (which increase with age, smoking history, and fluid overload), intersect with decreasing functional residual capacity (FRC) (associated with supine position, obesity, or abdominal surgery) to produce atelectasis, hypoxia, or predisposition to infection. (From Hall JB, Lawrence WD: Liberation of the patient from mechanical ventilation. JAMA 1987;257:1621–1627. Copyrighted 1987, American Medical Association.)

residual volume (RV) is the lung volume that remains in the lungs after a maximal expiration. In normal individuals, the FRC accounts for 50% of the total lung capacity, and the RV is approximately 25% of the total lung capacity. When pleural pressure exceeds the intraluminal pressure, airways close. The volume at which the airways close increases with age, smoking history, and fluid overload. In addition, FRC decreases with supine positioning and in patients with increased abdominal pressure including obesity, recent abdominal surgery, ascites, or peritonitis. Atelectasis and arterial hypoxemia in combination with the causes of neuromuscular weakness add up to produce severe hypoxemia and hypoventilation.

Preoperative Pulmonary Function Testing

Techniques

Airflow parameters during pulmonary function testing (PFTs) that are useful include the FEV_1 and the forced expiratory flow rate in the middle 50% of the forced expiratory flow curve. Clinical assessments are the 6-minute walking distance, stair climbing effort, and laboratory measurements of exercise capacity (e.g., maximum O_2 consumption during exercise). Measurements of preoperative PFTs are not routinely indicated in all patients. They should be reserved for high risk patients and patients undergoing thoracic and upper abdominal surgeries. In patients with chronic obstructive pulmonary disease (COPD) or asthma, PFTs are useful for estimating disease severity and identifying interventions that may decrease the risk of postoperative complications.

Arterial blood gases should be obtained preoperatively in patients with lung disease. Hypercapnia has been associated with an increased incidence of postoperative pulmonary complications, and hypercapnia in patients with COPD is associated with a shortened life expectancy. A chest radiograph is indicated in patients with evidence of new or deteriorating pulmonary disease, patients who have had no prior medical care, and those at high risk.

Functional residual capacity (FRC) is the volume that remains in the lung after expiration of a tidal volume. *Closure volume* (CV) is the lung volume at the time the flow from the dependent portions of the lungs stops during expiration due to airway closure. Under normal conditions, the FRC accounts for 50% and the CV for 30% of capacity. Reductions in FRC are significant in causing pulmonary complications: The FRC decreases by 10% to 15% after lower abdominal surgery, by approximately 30% after upper abdominal surgery, and by approximately 35% after thoracotomy and lung resection. Other factors that cause decreased FRC include supine positioning, obesity, the presence of ascites, the development of peritonitis, and exposure to general anesthesia.

Correction of Preoperative Deficiencies

For elective surgery in patients with evidence of severe pulmonary dysfunction, spirometry can be used to assess the need for a period of pulmonary rehabilitation to improve the preoperative pulmonary status. Decreased pulmonary complications have been reported in patients who stopped smoking at least 8 weeks before planned surgery. High risk patients benefit from preoperative pulmonary rehabilitation. Incentive spirometry for 15 minutes four times a day should be started preoperatively and continued for 3 to 5 days postoperatively. In patients with a new productive cough, antibiotic treatment should be given for 1 to 2 weeks and any elective surgery postponed. Patients should be instructed to stop smoking as soon as the operation is planned and be started on a transdermal nicotine replacement system if warranted. In patients with asthma, elective operations should be postponed until they are symptom-free.

Preoperative pulmonary rehabilitation is a multidisciplinary process that involves education, supervised exercise to improve cardiovascular fitness, medication compliance, and pulmonary hygiene. This approach may be useful in selected patients who are at high risk for pulmonary complications. Chest physical therapy includes deep breathing exercises along with chest percussion and postural drainage, perioperative intermittent positive-pressure breathing, and incentive spirometry. Chest therapy, particularly incentive spirometry, is a reasonable prophylactic measure in patients to prevent atelectasis.

Intraoperative Presentation of Respiratory Insufficiency

Bronchospasm is a common cause of respiratory failure and can be life-threatening in asthmatic patients. It can present intraoperatively and responds to bronchodilator treatment.

Phrenic nerve injury is a known complication of coronary artery bypass grafting (CABG) but may also occur in association with other cardiothoracic procedures, such as valve replacement or lung transplantation. Ten percent of patients undergoing CABG sustain phrenic nerve injury, usually involving the left phrenic nerve. It is due to thermal injury caused by the cold cardioplegia solution and results in demyelination and axonal degeneration of the phrenic nerve. Such injury should be suspected in the appropriate patient if attempts to wean the patient from the ventilator result in hypercapnia and/or atelectasis.

Venous air embolism can be a cause of respiratory insufficiency during the intraoperative period and may occur during various surgical procedures such as total hip arthroplasty, arthroscopy, hysteroscopy, laparoscopy, cesarean section, head and neck or neurologic surgery, liver transplantation, venous reconstruction, or peritoneovenous shunt. Venous embolism can mimic pulmonary thromboembolism and may present with cough, chest pain, wheezing, tachycardia, and hypotension. Treatment consists of immediately placing the patient in the Trendelenberg position (left lateral decubitus position). Severe cases may benefit from treatment with hyperbaric oxygen (if available).

Fat embolism can present intraoperatively. Although it is commonly associated with long bone fractures, it may be seen with a host of other entities, including pelvic fractures, total hip or knee replacement, median sternotomy, bone marrow transplant, renal transplant, cardiopulmonary bypass, burns, septic shock, and blood transfusions.

Postoperative Respiratory Insufficiency

Although the cause of respiratory failure is most often related to the lung parenchyma and interstitium, respiratory failure can result from simple mechanical causes such as pneumothorax, hydrothorax, obstruction of the endotracheal tube due to a mucous plug or kinking, or ascites. Depressed consciousness, inadequate postoperative analgesia, or ineffective cough can lead to decreased ability to clear secretions and may be complicated by atelectasis or pneumonia. Table 51–2 lists the causes of postoperative respiratory insufficiency. The following discussion focuses on these causes and highlights their relevance in the postoperative setting.

Atelectasis/Mucous Plugging

A common occurrence in the postoperative surgical patient, atelectasis and mucous plugging can lead to significant hypoxemia and respiratory distress. Atelectasis typically occurs in lung bases and is distributed segmentally.

Pneumonia

Ventilator-associated pneumonia (VAP) is a significant cause of morbidity in patients on mechanical ventilation, particularly after extensive traumatic injury. Risk factors specific for posttraumatic patients include severe chest injury, a need for abdominal and/or thoracic surgery, the presence of shock, and a high Injury Severity Score (ISS). In intensive care unit (ICU) patients, VAP may be due to prolonged endotracheal intubation, indiscriminate use of

Table 51–2
Causes of postoperative respiratory failure

Factors Extrinsic to the Lung

Depression of central respiratory drive (anesthetics, opioids, sedatives)

Phrenic nerve injury/diaphragmatic paralysis

Obstructive sleep apnea

Factors Intrinsic to the Lung

Atelectasis

Pneumonia

Aspiration

Acute lung injury (ALI)

Acute respiratory distress syndrome (ARDS)

Volume overload/congestive heart failure

Pulmonary embolism

Bronchospasm/COPD

Adapted from Kotloff RM: Acute respiratory failure in the surgical patient. In Fishman AP (ed): Fishman's Pulmonary Diseases and Disorders (3rd ed). New York: McGraw-Hill, 1998, with permission of The McGraw-Hill Companies.

broad-spectrum antibiotics, or the use of pharmacologic paralysis. Strict compliance with conscientious hand washing is a "low-tech" method to reduce the incidence of VAP.

Pulmonary Embolism

Pulmonary embolism (PE) is a significant cause of morbidity and mortality, particularly during the postoperative period. Most clinically significant PEs arise from a deep venous thrombosis (DVT) in the thigh and less often from clots originating below the knee. Pulmonary vascular obstruction results in a V/Q mismatch, gas exchange abnormalities, severe hypoxemia, and decreased cardiac output. In some patients, a PE can slowly progress to worsening pulmonary hypertension, eventually leading to *cor pulmonale*. Pulmonary embolism should be considered among the causes of respiratory failure if at any time the pulmonary artery systolic pressure suddenly exceeds 40 mmHg. The screening tests for pulmonary thromboembolism include a nuclear medicine V/Q scan and, more recently, spiral computed tomography (CT) scans of the chest. Pulmonary angiography remains the gold standard test for diagnosing PE. Most hospitals now implement guidelines for prevention of DVT. Prophylactic measures include elastic compression stockings, intermittent pneumatic compression of the lower extremities, and the use of low-dose subcutaneous heparin or low-molecular-weight heparin. Recurrent DVTs should prompt one to initiate a work-up for the many hypercoagulable states.

Pulmonary Edema

Pulmonary edema can result from some combination of increased capillary hydrostatic pressure, decreased plasma oncotic pressure, and increased pulmonary capillary permeability. As fluid collects in the lung interstitium, increased pulmonary vascular resistance and narrowing of bronchi occurs, resulting in decreased ventilation and perfusion. Because ventilation is decreased more than perfusion, the V/Q ratio is decreased. Long-standing pulmonary edema, especially the protein-rich edema due to capillary leakage, can lead to pulmonary fibrosis and can permanently alter lung function.

Aspiration

Aspiration of gastric contents significantly increases the risk for pneumonia. Even in the absence of pneumonia, severe chemical pneumonitis develops as a result of the inflammatory response, which results in severe respiratory failure. The inflammatory response is characterized by neutrophil and platelet infiltration, increased capillary permeability, alveolar flooding, decreased surfactant production, microvascular thrombosis, impaired gas exchange, and decreased compliance.

Measures should be taken to prevent aspiration in high risk patients by providing adequate nasogastric suction and raising the head of the bed to 30–45 degrees if possible. In patients with skeletal fractures, early fracture fixation, which decreases the time in skeletal traction (and thereby decreases the time spent in the supine position), can improve pulmonary mechanics and reduce the incidence of aspiration. In patients with gross aspiration, there is a role for early, aggressive bronchoscopy to remove particulate matter. Because bronchoscopy itself is associated with such complications as barotrauma, transient hypoxemia, hypercapnia,

increased intracranial pressure, and pneumothorax, it should be reserved for selected patients demonstrating hypoxia.

Obstructive Sleep Apnea

Obstructive sleep apnea (OSA) is a relatively common disorder, affecting 2% to 4% of the U.S. population. It is associated with obesity, anatomic narrowing of the upper airway passages, and snoring. OSA is characterized by episodes of upper airway obstruction, resulting in hypercapnia and cardiac arrhythmia. These patients are also at increased risk for postoperative pulmonary complications because anesthetics, sedatives, and opioid analgesics can relax the upper airway musculature and increase the frequency of apneic episodes. OSA patients should be started on nasal continuous positive airway pressure (CPAP) after extubation and be monitored closely during the perioperative period.

Acute Respiratory Distress Syndrome

The acute respiratory distress syndrome (ARDS) occurs in an estimated 150,000 patients in the United States every year and continues to be a significant etiology of morbidity and mortality in the ICU. Etiologies of ARDS can be divided into direct and indirect causes. The causes of direct lung injury include aspiration, pneumonia, near drowning, inhalation injury, and pulmonary contusion. The causes of indirect lung injury include factors "distant" from the lung, such as sepsis, systemic inflammatory response syndrome, multiple transfusions after shock and resuscitation, and other systemic processes such as pancreatitis. Table 51–3 outlines the clinical disorders associated with ARDS.

Acute respiratory distress syndrome may present as two distinct clinical entities: early and late forms. The early

Table 51–3
Recommended criteria for acute lung injury and acute respiratory distress syndrome diagnoses

Diagnosis	Timing	Oxygenation	Chest Radiograph	Pulmonary Artery Wedge Pressure
ALI	Acute onset	Pao$_2$/Fio$_2$ ≤ 300 mmHg (regardless of PEEP level)	Bilateral infiltrates seen on frontal chest radiograph	≤ 18 mmHg when measured or no clinical evidence of left atrial hypertension
ARDS	Acute onset	Pao$_2$/Fio$_2$ ≤ 200 mmHg (regardless of PEEP level)	Bilateral infiltrates seen on frontal chest radiograph	≤ 18 mmHg when measured or no clinical evidence of left atrial hypertension

Adapted from Bernard GR, Artigas A, Brigham KL, et al: Conference report: the American-European Consensus Conference on ARDS. Am J Respir Crit Care Med 1994;149:818–824. Official Journal of the American Thoracic Society. © American Lung Association.

form of ARDS occurs within 48 hours of injury and is often seen with profound hemorrhagic shock. The late form appears more than 48 hours after injury and is associated with pulmonary contusion and infection (pneumonia). Radiographically, ARDS appears as diffuse, patchy alveolar infiltrates on the chest film (Fig. 51–4). Table 51–4 categorizes several clinical disorders associated with ARDS.

Several classification schemes have been used to define ARDS. The terms "acute lung injury" and ARDS were recently clarified by a consensus conference to standardize the terminology in clinical studies and patient care (Table 51–4). ARDS can be difficult to distinguish from other pulmonary diseases, particularly when it occurs with a simultaneous or subsequent infection (e.g., bacterial or viral pneumonia). Bronchoscopy with bronchoalveolar lavage (BAL) can be a useful diagnostic test in patients with diffuse pulmonary infiltration and can help with the decision to initiate antibiotic therapy.

Much of the focus regarding treatment of ARDS has been on the mechanical ventilator. Although historically a high tidal volume of 12 to 15 cc/kg body weight has been advocated, recent studies from the ARDS network have shown decreased mortality rates at lower tidal volumes (6 cc/kg). The use of positive end-expiratory pressure (PEEP) purportedly increases the FRC by recruiting collapsed alveoli and potentially improves oxygenation in these patients. In patients with ARDS, a V/Q mismatch in the dependent portions of the lung can result in hypoxemia. As ARDS is an inhomogeneous process, the technique of prone positioning can help improve oxygenation by orienting the "healthy lung" to the dependent (and therefore better perfused) portions of the lung.

Nitric oxide is an inhaled vasodilator that redistributes blood flow from nonventilated lung units to ventilated units. A randomized trial of inhaled (by titration to a ventilator circuit) nitric oxide versus placebo in adults demonstrated clinically insignificant improvements in PaO_2 and a minor reduction in pulmonary artery pressures. There was no reduction in mortality with nitric oxide in this study, and its use in adults for treatment of respiratory failure cannot be advocated.

Prone positioning has been advocated as a technique to improve oxygenation in patients with respiratory failure, particularly ARDS. The mechanisms of this improvement are not entirely clear, but they involve changes in regional inflation, redistribution of tidal ventilation, a more homogeneous distribution of pulmonary blood flow, increased FRC, and a change in regional diaphragmatic motion. A recent study by Gattinoni and colleagues in Milan, Italy documented a significant increase in PaO_2 in the patients treated with prone positioning compared to conventionally treated (supine) patients, but the study failed to demonstrate an improvement in survival in the prone group.

The use of exogenously administered surfactant has shown promise for respiratory failure in newborns, but its utility in older patients has not been clearly defined. Clinical trials with administration of animal-derived and synthetic surfactant are currently underway to define the role of this therapy in adults.

Patients with preexisting lung disease are already at high risk for postoperative pulmonary complications. In addition, pathophysiologic changes that occur intraoperatively and postoperatively (e.g., bronchospasm, aspiration, atelectasis, pain, pulmonary edema) can increase the risk of complications. Adequate postoperative analgesia and institution of incentive spirometry are important for preventing atelectasis. Aggressive pulmonary toilet should be instituted, including bronchodilators (in the presence of wheezing), β-agonists, and atropine analogs in asthmatic patients. Patients on the ventilator have difficulty mobilizing

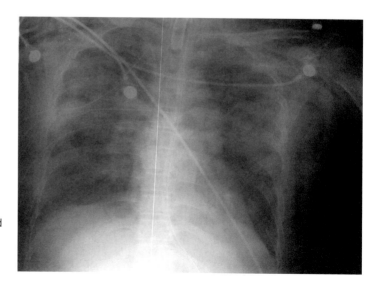

FIGURE 51–4 Top radiograph depicts an acute respiratory distress syndrome (ARDS) pattern in the lung fields of a 46-year-old man admitted after he fell from a tree, sustaining a pelvic fracture. He had a prolonged intensive care unit course, including ventilator-dependent respiratory failure and ARDS.

Table 51–4
Clinical disorders associated with the development of ARDS

Direct Lung Injury
Common Causes

  Pneumonia
  Aspiration of gastric contents

Less Common Causes

  Pulmonary ventilation
  Fat emboli
  Near-drowning
  Inhalational injury
  Reperfusion pulmonary edema after lung transplantation or
    pulmonary embolectomy

Indirect Lung Injury
Common Causes

  Sepsis
  Severe trauma with shock and multiple transfusions

Less Common Causes

  Cardiopulmonary bypass
  Drug overdose
  Acute pancreatitis
  Transfusions of blood products

secretions and require adequate airway suctioning periodically. However, airway suctioning should not be performed on a scheduled basis because it can be associated with a host of potential complications such as hypoxemia, airway trauma, cardiac arrhythmia, atelectasis, infection, increased intracranial pressure, and bronchospasm. If respiratory acidosis fails to correct with the usual ventilatory modes, causes of excess CO_2 production (e.g., overfeeding, fever, inadequate sedation) should be considered.

Mechanical Ventilation

Basics of Mechanical Ventilation

Mechanical ventilation serves two basic functions: ventilation and oxygenation support. Ventilatory support augments gas movement and exchange in the airways and alveoli by using positive airway pressure, and oxygenation support is given to reverse any V/Q mismatch. The common indications for starting mechanical ventilation include severely impaired

gas exchange, rapid onset of respiratory failure, and increased work of breathing with evidence of respiratory muscle fatigue. The goals of mechanical ventilation include improved gas exchange, reversed hypoxemia, relieved respiratory distress, decreased work of breathing, diminished respiratory muscle fatigue, corrected respiratory acidosis, and altered pressure-volume relations because of improved compliance of the lungs and reversal of atelectasis. Table 51–5 offers guidelines for instituting mechanical ventilation.

Endotracheal intubation serves to establish a secure airway and facilitate suctioning of oropharyngeal secretions. Gross aspiration of gastric secretions can be somewhat reduced by properly inflating the endotracheal tube cuff, however, microaspiration is not prevented by the endotracheal cuff. A sudden increase in peak airway pressures at the ventilator suggests obstruction of the endotracheal tube due to kinking or a mucous plug.

Defined as positive airway pressure at the end of expiration, PEEP may be useful in patients with hypoxemic respiratory failure such as ARDS or cardiogenic pulmonary edema. PEEP can be useful for preventing alveolar collapse and may redistribute alveolar fluid in pulmonary edema, thereby improving any V/Q mismatch. Low levels of PEEP should be maintained in patients with COPD. High levels of PEEP can cause an increase in peak and mean airway pressures and may result in barotrauma and hypotension due to decreased venous return. Weaning patients from high levels of PEEP should occur in 2- to 3-cm H_2O

Table 51–5
Guidelines for initiation of mechanical ventilation

Ventilation failure
  Respiratory acidosis with pH $\leq$ 7.25
  Evidence of progressive or impending ventilation failure
    Rising partial pressure of carbon dioxide
    Tachypnea with air hunger
    Diaphragmatic weakness or fatigue
      Paradoxical movement of the abdominal wall
    Vital capacity < 15 cc/kg
    Maximum inspiratory pressure $\geq$ −30 cm H_2O →
      $|IP_{Max}| \leq 30$ cm H_2O
    Maximum expiratory pressure $\leq$ 30 cm H_2O →
      $|EP_{Max}| \leq 30$ cm H_2O
Oxygenation failure
  Refractory hypoxemia

increments to prevent sudden atelectasis, which would lead to severe hypoxemia.

Modes of Mechanical Ventilation

Two of the major advances in critical care medicine have been (1) the ability to place and maintain an artificial airway and (2) the development and ongoing refinement of the mechanical ventilator. The commonly used modes of mechanical ventilation include assist control (AC), intermittent mandatory ventilation (IMV), and pressure control (PC). The AC and IMV modes are volume-cycled, whereas PC is pressure-cycled.

In the AC mode, the patient's spontaneous respirations trigger the ventilator to deliver a preset tidal volume with every breath. If there are no spontaneous respirations, the ventilator defaults to the preset tidal volume and preset respiratory rate. In the IMV mode, the ventilator coordinates the machine-delivered breaths with the patient's spontaneous breaths, ensuring at least the minimal rate and tidal volume. The patient is allowed to take additional, spontaneous breaths that are not assisted by the ventilator (except with the addition of pressure support, as described below). In the PC mode, ventilating gas is delivered at a high flow rate to achieve a preset pressure limit, thereby minimizing barotrauma. Barotrauma is thought to occur at airway pressures higher than 30 to 35 cm H_2O and is quickly damaging at pressures exceeding 50 cm H_2O.

Inverse ratio ventilation (IRV) is a method of ventilation useful in patients experiencing difficulty with oxygenation because of severe lung disease. The normal inhalation/exhalation ratio (I/E) is 1:3 to 1:4. By reversing the ratio (and increasing the time spent during inspiration), the mean airway pressure is increased. In patients with noncompliant ("stiff") lungs, oxygenation typically improves.

Mechanical ventilation should be used judiciously to minimize adverse effects. Potential complications of mechanical ventilation include barotrauma, "volutrauma" (due to alveolar stretch), pneumothorax, infection, aspiration of gastric contents, and bronchospasm. Pulmonary infections can result from impaired defense of the lung against the invading microorganisms, impaired cough and mucociliary clearance mechanisms, and atelectasis. Sudden hypotension in a patient on a ventilator may be due to a pneumothorax that has progressed to a tension pneumothorax.

Weaning Patients from Mechanical Ventilation

As patients recover from the physiologic derangements of anesthesia, a surgical procedure, or some other pathologic insult, it is important to discontinue ventilatory support at the earliest possible time. With the advances in medicine and the ability to keep critically ill patients alive even longer, standard weaning criteria are no longer applicable

to each and every patient. Premature discontinuation of mechanical ventilation can lead to severe stress on a patient's cardiovascular and respiratory system and so impede recovery. Traditional predictors of weaning—maximal negative inspiratory force, vital capacity, minute ventilation—have revealed mixed results. A more successful predictor has been the rapid shallow breathing technique, as reflected by the respiratory rate/tidal volume ratio (f/V_t) measured during spontaneous breathing. Weaning a patient on the ventilator involves the use of clinical judgment by the physician as well as knowledge of the underlying disease process along with the objective criteria, all of which help predict success at extubation. This may incorporate one or more of the following adjuncts.

1. *Synchronized intermittent mandatory ventilation (SIMV).* During the early 1970s, the SIMV mode was introduced with claims of an efficient weaning approach. This mode allows the patient to breathe spontaneously in concert with the mechanical ventilator.

2. *Pressure support ventilation.* Pressure support ventilation (PSV) was introduced during the 1980s. This method of weaning involves administering a set pressure to "assist" every inspiratory effort, which is slowly decreased as the patient improves, just prior to extubation. This method of ventilation should be optimized to overcome the resistance caused by the endotracheal tube and ventilator circuit tubing.

3. *Spontaneous breathing trials.* This method involves the institution of spontaneous breathing using only a T-piece connector to the endotracheal tube and gradually increasing the duration of the trial, working toward extubation. The goal is to recondition the respiratory muscles that may be debilitated from prolonged illness and mechanical ventilation. There is evidence from recent trials that once-a-day trials of spontaneous breathing are superior to SIMV and PS for weaning patients from ventilatory support.

Tracheostomy

Although some studies have advocated early tracheostomy (defined as being performed between days 3 and 7 after ICU admission) to reduce ventilator days, facilitate weaning, and decrease pneumonia rates in critically ill patients, others have failed to show any benefit. At this point, the timing and utility of tracheostomy in the ICU is speculative, and further prospective randomized trials are needed to determine if early tracheostomy is beneficial.

Noninvasive Ventilation

Noninvasive ventilation can be used to support patients after extubation who have COPD or hypercapneic respiratory failure. This is often accomplished by using tight-fitting masks and assisting the patient's respiratory effort. Gastric distention can occur and may result in vomiting and aspiration. CPAP can be delivered by nasal mask and can be effective in the management of obstructive sleep apnea. CPAP may also have a role in the management of pulmonary edema by improving any V/Q imbalance and restoring the FRC. The nasal mask is better tolerated than a face mask. Bilevel positive-pressure ventilation (BIPAP) is a mode of ventilation that requires a ventilator and a tight-fitting facial mask. It is often used to decrease respiratory muscle fatigue by providing a combination of PEEP and pressure support to assist spontaneous breaths.

Conclusions

Pulmonary complications are the most common cause of morbidity in the postoperative patient. It is imperative to identify the high risk patient and take adequate prophylactic measures to minimize such complications. Minimally invasive procedures (e.g., laparoscopic surgery and endoscopic stent grafts) have gained widespread acceptance, in part due to a decreased length of stay in the hospital for which a decrease in pulmonary complications is partly responsible. Understanding the pathophysiology of respiratory function and the various forms of respiratory failure can help the physician select the appropriate therapeutic interventions. Mechanical ventilation has evolved significantly in recent years, and management of the ventilatory patient is a science itself.

Despite these significant advances in ICU management and mechanical ventilation techniques, ARDS is associated with significant mortality. As the underlying pathophysiology of ARDS is better understood, it remains to be seen whether the new technology and other approaches can help decrease the mortality rate. As the population ages, primary care physicians and specialists should be more aware of the risk factors for pulmonary complications and take appropriate steps to minimize them.

Bibliography

ARDS Network: Ventilation with lower tidal volumes as compared with traditional tidal volumes for acute lung injury and the acute respiratory distress syndrome. N Engl J Med 2000;342:1301–1308.

Bartlett RH: Critical Care. *In* Greenfield LJ (ed): Surgery: Scientific Principles and Practice of Surgery. Philadelphia: Lippincott Williams & Wilkins, 1993.

Bernard GR, Artigas A, Brigham KL, et al: Conference Report: the American-European consensus conference on ARDS. Am J Respir Crit Care Med 1994;149:818–824.

Croce MA: Diagnosis of acute respiratory distress syndrome and differentiation from ventilator-associated pneumonia. Am J Surg 2000;179:26S–29S.

Croce MA, Fabian TC, Davis KA, et al: Early and late acute respiratory distress syndrome: two distinct clinical entities. J Trauma 1999;46:361–368.

Dellinger RP, Zimmerman JL, Taylor RW, et al: Effects of inhaled nitric oxide in patients with acute respiratory distress syndrome: results of a randomized phase II trial. Crit Care Med 1998;26:15–23.

Deppe AS, Thompson DR, Barrette RR: Other embolic syndromes. *In* Civetta JM, Taylor RW, Kirby RR (eds): Critical Care (3rd ed). Philadelphia: Lippincott Williams & Wilkins, 1997.

Doye RL: Assessing and modifying the risk of postoperative pulmonary complications. Chest 1999;115:77s–81s.

Esteban A, Frutos F, Tobin MJ, et al: A comparison of four methods of weaning patients from mechanical ventilation. N Engl J Med 1995;332:345.

Ferguson M: Preoperative assessment of pulmonary risk. Chest 1999;115:58S–63S.

Gattinoni L, Tognoni G, Presenti A: Effect of prone positioning on survival of patients with acute respiratory failure. N Engl J Med 2001;345:568–573.

Guyton AC, Hall JE: Textbook of Medical Physiology (10th ed). Philadelphia: WB Saunders, 2000.

Hall JB, Lawrence WD: Liberation of the patient from mechanical ventilation. JAMA 1987;257:1621–1627.

Kacmarek RM, Stoller JK: Principles of respiratory care. *In* Shoemaker WB, Ayers SM, Grenvik A, et al (eds): Textbook of Critical Care (3rd ed). Philadelphia: WB Saunders, 1995.

King MS: Preoperative evaluation. Am Fam Physician 2000;62:387–396.

Kotloff RM: Acute respiratory failure in the surgical patient. *In* Fishman AP (ed): Fishman's Pulmonary Diseases and Disorders (3rd ed). New York: McGraw-Hill, 1998.

Kreit JW, Rogers RM: Approach to the patient with acute respiratory failure. *In* Shoemaker WB, Ayers SM, Grenvik A, et al (eds): Textbook of Critical Care (3rd ed). Philadelphia: WB Saunders, 1995.

Livingston DH: Prevention of ventilator-associated pneumonia. Am J Surg 2000;179(Suppl 2A):12S–17S.

Mecca RS, Fragoso CV: The lungs and their function. *In* Civetta JM, Taylor RW, Kirby RR (eds): Critical Care (3rd ed). Philadelphia: Lippincott Williams & Wilkins, 1997.

Nierman E, Zakerzewski K: Recognition and management of preoperative risk. Rheum Dis Clin North Am 1999;25: 585–623.

Reilly J Jr: Preoperative and postoperative care of standard and high risk surgical patients. Hematol Oncol Clin North Am 1997;11:449–459.

Salzman SH: Pulmonary function testing: tips on how to interpret the results. J Respir Dis 1999;20:809–822.

Shapiro BA, Peruzzi WT: Pulmonary complications. *In* Civetta JM, Taylor RW, Kirby RR (eds): Critical Care (3rd ed). Philadelphia: Lippincott Williams & Wilkins, 1997.

Shapiro M, Anderson HL III, Bartlett R: Respiratory failure: conventional and high-tech support. Surg Clin North Am 2000;80:871–883.

Tobin MJ: Advances in mechanical ventilation. N Engl J Med 2001;344:1986–1995.

Tobin MJ: Mechanical ventilation. N Engl J Med 1994;330: 1056–1061.

Ware L, Matthay MA: The acute respiratory distress syndrome. N Engl J Med 2000;342:1335–1349.

CHAPTER 52

Myocardial Insufficiency, Failure, and Support

*D. Glenn Pennington, M.D., William H. Messerschmidt, M.D.,
and Marcus G. Williams, M.D.*

This chapter is designed to address the problems associated with operating upon patients with cardiac disease that may affect the outcome of the surgical procedure. It is directed toward surgeons of all disciplines, including cardiac surgeons, but deals more often with noncardiac surgical issues. However, much of the information regarding assessment, monitoring, and therapeutic measures derives from the experience of performing cardiac surgery. It is our belief that many of the same principles and protocols that are used in cardiac surgical patients apply to the patient undergoing noncardiac surgery.

Preoperative Cardiac Assessment

The role of cardiac function during the perioperative course of noncardiac procedures has become increasingly important because the surgical population has an increasing percentage of patients of older age with obesity, diabetes, and abnormal lipid patterns, which correlate with a high incidence of coronary artery disease. It is estimated that about one third of the 27 million patients undergoing surgical procedures annually in the United States have coexisting coronary artery disease. The noncardiac surgeon is sometimes faced with the disappointment of having performed successful surgical procedures in patients who have poor outcomes because of cardiac complications such as myocardial infarction and congestive heart failure. Some patients with severe problems, such as a perforated viscus or gangrenous extremity, may require surgery regardless of their cardiovascular status. However, it is extremely important that a careful preoperative cardiac assessment be done in all patients undergoing surgery. The decision as to whether to undertake high-risk procedures in patients with known cardiac disease is becoming increasingly difficult. In 1996, the American College of Cardiology and American Heart Association published guidelines for the perioperative cardiovascular evaluation of noncardiac patients. These guidelines have been extremely helpful in determining how to assess the preoperative patient.

The Cardiac Risk Index System (CRIS) was developed for cardiac risk assessment in patients undergoing noncardiac operations (Table 52–1). The CRIS demonstrates the high risk of perioperative cardiac complications in patients

Table 52-1

Cardiac Risk Index System (CRIS)

	Factors	Points
History	Age >70 yr	5
	Myocardial infarction in prior 6 mo	10
	Aortic stenosis	3
Physical examination	S_3 gallop, jugular venous distention, or congestive heart failure	11
Electrocardiogram	Any rhythm other than sinus	7
	> 0 PVCs/min	7
General information	Pao_2 <60 mm Hg	3
	$Paco_2$ >50 mm Hg	3
	K^+ <3 mEq/L	3
	BUN >50 mg/dL	3
	Creatine >3 mg/dL	3
	Bedridden	3
Operation	Emergency	4
	Intrathoracic	3
	Intra-abdominal	3
	Aortic	3

Risk of cardiac complications by CRIS class:

Class I (0–5 points):	1%	Class III (13–25 points):	11%
Class II (6–12):	5%	Class IV (≥ 26 points):	22%

BUN, blood urea nitrogen; $Paco_2$, arterial carbon dioxide tension; Pao_2, arterial oxygen tension; PVC, premature ventricular contraction.
Data from Goldman L, Caldera DL, Nussbaum SR, et al: Multifactorial index of cardiac risk in noncardiac surgical procedures. N Engl J Med 1977;297:845; and Mangano L, Goldman DT: Pre-operative assessment of patients with known or suspected coronary disease. N Engl J Med 1995;333:1750. Copyright 1977 and 1995 Massachusetts Medical Society. All rights reserved.

with congestive heart failure or recent myocardial infarction and in patients greater than 70 years of age. The most important aspect of the assessment is the history and physical examination, which may already have been performed by a referring internist or family physician. However, it is incumbent upon the surgeon to assess the patient carefully and make an independent determination of cardiac risk factors. In the absence of any positive history, men over age 35 and women over age 40 are considered at risk for coronary artery disease. Elevated plasma cholesterol and a history of cigarette smoking are significant predictors of coronary artery disease, as highlighted by the Multiple Risk Factor Intervention Trial, and may prompt an evaluation of cardiac function even in younger patients. Other factors that may prompt a full cardiac investigation are cardiac rhythm other than sinus or evidence of congestive heart failure (S_3 gallop or jugular venous distention). If the patient has a history of valvular disease, angina pectoris, or previous myocardial infarction, the need for preoperative

cardiac assessment is obvious. Most patients with significant valvular disease will have some symptoms, with the exception of patients with occult aortic valvular stenosis, which is associated with a significant incidence of sudden death in athletes and can be an insidious risk. The diagnosis of aortic stenosis may be suspected preoperatively by hearing a murmur on physical examination or detecting left ventricular hypertrophy on the electrocardiogram. These findings should lead to the performance of an echocardiogram to rule out valvular disease. Dysrhythmias also must be assessed in the preoperative period. It is particularly important to take a history of symptoms of palpitations or syncope, and, on physical examination, one should carefully note the rate and rhythm. If arrhythmias are suspected, 12- to 24-hour electrocardiographic monitoring should be performed. Significant dysrhythmias that should be investigated and treated preoperatively include atrial fibrillation with uncontrolled ventricular response, multifocal premature ventricular contractions, and nonsustained ventricular tachycardia.

Angina pectoris is an extremely important symptom to uncover in the preoperative assessment. Patients with angina pectoris usually can be detected on the basis of history, but it is important to note that as many as 70% of patients with chronic stable angina have silent (asymptomatic) ischemia. The surgeon must be particularly alert to the possibility of unstable angina, defined as (1) crescendo angina, (2) angina with minimal exertion and at rest, (3) angina of new onset, or (4) change in stable anginal pattern during the previous 6 weeks. Unstable angina, of course, may be a harbinger of impending myocardial infarction. The surgeon therefore must be certain of the absence of unstable angina before proceeding with the operation.

Further evaluation of angina in the preoperative patient can be accomplished with diagnostic testing. For example, the resting electrocardiogram may demonstrate a previous myocardial infarction by the presence of a Q wave 0.04 second or wider in any of the 12 electrocardiographic leads, although the absence of pathologic Q waves does not mean there is no ischemia. There may be findings of left ventricular hypertrophy or nonsinus rhythm, but the resting electrocardiogram is often normal in patients who have ischemic heart disease. The ambulatory electrocardiogram has low sensitivity and low specificity for the detection of ischemic heart disease in patients without previously diagnosed coronary artery disease. The exercise electrocardiogram is the most helpful test in evaluating patients in whom the presence of cardiac ischemia is not clear. Among large groups of patients collected from the Seattle Heart Watch, indications of ischemic heart disease in patients undergoing exercise electrocardiograms were (1) depression of the ST segment (≥ 2 mm); (2) exercise-induced hypotension (equal to a 10-mm Hg fall in systolic blood pressure); (3) complex ventricular ectopy (three or more consecutive premature ventricular depolarizations); and (4) symptomatic chest pain.

Although exercise stress testing is useful and quite specific for ischemic heart disease, many patients cannot perform on a treadmill and therefore cannot be evaluated in this manner. Radioisotopic imaging is useful in these patients. Thallium-201 (^{201}Tl), a potassium analog, is the isotope that has been used most frequently for cardiac imaging. Thallium-201 is introduced intravenously during a period in which cardiac images are obtained during exercise. Three or more hours later, delayed images are obtained to determine redistribution of the radioisotope. This is based on the concept that ^{201}Tl is almost completely extracted from coronary arterial blood by healthy myocardial cells and therefore ^{201}Tl uptake reflects zones of perfused and viable heart. Decreased or absent ^{201}Tl uptake indicates myocardial hypoperfusion. The ^{201}Tl images thus always provide comparisons of uptake in one region with that of an adjacent region. On 3-hour resting

scans, regions that fill in are interpreted as having been ischemic during exercise, while zones that do not fill in are presumed to be dead fibrotic tissue. More recently, technetium-99m (^{99m}Tc)-labeled sestamibi has been used more extensively than ^{201}Tl for myocardial perfusion imaging. Because many patients cannot exercise, ^{201}Tl can be combined with adenosine or dipyridamole, both of which produce maximum coronary vasodilation. These vasodilators lead to hyperperfusion of normal zones and therefore to relative hypoperfusion of regions fed by diseased coronary vessels. Dobutamine stress echocardiography also can be useful in identifying inducible ischemia. It can be performed with bicycle or treadmill exercise or by using pharmacologic stress with an agent such as dipyridamole.

Single-photon emission computed tomography (SPECT) is the predominant imaging technique for the myocardial perfusion stress studies performed with ^{201}Tl and ^{99m}Tc discussed above. A more advanced technique, the use of positron-emission tomography (PET), has the advantages of being able to label and image biologically active compounds and drugs and the ability to derive absolute quantitative measurements. The primary indications for PET studies are the identification of myocardial viability in patients with established coronary artery disease and regional or global left ventricular dysfunction and the noninvasive diagnosis of coronary artery disease. When SPECT studies are equivocal regarding myocardial viability, PET may give the definitive answer.

Cardiac catheterization and coronary angiography are indicated in patients in whom there is a strong suspicion of coronary artery disease. If exercise scans are positive, there is evidence of disease by electrocardiographic findings, or the patient has a history of angina that has not been evaluated, cardiac catheterization should be performed. If, indeed, severe coronary arterial occlusive disease is identified in preoperative patients in whom surgery for the noncardiac problem can be delayed, coronary revascularization is indicated. In some instances, such as carotid artery stenosis in patients with coronary artery disease, a combined procedure may be indicated. Careful evaluation and judgment by the cardiac surgeon and the noncardiac surgeon are required to determine the best course for the patient when there is severe coexisting coronary artery disease in patients with noncardiac surgical disease.

In patients who have had previous myocardial infarctions, the overall incidence of new perioperative infarction during noncardiac surgery is 7%, but, if the previous myocardial infarction occurred within 3 months of the procedure, the incidence of perioperative infarction is 27% to 37%. Furthermore, the mortality rate in patients with myocardial infarctions during surgical procedures is high. However, the reinfarction rate and the mortality rate can be markedly diminished with the proper monitoring and pharmacologic control in patients undergoing general anesthesia. A rather dramatic reduction of mortality rate was demonstrated by comparison of two groups of patients at the Mayo Clinic: those operated upon during the 1960s without proper monitoring and pharmacologic intervention, and those operated upon in the 1980s, who were aggressively monitored and vigorously controlled in the operating room with vasodilators, inotropic agents, vasopressors, β-blockers, and antiarrhythmic agents. It is important to continue or make substitutions for the appropriate medications for patients with known cardiac disease or recognized high risk of cardiac complications who are undergoing surgery. For example, most patients requiring β-blockers, antiarrhythmics, or antianginal medications should be continued on those medications until the time that they actually go into the operating room. This usually can be accomplished by allowing patients to take oral medications with small amounts of water on the day of surgery. It is also important to maintain insulin treatment in diabetics, with a common practice of allowing one-half the usual daily dose of insulin to be given before the operation and then augmenting this with intravenous insulin during the procedure. Patients on thyroid hormone do not require additional doses, but patients on long-term corticosteroids should receive supplemental doses before operation, intraoperatively, and postoperatively.

Physiologic Monitoring

During the operation and in the early postoperative period, appropriate physiologic monitoring is extremely important for rapid assessment of physiologic or pathologic changes to which quick responses can prevent complications. Currently patients with known cardiac problems should be monitored extensively using the following guidelines:

- Continuous electrocardiographic monitoring throughout the operative and immediate postoperative period is utilized to detect evidence of ischemic changes or irregular rhythm, which could be treated acutely.

- Continuous peripheral oxygen saturation measurements are used to determine the adequacy of oxygenation.

- Continuous urinary output measurement from an indwelling bladder catheter is essential to determine effects on peripheral perfusion.

- Intracardiac pressure measurements are necessary in order to determine volume requirements.

In younger patients who have reasonably good ventricular function, central venous pressure measurements may be all that are required. However, in older patients and patients with compromised left ventricular function, a Swan-Ganz pulmonary arterial catheter will give accurate and helpful information. This provides a direct measurement of systolic and diastolic pulmonary artery pressure as well as an opportunity to intermittently or continuously measure mixed venous oxygen saturation. Along with the measurements of arterial oxygen saturation, the end-tidal CO_2 measured by the anesthesiologist will be very useful in determining the adequacy of ventilation. The use of end-tidal CO_2 and continuous arterial oxygen saturation measurements markedly reduces the number of arterial blood gas measurements required.

- The measurement of continuous mixed venous oxygen saturation is a valuable tool in detecting abrupt changes in tissue oxygen delivery and often can detect change much sooner than continuous cardiac output measurements. Because the mixed venous oxygen saturation is an indirect measurement of oxygen delivery to the body, it may be decreased by reduced delivery of oxygen resulting from low cardiac output, by decreased oxygen content of the arterial blood, or by increased oxygen demand by increased activity, fever, or hypermetabolic state leading to increased extraction of oxygen from the blood by the tissues. The mixed venous oxygen saturation is also very useful in the immediate postoperative period.

- Continuous cardiac output monitoring is useful and is employed in many centers, but is probably not as essential as some of the other parameters listed. The continuous cardiac output measurement is often rather slow in responding to acute changes, and mixed venous oxygen changes occur before continuous cardiac output changes.

There is controversy about the use of pulmonary artery catheters because some previous studies have indicated that their use for perioperative monitoring has not significantly reduced mortality in critically ill patients. In spite of these criticisms, cardiac surgical units continue to use the pulmonary artery catheter because it simplifies patient management. However, patients with normal or near-normal ventricular function do not require pulmonary artery catheters and can be managed with intraoperative echocardiography, central venous pressure measurements, and the other monitoring systems described.

An extremely valuable monitoring device frequently used in cardiac surgical patients is transesophageal echocardiography (TEE). This modality is very helpful in the operating room because one can detect changes in ventricular contractility or ventricular volume, evidence of valvular regurgitation, and acute changes in regional or global myocardial function. This technique has not been widely employed in patients undergoing noncardiac surgical procedures. In some patients with esophageal or gastric disease it would be contraindicated. However, in patients undergoing repair of peripheral vascular disease and in many other procedures, TEE may be very useful. In cardiac surgical patients, echocardiography is often used in place of a pulmonary artery catheter because the detection of intraoperative cardiac events is as effective as the use of pulmonary artery catheters or more so. The availability of TEE has been markedly improved by the training of the anesthesiologists to perform these procedures without requiring a cardiologist in the operating room. In patients with cardiac disease undergoing noncardiac surgical procedures, it is often appropriate to ask the cardiac anesthesiologist to perform intraoperative TEE, and it may be desirable for noncardiac anesthesiologists to develop these skills as well.

Laboratory Monitoring

Surgical patients with cardiac disease represent a particular challenge to the surgeon and anesthesiologist, particularly regarding metabolic derangement. Most patients with heart failure receive diuretics and often have hypokalemic alkalosis when they enter the operating room. It is important to monitor the serum electrolytes as well as arterial blood gases to determine whether these changes persist or worsen during the operation. Hypokalemia and alkalosis beget arrhythmias and therefore should be corrected as soon as possible. Blood sugar levels are also of particular importance because there may be a relationship between hyperglycemia and central nervous system changes in postoperative cardiac patients. An intensive insulin protocol that tightly controls glucose levels in the intensive care unit is superior to any of the previous sliding scale techniques that have been employed and promises to markedly reduce complications related to glucose abnormalities in the perioperative period.

Arterial blood gases are particularly important when patients have compromised peripheral perfusion, which can lead to the development of metabolic acidosis. Rapid detection of metabolic acidosis and correction by administration of sodium bicarbonate, as well as correcting the cause of the acidosis, will markedly improve the intraoperative course of a severely ill patient. Failure to recognize the insidious onset of metabolic acidosis may result in hypotension, severe arrhythmias, poor organ perfusion, and cardiac arrest, all of which could have been corrected by earlier detection.

The measurement of serum magnesium and calcium levels is also important. Hypocalcemia is associated with decreased ventricular function and often occurs after the administration of multiple blood products. Hypomagnesemia is a common cause of cardiac arrhythmias and should be corrected as soon as abnormalities are detected. The serum magnesium should usually be maintained at a level of 2.0 mg/dL or greater, particularly in patients with a history of arrhythmias. This can be accomplished by the administration of 1 to 2 g of intravenous magnesium sulfate. The measurement of blood urea nitrogen and creatinine as well as liver enzymes can be extremely helpful in detecting progressive low cardiac output states and can help determine whether there is hypovolemia, poor perfusion, or local ischemia. In low cardiac output states, the perfusion is shifted preferentially toward the coronary and cerebral circulation and away from the liver and kidneys.

Measurements of coagulation are also important both intraoperatively and in the intensive care unit. Cardiac patients particularly have difficulty with intraoperative and postoperative bleeding because of induced coagulation disorders. For example, aspirin inhibits platelet aggregation by irreversible inhibition of platelet cyclooxygenase and thus inhibits the generation of thromboxane A_2, a powerful inducer of platelet aggregation and vasoconstriction. Glycoprotein IIb/IIIa inhibitors, abciximab (ReoPro), eptifibatide (Integrelin), and tirofiban hydrochloride (Aggrastat) cause severe platelet dysfunction, which may necessitate platelet transfusions to stop bleeding in spite of normal platelet counts. Clopidogrel and ticlopidine are structurally related thienopyridine derivatives that produce their antiplatelet effects by inhibiting the ATP-dependent pathway of platelet activation. These slow-acting agents require 5 to 8 days to clear after stopping the drugs. Patients may be receiving coumadin, unfractionated heparin, or low-molecular-weight heparins such as enoxaparin sodium prior to coming to the operating room. These may cause severe coagulation abnormalities and require reversal with protamine or fresh frozen plasma. Partial thromboplastin time, prothrombin time, and the international normalized ratio as well as platelet counts should routinely be measured in patients receiving any of these medications. More recently, platelet function assays are being used to detect alterations of platelet function. If bleeding persists, disseminated intravascular coagulation (DIC) assays should be performed and treatment strategies should be based upon the results. Because ε-aminocaproic acid (Amicar) should not be used when there is evidence of active intravascular coagulation, a dilemma arises when it is not clear whether bleeding is due to DIC or primary fibrinolysis. The following tests may be helpful:

- The platelet count is usually decreased in DIC but normal in primary fibrinolysis.

- The protamine paracoagulation test is positive in DIC and negative in primary fibrinolysis.

- The euglobulin clot lysis test is abnormal in primary fibrinolysis and normal in DIC.

Antifibrinolytic agents such as Amicar and anti-inflammatory agents such as aprotinin, (Trasylol), a nonspecific serine protease inhibitor, may be very effective if they are used prophylactically. Whereas Amicar has been used in noncardiac surgery, Trasylol use has been limited to cardiac surgical patients.

In some surgical patients with occult congestive heart failure, pulmonary dysfunction may occur and the cardiac status may not be immediately apparent. Sometimes it is difficult to perform TEE in these patients because of gastroesophageal pathology or coagulopathy. In these circumstances, measurement of the level of brain natriuretic peptide may be helpful. If markedly elevated, this is a strong indication that congestive heart failure is playing a role and appropriate measures can then be used to intervene.

Drug Therapy

Previous studies have demonstrated the effectiveness of appropriate monitoring and pharmacologic support in reducing the incidence of myocardial infarction and the mortality rate in surgical patients with cardiovascular diseases. It is extremely important to take a careful history and obtain information about preoperative drug regimens in order to make decisions about management of those drugs during the perioperative period. Drugs for cardiovascular management have been previously classified in five general categories: (1) antihypertensives and diuretics, (2) vasodilators used for chronic heart failure, (3) antianginal drugs, (4) inotropic drugs, and (5) antiarrhythmics. A large percentage of older surgical patients present with hypertension, and many of them are already receiving antihypertensive agents. These agents fall into four general classes: (1) diuretics, (2) adrenergic inhibitors, (3) vasodilators, and (4) angiotensin-converting enzyme (ACE) inhibitors.

The primary diuretics in use today are thiazides, which act at the distal convoluted renal tubules to inhibit sodium transport; furosemide, which acts at the ascending limb of

Henley's loop to inhibit chloride transport; and spironolactone, which competitively inhibits the binding of aldosterone to mineralocorticoid or type I receptors in the epithelial cells of the distal convoluted tubule and collecting duct. Because all of these drugs have the potential to produce hypovolemia and secondary dehydration, care must be taken in patients receiving these drugs to avoid profound hypotension induced by anesthetic agents that block reflex increases in cardiac output or peripheral vascular resistance. Furthermore, these diuretics induce hypokalemia (thiazides and furosemide) or hyperkalemia and acidosis (spironolactone), which may promote arrhythmias, so potassium management is important prior to surgery.

Adrenergic inhibitors are antihypertensive drugs that act by inhibiting function of the nervous system and include peripheral blocking agents such as reserpine and guanethidine, central blocking agents such as methyldopa and clonidine, β receptor inhibitors, and α receptor inhibitors. Peripherally acting agents are used less commonly, but, if they are being used, they should be discontinued prior to surgery because of their profound effect on cardiac output and tendency to cause hypotension. The centrally acting inhibitors such as clonidine and methyldopa also cause severe hypotension, but they should not be abruptly withdrawn because of severe reflex hypertension. Instead, they should be gradually weaned with substitution of other antihypertensive agents. The β-blocking agents are commonly used, and it is considered safer to continue these agents up until the surgical procedure and to utilize a specific β-agonist or atropine if hypotension or bradycardia develops. β-blockers also offer some protection from postoperative rhythm disturbance if they are continued in the immediate postoperative period. Patients with coronary artery disease or with risk factors often benefit from initiation of β-blockers perioperatively if they are not already on these drugs.

α-Receptor antagonists such as prazosin are uncommonly used for uncomplicated hypertension, but these drugs may induce relative volume depletion and loss of normal sympathetic vasoconstrictive response in the presence of surgically induced volume loss. Therefore, it is highly desirable to discontinue α-receptor antagonists prior to surgery.

Vasodilators

The most commonly used vasodilators are nitroprusside and nitroglycerin (Table 52–2). These drugs are particularly useful in acute perioperative situations because they are rapidly acting agents that can be quickly withdrawn. The drugs differ in that nitroglycerin has its predominant effect on preload reduction, whereas nitroprusside causes predominantly afterload reduction. Because of its coronary

Table 52–2
Vasodilator drugs

Drug	Afterload Reduction	Preload Reduction	Indications
Nitroprusside (IV)	+++	++	Acute hypertension
			Cardiac failure
			Valvar insufficiency
Nitrates (IV, PO, patch)	+	+++	Ischemic failure
Hydralazine (PO or IV)	+++	0	Chronic cardiac failure
			Hypertension
Prazosin (PO)	++	++	Hypertensive failure
			Pulmonary hypertension
			Chronic cardiac failure
Captopril (PO)	++	+	Chronic cardiac failure
Nifedipine (sublingual)	++	0	Acute left ventricular failure
Neseritide	+++		Cardiac failure

+, Present.
Values modified from Anderson RW: The use of cardiovascular pharmacologic agents in surgical patients. In Sabiston DC (ed): Textbook of Surgery—The Biological Basis of Modern Surgical Practice. Philadelphia: WB Saunders, 1986:2444.

vasodilatory effect, nitroglycerin is particularly useful in patients with coronary artery disease and myocardial ischemia. It is also effective in acutely reducing pulmonary arterial pressure in the treatment of acute right heart failure. Other vasodilator drugs such as minoxidil and diazoxide are reserved for severe hypertensive crises and are administered intravenously.

ACE inhibitors have become extremely important in the treatment of congestive heart failure and in the management of hypertension. They inhibit the enzyme responsible for conversion of inactive angiotensin I to the active peptide angiotensin II, a very potent vasoconstrictor. Captopril is a commonly used ACE inhibitor that lowers total peripheral resistance but causes little change in cardiac output, heart rate, or pulmonary arterial wedge pressure. It is useful to continue ACE inhibitors in the perioperative period because withdrawal may cause severe hypertension. They also may be instituted in the postoperative period with gradually increasing doses to control hypertension. Care must be used when administering ACE inhibitors in the presence of renal insufficiency, because the drugs can exacerbate already decreased renal function.

Agents for the Treatment of Congestive Heart Failure

The utility of drugs that produce relaxation of vascular smooth muscle leading to vasodilation has been well documented in the treatment of patients with chronic and acute congestive heart failure. The effect of these drugs is

to decrease the peripheral vascular resistance, which allows blood to shift from the central circulation into the peripheral venous capacitance; thus the preload of the left ventricle is reduced, as is the afterload. Physiologic benefits of this reduction of end-diastolic volume include (1) a reduction in myocardial wall stress and lowering of myocardial oxygen requirements, (2) a shift to the more effective portion of the diastolic pressure-volume curve, (3) a decrease in diastolic pressure in the left ventricle with a consequent decrease in pulmonary venous pressure, and (4) improved diastolic perfusion of the myocardium as a result of a lower transmyocardial pressure gradient between the epicardial and endocardial blood vessels.

The vasodilator drugs listed in Table 52–2 are useful in treating cardiac patients who have hypertension, myocardial ischemia, or congestive heart failure. Nesiritide, or human brain (B)-type natriuretic peptide, leads to increased intracellular concentrations of cyclic GMP and smooth muscle relaxation. In human studies, nesiritide produced dose-dependent reductions in pulmonary capillary wedge pressure (PCWP) and systemic arterial pressure in patients with heart failure. In the Vasodilation in the Management of Acute Congestive Heart Failure (VMAC) trials, nesiritide reduced PCWP and provided greater relief of dyspnea in patients with decompensated heart failure than did placebo. It is limited to the intravenous mode of delivery and should only be used when proper monitoring is maintained. It has no effect on myocardial contractility, but can cause hypotension. In general, patients with congestive heart failure who have been well maintained on vasodilating drugs will benefit greatly from the continuation of those drugs during the perioperative period. If the vasodilators have to be discontinued, they should be reinstituted as soon as possible in the postoperative period.

Spironolactone, a drug already discussed in the section on diuretics, has proven especially useful in patients with chronic congestive heart failure who are already receiving ACE inhibitors. In such a population of patients, spironolactone had beneficial effects on cardiac adrenergic tone and divalent cation balance (by elevating plasma magnesium levels), and it reduced ventricular arrhythmias. Echocardiographically determined measurements of systolic and diastolic function were unaltered by spironolactone, so there was no increase in myocardial oxygen demand.

Antianginal Drugs

The most common antianginal drugs are nitrates, β-blocking agents, and calcium channel blockers. It is well recognized that the incidence of coronary artery disease is high in the current noncardiac surgical population, particularly in patients with peripheral vascular disease. It is also known that the most important cardiovascular risk factor is a history of a recent myocardial infarction. The risk of another myocardial infarction or death during the perioperative period can be markedly reduced if the surgery can be delayed by 6 months after the myocardial infarction. Appropriate use and continuation of antianginal drugs is critical in reducing these risks.

Nitroglycerin is the most commonly used vasodilator in cardiac surgery and is a very effective antianginal and anti-ischemic agent that is safe to use in the perioperative period. The β-blocking drugs are also useful for the treatment of angina in patients who do not have profound left ventricular failure. β-Blockers have been suggested for use in patients with chronic congestive heart failure, but they are not recommended in patients with severe left ventricular failure during the immediate perioperative period. If patients are taking β-blockers preoperatively, there is a risk that abrupt withdrawal may lead to acute ischemia or the development of arrhythmias.

Calcium antagonists or calcium channel blockers also have been used as antianginal agents, as well as vasodilating drugs in some circumstances. They differ from β-blockers in that they cause relaxation of smooth muscle, whereas β-blockers tend to cause constriction of smooth muscle. Verapamil and diltiazem are effective in the management of supraventricular tachycardia, and nifedipine is used in the management of hypertension. All three of these agents may provide relief of coronary artery spasm and increase coronary blood flow. Diltiazem has little negative inotropic effect, and it is a very useful drug for the control of postoperative atrial fibrillation or other supraventricular

tachyarrhythmias. However, calcium channel blockers may produce problems in surgical patients because of their peripheral vasodilating effects, which may lead to profound hypotension if the patient is also hypovolemic. The combination of a β-blocker and a calcium antagonist can result in severe cardiac depression. In general, it is recommended that calcium antagonists be discontinued preoperatively and that β-blockers be continued up until the time of surgery and then resumed in the postoperative period.

Inotropic Drugs

Current inotropic agents used in the perioperative period include digitalis glycosides, which inhibit Na^+-K^+ ATPase activity; both α- and β-adrenergic sympathomimetic agents; and the phosphodiesterase inhibitors. The primary goal is to administer the various inotropic agents singly or in combination in order to provide optimal myocardial contractile force without excessive increase in oxygen demand produced by tachycardia or increased afterload of the heart.

Digitalis is an inotropic agent commonly used in patients with congestive heart failure. However, in the perioperative period digitalis can have adverse effects, including ventricular arrhythmias. It is often advisable to withhold digitalis for a period of time prior to the surgical procedure and during the operative and immediate postoperative period so that safer agents can be used. A common indication for digitalis in the perioperative period is a combination of congestive heart failure and atrial fibrillation, and in those circumstances it can be a useful agent.

The sympathomimetic stimulants are listed in Table 52–3. Isoproterenol has had modest use in the past but is now considered contraindicated in patients with ischemic heart disease, primarily because it causes tachycardia and hypotension and can induce severe arrhythmias. Epinephrine, which has both α and $β_1$ activity, is a classic inotropic drug used in cardiac surgery and continues to be used frequently because it is very inexpensive and is well known to most anesthesiologists and surgeons. Other commonly used inotropic agents are dopamine and dobutamine. The sympathomimetic agents are often limited in their effectiveness by their noncardiac effects (see Table 52–3). The α-receptor stimulants cause severe peripheral vasoconstriction, while $β_2$-receptors produce bronchial and peripheral vessel dilation. For example, norepinephrine increases cardiac contractility but causes severe peripheral vasoconstriction, which limits its usefulness, although it can be used effectively in combination with a vasodilating agent. Isoproterenol is effective because of its predominant β effect, but it also increases myocardial oxygen demand and may be deleterious in patients with

Table 52–3
Sympathomimetic agents with adrenergic receptor activity

Agent	α (Peripheral)	β1 (Cardiac)	β2 (Peripheral)
Isoproterenol	0	++++	++++
Epinephrine	++++	++++	++
Norepinephrine	++++	++++	0
Dopamine	+++	++++	++
Dobutamine	+	++++	++
Methoxamine	++++	0	0
Phenylephrine	++++	0	0

+, Present.
From Anderson RW: The use of cardiovascular pharmacologic agents in surgical patients. In Sabiston DC (ed): Textbook of Surgery–The Biological Basis of Modern Surgical Practice. Philadelphia: WB Saunders, 1986:2444, with permission.

ischemic heart disease. Dopamine is often the drug of choice for patients with acute myocardial failure because it is an excellent inotropic agent with widespread vasodilatory effects. Additionally, it may improve renal blood flow by selective stimulation of renal receptors. However, when dopamine is increased to doses above 10 μg/kg/min, the α effects dominate, and in that situation it must be combined with a vasodilator such as nitroprusside if hypotension is not present. Dobutamine is a synthetic analog of dopamine. It acts directly on $β_1$-adrenergic receptors, so it has a strong inotropic effect and causes peripheral vasodilation. It does not directly improve renal blood flow as dopamine is thought to do. Dobutamine also has been shown to be somewhat proarrhythmic, so it must be used with caution at higher doses. Combinations of dopamine and dobutamine have been very useful in the treatment of cardiogenic shock.

The phosphodiesterase inhibitors inamrinone and milrinone have similar laudatory effects in patients with heart failure by increasing cardiac output, lowering pulmonary vascular resistance, and producing peripheral vasodilation, greatly decreasing myocardial oxygen demand. They are also useful when combined with epinephrine or norepinephrine. These drugs have been extremely effective in the immediate perioperative period, but, in older patients with decreased renal perfusion, maintenance of these drugs has had deleterious effects on the kidneys, and inamrinone depletes platelets. We prefer to discontinue the phosphodiesterase inhibitors after 48 hours.

Antiarrhythmic Agents

The development of arrhythmias and conduction disturbances in surgical patients with cardiac disease is common

and has multiple etiologies. Many surgical patients with cardiac disease are already receiving diuretics and other drugs that produce hypokalemia and metabolic alkalosis, which beget supraventricular arrhythmias. Anesthetics and other drugs can cause ventricular irritability, and patients with myocardial infarction, cardiac trauma, or pericarditis are all prone to arrhythmias. Antiarrhythmics drugs are classified as follows:

- *Class I agents* (sodium channel blockers) include lidocaine, quinidine, procainamide, and mexiletine. The primary drug in this group is lidocaine, which is the standard for the initial treatment of ventricular arrhythmias. Toxicity related to these drugs is common.

- *Class II agents* (β-blocking drugs such as propranolol, esmolol, and labetalol) are reasonably rapid acting and useful in the perioperative period.

- *Class III agents* cause widening of the action potential duration. The most important drug in this group is amiodarone. The availability of intravenous amiodarone in the last several years has had a marked impact on the treatment of postoperative arrhythmias, including supraventricular and ventricular types. Amiodarone is effective in the management of atrial flutter and fibrillation. It has been used prophylactically in patients to prevent perioperative arrhythmias, although this use is controversial. It has very little negative inotropic effect. One of the potential complications of amiodarone is pulmonary toxicity. Current practice suggests that this can occur early after amiodarone treatment rather than being delayed several weeks or longer, as was previously thought. The risk of the pulmonary complications can be reduced by appropriate dosing.

- *Class IV agents* are the calcium channel blockers. The prototype of this group is verapamil. It has an important role in the control of supraventricular arrhythmias because it inhibits atrioventricular conduction, and has few side effects and a low incidence of toxicity. Diltiazem is also helpful in controlling supraventricular arrhythmias in patients with adequate blood pressure and can be used orally once the arrhythmia is controlled by intravenous infusions.

Patients not infrequently come to the operating room with a history of ventricular premature contractions but with current normal ventricular function. If there is no evidence of ventricular tachycardia or ventricular fibrillation, or if electrophysiologic studies have ruled out inducible ventricular tachycardia or fibrillation, there is probably no reason to treat such patients. Even if treated, the ventricular premature contractions tend to persist in the postoperative period. Patients with no known heart disease usually do not require specific antiarrhythmic drugs for sinus tachycardia, premature atrial beats, or unifocal premature ventricular beats.

The use of vasodilators is particularly important in patients undergoing coronary artery bypass grafting and specifically for those in whom the radial artery is employed. It is well recognized that the thickened muscular wall of the radial artery has a predilection for spasm, which must be treated effectively to avoid postoperative complications of graft spasm or closure. The calcium channel blocker diltiazem has been used extensively in patients intraoperatively as soon as the radial artery is harvested. Current data suggest, however, that nitroglycerin is preferable to diltiazem for prevention of coronary bypass spasm. Although others recommend using both nitroglycerin and calcium channel blockers, our practice is to use intraoperative and immediate postoperative intravenous nitroglycerin and, on the first or second postoperative day, begin oral nitrate in the form of isosorbide mononitrate. It is currently not clear how long the oral nitrate should be continued, but we believe it should be continued for 3 to 6 months. It has been suggested that intraoperative application of phenoxybenzamine may prevent long-term vasoconstriction in radial arterial grafts.

Use of Mechanical Circulatory Support Systems in Patients with Severe Cardiac Insufficiency

The above-described use of careful physiologic and laboratory monitoring, management of volume and metabolism, and the judicious use of drugs during the perioperative period lead to survival and successful outcomes in a large number of patients. However, in a small number of patients with heart failure in the perioperative period, these measures are insufficient and more complete circulatory support is required, such as mechanical circulatory support systems. These systems can be broadly categorized as follows: (1) intra-aortic balloon pump (IABP); (2) extracorporeal membrane oxygenation (ECMO); (3) externalized ventricular assist devices (VADs) for support for days or weeks; (4) implantable VADs, which can be used for several months or years, and (5) biventricular replacement systems (total artificial hearts), which may also be used for months or years.

Patients who are candidates for mechanical circulatory support systems vary widely, but include those in shock after cardiac operations, patients with acute myocardial infarction shock, and patients with chronic heart failure and deterioration who may be candidates for cardiac transplantation or permanent support. Hemodynamic inclusion criteria that help in the selection of patients for mechanical circulatory support systems include cardiac output index less than 2.0 $L/m^2/min$, mean arterial pressures less than 65 mm Hg, left or right atrial pressures greater than 20 mm Hg, urine output less than 20 mL/hr, and systemic vascular resistance greater than 2100 dynes/sec/cm^{-5}. Unless some dramatic intervention is made in patients with these parameters, they will not survive more than a few days. Pharmacologic criteria in patients meeting the above parameters include receiving two or more inotropic drugs at high doses (e.g., dopamine ≥10 µg/kg/min, dobutamine ≥10 µg/kg/min, and epinephrine ≥0.02 µg/kg/min) and receiving one inotropic drug at the above doses with use of an IABP.

Intra-aortic Balloon Pump

The most commonly used device for cardiac failure unresponsive to drug therapy is the IABP. It is almost always the first mechanical device chosen because of its relative ease of insertion, general effectiveness, and ease of removal. The IABP is mounted on a flexible catheter that most commonly is inserted through the femoral artery and positioned in the descending thoracic aorta. A predetermined volume of gas is pumped into the balloon during cardiac diastole and withdrawn during systole. The net result is an increase in diastolic arterial pressure and enhanced coronary perfusion pressure as well as decreased systolic arterial pressure, which decreases afterload resistance. As a result, the heart works more efficiently with less myocardial oxygen consumption (Table 52–4). The IABP usually can increase cardiac output by about 20%, which is frequently all that is required in patients with marginal cardiac function. However, patients with profound cardiac dysfunction require much more complete support.

In previous publications describing the IABP, its use in noncardiac surgical patients is indicated as rare. Indeed, that is still the case in current clinical practice, although it is probable that IABP could be utilized effectively much more often in noncardiac surgical patients. For example, patients with borderline cardiac function or those with ischemic myocardial disease might well benefit from a period of intra-aortic balloon pumping during or after the general surgical procedure. A possible contraindication would be the need for the use of heparin during intra-aortic balloon pumping, but anticoagulation is not essential to IABP use, and patients can be managed well for days without any anticoagulation without the fear of intravascular thrombosis. Therefore, a consideration in patients with known cardiac disease undergoing complex abdominal or peripheral vascular surgery might well be insertion of an IABP prior to beginning the operation.

Extracorporeal Membrane Oxygenation or Portable Cardiorespiratory Support

ECMO has been employed for cardiopulmonary support, usually as an acute resuscitative tool, but support can be prolonged for several days or even weeks. The ECMO circuit usually includes venous inflow and arterial outflow tubing with a connecting bridge, a bladder, and several regulators; various infusion ports; the roller head or centrifugal pump; the oxygenator; and the heat exchanger. Unlike the cardiopulmonary bypass circuit used in cardiac surgery, the ECMO circuit has no venous reservoir in which to collect volume and from which to distribute blood if venous return temporarily drops. Instead, the venous blood is collected in a small bladder that is pressure monitored to prevent the intake and pumping of air. The status of the bladder indicates whether the flow should be increased or decreased and acts as a servoregulator. The ECMO system provides only nonpulsatile flow. In cases of pulmonary insufficiency, it can be used in a venovenous mode, but, for cardiac support, venoarterial perfusion is required.

ECMO has been used in the support of cardiac and noncardiac surgical patients. One of its earlier applications was in support of a trauma patient, and it has had moderate use in postoperative cardiac surgical patients. Although ECMO is an important technique for acute resuscitation of patients in cardiogenic shock in the emergency room, cardiac catheterization laboratory, or operating room, it is not a system that provides long-term ventricular support. Its use in postcardiotomy patients has diminished with the development of more effective devices such as VADs. ECMO has been used as an acute measure to resuscitate severely ill patients and bridge them to a VAD. The noncardiac surgeon may be called upon at times to perform surgery on patients being supported with ECMO systems. Under these circumstances, patients usually remain quite stable from a cardiorespiratory standpoint. However, the surgeon must be prepared to deal with the likelihood of bleeding because continuous heparinization is essential in patients on ECMO. The heparin dose may be decreased to a minimum level, but it cannot be discontinued without risk of clotting the entire ECMO system.

Table 52–4
Physiologic effects of intra-aortic balloon pumping

Aortic systolic pressure	↓↓	Cardiac preload	↓
Aortic diastolic pressure	↑↑	Left ventricular wall tension	↓
Left ventricular systolic pressure	↓	Left ventricular volume	↓
Left ventricular end-diastolic pressure	↓	Left ventricular stroke work	↓
Cardiac output	↑	Coronary blood flow	↑
Cardiac afterload	↓↓	Renal blood flow	↑

From Chitwood RW: Use of the intra-aortic balloon counterpulsation technique. In Sabiston DC (ed): Textbook of Surgery–The Biological Basis of Modern Surgical Practice. Philadelphia: WB Saunders, 1986:2468, with permission.

Ventricular Assist Devices (VAD's)

While a complete description of VAD's is beyond the scope of this chapter, it is important to note that effective circulatory support for left, right, or biventricular failure can be provided with VAD's. Considerable experience has been gained in patients with postcardiotomy failure, bridge to transplantation, or as permanent or "destination" therapy. Although complications such as infections or thromboembolism are problematic, patients have been supported for a few weeks to up to four years with various types of VAD's. In long term patients with VAD's, noncardiac surgeons are often asked to perform noncardiac operative procedures and as the field progresses, thorough knowledge of these systems will be imperative for the success of such procedures.

Bibliography

Akins CW: Myocardial revascularization in the presence of carotid arterial disease. *In* Edmunds LH (ed): Cardiac Surgery in the Adult. New York: McGraw-Hill, 1997:597.

Al-Tabbaa A, Gonzalez RM, Lee D: The role of state-of-the-art echocardiography in the assessment of myocardial injury during and following cardiac surgery. Ann Thorac Surg 2001;72:S2214.

American College of Cardiology/American Heart Association Task Force Report: Guidelines for perioperative cardiovascular evaluation for non-cardiac surgery. Circulation 1996;93:1278.

Anderson RW: The use of cardiovascular pharmacologic agents in surgical patients. *In* Sabiston DC (ed): Textbook of Surgery—The Biological Basis of Modern Surgical Practice. Philadelphia: WB Saunders, 1986:2444.

Arom KV, Emery RW: Decreased postoperative drainage with addition of epsilon-aminocaproic acid before cardiopulmonary bypass. Ann Thorac Surg 1994;57:1108.

Barr CS, Lang CC, Garson J, et al: Effects of adding spironolactone to an angiotensin-converting enzyme inhibitor in chronic congestive heart failure secondary to coronary artery disease. Am J Cardiol 1995;76:1259.

Bruce RA, Hornstein TR: Exercise stress testing in evaluation of patients with ischemic heart disease. Prog Cardiovasc Dis 1969;11:371.

Chanda J, Brichkov BS, Canver CC: Prevention of radial artery graft vasospasm after coronary bypass. Ann Thorac Surg 2000;70:2070.

Chitwood RW: Use of the intra-aortic balloon counterpulsation technique. *In* Sabiston DC (ed): Textbook of Surgery—The Biological Basis of Modern Surgical Practice. Philadelphia: WB Saunders, 1986:2468.

Daylin JE, Bone RC: Is it time to pull the pulmonary artery catheter? JAMA 1996;276:916.

Goldberg LI: Dopamine—clinical uses of an endogenous catecholamine. N Engl J Med 1974;291:707.

Goldman L, Caldera DL, Nussbaum SR, et al: Multifactorial index of cardiac risk in noncardiac surgical procedures. N Engl J Med 1997;297:845.

Hillis LD, Cohn PF: Non-cardiac surgery in patients with coronary artery disease: risk, precautions, and perioperative management. Arch Intern Med 1978;138:972.

Kallis P, Tooze JA, Talbot S, et al: Aprotinin inhibits fibrinolysis, improves platelet adhesion and reduces blood loss: results of a double-blind randomized clinical trial. Eur J Cardiothorac Surg 1993;8:315.

Kawanishi DT, Rahimtoola SH: Silent myocardial ischemia. Curr Probl Cardiol 1987;12:509.

Koglin J, Peblivauli S, Schwaiblmair M, et al: Role of brain natriuretic peptide in risk stratification of patients with congestive heart failure. J Am Coll Cardiol 2001;38:1934.

Kumin L, Caldera D, Noosbaum S, et al: Multifactorial index of cardiac risk in non-cardiac surgical procedures. N Engl J Med 1977;297:845.

Lee S-H, Chang C-M, Lu M-J, et al: Intravenous amiodarone for prevention of atrial fibrillation after coronary artery bypass grafting. Ann Thorac Surg 2000;70:57.

Levy JH, Bailey JM, Deeb GM: Intravenous milrinone in cardiac surgery. Ann Thorac Surg 2002;73:325.

Magovern GJ: Extracorporeal life support following adult open-heart surgery. *In* Zwischenberger JB, Bartlett RH (eds): ECMO: Extracorporeal Cardiopulmonary Support in Critical Care. Ann Arbor, MI: Extracorporeal Life Support Organization, 1995:473.

Mangano DT, Goldman L: Pre-operative assessment of patients with known or suspected coronary disease. N Engl J Med 1995;333:1750.

Marcus LS, Hart D, Packer M, et al: Hemodynamic and renal excretory effects of human brain natriuretic peptide infusion in patients with congestive heart failure: a double-blind, placebo-controlled, cross-over trial. Circulation 1996;94:3184.

Marelli D, Laks H, Fazio D, et al: Mechanical assist strategy using the BVS 5000 i for patients with heart failure. Ann Thorac Surg 2000;70:59.

Martin TD, Craver JM, Gott JP, et al: Prospective, randomized trial of retrograde warm blood cardioplegia: myocardial benefit and neurologic threat. Ann Thorac Surg 1994;57:298.

Multiple Risk Factor Intervention Trial Research Group: Coronary heart disease, death, non-fatal acute myocardial infarction and other clinical outcomes in the multiple intervention trial. Am J Cardiol 1986;58:1.

Naunheim KS, Swartz MT, Pennington DG: Intra-aortic balloon pumping in patients requiring operations: risk analysis and long-term follow-up. J Thorac Cardiovasc Surg 1992;104:1654.

Noon GP, Morley D, Irwin S, et al: Clinical experience with the MicroMed DeBakey ventricular assist device. Ann Thorac Surg 2001;71:5133.

Owings JT: The coagulopathy of trauma. *In* Grenvik A, Ayers S, Holbrook PR, Shoemaker WC (eds): Textbook of Critical

Care Medicine (4th ed). Philadelphia: WB Saunders, 2000:306.

Pagani FD, Aaronson KD, Dyke DB, et al: Assessment of an extracorporeal life support to LVAD bridge to heart transplant strategy. Ann Thorac Surg 2000;70:1977.

Pennington DG, Swartz M, Codd JE, et al: Intra-aortic balloon pumping in cardiac surgical patients: a nine-year experience. Ann Thorac Surg 1983;36:125.

Pennington DG, Oaks TE, Hines MH, Lohman DP: Use of mechanical circulatory support systems in critically ill patients. *In* Grenvik A, Ayres S, Holbrook PR, Shoemaker WC (eds): Textbook of Critical Care Medicine (4th ed). Philadelphia: WB Saunders, 2000:1070.

Pennington DG, Oaks TE, Lohman DP: Extracorporeal support: the Thoratec device. *In* Goldstein DJ, Oz MC (eds): Cardiac Assist Devices. Armonk, NY: Futura, 2000:251.

Pennington DG, Swartz M, Codd JE, et al: Intra-aortic balloon pumping in cardiac surgical patients: a nine-year experience. Ann Thorac Surg 1983;36:125.

Rao TLK, Jacobs KH, El-Etr AA: Reinfarction following anesthesia in patients with myocardial infarction. Anesthesiology 1983;59:499.

Richard C, Ricome JL, Rimailiho A, et al: Combined hemodynamic effects of dopamine and dobutamine in cardiogenic shock. Circulation 1983;67:620.

Rose E, Gelijns AC, Moskowitz AJ, et al: Long-term use of a left ventricular assist device for end-stage heart failure. N Engl J Med 2001;345:1435.

Shapira OM, Alkon JD, Macron DSF, et al: Nitroglycerin is preferable to diltiazem for prevention of coronary bypass conduit spasm. Ann Thorac Surg 2000;70:883.

Tarhan S, Moffitt EZ, Taylor WF, et al: Myocardial infarction after general anesthesia. JAMA 1972;220:1451.

Tinker JH, Tarhan S: Discontinuing anticoagulant therapy in surgical patients with cardiac valve prostheses. JAMA 1978;239:738.

Tuman KJ, Roizen MF: Outcome assessment in pulmonary artery catheterization: why does the debate continue? Anesth Analg 1997;84:1.

Van den Bergh G, Wouters P, Weekers F, et al: Intensive insulin therapy in critically ill patients. N Engl J Med 2001;345:1359.

Velez DA, Morris CD, Muraki S, et al: Brief treatment of radial artery conduits with phenoxybenzamine prevents vasoconstriction long-term. Ann Thorac Surg 2001; 72:1977.

Wackers FJT, Soufer R, Zayet BL: Nuclear cardiology. *In* Braunwald E, Zipes DP, Libby P (eds): Heart Disease: A Textbook of Cardiovascular Medicine (6th ed). Philadelphia: WB Saunders, 2001:273.

CHAPTER 53

Perioperative Renal Dysfunction and Failure: Diagnosis and Management

Michael J. Casey, M.D. and Anthony J. Bleyer, M.D.

Renal failure is a major cause of morbidity and mortality in hospitalized patients. It is present in approximately 1% of all patients at hospital admission, and complicates approximately 5% of hospitalizations and 10% of all patients undergoing major vascular surgery. For patients undergoing cardiac bypass surgery, the development of renal failure is one of the strongest predictors of in-hospital mortality.

Evaluation of the Patient with Renal Failure

History

As in all of medicine, the evaluation of the patient with renal failure begins with a thorough history and physical examination. Once the presence of renal failure has been determined by one of the measurements described below, the goal is to establish the cause of renal failure and correct it promptly before permanent renal damage occurs. The time course of the renal failure should first be established. Renal failure is divided into categories of acute (days), subacute (weeks to months), and chronic (years).

The timing of the increase in the serum creatinine is of utmost importance, and it is of great benefit to have serum creatinine (SCr) values from prior to admission. If the SCr was elevated for some time before admission, the patient usually has chronic renal failure, which is unrelated to the admission. If the SCr was normal immediately prior to admission and elevated at the time of admission, the rise is usually related to the reason for admission. Most frequently, the SCr rises while the patient is in the hospital. This almost always means that the rise is related to some event that occurred in the hospital. Fortunately, during the hospital admission, careful recording of vital signs and medication administration frequently allows one to find a cause for the deterioration of kidney function. Most commonly, an operative procedure, administration of medication, or development of hypotension/sepsis results in a loss of renal function.

Acute renal failure is the most common type encountered in the hospital setting. Acute renal failure is subdivided into the categories of prerenal disease (hypoperfusion), postrenal disease (urinary tract obstruction), and intrinsic renal disease (primary glomerular or tubular dysfunction). The investigation should begin with the search for events that may result in acute renal failure, such as hypotension, intravenous (IV) contrast administration, arteriogram, new medications, or vascular, pelvic, or urologic surgery. The history should be reviewed for conditions that put patients at risk for the development of acute renal failure, such as diabetes, vascular disease, heart failure, cancer, liver disease, and prior chronic renal diseases. Previous chronic renal failure will place the patient at risk of developing further renal deterioration.

The review of systems should begin with the elements that determine the need for urgent dialysis. These include diminished mental status from uremic encephalopathy, intractable nausea and vomiting, angina or shortness of breath from volume overload, and chest pain consistent with uremic pericarditis. Other uremic symptoms include anorexia, weight loss, edema, and pruritus. Decreased urine stream, urinary frequency, incontinence, and nocturia can suggest bladder outlet obstruction. Foamy urine suggests proteinuria from a primary renal disease. Hematuria can be either from intrinsic renal disease, such as a glomerulonephritis, or postrenal disease, such as nephrolithiasis.

A thorough medication review is critical, especially for the identification of new medications. Antibiotics, especially penicillins, cephalosporins, sulfonamides, and quinolones, are notorious for causing acute allergic interstitial nephritis (AIN). Angiotensin-converting enzyme (ACE) inhibitors, angiotensin receptor blockers (ARBs), nonsteroidal anti-inflammatory drugs (NSAIDs), and pain medicines such as cyclooxygenase-2 (COX-2) inhibitors can all cause prerenal azotemia. These are very important to identify in patients who may have poor intravascular or effective circulatory volume. Lithium and gold are two less common drugs associated with renal failure. Over-the-counter cold remedies containing α-adrenergic antagonists can exacerbate prostatism and result in bladder outlet

obstruction (BOO). Many medications will need to require dosage adjustment because they are metabolized by the kidney.

Physical Examination

The blood pressure is critical in evaluating the patient with renal failure. All patients with significant hypotension (mean arterial pressure <60 mm Hg) will have impairment of renal perfusion and diminished glomerular filtration rate (GFR). Perhaps the reader will allow us to repeat an oft-cited, rather simple phrase from our consulting rounds that nonetheless succinctly summarizes this complex medical situation: "No BP, no PP!" Patients with long-standing hypertension or atherosclerotic vascular disease can have compromised renal blood flow at mean arterial pressures as high as 70 mm Hg. The "hunt for hypotension" is essential to finding the etiology of acute renal failure in the hospitalized patient. A patient's weight, intake, and output should be monitored closely every day while the patient has renal failure. Significant weight gain or loss in a short period of time is almost always secondary to fluid gain or loss. Discrepancies between weight changes in intake/output records should be investigated. Hypotension may be fleeting, and a careful review of the daily flow sheets is imperative.

The physical examination is crucial in determining the patients' volume status and cardiac function. The patient with tachycardia, fever, and the absence of jugular venous distention or edema is frequently volume depleted and requires fluid resuscitation. Obtaining orthostatic vital signs is of great importance. The heart rate and blood pressure should be measured in the supine and standing positions. If the patient cannot stand, having the patient sit over the edge of the bed may be adequate. A drop in the systolic blood pressure of 20 points or an increase in the heart rate of greater than 20 beats/min will frequently signify volume depletion.

The patient with edema, jugular venous distention, and rales on pulmonary auscultation probably has cardiac compromise as the cause of hypotension. The presence of a pericardial friction rub in the latter patient could suggest myocardial infarction or tamponade from uremic pericarditis. The presence of edema does not always mean that there is intravascular volume expansion. Patients who are critically ill can have significant edema and even anasarca from "third spacing" of fluids in the presence of significant intravascular volume depletion. The same is true for patients with right heart failure or liver disease. The presence of these conditions can usually be detected by the history and physical exam. However, these patients often require invasive monitoring with a Swan-Ganz catheter to elucidate their true volume status.

Other signs of renal failure can be detected on physical examination. Careful observation of the skin is important. Skin rashes may be associated with AIN from medications; purpuric or petechial rashes may be associated with vasculitis. Auscultation for vascular bruits is also important, as is abdominal auscultation for renal artery bruits. However, the latter are frequently difficult to hear, especially in the intensive care unit or in obese patients. Auscultation of carotid and femoral bruits is suggestive of diffuse atherosclerosis and also points to renal artery disease. Patients with cholesterol emboli syndrome (CES) will often have other sequelae of emboli, including retinal infarcts or hemorrhages, acute abdominal signs, and infarctions in the lower extremities, especially the toes. Examination of the toes for acral ischemia or digital emboli is of paramount importance.

One may also monitor for signs of uremia. One should test for asterixis by asking the patient to hold both hands forward and extend the wrists. It is helpful for the physician to demonstrate for the patient and to tell the patient to "make stop signs." When demonstrating, the physician should continue in this posture for as long as he or she wishes the patient to maintain it. This is helpful for two reasons: first, the patient is less inclined to lower his or her hands before the test is complete. Second, the patient may feel self-conscious when performing this act, and, if the physician performs it, virtually all eyes in the room will be on the physician instead of the patient. Within 30 seconds, a classic flap should be demonstrated. This may occur only once or several times. One should also listen for a pericardial friction rub. These rubs sound like Velcro separating and are not synchronous with the cardiac cycle; they are frequently evanescent. In addition, post–coronary artery bypass surgery patients will frequently have a rub from post-operative inflammation. Pleural rubs may also be due to uremia.

Laboratory Evaluation

Renal function is described in terms of the GFR. GFR is the theoretical volume of plasma that is completely filtered in a given unit of time, usually measured in milliliters per minute. The normal range for GFR is 100 to 150 mL/min, depending on age and sex. Patients are frequently asymptomatic until their GFR is less than 25 mL/min. GFR cannot be measured directly in humans, so numerous surrogate markers have been developed.

The renal clearance of a substance is equal to the amount filtered by the glomeruli plus tubular secretion minus tubular reabsorption. The clearance of any substance can be calculated by knowing the serum concentration and the amount of substance excreted in the urine in a given time period (Box 53–1). The ideal substance for measuring clearance should be completely filtered at the glomerulus and neither reabsorbed nor secreted in the tubule. To date, no such substance exists. We frequently perform clearances using urea and creatinine, though urea is reabsorbed in the tubule and creatinine is secreted. All estimations of GFR require that the patient be in a steady state.

Creatinine

The measurement of the SCr is the most widely used clinical measure of renal function. Creatinine is a breakdown product of muscle metabolism. Its production is primarily determined by muscle mass and varies little from day to day. However, the ingestion of large amounts of red meat can increase the serum creatinine level by up to 30%. Creatinine is primarily cleared by glomerular filtration, although a small proportion is actively secreted by the tubules. The secreted proportion increases as GFR falls. The secretion of creatinine is inhibited by drugs such as trimethoprim and cimetidine, resulting in an increased SCr without changing GFR.

The SCr in any given patient is inversely proportional to his or her GFR and directly proportional to lean body mass. In other words, for any given GFR, the creatinine decreases as lean body mass decreases. Assuming a patient's lean body mass does not change, the SCr increases as the GFR decreases. This relationship is important because a SCr of 1.5 mg/dL represents a much greater GFR in a 100-kg muscular male than in a 50-kg elderly female. In the setting of acute renal failure, the rise in SCr can lag the decrease in GFR by 12 to 24 hours and may not reach steady state for several days. This may result in an overestimation of GFR during the initial phase and an underestimation in the recovery phase of acute renal failure. For example, in the patient who undergoes bilateral nephrectomies, the SCr may be 1.0 mg/dL initially, but the following day it will have increased to 3 or 4 mg/dL. Even though the patient has no renal function, it will still take some time for creatinine to accumulate to steady state levels.

Several groups have developed formulas to estimate GFR using the SCr and other readily available parameters. The Cockroft and Gault equation (see Box 53–1) is the most widely used. It attempts to estimate creatinine clearance and thus GFR from the SCr using age, weight, and sex to estimate lean body mass. Like other estimations of GFR, it requires that the patient is in steady state. The Cockroft and Gault formula has not been validated in diabetics, amputees, or bed-bound patients. It likely underestimates renal function in African-Americans.

The urinary creatinine clearance (CCr) roughly estimates GFR in patients in a steady state. It can be measured using the standard formula for clearance of any substance (see Box 53–1). To obtain the CCr, one needs

---

Box 53–1

Calculation of Renal Function Indicators

Clearance of Substance X (C_x) $= (U_x \times V) / P_x$

U_x = concentration of X in the urine; V = urine flow, usually in mL/min; P_x = plasma concentration of X

Cockroft & Gault Formula*

$$\text{Estimated Creatinine Clearance} = \frac{[(140 - \text{age}) \times \text{Weight (kg)}] \times 0.85 \text{ for females}}{72 \times \text{Serum creatinine}}$$

$$\text{Creatinine Clearance} = \frac{\text{Urinary creatinine concentration} \times \text{Urine volume in 24 hr}}{\text{Serum creatinine}}$$

$$\text{Creatinine Clearance (mL/min)} = \frac{\text{Urine creatinine (g/24 hr)} \times 69}{\text{Serum creatinine (mg/dL)}}$$

$$\text{Urea Clearance} = \frac{\text{Urine urea nitrogen (g/24 hr)} \times 69}{\text{Blood urea nitrogen (mg/dL)}}$$

$$\text{Fractional Excretion of Sodium} = \frac{[\text{Urinary sodium}] \times [\text{Serum creatinine}]}{[\text{Urinary creatinine}] \times [\text{Serum sodium}]}$$

*From Cockroft DW, Gault MH: Prediction of creatinine clearance from serum creatinine. Nephron 1976;16:31.

---

to collect all of a patient's urine for a set time period and then measure the volume of urine and the concentration of creatinine in the urine and the plasma. The clinical standard is to collect the urine for 24 hours, though 8-, 12-, and 48-hour periods have been used. The longer the collection period, the smaller the chance for errors in the collection resulting in an over- or underestimation of CCr. For a 24-hour collection, there is a shortcut to the formula that allows easy approximation of the CCr (see Box 53–1).

Urea

Blood urea nitrogen (BUN) was the first endogenous substance measured to estimate renal function. Urea is a by-product of protein catabolism. It is completely renally cleared and is freely filtered by the glomerulus. It is also reabsorbed by the tubules, especially in volume-contracted states. BUN increases with worsening renal function, volume depletion, and states of high protein intake or breakdown. There is much more day-to-day variability in BUN than SCr. Patients who have poor protein intake can have minimal elevations in BUN in the presence of significant renal failure. Gastrointestinal (GI) bleeding, corticosteroid use, and volume depletion all can raise the BUN without significant renal insufficiency. Because urea is actively reabsorbed in the presence of volume depletion, the

BUN:Scr ratio is often used as a measure of volume status. A BUN:Scr ratio of greater than 20:1 is considered to be indicative of volume depletion, though this can be confounded in the situations described above.

The urea clearance (CUr) can be calculated from a 24-hour urine collection using the same formula as for CCR (see Box 53–1). Because of tubular reabsorption of urea, the urine CUr underestimates GFR. The average of the CUR and CCr is a good estimation of GFR because the overestimation of GFR by the CCr is balanced by the underestimation of GFR by the CUr.

Other measurements of GFR

Inulin is a naturally appearing fructose polymer that is completely filtered by the glomerulus. It is infused until a steady state is achieved and then its renal clearance is measured. Inulin clearance is the gold standard measurement of GFR. However, it is time consuming and of little use in clinical practice. Radionucleotides such as ^{125}I-iothalamate and ^{51}Cr-EDTA have been developed that can estimate GFR from a single IV bolus and serial plasma measurements. Some can be used with a gamma camera to estimate the function of each kidney individually. Again these studies are too cumbersome to find much use outside of research settings.

Urinalysis

"Study a factory by its products—study a kidney by its urine." In patients who have abnormalities of their kidney, we have direct and simple access to the product of this organ. It only makes sense that observation of the urine would be one of the first steps to determine the cause of kidney failure. For the renal consultant, the urinalysis provides a wealth of knowledge, and the performance of this test results in significant information in over half the cases examined. The urinalysis is one of the few laboratory tests that can elucidate the etiology of acute renal failure. A fresh urine specimen of at least 5 mL should be obtained for immediate dipstick and microscopic examination. Five milliliters of urine should be centrifuged at 2000 rpm and the supernatant poured off. The pellet is then resuspended and examined under the microscope for the presence of cellular elements and casts.

Patients with acute tubular necrosis (ATN) will typically have a sediment with "muddy brown" tubular casts and/or the presence of renal tubular epithelial cells (RTECs) or even RTEC casts. Patients with prerenal azotemia or early ATN will often have a concentrated urine with a high specific gravity but an otherwise bland sediment. Red blood cells are often found in the urine of patients after Foley catheterization and other urologic procedures. Patients with nephrolithiasis and bladder pathology also usually have hematuria. Small numbers of red blood cells can be present in patients with any renal disease. The presence of red blood cell casts suggests intrarenal pathology such as glomerulonephritis. The presence of white blood cells in the urine usually represents urinary tract infection or pyelonephritis. In the absence of bacteria or yeast, they may suggest the presence of interstitial nephritis. The urine should be tested for eosinophils if AIN or CES is suspected.

The urine dipstick is most useful for the assessment of proteinuria and hematuria. The presence of greater than "1+" proteinuria suggests a primary glomerular pathology. Most commonly this is seen in patients with chronic renal disease secondary to diabetes mellitus. High-level proteinuria is also often found in acute and chronic glomerulonephritis. Proteinuria less than or equal to "1+" can be from either glomerular or tubular origin. It may be present in any type of renal disease. The dipstick only detects albumin and can be negative in patients with myeloma kidney or other paraproteinemias.

Fractional Excretion of Sodium

The fractional excretion of sodium (FENa) (see Box 53–1) is a useful test in discriminating prerenal azotemia from ATN in oliguric patients. This is a common clinical dilemma because they represent the two most common causes of renal failure in the hospitalized patient. In volume-depleted states, the kidney avidly reabsorbs sodium in order to replete intravascular volume. The FENa is typically less than 1% in this situation. In ATN with oliguria, tubular injury prevents concentration of the urine and sodium reabsorption. In these situations, the FENa is usually greater than 2%. There is great overlap in these conditions. The FENa is less than 1% in about 15% of true ATN cases and in most cases of glomerulonephritis and obstructive nephropathy. The FENa is difficult to interpret if loop diuretics have been given in the past 6 to 12 hours or if thiazide diuretics have been given in the past 24 to 48 hours. These drugs can cause inappropriate sodium excretion and thus an elevated FENa despite the presence of a prerenal state. However, a FENa of less than 1% despite diuretics is an accurate indicator of a prerenal state. Also, the urine output should be less than 500 mL for the FENa to be accurate.

Urine Output

Urine output is a simple measurement of extreme importance in the diagnosis of kidney failure. First, of course, it is important to make sure that all the urine has been collected. A Foley catheter or condom catheter in males may be important if the patient is not totally alert. It is also important to ascertain that the nursing staff is collecting all urine and recording it. Patients with bathroom privileges may not collect all urine.

The urine output has become one of the most important "numbers" in the intensive care unit. The pisseprophets of old are replaced by the surgical intern who makes sure that the urine output is at least 30 mL/hr. If this is so, it is frequently assumed that all is right with the patient's (and intern's) world. However, it is important to realize that the urine output, while a good marker, must be taken into account with many other factors. It is important to make sure that the intake and output are evenly matched as well.

When the urine output drops, corrective actions must be taken that are in concert with the entire body homeostasis and not performed solely with the goal of increasing urine output. A decreased urine output does not mean that the kidney is functioning incorrectly. In many cases, the kidney is doing exactly what it should. For example, the surgical intern who is on call for 48 hours and missed breakfast, lunch, and dinner may have a urine output less than 30 mL/hour! When the urine output drops, it is important to first assess the volume status. If the patient is hypovolemic, he or she should be given fluid. If the patient appears euvolemic, a short trial of fluid may be given. However, if the patient is edematous (frequently short of breath), a trial of fluid should not be given—such fluid may place the patient in pulmonary edema and markedly worsen his or her status. In a similar manner, if the patient is volume overloaded, administration of a diuretic may be of benefit. This will not improve renal function, but will make the patient more comfortable, and improve overall body function. If the patient is euvolemic, administration of a diuretic may increase urine output and potentially prevent hypervolemia. However, establishing 50 mL of urine flow per hour by this method will not improve renal function. Administration of a diuretic to a patient who is volume depleted will result in worsening volume depletion and can precipitate renal failure.

Patients with less than 400 mL of urine output per 24 hours are defined as having oliguria. Patients with oliguric renal failure have a worse outcome than patients with nonoliguric renal failure. It is unclear whether administration of furosemide to convert the patient from oliguric to nonoliguric renal failure has an effect on renal recovery.

Daily Weights

Daily weights are often disregarded, but assume paramount importance especially on the hospital floor, where intake and output are frequently incorrectly recorded. In many hospitals, the determination of daily weights is difficult. While the graduate student in the next building may be accurately weighing a nanogram of a substance, the surgical intern is frequently perplexed by the lack of accurate weights on his or her patient. However, with careful perseverance and discussion with the nursing staff, it should be possible with diligence to obtain the weights. If weights are stable, this is in general a good sign indicating a sufficient urine output. By detecting an upward trend in weights, increased diuretics may be used and pulmonary edema avoided. Weights are especially important because of the frequent administration of large amounts of fluid intraoperatively, and the subsequent need for diuresis when these fluids enter the circulatory space a day or two after surgery.

Causes of Acute Renal Failure

In developing a differential diagnosis for the patient with acute renal failure, potential causes are divided into three categories: prerenal diseases, intrinsic renal diseases, and postrenal diseases. The typical approach is to rule out pre- and postrenal failure and then evaluate causes of intrinsic renal disease. By taking this approach, one tries to correct extrarenal problems before permanent intrinsic renal damage can occur.

Prerenal Azotemia

Prerenal azotemia is a reduction in GFR secondary to inadequate renal perfusion. It is the most common cause of renal failure in the hospitalized patient. The renal parenchyma remains intact, and, once perfusion is restored, the renal function normalizes. However, there is a continuum between prerenal azotemia and ischemic ATN. If prerenal azotemia is severe and prolonged, then subsequent interstitial ischemia can result in ATN and "intrinsic" renal failure.

Intravascular volume depletion is the most common cause of prerenal azotemia and is common in postoperative patients. This can occur from nasogastric suction, blood loss, insensible losses, or third spacing of fluids. Surgical patients are at high risk because they are frequently not receiving oral intake (nil per os, or NPO) and have drains, nasogastric suction, and limited access to fluids. Anesthesia can induce renal perfusion by expanding vascular beds and reducing blood pressure. Patients with preexisting renal disease, hypertension, or vascular disease may have renal failure with lesser degrees of hypotension or volume depletion than normal subjects. Patients with severe burns can have massive fluid losses that are difficult to quantitate, and they can rapidly become volume depleted. In outpatients, volume depletion typically presents as a history of poor intake and/or fluid losses such as vomiting, diarrhea, or bleeding. These patients typically have orthostatic hypotension, tachycardia, and flat neck veins. Patients with pancreatitis, trauma, sepsis, liver failure, and hypoalbuminemia can have massive capillary leak and third spacing of fluids. These patients may have significant edema and positive fluid balance despite intravascular volume depletion. Urine output is almost always diminished unless the patient is taking diuretics. The urine usually appears concentrated, with an elevated specific gravity and a FENa less than 1%. The sediment is bland except for the presence of hyaline casts or hematuria secondary to insertion of a urinary catheter.

For patients with intravascular volume depletion, fluid resuscitation with a crystalloid such as 0.9 N NaCl and/or a colloid such as blood (if appropriate) should be initiated. Lactated Ringer's solution should be avoided in patients with acute renal failure because of the risk of hyperkalemia. Hypotonic saline solutions are reserved until plasma volume has been restored because they are less effective volume expanders than 0.9 N NaCl. There is no good evidence that volume resuscitation with colloids such as Hespan, hetastarch, or albumin improves outcomes in most volume-depleted patients. The evidence supporting their use in patients with third spacing is only anecdotal and has not been supported in clinical trials. All NSAIDs, COX-2 inhibitors, ACE inhibitors, and ARBs should be discontinued until volume depletion and renal failure have resolved. Diuretics should not be used to "jump start" urine output because they will only exacerbate volume depletion. Once effective plasma volume is restored, urine output and renal function should return to baseline. If prerenal azotemia is prolonged and/or severe, then ATN can develop, which could delay recovery.

Patients with decreased cardiac output resulting from a variety of causes can develop prerenal azotemia. The most common cause is congestive heart failure (CHF). Most CHF patients have had long-standing ischemic, hypertensive, or valvular heart disease. These patients actually have an expanded plasma volume but poor renal blood flow because of low cardiac output. They typically present with orthopnea, shortness of breath, distended neck veins, rales, and peripheral edema. Like volume-depleted patients, they will usually have diminished urine output with a high specific gravity and FENa less than 1%. Therapy is focused on improving cardiac output with inotropes such as dopamine, dobutamine, and milrinone or correction of the valvular defect. In contrast to other causes of prerenal azotemia, these patients may benefit from diuretics and afterload reducers because they can improve cardiac output and thus renal blood flow. Some patients may actually have a combination of intravascular volume depletion and CHF. A common scenario is the patient with biventricular heart failure and pulmonary hypertension who has edema because of right heart failure. These patients are often given large doses of diuretics and become intravascularly volume depleted, with a subsequent drop in preload that reduces cardiac output. These patients may benefit from discontinuation of diuretics and the use of graded compression stockings to reduce the edema. A pulmonary artery catheter may be helpful in managing these patients.

Several classes of medications alter the normal renal responses to hypoperfusion and thus exacerbate prerenal azotemia. Diuretics result in renal sodium and fluid losses and exacerbate volume depletion.

A most important clinical situation that is encountered more and more frequently is the development of acute renal failure with ACE inhibitors and ARBs. An understanding of the effect of these medications is of critical importance. In the normal glomerulus, the afferent arteriole provides blood inflow, and the efferent arteriole allows for blood to exit the glomerulus. Several different conditions may decrease afferent arteriolar pressure. These include volume depletion, renal artery stenosis, cardiomyopathy, and any other condition causing hypotension. The normal response to this situation is constriction of the efferent arteriole, which raises intraglomerular pressure and allows for filtration. In contrast, ACE inhibitors cause efferent arteriolar vasodilatation, with the decrease in intraglomerular pressure being one mechanism by which they improve long-term renal function. Unfortunately, in low-flow states

in which the efferent arteriole would normally constrict, patients on ACE inhibitors do not have efferent vasoconstriction. The intraglomerular pressure then plummets, resulting in decreased glomerular filtration and renal failure. For this reason, the use of ACE inhibitors in heart failure must be monitored closely. ACE inhibitors should be avoided in renal artery stenosis or volume depletion. In general, with acute renal failure, we discontinue ACE inhibitors.

NSAIDs and COX-2 inhibitors block the prostaglandin-mediated afferent arteriole dilatation that preserves GFR in volume-depleted states and can also cause prerenal azotemia. These drugs can also exacerbate CHF and produce renal failure by that mechanism. These drugs have little or no effect on normal subjects with adequate blood pressure and volume status and thus are safe in most patients. They are most likely to cause renal failure in high-risk patients such as those with preexisting renal disease, CHF, hypertension, renovascular disease, or volume depletion. The combination of an ACE inhibitor or ARB with a NSAID or COX-2 inhibitor can be especially disastrous and should be avoided.

General anesthetics and antihypertensive medications can cause systemic vasodilatation that can result in renal hypoperfusion and prerenal azotemia. Anaphylaxis and sepsis can cause a similar syndrome. Volume resuscitation, discontinuation of the offending agent, and vasopressors restore adequate blood pressure and may improve renal function. Some vasopressors, such as norepinephrine, can cause renal arteriolar vasoconstriction and reduced blood flow, resulting in acute renal failure. Cirrhosis, hepatic failure, ergotamine ingestion, and hypercalcemia cause renal failure by the same mechanism.

Intrinsic Renal Disease

Intrinsic renal disease is the second most common cause of renal failure in the hospitalized patient. It accounts for approximately 40% of cases, 90% of which are ATN. Intrinsic renal disease can be divided into ATN, diseases of the renal vasculature, diseases of the glomeruli, and diseases of the interstitium. In the surgical setting, glomerular diseases and vasculitides are extremely rare. On vascular and cardiac surgery services, atheroembolic and occlusive large-vessel renovascular disease is frequently seen. Interstitial disease can be seen on any service where antibiotic use is common and on urologic services where patients have frequent nephrolithiasis, ureteral reflux, and recurrent pyelonephritis.

Acute tubular necrosis

ATN is caused by severe tubular injury resulting in loss of renal function. The injury can occur secondary to ischemia or a tubular toxin. Ischemic ATN is a part of the spectrum of prerenal azotemia. The lack of immediate recovery with restoration of renal perfusion differentiates it from prerenal azotemia. In its most severe form, there can be bilateral acute cortical necrosis and permanent renal failure. Typical clinical findings include a urinary sediment with numerous course granular (muddy brown) casts and RTECs. The presence of granular casts is highly suggestive of ATN. However, it is not uncommon that patients with ATN will not have granular casts. These patients will frequently have a bland sediment (which means that, on microscopic examination, there are no red cells, white cells, or casts).

Ischemic ATN is most commonly seen in cases of profound and prolonged hypotension in the setting of major surgery, trauma, burns, and sepsis. It is especially common in patients undergoing cardiac or aortic surgery. The risk of ATN correlates directly with the degree of cardiac dysfunction and the length of time on cardiopulmonary bypass. Patients undergoing valve repair have an even higher risk. Patients undergoing aortic surgery involving prolonged cross-clamping above the level of the renal arteries frequently develop ischemic ATN. It is important to note that, in half of the cases of postsurgical ATN, no documented hypotension is found. Trauma and sepsis patients often have multifactorial ATN, resulting from hypotension and renal ischemia but also from direct tubular toxicity from cytokines, endotoxin, myoglobin, and antibiotics.

The other mechanism of ATN is tubular injury secondary to a direct tubular toxin. These toxins can either be endogenous or exogenous. The kidney is especially susceptible to toxic injury because it receives 25% of total blood supply, and toxins and their metabolites are often concentrated in the urine. Table 53–1 lists drugs and other compounds associated with nephrotoxic ATN. By far the most common exogenous toxins are radiocontrast agents and aminoglycoside antibiotics. Although these agents can cause ATN in normal individuals, patients with preexisting renal disease, the elderly, and those with concurrent renal ischemia are at much higher risk.

Radiocontrast agents cause ATN by causing both renal vasoconstriction and direct tubular toxicity. Patients with diabetes mellitus, preexisting renal disease, and concurrent ischemia, volume depletion, or CHF are at especially high risk. It is generally accepted that larger doses of radiocontrast media increase the incidence and severity of contrast nephropathy, though conclusive evidence is lacking. The typical clinical course is the development of rising creatinine with or without oliguria 24 to 48 hours after the administration of radiocontrast medium. Patients typically have a bland urinary sediment, though coarse granular casts and RTECs may be present. The FENa may be less than 1% because of contrast-induced renal vasoconstriction. Renal failure and creatinine typically peak 3 to 5 days after contrast administration and resolve after 1 to 2 weeks. Permanent renal failure seldom occurs unless the patient had prior renal insufficiency or concomitant renal injury by another mechanism.

Hydration of patients with 0.45 N saline at 1 mL/kg/hr 12 hours before and after the procedure has been shown to be superior to "renal-dose" dopamine, mannitol, and loop diuretics in the prevention of contrast nephropathy.

Table 53–1
Exogenous nephrotoxins

Drugs		Other Compounds
Antibiotics	Gold	**Other Compounds**
Acyclovir/gancyclovir	Penicillamine	**Heavy Metals**
Aminoglycosides	Cyclosporin/FK-506	**Radiocontrast Dye**
Vancomycin	Interleukin-2	**Bacterial Endotoxins**
Pentamidine	**Chemotherapy**	**Poisons**
Foscarnet	Ifosphamide	Paraquat
Amphotericin	Cisplatin	Snake bites
Anti-Inflammatories/Immune Modulators	Methotrexate	**Solvents**
	Streptozocin	Ethylene glycol
NSAIDs	5-Fluorouracil	Toluene
COX-2 inhibitors		

COX-2, cyclooxygenase-2; NSAIDs, nonsteroidal anti-inflammatory drugs.

In patients with renal failure or CHF, fluids should be given carefully. These patients may be best served by simply temporarily discontinuing their diuretics and ACE inhibitor or ARB without the administration of additional fluids to prevent volume overload. The use of NSAIDs or COX-2 inhibitors and the development of hypotension should be avoided. Acetylcysteine given the day before and day of the procedure has been shown to reduce the incidence of contrast nephropathy in those undergoing computed tomography. Therapy for contrast nephropathy is avoidance of further nephrotoxins or renal injury and supportive care until the renal failure resolves.

Aminoglycoside antibiotics, amphotericin, acyclovir, and cyclosporin are the most common medications associated with ATN. Renal failure complicates between 10% and 30% of courses of aminoglycoside antibiotics. The renal failure usually begins after the first week of therapy, and the urinary sediment is frequently bland. Renal failure usually resolves with discontinuation of the medication. Ideally patients with renal failure should completely avoid the use of aminoglycosides. If they must be used in patients with prior renal insufficiency, the dose and frequency should be decreased. Patients with sepsis, hypotension, prior renal insufficiency, and advanced age should have antibiotic levels and renal function monitored daily, with immediate discontinuation of the drug if renal insufficiency develops. Amphotericin toxicity is almost ubiquitous in patients receiving greater than 1 g of drug, though the renal effects can be attenuated by saline infusion prior to drug administration. The new lipid formulations are associated with less renal toxicity in clinical trials. Patients with amphotericin toxicity frequently have tubular dysfunction and associated renal tubular acidosis, as well as magnesium and potassium wasting. The calcineurin

inhibitors cyclosporin and tacrolimus have been associated with both acute and chronic renal insufficiency. They can cause ATN by means of renal vasoconstriction and ischemia, though most of the time there is only a prerenal state that resolves when levels fall into a normal range. Acyclovir causes renal insufficiency by direct RTEC damage from crystallization of the drug in the tubules. Renal failure occurs in about one third of patients who are volume depleted and receive the drug as an IV bolus. Renal failure can be avoided by maintenance of volume status and appropriate adjustment of the drug dosage.

The most common endogenous toxins include myoglobin, hemoglobin, myeloma light chains, and uric acid crystals. Rhabdomyolysis is the most common cause of ATN secondary to myoglobinuria. It is most commonly seen in patients with trauma, seizures, and muscle ischemia. Other causes of rhabdomyolysis are listed in Table 53–2. Patients typically have a strongly heme-positive urinalysis in the absence of red blood cells by microscopy. Urine myoglobin is markedly positive, and the serum creatine kinase is often greater than 16,000 U/L. Hemolysis/hemoglobinuria rarely causes acute renal failure unless it is massive. This is usually associated with severe transfusion reactions or autoimmune hemolytic anemias. These patients will have a pink urine that dips strongly positive for blood in the absence of intact red blood cells by microscopy, an elevated serum lactate dehydrogenase (LDH), and low serum haptoglobin. In patients with a large tumor burden, especially lymphomas and leukemias, the administration of chemotherapy can result in the destruction of a large cell mass and the tumor lysis syndrome. These patients manifest with hyperkalemia, hypocalcemia, hyperphosphatemia, and hyperuricemia shortly after the administration of chemotherapy. Patients with multiple myeloma and cast

---

Table 53–2
Causes of rhabdomyolysis

Muscle Injury	Compartment syndrome	**Toxins**
Trauma	**Metabolic Disorders**	Ethanol
Electric shock	Hypokalemia	Isopropyl alcohol
Hyperthermia	Hypophosphatemia	Ethylene glycol
Muscle Exertion	Hyperosmolar states	Snake bites
Seizures	Inherited metabolic disorders	**Drugs**
Delerium tremens	**Infections**	Amphetamines
Extreme exercise	Influenza	Phencyclidine
Muscle Ischemia	Mononucleosis	Lysergic acid
Prolonged compression (coma)	Tetanus	Heroin
Embolism	Necrotizing fasciitis	Succinylcholine

nephropathy usually present with anemia, weight loss, bone pain/fractures, and hypercalcemia. The diagnosis is made by detecting monoclonal light chains in the serum or urine via immunoelectrophoresis and by bone marrow biopsy.

Treatment is reversal of the underlying disorder and volume administration to maintain urine output greater than 300 mL/hr. These patients may have significant third spacing of fluids and thus require large volumes to maintain intravascular volume. Diuretics can be used as needed to maintain urine output and volume status, but should be avoided until the patient is adequately volume replete. If urine output is adequate, then administration of sodium bicarbonate to alkalinize the urine and prevent cast/crystal formation has been tried with varying success. This has been best studied in crush injuries, for which therapy has been most successful if large volumes of saline and bicarbonate are administered prior to the release of the crushed limb. Mannitol has been theorized to reduce renal injury in pigment nephropathy by acting as a free radical scavenger, though clear evidence to support its use is lacking. Allopurinol should be given prophylactically in patients at risk for tumor lysis syndrome and in patients with rhabdomyolysis or hemolysis who develop significant hyperuricemia. Myeloma cast nephropathy is additionally treated with colchicine and chemotherapy. The management of the concomitant hyperkalemia and hyperphosphatemia is discussed later in the chapter.

Diseases of blood vessels

Any interruption of the blood supply to the kidneys will result in renal failure. By far the most common vascular cause of renal failure is atherosclerotic renovascular disease (ASRVD). Patients with renovascular disease are almost always hypertensive smokers with evidence of other atherosclerotic vascular disease on presentation. ASRVD often presents as difficult-to-control hypertension, flash pulmonary edema, and chronic renal failure. However, acute renal failure can develop if the patients is administered an ACE inhibitor, ARB, NSAID, or COX-2 inhibitor or develops relative hypotension. Either bilateral disease or other underlying renal disease is necessary for renal failure to be present. The diagnosis is made by imaging the renal arteries with either traditional renal arteriography, duplex ultrasonography, magnetic resonance angiography, or captopril renogram. Care must be taken in controlling blood pressure because a sudden drop in systemic blood pressure below the perfusion threshold of the stenosis can result in loss of renal perfusion, acute renal failure, and even permanent renal injury. Either percutaneous or surgical revascularization is warranted in patients with uncontrollable hypertension, recurrent pulmonary edema, or worsening renal function. Prevention of progression focuses on blood pressure control, treatment of concomitant hyperlipidemia, and smoking cessation.

Acute renal failure can also occur secondary to embolic events involving the renal vasculature. These can either be thromboemboli or atheroemboli. Thromboembolic events typically occur in the setting of a patient with acute myocardial infarction with left ventricular dysfunction and ventricular thrombus. It can also occur in patients with atrial fibrillation and endocarditis. Patients typically have flank pain, hematuria, and elevated LDH secondary to renal infarction. There is often evidence of embolic events to other parts of the body at the same time. Patient with atrial fibrillation or CHF after myocardial infarction should be anticoagulated with warfarin to prevent thromboembolic events. When emboli do occur, treatment is either with emergent surgical embolectomy or percutaneous administration of local thrombolytics. If therapy is not administered rapidly, infraction and permanent loss of renal function can occur. There are cases of patients with renal artery occlusion with blood supply adequate to prevent infarction but inadequate for renal function who have had restoration of renal function after revascularization.

CES is organ impairment caused by showers of cholesterol crystals from atherosclerotic plaques. CES usually affects elderly patients with diffuse atherosclerosis. It can also occur spontaneously or after the initiation of anticoagulation with warfarin or heparin. Renal failure results from a local inflammatory reaction in small to medium arteries and arterioles and not true vessel occlusion. Thus the presentation is often delayed. Typically it presents as subacute renal failure 2 to 8 weeks after manipulation of the aorta during arteriography, angioplasty, or surgery. If it is massive, it can present immediately with intestinal necrosis, peripheral limb infarction, livedo reticularis, and oliguria secondary to acute ischemia in those areas. Patients often have eosinophilia, eosinophiluria, and hypocomplementemia. The delayed onset of renal failure and the urinary findings distinguish CES from radiocontrast nephropathy. Patients must be watched closely for the development of intestinal or lower extremity gangrene. There is no specific therapy. Newer, smaller, and softer catheters and guidewires used in angioplasty may help reduce the incidence of CES.

Renal failure can also occur from reduced flow in the renal microvasculature. The most common cause is hypertension. Patients with long-standing severe hypertension develop hyalinosis of the small vessels, which results in reduced renal blood flow. Patients with malignant hypertension may develop a thrombotic microangiopathy and present with mental status changes, intracranial hemorrhage or pulmonary edema, and renal failure. Worsening of renal failure can ensue if these patients have their blood pressure abruptly lowered to normal, with an acute rise in creatinine and decreased urine output. The renal failure usually improves after several weeks as the kidney readjusts to the lower blood pressure.

However, aggressive treatment of the hypertension is necessary to prevent further end-organ damage.

The thrombotic microangiopathy that occurs with malignant hypertension must be differentiated from hemolytic uremic syndrome, systemic lupus erythematosus, eclampsia, and cyclosporin toxicity. These diseases can cause a thrombotic microangiopathy, renal failure, and secondary hypertension. The other primary causes of microvascular renal disease are glomerulonephritis and vasculitis. They can occur as a part of a systemic autoimmune disease such as systemic lupus erythematosus, scleroderma, or Wegener's granulomatosis, or they can be limited only to the kidney in diseases such as immunoglobulin A nephropathy or membranoproliferative glomerulonephritis. Patients with systemic disease typically present with fatigue, weight loss, anemia, and various other constitutional symptoms. Postinfectious glomerulonephritis can occur with subacute bacterial endocarditis and with chronic wound infections. The occurrence of vasculitis and glomerulonephritis is very rare, especially on the surgical services, and further discussion is beyond the scope of this chapter.

Interstitial disease

The final category of intrinsic renal disease is the interstitial nephritides. Typically these are inflammatory conditions of the interstitial compartment that result in renal tubular cell damage. The diagnosis is made by a renal biopsy revealing an inflammatory infiltrate in the interstitium that is causing the damage. By far the most common cause is AIN secondary to drugs such as β-lactam antibiotics and NSAIDs (Table 53–3). Patients with AIN typically present with acute renal failure with or without a rash developing 3 to 5 days after initiation of the culprit medication. Occasionally patients may have acute serum sickness with fever, rash, myalgias, and hemolysis and more rapid

renal failure. Eosinophilia and eosinophiluria are sometimes present. The condition is treated with corticosteroids and by withdrawal of the inciting medication. Occasionally patients with pyelonephritis can develop acute renal failure from interstitial disease. Other less common causes of interstitial renal disease are autoimmune diseases such as systemic lupus erythematosus and infiltrating leukemias and lymphomas. Treatment of these conditions is directed at the underlying illness.

Postrenal Azotemia

Disruption of the flow of urine anywhere from the renal pelvis to the urethra will result in renal failure and postrenal azotemia. Postrenal azotemia constitutes about 5% of cases of acute renal failure. In older adults, BOO is the most common cause. In young adult, urolithiasis is most common, and in children, congenital anatomic abnormalities are most common. All patients with acute renal failure in the postoperative setting should have a Foley catheter inserted to assess for BOO. Common causes of BOO include prostate disease (prostate cancer or benign prostatic hypertrophy [BPH]), neurogenic bladder, and anticholinergic drugs. Less common causes are blood clots, stones, and urethral spasm. BPH typically presents in a subacute manner unless an infection or the initiation of a drug with anticholinergic side effects causes sudden worsening and acute obstruction. Patients often complain of decreased urinary stream, difficulty voiding, incontinence, and suprapubic pain. Patients with BOO secondary to prostate disease can be treated medically with α-adrenergic blockers such as terazosin or by transurethral prostatectomy. Foley catheter trauma or obstruction and general anesthetics can cause BOO and renal failure in the postoperative patient. The diagnosis is made by insertion of a Foley catheter with immediate release of a large volume of urine and rapid

Table 53–3
Drugs associated with allergic interstitial nephritis

Antibiotics	**Antihypertensives**	Carbamazepine
β-Lactams	Chlorthalidone	Cimetidine
Cephalosporins	Furosemide	Clofibrate
Quinolones	Thiazides	Phenytoin
Rifampin	α-Methyldopa	Phenobarbital
Sulfonamides	**Other**	Phenylpropanolamine
Trimethoprim-sulfamethoxazole	Allopurinol	
NSAIDs–Almost all	Azathioprine	

NSAIDs, nonsteroidal anti-inflammatory drugs.

resolution of the renal failure. Neurogenic bladder can cause both acute and chronic renal failure. These patients typically have either spinal cord injury or long-standing diabetes mellitus. Patients with neurogenic bladder typically require either chronic indwelling catheters or intermittent catheterization. These treatments are complicated by recurrent urinary tract infections.

Renal failure secondary to upper urinary tract obstruction is less common because bilateral obstruction, solitary kidney, or other renal disease is necessary for renal failure to occur. Causes of upper tract obstruction include nephrolithiasis, blood clots, retroperitoneal fibrosis, malignant neoplasms, and inadvertent surgical ligature. Patients with acute ureteral occlusion typically have colicky abdominal pain and hematuria. Patients with subacute obstruction typically are asymptomatic. Diagnosis is made by demonstration of hydronephrosis on renal imaging studies such as renal ultrasound, spiral computed tomography, or IV pyelogram. Patients with retroperitoneal fibrosis or malignant neoplasm may have ureteral encasement and thus may not demonstrate hydronephrosis. If obstruction is suspected in these cases, the diagnosis can be made by either anterograde or retrograde pyelograms or a radionucleotide renogram. Treatment is relief of the obstruction by either percutaneous nephrostomy tubes or retrograde ureteral stenting. Patients with inadvertent surgical ligature typically develop renal failure and peritonitis postoperatively. The diagnosis can be made by measuring the creatinine concentration in the peritoneal fluid. Normally it will be equal to the SCr, but, with a ureteral leak, it will approach that of urine (at least 10-fold higher). Surgical repair is usually required.

Management of Patients with Renal Failure

Unfortunately, the number of specific therapies for renal failure is limited. Preventive measures and treatments for the various types of renal failure have been described earlier in this chapter. Much of the therapy involves supportive care and the prevention of complications while the patients' renal function recovers on its own. As one might suspect, the most common problems are those of fluid and electrolyte balance. Special care must also be paid to the dosing of medications that are excreted by the kidneys. These problems are discussed in detail below.

Volume Status

The kidney is the primary organ for the maintenance of intravascular volume status. Through modulation of the renin-angiotensin-aldosterone axis, sodium and plasma volume homeostasis is maintained. Patients with normal renal function can maintain plasma volume over a wide range of fluid intake. Renal failure often prevents the kidney from excreting and sometimes from retaining salt and water in appropriate concentrations. Therefore, great care must be taken in the administration of IV fluids in patients with renal insufficiency.

One of the most important first steps in caring for a patient with renal failure is determination and maintenance of intravascular volume. Methods for determining volume status have been described earlier in this chapter. If volume depletion is suspected, then the patient should receive intermittent boluses of either colloid or crystalloid until intravascular volume is restored. Isotonic fluids such as 0.9 N saline are more effective than hypotonic fluids in restoring plasma volume. Potassium-containing fluids such as lactated Ringer's should be avoided to prevent hyperkalemia. Boluses of 250 to 1000 mL should be given and the patient reassessed after each infusion in order to prevent "overshooting" and volume overload. This is a real concern in patients with renal failure because they may not be able to excrete the excess volume administered and can develop CHF and pulmonary edema.

Once plasma volume has been restored, maintenance fluids should be initiated at a rate that matches insensible losses and provides adequate urine output to excrete the daily solute and waste load. The average patient will require approximately 1500 mL of 0.45 N saline per day. Tachypnea and fever can significantly increase those requirements by increasing the insensible losses through the respiratory tract and skin. One must also take into account losses from the GI tract (nasogastric suction, diarrhea, or ostomy) and surgical drains. There can be large losses from these sites, and volume depletion can rapidly occur if they are not accounted for and replaced. Patients with trauma, sepsis, or pancreatitis can have massive third spacing of fluids and can require large volumes of fluids (>10 L/day) to maintain intravascular volume.

If a patient is oliguric or anuric, fluids should only be given in the amount needed to maintain intravascular volume status. With a few exceptions, there is no benefit to forcing urine output in patients with acute renal failure with the combination of IV fluids and diuretics. If the patient is euvolemic or marginally volume overloaded, no fluids may need to be given. If a patient is significantly volume overloaded, IV fluids should be stopped and a loop diuretic such as furosemide should be given in increasing doses (up to 200 mg IV) until an adequate diuresis is achieved. Once a dose has been reached that causes increased urine output, increased diuresis is best achieved by increasing the frequency of administration and not the dose. In some high-aldosterone states such as CHF, avid distal sodium reabsorption can limit the effectiveness of loop diuretics. In these situations, the coadministration of a thiazide diuretic such as metolazone (5 to 10 mg PO qd to bid) or chlorothiazide 30 minutes prior to administration of the loop diuretic can be helpful. Gastrointestinal absorption of furosemide is limited in some patients, and these patients may require higher doses of furosemide or the use of the better absorbed loop diuretics such as torsemide or bumetanide. If a patient has symptoms of pulmonary edema secondary to volume overload, topical nitroglycerin can increase venous capacitance and reduce symptoms until an adequate diuresis can be achieved. If the patient has severe volume overload not responsive to medical measures, ultrafiltration or hemodialysis may be required.

It is most important to discuss the universal question as to whether renal-dose dopamine has any beneficial effect on recovery of renal function. A number of well-done studies have failed to elicit any improvement in renal function with dopamine. The one situation in which low-dose dopamine may be effective is in patients with severe cardiomyopathy, who sometimes respond nicely to the low-dose (2 to 5 μg/kg/min) inotropic effect.

Water Balance

In the renal failure patient or the patient on dialysis, the ability to concentrate the urine is lost, and therefore the effects of antidiuretic hormone are muted or absent. When hyponatremia develops in these patients, it is usually the result of receiving excess water in relation to the amount of sodium received. Decreasing the amount of free water received (either enterally or parenterally) will improve hyponatremia. Increasing urine output will likely produce a dilute urine and will aid in increasing free water excretion.

Potassium Balance

The kidney is the primary organ for the maintenance of potassium balance. The majority of the total body potassium is intracellular. In the normal individual, 95% of the daily potassium load is excreted by the kidney. The rest is excreted by the GI tract, primarily in the colon. As one might suspect, disorders of potassium balance are extremely common in patients with renal failure. Hypokalemia often occurs in association with either GI losses or diuretic use in patients with renal failure. Also, administration of insulin, bicarbonate, or β-agonists can cause transient intracellular shifts of potassium and hypokalemia. In the absence of shifts, the patient with a plasma potassium (P_K) less than 3.0 mEq/L may have a total body K^+ deficit more than 300 mEq. A normal patient would require IV and oral supplementation for this deficit to be replaced. Replacement of potassium should be done carefully in patients with renal insufficiency because there is an impaired mechanism to excrete any excess. For any

given K^+ deficit, approximately 50% of the expected dose should be given to a patient with significant renal impairment. If the patient is anuric and being fed, the potassium may normalize on its own unless there are significant extrarenal losses.

Hyperkalemia is a much more common complication of renal insufficiency. It occurs primarily because of a reduction in potassium excretion. Patients with significant renal insufficiency should not be routinely administered potassium in their IV fluids. They often also require a potassium-restricted diet (2 g/day versus the normal 3 g/day) to prevent hyperkalemia. Drugs that impair renal potassium excretion, such as NSAIDs, COX-2 inhibitors, ACE inhibitors, ARBs, amiloride, triamterene, and spironolactone, should be avoided in patients with renal insufficiency and hyperkalemia. Because of the numerous beneficial effects of ACE inhibitors and ARBs on renal and cardiac diseases, potassium restriction should be attempted prior to their discontinuation as long as P_K is less than 5.5 mEq/L. Concomitant administration of loop diuretics can help increase potassium excretion and decrease the risk of hyperkalemia.

Severe hyperkalemia can be life threatening. It usually manifests as cardiac arrhythmias, so that an electrocardiogram (ECG) should be obtained in all patients with significant hyperkalemia (P_K >5.5mEq/L). The early ECG changes are peaked T waves. As the hyperkalemia worsens, the QRS complex widens, resulting in the classic "sine wave" ECG. This can progress further to complete heart block and asystole. Severe ECG changes typically do not occur unless P_K is greater than 6.0 mEq/L. If ECG changes are present, $CaCl_2$ or calcium gluconate, sodium bicarbonate, and insulin (with or without dextrose) should be given immediately. Calcium administration will stabilize the cardiac membrane and help prevent arrhythmias; it will not affect the serum potassium. Sodium bicarbonate and glucose/insulin temporarily shift potassium intracellularly. The cause of the hyperkalemia should then be sought out and corrected. If the patient is receiving IV or oral potassium, it should be stopped immediately.

Once the patient has been stabilized, the excess potassium must be excreted from the body. If the patient is hyperglycemic and/or acidotic, correcting those situations may be all the therapy that is necessary. If the patient is not oliguric, loop diuretics can be given to increase renal potassium excretion. Sodium polystyrene sulfate (30 to 90 g given orally or by enema) can be given to increase GI excretion. However, sodium polystyrene sulfate should be avoided in the postsurgical patient or patient with ileus because the sorbitol may result in intestinal necrosis. Such "medical management" is more likely to be effective in patients with fairly well preserved renal function and with easily reversible causes of hyperkalemia. If the patient has continued ECG changes or is oliguric, then hemodia-lysis is indicated.

Acidosis

The kidney is critical in maintaining the serum pH in the normal physiologic range of 7.35 to 7.45. It serves two main functions: to secrete the excess hydrogen ions and reclaim filtered bicarbonate. The normal dietary intake results in the production of approximately 1 mmol/kg of hydrogen ions from protein metabolism. The kidney must excrete the hydrogen ions to prevent their accumulation and the development of metabolic acidosis. As long as a patient has at least 30% of normal renal function, there is usually adequate ability to excrete this acid load and prevent metabolic acidosis. However, much more acid may need to be excreted if there is an acid-producing state in the body, such as diabetic ketoacidosis or tissue hypoperfusion. As a result, metabolic acidosis can occur at higher levels of renal function. In mild to moderate renal failure, the metabolic acidosis that occurs is caused by the accumulation of HCl from the daily dietary load, and thus there is a non–anion gap metabolic acidosis. The acidosis is seldom severe because of bone buffering (serum bicarbonate 15 to 20 mEq/L). If the serum bicarbonate is less than 15 mEq/L, then another cause of the acidosis should be entertained. If there is no anion gap, there may be GI bicarbonate losses or renal tubular acidosis. If there is an anion gap, then lactic acidosis, ketoacidosis, or ingested alcohols or salicylates may be present. With severe renal failure, an anion gap can develop as inorganic acids such as phosphates and sulfates accumulate. If the serum bicarbonate falls consistently below 20 mEq/L, therapy with oral sodium bicarbonate should be begun. If the acidosis is severe, or the patient cannot tolerate the sodium load associated with sodium bicarbonate therapy, then dialysis is indicated.

There is significant debate as to the benefit of correcting acidosis in the postoperative surgical patient. Correction of the acidosis has not been shown to improve survival. However, there are several situations in which correction may be indicated. First, if the patient is undergoing weaning from ventilation, correction of the acidosis will allow the patient to tolerate a higher partial pressure of CO_2 and require a lesser respiratory rate. Second, if the patient is hyperkalemic, correction of the acidemia should help decrease the serum potassium. Third, correction of severe acidemia may improve the function of cardiac inotropes.

Calcium/Phosphate Metabolism

The kidney is integral in the maintenance of calcium and phosphate homeostasis. It is the primary means of elimination for both calcium and phosphate. It also hydroxylates 25-hydroxy vitamin D to its 1,25-dihydroxy active form. In acute renal failure, vitamin D production and phosphate excretion are markedly reduced. The presence of hypocalcemia usually occurs only after prolonged renal failure because there is adequate bone buffering.

Most patients with renal failure and adequate protein intake will exhibit mild hyperphosphatemia as a result of dietary intake of protein and the inability of the kidney to excrete phosphate. The goal of short-term therapy is to maintain the serum calcium (mg/dL) × phosphate (mg/dL) product less than 70 to prevent metastatic calcification. Over longer periods, the goal is normalization of the serum phosphorus. The best way to treat hyperphosphatemia in patients with renal failure is with the administration of calcium-based phosphate (calcium carbonate or calcium acetate) binders given with each meal or every 6 hours to patient on tube feeding. For patients who are not receiving enteral alimentation and who are hyperphosphatemic in the setting of renal failure, hemodialysis may be the only means by which to lower the serum phosphorus concentration. Aluminum-based binders (aluminum hydroxide) have lost favor because of the risk of aluminum toxicity with chronic consumption. Dietary protein restriction is useful in reducing phosphate levels. However this practice is becoming increasingly controversial because of the high incidence of protein malnutrition in hospitalized patients with renal failure. The current trend is not to restrict protein intake and to maintain a normal serum phosphate through the use of phosphate binders.

Anemia

The kidney is the primary source for the production of erythropoietin, a hormone that regulates red blood cell production by the bone marrow. Once the GFR approaches 25 mL/min, there is usually deficient production and anemia occurs. Anemia secondary to renal failure can occur at higher GFRs if there is interstitial disease or in situations requiring increased red blood cell production. This anemia can also occur in acute renal failure of sufficient degree and duration. The primary therapy of anemia of chronic renal insufficiency is recombinant human erythropoietin, which is given subcutaneously or intravenously one to three times per week to maintain a hemoglobin between 11 and 12 g/dL. Erythropoietin is routinely given to all anemic patients on renal replacement therapy. Its use in patients with acute renal failure not requiring dialysis and anemia in other hospital settings is still controversial. If a patient is on erythropoietin, iron stores must be adequate for efficacy (serum ferritin >100 μg/L and transferrin saturation >20%).

Bleeding

Bleeding is common in patients with acute or chronic renal failure. It is a product of both the renal failure itself and the comorbidities in the population of renal failure patients. There are two primary mechanisms for increased bleeding in patients with renal failure. The first is the use of heparin anticoagulation during hemodialysis. In patients who have had recent surgery or have known bleeding, reduced or no heparin may be used during dialysis. It is most helpful for the surgeon to contact the nephrologist or nephrology fellow to ensure that heparin is withheld if surgery is planned or if there is concern regarding bleeding.

Anemia resulting from chronic renal failure also contributes to bleeding. Normally, because of cell mass, red blood cells force platelets to the endothelial surface, where they are more active. If the hemoglobin is less than 8 g/dL, the phenomenon does not occur and platelets are less effective. In addition, uremic platelet dysfunction may occur. The mechanism for this increased bleeding is unknown. In addition to the commonly associated anemia, it may be related to increased circulating levels of tissue-pathway activator inhibitor. The mainstay of treatment of acute bleeding in patients with renal disease is the administration of arginine vasopressin. This compound causes the release of von Willebrand's factor from the endothelial surface and improves platelet function. The administration of topical thromboplastin may be helpful for local bleeding. For chronic recurrent bleeding, the administration of estrogens can promote a procoagulant state and reduce bleeding, especially from the GI tract.

Medications

Patients with renal failure require close monitoring of their medications because there is great potential for side effects and drug-drug interactions. The potential for problems is made worse by the need for numerous medications in these patients. Many medications and/or their metabolites are cleared by the kidney and therefore require dosage adjustment. If adjustments are not made, side effects/toxicity can occur. Usually both the drug dosage and interval must be reduced. The most commonly used drugs requiring dosage adjustment are antibiotics, histamine$_2$-blockers, gabapentin, phenytoin, and allopurinol. Potentially nephrotoxic drugs (see Table 53–1) should be avoided if possible in patients who already have renal failure.

Some drugs can be lethal if administered in sufficient quantities in patients with renal failure (Table 53–4). Meperidine has a metabolite (normeperidine) that is excreted by the kidney and can build up to toxic levels, causing seizures and coma. Small or single doses are unlikely to have significant effects, however. In contrast, metformin (Glucophage) can accumulate rapidly to toxic levels in renal failure, resulting in a life-threatening lactic acidosis. It is absolutely contraindicated in patients with reduced GFR and should be withheld in patients prior to any procedure that confers a significant risk of renal failure.

Table 53–4
Drugs to avoid in renal failure

Antibiotics	Spironolactone[†]
Tetracycline	Triamterene[†]
Nitrofurantoin	**Other**
Aminoglycosides*	Chlorpropamide
Narcotics	Metformin
Meperidine	Sucralfate
Cardiovascular	Antacids containing
Nitroprusside	aluminum and
Amiloride[†]	magnesium

*Avoid unless end-stage renal disease or life-threatening infection exists.
[†]Can cause hyperkalemia and generally not effective if glomerular filtration rate is less than 50 mL/min.

The antihypertensive agent nitroprusside has a cyanide-like derivative that is renally excreted. It should be used with caution in patients with renal failure. Thiocyanate levels should be monitored to reduce the risk for toxicity. Digoxin and lidocaine can accumulate, resulting in heart block and seizures, respectively. Insulin and many sulfonylureas are eliminated by the kidneys, so prolonged hypoglycemia can occur if the dose is not reduced in renal failure.

Renal Replacement Therapy

The development of renal replacement therapy (RRT) over the past 30 years has revolutionized the care of patients with severe acute and chronic renal insufficiency. In the hospitalized patient, this primarily refers to hemodialysis, hemofiltration, or peritoneal dialysis. These modalities allow replacement of the native kidney's functions of waste product, solute and volume removal. Renal transplantation is an increasingly common option for RRT in the patient with chronic renal failure.

Indications

The indications for RRT vary depending on whether the patient has acute or chronic renal failure and on the likelihood and time period expected for the recovery of renal function. Regardless of the above factors, there are several emergent indications for initiation of RRT. These include uremic encephalopathy, uremic pericarditis, volume overload, and life-threatening hyperkalemia, hypercalcemia, or metabolic acidosis refractory to medical management.

It is frequently difficult to determine if the patient has uremic encephalopathy because there are many causes of altered mental status in the intensive care unit. Symptoms of this condition usually do not develop if the urea clearance is greater than 10 mL/min. In the questionable case, a trial of dialysis may be indicated. Uremic pericarditis requires urgent dialysis. Patients frequently have a pericardial friction rub on examination. Signs of pericardial effusion and cardiac tamponade may be present. Uremic pericarditis usually develops in the dialysis patient who has been poorly dialyzed. However, some dialysis patients may simply develop this condition even with adequate dialysis. The initial treatment involves pericardiocentesis if the patient is at risk of tamponade. The patient then is dialyzed on consecutive days to decrease uremic toxins. Patients with severe volume overload should be dialyzed if there is inadequate response to maximal diuretics (furosemide, 200 mg IV, combined with metolazone, 5 mg PO). It goes without saying that the IV fluids in such patients should be limited as much as possible. Patients with life-threatening hyperkalemia should undergo dialysis if serum potassium cannot be corrected rapidly—usually by controlling elevated blood sugar or correcting acidosis. In the interim, emergent medical measures to treat hyperkalemia should be undertaken (see above).

Another group of indications for hemodialysis are ingestions or drug overdoses such as methanol, ethylene glycol, lithium, and salicylates. The need for hemodialysis in these instances depends on drug levels and symptoms, not renal failure.

In hospitalized patients with acute renal failure, the initiation of RRT is typically based on the emergent criteria listed above. However, a lower threshold for initiation is used in order to prevent complications of uremia from developing. The longer the delay to effective recovery of renal function or the more severe the renal failure, the lower the threshold for initiation of RRT. RRT does not improve the recovery from renal failure; it only sustains the patient while natural recovery takes place. At this time there is no good evidence regarding the timing of initiation of RRT in the hospitalized patient. Some recommend early RRT to prevent malnutrition and improve mental and cardiovascular function. Others express concerns that intradialytic hypotension or immune system activation can cause further renal injury and delay recovery. Currently in the acute setting, hemodialysis, either intermittent or continuous, is most commonly performed. However, acute peritoneal dialysis can also be performed. Transplantation is not an option for patients with acute renal failure.

The initiation of RRT in the outpatient setting is also controversial. Some recommend initiation of RRT anytime the GFR is less than 10 mL/min regardless of symptoms. Others recommend initiation when the first uremic symptoms of anorexia, weight loss, protein malnutrition, and

volume overload occur. The choice of modality among transplantation, peritoneal dialysis, and hemodialysis depends on both medical criteria and patient preference. In many chronic patients, multiple modalities will be used over a lifetime.

Intermittent Hemodialysis

Intermittent hemodialysis (IHD) is the mainstay of RRT for both acute and chronic renal failure. It is the primary modality used for the removal of toxic ingestions. IHD involves the passage of blood via a pump across a semipermeable membrane against a countercurrent flow of dialysate. Solute removal occurs by diffusion and by ultrafiltration. Fluid removal (ultrafiltration) is controlled by varying the transmembrane pressure. With IHD, the patient typically receives 3- to 5-hour dialysis treatments 3 to 4 days a week. Frequency and duration vary with the amount of solute and volume removal required. If only volume and not solute is required, isolated ultrafiltration can be performed.

In the acute setting, blood access is obtained using dual-lumen large-bore central venous catheters placed in either the internal jugular vein or the femoral vein. Access size should be sufficient to allow blood flows of at least 250 mL/min. The subclavian vein should be avoided because of the high incidence of central venous stenosis. In patients with end-stage renal disease, blood access is usually in the form of a surgically created arteriovenous fistula or cortex loop graft. Some patients may have tunneled, cuffed central venous catheters as their only dialysis access because of poor circulation. Intravenous line insertions, phlebotomy, and blood pressure measurements should not be performed in an arm containing a hemodialysis access. Once the patient is connected to the hemodialysis machine, a roller pump pumps blood at flows of 200 to 500 mL/min through a hollow-filter dialyzer that separates the blood from the dialysate via a semipermeable membrane. Anticoagulation with heparin is standard to prevent clotting of the circuit. In patients at high risk of bleeding, the system can be periodically flushed with saline and thus less or no heparin can be used.

The most common complication of IHD is intradialytic hypotension caused by removal of plasma volume. If fluid is removed from the plasma compartment (ultrafiltration) faster it can equilibrate from the interstitial compartment, then hypotension can develop. This is a major problem with IHD because 48 to 72 hours of fluid intake must be removed in one 3- to 5-hour session. In hospitalized patients, poor cardiac output or low plasma oncotic pressure can exacerbate the situation. Colloids such as mannitol and albumin are frequently used to increase plasma oncotic pressure and improve volume and blood pressure during IHD. Longer and more frequent treatments reduce the rate of removal required to achieve a target volume status and can reduce the incidence of intradialytic hypotension. If hypotension is severe, vasopressor/inotropic support or slow continuous therapies may be required. Other hemodialysis complications include bleeding, access complications (infection or pneumothorax), dialysis disequilibrium syndrome, and anaphylactic reactions to the dialyzer membrane. Dialyzer disequilibrium occurs in patients who have advanced azotemia (BUN usually >150 mg/dL) if they are dialyzed too rapidly. Osmotic shifts resulting from a rapid lowering of the BUN can lead to cerebral edema resulting from retained solutes in the central nervous system. Over the course of the dialysis session, such patients become progressively obtunded; coma frequently develops that may resolve in several days. For this reason, the first dialysis treatment is typically only 2 hours, even in patients who do not have advanced uremia.

It is important to also consider the effects of dialysis on renal function. Immediately after dialysis, there is typically a decline in urine output for a day or two. Hemodialysis, especially with cuprophane membranes, may decrease the rate of recovery of renal function compared to that with newer synthetic membranes. Patients on outpatient hemodialysis frequently lose residual renal function over several months. This decline in renal function is likely due to release of cytokines from the membranes and hypotension. Such deterioration of renal function may be prevented by the use of synthetic membranes as well as by avoiding hypotension during dialysis.

Continuous Hemodialysis/Hemofiltration

Continuous hemodialysis therapies were designed to circumvent the problem of intradialytic hypotension by providing continuous RRT and therefore slower blood flow and ultrafiltration rates. They have now replaced peritoneal dialysis as the modality of choice in hemodynamically unstable patients. In these systems, an arterial cannula is inserted and the patient's own blood pressure forces the blood through the system and back through a venous cannula. Because the flows are slow, there is less stress on the cardiovascular system, and less hypotension. The initial therapies developed were continuous arteriovenous hemodialysis (CAVHD) and continuous arteriovenous hemofiltration. In CAVHD, the clearance occurs by the process of diffusion. In hemofiltration, a physiologic solution is infused into the system and an equal volume of plasma is removed, resulting in clearance by convection; no dialysate is used. The most common continuous therapy used now is continuous venovenous hemodialysis with hemofiltration. In this procedure, the same dual-lumen central venous access is used as with IHD, but blood

flows are 50 to 150 mL/min. Insertion of an arterial catheter and its inherent complications is avoided because an external pump forces the blood through the system. This system increases clearance by combining hemodialysis and hemofiltration in the same process. These modalities are especially useful in critically ill patients with unstable hemodynamics. They can provide excellent clearance and volume removal without altering a patient's tenuous hemodynamic status. For example, maintaining volume status in a patient with 2.5 L/day of net fluid intake would require an ultrafiltration rate of 1000 to 1250 mL/hour during a routine IHD treatment, whereas the ultrafiltration rate for a continuous therapy would be 100 mL/hour. This slower ultrafiltration rate allows excess volume to move from the interstitial compartment to replace the volume removed without intravascular volume depletion and hypotension. As with IHD, isolated continuous ultrafiltration can be performed if a patient needs only volume removal and no solute clearance. Drawbacks to this modality are the need for continuous anticoagulation and the fact that continuous hemodialysis hampers patient transport and therapies.

Peritoneal Dialysis

Peritoneal dialysis (PD) uses the peritoneum as the semipermeable membrane across which solutes and water can flow down the concentration gradients via diffusion. Typically 1.5 to 3.0 L of dialysate are infused into the abdominal cavity via a single-lumen tunneled catheter (Tenckhoff catheter) and allowed to dwell from 2 to 12 hours and then drained. Hypertonic concentrations of dextrose are used in the dialysate to create a gradient for ultrafiltration. The dextrose concentrations can be varied in order to achieve different ultrafiltration rates. With continuous ambulatory peritoneal dialysis, the patient or caregiver instills and drains fluid 3 to 5 times a day for 4 to 6 hours, followed by an overnight dwell. Another option is continuous cyclic peritoneal dialysis (CCPD). With CCPD, a machine performs three to six exchanges while the patient is sleeping, usually eliminating the need for the patient to perform a daytime exchange.

There are a number of contraindications to PD. In outpatients, PD is a home-based therapy, and thus the patient or a caregiver must have adequate mental and physical ability to perform the exchanges without assistance from medical personnel. Patients with a history of extensive abdominal surgery, adhesions, ostomies, or aortic grafts are usually not considered candidates for PD. Typically, the PD catheter is inserted 1 to 2 weeks prior to the initiation of PD to allow the catheter exit site to heal and prevent leakage. However, acute peritoneal dialysis can be performed in the hospitalized patient with acute renal failure. For acute PD, either a tunneled or straight

PD catheter is inserted depending on the anticipated length of time PD is needed. Frequent exchanges (every 2 to 3 hours) of small volumes of dialysate (1 to 1.5 L) are used with the patient strictly in the supine position to prevent leakage. Because PD is a continuous therapy, ultrafiltration rates can be low, allowing its use in hemodynamically unstable patients. PD also circumvents the need to systemically anticoagulate the patient. However, it can be difficult to achieve adequate solute clearance in large or hypercatabolic patients. The most common complications of PD are peritonitis and fluid leaks around the catheter.

Care of the Patient with Chronic Renal Failure

Care of the patient with chronic renal failure is similar to the management of patients with acute renal failure. For patients with a history of renal failure presenting for surgery, the focus should be on medications, volume status, and electrolytes. Special attention should also be given to the cause of the patient's underlying renal disease. Patients with renal disease often have numerous cardiovascular risk factors and should be carefully screened for cardiovascular disease prior to surgery. Patients with autoimmune diseases on chronic steroids may need "stress-dose" steroids for major procedures to prevent addisonian crisis. All patients with chronic renal failure are at increased risk of symptomatic acute renal failure. Therefore, nephrotoxic medications, IV contrast administration, and hypotension should be avoided. If the patient has end-stage renal disease, arrangements should be made with the patient's nephrologist to coordinate the procedure with his or her dialysis. It is frequently necessary to place the patient on a low-potassium diet instead of the regular diet. In addition, postoperatively it is important not to give maintenance fluids, but rather to use as little fluid as possible to avoid volume overload and urgent dialysis.

Bibliography

Anderson RJ, Linas SL, Berns AS, et al: Nonoliguric acute renal failure. N Engl J Med 1977;296:1134.

Bakris GL, Weir MR: Angiotensin converting enzyme inhibitor associated elevations in serum creatinine. Arch Intern Med 2000;160:685.

Better OS, Stein JH: Early management of shock and prophylaxis of acute renal failure in traumatic rhabdomyolysis. N Engl J Med 1990;322:825.

Brady HR, Brenner BM, Clarkson MR, et al: Acute renal failure. *In* Brenner BM (ed): The Kidney (6th ed). Philadelphia: WB Saunders, 2000:1209.

Branch RA: Prevention of amphotericin B induced renal impairment: a review on the use of sodium supplementation. Arch Intern Med 1988;148:2389.

Chasis H, Smith HW: The excretion of urea in normal man and in subjects with glomerulonephritis. J Clin Invest 1938;17:285.

Clive DM, Stoff JS: Renal syndromes associated with nonsteroidal anti-inflammatory drugs. N Engl J Med 1984;310:563.

Cockroft DW, Gault MH: Prediction of creatinine clearance from serum creatinine. Nephron 1976;16:31.

Conger JD: Acute uric acid nephropathy. Semin Nephrol 1981;1:69.

deMattos AM, Olyaei AJ, Bennett WM: Nephrotoxicity of immunosuppressive drugs: long term consequences and challenges for the future. Am J Kidney Dis 2000;35:333.

Denton MD, Chertow GM, Brady HR: "Renal-dose" dopamine for the treatment of acute renal failure: scientific rationale, experimental studies and clinical trials. Kidney Int 1996;50:4.

Forni LG, Hilton PJ: Continuous hemofiltration in the treatment of acute renal failure.N Engl J Med 1997;336:1303.

Gornick CCJ, Kjelstrand CM: Acute renal failure complicating aortic aneurysm surgery. Nephron 1983;35:145.

Greco BA, Breyer JA: Atherosclerotic ischemic renal disease. Am J Kidney Dis 1997;29:167.

Hammermeister KE, Burchfiel C, Johnson R, et al: Identification of patients at greatest risk for developing major complications at cardiac surgery. Circulation 1990;82 (Suppl IV):IV-380.

Heymsfield SB, Arteaga C, Mcmanus C, et al: Measurement of muscle mass in humans: validity of the 24-hour urinary creatinine method. Am J Clin Nutr 1983;37:478.

Himmelfarb J, Tolkoff Rubin N, Chandran P, et al: A multicenter comparison of dialysis membranes in the treatment of acute renal failure requiring dialysis. J Am Soc Nephrol 1998;9:257.

Hou SH, Bushinskey DA, Wish JB, et al: Hospital-acquired renal insufficiency: a prospective study. Am J Med 1983; 74:243.

Humes HD: Aminoglycoside nephrotoxicity. Kidney Int 1988;33:900.

Jacobsen FK, Christensen CK, Mogensen CE, et al: Pronounced increase in the serum creatinine concentration after eating cooked meat. Br Med J 1970;1:1049.

Kron IL, Joob AW, Meter CV: Acute renal failure in the cardiovascular surgical patient. Ann Surg 1985;39:590.

Lessman RK, Johnson SF, Coburn JW, et al: Renal artery embolism: clinical features and long term follow-up of 17 cases. Ann Intern Med 1978;89:477.

Levy AS: Measurement of renal function in chronic renal disease. Kidney Int 1990;38:167.

Luke RG, Boyle JA: Renal effects of amphotericin B lipid complex. Am J Kidney Dis 1998;31:780.

Michel DM, Kelly CJ: Acute interstitial nephritis. J Am Soc Nephrol 1998;9:506.

Peterslund NA, Beach FT, Tauris T: Impaired renal function after bolus injections of acyclovir. Lancet 1983;1:243.

Rascoff JH, Golder RA, Spinowitz BS, et al: Non-dilated obstructive nephropathy. Arch Intern Med 1983;143:696.

Rose BD: Clinical Physiology of Acid-Base and Electrolyte Disorders (4th ed). New York, McGraw-Hill, 1994:823.

Rose BD: Diuretics. Kidney Int 1991;39:336.

Schierhout G, Roberts I: Fluid resuscitation with colloid or crystalloid solutions in critically ill patients: a systematic review of randomized trials. BMJ 1998:316:961.

Scolari F, Tardanico R, Zani R, et al: Cholesterol crystal embolization: a recognizable cause of renal disease. Am J Kidney Dis 2000;36:240.

Solomon R: Contrast media induced acute renal failure. Kidney Int 1998;53:230.

Soloman R, Werner C, Mann D, et al: Effects of saline, mannitol and furosemide on acute decreases in renal function induced by radiocontrast agents. N Engl J Med 1994;331:1416.

Swan SK, Rudy DW, Lasseter KC, et al: Effect of cyclooxygenase-2 inhibition on renal function in elderly persons receiving a low salt diet: a randomized controlled trial. Ann Intern Med 2000;133:1.

Tepel M, van der Geit M, Scharzfeld C, et al: Prevention of radiocontrast agent induced reductions in renal function by acetylcysteine. N Engl J Med 2000;343:180.

Thadhani R, Pascula N, Bonventre JV: Acute renal failure. N Engl J Med 1996;334:1448.

Valtin H, Schafer JA: Renal Function (3rd ed). Boston, Little, Brown, 1995:50.

Ward MM: Factors predictive of acute renal failure in rhabdomyolysis. Arch Intern Med 1988;148:1553.

CHAPTER 54

Recognition and Treatment of Perioperative Arrhythmias

Warren Holshouser, M.D., John Hoyle, M.D., Matthew Sackett, M.D., and David M. Fitzgerald, M.D.

Cardiac rhythm disturbances are frequently encountered in the perioperative period. It is important to recognize arrhythmias early and to initiate therapy or arrange consultation when appropriate. In this chapter, a brief overview of the various heart rhythm disturbances is provided, as well as a general approach to treatment with emphasis on the perioperative period. An outline of the various perioperative arrhythmias most likely to be encountered is provided in Box 54–1.

Supraventricular arrhythmias are the most common rhythm disturbance encountered in the perioperative period. In a group of 4181 consecutive patients undergoing major, nonemergency, noncardiac surgery, 83 patients (2.0%) experienced an intraoperative supraventricular arrhythmia and 256 patients (6.1%) experienced a supraventricular arrhythmia in the postoperative period. The presence of such an arrhythmia was associated with a 33% increase in hospital length of stay. Ventricular arrhythmias may also occur in the perioperative setting and are often associated with preexisting heart disease or myocardial ischemia.

As the population increases in age and more elderly patients undergo surgical procedures, more patients with a history of heart rhythm disturbances are likely to undergo elective surgery. These patients are subject to an exacerbation of stable arrhythmias or recurrence of a paroxysmal arrhythmia. They may also require special considerations such as management of chronic anticoagulation in the perioperative setting. Increasing numbers of patients with heart rhythm disturbances are treated with implanted cardiac assist devices such as permanent pacemakers and implantable cardiac defibrillators (ICDs). These patients represent an additional challenge both from concerns over perioperative management of the device and from the potential for exacerbation of arrhythmias from the stress of surgery.

Identification of Patients at Risk for Perioperative Arrhythmias

Preoperative Assessment

A thorough preoperative evaluation should include an evaluation of prior arrhythmias, because such patients are at increased risk for recurrence with the stress of surgery. Knowledge of preexisting structural heart disease (coronary artery disease, valvular or congenital heart disease, congestive heart failure, etc.) is critical for choosing appropriate therapies for various arrhythmias. If available, an assessment

Box 54–1
Perioperative Arrhythmias

Supraventricular arrhythmias
- Tachyarrhythmias (heart rate >100bpm)
  - Atrial fibrillation/atrial flutter with rapid ventricular response
  - AV nodal re-entrant tachycardia (SVT or PSVT)
  - Atrial tachycardia/premature atrial contractions
    - Multifocal
    - Ectopic
  - Accessory pathway mediated tachycardia (AVRT)
- Brady arrhythmias (heart rate < 60 bpm)
  - Sinus bradycardia
  - Junctional bradycardia
  - Complete heart block/high degree AV block

Ventricular arrhythmias
- PVCs
- Ventricular tachycardia (sustained and nonsustained)
  - Monomorphic
  - Polymorphic
- Ventricular fibrillation

of left ventricular function not only is important for the intraoperative management of the patient with structural heart disease but also is essential when choosing various rate control and antiarrhythmic medications.

The preoperative electrocardiogram (ECG) is a powerful tool for the potential identification of both previously undiagnosed asymptomatic arrhythmias and structural heart disease. It is also invaluable as a baseline should cardiac complications develop in patients regardless of whether there is any history of heart disease or rhythm disturbances. A new diagnosis of atrial fibrillation on the preoperative ECG should prompt further assessment before elective noncardiac surgery is performed. Similarly, electrocardiographic abnormalities suggesting prior myocardial infarction should prompt further cardiac risk assessment. One important but uncommon condition that can be identified on the preoperative ECG is the presence of ventricular preexcitation, or Wolff-Parkinson-White (WPW) syndrome. Additional discussion of WPW syndrome and management in the perioperative period is provided later in the chapter.

Risk Factors for Perioperative Arrhythmias

Supraventricular tachyarrhythmias

Several studies have attempted to identify clinical characteristics that predict perioperative supraventricular

arrhythmias, particularly supraventricular tachycardias (SVTs). The predominant rhythm noted in these studies was atrial fibrillation, accounting for approximately 90% of perioperative SVTs. Three independent risk factors have been identified for the development of perioperative SVT: age greater than 70 years, type of surgery (intra-abdominal, intrathoracic, or major vascular surgery), and presence of pulmonary rales from either heart failure or chronic lung disease. Interestingly, a history of prior myocardial infarction, congestive heart failure, chronic lung disease, angina, valvular heart disease, and hypertension were not *independent* predictors of increased risk in this study. The majority of the arrhythmias occurred in the setting of blood loss, electrolyte abnormalities, infection, myocardial infarction, or hypoxia. A second study also found that the only independent predictors for perioperative SVT were blood loss (>1 L) or a postoperative rise in pulmonary arterial pressure. In both studies, the mean time of onset was 48 to 72 hours after surgery. Another study evaluated the effects of preoperative characteristics, the type of surgery, and perioperative events on development of supraventricular arrhythmias in patients undergoing noncardiac surgery. Age (>70 years), male sex, history of congestive heart failure, evidence of clinically significant valvular disease, history of prior supraventricular arrhythmia, history of asthma, presence of premature atrial contractions on the preoperative ECG, and American Society of Anesthesiologists clinical class III and IV were independent correlates of supraventricular arrhythmias in the perioperative setting. Patients undergoing vascular, intrathoracic and abdominal surgery were at increased risk for development of supraventricular arrhythmias. Perioperative events associated with these arrhythmias included acute cardiac events (congestive heart failure, ischemia with or without infarction, ventricular tachycardia, or cardiac arrest), bacterial pneumonia, bacteremia, wound infection, urinary tract infection, cerebrovascular accident, pulmonary embolism, and gastrointestinal bleeding. In summary, supraventricular arrhythmias occur mainly in the setting of some hemodynamic event that results in increased circulating catecholamines. Preoperative clinical predictors for a perioperative SVT include age and a previous history of SVTs. Other predictors, such as preexisting structural heart disease and lung disease, have been shown to have an association in some but not in all studies.

Prophylactic β-blocker administration has been shown to decrease the incidence of postoperative atrial fibrillation after cardiac surgery in numerous studies. Withdrawal of β-blockers has also shown to increase postoperative atrial fibrillation in this same population. The prophylactic use of these medications in patients undergoing noncardiac surgery has not been studied. β-Blockers should be considered in all patients with cardiac risk factors undergoing major surgery because of the decreased number of adverse cardiac events demonstrated in two prospective randomized trials of patients undergoing noncardiac surgery. Patients on β-blockers preoperatively should be maintained on these agents in the perioperative setting to reduce the incidence of atrial fibrillation, to avoid β-blocker withdrawal, and for their potential cardioprotective effects. No firm recommendation can be made for initiation of β-blocker therapy in patients undergoing noncardiac surgery solely for the purpose of preventing arrhythmias. Various antiarrhythmic drugs have been studied in the pre- and intraoperative setting to prevent atrial fibrillation after cardiac surgery, with mixed results, but cannot be recommended for prevention of atrial fibrillation after noncardiac surgery. However, all patients on antiarrhythmic medications preoperatively should have these continued in the postoperative setting to prevent recurrence of the arrhythmia.

Bradyarrhythmias

These arrhythmias are rarely significant problems in the perioperative period and can be managed just as they would be in a nonoperative setting. Patients with asymptomatic bradycardia, whether from sinus bradycardia, junctional rhythm, or atrial fibrillation, infrequently have problems with perioperative symptomatic bradycardia because of the hyperadrenergic state associated with surgery. Patients with symptomatic bradycardia should be evaluated for permanent pacing prior to elective surgery. The major bradycardic rhythm that must be anticipated perioperatively is heart block. Those patients with underlying conduction system disease are at highest risk of progression to complete heart block, but that risk remains low. Several studies have looked at the role of perioperative temporary transcutaneous or transvenous pacing in patients with underlying bifascicular block (right bundle branch block [RBBB] with left anterior fascicular block with or without first-degree atrioventricular [AV] block, or left bundle branch block [LBBB] with first-degree AV block), and all have found that prophylactic pacing was not necessary. Patients with preexisting LBBB who require pulmonary artery catheterization for hemodynamic monitoring are also at low risk for temporary complete heart block by induction of RBBB (mechanical trauma to the proximal right bundle) with catheter insertion and do not require prophylactic temporary pacing.

Ventricular arrhythmias

Perioperative ventricular arrhythmias are strongly associated with the presence of underlying structural heart disease. Patients with coronary artery disease and left ventricular dysfunction are at the highest risk. In a prospective cohort of 1001 patients undergoing major noncardiac surgery, the presence of more than five premature ventricular contractions (PVCs) per minute at any time before the operation was an independent predictor of cardiac complications. No information was given regarding the relationship of these PVCs to symptoms or the existence of heart disease. Another study monitored for intra- and postoperative arrhythmias prospectively in 60 patients with structural heart disease and ventricular couplets or nonsustained ventricular tachycardia (NSVT) on preoperative Holter monitoring. These same arrhythmias were noted intraoperatively in 35% and postoperatively in 87% of the patients. None of these patients experienced sustained ventricular tachycardia (VT) or ventricular fibrillation (VF) during observation after surgery. Eight percent experienced an adverse outcome ($n = 5$; unstable angina, $n = 1$, congestive heart failure, $n = 4$). There was no difference in the frequency of arrhythmias on monitoring at any time between the group with an adverse outcome and those with a good outcome. The authors concluded that, in noncardiac surgery involving patients with structural heart disease and couplets or NSVT, the frequency of ventricular arrhythmias was not associated with an adverse cardiac outcome.

Preoperative assessment is targeted at identifying patients at risk for perioperative ischemia and those with poorly controlled heart failure. This can be accomplished by a symptom review looking for unstable angina, paroxysmal nocturnal dyspnea, orthopnea, and resting or exertional dyspnea. Any recent worsening of symptoms or symptoms at rest should be evaluated by medicine or cardiology consultation. In general, those patients with preoperative ventricular arrhythmias are at the highest risk of perioperative ventricular arrhythmias, but the majority of these represent a recurrence of chronic arrhythmias that are hemodynamically benign. In the rare instance of identification of a patient with recurrent or unstable VT, surgery should be postponed until this can be evaluated. As with supraventricular arrhythmias, perioperative ventricular arrhythmias most often occur in the setting of hemodynamic stressors of ischemia, decompensated congestive heart failure, hypoxia, blood loss, or electrolyte imbalance. Initial therapy should be directed at correction of the underlying problem, rather than at the arrhythmia itself.

Diagnosis and Management of Perioperative Arrhythmias

Supraventricular Tachyarrhythmias

Atrial fibrillation and atrial flutter

Atrial arrhythmias have been observed in 11% to 40% of patients after coronary artery bypass graft surgery and over 50% of patients after valvular heart surgery. However, in the general surgery population, atrial fibrillation and atrial flutter are still clinically important, occurring in 4.1% and 1.2% of patients, respectively, in the perioperative period.

ATRIAL FIBRILLATION. Atrial fibrillation is the most common arrhythmia in patients undergoing both cardiac and noncardiac surgery. Atrial fibrillation can result in an overall decrease in cardiac output secondary to loss of atrial contribution to ventricular filling and inappropriately fast heart rates that reduce overall ventricular ejection volumes. In addition to these hemodynamic problems, persistent atrial fibrillation (duration longer than 48 hours) is associated with an increased risk of stroke and thromboembolism that can be reduced with anticoagulant therapy. Therefore, prevention and early identification are important in reducing patient morbidity.

Identification. Atrial fibrillation is characterized by an irregularly irregular cardiac rhythm. The ventricular response is variable but may reach 180 to 200 beats/min and is affected by the presence of medications that slow conduction in the AV node. The loss of organized atrial activity is signified by an irregular baseline (the fibrillating atria) and an absence of P waves. The morphology of the QRS complex is usually the same as that in sinus rhythm but can appear different if conduction is aberrant, which may occur when the ventricular rate is fast or in response to sudden rate changes caused by irregular conduction (Fig. 54–1).

Management. Treatment of atrial fibrillation is directed at controlling the rate and ultimately restoring sinus rhythm. Atrial fibrillation associated with a rapid ventricular response, and hypotension should be treated with urgent synchronized direct current (DC) cardioversion. However, atrial fibrillation that is hemodynamically tolerated should be initially controlled with drugs that slow conduction through the AV node if the ventricular rate remains elevated. Intravenous calcium channel blockers or β-blockers are very effective in slowing conduction through the AV node and can rapidly provide control of the ventricular response in atrial fibrillation. These drugs may be administered by bolus infusion but require maintenance infusions or follow-up oral dosing to maintain adequate rate control (Table 54–1). When continuous infusions are administered, blood pressure and heart rate must be closely monitored because these medications have the potential for hypotension and bradycardia. Patients with a depressed ejection fraction should be monitored for exacerbation of congestive heart failure because these medications also have negative inotropic effects. Intravenous and/or oral digoxin has been used extensively in the past for postoperative atrial fibrillation. The pharmacology of digoxin is suited for its use in chronic atrial fibrillation because it increases parasympathetic tone to the AV node, with a resultant slowing of AV nodal conduction. In the postoperative setting, where atrial fibrillation is often associated with excessive sympathetic tone, it is less effective and should not be considered first-line treatment.

It is important to assess each patient for a potential etiology of atrial fibrillation, with specific attention to ischemia, volume overload, undiagnosed thyroid disease, electrolyte abnormalities, and enhanced sympathetic stimulation (e.g., pain, use of pressors or cardiac stimulants). All patients should have the abnormal rhythm documented on a 12-lead ECG (rather than a single-lead rhythm strip) to assure the diagnosis. Additionally, these patients should be placed on a cardiac monitor. A significant number of patients will spontaneously convert to sinus rhythm without electrical or pharmacologic intervention. These patients should still be evaluated for causative factors. If atrial fibrillation is believed to be secondary to identified factors that have resolved, then these patients may be discharged without anticoagulation with follow-up only if their arrhythmia recurs.

For those patients who remain in atrial fibrillation, restoration of sinus rhythm is generally desired because patients in persistent atrial fibrillation are at increased risk of stroke. In addition, the longer the patient remains in atrial fibrillation, the more difficult it is to subsequently restore sinus rhythm. No conclusive evidence has suggested that maintenance of sinus rhythm with drugs or electrical cardioversion is superior to rate control and anticoagulation for *chronic* atrial fibrillation. However, restoration of sinus rhythm is usually pursued when associated with a transient condition such as surgery to avoid anticoagulation in the postoperative setting and improve hemodynamic stability.

If patients have been in atrial fibrillation for less than 48 hours, then an attempt to restore sinus rhythm may be made without the need for subsequent anticoagulation. If patients have been in atrial fibrillation for greater than 48 hours, then anticoagulation should be initiated if safe from the surgical standpoint. One approach is to use transesophageal echocardiography to exclude atrial

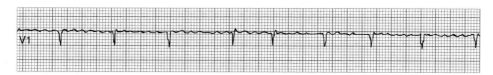

FIGURE 54–1 Atrial fibrillation. A single-lead rhythm strip of precordial lead V₁ in which an irregularly irregular ventricular rate is seen. Note that there are fine fibrillatory waves with varying morphology at very rapid rates of 350 to 400 msec forming the baseline, which is characteristic of atrial fibrillation.

Table 54–1
Drugs used for rate control in atrial fibrillation

Drug	Acute Therapy	Maintenance Therapy	Notes
Beta-blockers			
Esmolol	0.5-mg/kg IV bolus, then 0.05-mg/kg/min infusion; may be increased to 0.2 mg/kg/min if needed	None	Poor efficacy if concomitant β-agonists required because of antagonistic actions
Metoprolol	5-mg IV push; may repeat q2–5 min for a total of 15 mg No data on continuous infusion	25–200 mg orally q12h	May induce bronchospasm. Monitor for hypotension and bradycardia
Atenolol	5-mg IV push; may repeat in 5–10 min for a total of 10 mg No data on continuous infusion	25–200 mg orally q24h	May induce bronchospasm. Monitor for hypotension and bradycardia. Dose adjustment may be needed in renal impairment
Calcium channel blockers			
Diltiazem	10- to 20-mg bolus over 2 min, then continuous infusion at 5–15 mg/min	120–360 mg orally divided q6h or once a day as a sustained-release preparation	Monitor for hypotension and bradycardia. May exacerbate congestive heart failure if reduced left ventricular function
Verapamil	5- to 10-mg bolus over several minutes; IV continuous infusion not recommended	120–480 mg orally divided q6–8h or once daily as a sustained-release preparation	Same as diltiazem.
Digoxin	0.75–1.5 mg IV or orally divided q6–8h	0.125–0.375 mg orally q24h	Less efficacious in states of elevated sympathetic tone. Dosage adjustment required in renal failure. Numerous drug interactions.

thrombi, with cardioversion if none are identified. However, anticoagulation should be continued for at least 4 weeks after conversion if sinus rhythm is maintained. Also acceptable is the approach of discharge on anticoagulant therapy with outpatient cardioversion if the patient remains in atrial fibrillation after 3 to 4 weeks of therapeutic anticoagulation (international normalized ratio 2 to 3). These patients should be anticoagulated for at least 4 weeks after cardioversion if sinus rhythm is maintained during follow-up. Antiarrhythmic therapy may be utilized both in acute cardioversion and as an adjunct for maintenance of sinus rhythm. Drugs potentially useful include flecainide, propafenone, quinidine, procainamide, amiodarone, sotalol, ibutilide, and dofetilide. All of these have specific situations in which their use is contraindicated, and initiation should only be done by physicians familiar with their administration. Table 54–1 lists these medications, routes of administration, and various concerns with initiation.

ATRIAL FLUTTER. Atrial flutter is similar to atrial fibrillation in many respects except that the ECG shows an organized pattern of atrial activation from beat to beat (Fig. 54–2). It is recognized as sudden onset of a tachycardia with a ventricular rate of 140 to 160 beats/min. A saw-toothed pattern of "flutter" waves is often present in the inferior leads (ECG leads II, III, and aVF). The atrial rate in atrial flutter is usually 280 to 320 beats/min, so that a ventricular rate of 140 to 160 beats/min reflects 2:1 conduction through the AV node, which is often regular. Variable conduction may be present, with evidence of 2:1, 3:1, 4:1, and even slower conduction, especially if the patient is taking medications that slow AV nodal conduction or if there is preexisting conduction system disease. Management is similar to that for atrial fibrillation, although rate control is sometimes more difficult. Atrial flutter also carries a risk of thromboembolism, and anticoagulation should be considered for persistent atrial flutter.

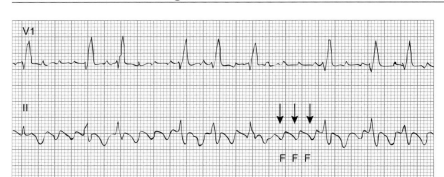

FIGURE 54–2 Atrial flutter. A rhythm strip including surface leads V₁ and III demonstrates the rapid but regular flutter waves (F). Common atrial flutter is characterized by negative flutter waves in the inferior leads (II, III, and aVF), marked by *arrows* in lead III.

AV nodal reentrant tachycardia or SVT/Paroxysmal SVT

BACKGROUND. AV nodal reentrant tachycardia (AVNRT) is a supraventricular tachyarrhythmia likely to be initiated in the perioperative setting, with a reported prevalence of 3.7%. AVNRT may occur in any age group and is unrelated to the presence of structural heart disease. It is due to the presence of two pathways of conduction within the AV node, which allows for the establishment of a reentry circuit and tachycardia. Initiation of the tachycardia is abrupt and usually associated with enhanced adrenergic tone and triggers such as premature atrial contractions (PACs) or PVCs. Identification of AVNRT can usually be made with a 12-lead ECG and review of the manner in which the arrhythmia was initiated and terminated. The rate is variable but often 140 to 160 beats/min, and may exceed 200 beats/min. The QRS morphology is typically normal or the same as the underlying sinus QRS complex; however, aberrant conduction (with a LBBB or RBBB) may occur, making it difficult to differentiate from VT. No P waves are present preceding the QRS complexes, and the baseline appears flat. This is in contrast to atrial fibrillation or atrial flutter, which have an irregular or saw-toothed baseline. A retrograde inverted P wave can sometimes be seen in the terminal portion of the QRS complex (Fig. 54–3).

MANAGEMENT. Treatment of AVNRT involves maneuvers or agents that temporarily alter AV nodal conduction and break the reentrant cycle. Infrequently, AVNRT can cause hemodynamic compromise and may require prompt synchronized DC cardioversion. Most patients, however, are hemodynamically stable. Maneuvers to increase vagal tone, such as a carotid sinus massage or Valsalva maneuver, can be successful. When these are unsuccessful or cannot be performed, pharmacologic treatment is appropriate. Adenosine is considered the first-line treatment because it is highly effective in terminating AVNRT. It works by temporarily blocking AV nodal conduction, interrupting the reentrant circuit. Other drugs that may be effective include intravenous diltiazem, verapamil, and esmolol (Table 54–2). These medications are given as a bolus to terminate the tachycardia. Maintenance therapy with oral agents such as diltiazem, verapamil, or β-blockers is only necessary in patients with recurrent episodes.

Multifocal and ectopic atrial tachycardia

Multifocal atrial tachycardia (MAT) and ectopic atrial tachycardia (EAT) are atrial arrhythmias also occurring in the perioperative setting, although less commonly than atrial fibrillation and AVNRT. MAT has a low prevalence in the hospitalized population (0.05% to 0.32%) and a postoperative prevalence of approximately 0.2%, with a mortality rate as high as 45%. The diagnosis is made on the basis of electrocardiographic criteria and is defined as an atrial rate of greater than 100 beats/min with at least three different, nonsinus P-wave morphologies identified

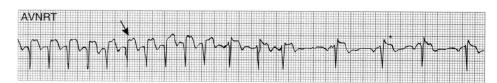

FIGURE 54–3 AV nodal reentry. A single-lead rhythm strip demonstrates termination of an episode of AV nodal reentry following administration of adenosine. A narrow-complex tachycardia with a small deflection noted at the end of the QRS complex *(arrow)* indicates retrograde atrial activation in this reentrant tachycardia. Note the sharp peak at the end of the QRS complex (*) in sinus rhythm and compare this region to the QRS complex during tachycardia to more clearly see the retrograde P wave in tachycardia.

Table 54–2

Drugs for termination of AVNRT

Drug	Dosage	Side Effects
Adenosine	6 to 12 mg rapid IV push	Chest pain, flushing, dyspnea, brief period of prolonged AV block
Diltiazem	10 to 20 mg IV push over 2-3 min	Hypotension and bradycardia
Verapamil	5 to 10 mg IV push over 2-3 min	Hypotension and bradycardia
Esmolol		

on a 12-lead ECG (Fig. 54–4). Both the atrial rate and the ventricular response are irregular, resulting in variable P-P, P-R, and R-R intervals. A flat baseline with distinct atrial activation waves is required to exclude atrial fibrillation. MAT is strongly associated with chronic obstructive lung disease and more common in patients with pulmonary infection and heart disease. Diabetes and electrolyte abnormalities are common in patients with MAT, and pulmonary embolism has been associated with it. Use of theophylline preparations may increase the incidence of MAT.

Treatment of MAT is directed at addressing the underlying etiology. β-Blocking agents have been reported to improve the ventricular rate and may convert MAT to sinus rhythm. Concern over exacerbation of concomitant severe lung disease and hypotension are potential contraindications. Metoprolol has been shown to decrease the ventricular rate compared to verapamil and placebo in a prospective, double-blind study. Verapamil has been observed in several studies to decrease the rate and possibly the incidence of MAT. It may worsen hypoxemia by antagonizing hypoxic pulmonary vasoconstriction. Patients should be monitored for hypotension. Intravenous magnesium therapy has been observed to suppress atrial ectopy acutely, even in patients with magnesium levels in the normal range. There is no role for electrical cardioversion, and the role of membrane-stabilizing antiarrhythmic agents is poorly defined.

EAT is recognized as a rapid, regular tachycardia with a single P-wave morphology different from the sinus P wave (Fig. 54–5). It could reflect any area of abnormal automatic behavior in the atrium or, less commonly, a reentrant circuit in the atrium. Atrial tachycardia associated with AV block is not pathognomonic for but should raise the question of digitalis excess. Brief episodes of atrial tachycardia do not require specific treatment unless they become symptomatic or frequent. Various drug therapies, including β-blockers, calcium channel blockers, and membrane-stabilizing antiarrhythmic drugs, are appropriate depending on the underlying mechanism. Reentrant atrial tachycardia responds to membrane-stabilizing antiarrhythmic drugs, while automatic atrial tachycardias may respond to calcium channel blockers and β-blockers. Medical therapy to control the ventricular rate or suppress the arrhythmia is appropriate in the acute setting. Anticoagulation is not indicated.

Accessory pathway or AV reentrant tachycardia

BACKGROUND. Accessory pathway–mediated tachycardia is a special category of supraventricular tachycardia that merits discussion because of important differences in management. Sometimes referred to as AV reentrant tachycardia, this form of SVT results from the presence of an "accessory" bundle of myocardial tissue that electrically connects the atria and ventricles in addition to the normal AV node/His-Purkinje system. Some, but not all, patients with accessory pathways may be identified by the presence of a "delta" wave on the ECG.

FIGURE 54–4 Multifocal atrial tachycardia. A rhythm strip including surface leads V_1 and II shows runs of an irregular atrial tachycardia. The varying P-wave morphology (P_1, P_2, P_3, and P_4) suggests a multifocal atrial tachycardia. The wide complex beat between P_3 and P_4 is a premature ventricular complex.

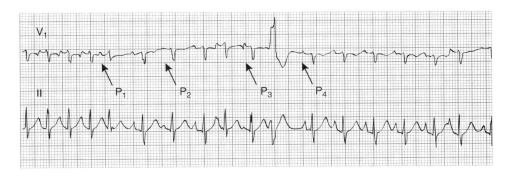

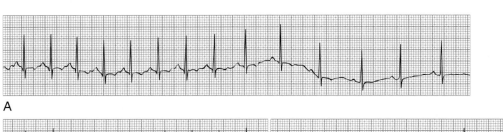

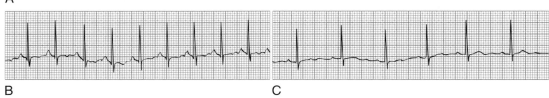

A

B   C

FIGURE 54–5 Ectopic atrial tachycardia. **A,** A narrow-complex tachycardia at approximately 120 beats/min slows and abruptly stops after the 10th beat (*), with change in the P-wave amplitude and morphology indicating shift from an ectopic focus to sinus rhythm. **B,** The atrial tachycardia preceding termination is displayed for comparison of the P-wave amplitude and morphology to that of a sinus rhythm tracing recorded upon termination of ectopic atrial tachycardia (**C**).

Recognized as an early upsloping of the QRS, the delta wave represents early activation or preexcitation of the ventricle via the accessory pathway (Fig. 54–6). The WPW syndrome describes patients with evidence of (1) preexcitation (delta waves) on the ECG, (2) a shortened P-R interval, and (3) paroxysmal tachycardias.

When conducted antegrade over the native conduction system and retrograde over the accessory pathway, the tachycardia usually has a QRS complex similar to that in normal sinus rhythm (Fig. 54–7). The baseline is flat, and a retrograde P wave is occasionally seen in the ST segment or the T wave, similar to and often indistinguishable from AVNRT. Infrequently the tachycardia may conduct antegrade over the accessory pathway and retrograde over the native conduction system, with a resulting wide QRS complex, and may be difficult to distinguish from VT.

IDENTIFICATION AND MANAGEMENT. Patients in normal sinus rhythm with evidence of preexcitation on the ECG and no symptoms of tachycardia need no specific treatment. It is important, however, to recognize patients with preexcitation on an ECG or a known history of WPW because this will affect treatment if the patient has tachycardia. Onset of a regular narrow-complex tachycardia in a patient with a history of WPW suggests orthodromic reentry using the AV node for antegrade conduction to the ventricle and the accessory pathway for retrograde activation of the atrium. This tachycardia can be terminated by slowing conduction through the AV node. Acutely unstable patients respond to synchronized DC cardioversion. Most patients are hemodynamically stable, and vagal maneuvers such as carotid sinus massage and Valsalva maneuver may be attempted before pharmacologic therapy.

Adenosine, 6 to 18 mg as a rapid intravenous push, is very effective in terminating the tachycardia.

Development of a regular wide-complex tachycardia in a patient with preexcitation may represent antegrade conduction over the accessory pathway with retrograde conduction over the AV node or another accessory pathway. In a patient with preexisting structural heart disease, differentiating ventricular tachycardia from a preexcited tachycardia can be difficult. Hemodynamically unstable patients should be treated with synchronized DC cardioversion. Stable patients merit a trial of medical therapy, which is directed at slowing conduction through the accessory pathway and terminating the tachycardia. Procainamide at 15 mg/kg (up to 1000 mg) administered over 30 to 60 minutes usually results in acute termination of the tachycardia. Blood pressure must be monitored closely because intravenous procainamide may cause hypotension. Only a bolus administration is needed for termination of the tachycardia.

Atrial fibrillation in a patient with preexcitation is a potentially dangerous condition. Blockade of the AV node with drugs such as diltiazem, verapamil, digoxin, or β-blockers can result in preferential ventricular activation through the accessory pathway. These pathways are typically able to conduct faster than the AV node/His-Purkinje system, and atrial fibrillation may be conducted to the ventricle in a 1:1 fashion at rates greater than 250 beats/min and may cause VF. Accordingly, acute-onset atrial fibrillation in patients with preexcitation should be managed with DC cardioversion if the patient is unstable. Stable patients may be managed with antiarrhythmic medications such as amiodarone or procainamide, which are effective both in slowing accessory pathway conduction and in the management of atrial fibrillation.

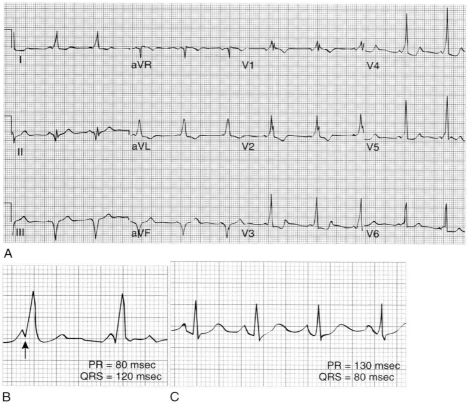

FIGURE 54–6 Wolff-Parkinson-White syndrome and ventricular preexcitation. **A,** Twelve-lead ECG of a patient with evidence of ventricular preexcitation as demonstrated by the short P-R interval, upsloping of the P wave into the QRS complex without an isoelectric line, and widened QRS complex. The apparent right bundle branch pattern of activation suggests a left-sided accessory pathway connecting the left atrium to the left ventricle. **B,** Rhythm strip showing delta wave *(arrow)* in a patient with preexcitation. **C,** Following ablation of the accessory pathway in this same patient, there is an isoelectric interval between the P wave and the QRS complex. The QRS complex has narrowed.

Supraventricular Bradyarrhythmias

Sinus and junctional bradycardias

Sinus bradycardia is defined as sinus rhythm less than 60 beats/min. It is a common finding in people who are well conditioned and in patients taking medications that slow the sinus rate. In the absence of symptoms or hemodynamic compromise, it is generally not treated. In the perioperative setting, however, it may signify a serious underlying problem that requires immediate attention. Etiologies in this setting include hypoxemia, cardiac ischemia, hyperkalemia, vagal surges, and drug toxicity. Drugs implicated include digitalis, β-blockers, calcium

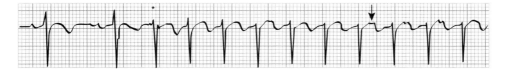

FIGURE 54–7 Supraventricular tachycardia associated with an accessory pathway. The common tachycardia seen in patients with accessory pathways is a reentrant tachycardia as a result of antegrade ventricular activation over the AV node and retrograde atrial activation using the accessory pathway. A single-lead rhythm strip shows sinus rhythm in the first two beats with a premature atrial complex (*) initiating a regular tachycardia with a retrograde P wave in the ST segment *(arrow)*. Note the change in the ST-T wave in tachycardia as a result of deformation of this segment by the retrograde P wave when compared to the ST-T wave of the first sinus beat. The retrograde P wave is usually 120 msec or more after the onset of the QRS complex, whereas, with AV nodal reentry, the retrograde P wave occurs at less than 110 msec from the onset of the QRS complex.

channel blockers, clonidine, and antiarrhythmic agents. Sinus bradycardia and even asystole have been reported in association with spinal anesthesia.

Other than correcting the reversible causes, specific treatment of sinus bradycardia is required only when it causes hemodynamic problems. Atropine, 0.5 to 1 mg intravenously, usually results in a prompt increase in the sinus rate because of its vagolytic effect, which will persist for 20 to 40 minutes. Alternatively isoproterenol, a β-agonist, can be administered as a continuous drip at 1 to 3 μ/min to increase the sinus rate. Dopamine and aminophylline infusions may also be considered. Pacing is rarely necessary for isolated sinus bradycardia in the perioperative setting.

Junctional bradycardia or junctional rhythm is recognized as a regular rhythm with rates usually 30 to 60 beats/min, with no P wave or a very short P-R interval preceding the normally conducted beat (Fig. 54–8). Its causes are similar to those for sinus bradycardia because it often reflects a condition wherein the junctional rate exceeds the sinus rate in association with sick sinus syndrome. As with sinus bradycardia, management is directed to treating reversible causes and withholding medications that slow conduction until normal sinus rhythm returns. If the junctional rhythm results in significant symptoms or hemodynamic compromise, temporary pacing is warranted.

Complete heart block

Complete heart block or third-degree heart block is a condition in which atrial and ventricular activity are completely dissociated as a result of an inability of the atrial impulses to conduct to the ventricle. The 12-lead ECG demonstrates a regular P wave and QRS complex, each with an independent rate with no evidence of conduction (Fig. 54–9). The ventricular rate and QRS morphology are determined by the level where the impulse is blocked in the specialized conduction tissues. A narrow QRS complex and a ventricular rate of 40 to 60 beats/min implies block at or near the AV node, and a wide QRS complex and slower ventricular rate implies block below the AV node in the His-Purkinje system.

The most common cause of complete heart block is degeneration of the conduction system with age. Numerous other etiologies exist and are beyond the scope of this discussion. Perioperative causes of complete heart block include hyperkalemia, drug toxicity (the same drugs as those listed for sinus bradycardia), hypoxemia, ischemia, infarction, and trauma from intracardiac catheters. Heart block can occur after cardiac surgery. Complete heart block may be associated with endocarditis but is usually preceded by progressive conduction system abnormalities. Transient complete heart block or high-degree AV block may be seen during vagal surges associated with pain, hypoxemia, or volume depletion.

Treatment of complete heart block is dictated by the duration, etiology, and hemodynamic significance. Transient episodes of complete heart block, such as vagal surges during suctioning, do not usually require treatment. Temporary pacing may be required for causes such as drug toxicity or metabolic abnormalities while the underlying

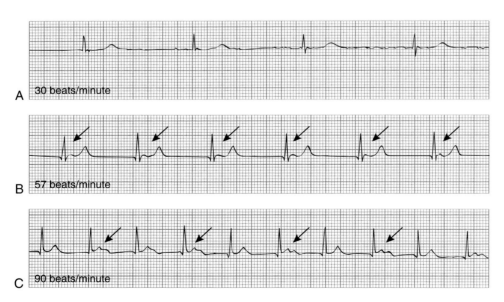

FIGURE 54–8 Junctional rhythm. Junctional rhythm reflects activation of the AV nodal region either as a default escape pacemaker when the atrium fails to control activation or when the AV node is stimulated by changes in autonomic tone. **A,** Junctional bradycardia controls the rate with no evidence of atrial activation. **B,** A junctional rhythm is present with consistent retrograde atrial activation *(arrows).* **C,** An accelerated junctional rhythm is present with 2:1 retrograde atrial activation *(arrows).*

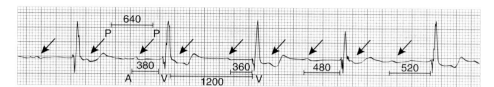

FIGURE 54–9 Complete heart block. A rhythm strip demonstrates a stable atrial rate of 640 msec *(arrows)* and a stable ventricular rate (V-V) of 1200 msec. There is a varying AV interval with no change in the ventricular rate, indicating dissociation of the ventricle from the atrium and complete heart block.

etiology is being corrected. Acutely, temporary pacing may be performed transcutaneously, although not all patients can be effectively paced because of high chest wall impedance. Transcutaneous pacing is also uncomfortable. Transvenous pacing is more reliable and may be utilized as a bridge to permanent pacing if normal conduction does not return.

Ventricular Arrhythmias

Postoperative ventricular tachyarrhythmias may include relatively benign conditions such as PVCs or potentially lethal conditions including sustained VT and VF. If not recognized and treated promptly, these arrhythmias may lead to permanent end-organ dysfunction, especially cerebral hypoperfusion, with substantial morbidity and mortality. They may also signify an underlying major complication such as myocardial ischemia/infarction. This section reviews the identification and treatment of the various ventricular arrhythmias that may be encountered in the perioperative period.

Clinical settings for ventricular arrhythmias

New-onset sustained VT is relatively uncommon after cardiac surgery, and is even less common after noncardiac surgery. Two hundred thirty consecutive male patients at high risk for coronary artery disease (54%) or known coronary artery disease (46%) who were undergoing major noncardiac surgery were evaluated for the presence of perioperative arrhythmias and the relationship to nonfatal myocardial infarction and death. Frequent or major ventricular arrhythmias (>30 PVCs/hr or VT) occurred in 44% of the patients. In 21% of patients, the ventricular arrhythmia was noted preoperatively, while in 16% it occurred intraoperatively, and in 36% it was a postoperative problem. Nine patients (4%) suffered an adverse cardiac outcome. Adverse outcomes were not associated with arrhythmias occurring in any of the three monitoring periods. The authors concluded that these arrhythmias may not require aggressive monitoring or treatment in the perioperative period in the absence of signs or symptoms of myocardial ischemia.

Certain perioperative clinical factors may incite ventricular arrhythmias in patients with both structurally

normal and abnormal hearts. These include hypoxemia, hypercarbia, electrolyte disturbances, and drug toxicity resulting from altered pharmacologic metabolism (particularly in cases of altered drug metabolism caused by changing renal or hepatic function). Further, catecholamine elevation as a result of physical or psychological stressors can also adversely affect ventricular function and lead to VT.

Diagnosis and classification of ventricular arrhythmias

PVCs are identified as periodic wide-complex beats of a morphology different from the native QRS complex. There is frequently a "compensatory pause" after a PVC in sinus rhythm as a result of retrograde conduction of the PVC into the His-Purkinje region, with either block of the subsequent sinus beat or retrograde conduction to the atrium resetting the sinus beat. PVCs may be difficult to distinguish from aberrantly conducted supraventricular beats resulting from sudden rate changes in atrial fibrillation or PACs with aberrant conduction.

VT is defined as at least three or more consecutive beats originating from the ventricle with a rate of at least 100 beats/min. When its duration is 30 seconds or more, it is considered sustained. VT may be further defined as monomorphic or polymorphic. The QRS complex in monomorphic VT is uniform (Fig. 54–10), whereas in polymorphic VT the complex is variable (Fig. 54–11). Electrocardiographic clues favoring the diagnosis of VT include (1) AV dissociation (P waves occurring independently of QRS complexes); (2) a wide QRS interval (>160 msec); (3) a QRS axis between −90 and 180 degrees; and (4) fusion complexes (ventricular activation by both a sinus beat and the tachycardia simultaneously, with resulting change in the QRS). VT must be distinguished from a SVT with preexisting bundle branch block, aberrant ventricular conduction, or antegrade conduction via an accessory pathway (WPW syndrome). VF is easily recognized as a rapid, chaotic wide-complex rhythm with hemodynamic compromise. Artifact from seizure activity, tremor, repetitive movements, or electrical interference can appear similar to VT or VF. This may be confirmed by assessment of the heart rate by palpation or oximetry and overall clinical status during the period of suspected artifact.

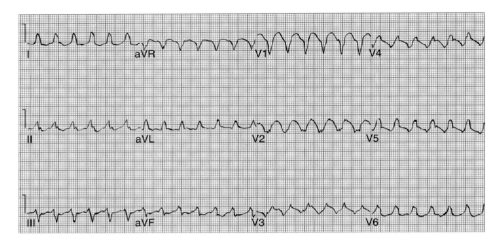

FIGURE 54–10 Monomorphic ventricular tachycardia. A twelve-lead ECG of a regular monomorphic wide-complex tachycardia that is ventricular tachycardia.

Management of ventricular arrhythmias

GENERAL. Ventricular tachyarrhythmias in the postoperative setting have variable levels of severity. Isolated PVCs or short runs of nonsustained VT on a rhythm strip in an otherwise healthy patient with a structurally normal heart and no symptoms to suggest underlying ischemia require evaluation of serum electrolytes to exclude hypokalemia or hypomagnesemia and a 12-lead ECG to exclude ischemia or infarction. Patients with history of structural heart disease represent a higher risk group. If ischemia is suspected as an etiologic factor for VT, additional testing should include serial cardiac enzyme levels (creatine kinase with MB isoenzymes and/or troponin). A transthoracic echocardiogram can provide additional useful information regarding overall left ventricular function, presence or absence of significant valvular heart disease, and an assessment of left ventricular wall motion, which can be compromised during ischemia or infarction. Occasionally, imaging by surface echocardiography can be limited because of anatomic variation, surgical intervention to the chest wall, or lung disease. In these situations, transesophageal echocardiography or magnetic resonance imaging may be employed for functional assessment of the left ventricle. Patients with evidence of active ischemia/acute coronary syndrome should be treated with β-blockers and nitrates under the supervision of an internist/cardiologist. Patients should be considered for antithrombotic therapy such as aspirin and heparin if it is deemed safe from a surgical standpoint. Patients with refractory symptoms or infarction should be evaluated for emergent cardiac revascularization.

SUSTAINED MONOMORPHIC VT. Sustained monomorphic VT usually occurs in the setting of structural heart disease. Monomorphic VT is rarely a manifestation of an acute myocardial infarction but can occur in patients with prior myocardial infarction and depressed left ventricular function. The immediate management of sustained

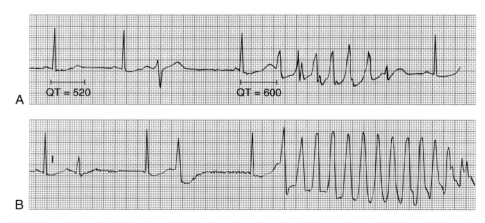

FIGURE 54–11 Polymorphic ventricular tachycardia. Rhythm strips of a patient with a prolonged Q-T interval. Note the marked lengthening of the Q-T interval in response to pauses (**A**) that lead to short runs of polymorphic ventricular tachycardia. **B,** A sustained run of polymorphic ventricular tachycardia occurs.

monomorphic VT is dictated by the clinical status of the patient. An arrhythmia that results in hemodynamic compromise (hypotension or hypoperfusion) should be treated with prompt DC cardioversion. Specific antiarrhythmic drug therapy can be given to prevent recurrences or as the initial therapy to terminate the arrhythmia in hemodynamically stable patients who are at risk for progression to hemodynamic compromise. Lidocaine is the initial agent of choice, and procainamide is an alternative, especially if the diagnosis of the wide-complex tachycardia is uncertain (i.e., in rhythms that could potentially be bundle branch block with aberrant conduction of a SVT). Amiodarone can also be administered intravenously and may be the agent of choice in patients with reduced left ventricular function. Antiarrhythmic medications most frequently used to treat ventricular arrhythmias are listed in Table 54–3. After the patient is stabilized, an evaluation for recent myocardial infarction, heart failure, electrolyte abnormality, hypoxia, and the like is appropriate.

POLYMORPHIC VT/VF. Polymorphic VT represents a particularly dangerous form of VT because it often quickly degenerates into VF. Sustained polymorphic VT rapidly becomes symptomatic and requires prompt, unsynchronized DC cardioversion. Upon restoration of sinus rhythm, the initial step is a clinical evaluation for signs of ischemia and/or infarction. The ECG is an important part of the ischemia assessment and is necessary for determination of the corrected Q-T interval (Q-Tc). Evidence of an acute coronary syndrome should prompt immediate treatment as noted above.

Polymorphic VT may also occur in association with prolongation of the Q-Tc interval. The Q-Tc interval is calculated by dividing the measured Q-T interval by the square root of the R-R interval in seconds (Q-Tc = Q-T/$\sqrt{R\text{-}R}$). This corrects the Q-T interval for differences in heart rate. The upper limit for a normal Q-Tc is debated but ranges from 440 to 460 msec. It has been reported that the upper normal Q-Tc may be 460 msec for men and 470 msec for women. Prolongation of the Q-Tc interval may be acquired or congenital. Many abnormalities can cause the acquired form of polymorphic VT associated with a prolonged Q-Tc, including hypokalemia, hypomagnesemia, hypothermia, antiarrhythmic drugs (quinidine, procainamide, and sotalol), antibiotics (erythromycin and pentamidine), and tricyclic antidepressants. Bursts of polymorphic VT often precede the development of sustained arrhythmias, such that the distinction between sustained and nonsustained polymorphic VT can be clinically unimportant (see Fig. 54–11). Polymorphic VT may also occur in the setting of the familial or hereditary long Q-T syndrome, wherein congenital abnormalities in myocardial cell ion channel function result in abnormal repolarization and a predisposition for cardiac arrhythmias. A prolonged Q-Tc interval at baseline and a syndrome of rapid VT with a phasic continuous alteration of QRS morphology comprises the syndrome of torsade de pointes. Patients usually have a prolonged Q-Tc interval at baseline but may have marked prolongation of the Q-Tc interval and an exacerbation of their arrhythmias with stress and any of the factors that cause the acquired form of polymorphic VT. Acquired polymorphic VT should be treated with intravenous magnesium

Table 54–3
Antiarrhythmic drugs most commonly utilized the acute management of VT/VF

Drugs	Loading Dose	Maintenance Dose	Notes
Lidocaine	75- to 100-mg bolus	1–4 mg/min as continuous infusion	Monitor drug levels. Dose adjust in patients with impaired hepatic function. High doses/levels may cause CNS side effects.
Procainamide	500–1000 mg IV over 30–60 min; 1000 mg PO for loading and acute conversion	1–6 mg/min continuous IV; 1000–4000 mg daily in divided doses (q3–6h)	Prolongs Q-T interval. Hypotension associated with IV administration. Lupus associated with prolonged administration. Dose adjustment required in renal impairment—follow drug levels. Not FDA approved for atrial fibrillation but widely used.
Amiodarone	150 mg over 10 min, then 1 mg/min over 6 hr, then 0.5 mg/min for 18 hr; 800–1600 mg daily in divided doses for 7–14 days	400–600 mg qd	Repeat bolus of 150 mg over 10 min and extension of infusion may be done when recurrent/refractory VT/VF present. Agent of choice in patients with severe LV dysfunction.

CNS, central nervous system; FDA, Food and Drug Administration; LV, left ventricular; VF, ventricular fibrillation; VT, ventricular tachycardia.

and correction of other electrolyte abnormalities and discontinuing potentially offending drugs. Because the Q-T interval lengthens as the ventricular rate slows, both the acquired and congenital forms of polymorphic VT are more likely to occur in association with pauses or bradycardia. When VT is pause dependent, medications such as isoproterenol and temporary transvenous pacing may be used to increase the heart rate and shorten the Q-T interval, thus suppressing further episodes of polymorphic VT. Raising the heart rate to 100 beats/min will usually suppress triggering of VT. Recurrences of polymorphic VT should prompt cardiac consultation.

VF primarily occurs in association with an acute myocardial infarction but may occur as a result of degeneration of VT caused by induced ischemia. Ventricular fibrillation may present spontaneously in patients with depressed left ventricular function. Patients require prompt unsynchronized DC cardioversion and the assessment of the etiology. Recurrent VF merits adjunctive antiarrhythmic therapy similar to that for VT.

Special Considerations

Perioperative Management of the Patient with a Permanent Pacemaker or Cardioverter/Defibrillator

Background

Patients with implanted electronic pacemakers or ICDs provide additional concerns for medical management during the perioperative period. Because they have an implanted device, these patients have been identified as

having underlying arrhythmias. It is important to be aware of the severity of these problems and the status of the associated cardiac disease. In general, pacemakers provide treatment for symptomatic bradyarrhythmias while defibrillators provide therapy for symptomatic tachyarrhythmias, although current ICDs also function as backup pacemakers.

Since the first pacemakers were implanted in 1962, advances in technology have resulted in pacemakers that are fairly sophisticated in their function. With the development of efficient and reliable circuitry, a dependable energy supply (lithium-powered battery), and lead technology allowing placement in multiple chambers with reliable long-term pacing thresholds, their complexity has increased significantly over the last 20 years. A special coding system has been developed to describe the function of a pacemaker. This pacemaker code was originally developed by the Intersociety Commission for Heart Disease Resources in 1974 and subsequently modified on several occasions to keep up with changes in pacemakers. Currently, this five-letter coding system (Table 54–4) can be used to describe how a pacemaker is programmed to function. Codes representing the first three letters are most commonly used and refer to the chamber(s) paced (letter I code), the chamber(s) sensed (letter II code), and the response to sensing (letter III code). The letter IV code refers to the programmability of the device (including whether it provides some type of rate response), and the letter V code indicates whether anti-tachycardia functions such as rapid pacing or shocks can be programmed.

A pacemaker with a single lead in the right ventricle programmed to pace if the heart rate drops below a certain rate would be described as a VVI pacemaker that is inhibited (I) if the patient's intrinsic ventricular rate

Table 54–4

NASPE/BPEG (NBG) generic pacemaker codes

I	II	III	IV	V
Chamber(s) Paced	**Chamber(s) Sensed**	**Response to sensing**	**Programmability, Rate Modulation**	**Anti-tachyarrhythmia Function(s)**
0 = None	0 = None	0 = None	0 = None	0 = None
A = Atrium	A = Atrium	T = Triggered	P = Simple programmable	P = Pacing (tachyarrhythmia)
V = Ventricle	V = Ventricle	I = Inhibited	M = Multiprogrammable	S = Shock
D = Dual (atrium and ventricle)	D = Dual (atrium and ventricle)	D = Dual (trigger and inhibit)	C = Communicating	D = Dual (pacing and shock)
S = Single (atrium or ventricle)	S = Single (atrium or ventricle)		R = Rate modulation	

From Bernstein AD, Camm AJ, Fletcher R, et al: The NASPE/BPEG generic pacemaker code for antibradyarrhythmia and adaptive-rate pacing and anti-tachyarrhythmia devices. Pacing Clin Electrophysiol 1987;10:794, permission from Futura Publishing Company, Inc.

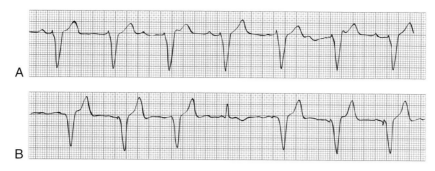

FIGURE 54–12 Ventricular demand pacemaker. **A,** A ventricular demand pacemaker controls the rate. Note that atrial activation continues in a regular fashion out of synchrony with the slower ventricular pacing rate. **B,** During atrial fibrillation, a ventricular demand pacemaker controls the rate unless a spontaneous conducted complex occurs at a rate faster than the programmed ventricular pacing rate, which will suppress ventricular pacing.

is greater than the programmed rate and would pace the right ventricle if the intrinsic rate drops below the programmed rate (Fig. 54–12). A dual-chamber pacemaker typically has leads in the right atrium and in the right ventricle (Fig. 54–13). This pacing configuration can maintain synchrony between atrial and ventricular activation. When programmed in the DDD mode, the pacemaker will first look at the intrinsic atrial rate; if above the programmed rate, it will inhibit atrial pacing but, if below the lower pacing rate, it will pace the atrium at the lower programmed rate. Next, after an atrial sensed or paced event, an AV interval occurs during which the pacemaker looks for a ventricular event. If no intrinsic ventricular rhythm is detected, a ventricular paced event occurs. If an intrinsic ventricular event occurs, ventricular pacing is inhibited. After a ventricular paced or sensed event, a postventricular refractory period occurs during which time atrial and ventricular events are not sensed. At the end of this period, the pacemaker is ready to respond to the next atrial event with either sensing or pacing. The combination of the AV interval and the postventricular refractory period determines the upper tracking rate of the device.

ICDs have similar pacing parameters and responses for antibradycardia therapies. However, ICDs also will provide therapy for rapid heart rates. A programmable tachycardia detection interval will determine the heart rate that will be treated with anti-tachycardia therapy. The anti-tachycardia therapy may include attempts at rapid pacing or shock delivery to terminate rhythms above the detection interval. Different anti-tachycardia therapies can be used for different ranges (zones) of rapid heart rates.

Preoperative assessment

With regard to the perioperative period, because of physiologic changes in heart rate in response to operative stress, it is important to know the programmed parameters of a pacemaker or ICD to assure adequate function. If a patient has a limited heart rate response to stress, the pacemaker may require some adjustment in the lower rate to cover increased metabolic needs in the perioperative period. Sinus tachycardia or atrial fibrillation may result in heart rates above the tachycardia detection rate of an ICD, with subsequent delivery of anti-tachycardia pacing or shocks that may not be warranted. Therefore, preoperative evaluation of these patients should include device interrogation by a cardiologist or technician so that the ranges of heart rates and therapies for rhythms will be known prior to surgery. This is done on a periodic basis, and information from a recent office interrogation may be satisfactory. All of these patients should be monitored during the intraoperative and postoperative period so that any problems with device function or rhythm management can be promptly recognized and dealt with.

Intra- and postoperative management

The principal concern with the function of a rhythm control device during the perioperative period is related to the effects of external devices that generate electrical fields that could interfere with the sensing function of the pacemaker or ICD. Additionally, there are concerns that the energy generated by some of these external devices could damage the circuitry of pacemakers or ICDs.

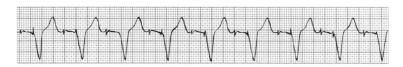

FIGURE 54–13 Dual-chamber pacemaker. A dual-chamber pacemaker provides AV sequential pacing in this rhythm strip.

Electrocautery is the common source of electromagnetic interference (EMI) encountered during surgical procedures. When delivered in a monopolar fashion between an active electrode and a dispersing skin electrode, it can result in electrical signals that can be sensed by the device, resulting in inhibition of pacing during cautery. If the signals are of very high frequency, the device may sense it as noise and pace in an asynchronous fashion, which could cause problems. To avoid sensing issues with use of cautery, the dispersive ground patch should be placed as far away from the pacemaker generator as possible and the active electrode should not be used in a monopolar fashion if the incision is near the pacemaker pocket. Cautery should be used in short bursts with long pauses in between. In cases in which cautery in proximity to the device cannot be avoided, bipolar cautery systems should be used.

EMI from electrocautery can result in sensing of electrical signals above the tachycardia detection interval in patients with ICDs. This could result in either shock delivery or anti-tachycardia pacing. Precautions similar to those described above should be employed, with the additional option of turning the ICD tachycardia therapies off to prevent inappropriate shocks during cautery. Pacemakers and ICDs should be interrogated after exposure to electrocautery to assure that no programming changes have occurred.

Magnet application over a pacemaker results in asynchronous pacing (Fig. 54–14). The magnet behavior

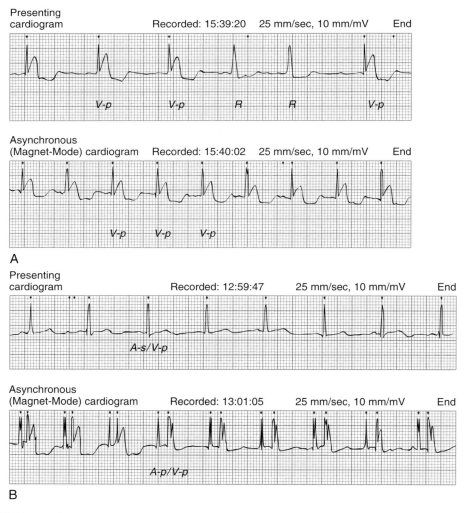

FIGURE 54–14 Magnet effect on single- and dual-chamber pacemakers. **A,** A transtelephonic monitor check of a single-chamber pacemaker shows an upper tracing of the patient's native rhythm and a lower tracing of the effect of magnet application to the pacemaker. In the upper tracing, ventricular demand pacing (Vp) is seen in the absence of spontaneous QRS complexes (R). In the lower tracing, with magnet application, the pacemaker functions in an asynchronous mode, pacing at a prescribed "magnet" rate. **B,** A similar display of a dual-chamber pacemaker shows a spontaneous rhythm that senses atrial activation (A sense) and then senses ventricular depolarization (V sense), suppressing pacemaker activity. With magnet application in the lower tracing, asynchronous AV pacing occurs at the "magnet" rate.

of a pacemaker is manufacturer and model dependent. If a magnet is applied, the physician should be aware of the expected heart rate response. This can be employed at surgery to prevent pacemaker inhibition during electrocautery in patients who are pacemaker dependent. In patients with ICDs, magnet application will prevent tachycardia detection and therapy delivery. If tachycardia therapy cannot be turned off by the programmer prior to surgery, magnet application will disable tachycardia detection and prevent tachycardia therapy delivery. Magnet application over an ICD has no effect on bradycardia sensing or pacing. Therefore, bradycardia pacing inhibition could still occur in response to EMI. If a magnet is applied to an ICD or if anti-tachycardia therapies and/or detection are turned off, life-threatening ventricular arrhythmias will need to be treated with external shocks until the magnet is removed or tachycardia therapies are restored. The device should be interrogated postoperatively to assure that it has been restored to normal function.

In addition to EMI as a source of interference with device function in the operating room, the physician must be aware of the potential problems caused by certain diagnostic tests or treatments. Magnetic resonance imaging is contraindicated in patients with pacemakers and ICDs. The large magnetic fields produced by these scanners can result in magnet-like behavior of pacemakers that are within several feet of the scanner. The device itself could be physically moved in the subcutaneous tissue of the patient by the strong magnetic fields. Rapid pacing has been induced by these strong magnetic fields. Sensing may also be adversely affected in a magnetic resonance imaging scanner.

Lithotripsy uses electrical discharges to create shock waves that are focused on a point in the body. The shock waves are timed to the cardiac cycle. If a pacemaker or ICD is near the shock field, it could be damaged. However, this is rare, especially if the device and the target zone for shock wave therapy are more than 18 cm apart. Transcutaneous electrical nerve stimulators used for relief of chronic pain release bursts of pulses that can result in pacemaker inhibition but rarely do. No data are available regarding potential interactions with ICDs.

Some pacemakers provide rate-responsive pacing using specific sensors that will increase the heart rate in response to activation. The two common types of sensors used are an activity sensor and a respiratory sensor. The activity sensor is a small piezoelectric crystal that oscillates in response to body movement. The pacemaker can increase the pacing rate in response to the oscillating crystal. The respiratory sensor uses a small current delivered through the pacing lead to measure the lead impedance on a constant basis. The impedance changes with respiration, and the pacemaker tracks these changes in respiratory rate to increase the pacing rate. Other sensors less commonly

encountered include sensors that monitor Q-T interval, temperature, right ventricular contractility (*dp/dt*), oxygen saturation, and pH. Because the perioperative period might be associated with inappropriate activation of a sensor, it may be of value to turn off the rate-responsive sensor until after surgery.

In summary, patients with pacemakers or ICDs should have the device evaluated preoperatively to assess programmed parameters and to develop a plan of management. These patients should have their heart rhythm monitored throughout the perioperative period. ICDs should have therapy inhibited during the surgical procedure to avoid inappropriate administration of anti-tachycardia therapy during surgery. All devices should be evaluated postoperatively to assure proper device function.

Management of Perioperative Anticoagulation in Patients with Chronic Atrial Fibrillation/Flutter

One challenge in patients with chronic atrial fibrillation is management of anticoagulation in the perioperative setting. This risk of thromboembolism during the time anticoagulation is withheld must be balanced with the safety of resuming therapy in a patient recently having undergone surgery, given the inherent risk of bleeding. There is no consensus regarding the management of anticoagulation in the pre- and postoperative period. Practice patterns vary widely. Some physicians hospitalize patients and bridge the period during which anticoagulants are withheld with full heparin/low-molecular-weight heparin (LMWH) pre- and postsurgery. This method would seem to potentially reduce the small and poorly defined thromboembolic risk, but with an increase in hospital stay, cost, and patient inconvenience. Other physicians pursue a less intensive approach and withhold oral anticoagulation therapy 3 to 4 days prior to surgery and resume therapy after surgery with or without bridging heparin therapy. This approach would offer a shorter hospital stay with a potential increased thromboembolic risk. No prospective randomized trials have been conducted to address this issue.

A survey of physicians who managed patients with chronic atrial fibrillation undergoing elective surgery attempted to identify practice patterns in two clinical scenarios of risk. Physicians were surveyed regarding various pre- and postoperative strategies for high-risk (a patient with chronic rheumatic atrial fibrillation undergoing surgery for colon cancer) and low-risk (lone atrial fibrillation in an elderly patient undergoing hernia repair) scenarios. Preoperative management options included simply stopping warfarin preoperatively, full-dose in-hospital or outpatient heparin/LMWH, or other (not defined) strategy. Postoperative management included resuming warfarin therapy with no bridging heparin/LMWH, full dose in-hospital or outpatient heparin/LMWH, in-hospital low-dose heparin/LMWH while restarting warfarin, or other (not defined). In the high-risk scenario preoperatively, 54% chose withholding oral anticoagulation without bridging therapy, while 44% chose in-hospital or outpatient full-dose anticoagulation during the period that warfarin was withheld. In the low-risk scenario, 80% chose to hold warfarin with no bridging therapy preoperatively. In the high-risk postoperative setting, 35% resumed warfarin without bridging therapy, 48% chose full-dose heparin/LMWH, and 15% chose low-dose heparin/LMWH. These rates were 68%, 20%, and 10%, respectively, in the low-risk scenario.

A review of patients with multiple reasons for anticoagulation addressed this issue of perioperative anticoagulation. For patients with atrial fibrillation not associated with valvular heart disease, the authors recommended withholding warfarin therapy preoperatively and using subcutaneous heparin postoperatively as long as the patient was hospitalized until warfarin was therapeutic. Their recommendations were based on the estimated low stroke risk in chronic atrial fibrillation over the brief time that anticoagulation was held and the increased risk of bleeding associated with full-dose heparin in the postoperative setting.

Given no clear consensus, consultation with the patient's primary physician should be considered and treatment individualized. It would appear prudent for patients at very high risk with atrial fibrillation (i.e., prior thromboembolic events, mechanical heart valves, known intracardiac thrombi) to be managed more aggressively with bridging therapy. Low-risk patients may be considered for a more conservative approach.

Bibliography

Amar D, Roistacher N, Burt M, et al: Clinical and echocardiographic correlates of symptomatic tachydysrhythmias after noncardiac thoracic surgery. Chest 1995;108:349.

Andrews TC, Reimilod SC, Berlin JA, Antman EM: Prevention of supraventricular arrhythmias after coronary artery bypass surgery: a meta-analysis of randomized control trials. Circulation 1991;84(Suppl III):III-236.

Arsura EL, Lefkin AS, Scher DL, et al: A randomized double-blind placebo-controlled study of verapamil or metoprolol in multifocal atrial tachycardia. Am J Med 1988;85:519.

Bernstein AD, Camm AJ, Fletcher R, Gold RD, et al: The NASPE/BPEG generic pacemaker code for antibradyarrhythmia and adaptive-rate pacing and antitachyarrhythmia devices. Pacing Clin Electrophysiol 1987;10:794.

Chauvin M, Crenner F, Brechenmacher C: Interaction between permanent cardiac pacing and electrocautery: the significance of electrode position. Pacing Clin Electrophysiol 1992;15:2028.

Cooper D, Wilkoff B, Masterson M, et al: Effects of extracorporeal shock wave lithotripsy on cardiac pacemakers and its safety in patients with implanted cardiac pacemakers. Pacing Clin Electrophysiol 1988;11:1607.

Douketis JD, Crowther MA, Cherian SS: Perioperative anticoagulation in patients with chronic atrial fibrillation who are undergoing elective surgery: results of a physician survey. Can J Cardiol 2000;16:326.

Feldman RM: The use of diathermy in the presence of metal implants and cardiac pacemakers. Can Med Assoc J 1980;123:16.

Furman S: Rate-modulated pacing. Circulation 1990;82:1081.

Gauss A, Hubner C, Meierhenrich R, et al: Perioperative transcutaneous pacemaker in patients with chronic bifascicular block or left bundle branch block and additional first degree atrioventricular block. Acta Anaesthesiol Scand 1999;43:731.

Goldman L: Supraventricular tachyarrhythmias in hospitalized patients after surgery: clinical correlates in patients over 40 years of age after major noncardiac surgery. Chest 1978;73:450.

Goldman L, Caldera DL, Nussbaum SR, et al: Multifactorial index of cardiac risk in noncardiac surgical procedures. N Engl J Med 1977;297:845.

Hayes DL: Pacemaker timing cycles and pacemaker electrocardiography. *In* Lloyd MA, Friedman PA (eds): Cardiac Pacing and Defibrillation: A Clinical Approach (2nd ed). Armonk NY: Futura, 2000:201.

Hollenberg SM, Dellinger RP: Noncardiac surgery: postoperative arrhythmias. Crit Care Med 2000;28(Suppl):N145.

Holmes DR, Hayes DL, Gray JE, Meredeth J: The effects of magnetic resonance imaging on implantable pulse generators. Pacing Clin Electrophysiol 1986;9:360.

Iberer F, Justich E, Tscheliessnigg KH, Wasler A: Nuclear magnetic resonance imaging in pacemaker patients. In Atlee JL, Gombotz H, Tscheliessnigg KH (eds): Perioperative Management of Pacemaker Patients. Berlin: Springer-Verlag, 1992:86.

Kartritisis D, Shakespeare CF, Camm AJ: New and combined sensors for adaptive-rate pacing. Clin Cardiol 1993;16:240.

Kastor JA: Multifocal atrial tachycardia. N Engl J Med 1990;322:1113.

Kearon C, Hirsh J: Management of anticoagulation before and after elective surgery. N Engl J Med 1997;336:1506.

Kowey PR, Taylor JE, Rials SJ, Marinchak RA: Meta-analysis of the effectiveness of prophylactic drug therapy in preventing supraventricular arrhythmia after coronary artery bypass grafting. Am J Cardiol 1992;69:863.

Laupacis A, Albers G, Dalen J, et al: Antithrombotic therapy in atrial fibrillation. Chest 1995;108(Suppl 4):352S.

Mackey DC, Carpenter RL, Thompson GE, et al: Bradycardia and asystole during spinal anesthesia: a report of three cases without morbidity. Anesthesiology 1989;70:866.

Mahla E, Rotman B, Rehak P, et al: Perioperative ventricular arrhythmias in patients with structural heart disease undergoing noncardiac surgery. Anesth Analg 1998;86:16.

Mangano DT, Layug EL, Wallace A, Tateo I: Effect of atenolol on mortality and cardiovascular morbidity after noncardiac surgery. N Engl J Med 1995;333:1750.

Manning WJ, Silverman DI, Keighley CS, et al: Transesophageal echocardiographically facilitated early cardioversion from atrial fibrillation using short term anticoagulation: final results of a prospective 4.5 year study. J Am Coll Cardiol 1995;25:1354.

McCord J, Borzac S: Multifocal atrial tachycardia. Chest 1998;113:203.

Morris D, Mulvihill D, Lew WY: Risk of developing complete heart block during bedside pulmonary artery catheterization in patients with left bundle branch block. Arch Intern Med 1987;147:2005.

Moss AJ: Measurement of the QT interval and the risk associated with QT_c interval prolongation: a review. Am J Cardiol 1993:23B.

O'Kelly B, Browner WS, Massie B, et al: Ventricular arrhythmias in patients undergoing noncardiac surgery. JAMA 1992;268:217.

Ommen SR, Odell JA, Stanton MS: Atrial arrhythmias after cardiothoracic surgery. N Engl J Med 1997;336:1429.

Pastore JO, Yurchak PM, Janis KM, et al: The risk of advanced heart block in surgical patients with right bundle branch block and left axis deviation. Circulation 1978;57:677.

Polanczyk CA, Goldman L, Marcantonio ER, et al: Supraventricular arrhythmia in patients having noncardiac surgery: clinical correlates and effect on length of stay. Ann Intern Med 1998;129:279.

Poldermans D, Boersma E, Bax JJ, et al: The effect of bisoprolol on perioperative mortality and myocardial infarction in high-risk patients undergoing vascular surgery. N Engl J Med 1999;341:1789.

Prystowsky EN, Klein GJ: Cardiac Arrhythmias. New York: McGraw-Hill, 1994:171.

Ramaswamy K, Hamdan MH: Ischemia, metabolic disturbances and arrhythmogenesis: mechanisms and management. Crit Care Med 2000;28(Suppl):N151.

Rasmussen MJ, Hayes DL, Vlietstra RE, Thorsteinsson G: Can transcutaneous electrical nerve stimulation be safely used in patients with permanent cardiac pacemakers? Mayo Clin Proc 1988;63:443.

Risk factors for stroke and efficacy of antithrombotic therapy in atrial fibrillation: analysis of pooled data from five randomized controlled trials. Arch Intern Med 1994; 154:1449.

CHAPTER 55

Acute Cardiopulmonary Resuscitation

Jeffrey S. Kelly, M.D., F.A.C.E.P. and Peter C. Brath, M.D.

▸ Epidemiology of Cardiac Arrest and CPR
▸ Physiology of CPR
▸ Initial Assessment and Treatment of the Adult
  Cardiac Arrest Victim
▸ Advanced Resuscitation Techniques
  Electrical Therapy
  Pharmacology of Resuscitation
  Percutaneous Cardiopulmonary Support and
  Suspended Animation
▸ Mediocolegal and Ethical Aspects of CPR
▸ Conclusion
▸ Bibliography

Cardiac arrest from coronary heart disease (CHD) remains the leading cause of death in the United States. Since first described over 40 years ago, cardiopulmonary resuscitation (CPR) using closed chest compressions (CCC), airway support with 100% oxygen, defibrillation or cardioversion of electrically responsive arrhythmias, and intravenous administration of antiarrhythmic and/or vasopressor medications has become the de facto standard of care for patients suffering such events. Resuscitation guidelines have evolved during this time from initial application of anecdotal human data and controlled animal research to the most recent consensus recommendations using an evidence-based approach. Although the majority of cardiac arrests occur in medical patients secondary to acute coronary syndromes, cardiac arrest may occur in the surgical population from causes such as trauma, intraoperative anesthetic events, perioperative arrhythmias or myocardial infarction, or pulmonary embolus. Thus it is important that surgical practitioners

be able to identify patients at risk for cardiac arrest and have familiarity with the basic principles of CPR.

Because this topic has been recently reviewed both briefly and extensively in well-known journals, we have chosen to synthesize this chapter from these sources, which are listed in the bibliography. Additional references listed there will direct the reader to quality supporting peer-review literature. In the interest of space, we have also elected to focus solely on adult cardiac arrest and do not address cardiac arrest in the pediatric patient, special arrest situations such as drug overdose or hypothermia, or postresuscitation care.

Epidemiology of Cardiac Arrest and CPR

An estimated 12 million Americans have CHD, of whom 1.1 million were predicted to have a CHD event (acute myocardial infarction, angina pectoris, or myocardial ischemia) during 2001. CHD resulted in approximately 460,000 deaths in 1998, 44% of which were attributed to acute myocardial infarction. Of these deaths, 99.5% took place in patients greater than 35 years of age, with approximately half occurring suddenly in unhospitalized patients. Age-adjusted death rates reported in 1998 were men > women, Caucasian > African-American > Hispanic in men, and African-American > Caucasian > Hispanic among women. Prevention remains the key strategy for reducing death from CHD. Modifiable risk factors include appropriate control of hypertension, diabetes, and hypercholesterolemia; smoking cessation; and increased physical activity.

Survival data in cardiac arrest victims receiving CPR depend on variables such as setting (witnessed vs. unwitnessed), location (hospitalized vs. public), and time from arrest to administration of appropriate electrical therapy. Up to 90% of patients have survived neurologically intact to hospital discharge when defibrillation occurs within the first minute after publically witnessed cardiac arrest. Under such circumstances, meaningful survival rates decrease approximately 7% to 10% per additional minute of untreated ventricular fibrillation (VF), reaching 10% at 10 minutes and 2% to 5% beyond 12 minutes. This leads to a cumulative neurologically intact survival rate as high as 20% to 25% when applied to large patient series under similar conditions. Because hospitalized patients usually suffer cardiac arrest as an end-stage sequela of their comorbid disease state(s), survival to discharge seldom exceeds 15% in this population.

Physiology OF CPR

Because untreated VF degenerates to asystole within a few minutes, the goal of CCC is twofold: (1) to extend (up to 10 minutes) the duration of VF until a defibrillator becomes available, and (2) to maintain adequate cerebral perfusion with oxygenated blood and prevent brain damage during this same interval. When properly performed (as described in the following section), CCC generates a cardiac output approximately 25% to 35% of normal, systolic blood pressures of 60 to 80 mm Hg, and central mean arterial pressures seldom greater than 40 mm Hg. At first, blood flow depends on direct cardiac compression between the sternum and thoracic spine (so-called cardiac pump mechanism). With more prolonged resuscitation, the heart becomes ischemic and blood flow becomes dependent on manipulations of intrathoracic pressure (so-called thoracic pump mechanism). Cardiac output under the latter mechanism decreases significantly. With both mechanisms, blood is ejected from the heart during the compression phase and returns back to the heart during the relaxation phase. Effective cerebral and coronary perfusion occurs when both chest compression and relaxation phases occupy 50% of the total ("duty") cycle.

More recent research efforts have focused on improving the hemodynamic profile provided by standard CCC using a variety of adjunctive techniques. Interposed abdominal compression CPR (IAC-CPR) utilizes a second rescuer applying manual pressure halfway between the xiphoid process and umbilicus during the relaxation phase of simultaneous chest compressions. The force applied should be sufficient to generate approximately 100 mm Hg of external pressure on the intra-abdominal great vessels. When properly performed, mathematical models suggest that cardiac output is as much as twice that of standard CCC. IAC-CPR appears as safe as CCC, with no increase in the incidence of emesis or aspiration. Pooled data from all randomized trials comparing IAC-CPR with standard CCC demonstrate improved rates of initial

resuscitation ("return of spontaneous circulation") with no improvement in ultimate outcome. However, subset analysis suggests that early application of IAC-CPR during in-hospital cardiac arrest results in both improved resuscitation and improved neurologically intact survival rates. A similar benefit has not been demonstrated in prehospital studies. Thus IAC-CPR is considered an acceptable alternative to CCC for in-hospital cardiac arrest if applied early by sufficient numbers of appropriately trained providers. "Last-ditch" use of IAC-CPR after prolonged unsuccessful resuscitation is not recommended.

Another adjunctive method actively under investigation is active compression-decompression CPR (ACD-CPR). In this technique, a handheld suction device ("plunger") is attached to the anterior chest, forming an airtight seal. Positive pressure and negative pressure are then alternately applied to the chest wall via this plunger in an active fashion. When compared with standard CCC, ACD-CPR improves venous return and augments minute ventilation (assuming a patent upper airway) by decreasing intrathoracic pressure during the active decompression phase. The increased venous return theoretically improves cardiac stroke volume during the subsequent active compression. While animal models of ACD-CPR demonstrate improved hemodynamics compared to standard CCC, results in humans have been mixed. Some comparative human studies demonstrate improvements in short-term survival, while others report survival rates similar to those utilizing CCC. The most promising study reported an improvement in 1-year survival from 2% with CCC to 5% with ACD-CPR.

Open cardiac massage (OCM) using direct anteroposterior compression of the heart by the resuscitator's hand generates hemodynamics superior to CCC and provides near-normal perfusion to the brain as well as the heart. The obvious limitation to its routine application is the inherent morbidity associated with the requisite emergency left thoracotomy. Thus most of the available literature supports the initial application of CCC with appropriate electrical and pharmacologic therapy to all patients. If unsuccessful, OCM may be considered *early* in specific circumstances, such as penetrating thoracoabdominal trauma, hypothermia, pulmonary embolism, pericardial tamponade, severe aortic stenosis, severe chest wall deformities, and after open heart surgery. It is inappropriate to use OCM as a terminal last-ditch intervention at the end of a prolonged resuscitation sequence.

Another recent proposal aimed at improving layperson CPR is application of CCC without mouth-to-mouth assisted ventilation, particularly in the setting of witnessed cardiac arrest. This concept is based on a number of factors, including (1) aortic oxygenation is normal prearrest, (2) the low cardiac output generated by CCC limits peripheral oxygen utilization, (3) the relaxation phase of

CCC generates negative intrathoracic pressure and (assuming a patent upper airway) entrains oxygen-containing ambient air into the lungs, and (4) active, gasping respiratory effort commonly occurs during the initial phase of resuscitation. Such a technique theoretically increases the effectiveness of bystander CPR by improving skill acquisition/retention, alleviating fears of mouth-to-mouth contact with a stranger, and ultimately encouraging earlier application of effective CCC. One recent randomized study from Seattle comparing CCC with assisted mouth-to-mouth ventilation to CCC without assisted ventilation showed no difference in the rate of survival to hospital discharge. These results, however, may not be reproducible in areas lacking the rapid (<5 minutes) emergency medical services (EMS) response times found in the suburban Seattle area. The "no ventilation" concept is also not applicable to asphyxial cardiac arrest (i.e., cardiac arrest caused by profound hypoxemia). In this case, extreme depletion of oxygen stores leading to lactic acidosis and inadequate myocardial oxygen delivery is the primary causative factor. Assisted ventilation to restore arterial oxygenation and improve pH by eliminating carbon dioxide is indicated, and should be applied along with CCC in the standard fashion.

Initial Assessment and Treatment of the Adult Cardiac Arrest Victim

Given the audience toward which this text is oriented, the following describes the basic resuscitation sequence appropriate for an experienced health care provider in the setting of adult cardiac arrest within a health care facility. We assume for the purpose of discussion that advanced resuscitation capabilities are not immediately available, but become available within 5 minutes.

The initial step involves assessing patient responsiveness to moderate physical and verbal stimulation. After confirming unresponsiveness, the provider should immediately activate the appropriate emergency response team (EMS or the facility's code team) while simultaneously establishing a patent upper airway (using either the head tilt–chin lift or jaw thrust maneuver) and evaluating the patient for spontaneous breathing. In the presence of spontaneous breathing, the patient should be positioned in the lateral "recovery" position and assessed for signs of circulation as described below. The apneic patient should receive two mouth-to-mouth "rescue" breaths of approximately 10 mL/kg each delivered slowly over 2 seconds to minimize gastric insufflation. The patient should then be quickly reevaluated for return of spontaneous respiratory activity (the provider can hear or feel air movement

through the mouth, rise and fall of the chest, and/or coughing) and circulation (e.g., palpable carotid or femoral pulse, spontaneous patient movement).

In the absence of clear-cut evidence supporting the return of spontaneous ventilation and circulation, basic CPR should be initiated. The patient should be placed supine on a firm surface and chest compressions initiated. The provider should place the heel of his or her hand over the lower half of the victim's sternum with the other hand placed on top in a parallel fashion. With the elbows locked, the sternum should be compressed 4 to 5 cm in a direct anteroposterior direction at a rate of 100 compressions per minute. Two rescue mouth-to-mouth breaths should be administered after every 15 compressions irrespective of whether one-person or two-person CPR is occurring. This should be continuously performed until advanced resuscitation equipment arrives.

Advanced Resuscitation Techniques

When advanced resuscitation capabilities become available, the first priority is application of the multifunction automatic external defibrillator (AED) pads to the patient anteriorly and posteriorly. Diagnosis of electrically responsive arrhythmias should be immediately followed by sequential defibrillation or synchronized cardioversion (as detailed below). Diagnosis of electrically unresponsive arrhythmias or failure to restore spontaneous circulation with appropriate electrical therapy should be followed by algorithmic, arrhythmia-specific pharmacologic and electrical therapy (see below) as well as active airway management. Assisted ventilation with high-flow (15 L/min) 100% oxygen utilizing a self-inflating bag-valve-mask (BVM) and establishment of intravenous access should be initiated. Insertion of an oropharyngeal or nasopharyngeal airway may help maintain upper airway patency during BVM-assisted ventilation. This should be followed by performance of advanced airway techniques when experienced personnel are present. Definitive airway control via endotracheal intubation with an appropriately sized (7.0 to 7.5 mm in the average-size adult) cuffed endotracheal tube (ETT) remains the procedure of choice in this setting. Because intubation skills are difficult to maintain when used infrequently, the most recent guidelines recommend that only providers who perform 6 to 12 intubations per year should attempt emergency intubation. Proper endotracheal tube position should be confirmed using a combination of physical exam findings (symmetrical chest rise, bilateral and symmetrical breath sounds, and absence of breath sounds over the stomach) and nonphysical exam techniques (esophageal detector device, colorimetric carbon dioxide detector, capnometry, or capnography).

The ETT should be securely taped at the corner of the mouth to prevent dislodgement during subsequent application of CCC, with strong consideration for the use of a commercially produced tracheal tube holder if available. A useful rule of thumb in this regard is the mnemonic "22 teeth to trachea"; that is, securing the ETT with the 22-cm mark at the teeth in an average-sized patient will usually result in the ETT tip lying in the midtrachea. The role of newer, invasive airway adjuncts (such as the laryngeal mask airway and esophageal-tracheal combitube) is not well defined, although their use may be preferable to prolonged BVM-assisted ventilation in less experienced hands.

While skilled airway management is crucial to maintain arterial oxygenation and protect the airway, electrical therapy of malignant arrhythmias (the most common cause of sudden cardiac death) is the first priority. Immediate return of a stable rhythm and restoration of adequate coronary perfusion pressure is the goal of such initial interventions. We have chosen to cover the electrical and pharmacologic treatment of immediately life-threatening arrhythmias (e.g., ventricular tachycardia [VT], ventricular fibrillation [VF], pulseless electrical activity [PEA], and asystole) here since other arrhythmias have been extensively covered in Chapter 54.

Electrical Therapy

Electrical therapy for cardiac arrest involves either unsynchronized defibrillation for VF/pulseless VT or synchronized cardioversion for termination of VT with a pulse (also referred to as hemodynamically stable VT). In addition to the short arrest-to-defibrillation time noted above, successful defibrillation also depends upon the balance between adequate transmyocardial current generation and associated electrically-induced myocardial injury. Myocardial action potentials during fibrillation sequentially follow one another, generally without a period of electrical diastole in between. As a result, cells in different regions of the myocardium are in different phases of the cardiac action potential at any given time. Successful defibrillation, therefore, depends upon generating a uniform post-shock electrical response (or pause) to allow for restoration of a more stable electrical rhythm. The electrical energy (in Joules or J) can be delivered to the arrest victim through either manual paddles or through application of self-adhesive monitor/defibrillator pads. The current ultimately transmitted to the myocardium from these devices depends upon both the energy selected (J) and the intrinsic resistance of the chest wall to the delivered energy (i.e., impedance). Transthoracic impedance is affected by many factors, including the selected energy level, paddle/pad size, paddle-skin interface, phase of ventilation, chest size, previous shocks, and applied paddle electrode pressure.

Electrical energy can be delivered either as a monophasic waveform (a single burst of energy flowing in one direction) or a biphasic waveform (a burst of energy that briefly flows in one direction, then reverses its path for the remainder of the discharge cycle). Monophasic defibrillators are the most common and remain the historical standard. Interest in biphasic defibrillation has grown in recent years because of research suggesting that repetitive biphasic shocks at lower energy levels (<200 J) are at least as effective as three traditional escalating monophasic shocks (200, 300, 360 J). To date, neither the optimal energies nor shape of the biphasic waveform have been conclusively determined. It is also unclear whether improved resuscitation rates from biphasic defibrillation will translate into beneficial long-term outcomes.

When VF is diagnosed, immediate, "stacked," unsynchronized, monophasic defibrillation at 200 J, 300 J, and 360 J is recommended. Reassessment for return of spontaneous respiration and a palpable pulse should occur between shocks, and the shock sequence discontinued if detected. All airway interventions are deferred until the last defibrillation attempt at 360 J proves unsuccessful. The initial energy level chosen for VT depends somewhat on its morphology. Monomorphic VT (with or without a pulse) typically responds to monophasic shocks of 100 J, while polymorphic VT behaves much like VF and is treated identically (as noted above). For treatment of hemodynamically stable VT, the defibrillator must be placed in the synchronized mode to avoid inducing VF from shock delivery during the relative refractory period of the cardiac action potential.

The automated external defibrillator (AED) has been recently developed to facilitate early defibrillation by relatively unskilled initial responders. These devices incorporate rhythm recognition software capable of analyzing multiple features of the patient's underlying cardiac rhythm. Should the AED's software detect a "shockable" rhythm (VF or VT), a prompt (digital display, audio or visual alarm, audio display) directs the responder to defibrillate by pressing the "shock" button. AEDs should only be utilized on apneic, pulseless, unresponsive patients and may discharge inappropriately in patients who have seizures, agonal respirations, or perfusing tachyarrhythmias. Such events typically do not represent AED malfunction and emphasize the importance of a complete physical assessment prior to AED utilization. The proper steps for AED use are:

1. Assess the patient for signs of circulation (responsiveness, respiratory effort, pulse palpation)

2. Power up the AED

3. Attach the self-adhesive electrodes as diagrammed on the pads (upper-right sternal border just below the clavicle and lateral to the left nipple in the mid-axillary line)

4. Analyze the rhythm (performed automatically by some units; others require pressing the "analyze" button)

5. Clear the patient and press the "shock" button if prompted to do so by the AED

6. Reevaluate the rhythm (as in step 4 above) twice more, if necessary, for a total of three shocks

7. Failure to restore a palpable pulse and spontaneous respiratory activity after delivery of the third shock mandates institution of CPR and appropriate ACLS interventions.

Should the AED recommend no shock be administered, the patient should be immediately assessed for signs of spontaneous circulation. If absent, CPR and therapy for asystole should be initiated and the patient reevaluated at 1-2 minute intervals. If present, airway obstruction should be established. While recent data suggest that 90 seconds of CPR prior to defibrillation may increase its success rate (possibly by improving pre-shock coronary blood flow), CPR should not delay AED application and utilization when one is immediately available.

Pharmacology of Resuscitation

The recent emphasis on evidence-based medicine has caused resuscitation researchers to reevaluate the role of pharmacologic therapy in advanced cardiac life support (ACLS). The updates in drug treatment for various arrhythmias resulting from such reevaluation will be highlighted in this section.

Hemodynamically stable ventricular tachycardia

For any hemodynamically stable wide-complex tachycardia of unknown etiology, the current antiarrhythmic recommendation is intravenous (IV) administration of either amiodarone or procainamide. Amiodarone is a complex drug with many actions, but primarily acts as a class III antiarrhythmic agent. It is dosed as a 150 mg IV load over 10 minutes (repeated as necessary) followed by a differential infusion of 1.0 mg/min for 6 hours and 0.5 mg/min thereafter. Procainamide is a class IA antiarrhythmic agent

that can either be administered as a 100 mg IV bolus at 20 to 30 mg/min or as a loading dose of 12 to 17 mg/kg over 45 to 60 minutes followed by an infusion of 1 to 4 mg/min. One potential side effect of procainamide is QT prolongation and precipitation of *torsades de pointes*. Blood concentrations of both procainamide and its primary metabolite N-acetyl procainamide should be monitored during continuous infusion therapy. Current guidelines for the treatment of hemodynamically stable VT of any morphology include either amiodarone (dosed as above) or sotalol (which is not currently FDA approved for intravenous use in the United States).

Ventricular fibrillation and pulseless ventricular tachycardia

The pharmacological treatment of VF and pulseless VT has also undergone evidence-based modification. Should the initial defibrillation sequence outlined above prove unsuccessful, the most recent VF/pulseless VT algorithm suggests the provider "consider antiarrhythmics" and directs them to several options. The traditional use of lidocaine (1 to 1.5 mg/kg IV followed by an infusion of 1 to 4 mg/min) lacks compelling data demonstrating a positive impact on outcome. While lidocaine administration for VF/pulseless VT remains acceptable, the American Heart Association (AHA) currently gives it an "indeterminate" level of recommendation. Conversely, a recent investigation of amiodarone administration for initial treatment of VF/pulseless VT demonstrated a favorable impact on the rate of successful resuscitation. This data has led many practitioners to consider amiodarone (dosed identical to hemodynamically stable VT) as the first line antiarrhythmic for shock-refractory VF/VT. Increased survival associated with amiodarone administration under such circumstances has not yet been demonstrated. Magnesium (1 to 2 g IV) may be considered for shock-refractory VF/VT, but is only truly indicated for known hypomagnesemic states and *torsades de pointes*. Bretylium, the historic second line agent of choice after lidocaine, is still listed as acceptable for VF/pulseless VT. However, bretylium is no longer manufactured due to a worldwide lack of raw materials required for its production.

The vasoactive drug recommendations for VF/pulseless VT have similarly undergone evidence-based change. Epinephrine 1 mg IV every 3 to 5 minutes has been the standard vasoconstrictor administered to improve coronary perfusion and (hopefully) make the myocardium more responsive to subsequent defibrillation. However, upon closer scrutiny, the evidence supporting positive outcomes from epinephrine administration for VF/pulseless VT is sparse. This is particularly true for "high dose" (up to 0.2 mg/kg) and escalating dose (1 mg up to 3 to 5mg) epinephrine regimens advocated in the late 1980s and early 1990s. Clinical trials performed at that time demonstrated improved resuscitation rates with such techniques, but no increased survival to hospital discharge. Higher cumulative doses of epinephrine may contribute to a post-resuscitative hyperadrenergic state, leading to increased myocardial oxygen demand in the face of limited myocardial oxygen supply. The end result would be poor left ventricular function, unstable hemodynamics, and poorer neurologic outcome (although a direct cause-and-effect relationship has not been definitively established). In the absence of IV access, epinephrine may also be administered intratracheally at 2.5 to 3 times the IV dose.

The equivocal data associated with epinephrine use in VF/pulseless VT has caused investigators to study alternative vasoconstrictors, primarily vasopressin. When administered in dosages higher than required for its antidiuretic action, vasopressin causes direct smooth muscle contraction and increases coronary perfusion pressure. In contrast to epinephrine, which increases myocardial oxygen consumption via its beta-adrenergic actions, vasopressin is devoid of such effects and more favorably influences the myocardial oxygen supply-demand balance. While large, randomized trials comparing epinephrine and vasopressin have not yet been published, preliminary studies have led the AHA to recommend vasopressin (40 units IV given once) as an acceptable alternative to epinephrine for shock-refractory VF/VT in adults.

Pulseless electrical activity (PEA) and asystole

The non-VF/VT rhythms (PEA and asystole) represent a continuum of terminal electrical activity emanating from a profoundly injured myocardium and, as such, carry a uniformly poor prognosis. PEA is non-VF/VT electrical activity that may stimulate mechanical contraction, but is insufficient to generate a palpable pulse or detectable blood pressure. Asystole is, by definition, myocardial electrical silence demonstrated in at least two leads.

Because these agonal rhythms are typically due to similar physiologic causes, their treatment algorithms are essentially identical. Successful resuscitation from PEA depends almost entirely upon prompt diagnosis and treatment of the underlying cause(s) (commonly referred to as the 5 H's and the 5 T's and detailed in Table 55-1). Pharmacologic therapy of PEA attempts to preserve myocardial viability during the period of emergency definitive therapy and includes IV epinephrine (dosed as per VF/pulseless VT above), atropine 1 mg IV every 3 to 5 minutes up to 0.04 mg/kg (for bradycardic PEA rhythms < 60), and transcutaneous pacing (for witnessed arrest). While a similar evaluation for reversible causes should occur with asystole, a simultaneous assessment for the appropriateness of resuscitative efforts is warranted. Absent sure signs of death, pharmacologic therapy for asystole is identical to PEA, with the exception of routine atropine

Table 55-1
Reversible causes of pulseless electrical activity and asystole

The Five Hs	The Five Ts
Hypovolemia	Tamponade (cardiac)
Hypothermia	Tablets (drug overdose or accidents)
Hyper-/hypokalemia	Thrombosis (pulmonary embolus)
Hydrogen ion (acidosis)	Thrombosis (acute coronary syndrome)
Hypoxia	Tension pneumothorax

administration to all asystolic patients. Should the provider detect irrefutable evidence of death (such as dependent livedo or rigor mortis), further resuscitative efforts should be withheld except in extremely rare circumstances (such as profound hypothermia).

Percutaneous Cardiopulmonary Support and Suspended Animation

Percutaneous cardiopulmonary support (PCPS) has been available for almost 20 years and is advocated by some as an emergency alternative to more traditional ACLS interventions. The technique is essentially identical to veno-arterial extracorporeal membrane oxygenation, with the femoral artery and vein undergoing rapid, large bore cannulation and the patient's blood subsequently circulated through an oxygenator/heat exchanger circuit using a roller or centrifugal pump. While PCPS can potentially be implemented within 15 minutes, its ultimate success depends upon a variety of factors (arrest cause, arrest location, personnel numbers/skill, arrest-to-perfusion time, etc.). When emergently utilized in cardiac arrest from reversible causes (cardiogenic shock amendable to revascularization, pulmonary embolus), survival rates of 48% to 69% have been reported.

Suspended animation has evolved from a science fiction fantasy into the latest "cutting edge" area of resuscitation research. This concept involves rapidly placing an unresuscitatable patient into a temporary suspended state in which core organ viability is maintained. Reversible causes can then be diagnosed and treated during this period of "clinical death," followed by carefully controlled, methodical resuscitation to avoid reperfusion injury to vital organs (particularly the brain). Suspended animation treatment specifically involves IV infusion of hypothermic fluid (typically normal saline) with or without pharmacologic adjuncts (such as antioxidants) within 5 minutes of arrest, followed by transport to an appropriate care facility/area. Definitive treatment of the underlying cause ensues, followed by controlled rewarming/resuscitation utilizing cardiopulmonary bypass. Patient populations theoretically benefitting from suspended animation techniques may include battlefield casualties, exsanguinating traumatic arrest, and sudden cardiac death victims. Initial animal studies utilizing this technique demonstrate mixed results, with a few centers actively considering human studies.

In summary, extensive scrutiny of resuscitation methods using an evidence-based approach has demonstrated little support for many traditional ACLS interventions and spawned a plethora of new resuscitation research. Rapid delivery of appropriate electrical therapy combined with maintenance of coronary perfusion via CPR and pharmacologic agents remain the key to successful resuscitation. The International Liaison Committee on Resuscitation algorithm reproduced below succinctly emphasizes these principles (see Fig. 55-1).

Mediocolegal and Ethical Aspects of CPR

Given the current litigious nature of American society, a basic understanding of the medicolegal and ethical considerations involved in the resuscitation of cardiac arrest victims is perhaps as important as the proper application of appropriate resuscitation techniques.

So-called Good Samaritan laws, originally developed to protect the layperson administering on-scene basic life support, have quickly become antiquated with the increasing emphasis on rapid (within 5 minutes) defibrillation of cardiac arrest victims by nonmedical personnel properly trained to use an AED. Groups studied to date include public servants, airline attendants, and casino security personnel. This focus on so-called public access defibrillation (PAD) has led to additional "Good Samaritan" issues regarding appropriate layperson qualifications, legal liability (layperson provider, AED owner/acquirer, AED manufacturer), and oversight/monitoring of such PAD programs. American Heart Association–sponsored conferences on PAD have suggested that all individuals who successfully complete a physician-monitored AED program be allowed to defibrillate. Furthermore, the federal government and the majority of states have instituted legislation conferring provider immunity for AED use in physician-authorized PAD programs. Some states extend this protection to other relevant parties (AED trainers, acquirers, and owners).

An important ethical point to consider is the appropriateness of applying CPR techniques to cardiac arrest victims with terminal, irreversible, and incurable disease (such as end-stage Alzheimer's disease or widely metastatic carcinoma). "Do not attempt resuscitation" (DNAR) orders must be viewed in the context of the basic principles of patient autonomy and medical futility.

Patient autonomy means that mentally competent adults capable of communicating their wishes (either verbally to surrogates/physicians or through legal documents such as living wills, advance directives, or health care powers of attorney) have received sufficient medical information from a physician regarding therapeutic options and refused further treatment. Such autonomy issues led to passage of the Patient Self-Determination Act of 1991, which requires health care institutions and managed care organizations to inquire whether patients have advance directives. This legislation also requires health care institutions to assist any patient desiring completion of advanced directive documents. Although good in theory, this act has not resulted in increased use of advance directives or had a significant impact on patient care decisions regarding resuscitation from cardiac arrest. Medical futility in the setting of cardiac arrest is qualitatively defined as both a low chance of survival *and* a low quality of life if successfully resuscitated. Key variables here include the underlying disease(s) before cardiac arrest as well as the expected state of health postresuscitation. Given the difficult nature of these discussions and the unavoidable projection of the value systems of others (e.g., health care providers, family members) into the decision, most hospitals have ethics advisors or committees available for consultation should conflicts arise.

Because CPR in the United States may be initiated without a physician's order under the theory of implied consent for emergency treatment, a written physician order is necessary to withhold resuscitative efforts. Such DNAR orders should specify as closely as possible the patient's desires and be reviewed/renewed at regular intervals. Efforts should be made to educate the patient/surrogate that a limited "menu" approach to resuscitation options (e.g., chest compressions and electrical therapy, but no intubation or ventilation) is seldom appropriate and will only be ordered with the understanding of a diminished chance for successful resuscitation. Furthermore, the patient/surrogate should be reassured that DNAR orders do not include discontinuation or limitation of appropriately indicated medical treatment, nursing care, and comfort measures (such as sedation/analgesia, nutrition, and hydration). Patients with DNAR orders undergoing surgical procedures present an additional dilemma. In this environment, such patients may require elective endotracheal intubation and mechanical ventilation or become unstable from readily correctable physiologic derangements such as hypovolemia, hypotension, or nonmalignant arrhythmias. Because many of these disturbances may predictably occur in any patient under the same circumstances and have effective, commonly used therapies, most clinicians do not view treatment of such conditions as "resuscitation." Although this philosophy initially led to policies automatically suspending DNAR

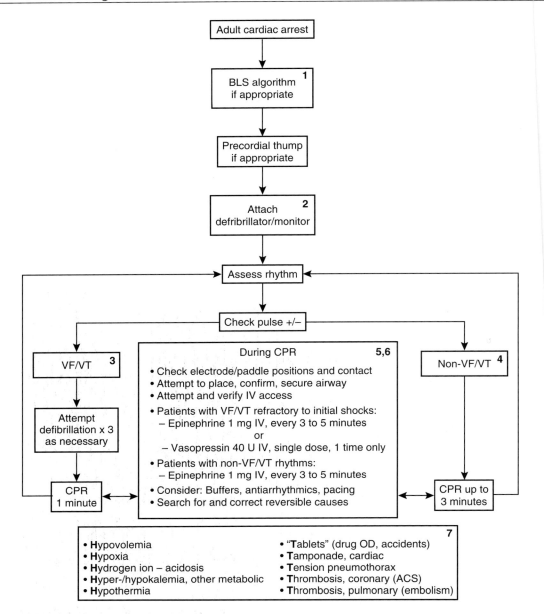

FIGURE 55–1 ACLS algorithm. (From American Heart Association in Collaboration with the International Liaison Committee on Resuscitation [ILCOR]: Guidelines 2000 for cardiopulmonary resuscitation and emergency cardiovascular care. Circulation 2000;102:I-143, with permission. © 2000 copyright American Heart Association.)

orders for patients requiring surgery, such an approach is no longer supported by either the American Society of Anesthesiologists or the American College of Surgeons. Many institutions have adopted a goal-directed, procedure-specific approach to this problem, with the DNAR form located in the front of the patient's chart for easy access. It is also recommended that CPR not be initiated in patients with clear signs of irreversible death (rigor mortis or dependent lividity) or in situations where resuscitation team members are at risk for personal injury.

A decision to discontinue unsuccessful resuscitative efforts should consider factors such as time to CPR, time to defibrillation, prearrest patient condition, comorbid disease(s), and initial arrest rhythm. The chance of surviving neurologically intact to hospital discharge is inversely related to cumulative resuscitation time. A recent retrospective study in hospitalized patients suggests that unwitnessed arrest victims whose initial rhythm is not VT or VF and who do not regain a pulse within the first 10 minutes of resuscitation have a 1% survival rate to hospital discharge. Cardiac arrests occurring in the operating room were excluded from this analysis. Consensus evidence indicates that, in the absence of mitigating factors, CPR failing to restore any spontaneous circulation within the first

30 minutes is unlikely to be successful if continued longer, and may be terminated.

An equally difficult decision involves withdrawal of life support in successfully resuscitated patients who fail to regain consciousness. Unfortunately, no reliable criteria exist that can predict a given patient's neurologic outcome in the midst of his or her resuscitation. Cardiac arrest survivors who remain deeply comatose (Glasgow Coma Scale score <5) without either a pupillary response to light or a motor response to pain by the third postresuscitation day carry a poor prognosis. Nationally accepted brain death criteria (utilizing any combination of complete neurologic exam, cerebral blood flow imaging, and/or absence of respiratory effort in response to hypercarbia, i.e., the "apnea test") may also be met in some comatose resuscitation survivors. Withdrawal of life support in these two patient populations is both reasonable and ethically permissible. In the case of brain death, seeking consent for organ donation from the patient's surrogates should be strongly considered. Donor transfer to a tertiary care center is often necessary, and donors themselves frequently require aggressive therapeutic interventions (hemodynamic support with fluids/vasopressors, treatment of diabetes insipidus, and so forth) to maintain donor organ function.

Because the majority of cardiac arrest victims cannot be successfully resuscitated, notifying family about a loved one's death from cardiac arrest is a difficult, but vitally important part of the CPR continuum. This task should ideally be performed by a knowledgeable health care provider who was a member of the resuscitation team. A sensitive, compassionate approach using careful word selection and appropriate body language often reassures survivors that good care was given and suffering minimized. Involvement of the hospital chaplain or family pastor can help friends and family cope with their immediate grief. Similarly, viewing the body as soon as feasible can bring a sense of closure and allow survivors to move ahead with decisions regarding funeral and burial arrangements. The physician should then focus on reviewing/correcting code sheet documentation, writing a death note in the patient's medical record sufficiently detailing the precise sequence of code events, completing the death certificate, and notifying the medical examiner or organ donation team as appropriate. The nursing supervisor on duty will typically be responsible for transporting the body to the morgue, obtaining funeral home information from the family, and transferring the patient's personal articles to family members.

Conclusion

Knowledge and experience in CPR is a vital skill for all surgical trainees to acquire. Prompt and appropriate

application of these techniques to patients with reversible causes of cardiac arrest can potentially save lives.

Bibliography

American College of Surgeons: Statement on advance directives by patients: "do not resuscitate" in the operating room. Bull Am Coll Surg 1994;79:29.

American Heart Association in Collaboration with the International Liaison Committee on Resuscitation (ILCOR): Guidelines 2000 for cardiopulmonary resuscitation and emergency cardiovascular care. Circulation 2000;102(8).

American Heart Association in Collaboration with the International Liaison Committee on Resuscitation (ILCOR): Proceedings of the Guidelines 2000 Conference for Cardiopulmonary Resuscitation and Emergency Cardiovascular Care: an international consensus on science . Ann Emerg Med 2001;37(4 Suppl).

American Society of Anesthesiologists: Ethical guidelines for the anesthesia care of patients with do-not-resuscitate orders or other directives that limit treatment. Approved by the House of Delegates, October 13, 1993 and last amended October 17, 2001. Available at *www.asahq.org/publicationsAndServices/Standards/09.html*

Auble TE, Menegazzi JJ, Paris PM: Effect of out-of-hospital defibrillation by basic life support providers on cardiac arrest mortality: a metaanalysis. Ann Emerg Med 1995;25:642.

Badner NH, Knill RL, Brown JE, et al: Myocardiac infarction after noncardiac surgery. Anesthesiology 1998;88:572.

Behringer W, Kittler H, Sterz F, et al: Cumulative epinephrine dose during cardiopulmonary resuscitation and neurologic outcome. Ann Intern Med 1998;129:450.

Brown CG, Martin DR, Pepe PE, et al: A comparison of standard-dose and high-dose epinephrine in cardiac arrest outside the hospital. The Multicenter High-Dose Epinephrine Study Group. N Engl J Med 1992; 327:1051.

Callaham M, Madsen CD, Barton CW, et al: A randomized clinical trial of high-dose epinephrine and norepinephrine vs standard-dose epinephrine in prehospital cardiac arrest. JAMA 1992;268:2667.

Caplan RA, Ward RJ, Posner K, et al: Unexpected cardiac arrest during spinal anesthesia: a closed claims analysis of predisposing factors. Anesthesiology 1988;68:5.

Centers for Disease Control and Prevention: Mortality from coronary heart disease and acute myocardial infarction— United States, 1998. MMWR Morb Mortal Wkly Rep 2001;50:90.

Ewy GA, Ornato JP: Bethesda Conference Report. 31st Bethesda Conference: Emergency Cardiac Care (1999). J Am Coll Cardiol 2000;35:825.

Hallstrom A, Cobb L, Johnson E, et al: Cardiopulmonary resuscitation by chest compression alone or with mouth-to-mouth ventilation. N Engl J Med 2000;342:1546.

Hyers TM: Venous thromboembolism. Am J Respir Crit Care Med 1999;159:1.

Hyers TM, Agnelli G, Hull RD, et al: Antithrombotic therapy for venous thromboembolic disease. Chest 1998;114 (5 Suppl):561S.

Karch SB, Graff J, Young S, et al: Response times and outcomes for cardiac arrests in Las Vegas casinos. Am J Emerg Med 1998;16:249.

Keenan RL, Boyan CP: Cardiac arrest due to anesthesia: a study of incidence and causes. JAMA 1985;253:2373.

Kern KB, Halperin HR, Field J: New guidelines for cardiopulmonary resuscitation and emergency cardiac care: changes in the management of cardiac arrest. JAMA 2001;285:1267.

Kouwenhoven WB, Jude JR, Knickerbocker GG: Closed-chest cardiac massage. JAMA 1960;173:94.

Kouwenhoven WB, Milnor WR, Knickerbocker GG, et al: Closed chest defibrillation of the heart. Surgery 1957; 42:550.

Kudenchuk PJ, Cobb LA, Copass MK, et al: Amiodarone for resuscitation after out-of-hospital cardiac arrest due to ventricular fibrillation. N Engl J Med 1999;341:871.

Lindner KH, Prengel AW, Brinkman A, et al: Vasopressin administration in refractory cardiac arrest. Ann Intern Med 1996;124:1061.

Luce JM, Weil MH, Tang W: Wolf Creek V Conference on Cardiopulmonary Resuscitation. Crit Care Med 2000; 28(11 Suppl).

Morris DC, Dereczyk BE, Grzybowski M, et al: Vasopressin can increase coronary perfusion pressure during cardiopulmonary resuscitation. Acad Emerg Med 1997;4:878.

Mosesso VN Jr, Davis EA, Auble TE, et al: Use of automated external defibrillators by police officers for treatment of out-of-hospital cardiac arrest. Ann Emerg Med 1998;32:200.

O'Rourke MF, Donaldson E, Geddes JS: An airline cardiac arrest program. Circulation 1997;96:2849.

Overlie PA, Walter PD, Hurd HP II, et al: Emergency cardiopulmonary support with circulatory support devices. Cardiology 1994;84:231.

Plaisance P, Lurie KG, Vicaut E, et al: A comparison of standard cardiopulmonary resuscitation and active compression-decompression resuscitation for out-of-hospital cardiac arrest. N Engl J Med 1999;341:569.

Rivers EP, Wortsman J, Rady MY, et al: The effect of the total cumulative epinephrine dose administered during human CPR on hemodynamic, oxygen transport, and utilization variables in the postresuscitation period. Chest 1994;106:1499.

Safar P, Tisherman SA, Behringer W, et al: Suspended animation for delayed resuscitation from prolonged cardiac arrest that is unresuscitable by standard cardiopulmonary-cerebral resuscitation. Crit Care Med 2000;28(11 Suppl):N214.

Sprung J, Abdelmalak B, Gottlieb A, et al: Analysis of risk factors for myocardial infarction and cardiac mortality after major vascular surgery. Anesthesiology 2000;93:129.

Stiell IG, Hebert PC, Weitzman BN, et al: High-dose epinephrine in adult cardiac arrest. N Engl J Med 1992;327:1045.

Truog RD, Waisel DB, Burns JP: DNR in the OR: a goal-directed approach. Anesthesiology 1999;90:289.

Urbanek P, Bock H, Vicol C: Percutaneous cardiopulmonary support (PCPS). Cardiology 1994;84:216.

Valenzuela TD, Roe DJ, Nichol G, et al: Outcomes of rapid defibrillation by security officers after cardiac arrest in casinos. N Engl J Med 2000;343:1206.

van Walraven C, Forster AJ, Parish DC, et al: Validation of a clinical decision aid to discontinue in-hospital cardiac arrest resuscitations. JAMA 2001;285:1602.

CHAPTER 56

Alternatives in Physiologic Monitoring

Michael C. Chang, M.D., F.A.C.S.

Effective therapeutic decision making during resuscitation of critically ill patients depends upon both accurate physiologic monitoring and an ability to interpret the obtained information within the correct physiologic context. Several conditions unique to critically ill patients may make the information from these monitoring systems misleading or difficult to interpret. The complex, often multisystemic nature of the critical surgical illness, coupled with the multiple sequential physiologic insults often sustained by these patients, perpetuates and upregulates the inflammatory response to injury. This state of massive sustained inflammation can, both directly and indirectly, lead to the development of multiple extrinsic forces that can affect the quality of the information obtained from any given monitoring system.

Over the past 20 years, continued development has led to the introduction of several new and modified monitoring systems. Advances in pulmonary artery catheter technology, regional perfusion monitoring, and respiratory monitoring now make it possible to assess systemic and regional perfusion comprehensively at the bedside, and evaluate the physiologic determinants of problems at each of these levels.

The intent of this chapter is to review recent developments in monitoring techniques that have been demonstrated to provide useful clinical information in critically ill patients. Cardiac, pulmonary, and splanchnic monitoring are addressed, as well as interpretation of laboratory blood tests that assess acid-base and perfusion status.

Cardiovascular Monitoring

Since 1970, with the introduction of the flotation pulmonary artery catheter (PAC), right heart catheterization has been the accepted method of monitoring cardiac preload and myocardial performance in the intensive care unit (ICU). Thermodilution cardiac output has been used to intermittently quantify ventricular energy output and calculate oxygen delivery and consumption. Information from the PAC has also been used to assess the independent determinants of ventricular function (preload, contractility, and afterload). Ventricular preload has been estimated indirectly by transducing central venous pressure (CVP) and pulmonary artery occlusion pressure (PAOP). Afterload has been assessed by calculating systemic and pulmonary vascular resistance. Estimates of contractility have been inferred by changes in ventricular stroke work.

Unfortunately, several extrinsic factors common in critically ill patients may, alone or in combination, adversely affect the information obtained from these variables. Increased airway and pleural pressure secondary to increased positive end-expiratory pressure (PEEP) therapy for acute respiratory distress syndrome (ARDS) can elevate transduced values of CVP and PAOP, leading the unsuspecting clinician to believe that intravascular volume status is adequate, when actually it is not. Intra-abdominal hypertension (intra-abdominal pressure > 25 mm Hg) caused by perihepatic packing, retroperitoneal swelling, or bowel edema can affect CVP and PAOP similarly.

Fortunately, several advances have been made in PAC technology over the past 25 years that help overcome several of these shortcomings. The volumetric oximetry PAC (93A-754H-7.5F; Baxter Edwards Critical Care, Irvine, CA), which measures right ventricular volumes, has proven to be very useful in the care of critically ill patients. This modified PAC measures beat-to-beat temperature changes with sampling, from which the right ventricular ejection fraction (RVEF) is calculated. Right ventricular end-diastolic volume index (RVEDVI) is then derived via the following formula:

$$RVEDVI = SVI/RVEF$$

where SVI represents the stroke volume index, calculated from cardiac index (CI) and heart rate. Adding the volumetric measurements available with this technology improves the clinician's ability to estimate preload, contractility, and afterload.

Assessing the Independent Determinants of Ventricular Function

Measuring preload

Cardiac preload is defined physiologically as myocardial fiber length; in the intact heart, this is represented by ventricular volume at end-diastole. Because it is a measure of ventricular volume, the RVEDVI, by definition, is a better estimate of preload than indirect estimates based upon transduced pressure. Furthermore, extrinsic forces acting upon the ventricle and pulmonary artery, such as pleural pressure and abdominal pressure, do not affect volumetric measurements. Therefore, RVEDVI should theoretically be more closely related to preload than either CVP or PAOP.

Clinical studies have demonstrated this logic to be correct. By convention, preload is often defined in terms of its relationship with ventricular energy output, usually either cardiac output or stroke work. Several authors have demonstrated, in mixed populations of critically ill patients, that the RVEDVI is a better predictor of preload and preload-recruitable increases in CI than either PAOP or CVP (Table 56–1). They have further demonstrated this to be the case in several different populations of trauma patients, such as patients who receive large volumes of resuscitation fluid, patients on increased levels of PEEP, and patients with intra-abdominal hypertension. An early criticism of estimating preload with the RVEDVI, noting that the better correlations between RVEDVI and CI (when compared with PAOP) were due to mathematical coupling, has been addressed with a clinical study specifically designed to eliminate mathematical coupling from the data analysis.

These studies also uniformly demonstrate the poor correlation between PAOP and CI (Table 56–1). These findings illustrate the effects that extrinsic forces acting upon the pressure transduced in the proximal pulmonary artery can have on the meaning of specific values of the PAOP. Increased levels of PEEP and intra-abdominal hypertension are associated with a negative correlation between PAOP and CI, illustrating the effects of increased pleural and abdominal pressure on transduced intracavitary pressures within the heart and proximal pulmonary vasculature.

Table 56–1
Correlation of CVP, PAOP, and RVEDVI versus cardiac index

Study	Population	CVP	PAOP	RVEDVI
Martyn et al. (1981)	Burns	0.27	0.36	0.75
Diebel et al. (1992)	Surgery/trauma	0.51	0.42	0.61
Diebel et al. (1994)	Trauma	0.16	0.12	0.64
Durham et al. (1995)	Surgery/trauma	0.03	0.10	0.60
Chang, Black, et al. (1996)	Trauma	—	0.05	0.39
Diebel et al. (1997)	Trauma (increased PEEP)	—	−0.06	0.40
Chang, Blinman, et al. (1996)	Trauma	0.07	0.03	0.48
Chang, Miller, et al. (1998)	Trauma (abdominal hypertension)	−0.19	−0.16	0.49
Cheatham et al. (1998)	Surgery/trauma (increased PEEP)	−0.76	−0.04	0.39–0.94

In fact, in patients with intra-abdominal hypertension, PAOP and CVP correlate better with abdominal pressure than with CI, and abdominal pressure accounts for 20% to 24% of the variability observed in end-diastolic pressure. The PAOP and CVP should not be ignored, however, but rather should be interpreted in the context of the extrinsic intracavitary pressure surrounding the catheter tip.

In summary, the clinician estimating intravascular volume status and preload should take into account all available information, including RVEDVI, CVP, and PAOP. The vast majority of extrinsic forces that affect CVP and PAOP tend to increase their values; thus increased values may reflect increased volume status, increased extrinsic pressure on the heart and pulmonary artery, or some combination of both. Low values of PAOP or CVP, however, likely indicate the potential for increasing cardiac output with fluid administration. Transduced pressures should be interpreted in the context of airway, pleural, and abdominal pressure, even if a volumetric PAC is not used in these patients.

Estimating preload by measuring the RVEDVI has been demonstrated to provide useful information that affects patient care. One study examined the relationship between cardiac preload and gut perfusion, estimated by gastric tonometry. This study demonstrated that occult hypovolemia (detected as a lower RVEDVI) was associated with decreased intestinal perfusion and the patients with a lower RVEDVI and gastric intramucosal pH had a higher rate of death and multiple organ failure (MOF). Systemic perfusion, indicated by CI and oxygen delivery, was not different between the two groups. A subsequent randomized prospective evaluation of the effects of maintaining various levels of RVEDVI on pulmonary function and gut perfusion was performed. The patients maintained at a RVEDVI greater than 120 mL/m^2 had significantly better intestinal perfusion than the patients maintained at lower levels of RVEDVI (90 to 100 mL/m^2), who were supported with inotropic agents. Furthermore, these higher levels of preload were not associated with any differences in oxygenation function, ventilator days, or an increased incidence of ARDS.

Thus the ability to measure ventricular volumes has led to a new definition of adequate levels of preload. Whereas preload has traditionally been defined in terms of its relationship with cardiac function and the Frank-Starling relationship, increasing preload beyond levels that result in increased cardiac output may replenish blood flow to regional tissue beds, such as the gut (Fig. 56–1). This may occur either as a result of replenishing occult intravascular volume deficits, or by ameliorating the need for shunting of blood away from the gut via other mechanisms.

Contractility and afterload

Myocardial contractility is defined as that determinant of intrinsic ventricular performance that is independent of

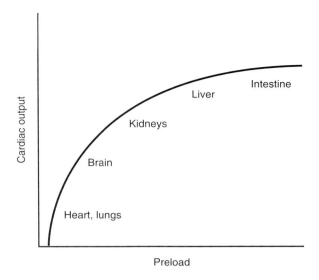

FIGURE 56–1 Representative Starling ventricular function curve illustrating the effects of various levels of preload on cardiac output and regional perfusion.

preload and afterload. Afterload is defined as the impedance to ejection of blood by the ventricle. Commonly used variables describing these independent determinants of ventricular function have several potential shortcomings. Variables such as ejection fraction and stroke work have been used in the past as clinical estimates of contractility, but they are preload and/or afterload dependent, and thus do not represent contractility per se. Vascular resistance indices, based on mean systemic and pulmonary arterial pressure, are also less than ideal. They do not account for oscillatory pressure, pulsatile load, or reflected pulse waves. This may be a problem in older patients, in whom oscillatory pressure proportionally accounts for a greater amount of afterload. Furthermore, each of these clinical indices of contractility and afterload are expressed in different units, or have no units at all, and the relationship of each of these variables with each other and how these relationships affect clinical cardiac function is unclear, at best.

The ventricular pressure-volume diagram

Given these limitations in current monitoring techniques, the ventricular pressure-volume diagram, as described by Suga, Sagawa, and others in the 1970s, presents itself as a potential monitoring technique free of many of the above limitations. Figure 56–2 shows a hypothetical ventricular pressure-volume diagram. Preload is represented on the abscissa by end-diastolic volume. The slope of the ventricular end-systolic pressure-volume relationship, or end-systolic elastance (E_{es}), represents myocardial contractility. This parameter has long been used as a load-independent measure of contractility in the cardiovascular laboratory, and a clinical adaptation of this variable has recently been described and tested in trauma patients.

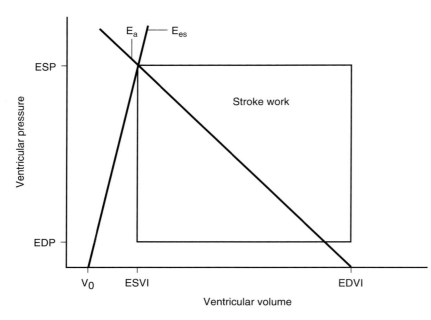

FIGURE 56–2 Ventricular pressure-volume diagram. E_{es} represents ventricular end-systolic elastance, a load-independent measure of ventricular contractility. E_a represents effective arterial elastance, a rate-independent measure of afterload that accounts for oscillatory pressure as well as steady-flow pressure. ESP represents end-systolic ventricular pressure, derived from peak systolic pressure. V_0 represents ventricular volume at zero pressure. ESVI represents ventricular end-systolic volume index, EDVI represents ventricular end-diastolic volume index, and EDP represents ventricular end-diastolic pressure.

Afterload can also be estimated within the pressure-volume framework. Effective arterial elastance (E_a), calculated as end-systolic pressure divided by SVI, is represented by the slope of a line drawn from the end-diastolic volume axis intercept through the end-systolic point. As the slope of this line increases, impedance to ventricular ejection increases, and as the slope decreases, afterload decreases. There are several theoretical reasons why this term is a better measure of afterload than vascular resistance. First, E_a is rate independent, whereas systemic vascular resistance is not. Second, E_a accounts for oscillatory pressure. This is important when estimating afterload in older patients, in whom pulsatile load has an increasing effect on both myocardial performance and the development of subsequent cardiac complications. Finally, E_a can be examined in conjunction with E_{es} on the pressure-volume diagram to evaluate the relationship between the heart and the arterial system, or ventricular-vascular coupling.

Ventricular-Vascular Coupling

The interactions between any physical energy source and its output environment are critical in determining the amount of useful work and power output the system is able to generate. In cardiovascular physiology, the efficacy of circulation is closely related to the coupling of the heart and the arterial system. Because cardiac contractility is represented by E_{es} and afterload by E_a, the relationships between E_{es} and E_a on the ventricular pressure-volume diagram can be used to estimate ventricular-vascular coupling status, and the effects of each of these variables on resultant stroke work and power output can be examined. Relationships between E_{es} and E_a have been studied in

various patient populations, including trauma patients. One study found that survivors of post-traumatic shock have better ventricular-vascular coupling than nonsurvivors, and described the effects that the better ventricular-vascular coupling in survivors had on stroke work and power output.

Ventricular Stroke Work and Power

Referring again to Figure 56–2, end-diastolic volume, E_{es}, and E_a define the boundaries of ventricular stroke work, a term classically described by both Starling and Sarnoff as the most appropriate measure of ventricular energy output. Stroke work and ventricular power output (stroke work performed over time) are both more closely related to cardiovascular performance and perfusion in trauma patients than CI, oxygen delivery, or oxygen consumption. Using the ventricular pressure-volume diagram, preload, contractility, and afterload can be evaluated in a common, integrated framework, and the effects of changes in any one variable on stroke work and power output can be predicted. Furthermore, by constructing pressure-volume diagrams at the bedside using measurements from the volumetric PAC, inadequate perfusion resulting from cardiac dysfunction can be evaluated in terms of the independent determinants of ventricular function, and specific therapy can be applied in a goal-directed fashion (Figs. 56–3 and 56–4).

Mixed Venous Oxygen Saturation Monitoring

Continuous mixed venous oxygen saturation (SvO_2) monitoring using fiberoptics incorporated into the PAC has been available since 1980, and monitoring SvO_2

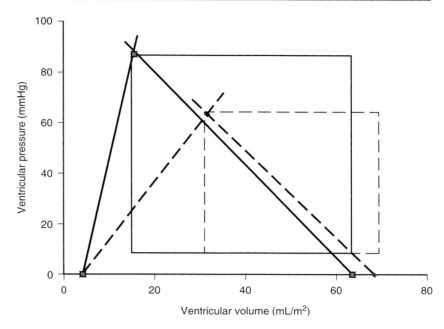

FIGURE 56–3 Ventricular pressure-volume diagram of a patient with hypotension caused by inadequate contractility after initial fluid resuscitation *(dashed lines)*. Blood pressure and stroke work increased after administration of 5 mcg/kg/min dobutamine *(solid lines)*. Increase in contractility is represented by the increase in the slope of E_{es}. Note that E_a did not change. The *x* axis represents left ventricular end-diastolic volume index; the *y* axis represents left ventricular pressure.

on a minute-to-minute basis has become popular in the care of complex, critically ill patients. This subject matter is covered extensively elsewhere. In the presence of adequate arterial O_2 saturation (SaO_2), the SvO_2 provides an indicator of oxygen utilization, or the balance between oxygen delivery and consumption. Acute decreases in SvO_2 represent either an increase in oxygen demand and consumption, or a decrease in oxygen delivery resulting from a change in one or more of the determinants of oxygen delivery (SaO_2, cardiac output, or hemoglobin concentration).

Continuous Cardiac Output Monitoring

The ability to continuously monitor cardiac output represents a recent advance in PAC technology. Monitoring systems that measure cardiac output as often as every 15 seconds are now available, and have been demonstrated to agree closely with conventional cardiac output values obtained on an intermittent basis. Continuous monitoring of cardiac output has theoretical advantages over intermittent measurements. The measurements are performed without injectate, and are therefore free of inaccuracies

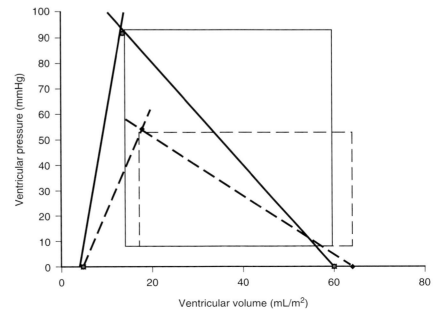

FIGURE 56–4 Ventricular pressure-volume diagram of a patient with inadequate perfusion and hypotension caused by both inadequate afterload and inadequate contractility after initial fluid resuscitation *(dashed lines)*. Blood pressure and stroke work increased after administration of dopamine, 10 μg/kg/min *(solid lines)*. The increase in contractility is represented by increase in slope of E_{es}, and the increase in afterload is represented by increase in slope of E_a.

associated with injectate temperature and volume, and timing within the respiratory cycle. Furthermore, the displayed value represents a time-averaged value obtained over the previous few minutes, and therefore may be more representative of ongoing changes than intermittent values. Finally, continuous measurement of cardiac output may allow the clinician to titrate therapy in a more timely fashion, and to observe the effects of sequential interventions without depending upon intermittent samples in between interventions. PACs are now available that monitor cardiac output, mixed venous saturation, and RVEDVI on a continuous basis.

Monitoring Acid-Base Status

Lactate

Impaired oxygen utilization with concomitant anaerobic respiration after injury and critical illness may result in the development of postinsult metabolic acidosis, and this acidosis is primarily due to increased levels of lactate in the blood. Lactate is the metabolic by-product of anaerobic metabolism, and increasing levels of lactate indicate increasing oxygen debt. In a prospective resuscitation study involving trauma patients, all patients who normalized lactate within 24 hours survived, whereas those who required 24 to 48 hours to clear lactate had a mortality of 25%, and those that required greater than 48 hours had a mortality of 86%. Furthermore, one randomized prospective study in a mixed population of surgical patients demonstrated that normalization of lactate is a useful goal during resuscitation.

Recent developments have led to the availability of point-of-care bedside testing of serum lactate levels, and this has been demonstrated to be an effective clinical method of determining perfusion status through serial measurements of lactate at the bedside in critically ill patients. Rapid determination of lactate levels, coupled with invasive monitoring of hemodynamics and oxygen transport status, enable the clinician caring for critically ill patients to comprehensively assess the adequacy of circulation and interventions directed toward ameliorating the effects of post-traumatic shock.

Arterial Base Deficit

The arterial base deficit (BD) represents a rapid, widely available measure of post-traumatic metabolic acidosis. This variable is calculated from directly measured values of arterial pH and arterial carbon dioxide tension ($PaCO_2$) from an arterial blood gas sample, and provides the clinician with a nonspecific marker of lactate, and therefore anaerobic metabolism and oxygen debt. Several investigators

have retrospectively demonstrated that the BD is a powerful predictor of survival in critically ill patients. BD is also related to the amount of fluid and blood administered during resuscitation, post-traumatic complications, and the subsequent development of MOF.

The majority of these studies focus upon the admission value or largest BD during the first 24 hours after admission. However, subsequent BD measurements during the later phases of resuscitation (up to 96 hours after admission) are also related to outcome. Persistently elevated values of BD throughout the resuscitation period have been correlated with impaired oxygen utilization, and may provide insight into the adequacy of ongoing resuscitation and therapy. Thus measuring the BD is a rapid, practical way to estimate ongoing and cumulative dysoxia throughout resuscitation in critically ill patients.

Tissue Perfusion Monitoring

Monitoring various indices of tissue perfusion provides many theoretical advantages over measuring the central supply of oxygen, energy, and nutrients to the periphery. First, different tissue beds may have varying levels of metabolic activity during post-traumatic shock. Second, the perfusion status of specific tissue beds, such as the gut or the brain, may be selectively important beyond simply estimating blood and nutrient flow. For example, gut ischemia is thought to be an important determinant of the subsequent development of post-traumatic proinflammatory state and MOF. Finally, tissue-specific monitoring capabilities may allow the detection of otherwise occult perfusion deficits.

Gastric Tonometry

Intestinal ischemia and reperfusion play an important role in the development of postinjury MOF. Gut perfusion can be indirectly assessed using tonometric techniques to measure the gastric intramucosal pH (pHi). This technique involves instilling saline into a semipermeable balloon at the end of a modified nasogastric tube, followed after a period of equilibration by removing the saline and measuring the carbon dioxide tension (PCO_2) of the saline sample. Mucosal ischemia leads to the production of increased CO_2 within the stomach lumen, which is detected as an increased PCO_2 in the saline sample. This gastric mucosal PCO_2 is then used, along with simultaneously measured arterial bicarbonate, in a modified version of the Henderson-Hasselbalch equation to calculate the pHi.

Trauma patients with a pHi less than 7.32 and otherwise adequate central hemodynamics and oxygen transport 24 hours after ICU admission have a higher rate of MOF and death than a comparable group of patients with both adequate central and intestinal perfusion. This observation has fueled hope that measuring the pHi would enable clinicians to detect and correct intestinal hypoperfusion during resuscitation. Although several investigators have attempted to improve the pHi in critically ill patients by improving global perfusion status, none to date have been able to demonstrate an improvement in either mortality or the incidence of MOF using these strategies.

One drawback to this approach has been the inability to selectively improve intestinal perfusion in the setting of otherwise adequate systemic perfusion. Most studies to date directed toward improving the pHi have done so by improving CI and systemic acid-base status. These studies failed to selectively study the patients in whom tonometry would be most useful, that is, patients with selective gut hypoperfusion and otherwise adequate systemic perfusion. Although there are some preliminary data that suggest that it may be possible to selectively improve gut perfusion with focused therapy, no one has demonstrated the ability to reliably correct selective gut malperfusion on demand. This makes performing a prospective study examining whether improving gut perfusion affects outcome very difficult.

Capnometric Recirculating Gas Tonometry

Recent technical innovations have led to the development of a semicontinuous gas tonometer, and a model of this device is now available for clinical use. This machine works on the same principle as saline tonometry, but samples mucosal CO_2 intermittently at short intervals, rather than depending on manual sampling of a saline sample in the tonometer balloon. Gut perfusion using this technique is detected by an elevated mucosal-arterial CO_2 gap (GAP), rather than by calculating the pHi. This technique has several theoretical advantages over conventional saline tonometry. Gas tonometry is automated and less prone to sampling error. Furthermore, GAP measurements should more accurately reflect gastric mucosal ischemia than saline tonometry because systemic bicarbonate is not used in calculating GAP.

Despite these theoretical advantages, however, there are still important shortcomings of this technique. Until recently, critical values for GAP in any patient population had not been described. A recent clinical study, however, describes a GAP of 18 mm Hg and a pHi of 7.25 as appropriate threshold values for identifying trauma patients at risk for MOF and death. Furthermore, in trauma patients, GAP does not predict MOF and death as well as conventional tonometry. Theoretically, this is not surprising, because gut perfusion would not be expected to account for all organ failure and mortality in these patients, and the pHi contains a systemic component (arterial bicarbonate) that reflects whole-body oxygen debt, as well as the gut-specific mucosal CO_2.

Other Applications of Tonometry

Although there are no prospective data demonstrating that monitoring and attempting to improve gut perfusion improve outcome, the ability to detect gut ischemia has produced several findings of potential importance. Gut perfusion is closely related to preload status, and it has been prospectively demonstrated that maintaining patients at higher levels of preload (RVEDVI >120 mL/m^2) improves the pHi during shock resuscitation. Administration of angiotensin-converting enzyme inhibitors to trauma patients during resuscitation has been associated with increased values of pHi. Abdominal decompression in patients with intra-abdominal hypertension improves pHi. A recently published article comprehensively reviews the current literature describing the effects of numerous vasoactive agents on pHi and intestinal perfusion. One clinical study in trauma patients demonstrates that dopamine and epinephrine lower pHi, whereas dobutamine administration does not affect pHi. Thus the clinician caring for critically ill patients now has available a list of helpful and harmful therapeutic maneuvers with regard to pHi and intestinal perfusion.

Ventilation Monitoring

Several recent advances have been made in the field of respiratory monitoring. On-line monitoring of SaO_2 and SvO_2 has been available for several years. Continuous monitoring of end-tidal CO_2, pulmonary pressure-volume loops, work of breathing, and esophageal pressure all represent newer respiratory monitoring techniques that have been described and clinically tested. These techniques can potentially help clinicians evaluate oxygenation, ventilation, and weaning from mechanical ventilation more effectively. Furthermore, they provide direct and immediate feedback of the results of bedside changes in ventilator therapy.

Pulse Oximetry and Dual Oximetry

Continuous, transcutaneous real-time monitoring of SaO_2 is possible via pulse oximetry. This is important for several reasons. When compared to partial pressure of arterial oxygen (PaO_2), SaO_2 represents functional oxygenation much more accurately because oxygen bound to hemoglobin is a primary determinant of arterial oxygen content, whereas the PaO_2 only represents the amount of oxygen dissolved in plasma. Also, the ability to measure SaO_2 noninvasively and continuously allows the clinician to titrate ventilator therapy in real time, without having to check multiple arterial blood measurements to assess the efficacy of therapy.

Established oxygenation support algorithms for ARDS in critically ill patients involve titrating PEEP in a goal-directed fashion to a predefined value of intrapulmonary shunt fraction (Qs/Qt). In patients being monitored with an oximetry PAC, Qs/Qt can be continuously estimated by calculating the ventilation-perfusion index (VQI) using simultaneous measurements of SaO_2 and SvO_2. This variable, calculated as

$$VQI = 1 - SaO_2/1 - SvO_2$$

closely approximates Qs/Qt (Fig. 56–5). By continuously estimating VQI with dual oximetry, the clinician treating a patient with hypoxemic respiratory failure can continuously assess the effects of titrating PEEP and other changes in oxygenation support on patients without having to measure arterial blood gases and calculate Qs/Qt by hand. Thus changes in critical support can be made more frequently and at lower cost with this technique. Furthermore, the effects of adding other therapy not primarily directed at pulmonary function, such as inotropic agents or vasoactive drugs, on oxygenation function can be monitored in real time.

End-Tidal Carbon Dioxide Monitoring

Continuous on-line measurement of end-tidal carbon dioxide tension ($PetCO_2$) levels in mechanically ventilated patients is now widely available. Originally, it was hoped that values of $PetCO_2$ and $PaCO_2$ would correlate closely, and that using this technique would help decrease the frequency of arterial blood gas measurements. However, the correlation between these two values has been fair, at best, and trends between $PaCO_2$ and $PetCO_2$ were found to be unreliable in trauma patients, most likely as a result of variability in the $PetCO_2$ secondary to dead space and pulmonary disease.

Recently, however, the difference between arterial and end-tidal CO_2 has been described as a measure of the adequacy of cardiac output and perfusion. The $PaCO_2/PetCO_2$ difference increases with increasing pulmonary dead space. As cardiac output and pulmonary blood flow improve in patients in shock, alveolar perfusion improves, dead space decreases, and the $PaCO_2/PetCO_2$ difference decreases. This relationship has been examined retrospectively in critically ill patients, and an intraoperative difference of greater than 8 torr was associated with increased mortality.

Work of Breathing

Prolonged ventilator dependence is an important problem in trauma patients, as well as other patient populations, in terms of incidence, resource utilization, cost, and complications. Several weaning algorithms based upon such parameters as respiratory rate, tidal volume, and oxygenation have been proposed, though none has earned universal acceptance. Recently, measurements of work of breathing have been used to help determine when patients are ready for rapid weaning from ventilatory support and/or extubation. Microprocessor-based pulmonary monitors enable the clinician to measure total, physiologic, and imposed work of breathing (WOB_{TOT}, WOB_{PHYS}, and WOB_{IMP}, respectively). WOB_{TOT} represents the sum of WOB_{PHYS} and WOB_{IMP}. Many patients who fail conventional extubation criteria may do so because they have an increased WOB_{TOT}. Measuring WOB_{PHYS} and WOB_{IMP} helps differentiate between those patients who fail because of their disease process and those who fail as a result of increased WOB_{IMP} from mechanical factors such as the endotracheal tube or ventilator circuit. This was evaluated prospectively in a

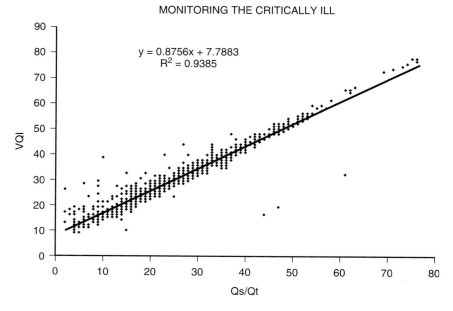

MONITORING THE CRITICALLY ILL

$y = 0.8756x + 7.7883$
$R^2 = 0.9385$

FIGURE 56–5 XY scatter diagram of 1219 simultaneously measured values of Qs/Qt (intrapulmonary shunt fraction) versus VQI (ventilation-perfusion index) over a 1-year period in 46 trauma patients treated with approximately 10 cm PEEP at a level I trauma center.

predominantly trauma population by Kirton and colleagues. They found that 18% of patients who failed conventional weaning criteria were actually extubatable based upon work-of-breathing measurements, and that these findings could potentially lead to a significantly decreased number of ventilator days in the studied population. This strategy has not, however, been compared to conventional, more widely employed extubation criteria.

Conclusion

The complex, multisystem pathology characteristic of critically ill patients makes delivery of optimal critical care to these patients challenging and often complex. New advances in cardiac, pulmonary, and systemic and regional perfusion monitoring now make it possible to recognize and evaluate problems in these areas that were previously unrecognized. Only through a comprehensive understanding of the monitoring systems available, and through the application of sound physiologic principles in conjunction with these techniques, can the physician caring for these patients take maximum advantage of these new advances and apply them in a way that is beneficial to the well-being of critically ill patients.

Bibliography

Abrams JF, Cerra F, Holcroft JW: Cardiopulmonary monitoring. *In* Wilmore DW, Brennan MF, Harken AH, et al (eds): Care of the Surgical Patient: Perioperative Management and Techniques. New York: Scientific American, 1988–1998:1.

Abramson D, Scalea TM, Hitchcock R, et al: Lactate clearance and survival following injury. J Trauma 1993;35:584.

Asanoi H, Sasayama S, Kameyama T: Ventriculoarterial coupling in normal and failing heart in humans. Circ Res 1989;65:483.

Barquist E, Kirton O, Windsor J, et al: The impact of antioxidant and splanchnic-directed therapy on persistent uncorrected gastric mucosal pH in the critically ill patient. J Trauma 1998;44:355.

Botha AJ, Moore FA, Moore EE, et al: Early neutrophil sequestration after injury: a pathologic mechanism for multiple organ failure. J Trauma 1995;39:411.

Boyd O, Grounds RM, Bennett ED: A randomized clinical trial of the effect of deliberate perioperative increase of oxygen delivery on the mortality in high-risk surgical patients. JAMA 1993;270:2699.

Burchell SA, Yu M, Takiguchi SA, et al: Evaluation of a continuous cardiac output and mixed venous oxygen saturation catheter in critically ill surgical patients. Crit Care Med 1997;25:388.

Chang MC, Black CS, Meredith JW: Volumetric assessment of preload in trauma patients: addressing the problem of mathematical coupling. Shock 1996;6:326.

Chang MC, Blinman TA, Rutherford EJ, et al: Preload assessment during large volume resuscitation in trauma patients. Arch Surg 1996;131:728.

Chang MC, Cheatham MC, Nelson LD, et al: Gastric tonometry supplements information provided by the systemic indicators of oxygen transport. J Trauma 1994;37:488.

Chang MC, Meredith JW: Cardiac preload, splanchnic ischemia, and their relationship during resuscitation in trauma patients. J Trauma 1997;42:577.

Chang MC, Miller PR, D'Agostino R Jr, Meredith JW: Effects of abdominal decompression on cardiopulmonary function and visceral perfusion in patients with intra-abdominal hypertension. J Trauma 1998;44:440.

Chang MC, Mondy JS III, Meredith JW, Holcroft JW: Redefining cardiovascular performance during resuscitation: ventricular stroke work, power, and the pressure-volume diagram. J Trauma 1998;45:470.

Chang MC, Mondy JS III, Meredith JW, et al: Clinical application of ventricular end-systolic elastance and the ventricular pressure-volume diagram. Shock 1997;7:413.

Cheatham ML, Nelson LD, Chang MC, Safcsak K: Right ventricular end-diastolic volume index as a predictor of preload status in patients on positive end-expiratory pressure. Crit Care Med 1998;26:1801.

Chernow B, Aduen J, Bernstein WK, Wiese J: Lactate: the ultimate blood test in critical care? *In* Parker MM, Shapiro MJ, Porembka DT (eds): Critical Care: State of the Art, Vol 15. Anaheim, CA: Society of Critical Care Medicine, 1995:253.

Civetta JM: Bedside use of arterial and venous oximetry. *In* Civetta JM, Taylor RW, Kirby RR (eds): Critical Care (2nd ed). Philadelphia: JB Lippincott, 1992:313.

Creteur J, De Backer D, Vincent JL: Monitoring gastric mucosal carbon dioxide pressure using gas tonometry: in vitro and in vivo validation studies. Anesthesiology 1997;87:504.

Davis JW, Kaups KL: Base deficit in the elderly: a marker of severe injury and death. J Trauma 1998;45:873.

Davis JW, Parks SN, Kaups KL, et al: Admission base deficit predicts transfusion requirements and risk of complications. J Trauma 1996;41:769.

Davis JW, Shackford SR, Holbrook TL: Base deficit as a sensitive indicator of compensated shock and tissue oxygen utilization. Surg Gynecol Obstet 1991;173:473.

Deitch EA: The role of intestinal barrier failure and bacterial translocation in the development of systemic infection and multiple organ failure. Arch Surg 1990;125:403.

Diebel LN, Myers T, Dulchavsky S: Effects of increasing airway pressure and PEEP on the assessment of cardiac preload. J Trauma 1997;42:585.

Diebel L, Wilson RF, Heinz J, et al: End-diastolic volume versus pulmonary artery wedge pressure in evaluating cardiac preload in trauma patients. J Trauma 1994;37:950.

Diebel LN, Wilson RF, Tagett MG, Kline RA: End-diastolic volume: a better indicator of preload in the critically ill. Arch Surg 1992;127:817.

DiRusso SM, Nelson LD, Safcsak K, Miller RS: Survival in patients with severe adult respiratory distress syndrome treated with high-level positive end-expiratory pressure. Crit Care Med 1995;23:1485.

Domsky M, Wilson RF, Heins J: Intraoperative end-tidal carbon dioxide values and derived calculations correlated with outcome: prognosis and capnography. Crit Care Med 1995;23:1497.

Ducey JP, Lamiell JM, Gueller GE: Arterial–venous carbon dioxide tension difference during severe hemorrhage and resuscitation. Crit Care Med 1992;20:518.

Durham R, Neunaber K, Vogler G, et al: Right ventricular end-diastolic volume as a measure of preload. J Trauma 1995;39:218.

Fiddian-Green RG: Studies in splanchnic ischemia and multiple organ failure. In Marston A, Bulkley GB, Fiddian-Green RG, et al (eds): Splanchnic Ischemia and Multiple Organ Failure. St. Louis: CV Mosby, 1989:349.

Gutierrez G, Palizas F, Doglio G: Gastric intramucosal pH as a therapeutic index of tissue oxygenation in critically ill patients. Lancet 1992;339:195.

Guzman JA, Kruse JA: Development and validation of a technique for continuous monitoring of gastric intramucosal pH. Am J Respir Crit Care Med 1996;153:694.

Haller M, Zollner C, Briegel J, et al: Evaluation of a new continuous thermodilution cardiac output monitor in critically ill patients: a prospective criterion standard study. Crit Care Med 1995;23:860.

Ivatury RR, Simon RJ, Havriliak D, et al: Gastric mucosal pH and oxygen delivery and oxygen consumption indices in the assessment of adequacy of resuscitation after trauma: a randomized, prospective study. J Trauma 1995;39:128.

Ivatury RR, Simon RJ, Islam S, et al: A prospective randomized study of end points of resuscitation after major trauma: global oxygen transport indices versus organ-specific gastric mucosal pH. J Am Coll Surg 1996;183:145.

Kincaid EH, Miller PR, Meredith JW, Chang MC: Enalaprilat improves gut perfusion in critically ill patients. Shock 1998;7:79.

Kincaid EH, Miller PR, Meredith JW, et al: Elevated arterial base deficit in trauma patients: a marker of impaired oxygen utilization. J Am Coll Surg 1998;187:384.

Kirton OC, DeHaven B, Hudson-Civetta J, et al: Re-engineering ventilatory support to decrease days and improve resource utilization. Ann Surg 1996;224:396.

Kirton OC, DeHaven B, Morgan JP, et al: Elevated imposed work of breathing masquerading as ventilator weaning intolerance. Chest 1995;108:1021.

Martyn JA, Snider MT, Farago LF, Burke JF: Thermodilution right ventricular volume: a novel and better predictor of volume replacement in acute thermal injury. J Trauma 1981;21:619.

Mihm FG, Gettinger A, Hanson CW III, et al: A multicenter evaluation of a new continuous cardiac output pulmonary artery catheter system. Crit Care Med 1998;26:1346.

Miller PR, Kincaid EH, Meredith JW, Chang MC: Threshold values of intramucosal pH and mucosal-arterial CO_2 gap during shock resuscitation. J Trauma 1998;45:868.

Miller PR, Meredith JW, Chang MC: Randomized, prospective comparison of increased preload versus inotropes in the resuscitation of trauma patients: effects on cardiopulmonary function and visceral perfusion. J Trauma 1998;44:107.

Miller RS, Nelson LD, DiRusso SM, et al: High-level positive end-expiratory pressure management in trauma-associated adult respiratory distress syndrome. J Trauma 1992;33:284.

Moore EE, Moore FA, Francoise RJ, et al: Postischemic gut serves as a priming bed for circulating neutrophils that provoke multiple organ failure. J Trauma 1994;37:881.

Nelson LD: Continuous venous oximetry in surgical patients. Ann Surg 1986;203:329.

Nelson LD: The new pulmonary artery catheters: continuous venous oximetry, right ventricular ejection fraction, and continuous cardiac output. New Horizons 1997;5:251.

Rasanen J, Downs JB, Malec DJ, et al: Real time continuous estimation of gas exchange by dual oximetry. Intensive Care Med 1988;14:118.

Ridings PC, Bloomfield GL, Blocher CR, et al: Cardiopulmonary effects of raised intra-abdominal pressure before and after intravascular volume expansion. J Trauma 1995;39:1071.

Russell GB, Graybeal JM: Reliability of the arterial to end-tidal carbon dioxide gradient in mechanically ventilated patients with multisystem trauma. J Trauma 1994;36:317.

Rutherford EJ, Morris JA, Reed GW, et al: Base deficit stratifies mortality and determines therapy. J Trauma 1992;33:417.

Sarnoff SJ, Berglund E: Ventricular function: Starling's law of the heart studied by means of simultaneous right and left ventricular function curves in the dog. Circulation 1954;71:994.

Sauia A, Moore FA, Moore EE, et al: Early predictors of postinjury multiple organ failure. Arch Surg 1994;129:39.

Siegel JH, Fabian M, Smith JA, et al: Use of recombinant hemoglobin solution in reversing lethal hemorrhagic hypovolemic oxygen debt shock. J Trauma 1997;42:199.

Silva E, DeBacker D, Creteur J, Vincent JL: Effects of vasoactive drugs on gastric intramucosal pH. Crit Care Med 1998;26:1749.

Starling EH: The Linacre Lecture on the Law of the Heart. London: Longmans, Green, 1918.

Suga H, Sagawa K: Instantaneous pressure-volume relationships and their ratio in the excised, supported canine left ventricle. Circ Res 1974;35:117.

Suga J, Sagawa K, Shoudas AA: Load independence of the instantaneous pressure-volume ratio of the canine left ventricle and effects of epinephrine and heart rate on the ratio. Circ Res 1973;32:314.

Sunagawa H, Maughan WL, Burkoff D, Sagawa K: Left ventricular interaction with arterial load studied in isolated canine ventricle. Am J Physiol 1983;245:H773.

CHAPTER 57

Shock: Differential Diagnosis and Management

Michael C. Chang, M.D., F.A.C.S.

Shock can be defined as inadequate delivery of oxygen and nutrients to the tissues during times of metabolic stress. This inadequate delivery may be due to decreased supply, increased demand, or some combination of both. Hypoperfusion can occur at the regional or systemic level, and, although in its extreme form can be evident on physical examination, it also can occur with no obvious findings on clinical examination. Through several inflammatory and dysoxic pathways that are only recently becoming understood, untreated or uncompensated shock of any sort is closely associated with the late development of a hyperinflammatory septic state, multiple organ failure, and death. Multiple organ failure has been and continues to be the leading cause of late mortality in the surgical intensive care unit.

Fortunately, through early detection of shock and aggressive resuscitation and removal of the underlying source, late organ failure and mortality are to some degree avoidable. The combination of early and immediate removal of the stimulus for ongoing shock, plus aggressive resuscitation after diagnosis and removal of the stimulus, has resulted in improved outcome in critically ill surgical patients.

The conceptual outline of this chapter includes defining shock and the traditional categories of shock, discussing the molecular mechanisms of shock in terms of the inflammatory response to metabolic stress, and the presentation of a deterministic approach to the diagnosis and clinical treatment of shock.

Mechanisms of Tissue Damage in Shock

The general term *shock* implies inadequate perfusion of tissues. This could occur at the systemic level with obvious clinical findings or at the regional level with more subtle or absent clinical findings. Perfusion is defined as the delivery of oxygen and nutrients to the tissues with adequate flow and pressure. Furthermore, in addition to the adequate delivery of oxygen, the tissues must be able to consume the oxygen delivered, in accordance with the peripheral tissue oxygen demand. An imbalance between oxygen consumption and oxygen demand leads to tissue acidosis. Rapid restoration of tissue perfusion will result in restoration of aerobic metabolic pathways, and a resolution of the shock-related acidosis.

Untreated or uncompensated shock, if not identified and corrected, is associated with late organ failure and death. This occurs through regulation of the metabolic response to injury, with a predominant systemic upregulation of the inflammatory response seen in the host with prolonged shock and/or upon reperfusion. This dysregulated inflammatory response, sometimes referred to as "autodestructive inflammation" is a major contributor to the progressive organ failure seen with uncompensated shock.

Physiologic insults that stimulate the inflammatory response to stress and shock can be broken down into three broad categories: ischemia/reperfusion, infection, and dead/injured tissue. Uncontrolled stimulation from one or more of these categories leads to a multilevel inflammatory response at the cellular level, the end result of which, if untreated, leads to an exuberant autoinflammatory host response, with resultant organ failure and death.

Inflammatory Mediators in Shock

This autoinflammatory host response is due to the release and loss of regulation of a variety of soluble inflammatory mediators, which include cytokines, eicosanoids, complement, and adhesion molecules, among others. These substances are produced by a wide variety of cells, including white blood cells, vascular endothelial cells, and platelets. Inflammatory mediators can be grouped into two broad categories: proinflammatory substances, which upregulate the inflammatory response to injury and sepsis, and anti-inflammatory mediators, which work opposite the proinflammatory substances and downregulate the immune inflammatory response.

Examples proinflammatory cytokines include interleukin (IL)-1, IL-2, IL-6, and tumor necrosis factor (TNF). IL-1, IL-2, and IL-6 are produced by a variety of cells, including T cells, macrophages, and endothelial cells, and persistently increased levels of these substances are associated with organ failure and death in septic and injured patients. These substances stimulate other cells in the inflammatory pathways to multiply and grow, cause migration of white blood cells to wounds, and cause increased vascular permeability. TNFs such as TNF-α and TNF-β are produced by lymphocytes and macrophages, respectively, and are associated with local and systemic inflammation and endothelial activation.

Interleukin-10 is an example of a potent anti-inflammatory cytokine. IL-10 suppresses white cell function and antigen processing by macrophages. The balance between pro- and anti-inflammatory cytokines at any given time after shock or metabolic stress is thought to play a large role in the systemic response to shock, characterized clinically by tachycardia, hypotension, increased capillary permeability, and decreased organ perfusion. Failure of downregulation of the proinflammatory response is thought to lead ultimately to persistent sepsis syndrome, reactivation hypermetabolism, organ failure, and death.

At the time of this writing, exogenous attempts to manipulate this inflammatory cascade have been largely unsuccessful, although a recent Phase III trial demonstrated improved survival after severe sepsis with the administration of drotrecogin alfa (activated), an analogue of activated protein C, which is an endogenous antithrombotic and anti-inflammatory mediator. For septic and other types of shock, however, removal of the underlying stimulus for shock, along with adequate and aggressive resuscitation, can help downregulate the systemic inflammatory response, thus ameliorating the mechanisms of organ failure in these stressed patients.

Oxidative Injury in Shock

Reactive oxygen free radicals are an important part of normal host immune systems. However, after periods of shock and reperfusion, these normally well-controlled oxygen metabolites may work against host systems and harm rather than help the patient in shock. Oxygen free radicals of clinical importance include superoxide anion, hydroxyl radicals, peroxynitrite anion, and nitrogen dioxide radicals. These reactive species cause cell damage and inhibit normal enzymatic pathways, mostly through lipid peroxidation of cell membranes. This may be manifest as organ dysfunction, impaired oxygen consumption, and immunosuppression.

Differentiating Types of Shock

Classically, shock is categorized as being of one of four types: hypovolemic (hemorrhagic) shock, septic shock, cardiogenic shock, and neurogenic shock. All of these different types of shock have a final common pathway, as described above: inadequate perfusion of regional and systemic tissue beds. This classic categorization of shock provides a convenient framework upon which to diagnose and treat patients with systemic shock. However, the clinician must be careful not to "pigeonhole" patients into one type of shock versus another, thus potentially failing to treat other major sources for ongoing tissue hypoperfusion.

Hypovolemic (Hemorrhagic) Shock

The term *hypovolemic (hemorrhagic) shock* refers to any episode of hypoperfusion that is related to decreased circulating blood volume. This decrease in circulating blood volume can come from any of a number of sources, including hemorrhage, capillary leak syndrome after infection or tissue damage, reperfusion injury after significant hemorrhage, and dehydration/malnutrition. The underlying cause of the hypoperfusion in this type of shock is decreased circulating blood volume, which leads to decreased cardiac preload and end-diastolic volume. This in turn causes a decrease in stroke volume, cardiac output, and blood pressure. This decrease in pressure and flow from the heart results in tissue hypoperfusion.

The treatment of hypovolemic shock involves restoring circulating blood volume. This is done first with isotonic crystalloid solution, followed with or in conjunction with restoration of red blood cell mass with transfusion of packed red blood cells. Restoring red blood cell mass alone is not adequate, as demonstrated in a series of animal experiments from the 1960s. Resuscitation of the extracellular fluid space is a necessary component of resuscitation from hemorrhagic shock. In an effort to maintain circulating blood volume in times of stress, interstitial fluid is recruited into the vascular space during hemorrhage. This fluid must be replaced, and replacement can be carried out with isotonic crystalloid solutions such as normal saline or lactated Ringer's solution.

End points for fluid administration during resuscitation from hypovolemic shock include physical examination, urine output, heart rate and blood pressure, and improvement of neurologic status. Invasive hemodynamic monitoring provides other indicators of circulating blood volume, such as pulmonary artery occlusion pressure, central venous pressure, end-diastolic volume index, and cardiac output. It is currently unclear as to whether an optimal "transfusion trigger" exists as a target for blood administration; recent literature demonstrates that hemoglobin levels of 8.0 mg/dL are well tolerated in critically ill patients.

Septic Shock

The term *septic shock* refers to decreased hypoperfusion as a result of a drastically upregulated systemic inflammatory response, most commonly from overwhelming infection, but also from cytokines released by dead or injured tissues. Infection and dead/injured tissue causes a regional and systemic upregulatory release of proinflammatory mediators. This response to insult is known as the systemic inflammatory response syndrome (SIRS), as defined in a recent consensus statement. The presence of two or more SIRS criteria constitute a diagnosis of SIRS, and SIRS caused by infection with hypotension constitutes the definition of septic shock.

Classically, the primary hemodynamic derangement in septic shock has been thought to be uncontrolled vasodilatation. The vasodilatation leads to decreased blood pressure, decreased preload, and subsequent decreased tissue perfusion. Recent laboratory and clinical data suggest that myocardial depression with decreased myocardial contractility is another major contributor to hypoperfusion during septic shock. Thus severe overwhelming sepsis affects all the major determinants of cardiovascular function, providing a potentially difficult management problem in patients with severe sepsis.

The primary therapeutic goal in septic shock is to remove the source of the sepsis and systemic inflammation. Once this is done, either with surgical débridement of infected or dead tissue or adequate antibiotic therapy for soft tissue infections, treatment is primarily supportive. Cardiovascular function must be optimized, and nutritional status must be optimized as well. In terms of cardiovascular function, invasive hemodynamic monitoring or advanced noninvasive techniques may be necessary to identify which of the independent determinates of cardiac function (preload, contractility, and afterload) are involved. Often, patients will suffer from derangements of all three. The particular cardiac interventions necessary then should be based upon bedside assessment of preload, contractility, and afterload. Derangements in any or all of these determinants should be corrected to restore perfusion, starting with preload.

Because septic shock can affect preload, contractility, and afterload, the danger is in treating the symptoms of the problem rather than its root. For example, hypotensive patients with septic shock are often started on vasopressor agents, when actually the underlying problem may be decreased preload or poor contractility. Obviously, an approach like this will not restore perfusion to adequate levels. Thus support algorithms for septic shock should always involve restoration of preload, followed by assessment and restoration of contractility and afterload.

Nutritional support in septic shock is also vitally important. During these times of upregulated systemic inflammation the body, uses protein as a primary energy source. Because excess dietary protein is not stored in the body, the response to systemic inflammation is best characterized as a hypercatabolic response. Protein is scavenged from smooth and skeletal muscle, solid and hollow visceral organs, and the blood stream. Protein from these sources is then broken down into short peptides, which are then deaminated, and these carbon fragments are then used as fuel. The nitrogen is excreted in the urine, and can be measured as urinary urea nitrogen.

Use of the body's current storage of protein results in subsequent organ failure, immunosuppression, and decreased muscle mass. If unchecked or unsupported, this actually can result in multiple organ failure, the leading cause of late death in surgical intensive care units. Support for the malnutrition associated with septic shock involves administration of adequate levels of protein, preferably via an enteral route. Protein needs generally run between 1.5 and 2.5 g/kg body weight per day, and can be fine tuned by measurements of urinary urea nitrogen to estimate protein loss during sepsis.

Cardiogenic Shock

The term *cardiogenic shock* refers to hypoperfusion that is due solely to cardiac and insufficiency and failure.

Inability of the heart to generate adequate pressure and flow of blood in aortic route for whatever reason results in systemic hypoperfusion, and subsequent entrance into the pathologic pathways described above. Cardiogenic shock, by definition, involves myocardial failure. Ventricular failure can occur for any of several reasons, including ischemia, myocardial suppression from systemic inflammation, cardiac tamponade, and dysrhythmias.

Support for cardiogenic shock involves first removing the extrinsic forces that may be affecting myocardial function, such as cardiac tamponade; correcting any rhythm abnormalities; and then improving the inotropic status of the heart. Inotropic state can be improved by correcting systemic pH; correcting potassium, calcium, magnesium, and other electrolyte abnormalities; and addition of inotropic agents guided by appropriate monitoring techniques.

Neurogenic Shock

Neurogenic shock is characterized clinically by slow heart rate, low blood pressure, and warm skin. This is in contradistinction to the other forms of essentially mediated shock, which usually manifest with cool, clammy skin and/or tachycardia. The mechanism of neurogenic shock involves high spinal cord injury with loss of normal autoregulatory vasomotor responses as a result of the injury.

The mechanisms of inadequate systemic perfusion caused by neurogenic shock occur at several levels. Uncontrolled vasomotor autoregulation leads to inappropriate peripheral vasodilatation. High spinal cord injuries often occur above the level of the sympathetic innervation to the heart, removing the neurogenic stimulus for tachycardia in these disease states. Increased venous capacity causes pooling of blood in the venous system, with subsequent decreased preload and cardiac output. Systemic acidosis occurs as a result of this malperfusion and loss of autoregulation.

Treatment of neurogenic shock involves resuscitation at several different levels. Initially, venous volume should be restored so that a pressure gradient exists between the venous system and right atrium. This will compensate for the increase in venous capacity, improving preload and therefore cardiac output. Once adequate preload has been achieved, the next steps should work toward achieving some degree of peripheral vasodilatation to increase central blood pressure, as well as increasing heart rate in cases of inappropriate bradycardia. β-Adrenergic agents such as dopamine and epinephrine work well in this regard. These would be preferable to the predominantly α-adrenergic drugs such as phenylephrine and norepinephrine, which have primarily peripheral vasomotor effects, without much chronotropic effect on the heart.

Resuscitation Strategies for Patients in Shock

Efficacious treatment for shock primarily involves removal of the underlying stimulus for the metabolic stress response, if possible, followed by optimization of cardiovascular function, with the goal being restoration of perfusion to vital tissue beds. Resuscitation involves restoring and maintaining an adequate level of global cardiovascular performance until systemic and regional perfusion has been restored. Optimal resuscitation strategies, as well as optimal resuscitation end points, have been the focus of a tremendous amount of research over the past three decades.

Traditional resuscitation involves measures aimed at restoring central circulating blood volume and cardiac output (CO), as evidenced by improvement in clinical indicators of shock, such as mental status, urine output, skin turgor, blood pressure, and heart rate. However, resuscitation targeted to these variables has been associated with increased organ failure and mortality when compared with other, more invasive and comprehensive methods of resuscitation, such as monitoring of mixed venous oxygen saturation (SvO_2), oxygen delivery (DO_2), and oxygen consumption (VO_2). Oxygen delivery and consumption are calculated from the following formulas:

$$DO_2 = CO \times [Hgb \times 1.34 \times SaO_2]$$

$$VO_2 = CO \times [Hgb \times 1.34 \times ([SaO_2 - SvO_2)]$$

where Hgb represents serum hemoglobin concentration (in mg/dL), SaO_2 represents arterial oxygen saturation, and 1.34 is a constant describing milliliters of oxygen carried per milligram of Hgb.

Normal SvO_2 is 75%. In situations of decreased oxygen delivery resulting from anemia, decreased cardiac output, or decreased oxygen saturations, peripheral tissues extract more than one oxygen molecule from the fully saturated hemoglobin tetramer, resulting in a decrease in SvO_2. SvO_2 also decreases in situations where DO_2 may be normal, but peripheral oxygen demand may be very high.

Survivors of high-risk surgical procedures and other populations of critically ill patients have been observed to have higher levels of DO_2 and VO_2 than comparable nonsurvivors. This has led to several randomized controlled clinical trials over the past three decades comparing goal-directed resuscitation to predefined levels of DO_2 and VO_2 to conventional resuscitation. Although early studies suggested an improvement in mortality and organ failure in patients resuscitated to oxygen transport goals, larger, more recent studies have not. However, in spite of these negative clinical trials, monitoring of these variables in individual patients may have value in terms of diagnosis and treatment of specific disease states.

Improving Global Cardiac Function

Optimizing global cardiovascular function requires a working knowledge of the independent determinants of cardiac function, and the ability to manipulate these determinants clinically. The three independent determinants of cardiac function are preload, afterload, and myocardial contractility. Optimizing cardiac performance can be simplified at the first approximation by taking the following steps:

1. Assess preload status

2. Optimize preload

3. Assess myocardial contractility

4. Improve contractility as appropriate (afterload and contractility often can be optimized through the use of a single agent with effects on both properties)

5. Assess afterload

6. Increase or decrease afterload as appropriate

In order to follow this algorithm, the reader must have a working knowledge of the definitions of preload, contractility, and afterload; understand the appropriate choices of fluids available for administration; and understand the relative inotropic and afterload effects of the commonly used inotropic agents.

Preload

With respect to the heart, preload is defined as end-diastolic volume. Preload is estimated by two different methods using the pulmonary artery catheter: pulmonary artery occlusion pressure (PAOP) and right ventricular end-diastolic volume index (RVEDVI). Measuring the PAOP gives an indirect estimate of left ventricular end-diastolic pressure, which then gives an indirect estimate of left ventricular end-diastolic volume. The PAOP is subject to several extrinsic forces that may affect its reliability as a measure of preload. Nonetheless, values of PAOP are very

useful, especially when extrinsic factors such as intrathoracic and intra-abdominal pressure are taken into account.

The volumetric pulmonary artery catheter equipped with a fast-response thermistor allows for calculation of the RVEDVI, which predicts preload better than the PAOP in critically ill patients. Normal values for the RVEDVI in spontaneously breathing patients range from 80 to 100 mL/m^2, but several investigators have found that the optimum cardiac index may be reached with values as high as 140 mL/m^2, depending on the level of intrinsic myocardial performance. For example, patients with good myocardial performance reach their best cardiac index (CI) at 80 to 100 mL/m^2, whereas patients with impaired ventricular function reach their best CI at approximately 120 mL/m^2.

Unfortunately, there are presently no clinical methods available to measure left ventricular end-diastolic volume directly in a rapid and clinically useful way.

Contractility

Ventricular contractility is defined as that element of myocardial performance that is independent of loading conditions on the heart (preload and afterload). Contractility is thus a difficult term to understand conceptually, and even more difficult to measure clinically. The most commonly used clinical estimate of contractility, ejection fraction, is preload dependent, and thus by definition is not a "pure" descriptor of contractility. Relative changes in ejection fraction may be useful at constant loading conditions, but these concessions are difficult to make in the clinical setting.

The end-systolic ventricular elastance (E_{es}) has been shown by several investigators to be independent of preload and afterload, but to vary with changes in inotropic state. E_{es} thus meets the criteria to be considered a measure of contractility. The derivation of E_{es} for the left ventricle is complex, but E_{es} can be calculated according to the following formula:

$$E_{es} = ESP/ESVI - V_0$$

where ESP represents left ventricular end-systolic pressure, ESVI represents left ventricular end-systolic volume index, and V_0 represents the left ventricular volume at zero pressure. Increases in contractility are represented by an increase in E_{es}, and decreases in contractility are represented by a decrease in E_{es}.

Afterload

Afterload can be defined as the total impedance to cardiac ejection. This is a difficult concept to translate into a descriptive, quantifiable variable; thus systemic afterload is usually expressed as the systemic vascular resistance index (SVRI).

Resistance expressed in this fashion is a major component of afterload, but by no means does it completely describe afterload. SVRI is calculated analogously to resistance in a direct current circuit from the following formula:

$$SVRI = (MAP - CVP)/CI \times 80$$

where MAP represents mean arterial pressure and CVP represents central venous pressure.

There are shortcomings to using the SVRI as an indicator of afterload. For example, the SVRI does not account for changes in oscillatory pressure (the difference between MAP and peak systolic pressure), which certainly must be a consideration in older patients. Furthermore, SVRI is time, or rate, dependent. An alternative variable expressing afterload that accounts for these shortcomings to some degree is the effective arterial elastance (E_a), which is calculated by the following formula:

$$E_a = ESP/SVI$$

where SVI represents the stroke volume index. Increases in afterload are indicated by an increase in E_a, and decreases by a decrease in E_a.

The Ventricular Pressure-Volume Diagram

Ideally, the clinician should be able to assess each of the primary determinants of myocardial performance (preload, contractility, and afterload) both independently and in relation to one another. Unfortunately, conventional methods of using PAOP, ejection fraction, and SVRI do not allow the clinician to relate values of these variables with each other, or predict how changes in one variable affect the other two. However, ventricular end-diastolic volume index (EDVI), E_{es}, and E_a can all be plotted on the ventricular pressure-volume diagram and used as tools to identify problems and improve cardiac performance in a goal-directed fashion. Figure 57–1 represents a hypothetical

ventricular pressure-volume diagram with EDVI, E_{es}, and E_a plotted on the diagram. The area enclosed within the pressure-volume loop represents external stroke work.

Preload, or the end-diastolic point, has EDVI as its x value and PAOP as its y value. (For the purposes of this example, right ventricular volumes are substituted for left ventricular volumes, recognizing that this is not necessarily the case.) Contractility is represented as the slope of ventricular end-systolic elastance, and is drawn as a line from V_0 (assumed to be 5 mL/m²) through the end-systolic point. Afterload is represented as E_a, having SVI (the difference between EDVI and ESVI) as its "run" on the x axis and ESP as the y coordinate. E_a is the line drawn from EDVI on the x axis through the end-systolic point, which has ESVI as its x coordinate, and ESP as its y coordinate.

The pressure-volume loop is thus defined by ESVI and EDVI on the x axis and ESP and PAOP on the y axis. The area within the loop represents ventricular stoke work, a very useful variable describing ventricular energy output and perfusion.

Clinical Application

Using the above-outlined methods, pressure-volume diagrams can be constructed for any patient being monitored with an arterial catheter and a volumetric pulmonary artery catheter. These loops, in turn, can be used to diagnose the reasons behind inadequate cardiac performance, and can also be used to select interventions and predict hemodynamic responses. For example, Figure 57–2 shows low blood pressure and stroke work caused by inadequate preload (solid lines) versus increased blood pressure and stroke work after increasing preload (dotted lines) with fluid administration (note that the slopes of E_a and E_{es} stay constant). Figure 57–3 illustrates low blood pressure and stroke work caused by low contractility (E_{es}, solid lines). Note the increase in blood pressure and stroke work with increased contractility (dotted lines), and that

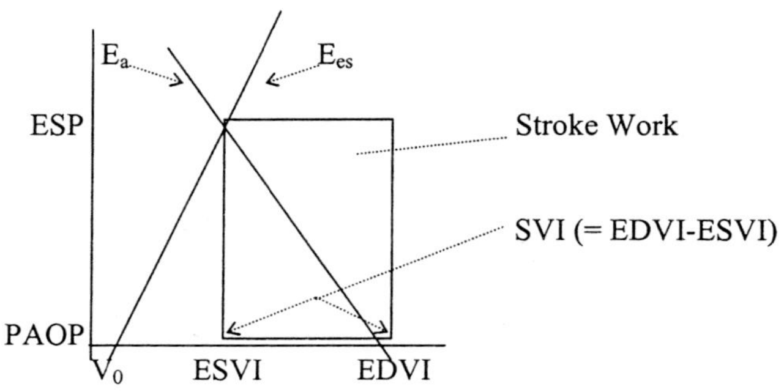

FIGURE 57–1 A hypothetical ventricular pressure-volume diagram with EDVI, E_{es}, and E_a plotted on the diagram.

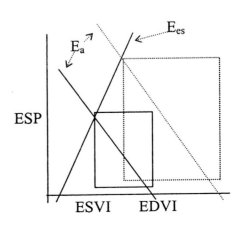

FIGURE 57–2 Inadequate preload.

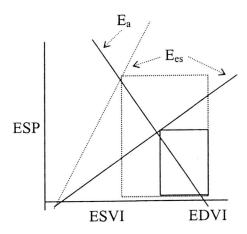

FIGURE 57–3 Inadequate contractility.

E_{es} and EDVI stay constant. Similar calculations of the hemodynamics of inadequate afterload are shown in Figure 57–4.

Using the pressure-volume diagram also aids in picking the appropriate inotrope once preload has been optimized. For example, if blood pressure and stroke work remain low because of a combination of low contractility and low afterload, an "inoppressor" (e.g., dopamine or epinephrine) can be used to increase both with one drug. If blood pressure and stroke work are inadequate as a result of contractility only, a drug with predominately β-adrenergic effects, such as dobutamine, may be more appropriate.

Endpoints of Resuscitation from Shock

Optimal end points of resuscitation remain the subject of intense clinical research as well. Arterial lactate, a product of anaerobic metabolism, has been shown to be elevated in various populations of patients in shock. Furthermore, rate of normalization of lactate with resuscitation is directly related to subsequent development of multiple organ failure and death. Patients whose lactate levels normalize within 24 hours of the onset of shock have a lower mortality and lower incidence of organ failure and other complications than patients in whom lactate remains persistently elevated.

The arterial base deficit (BD) is a nonspecific marker of metabolic acidosis. Persistently elevated levels of BD have been related to inadequate oxygen consumption, and the BD has been used much like lactate, as a measure of postshock metabolic acidosis. Multiple clinical studies in injured patients have demonstrated that inability to normalize BD with resuscitation is closely related to the subsequent development of multiple organ failure and death. Levels of BD must be interpreted with caution, however, because BD is a nonspecific marker of metabolic acidosis, and other conditions, such as diabetic ketoacidosis, methanol toxicity, and uremia from renal failure, may cause elevations in BD independent of anaerobic glycolysis and shock.

Bibliography

Bone RC, Balk RA, Cerra FB, et al: American College of Chest Physicians/Society of Critical Care Medicine consensus conference: definitions for sepsis and organ failure and guidelines for the use of innovative therapies in sepsis. Crit Care Med 1992;20:864.

Chang MC, Mondy JS III, Meredith JW, Holcroft JW: Redefining cardiovascular performance during resuscitation: ventricular stroke work, power, and the pressure-volume diagram. J Trauma 1998;45:470.

Fabian TC: Inflammatory mediators. *In* Trunkey DD, Lewis FR (eds): Current Therapy of Trauma (4th ed). St. Louis: Mosby, 1999:317.

Holcroft JW: Shock: ICU management. *In* Wilmore DW, Brennan MF, Harken AH, et al (eds): Care of the Surgical Patient: Perioperative Management and Techniques. New York: Scientific American, 1988–1999:1.

Kincaid EH, Miller PR, Meredith JW, et al: Elevated arterial base deficit in trauma patients: a marker of impaired oxygen utilization. J Am Coll Surg 1998;187:384.

Moore FA, Haenel JB, Moore EE, Whithell TA: Incommensurate oxygen consumption in response to maximal oxygen availability predicts postinjury multiple organ failure. J Trauma 1992;33:58.

Shoemaker WC, Montgomery ES, Kaplan E, Elwyn DH: Physiologic patterns in surviving and nonsurviving shock patients. Arch Surg 1973;106:630.

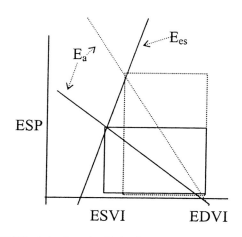

FIGURE 57–4 Inadequate afterload.

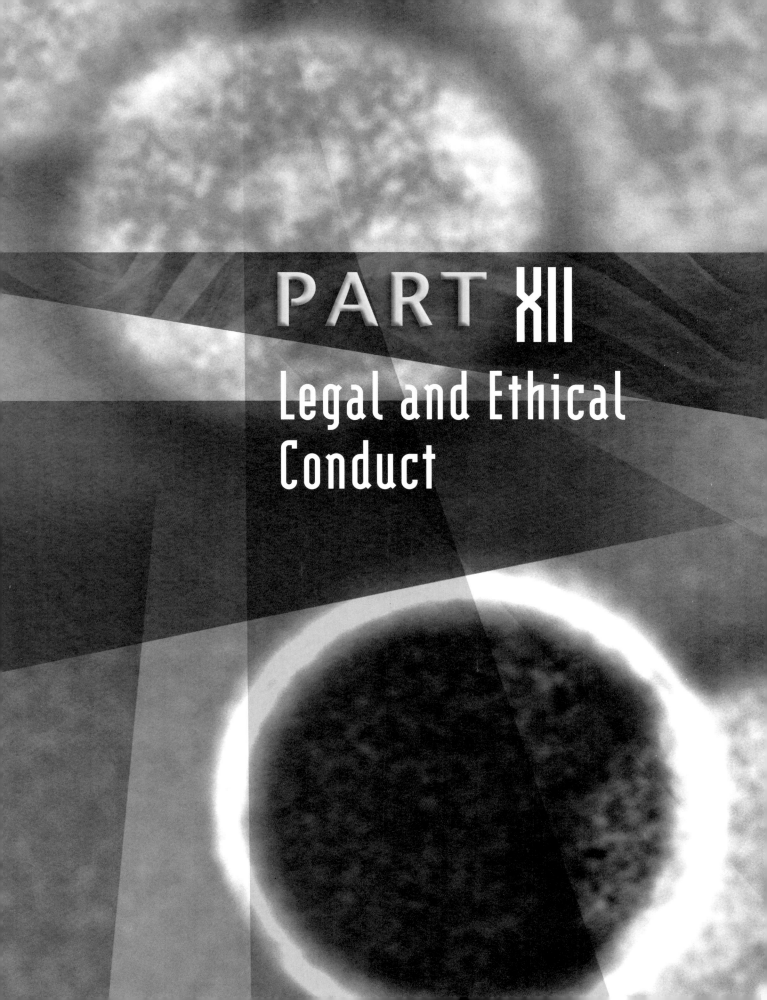

PART XII
Legal and Ethical Conduct

CHAPTER 58

Legal Medicine, Medical Ethics, and Professional Behavior

Erle E. Peacock, Jr., M.D., J.D.

▶ Medical Records
▶ Medical Malpractice
▶ End-of-Life Decisions
▶ Fraud and Abuse
▶ Peer Review
▶ Bibliography

As the practice of medicine has taken on more of the characteristics of business practice during the last two decades, the need for some formal education in business law and health care law has become painfully apparent to most physicians. Although most health care providers jealously guard their calling as a service-oriented learned profession, the consumer public seems to view medical care as a business enterprise dispensing service as its product, and insists that the product be dispensed under warranty. Economic considerations seem to drive most industrial engines, and they in turn require controlling factors such as legislative and legal restraints. Hence the need for some modicum of formal education in business law in order to comply with the ever-tightening regulations of what has become another industrial giant. Failure to learn basic principles and some specific applications of business law to the delivery of health services by professional providers invites serious problems in being productive and reasonably happy, in spite of the fact that patients still need and deserve professional dedication more than business and legal administration. This chapter outlines and covers briefly five areas in which business and legal knowledge enriched by basic ethical considerations is necessary to maintain professional standards in the practice of surgery. These areas are medical records, malpractice, end-of-life decisions, fraud and abuse, and peer review; however, knowledge needs are not limited to these five areas.

Medical Records

The Medical Practice Act requires physicians in all states to keep adequate medical records. Thus what was once only good medical practice has become a legal duty. The noble goal behind imposing such a duty is to assure the best available care for patients; the not-so-noble but increasingly imperative goal is to protect the physician from a variety of allegations ranging from civil negligence to criminal allegations such as fraud and even murder. In medical malpractice issues, it is almost always the record that ends up being tried; the medical record is always the most dispositive piece of evidence either side can introduce.

Accuracy, of course, is the single most important goal in keeping a medical record. The record, from a legal standpoint, should record facts as clearly as possible and only rarely record unsubstantiated opinions and speculations. It is very important to record intent clearly when there is any possibility that intent can be misinterpreted, such as in some end-of-life treatment plans. Second, *confidentiality* should be an obsession. Attempts to establish a federal medical record confidentiality statute have not succeeded so far. Congress failed to pass a law in the time frame dictated by the Health Insurance Portability and Accountability Act of 1996 (the Kennedy-Kassebaum bill), so the Secretary of Health and Human Services recommended confidentiality rules and regulations as she was directed to do if Congress failed to enact a medical records confidentiality statute. The result is so complex and ambiguous that it has seemed unworkable and, therefore, unlikely to replace the various state legislative efforts that also are underway. As of April 2003, the first attempt is being enforced even though litigation to render federal legislation unconstitutional is making its way through the courts. Various state medical record confidentiality statutes are not completely satisfactory for general use at this time.

Until further refinements appear, a good rule for practicing physicians is to maintain absolute confidentiality except when patients sign a legally binding release or a court of proper jurisdiction issues a subpoena. Other exceptions often utilized vary between states and should be followed according to state law where a physician practices. Physicians should periodically warn all of their staff to make confidentiality paramount in their approach to the medical record. In addition, it should be remembered that not all states give patients the right to inspect their own medical records.

The third general legal principle involving medical records is called *spoliation*. Spoliation means intentional destruction or alteration of medical records, and most states now have statutes making spoliation a tort and/or a crime. Destruction or alteration of a record that may be entered as evidence in a trial, of course, is a crime. Because errors can and do occur in medical records, a careful, disciplined method for correcting errors in all medical records is essential. One should never change or attempt to change the medical record; it is virtually impossible to do so without detection later. Once a jury determines that a medical record has been altered, the odds are heavily against being able to mount an effective defense for other allegations such as malpractice. When a mistake is discovered, the proper way to correct it usually is to go to the end of the record and make a completely new and presently dated entry describing the error and stating the correct information. It is legally permissible to highlight an error in a medical record by drawing a thin fine line through the mistake, labeling it an error and then initialing and dating the correction. The line must never obliterate the error, however, or keep it from being easily deciphered by anyone reviewing the document. Even though space may remain between previous entries in a medical record, or at the bottom of a page, one should never insert or backdate an entry that was not made in proper sequence at the time the record was being constructed.

In summary, the function of a medical record is to document accurately, completely, and objectively what happened during diagnosis and treatment of a patient. Everything in a medical record is discoverable in a court of law; the fact that the record was introduced in the course of peer review or other such functions does not protect it from legal discovery. The duty to keep accurate records has passed from ethical self-regulation to enforceable legal duty, including statutory regulations and statements of a patient's right to privacy. A patient's control of disclosure overrides all other considerations except a subpoena from a court of law. There are a few exceptions, of course, such as reporting communicable diseases, including human immunodeficiency virus (HIV) (particularly for infants); reporting gunshot wounds; and the Tarsoff rule, which defines a duty to warn potential third-party victims when

a physician has uncovered potential peril. However, such exceptions vary with state law and should be investigated and followed according to the statutes and department of health regulations of the state where practice is conducted.

Medical Malpractice

Most physicians believe that the modern medical malpractice burden is primarily the result of greedy, unethical lawyers and patient avarice. Therefore, they see tort reform as the most logical and efficient solution to the problem. The author does not agree. First, the causes of an escalating number of frivolous lawsuits as well as some increase in genuine medical malpractice claims are more related to technical advancements and cultural and social changes than to lawyers' and patients' greed. Second, tort reform, to be of any significance as far as medical malpractice insurance premiums are concerned, must place significant caps on damage awards, particularly noneconomic damages such as for mental anguish, emotional harm, pain and suffering, and loss of consortium. In the 16 states that have passed such legislation, the state supreme court in 9 has found economic caps on damages to be unconstitutional under the state constitution. Although the question has never reached the U.S. Supreme Court, the author does not believe there is any doubt that the High Court would strike down legislation favoring any professional group as being unconstitutional under the "equal treatment under the law" clause of the 14th amendment to the U.S. Constitution.

A far more practical approach now would seem to be recognition that medical practice is being conducted as a business enterprise and that business principles include warranty of service. In many respects, practicing medicine at this time has some liability resemblance to being president of a diving board company. Being sued for medical malpractice, including frivolous allegations, is almost a certainty now, and physicians simply have to accept the risk as part of the total package of rewards and costs for practicing medicine. Approximately one in five physicians on average will be sued in the United States each year. Actually, the courts have been very fair to physicians; less than 30% of malpractice cases going to trial result in any award to plaintiffs. If a physician knows that he or she has fallen below the standard of practice and injury to a patient resulted, that physician should move as quickly as possible to help settle claims fairly and reasonably. When this is impossible because of unrealistic demands or when the allegations are frivolous, legal redress may be unavoidable and should be accepted with grace as part of the conditions that prevail in the business community. Once a physician pays a premium for medical malpractice insurance, he or she is viewed as a "deep pocket" for liability claims.

Unless there is criminal negligence, fraud, or malicious intent to hurt another, medical malpractice is classified as the tort of *negligence*. Negligence is usually a civil court complaint. Criminal negligence requires proof of intent to harm, prosecution is by the district attorney representing the state, and the defendant is tried in criminal court. Conviction requires a standard of proof beyond a reasonable doubt and is punishable by imprisonment, fine or both. The victim in a criminal case is not compensated. In contrast, tortuous claims such as negligence are tried in civil court, where the standard for conviction is a preponderance of the evidence (51%) and the remedy is monetary compensation for the victim. To be successful in medical malpractice litigation, a plaintiff must prove five issues, as shown in Box 58–1. Failure to prove any of these five prima facie items results in a directed verdict, as a matter of law, in favor of the defendant physician. Definition of the duty that the patient had a legal right to expect, proof of breach of that duty by the patient's physician, and determination of both direct and proximate causation require testimony from an expert witness, usually another physician. In many states, any physician can be accepted by the court as an expert witness. The most enlightened state laws, however, define the qualifications for an expert witness in a medical malpractice proceeding. Some states require that a potential expert witness be identified and review the medical record before a summons and complaint can be issued. Other states require that a medical expert witness be practicing at least 50% of the time and be certified in the same specialty as the defendant. Failure by the plaintiff to acquire an expert witness will result in a directed verdict in favor of the defendant physician except when the doctrine of *res ipsa loquitur* applies. *Res ipsa loquitur* means "the thing speaks for itself," and applies when breach of duty and causation are so obvious that an expert witness is not needed to explain technical matters to a jury. *Res ipsa* cases in surgical malpractice are pretty much limited to operating room explosions, operating upon the wrong part of the body, or leaving foreign bodies

such as sponges or instruments in a patient. The test for *res ipsa* is sometimes stated as the "Oh my God" test. This does not mean that a *res ipsa* case should not be defended vigorously. Many such cases are won by defendants.

Damages can be economic damages, which require receipts or bills to document, and noneconomic damages such as mental anguish, anxiety, pain and suffering, and loss of consortium (right to the company, society, and affection of a spouse, parent, or child.) Punitive damages are awarded rarely in medical malpractice cases because punitive damages are supposed to be awarded as a deterrent to others and, therefore, can be awarded only when there has been gross or willful misconduct, fraud, or malice. Because punitive damages are not covered by medical malpractice insurance, unethical plaintiffs' lawyers may include a request for punitive damages in the original complaint to frighten an unsophisticated physician into making a quick, personal settlement, ostensibly in return for dropping the punitive damage demands. This is why it is imperative for physicians to notify their insurance carrier as early as possible when threatened and certainly when actually served with a malpractice summons and complaint.

A huge disappointment to unsuspecting physicians is the realization that their malpractice insurance is not necessarily written to provide defense against claims of malpractice but rather to indemnify them against financial loss. Actually, an insurance carrier has a legal duty to "investigate and settle expeditiously" medical malpractice claims. Inserting a clause in a malpractice insurance policy that prevents settlement without the insured physician's approval offers little solace to physicians defending frivolous malpractice lawsuits. The reason is that, if the insurance company makes a bona fide offer of settlement that the plaintiff is willing to accept, but the offer is thwarted by the defendant physician demanding to be defended at trial, there is significant risk that a jury may award more than the settlement offer. If this happens, the defendant physician will be legally responsible for the difference, and, possibly just as devastating, be responsible for attorney's fees for the plaintiff after the settlement was rejected. Settlement of a frivolous claim is a bitter pill for a physician, however, because of mandatory reporting of payment of any settlement award to the National Physician's Databank. Insurance company–assigned lawyers often overlook the fact that the physician defendant is entitled to include a statement of *his or her* composition indicating that the settlement was not an admission of negligence but was made for economic practicality. A personal attorney, experienced in Databank forms and regulations, may be extremely helpful and well worth a relatively small personal expense during settlement stages of a frivolous lawsuit.

Another form of medical malpractice negligence is failure to obtain informed consent. Failure to obtain any consent is cause for the intentional tort or crime of battery,

Box 58–1

Five Prima Facie Points the Plaintiff Must Prove in a Malpractice Suit

1. A duty that the defendant physician must meet
2. Breach of that duty by the defendant physician
3. That breach of duty directly caused damage to the plaintiff ("but for" test)
4. That breach of duty could be reasonably foreseen to cause the plaintiff's damage (proximate causation)
5. Actual damage

but failure to inform the patient sufficiently while obtaining consent so that the patient can make the best possible decision has been classified in all states but Pennsylvania as negligence. The standard in some states is called a "reasonable prudent person standard"; other states have what is called a "community standard." Plaintiffs' attorneys favor the reasonable prudent person standard to determine what the patient should have been informed of because a physician expert witness is not needed to testify as to what the local physician's standard is in that community. Courts have determined that a reasonable, prudent person is entitled to know the diagnosis, prognosis with and without treatment, complications that may occur often enough or be serious enough to influence a decision to have or not to have treatment, alternative forms of treatment, and the results of laboratory tests. The competency of the physician or surgeon to perform treatment is more properly assigned to hospital credentialing and state medical boards, but infectious diseases such as acquired immunodeficiency syndrome and hepatitis carried by providers are beginning to creep into informed consent legal requirements in some jurisdictions. Both the American Medical Association and the American Dental Association have published ethical statements saying that surgeons should reveal HIV-positive status to preoperative patients. A Wisconsin court decision (*Johnson v. Kohamoor*, 1994) held that a neurosurgeon was required to inform a patient giving consent for aneurysm surgery that he had not had extensive experience performing the procedure. Because another neurosurgeon in the immediate vicinity had extensive aneurysm experience, the court ruled that informed consent required this patient be told of readily available more experienced medical care. Waiver by a patient to participate in informed consent procedure is very dangerous for the physician; legal aid should be obtained when such problems are encountered.

The single most frequent cause of medical malpractice litigation is financial dispute. The second most frequent cause is miscommunication, particularly failure to spend time and effort in trying to communicate. Many suits from both causes are preventable; some are not, but courts, on the whole, have been fair to physicians, and the best answer to the number of medical malpractice lawsuits at this time probably is to take risk management seriously, avoid financial disputes, spend as much time and effort as possible communicating with patients, and, finally, recognize that some medical malpractice claims are unavoidable now and should not be a cause for developing a discouraged or vengeful attitude toward what is left of a once highly respected profession. As long as the courts continue to support hospitals' requiring their medical staff to carry malpractice insurance, surgeons, in particular, will be forced to carry substantial malpractice insurance and will be viewed, therefore, as "deep pocket targets" by plaintiffs' attorneys.

End-of-Life Decisions

The most important general principle for physicians caring for dying patients is to remember that there are no legal obstacles to providing the best care that can be rendered, regardless of whether such care hastens or even causes death. No physician has ever been successfully prosecuted for any act or any omission of an act that hastened or led to the death of a terminally ill patient. To the contrary, dictum in *Cruzan v. Director, Missouri Dept. of Health* (1990) served notice to health care providers that not only was there no legal obstacle to providing whatever is necessary to relieve pain and anxiety in dying patients, but, if the question were more narrowly framed in any subsequent case reaching the U.S. Supreme Court, the court might well find that dying patients have a constitutional right to death with dignity, specifically, without preventable pain and suffering.

The problem, however, has been to achieve such an objective without being accused of neglect at one end of the spectrum or murder at the other. The key legal word in this issue is *intent*. When intent is to relieve pain and suffering, any reasonable treatment, including prescribing any dose of any approved drug, is legally permissible; it is only necessary to be certain that the patient's desires are being followed when they can be determined, or that the desires of the patient's next of kin are followed when the patient's desires have not been expressed or are unknown. Intent and the basis for intent should be clearly documented in the medical record.

There are two generally recognized legal methods for patients to provide end-of-life preferences. One is called a living will or advance directive. The other is the appointment of a surrogate who has durable power of attorney for health care. Durable power of attorney for health care is the superior method. Advance directives suffer from all of the problems of any will. Health care language may either be ambiguous relative to the specific problem at hand or too narrow to provide clear direction. Technological advances, not anticipated at the time the will was written, may improve the odds for aggressive treatment, and changing family and social values can make a written document obsolete. By designating a surrogate decision maker, a patient provides the best assurance that health care providers will have accurate direction based upon the patient's wishes no matter how circumstances change.

Do-not-resuscitate (DNR) orders are legal disasters waiting to happen throughout most of the country. Some states, such as New York and Montana, have codified DNR orders; most states have not. DNR orders are often written by a variety of professionals and frequently do not include recent input from the family or even from the patient when such input was possible. Until there are more uniform state laws or a federal law covering DNR orders, physicians should be the only health care providers who write them, and such orders should be reviewed by the physician at least every 2 weeks and only rewritten after consultation with the patient or close family members. Nothing short of this is really legally safe, in the judgment of the author. Quality of life and age are dangerous reasons to impose a DNR order. Prognosis is the safest reason.

Designating a surrogate should be defined taking into consideration the legal difference between competency and capacity. A patient may be competent generally but not have the capacity to make special decisions, or the reverse may be true. When any doubt exists, psychiatric and legal consultation should be obtained.

The definition of death is delineated by state law, and most states include in the definition the concept that death is a diagnosis. A patient is dead when a licensed physician says that death has occurred. In these states, there is legal significance, therefore, in whether a ventilator is removed and the patient subsequently pronounced dead as opposed to pronouncing a patient dead and then removing the ventilator. From an ethical standpoint, it is important to avoid crude expressions such as "pull the plug," and it is extremely important when ventilators are removed that the physician be present to administer or discontinue paralytic drugs or sedatives if needed, suppress or aspirate secretions, and reassure the family that agonal sounds and movements do not mean dying loved ones are suffering respiratory distress.

Discontinuing food and hydration should be ordered only after careful consideration and documentation of the patient's and the family's wishes. It is prudent to have the concurrence of a second physician who has not been associated with the case and who has nothing to gain regardless of the outcome. If there is any disagreement among family members, every attempt to resolve the disagreement should be made and, if that is not possible, supportive treatment should be continued until legal clarification can be obtained. When a patient decides to refuse treatment, including food and water, it may be considered battery to force artificial nutrition and hydration upon him or her.

Assisted suicide is legal in five states; it is a crime in the remaining states. The objective of patients requesting assisted suicide usually is to keep control of their medical treatment and conduct of their affairs until the very end. There are ample ways to accomplish this without breaking the law. Again, intent is key from a legal standpoint. Intent to help patients kill themselves is illegal in 45 states. It is not illegal in these states, however, to prescribe sedatives and analgesics sufficient to assure a patient adequate rest and freedom from pain, even though there may be some risk that an occasional patient may use such prescriptions for another purpose. This seldom happens, however, because, once patients realize that they are not alone and

they are maintaining control over their own health, the desire to commit suicide usually diminishes or disappears.

The function of the medical examiner and/or coroner is controlled by state law and varies somewhat between states. Every physician should be familiar with state law and accept responsibility to abide by it. The death certificate is a legal document and must be as accurate as it is possible for a physician to make it, including stating clearly what the cause of death is when it can be determined with a reasonable degree of medical certainty. Speculation, evasion of truth, protecting a patient's reputation, and the like are illegal when accuracy is called for as a matter of law. Perjury in filling out a death certificate can be a criminal offense.

Fraud and Abuse

Fraud and abuse are considered by many health care economists to be one of the primary causes of escalating health costs. Physicians should understand three relevant laws and take whatever measures are necessary to prevent even an appearance of noncompliance. These are laws related to (1) false claims against the government, (2) anti kickback statutes, and (3) Stark anti–self-referral laws. The false claims act was passed during the civil war to punish Northern munition makers who defrauded the government by selling gunpowder diluted with sawdust. The original law has been revised to include Medicare and Medicaid fraud, which primarily has consisted of charging the government for services not "medically necessary," improperly coded, or never rendered. Anti kickback law was enacted in 1972 by Congress specifically targeting physicians receiving anything of value, in cash or in kind, in exchange for a referral to another medical entity. Anti kickback law prohibited outright payments in exchange for referrals but did not address other potential conflicts, such as when physicians have an investment interest in medical facilities to which they refer, becoming enriched by an increased return on their investment. Stark laws prohibit a physician from referring a patient to any entity in which the physician or his or her family has a financial interest. Owning common stock in a relatively large company is excluded.

Violations of fraud and abuse laws resulted in more than $20 billion being paid out for improper claims in 1997. Cases are heard in criminal courts, civil courts, or before an administrative law judge, depending upon whether violations were made knowingly or with intent. Conviction requires evidence beyond a reasonable doubt in criminal court, preponderance of the evidence (51%) in civil court, and whatever an administrative law judge or board of appeals may require to satisfy burden of proof.

Investigation of fraud and abuse can be by state Medicaid officials (who are 90% federally funded), intermediate managed care organizations, the Office of the

Inspector General of the Health Care Financing Agency, the Department of Justice (Federal Bureau of Investigation), and, finally, the public at large in what is called a *qui tam* investigation. *Qui tam* is short for *qui tam pro domino rege quam pro se imposo sequitur*, which means "who brings the action as well for the King as for himself." This doctrine enables any citizen who suspects a physician of violating fraud and abuse statutes to file a claim in civil court. The United States then has 60 days to make investigations and decide whether to take over prosecution of the case or to withdraw and allow the plaintiff (called the "relator" in *qui tam* actions) to pursue litigation alone. If the government intervenes, the original relator is entitled to a minimum of 15% but not more than 25% of the proceeds. If the relator wins the case without government prosecution help, he or she is entitled to not less than 25% nor more than 30% of the proceeds. More than $800 million has been paid to relators in *qui tam* cases in recent years. If allowed to stand, a recent Fifth Circuit Court decision that *qui tam* prosecution is unconstitutional will reduce substantially the number of fraud and abuse cases.

Remedies for conviction of various fraud and abuse violations include an automatic 5-year exclusion from Medicare or Medicaid programs if there is criminal intent or if a patient is hurt significantly. Fines, penalties, and temporary exclusion can be levied in administrative and civil cases. Imprisonment following criminal conviction can be for up to life; however, only conviction by a jury can result in imprisonment.

A major problem, of course, has been determining whether guilty physicians merely committed simple error or they actually intended to defraud the government. In the past, the causation standard for criminal conviction was "known or should have known," which allowed very little room for making an honest mistake. Recently, the standard has been softened to "reckless disregard or deliberate ignorance," which allows a wider consideration for possibilities of honest mistakes.

The Department of Health and Human Services, Office of the Inspector General, has recently released voluntary compliance standards intended to develop a voluntary compliance program that best fits the needs of individual practitioners and provides health care attorneys with insight into the Office's standards for complying with fraud and abuse law. Adopting or developing a compliance plan and, even more importantly, actual implementation of a plan are the most significant steps in avoiding fraud and abuse allegations. If a health care provider is investigated, an attorney should be engaged immediately. A physician has 24 hours to obtain legal assistance before turning over any documents unless, of course, a search warrant is produced. Anyone claiming to be a legitimate investigator should be required to identify themselves fully

and should be required to identify in writing exactly what they want and sign a receipt for anything they take. Large organizations should appoint a senior employee to stay current about and handle such matters when they arise. Nothing should ever be turned over to an investigator that an attorney does not authorize unless a search warrant has been issued and is produced at the time of the investigation.

Improper payments, when recognized, should be returned without cashing checks. If a long-standing error in the past is discovered, an attorney should be consulted about the proper way to correct and report the problem. Recent developments in the Department of Health and Human Services have suggested a more tolerant and understanding attitude for honest mistakes in coding and billing then has been practiced in the past. Every effort should be made to comply with "medically necessary" restrictions, proper coding, and other compliance procedures, which are available now to protect physicians against harassment or false accusations of fraud and abuse.

Peer Review

Flawed peer review is an increasingly prevalent problem for health care providers. The economic realities of managed care, which is really managed competition now, plus the limited immunity provided to institutions and peer review participants under the Quality Assurance Act of 1986 offer attractive opportunities to eliminate a nonconformist or rugged individualist from institutional membership or, even worse, to protect economic advantages of those in power.

The Quality Assurance Act of 1986 (Public Law 99-660) grants limited immunity to physicians sitting on peer review panels provided that (1) action is taken in the reasonable belief that it was in the furtherance of quality health care, (2) there has been a reasonable effort to obtain facts, (3) there has been adequate notice and hearing, and (4) there is reasonable belief that the action was warranted by the facts. Such immunity is not absolute; there are dangerous holes a clever attorney can exploit for a physician. It is essential, therefore, that any surgeon sitting on a peer review committee be assured that the hospital provides specific indemnity for that service, or personal insurance should be obtained in the event of later allegations of unwarranted action.

The Medical Practice Act grants the trustees of hospitals in all states the right to control appointment and discharge of medical staff for any reasonable purpose, including economic credentialing. All administrative remedies, such as informal and formal hearings and appeals at all levels, must be exhausted before turning to the courts. Courts will only hear hospital credentialing cases when there is some evidence that the institution's action was malicious or that it was arbitrary and capricious. Malice is extremely difficult to prove. To be arbitrary, actions have to have been taken without any reasonable basis; to be capricious, the action taken must be based upon something other than the evidence presented. Hospital staff membership, under the law, is a privilege that can be extended or withdrawn fairly freely as long as it is done correctly. Correctly, for the most part, means according to the institution's own rules and regulations, including the medical staff bylaws. A hospital administration that flagrantly disregards its own rules and regulations often can be ordered by a judge to conform to those regulations by filing for a *writ of mandamus*. Some courts have ruled that a hospital has a legally binding contract with members of the medical staff and that failure to follow its own rules is breach of that contract. The peer review then must start over and follow the institution's rules. Damages usually are not awarded for breach of contract.

Every way possible should be explored to avoid legal redress in a hospital credentialing dispute. The physician is at a serious disadvantage in that the burden of proof rests on the plaintiff (the physician) to prove that he or she was treated unfairly. Litigation takes 4 to 6 years, costs upward of $100,000, and takes a massive toll on a physician's family and medical practice. About all that can be achieved is award of damages, and the likelihood of being awarded substantial damages is so small that litigation should only be resorted to in cases of outrageous institutional behavior. It is almost never possible to gain reinstatement to the medical staff by a court order; courts are extremely reluctant to second-guess medical staff decisions. The best course for physicians facing credentialing problems is to try every possible way to conform to the institution's requirements. If that is not possible, settlement negotiations should be undertaken to try to allow physicians to resign from the staff without suffering undeserved embarrassment or lost of professional dignity.

Bibliography

42 U.S.C.A. §§ 11101–11152.

Contone L: Corporate compliance: critical to organizational success. Nurs Econ 1999;17:15.

Cruzan v. Director, Missouri Dept. of Health, 497 U.S. 261 (1990).

Curran WJ, Hall MA, Bobinski MA, Orentlicher D: Confidentiality of Medical Information in Health Care Law and Ethics (5th ed). Gaithersburg, MD: Aspen Publishers, 1998:189.

Daniels S: Tracing the shadow of the law: jury verdicts in medical malpractice cases. Justice System J 1990;14:4.

Department of Health and Human Services. Confidentiality of individually identifiable health information (recommendations of the Secretary of Health and Human Services, pursuant to section 264 of the Health Insurance Portability and Accountability Act of 1996). Available at: *aspe.os.dhhs.gov./admorsimp/pvcreo.htm*

DeVille K: Medical malpractice in twentieth century United States: the interaction of technology, law and culture. Int J Technol Assess Health Care 1998;14:197.

Foster HW: The Supreme Court speaks: not assisted suicide but a constitutional right to palliative care. N Engl J Med 1997;337:1234.

Furrow BR, Greaney TL, Johnson SH, et al: Reforming Tort System for Medical Injuries in Health Law, Vol 1. St. Paul, MN: West Publishing Co., 1995:518.

Health Insurance Portability and Accountability Act of 1996 (P.L. 104-191).

Johnson v. Kohamoor, 525 N.W. 2d 71 (Wisc. App. 1994).

King N: Patient waiver of informed consent. N C Med J 1993;54:399.

Klein SA: Doctors not being targeted, fraud enforcers say they're not going to jump on simple errors. AMA News, 1998;March 16:3.

Kridelbaugh WW, Palmisano DJ: Compensation caps for medical malpractice. ACS Bulletin 1993;78:27.

McKinney's Public Health Law, N.Y.G.S. § 2962.

Olson SM, Howard-Martin J: Controversy brews over guidelines for AIDS-infected health care worker. Healthspan 1991;8:13.

Riley v. St. Luke's Episcopal Hospital, No. 97-20948 (5th Cir. November 15, 1999).

Thomas SS: An insurer's right to settle versus it's duty to defend non-meritorious medical malpractice claims. J Legal Med 1995;16:545.

Tsai VW: Cheaper and better. J Legal Med 1998;19:549.

Virmoni v. Presbyterian Health Services Corp., 127 N.C. App. 629, 648, 493 S.E.2d 310, 323 (1997).

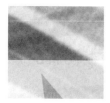

Index

Note: Page numbers followed by f refer to figures; page numbers followed by t refer to tables; page numbers followed by b refer to boxes.

Rifamycin, 544
Right ventricular end-diastolic volume index, 772, 772t, 773
   in shock, 785
Rituxumab, in cancer, 634
RNA polymerase, 10-11
Rocuronium, for anesthesia, 588, 590t
Ropivacaine, 598t
Roseola, 574t
Round ligament, 218
Roux-en-Y gastric bypass, in morbid obesity, 367f, 368, 368t
RSR13, radiation therapy and, 653
RU-486, 271
Rubella, fetal exposure to, 187
Ruffini's endings, in nerve injury, 154
Ryanodine receptor, 143

Saethre-Chotzen syndrome, 73-74, 73f-75f, 169
Saliva, electrolyte composition of, 508t
Salivary glands
   amylase of, 306
   cancer of, 658. See also Cancer.
   embryology of, 182
Saltatory conduction, 235
Sarcolemma, 278, 279f
Sarcoma, soft-tissue, radiation therapy in, 658
Sarcomere, 278, 279f
Sarcopenia, 141-142
Sarcoplasmic reticulum, 278, 279f, 280
Scaphocephaly, 175-176, 175f
Scarring
   connective tissue growth factor in, 34
   hypertrophic, 59-60
   in fetal wound healing, 66
   transforming growth factor-β effect on, 32
Schizencephaly, 168
Schwann cell, 148, 148f
   in end-to-side neurorrhaphy, 159
   nerve, 149f
   proliferation of, 153
Sciatic nerve block, 606-607, 607f
Sclera, embryology of, 185
Scrotum, development of, 216
Sebaceous glands, 123, 125
Sebum, 123, 125
Second messengers, 19, 21t
Secretin, 311
Secretin receptors, of acinar cell, 310
Sedation, 599-600, 600t. See also Anesthesia.
Seizures, 675-676, 675b
Selectins, in bacterial infection, 538-539, 538t
Selenium deficiency, in parenteral nutrition, 471
Semen, 271
Semilunar valves, formation of, 195-196
Seminal vesicles
   development of, 215f
   formation of, 213
Seminoma, radiation therapy in, 655
Senescence, replicative, 23
Sensory receptors
   in skin, 122-123
   reinnervation of, 154

Sepsis. See also Infection.
   coagulation in, 483
   in trauma, 393
   insulin in, 358
   insulin resistance in, 390
   parenteral nutrition in, 470
   postsplenectomy, 84-85
   thrombocytopenia with, 485
   with parenteral nutrition, 472
Septic shock, 783
Septum primum, 193, 193f
Septum secundum, 193, 193f
SERCA2 pump, 280
Serotonin, 235t
Sertoli cells, 212-213, 264-265
Serum bactericidal titer (SBT), 542
Severe combined immunodeficiency disorder, 94t
Sevoflurane, 587-588, 588t
Sexual differentiation, 219-220, 219f, 261-263
   disorders of, 262-263, 262t, 263b
SF1 gene, 219-220, 219f
SGLT-1 transport protein, 306, 306f
Shake test, 337t
Shear stress, 20t, 297, 298f
Shed-antigen vaccine, in melanoma, 635
Shivering, in thermoregulation, 446-447
Shock, 781-787
   afterload in, 785-786, 787, 787f
   anaphylactic, 93
   arterial base deficit in, 787
   arterial lactate in, 787
   burn-related, 406-410, 407f
      pathophysiology of, 406-408, 407f
      resuscitation for, 408-410
   cardiac function in, 785-786
   cardiogenic, 783-784
   cytokines in, 782
   hypovolemic (hemorrhagic), 782-783
   in children, 350-351
   neurogenic, 784
   oxidative injury in, 782
   oxygen therapy in, 784-785
   pathophysiology of, 781-782
   preload in, 785, 786, 786f
   resuscitation strategies for, 784-785, 787
   septic, 783
   thrombocytopenia with, 485
   ventricular contractility in, 785, 786-787, 787f
   ventricular pressure-volume diagram in, 786-787, 786f
Short-bowel syndrome, 469, 686-687, 686b, 686t
Short-chain fatty acids, for enteral nutrition, 467
Shunt, for cerebrospinal fluid, 673
Signal peptide, 13
Signal recognition particle, 13
Signal transduction, 17-21, 19f, 20t
   in chemokine receptors, 29f, 30
   in cytokine receptors, 28-30, 29f
   in growth factor receptors, 28, 29f
   in muscle, 142
   inhibitors of, 636
   postreceptor component of, 19-20
   receptor component of, 18-19
   signal component of, 18, 19f

Silent mutation, 76f
Silver nitrate, in burn injury, 422-423
Silver sulfadiazine, in burn injury, 423
Silver-enhanced dressings, in burn injury, 423
Simon nitinol filter, 525-526, 525t
Single-photon emission computed tomography, preoperative, 709
Sinoatrial node, 277-278
Sinovaginal bulbs, 215
Sinus bradycardia, 749-750
Sinusitis, fungal, 559
Sirolimus, 381-382, 381t
   in transplantation, 98t, 105-106, 105t
Skin, 115-126
   apocrine glands of, 124
   artificial, 125-126
   basement membrane zone of, 119
   biosynthetic, 126
   Blastomyces dermatitidis infection of, 557
   blood supply to, 121, 122f
   cadaver, 125-126
   cancer of, 658-659. See also Cancer.
   cold receptors of, 445
   dermis of, 119-120
   eccrine glands of, 123-124
   epidermal appendages of, 123-125, 124f
   epidermis of, 115-119, 116f
   fungal infection of, 551-553
   hair of, 124-125, 124f
   hypodermis of, 120-121
   innervation of, 122-123
   Langer's lines of, 125
   lymphatics of, 122
   nerve endings in, 122-123
   radiation injury to, 660-661
   receptors in, 122-123
   sebaceous glands of, 125
   thermoregulatory function of, 121-122
   warm receptors of, 445
Skin graft, 49
Skull
   dysmorphogenesis of, 168-169, 175-176, 175f
   embryology of, 166-167, 174-176
Sleep apnea
   in morbidly obese, 369
   obstructive, 700
Small intestine, 305-310
   calcium absorption by, 308, 309f
   carbohydrate absorption by, 305-306, 306f
   digestion in, 305-307, 306f-308f
   dysmotility of, 684-685
   fat absorption by, 307, 308f
   fluid/electrolyte composition of, 508t
   iron absorption by, 308-309
   motility of, 309
   protein absorption by, 306-307, 307f
   radiation injury to, 470, 662
   vitamin B_{12} absorption by, 309
   water absorption by, 307-308
Smoke inhalation injury, 410-415. See also Inhalation injury.
SNARE proteins, 15
Sodium
   cardiac, 275-277, 276t
   deficiency of, 509
      in children, 354-355
   excess of, 509-510